MEDICAL GUIDE

MAGILL'S

MEDICAL GUIDE

Fourth Revised Edition

Volume II
Corticosteroids — Heel spur removal

Medical Consultants

Anne Lynn S. Chang, M.D.
Stanford University

Laurence M. Katz, M.D.
University of North Carolina, Chapel Hill

H. Bradford Hawley, M.D.
Wright State University

Nancy A. Piotrowski, Ph.D.
University of California, Berkeley

Connie Rizzo, M.D., Ph.D.
Columbia University

Project Editor
Tracy Irons-Georges

SALEM PRESS, INC.
Pasadena, California   Hackensack, New Jersey

Editor in Chief: Dawn P. Dawson

Editorial Director: Christina J. Moose	*Production Editor:* Joyce I. Buchea
Project Editor: Tracy Irons-Georges	*Acquisitions Editor:* Mark Rehn
Editorial Assistant: Dana Garey	*Page Design:* James Hutson
Photo Editor: Cynthia Breslin Beres	*Layout:* William Zimmerman

Cover Design: Moritz Design
Illustrations: Hans & Cassady, Inc., Westerville, Ohio

Magill's Medical Guide: Health and Illness, 1995
Supplement, 1996
Magill's Medical Guide, revised edition, 1998
Second revised edition, 2002
Third revised edition, 2005
Fourth revised edition, 2008

∞ The paper used in these volumes conforms to the American National Standard for Permanence of Paper for Printed Library Materials, Z39.48-1992 (R1997).

Note to Readers
The material presented in *Magill's Medical Guide* is intended for broad informational and educational purposes. Readers who suspect that they suffer from any of the physical or psychological disorders, diseases, or conditions described in this set should contact a physician without delay; this work should not be used as a substitute for professional medical diagnosis or treatment. This set is not to be considered definitive on the covered topics, and readers should remember that the field of health care is characterized by a diversity of medical opinions and constant expansion in knowledge and understanding.

Library of Congress Cataloging-in-Publication Data
Magill's medical guide. — 4th rev. ed. / medical consultants, Anne Lynn S. Chang . . . [et al.] ; project editor, Tracy Irons-Georges.
   p. ; cm.
  Includes bibliographical references and index.
  ISBN 978-1-58765-384-1 (set : alk. paper)
  ISBN 978-1-58765-385-8 (vol. 1 : alk. paper)
  ISBN 978-1-58765-386-5 (vol. 2 : alk. paper)
  ISBN 978-1-58765-387-2 (vol. 3 : alk. paper)
  ISBN 978-1-58765-388-9 (vol. 4 : alk. paper)
  ISBN 978-1-58765-407-7 (vol. 5 : alk. paper)
1. Medicine—Encyclopedias. I. Chang, Anne. II. Title: Medical guide.
  [DNLM: 1. Medicine — Encyclopedias — English.   W 13 M194 2008]
RC41.M34   2008
610.3—dc22

        2007033818

Second Printing

PRINTED IN THE UNITED STATES OF AMERICA

CONTENTS

COMPLETE LIST OF CONTENTS

VOLUME 1

VOLUME 2

VOLUME 3

VOLUME 4

VOLUME 5

MAGILL'S

MEDICAL GUIDE

CORTICOSTEROIDS

BIOLOGY

ALSO KNOWN AS: Glucocorticoids, mineralcortcoids

ANATOMY OR SYSTEM AFFECTED: Endocrine system, immune system

SPECIALTIES AND RELATED FIELDS: Biochemistry, endocrinology, family medicine, immunology

DEFINITION: Steroid hormones such as cortisol and aldosterone synthesized and secreted by the adrenal cortex, or their synthetic equivalents.

KEY TERMS:

Addison's disease: a disease characterized by hypoadrenalism caused by cortisol deficiency

cortisol: a steroid hormone of the adrenal cortex that has many physiological actions

Cushing's syndrome: a disease characterized by hyperadrenalism caused by an excess secretion or exogenous administration of cortisol

glucocorticoid: a steroid hormone such as cortisol from the adrenal cortex that has many physiological actions, including the regulation of glucose metabolism

mineralocorticoid: a steroid hormone from the adrenal cortex that regulates salt and water balance

STRUCTURE AND FUNCTIONS

Corticosteroids are steroid hormones produced by the cortex of the adrenal glands. They have several physiological actions, including regulation of glucose, lipid and protein metabolism, regulation of inflammation and the immune response, maintenance of homeostasis during stress, and control of water and electrolyte balance and blood pressure.

Corticosteroids that have their primary effects on glucose metabolism are glucocorticoids, whereas those that have the control of electrolyte and water balance as their main functions are mineralocorticoids. Cortisol is the primary glucocorticoid, although significant amounts of corticosterone and cortisone are secreted. Aldosterone is the primary mineralocorticoid.

Glucocorticoids promote an increase in blood glucose by stimulating the synthesis of glucose (gluconeogenesis). They also stimulate the catabolism of lipids and proteins. Thus, glucocorticoids increase blood glucose and are antagonistic to insulin.

The synthesis of corticosteroids is controlled by adrenocorticotropic hormone (ACTH) produced by the pituitary gland. Corticotropin-releasing hormone (CRH) produced by the hypothalamus controls the secretion of ACTH. A feedback loop exists so that when cortisol levels are high, the release of CRH and ACTH are inhibited, and when cortisol levels are low, CRH and ACTH are released.

Aldosterone is primarily responsible for the control of salt and water balance by promoting the excretion of potassium and the retention of sodium and water. Through its effect on salt and water balance, aldosterone can increase blood pressure. Plasma levels of aldosterone are controlled by a variety of mechanisms, including plasma volume and potassium ion concentration.

DISORDERS AND DISEASES

Addison's disease results from adrenal insufficiency (hypocortisolism). Although most cases are caused by a disorder of the adrenal glands (primary adrenal insufficiency), some cases are caused by a disorder of the pituitary gland (secondary adrenal insufficiency). An autoimmune disorder that destroys the adrenal cortex is the major cause of primary adrenal insufficiency. Secondary adrenal insufficiency is usually caused by a lack of ACTH. Pituitary tumors, surgical removal of the pituitary, and loss of blood flow to the pituitary are the major causes of secondary adrenal insufficiency. Major symptoms of adrenal insufficiency include loss of appetite, weight loss, fatigue, muscle weakness and hypotension. Addison's disease can be diagnosed by administering ACTH and monitoring the adrenal gland's response by measuring serum and urine cortisol levels. Adrenal insufficiency is treated by oral administration of hydrocortisone, a synthetic form of cortisol. If aldosterone is also deficient, then fludrocortisone is administered.

Adrenal insufficiency is often caused by a mutation in one of the enzymes synthesizing cortisol. These cases are referred to as congenital adrenal hyperplasia (CAH). Since serum cortisol is low or absent, the pituitary gland stimulates the adrenal gland to produce more cortisol. The precursor steroids and their metabolic products that accumulate can cause varying degrees of virilization of female fetuses and infants. Replacement therapy is the treatment of choice. Surgery to reconstruct the genital organs may be necessary in severe cases.

Hypercortisolism can lead to Cushing's syndrome. Major symptoms include obesity, osteoporosis, fatigue, hypertension, hyperglycemia, and amenorrhea (absence of menstruation). Cushing's syndrome may be caused by prolonged use of glucocorticoids or by an overproduction of glucocorticoids by the adrenal glands. The major causes of an overproduction of glucocorticoids are pituitary and adrenal tumors. Diagnosis of Cushing's syndrome is most commonly made by determining the amount of cortisol in the urine. Cushing's syndrome can be treated by reducing administered glucocorticoids or by treatment of the tumor causing the disease through surgical removal, radiation, and/or chemotherapy.

Hypoaldosteronism is a condition in which the adrenal cortex does not produce an adequate amount of aldosterone, which results in an inability to control and regulate blood volume and blood pressure. Blood pressure can fall to dangerously low levels.

Synthetic corticosteroids such as prednisone, prednisolone, methylprednisolone, hydrocortisone, and dexamethasone have an immunosuppressive effect and are used to treat a variety of chronic autoimmune and inflammatory diseases. They can reduce the pain, swelling, itching, inflammation, and redness associated with arthritis, bursitis, asthma, dermititis, eczema and psoriasis, lupus erythematosus, Crohn's disease, and various ear, eye, and skin infections and allergic reactions.

Prolonged use of corticosteroids can lead to medically induced Cushing's syndrome, suppression of the immune system, hypertension, hypokalemia (low serum potassium), and hypernatremia (high serum sodium).

PERSPECTIVE AND PROSPECTS

In 1855, Thomas Addison became the first physician to describe the clinical symptoms of adrenal insufficiency. In the early 1930's, Frank Hartman, Wilbur Swingle, and Joseph Pfiffner were the first to prepare active adrenal extracts capable of treating the symptoms of adrenal insufficiency. By the mid-1930's, Pfiffner, Edward Calvin Kendall, Oskar Wintersteiner, and Tadeus Reichstein had isolated and crystallized some of the adrenal hormones. In 1944, Lewis Sarett became the first to synthesize cortisone. In the late 1940's, Philip Showalter Hench discovered that the administration of cortisone could alleviate the symptoms of arthritis.

In recent years, it has been shown that corticosteroids express their effect by modulating the expression of a variety of genes involved in many physiological functions, including metabolism and the immune or inflammatory response.

—*Charles L. Vigue, Ph.D.*

See also Addison's disease; Adrenalectomy; Cushing's syndrome; Endocrine disorders; Endocrinology; Endocrinology, pediatric; Glands; Hormones; Kidneys; Osteonecrosis.

FOR FURTHER INFORMATION:

Griffin, James E., and Sergio R. Ojeda, eds. *Textbook of Endocrine Physiology.* 5th ed. New York: Oxford University Press, 2004. An examination of endocrine physiology with several chapters devoted to adrenal physiology and disorders. Each chapter is by a different expert in the field.

Lüdecke, Dieter K., George P. Chrousos, and George Tolis, eds. *ACTH, Cushing's Syndrome, and Other Hypercortisolemic States.* New York: Raven Press, 1990. The proceedings of a 1989 conference. Several contributors who are specialists in adrenal disorders.

Vaughan, Darracott E., and Robert M. Carey. *Adrenal Disorders.* New York: Thieme Medical, 1989. Specifically addresses the various disorders of the adrenal gland. Several specialists have contributed chapters.

Vinson, Gavin P., Barbara Whitehouse, and Joy Hinson. *The Adrenal Cortex.* Englewood Cliffs, N.J.: Prentice-Hall, 1992. Addresses the adrenal cortex and its associated disorders.

COSMETIC SURGERY. *See* PLASTIC SURGERY.

COUGHING

DISEASE/DISORDER

ANATOMY OR SYSTEM AFFECTED: Chest, immune system, lungs, respiratory system

SPECIALTIES AND RELATED FIELDS: Family medicine, internal medicine, pulmonary medicine

DEFINITION: A physiological act in which air is forcibly expelled from the lungs.

CAUSES AND SYMPTOMS

The energy that is consumed during the breathing process is used to stretch the chest cavity and allow air to flow into the lungs. This amounts to about 1 percent of the basic energy requirements of the body but increases considerably during periods of exercise or respiratory system illness.

When the respiratory tract is invaded by irritants (such as smoke, perfume, and pollen) or there is an excessive accumulation of secretions, coughing takes place. It arises via a reflex mechanism that starts with the stimulation of the nerves that supply the larynx, trachea (windpipe), and bronchial tubes. The pressure within the chest cavity is increased by the action of chest muscles and the diaphragm. The glottis, the opening of the windpipe at the back of the mouth, remains closed in order to allow the pressure to rise. Within a few seconds, the glottis

---

INFORMATION ON COUGHING

CAUSES: Various diseases, allergens, lung infection, environmental factors
SYMPTOMS: Breathlessness, chest and lung pain
DURATION: Ranges from short-term to chronic
TREATMENTS: Antibiotics, anti-inflammatory drugs

---

opens again and a rapid, noisy release of air is allowed through the bronchial tubes and the windpipe. Any invading foreign substance is expelled through the mouth.

TREATMENT AND THERAPY

Coughing is an important symptom of diseases that affect any part of the respiratory system, such as the nasal cavities, the pharynx (throat), the larynx, the trachea, the bronchi, and lung tissue. Sputum formation during coughing is an important evidence of a disease, such as bronchitis. In this case, the lining of the bronchi enlarges dramatically and sputum production may increase to 60 milliliters per day. An irritative cough without sputum may be due to the extension of the disease to the bronchial tube and eventually to nearby organs. The use of antibiotics and anti-inflammatory agents to reduce the discomfort is part of the standard treatment.

The presence of blood in the sputum (called hemoptysis) is important and should alert patients or their caregivers to call a doctor. This symptom often arises from an existing infection, inflammation, or tumor. It is also a sign of tuberculosis. In this case, extensive and reliable tests will identify the real cause of the bleeding.

Polluted air increases the possibility of chronic bronchitis. Common air pollutants include vehicle exhaust, chemical fumes, smoke, smog, molds, and pollen. They are all responsible for a decrease in arterial oxygen and an increase in carbon dioxide tension in the lungs. The use of air-conditioning, air filters, and inhalers and an increased-oxygen environment can provide relief for people with respiratory problems.

—*Soraya Ghayourmanesh, Ph.D.*

See also Allergies; Asbestos exposure; Aspergillosis; Avian influenza; Bronchitis; Choking; Common cold; Croup; Cystic fibrosis; Diphtheria; Immune system; Influenza; Laryngitis; Lung cancer; Lungs; Otorhinolaryngology; Over-the-counter medications; Pneumonia; Pulmonary diseases; Pulmonary medicine; Pulmonary medicine, pediatric; Respiration; Sore throat; Tuberculosis; Wheezing; Whooping cough.

FOR FURTHER INFORMATION:
Adelman, Daniel C., et al., eds. *Manual of Allergy and Immunology.* 4th ed. Philadelphia: Lippincott Williams & Wilkins, 2002.
Braga, Pier Carlo, and Luigi Allegra, eds. *Cough.* New York: Raven Press, 1989.
Chung, Kian Fan, John G. Widdicombe, and Homer A. Boushey, eds. *Cough: Causes, Mechanisms, and Therapy.* Malden, Mass.: Blackwell, 2003.
Glenn, Jim. *Colds and Coughs.* Springhouse, Pa.: Springhouse, 1986.
Kimball, Chad T., ed. *Colds, Flu, and Other Common Ailments.* New York: Omnigraphics, 2002.
Korpás, Juraj, and Z. Tomori. *Cough and Other Respiratory Reflexes.* New York: S. Karger, 1979.
Woolf, Alan D., et al., eds. *The Children's Hospital Guide to Your Child's Health and Development.* Cambridge, Mass.: Perseus, 2002.

CRANIOSYNOSTOSIS
DISEASE/DISORDER

ANATOMY OR SYSTEM AFFECTED: Bones, head
SPECIALTIES AND RELATED FIELDS: Orthopedics, plastic surgery
DEFINITION: The premature closing of the open areas between the bones in an infant's skull.

CAUSES AND SYMPTOMS

Craniosynostosis is an important craniofacial abnormality that occurs in a variety of forms. The skull of a newborn infant contains several open areas between the bones that make up the skull. These areas, called fontanelles, allow the skull to expand as the child's brain grows. Craniosynostosis is the premature closure of one or more of these open areas, resulting in the abnormal shaping of the head and face. Craniosynostosis may occur alone or in association with other defects.

TREATMENT AND THERAPY

During the 1960's the French surgeon Paul Tessier developed improved techniques for treating craniosynostosis. Treatment of craniosynostosis is often done with a surgical procedure known as fronto-orbital advancement. This technique involves cutting the skull in such a way that the frontal bone (the portion of the skull behind the forehead) and the supraorbital rim (the portion of the skull above and to the sides of the eyes) can be moved forward. These portions of the skull are then attached to the rest of the skull in their new positions with surgical wire. For some types of craniosynostosis, it may also be necessary to cut the frontal bone and the supraorbital rim down the middle to allow them to be reshaped. Fronto-orbital advancement usually takes place after the patient is three months old.

Correction of craniosynostosis is a complicated procedure, requiring the patient to be monitored in a special hospital bed for at least four or five days after surgery. After the plastic surgery, the patient will experience severe swelling of the eyelids and scalp. Most patients will be unable to open their eyes until several days after surgery, and the swelling may not completely disappear for a few months. Care must be taken to keep the incision clean.

—Rose Secrest

See also Birth defects; Bone disorders; Bones and the skeleton; Growth; Surgery, pediatric.

FOR FURTHER INFORMATION:

Cohen, M. Michael, Jr., and Ruth E. MacLean, eds. *Craniosynostosis: Diagnosis, Evaluation, and Management.* 2d ed. New York: Oxford University Press, 2000.

Galli, Guido, ed. *Craniosynostosis.* Boca Raton, Fla.: CRC Press, 1984.

Hayward, Richard, et al., eds. *The Clinical Management of Craniosynostosis.* New York: Cambridge University Press, 2004.

McCarthy, Joseph G., ed. *Distraction of the Craniofacial Skeleton.* New York: Springer, 1999.

Moore, Keith L., and T. V. N. Persaud. *The Developing Human.* 7th ed. Philadelphia: W. B. Saunders, 2003.

Sadler, T. W. *Langman's Medical Embryology.* 10th ed. Philadelphia: Lippincott Williams & Wilkins, 2006.

Turvey, Timothy A., Raymond J. Fonseca, and Katherine W. Vig, eds. *Facial Clefts and Craniosynostosis: Principles and Management.* Philadelphia: W. B. Saunders, 1996.

CRANIOTOMY

PROCEDURE

ANATOMY OR SYSTEM AFFECTED: Brain, head
SPECIALTIES AND RELATED FIELDS: Critical care, neurology
DEFINITION: A means of exposing or gaining access to the brain and cranial nerves so that intracranial disease can be treated surgically.

INDICATIONS AND PROCEDURES

Problems requiring craniotomy include tumors, abscesses, hematomas, and vascular lesions. The cranium may also be opened to excise an area of cortex or to disrupt various nerves and fiber tracts for the relief of pain, seizures, tremors, or spasms that do not respond to pharmacologic therapy. Skull fractures and other traumatic head wounds may be repaired by opening the cranium. Bony defects, dural tearing, bleeding, and removal of penetrating objects are also treated with this procedure. In case of a neoplasm (tumor), the goal of surgery is to remove the pathology completely while preserving the normal neural and vascular structures.

In craniotomy, the skin is cut to the skull bone. Small bleeding arteries are sealed with electric current, and the skin is pulled back. Three burr holes are drilled into the skull, and a fine-wire Gigli's saw is used to connect the holes. The skull piece is hinged open, and the dura mater, a tough membrane covering the brain, is dissected away. After the required procedure on the brain is completed, the dura mater is stitched together, the bone flap is replaced and secured with soft wire, and the scalp incision is closed.

An intracranial operation can be considered a planned head injury, and the complications are similar. Postoperatively, the degree of impairment depends on the extent of damage to neural tissue caused both by the neurological disorder and by surgical manipulation. Damage may be transient or permanent.

USES AND COMPLICATIONS

With craniotomy, complications include cerebral edema (swelling), which is a normal reaction to the manipulation and retraction of brain tissue. Periorbital edema and ecchymosis (bleeding under the skin) usually follow frontal and temporal surgery. Focal motor deficits result from cerebral edema and are transitory. Permanent focal motor deficits may occur and are a direct and predictable consequence of the surgical procedure or the result of a complication such as stroke. Hematomas are the most devastating and dreaded complication. The clots may be extradural, intradural, or both and usually are caused by a single bleeding vessel rather than a generalized bleed.

Pain and discomfort are expected following cranial surgery, with headache being most common. Pain control may be accomplished with mild analgesics. Fever may occur following operations in the region of the upper brain stem and hypothalamus, and it requires vigorous treatment. Infection may occur, with the risk being greater following open head trauma and if a cerebrospinal fluid leak is present. Postoperative seizure risk is related to the underlying pathological condition and the degree of damage caused by surgery. Diabetes insipidus and the syndrome of inappropriate antidiuretic hormone (SIADH) secretion are also possible complications of craniotomy. These endocrine disorders may be transient or permanent. If unchecked, either may be life-threatening because of the severity of the fluid and electrolyte imbalance precipitated.

A cerebrospinal fluid leak may occur immediately following surgery but usually appears later in the postoperative course. Fluid seeps from the wound edges. Discharge from the nose (rhinorrhea) or ears (otorrhea) of cerebrospinal fluid is frequent with basal skull fractures, but these conditions may also occur following surgery in the frontal sinus or mastoid cavity. Anosmia (loss of sense of smell) frequently occurs following head injury or frontal craniotomy. Visual loss may be caused by damage to the optic nerve, resulting in blindness and lack of response to direct light. Hydrocephalus may develop as a result of postoperative adhesions secondary to blood sealing the subarachnoid space. Postoperative meningitis, abscess formation, and osteomyelitis of the bone flap occur as complications of a break in sterility or the introduction of organisms as a result of a contaminated open wound.

—*Jane C. Norman, R.N., Ph.D.*

See also Bones and the skeleton; Brain; Brain disorders; Hydrocephalus; Neuroimaging; Neurology; Neurology, pediatric; Neurosurgery.

FOR FURTHER INFORMATION:

Aminoff, Michael J., David A. Greenberg, and Roger P. Simon. *Clinical Neurology*. 6th ed. New York: McGraw-Hill Medical, 2005.

Bakay, Louis. *An Early History of Craniotomy: From Antiquity to the Napoleonic Era*. Springfield, Ill.: Charles C Thomas, 1985.

Rowland, Lewis P., ed. *Merritt's Textbook of Neurology*. 11th ed. Philadelphia: Lippincott Williams & Wilkins, 2005.

Samuels, Martin A., ed. *Manual of Neurologic Therapeutics*. 7th ed. New York: Lippincott Williams & Wilkins, 2004.

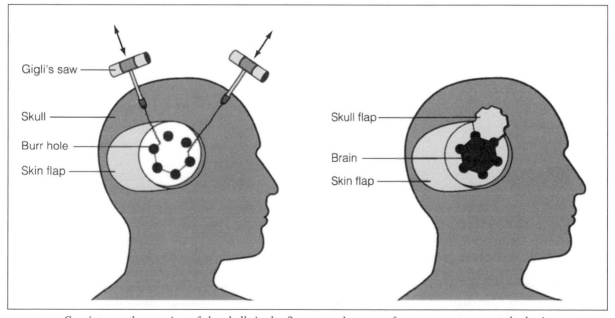

Craniotomy, the opening of the skull, is the first step taken to perform neurosurgery on the brain.

CRETINISM

DISEASE/DISORDER

ALSO KNOWN AS: Infantile hypothyroidism

ANATOMY OR SYSTEM AFFECTED: Endocrine system, musculoskeletal system, neck, nervous system

SPECIALTIES AND RELATED FIELDS: Endocrinology, internal medicine, perinatology, preventive medicine

DEFINITION: Retardation of mental and physical growth arising from prenatal or neonatal hypothyroidism.

KEY TERMS:

goiter: the sometimes gross enlargement of the thyroid gland in an effort to produce hormones when insufficient iodine is available

L-thyroxine (T4): a less potent thyroid hormone than the T3 form that can be converted in the cells to T3

L-triiodothyronine (T3): the most potent of the thyroid hormones

myxedema: a hypothyroid disorder that can develop in children or adults; characterized by thick, dry skin, slow reflexes, and low body temperature

thyroid gland: the endocrine gland in humans that produces the hormones that control metabolism

CAUSES AND SYMPTOMS

In humans, the thyroid gland consists of two connected lobes in the front of the neck, on either side of the thyroid cartilage or Adam's apple. It produces the thyroid hormones, the most important of which are L-triiodothyronine (T3) and L-tetraiodothyroxine or L-thyroxine (T4). These compounds circulate in the blood serum to the body's cells and regulate virtually all metabolism: the production and consumption of proteins, carbohydrates, fats, and vitamins and the generation of energy that makes body heat. In these activities, the T3 molecule (which can be derived in the cells from T4)

INFORMATION ON CRETINISM

CAUSES: Thyroid disorder

SYMPTOMS: Mental retardation, low body temperature, poor appetite, decreased activity, flabbiness, low pulse rate, delayed union of skull bones, feeding difficulties, off-color skin

DURATION: Lifelong

TREATMENTS: Thyroid replacement therapy from birth

---

has two to four times the effectiveness of T4. Because of the high iodine content of both T3 and T4, sufficient dietary iodine must be supplied to maintain normal thyroid function.

Abnormal levels of T3 and T4 have a profound effect on all bodily functions. In adults, the low production of T3 and T4, or hypothyroidism, leads to reduced mental and physical activity, weight gain, general weakness, and other symptoms. Elevated thyroid activity, or hyperthyroidism, produces restlessness and irritability, weight loss, and symptoms generally the opposite of those seen with hypothyroidism. When either of these conditions develops in adults, drug regimens are available to control them and to produce normal metabolism in the patient. When they occur in utero, however, there is almost no way to counteract their effects.

If the problem is hypothyroidism, the resulting child will be born with cretinism. A cretin is mentally retarded with little or no chance of improvement and, unless immediately treated with thyroid hormones, also physically retarded or dwarfed, with the bone ends not growing or maturing normally. The typical cretin infant can show a variety of symptoms: low body temperature, poor appetite, decreased activity, flabbiness, low pulse rate, delayed union of bones of the skull, feeding difficulties even to the point of choking and cyanosis (turning blue from lack of oxygen), and thickened, off-color skin.

TREATMENT AND THERAPY

For the child born a cretin, no treatment is available for the mental damage that has taken place. Thyroid replacement therapy from birth, using either natural or synthetic hormones, will avert most physical effects, but the mental retardation is irreversible.

The most effective way to avoid this problem is to ensure that a pregnant woman consumes enough iodine to be made into the T3 and T4 molecules by her fetus. The thyroid hormones do not transfer readily from the placental blood supply to that of the fetus, but the iodide ion does. This alone is enough, when made available before the end of the second trimester of pregnancy, to allow the fetal thyroid gland to develop normally and the unborn fetus to have proper neurological and musculoskeletal function. Iodide ions are most easily supplied in iodized salt, but they can also be given as an injection of iodized oil or by the oral administration of a number of iodine-containing medicines, such as Lugol's iodine solution.

When hypothyroidism develops in the older child or

adolescent—often appearing as a goiter, in addition to the other symptoms described above—iodine therapy is sometimes sufficient to return thyroid function to normal levels. Oddly, such therapy can also be counterproductive. The complex mechanisms that maintain proper hormone levels in blood serum can be misled by artificially high iodine concentrations and may close down hormone production because it appears high. For this condition, only thyroid hormone administration is effective.

PERSPECTIVE AND PROSPECTS

Hypothyroidism, goiter, and cretinism are worldwide health problems because of the body's dependence on dietary iodine. Many places on Earth have low soil levels of iodine, leading to low iodine levels in crops and thus inadequate iodine intake from food. Such areas include high mountain country, such as the Himalayas, where glacial meltwater leaches iodine from the soil with no replacement from higher geologic formations; and the Ganges basin, where the sheer volume of water removes iodine from croplands. Some mountainous areas of the United States—such as the hill country of West Virginia, Kentucky, and Tennessee—have been, historically, centers of endemic goiter formation. Supplying iodine to inhabitants of these areas is a medical necessity but, like so many such problems, is complicated by logistic and political considerations.

—*Robert M. Hawthorne, Jr., Ph.D.*

See also Birth defects; Dwarfism; Endocrine system; Endocrinology, pediatric; Growth; Malnutrition; Mental retardation; Nutrition; Vitamins and minerals.

FOR FURTHER INFORMATION:

"Another Reason for Iodine Prophylaxis." *The Lancet* 335, no. 8703 (June 16, 1990): 1433-1434. Despite iodine supplementation programs, severe iodine deficiency persists in several parts of Europe and the developing countries. The failure of iodine supplementation programs is discussed in an editorial.

Cao, Xue-Yi, et al. "Timing of Vulnerability of the Brain to Iodine Deficiency in Endemic Cretinism." *New England Journal of Medicine* 331, no. 26 (December 29, 1994). Iodine was administered to children from birth to three years of age and women at each trimester of pregnancy in an iodine-deficient area of the Xinjiang region of China. According to the results, iodine treatment protects the fetal brain from the effects of iodine deficiency.

Gomez, Joan. *Thyroid Problems in Women and Children.* Alameda, Calif.: Hunter House, 2003. Discusses current research, incorporates case studies, and includes special chapters for pregnant women and about babies and children with the disease.

Hetzel, Basil S. "Iodine and Neuropsychological Development." *The Journal of Nutrition* 130, no. 2S (1999): 493S-495S. The establishment of the essential link among iodine deficiency, thyroid function, and brain development has emerged from a fascinating combination of clinical, epidemiologic, and experimental studies.

Larsen, P. Reed, et al., eds. *Williams Textbook of Endocrinology.* 10th ed. Philadelphia: W. B. Saunders, 2003. Text that covers the spectrum of information related to the endocrine system, including thyroid disorders, diabetes, endocrinology and aging, female reproduction and fertility control, sexual function and dysfunction, kidney stones, and endocrine hypertension.

Maberly, Glen F. "Iodine Deficiency Disorders: Contemporary Scientific Issues." *Journal of Nutrition* 124, no. 8 (August, 1994): 1473-1478S. Iodine deficiency is the leading cause of preventable intellectual impairment and is associated with a spectrum of neurologic pathology. Although some 1 billion people are at risk, developing fetuses and infants are most susceptible to the intellectual impairment caused by iodine deficiency.

March of Dimes. http://www.marchofdimes.org/. Web site offers a range of excellent fact sheets on myriad birth defects, information about prenatal testing, and special sections for pregnant women and researchers and professionals.

Rosenthal, M. Sara. *The Thyroid Sourcebook.* 4th ed. New York: McGraw-Hill, 2000. Wide-ranging examination of thyroid disorders from hyperthyroidism to cancer.

Woeber, K. A. "Iodine and Thyroid Disease." In *The Medical Clinics of North America: Thyroid Diseases* 75, no. 1 (January, 1991): 169-178. Environmental iodine deficiency continues to be a significant public health problem worldwide, compounded in some geographic regions by the presence of other goitrogens in some staple foods.

CREUTZFELDT-JAKOB DISEASE (CJD)

DISEASE/DISORDER

ANATOMY OR SYSTEM AFFECTED: Brain, nervous system

SPECIALTIES AND RELATED FIELDS: Environmental health, epidemiology, microbiology, neurology, public health, virology

DEFINITION: Creutzfeldt-Jakob disease (CJD) is a human central nervous system disorder that is characterized by distinctive lesions in the brain, progressive dementia, lack of coordination, and eventual death. Although uncommon, it is the most prevalent of the human spongiform encephalopathies, inherited or transmissible illnesses of uncertain etiology associated with proteinaceous molecules called prions. Mad cow disease is a spongiform encephalopathy that affects cattle but may be transmissible to humans, leading to a new variant of CJD.

KEY TERMS:

dementia: an organic mental disorder characterized by personality disintegration, confusion, disorientation, stupor, deterioration of intellectual function, and impairment of memory and judgment

encephalopathy: any abnormality in the structure or function of the brain

knockout mouse: a mouse in which a specific gene has been inactivated or "knocked out"

myoclonus: involuntary twitching or spasm of muscle

spongiform: shaped like or resembling a sponge

CAUSES AND SYMPTOMS

Spongiform encephalopathies are inherited or transmissible neurological diseases that are associated with abnormalities in proteinaceous molecules called prions, which can aggregate, leading to spongelike lesions in the brain and causing disruptions in brain function. Prions are found in all species from yeast to humans, but their normal role is not known. Their evolutionary persistence in so many species implies an important purpose, although knockout mice lacking prions do not appear to be deleteriously affected.

Inherited spongiform encephalopathies are primarily attributed to mutations in the prion gene, producing abnormal prions that adopt an unusual conformation and clump together over time to cause the brain pathology and neurological symptoms characteristic of this type of disease. The diseases can be transmitted to a susceptible animal by inserting a fragment or extract from diseased tissue into the brain or blood or, much less efficiently, by oral ingestion. The infectious agent

seems to be the abnormal prion itself, which apparently recruits normal prions in the brain to adopt the abnormal conformation, leading to their aggregation and the disruption of brain function. This is an unorthodox etiology, in that the infectious agent appears to be devoid of nucleic acid (RNA or DNA); its mode of action is not fully understood, nor is this etiology universally accepted.

Creutzfeldt-Jakob disease (CJD), known since the 1920's, is the major spongiform encephalopathy in humans, although it occurs only in one per million persons worldwide. It has different forms, namely sporadic, inherited, infectious, and, recently, new variant.

The sporadic form has no known basis, accounts for 85 percent of the cases, and usually affects individuals aged fifty-five to seventy years of age. The pathologic findings are limited to the central nervous system, although the transmissible agent can be detected in many organs. Researchers noted in 2002 that psychiatric and neurological symptoms are often present within four months of the disease's onset. Common symptoms include withdrawal, anxiety, irritability, insomnia, and a loss of interest. Within a few weeks or months, a relentlessly progressive dementia becomes evident, and myoclonus is often present at some point. Deterioration is usually rapid, with 90 percent of victims dying within one year. CJD patients do not have fevers, and their blood and cerebrospinal fluid are normal.

The inherited or familial form has been noted in some one hundred extended families, accounting for 15 percent of the cases of CJD. At least seven different point mutations and one insertion mutation in the prion gene have been identified. Some prion mutations result in slightly different symptoms and are classified as different diseases. Other mutations may lead to the sporadic, infectious, or new variant forms.

The infectious form is rare and has generally been associated with medical procedures, such as organ

---

INFORMATION ON CREUTZFELDT-JAKOB DISEASE (CJD)

CAUSES: Prion disease; can be acquired through ingestion of infected cow tissue

SYMPTOMS: Dementia, lack of coordination, personality change

DURATION: Weeks to months; death typically occurs within one year

TREATMENTS: None

transplants, inadvertent infection from contaminated surgical instruments, or treatment with products derived from human brains. Because the infectious agent is highly resistant to denaturation, thorough decontamination of surgical instruments has proven essential in minimizing transmission. A number of cases occurred in individuals receiving growth hormone extracts derived from human pituitary glands, a practice discontinued in the United States in 1985. The infectious form also appears to be the basis for kuru, a disease previously endemic among the Fore people of the eastern highlands of Papua New Guinea. Typically, it was characterized by cerebellar dysfunction, dementia, and progression to death within two years. Evidence indicates that the kuru agent was transmitted through the ritual handling and consumption of affected tissues, especially brains, from deceased relatives. With discontinuation of these cultural practices, kuru has virtually disappeared.

A new variant CJD (nvCJD) was first reported in Britain in 1996. It differed from sporadic CJD in affecting younger persons (aged sixteen to thirty-nine) and in its behavioral symptoms, pathology, and longer course. This variant followed the British epidemic of bovine spongiform encephalopathy (BSE), known as mad cow disease. Contaminated beef consumption was suspected as the source of nvCJD, which has subsequently been shown to have a molecular signature similar, if not identical, to that for BSE. Furthermore, nvCJD has been observed only in countries with BSE.

BSE first appeared in Britain in 1986 and has subsequently been diagnosed in nine other European countries. It occurs in adult cattle between two and eight years of age and is fatal. In the course of the disease, the animals lose coordination and show extreme sensitivity to sound, light, and touch. While it may be transmitted from mother to calf, the major cause of the BSE epidemic in Britain is attributed to feed containing contaminated ruminant-derived protein. Following a ban on incorporating such protein into cattle feed, the incidence has decreased. Since the beginning of the epidemic, a total of two hundred thousand cattle have been diagnosed with the disease; fewer than one thousand new cases are currently reported per year. In the United States, a surveillance program is in effect, importation of beef from affected countries is prohibited, and incorporating ruminant-derived protein into cattle feed has been banned. Nevertheless, an infected cow was discovered in 2003 on a farm in Washington State. It had been imported from Canada.

When the British BSE outbreak occurred, concern arose for its human health implications, despite the fact that scrapie, the comparable condition in sheep, was long known not to be a risk to human consumers. A surveillance unit was established in 1990, and ten cases of the new variant form of CJD were reported in 1996. As of August, 2000, a cumulative total of eighty such cases had been identified. Its incidence in Britain showed an upward trend: For the year ending June 30, 2000, twenty-two deaths were reported, compared to nineteen for the previous year. In view of uncertainties in its etiology and its long incubation period, it is unknown how high the toll will eventually be.

TREATMENT AND THERAPY

Research on experimental animals has been crucial to understanding the unusual etiology of these diseases. Brain tissue from patients dying of kuru was inoculated into the brains of chimpanzees that, after a prolonged incubation period, developed a similar disease. CJD, BSE, and scrapie have been similarly transmitted to a wide variety of laboratory animals. Mouse models have been particularly useful. Knockout mice lacking their normal prion gene are not susceptible to transmissible disease, indicating the importance of endogenous brain prions in the etiology. Transgenic mice, in which their own prions have been replaced with those from other species or with specific mutations, exhibit different susceptibilities to various infectious particles.

Because none of the spongiform encephalopathies stimulates a specific immune response, diagnosis of these diseases in living persons or animals is difficult. Postmortem identification of brain lesions is necessary to verify the diagnosis. The use of antibodies to prions is permitting rapid confirmation of the diagnosis from specimens obtained by brain biopsy or postmortem examination. As of 2000, no effective treatment was available for these diseases, which are uniformly fatal. Although these diseases can be transmitted to health care workers and others having contact with CJD patients, the risk is no higher than for the general population. Isolation of patients is not suggested, but reasonable care should be exercised. No organs, tissues, or tissue products from these patients or others with an ill-defined neurologic disease should be used for transplantation, replacement therapy, or pharmaceutical manufacturing.

PERSPECTIVE AND PROSPECTS

Clinically, Creutzfeldt-Jakob disease can be mistaken for other disorders that cause dementia in the elderly, especially Alzheimer's disease. CJD, however, usually has a shorter clinical course and includes myoclonus. While nvCJD has a longer clinical course, it generally affects younger persons.

Continued monitoring of CJD and especially nvCJD in Britain is warranted. In addition, surveillance of the food supply in the United States and other countries should persist to prevent meat from BSE cattle from reaching consumers. Above all, further research into the etiology of these pathologies is needed. Research into prion biology and disease epidemiology, including studies of nvCJD clusters, must be pursued until the progression of these diseases is fully understood. Early detection and effective treatment await this understanding.

—*James L. Robinson, Ph.D.*

See also Brain; Brain disorders; Dementias; Food poisoning; Prion diseases; Viral infections; Zoonoses.

FOR FURTHER INFORMATION:

Balter, Michael. "Tracking the Human Fallout from Mad Cow Disease." *Science* 289 (September, 2000): 1452-1453. This news report presents the history, current status, and future prospects of nvCJD, the new variant of Creutzfeldt-Jacob disease that is associated with consumption of cattle affected by mad cow disease.

Bloom, Floyd E., M. Flint Beal, and David J. Kupfer, eds. *The Dana Guide to Brain Health.* New York: Simon & Schuster, 2003. An easy-to-understand health guide to the brain from neuroscience, neurology, and psychiatry perspectives. More than seventy psychiatric and neurological disorders, their diagnoses, and their treatments are covered.

Dana.org. http://www.dana.org/. A nonprofit organization of neuroscientists, which was formed to provide information about the personal and public benefits of brain research. The Web site is research oriented and gives excellent information and links on current brain studies, new diagnosis and treatment technology, and brain-related news stories.

Marieb, Elaine N., and Katja Hoehn. *Human Anatomy and Physiology.* 7th ed. San Francisco: Pearson Benjamin Cummings, 2007. Several chapters explore the fundamentals of the nervous system and nervous tissue, the central nervous system, and neural integration. Well illustrated and includes many applications in the fields of physical education and medical science.

Nolte, John. *Human Brain: An Introduction to Its Functional Anatomy.* 5th ed. New York: Elsevier, 2001. Text covering major concepts and structure-function relationships in the human neurological system.

Prusiner, Stanley B. "The Prion Diseases." *Scientific American* 272, no. 1 (January, 1995): 48-57. The author explains the history and basis for the prion theory, which he developed and for which he was awarded a Nobel Prize in 1997.

_____, ed. *Prion Biology and Diseases.* 2d ed. Cold Spring Harbor, N.Y.: Cold Spring Harbor Laboratory Press, 2004. The originator of the prion theory edits this book, which presents the latest scientific information about prions and the diseases with which they are associated.

Schwartz, Maxime. *How the Cows Turned Mad.* Translated by Edward Schneider. Berkeley: University of California Press, 2003. Traces the history of mad cow disease and related infectious brain diseases of livestock and people and outlines advances in understanding the disease.

Spencer, Charlotte A. *Mad Cows and Cannibals: A Guide to the Transmissible Spongiform Encephalopathies.* Upper Saddle River, N.J.: Prentice Hall, 2004. Explores the biology of and issues surrounding mad cow disease and related conditions, including discussions of ritualistic cannibalism in New Guinea and modern agricultural feeding practices that triggered the mad cow disease epidemic in Great Britain.

Transmissible Spongiform Encephalopathies in the United States. Ames, Iowa: Council for Agricultural Science and Technology, 2000. This report of a scientific task force organized to evaluate mad cow disease and related disorders provides a factual, balanced, and succinct summary of these conditions.

CRITICAL CARE

SPECIALTY

ANATOMY OR SYSTEM AFFECTED: All

SPECIALTIES AND RELATED FIELDS: Anesthesiology, cardiology, emergency medicine, gastroenterology, geriatrics and gerontology, neurology, nursing, obstetrics, pharmacology, pulmonary medicine, radiology, sports medicine, toxicology

DEFINITION: The care of patients who are experiencing severe health crises—short-lived or prolonged, accidental or anticipated—that require continuous monitoring.

KEY TERMS:

asphyxia: an impaired exchange of oxygen and carbon dioxide in the lungs; if prolonged, this condition leads to death

aspirate: to suck fluid or a foreign body into an airway of the lungs, which frequently leads to aspiration pneumonia

debridement: the excision of bruised, injured, or otherwise devitalized tissue from a wound site

electrocardiogram (EKG or ECG): a graphic record of the electrical activity of the heart, obtained with an electrocardiograph and displayed on a computer screen or paper strip

emphysema: an increase in the size of air spaces at the terminal ends of bronchioles in the lungs; this damage reduces the ability of the lungs to exchange oxygen and carbon dioxide

esophagus: the portion of the digestive system connecting the mouth and stomach; it is muscular, propelling food during the act of swallowing

hypothermia: a subnormal body temperature; clinically, it is a sustained cooling of the body to lower-than-normal temperatures

resuscitation: the restoration to life after apparent death; the methods used to restore normal organ functioning, primarily referring to the heart

sternum: the breastbone; found in the midline of the chest cavity and lying over the heart

trauma: an injury caused by rough contact with a physical object; it can be accidental or induced

SCIENCE AND PROFESSION

Critical care is the branch of medicine that provides immediate services, usually on an emergency basis. It also encompasses some forms of ongoing care provided in a hospital setting for patients who are so sick that they are medically unstable and must be monitored constantly. Such patients are at an ongoing high risk for disastrous complications.

Critical care personnel must be specially trained, and standards for training and evaluation in this field have been prepared for physicians, nurses, and other hospital personnel. Ninety percent of hospitals in the United States with fewer than two hundred beds have a single critical care unit, usually called an intensive care unit (ICU). Only 9 percent of these hospitals have a second intensive care facility, typically dedicated solely to the care of heart attack victims. In total, 7 to 8 percent of all hospital beds in the United States are used for intensive care. Because ICU facilities are at a premium and are expensive to operate, patients are transferred to a regular hospital bed as quickly as possible, given their specific medical condition. Of the physicians who are certified in critical care, most are anesthesiologists, followed by internists. A shortage of trained critical care physicians has existed in the United States for many years.

Critical care facilities are available in several varieties, providing specialized care to particular patients. The most common type of ICU is for individuals who require care for medical crises. These patients frequently have a short-term condition or disease that can be treated successfully. Others are admitted to a medical ICU for multiple organ system failure. These people are often very sick with conditions that overwhelm even the best available care and equipment. Heart attack victims are often admitted to a coronary ICU, which has specialized equipment for support and resuscitation if needed. Once medically stable, coronary ICU patients are transferred to a regular hospital bed.

Larger hospitals may have an ICU for surgical patients. Typically, these individuals are admitted to the surgical ICU from the operating room after a procedure. In the ICU, they are stabilized while the effects of anesthesia wear off. They, too, are transferred to a normal hospital room as soon as is medically safe. Neonatal ICUs exist in some larger hospitals to provide care for premature and very sick infants. Such infants may stay in neonatal ICUs for extended periods of time (weeks to months) depending on their specific condition. There may also be a pediatric ICU specially designed for very sick children.

DIAGNOSTIC AND TREATMENT TECHNIQUES

Critical care is synonymous with immediate care: Swift action is required on an emergency basis to sustain or save a life. The most immediate of critical care needs are to establish and maintain a patent airway for ventilation and to maintain sufficient cardiac functioning to provide minimal perfusion or blood supply to critical organs of the body.

Resuscitation is the support of life by external means when the body is unable to maintain itself. Basic life support is for emergency situations and consists of delivering oxygen to the lungs, maintaining an airway, inflating the lungs if necessary, and assisting with circulation. These methods are collectively known as cardiopulmonary resuscitation (CPR). Oxygen can be transferred from one mouth to another by forceful breathing or by the means of pumps and pure oxygen from a container. The airway is commonly maintained by positioning the head and neck so as to extend the chin and open the trachea. It is also possible to make an incision in the trachea, insert a tube, and provide oxygen through the tube. The lungs may be inflated by using the force of exhaled air from one person breathing into another's mouth or by utilizing a machine that inflates the lungs to a precise level and delivers oxygen in accurate, predetermined amounts. When a victim's heart is not working, the circulation of blood is provided by external compression of the chest. This action squeezes the heart between the sternum and the spine, forcing blood into the circulatory system.

Advanced life support includes attempts to restart a nonfunctioning heart. This goal is commonly accomplished by electrical means (defibrillation). The heart is given a brief shock that is sufficient to start it beating on its own. Drugs can also be used to restore spontaneous circulation in cardiac arrest. Epinephrine (adrenaline) is the most commonly used drug, although sodium bicarbonate is used for some conditions. A heart can be restarted by manual compression. This technique requires direct access to the heart and is limited to situations in which the heart stops beating during a surgical procedure involving the thorax, when the heart is directly accessible.

Prolonged life support is administered after the heart has been restarted and is concerned chiefly with the brain and other organs such as the kidneys that are sensitive to oxygen levels in the blood. Drugs and mechanical ventilation are used to supply oxygen to the lungs. Prolonged life support uses sophisticated technology to deliver oxygenated blood to the organs continuously. The body can be maintained in this manner for long periods of time. Once begun, prolonged life support is continued until the patient regains consciousness or until brain death has been certified by a physician. A patient's state of underlying disease may be determined to be so severe that continuing prolonged life support be-

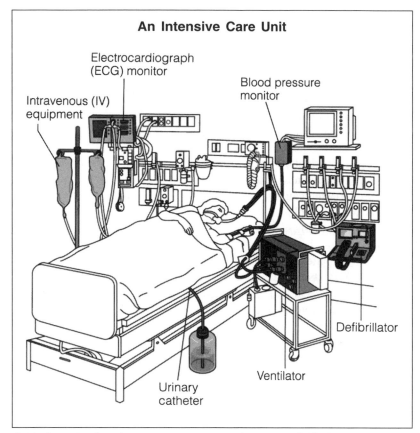

Critical care involves the constant monitoring of patients with life-threatening conditions. This care is usually provided in an intensive care unit (ICU).

comes senseless. The factors entering into a decision to terminate life support are complex and involve a patient's family, the physician, and other professionals.

Individuals who are critically ill must be closely monitored. Many of the advancements in the care of these patients have been attributable to improvements in monitoring. While physiologic measurements cannot replace the clinical impressions of trained professionals, monitoring data often provide objective information that reinforces clinical opinions. More people die from the failure of vital organs than from the direct effects of injury or disease. The most commonly monitored events are vital signs: heart rate, blood pressure, breathing rate, and temperature. These are frequently augmented by electrocardiograms (ECGs or EKGs). Other, more sophisticated electronic methods are available for individuals in intensive care units.

Vital signs are still frequently assessed manually, although machinery is available to accomplish the task. Modern intensive care units are able to store large amounts of data that can be analyzed by computer programs. Data can be transmitted to distant consoles, thus enabling a small number of individuals to monitor several patients simultaneously. Monitoring data can also be displayed on computer screens, allowing more rapid evaluation. Automatic alarms can be used to indicate when bodily functions fall outside predetermined parameters, thus rapidly alerting staff to critical or emergency situations.

Breathing—or, more correctly, ventilation—can be monitored extensively. The volume of inspired air can be adjusted to accommodate different conditions. The amount of oxygen can be changed to compensate for emphysema or other loss of oxygen exchange capacity. The rate of breathing can also be regulated to work in concert with the heart in order to provide maximum benefit to the patient. The effectiveness of pulmonary monitoring is itself monitored by measuring the amount of oxygen in arterial blood. This, too, can be accomplished automatically, with adjustments made by instruments.

Common situations that require critical care are choking, drowning, poisoning, physical trauma, psychological trauma, and environmental disasters.

Choking. Difficulty in either breathing or swallowing is termed choking. The source of the obstruction may be either internal or external. Internal obstructions can result from a foreign body becoming stuck in the mouth (pharynx), throat (esophagus or trachea), or lungs (bronchi). The blockage may be partial or total. A foreign body that is caught in the esophagus will create difficulty in swallowing; one that is caught in the trachea will obstruct breathing. Any foreign body may become lodged and create a blockage. Objects that commonly cause obstructions include teeth (both natural and false), food (especially meat and bones from fish), and liquids such as water and blood.

Obstructions can occur externally. Examples of external causes of choking include compression of the larynx or trachea as a result of blunt trauma (a physical blow or other injury sustained in an accident), a penetrating projectile such as a bullet or stick, and toys or small items of food that are swallowed accidentally. Foods such as nuts or candy are frequently aspirated as the result of trying to catch one in the mouth after tossing it in the air. An object that becomes stuck in the lungs frequently does not cause an acute shortage of breath, but this situation can lead to aspiration pneumonia, which is extremely difficult to treat.

The symptoms of choking are well known: gagging, coughing, and difficulty in breathing. Pain may or may not be present. Frequently, there is a short episode of difficulty in breathing followed by a period when no symptoms are experienced. The foreign body may be moved aside or pushed deeper into the body by the victim's initial frantic movements. A foreign body lodged in the esophagus will not interfere with breathing but may cause food or liquids to spill into the trachea and become aspirated; as with an object in the lungs, this usually leads to pneumonia or other serious respiratory conditions.

Drowning. Drowning is defined as the outcome (usually death) of unanticipated immersion into a liquid (usually water). Consciousness is an important determinant of how an individual reacts to immersion in water. A person who is conscious will attempt to escape from the fluid environment, which involves attempts to regain orientation and not to aspirate additional liquids. An unconscious person has none of these defenses and usually dies when the lungs fill rapidly with water. Normal persons can hold their breath for thirty seconds or more. Frequently, this is sufficient time for a victim to escape from immersion in a fluid environment. When a victim exhales just prior to entering water, this time period is not available; indeed, panic frequently develops, and the victim aspirates water.

Most but not all victims of drowning die from aspirating water. Approximately 10 percent of drowning victims die from asphyxia while underwater, possibly because they hold their breath or because the larynx goes into spasms. The brain of the average person can survive without oxygen for about four minutes. After that time, irreversible damage starts to occur; death follows in a matter of minutes. After four minutes, survival is possible but unlikely to be without the permanent impairment of mental functions.

The physical condition of the victim exerts a profound influence on the outcome of a drowning situation. Physically fit persons have a far greater chance of escaping from a drowning environment. Individuals who are in poor condition, who are very weak, or who have handicaps must overcome these conditions when attempting to escape from a drowning situation; frequently, they are unable to remove themselves and die in the process.

Another physical condition such as exhaustion or a heart attack may also be present. An exhausted person is weak and may not have the physical strength or endurance to escape. A person who experiences a heart attack at the moment of immersion is at a severe disadvantage. If the heart is unable to deliver blood and nutrients to muscles, even a physically fit person is weakened and may be less likely to escape a drowning situation.

The temperature of the water is critical. Immersing the face in cold water (below 20 degrees Celsius or 56 degrees Fahrenheit) initiates a reflex that slows the person's heart rate and shunts blood to the heart and brain, thus delaying irreversible cerebral damage. Immersion in water even colder leads to hypothermia (subnormal body temperature). In the short term, hypothermia reduces the body's consumption of oxygen and allows submersion in water for slightly longer periods of time. There have been reports of survival after immersion of ten minutes in warm water and forty minutes in extremely cold water. Age is also a factor: Younger persons are more likely to tolerate such conditions than older persons.

Poisoning. Whether intentional or accidental, poisoning demands immediate medical care. Intoxication can also initiate a crisis that requires critical care. Alcohol is the most common intoxicant, but a wide range of other substances are accidentally ingested. Accidental poisoning is the most common cause of death in young children. When an individual is poisoned, the toxic substance must be removed from the body. This removal may be accomplished in a variety of ways and is usually done in a hospital. Supportive care may be needed during the period of acute crisis. The brain, liver, and kidneys are usually at great risk during a toxic crisis; steps must be taken to protect these organs.

Physical trauma. In the United States, more than 1.5 million persons are hospitalized each year as a result of trauma; some 100,000 of these patients die. Trauma is the leading cause of death in persons under the age of forty and, overall, is the third most common cause of death. Approximately three million people have died as a result of motor vehicle accidents alone in the United States; the first such death occurred in 1899. Trauma is commonly characterized as either blunt or penetrating.

Blunt trauma occurs when an external force is applied to tissue, causing compression or crushing injuries as well as fractures. This force can be applied directly from being hit with an object or indirectly through the forces generated by sudden deceleration. In the latter event, relatively mobile organs or structures continue moving until stopped by adjacent, relatively fixed organs or structures. Any of these injuries can result in extensive internal bleeding. Damage may also cause fluids to be lost from tissues and lead to shock, circulatory collapse, and ultimately death.

The most frequent sources for penetrating wounds are knives and firearms. A knife blade produces a smaller wound; fewer organs are likely to be involved, and adjacent structures are less likely to sustain damage. In contrast, gunshot wounds are more likely to involve multiple tissues and to damage adjacent structures. More energy is released by a bullet than by a knife. This energy is sufficient to fracture a bone and usually leads to a greater amount of tissue damage.

The wound must be repaired, typically through surgical exploration and suturing. Extensively damaged tissue is removed in a process called debridement. Any visible sources of secondary contamination must also be removed. With both knife and firearm wounds often comes contamination by dirt, clothing, and other debris; this contamination presents a serious threat of infection to the victim and is also a problem for critical care workers. The wound is then covered appropriately, and the victim is given antibiotics to counteract bacteria that may have been introduced with the primary injury.

Psychological trauma. Critical care is often required in situations that lead to psychological stress. Individuals taking drug overdoses require critical supportive care until the drug has been metabolized by or removed from the body. Respiratory support is needed when the drug depresses the portion of the brain that controls breathing. Some drugs cause extreme agitation, which must be controlled by sedation.

Severe trauma to a loved one can initiate a psychological crisis. Psychological support must be provided to the victim; frequently, this is done in a hospital setting. An entire family may require critical care support for brief periods of time in the aftermath of a catastrophe. Severe trauma, disease, or the death of a child may require support by outsiders. Most hospitals have professionals who are trained to provide such support. In addition, people with psychiatric problems sometimes fail to take the medications that control mental illness. Critical care support in a hospital is often needed until these people are restabilized on their medications.

Environmental disasters. The need for psychological support, as well as urgent medical care, is magnified with natural or environmental disasters such as earthquakes, hurricanes, floods, or tornadoes. Environmental disasters seriously disrupt lives and normal services; they arise with little or no warning. The key to providing critical care in a disaster situation is adequate prior planning.

Responses to disasters occur at three levels: institutional (hospital), local (police, fire, and rescue), and regional (county and state). The plan must be simple and evolve from normal operations; individuals respond best when they are asked to perform tasks with which they are familiar and for which they are trained. The response must integrate all existing sources of emergency medical and supportive services. Those who assume responsibilities for overall management must be well trained and able to adapt to different conditions that may be encountered. Because no two disasters are ever alike, such flexibility is essential. Summaries of individual duties and responsibilities should be available for all involved individuals. Finally, the disaster plan should be practiced and rehearsed using specific scenarios. Experience is the single best method to ensure competency when a disaster strikes.

Environmental disasters such as earthquakes, hurricanes, floods, or tornadoes cause loss of life and extensive loss of property. Essential services such as water, gas, electricity, and telephone communication are often lost. Victims must be provided food, shelter, and medical care on an immediate basis. Critical care is usually required at the time of the disaster, and the need for support may continue long after the immediate effects of the disaster have been resolved.

PERSPECTIVE AND PROSPECTS

One of the most important issues with regard to critical care is sometimes controversial: when to discontinue life support. Life-support equipment is usually withdrawn as soon as patients are able to function independent of the machinery. These patients continue to recover, are discharged from the hospital, and complete their recovery at home. For some, however, the outcome is not as positive. Machines may be used to assist breathing. For a patient who does not improve, or who deteriorates, there comes a point in time when a decision to stop life support must be made. This is not an easy decision, nor should it be made by a single individual.

The patient's own wishes must be paramount. These wishes, however, must have been clearly communicated while the individual was in good health and had unimpaired thought processes. A patient's family is entitled to provide input in the decision to terminate care, but others are also entitled to provide input: the patient's physician, representatives of the hospital or institution, a representative of the patient's religious faith, and the state.

Medical science has developed criteria for death. The application of these criteria, however, is not uni-

form. The final decision to terminate life support is frequently a consensus of all the parties mentioned above. When there is a dispute, the courts are often asked to intervene. Extensive disagreements exist concerning the ethics of terminating critical care. It is beyond the scope of this discussion to provide definitive guidelines. This logical extension of critical care may not have a uniform resolution; the values and beliefs of each individual determine the outcome of each situation.

—*L. Fleming Fallon, Jr., M.D., Ph.D., M.P.H.*
See also Accidents; Aging: Extended care; Choking; Coma; Critical care, pediatric; Death and dying; Disease; Drowning; Electrocardiography (ECG or EKG); Electroencephalography (EEG); Emergency medicine; Ethics; Euthanasia; Hospitals; Hyperbaric oxygen therapy; Nursing; Paramedics; Poisoning; Psychiatric disorders; Respiration; Resuscitation; Surgery, general; Terminally ill: Extended care; Tracheostomy; Unconsciousness; Wounds.

FOR FURTHER INFORMATION:

Bongard, Frederick, and Darryl Y. Sue, eds. *Current Critical Care Diagnosis and Treatment.* 2d ed. New York: Appleton & Lange, 2002. A medical text that combines medical and surgical perspectives with diagnostic and treatment knowledge. Covers forty topics in critical care basics, medical critical care, and essentials of surgical intensive care and includes information on pregnancy, psychiatric disorders, imaging procedures, and transport, among other topics.

Fink, Mitchell P., et al. *Textbook of Critical Care.* 5th ed. Philadelphia: Elsevier Saunders, 2005. This medical text, written by experts in the field, represents the views of the Society of Critical Care Medicine. The general reader will find it interesting but may elect to skip some sections containing highly technical details.

Hogan, David E., and Jonathan L. Burstein. *Disaster Medicine.* Philadelphia: Lippincott Williams & Wilkins, 2002. Examines a wide range of relevant topics including natural, industrial, transportation and conflict-related disasters; and infectious diseases, winter storms, fires and mass burn care, intentional chemical disasters, and mass shootings.

Markovchick, Vincent J., and Peter T. Pons. *Emergency Medicine Secrets.* 4th ed. Philadelphia: Mosby Elsevier, 2006. A clinical reference book that covers decision making in emergency medicine, hematology and oncology, metabolism and endocrinology, infectious disease, environmental emergencies, neonatal and childhood disorders, toxicologic emergencies, and behavioral emergencies, among many other topics.

Safar, Peter, and Nicholas G. Bircher. *Cardiopulmonary Cerebral Resuscitation: Basic and Advanced Cardiac and Trauma Life Support—An Introduction to Resuscitation Medicine.* 3d ed. Philadelphia: Saunders, 1988. A text that completely describes the process of cardiopulmonary resuscitation (CPR). The general reader can learn much from it but is cautioned to take a training course taught by the Red Cross or American Heart Association before attempting to use CPR.

CRITICAL CARE, PEDIATRIC

SPECIALTY

ANATOMY OR SYSTEM AFFECTED: All

SPECIALTIES AND RELATED FIELDS: Anesthesiology, cardiology, emergency medicine, gastroenterology, neonatology, neurology, nursing, pediatrics, pharmacology, pulmonary medicine, radiology, toxicology

DEFINITION: The hospital care of seriously ill or injured infants and children.

KEY TERMS:

computed tomography (CT) scanning: a radiographic technique using computer-enhanced X-ray images to show the anatomy of cross sections of the body

magnetic resonance imaging (MRI): a technique using strong electromagnets to show the anatomy of cross sections of the body in great detail

SCIENCE AND PROFESSION

When a serious illness or injury occurs to children, they cannot simply be treated as small adults. The serious illnesses from which they suffer are different from those of adults. Children's bodies respond differently to illness and injuries and require different types of resuscitative fluids and medications. The critical care pediatrician is specially trained to provide this special care.

A critical care pediatrician has undergone, in addition to four years of medical school, three years of pediatric residency and three years of fellowship training in the care of critically ill or injured children. Critical care pediatricians usually practice in large referral hospitals or children's hospitals.

The care of a seriously ill or injured child requires many skills, including the resuscitation and stabilization of the patient's condition, consultation with other specialists, and the establishment and execution of a plan of action. The plan is often complicated, especially if more than one organ system is involved. The critical care pediatrician coordinates the work of the patient's health team.

Resuscitation usually begins in the emergency room and is directed by the emergency room physician. The critical care pediatrician may take over care in the emergency room or when the patient is moved from there or from the operating room to the intensive care unit (ICU).

On the patient's arrival at the hospital, the team first ensures that the patient is able to breathe adequately, and, if not, begins to ventilate the patient's lungs. The patient's cardiac output is quickly evaluated, and chest compression is begun if it is inadequate. The degree of shock is evaluated next and is treated with intravenous fluid. As this resuscitation is being carried out, the critical care pediatrician obtains a history of the illness or injury and conducts a thorough examination of the patient. Based on this information, the physician orders appropriate laboratory and radiographic tests and calls on other specialists, as needed, for help and advice.

Once the patient arrives in the ICU, the critical care pediatrician must continue to treat the initial problem as well as any complications and difficulties added by surgery or other therapies. The physician must be able to relate these problems to his or her knowledge of anatomy and physiology. A quick and accurate assessment of a large number of factors is required, as is the ability to gain an overview of all the conditions faced in the care of the patient.

The critical care pediatrician's day is largely spent in a hospital emergency room and its intensive care areas. This type of specialist does not usually practice in a clinic except for occasional follow-up examinations of patients who have been discharged from the hospital.

DIAGNOSTIC AND TREATMENT TECHNIQUES

The critical care pediatrician utilizes a wide variety of diagnostic techniques. Complete blood counts, blood chemistry tests, and cultures of blood, urine, and cerebrospinal fluid are initially helpful, especially in looking for bacterial infections. These tests must be performed periodically to assess the patient's progress. Depending on the patient's problem, more specific tests may be necessary. Imaging studies, such as X rays, ultrasonography, and computed tomography (CT) or magnetic resonance imaging (MRI) scans, are often critical to this evaluation.

Besides closely monitoring the patient's condition, the critical care pediatrician must be able to perform a number of procedures. One is the management of ventilators, machines that can breathe for a child who is too ill or injured to breathe adequately on his or her own. The critical care physician is also expert at inserting a number of intravascular devices, such as central intravenous catheters, for intravenous (IV) fluids and for monitoring the function of the heart, and intra-arterial catheters, for monitoring blood pressure and conducting blood gas tests, which are used to evaluate the function of the lungs.

A complicated form of cardiopulmonary support for some critically ill children is called extracorporeal membrane oxygenation (ECMO). It is the circulation of the child's blood through an artificial lung machine using large intravenous tubes, generally inserted in the neck. This machine adds oxygen to and removes carbon dioxide from the child's circulation. ECMO requires a team of highly trained technicians. Its use is overseen by the critical care pediatrician when the patient is older than a newborn. ECMO is available only in the largest referral hospitals.

The care of critically ill children requires much emotional maturity on the part of the physician. The child's family is frightened and anxious, and the child is under great emotional stress. The team of caregivers feels the stress of working with these children as well. The critical care pediatrician must be able to provide empathetic support to all people involved in the health crisis. Despite its share of tragedies, critical care pediatrics is a richly rewarding field. The outcome for critically ill children is better than that for equally ill adults.

PERSPECTIVE AND PROSPECTS

While there have always been pediatricians with an interest in critical pediatric care, fellowships in the specialty were first developed in the last quarter of the twentieth century. Critical care was recognized as a subspecialty of pediatrics in 1987. By 1994, there were only sixty-five pediatricians who had been accepted as fellows of the American College of Critical Care Medicine. By then, there was a rapidly increasing demand for these specialists, with four to six positions being advertised for pediatric critical care doctors for every one adult position.

—*Thomas C. Jefferson, M.D.*

See also Accidents; Choking; Coma; Critical care; Death and dying; Disease; Drowning; Electrocardiography (ECG or EKG); Electroencephalography (EEG); Emergency medicine; Ethics; Euthanasia; Hospitals; Nursing; Paramedics; Pediatrics; Poisoning; Psychiatric disorders; Respiration; Resuscitation; Surgery, pediatric; Terminally ill: Extended care; Tracheostomy; Unconsciousness; Wounds.

FOR FURTHER INFORMATION:

Behrman, Richard E., Robert M. Kliegman, and Hal B. Jenson, eds. *Nelson Textbook of Pediatrics*. 17th ed. Philadelphia: Saunders, 2004. Text covering all medical and surgical disorders in children with authoritative information on genetics, endocrinology, aetiology, epidemiology, pathology, pathophysiology, clinical manifestations, diagnosis, prevention, treatment, and prognosis.

Fuhrman, Bradley P., and Jerry J. Zimmerman, eds. *Pediatric Critical Care*. 3d ed. Philadelphia: Mosby-Elsevier, 2006. A manual of pediatric intensive and emergency care. Includes bibliographical references and an index.

Merenstein, Gerald B., and Sandra L. Gardner, eds. *Handbook of Neonatal Intensive Care*. 6th ed. St. Louis: Mosby Elsevier, 2006. A text covering clinical issues such as nutritional and metabolic support and diseases of the neonate.

Todres, I. David, and John H. Fugate, eds. *Critical Care of Infants and Children*. Boston: Little, Brown, 1996. Written from the necessarily pragmatic point of view of the busy clinician, this invaluable volume is filled with practical information without digressions into obscure basic science. A comprehensive section of procedures opens the book, with systems forming its basic organization.

CROHN'S DISEASE

DISEASE/DISORDER

ALSO KNOWN AS: Regional enteritis

ANATOMY OR SYSTEM AFFECTED: Gastrointestinal system, intestines

SPECIALTIES AND RELATED FIELDS: Gastroenterology, immunology, nutrition, pediatrics

DEFINITION: A chronic disease process in which the bowel becomes inflamed, leading to scarring and narrowing of the intestines.

KEY TERMS:

abscess: a localized collection of pus (dead cells and a mixture of live and dead bacteria)

antigen: a foreign substance in the body causing an immunological response that produces antibodies

fissure: a break in the surface tissue of the anal canal or the wall of the gastrointestinal tract

fistula: an abnormal connection between two hollow structures or between a hollow structure and the skin surface

CAUSES AND SYMPTOMS

Crohn's disease is a chronic disease of the digestive system. It is one of two diseases labeled as inflammatory bowel disease (IBD); the other is ulcerative colitis. With both diseases, patients suffer from diarrhea, abdominal pain, bleeding from the rectum, and fever. The cell lining of the bowel (usually the small intestine) becomes inflamed, leading to erosion of tissues and bleeding.

Crohn's disease may affect areas of the gastrointestinal system from the mouth to the exit of the body, the anus. The inflammatory process may spread to include the joints, skin, eyes, mouth, and sometimes liver. In children, IBD involves a substantial risk of slow or interrupted growth.

The most common early sign is abdominal pain, often felt over the navel or on the right side. Diarrhea and subsequent weight loss often follow. Other early signs of Crohn's disease include sores in the anal area (skin tabs), hemorrhoids, fissures (cracks), fistulas (abnormal openings from the intestines to the skin surface or other organs), abscesses (uncommon in children), and nausea and vomiting, especially in young children. Children as young as ten may develop this disease; however, in the majority of cases the onset is between the ages of sixteen and twenty-five. Some sources report that Crohn's disease is slightly more common in females. The incidence is greater in persons of Jewish ethnic origin.

Diagnosis often is made after a series of abdominal X rays, an upper gastrointestinal series, or a colonoscopy (visual inspection of the intestines with a camera). The gastrointestinal (GI) tract is best pictured as a continuous tube that begins at the mouth and ends at the anus. The mucosal layer of intestine that absorbs nutrients contains immune cells that act as defenders of the body (antibodies). Sometimes, this mucosal layer breaks down, and harmful bacteria enter the deep layers of the intestine. The resulting inflammatory process can entail swelling (edema), increased blood flow, and ulcerations (disruptions in the intestinal lining). In Crohn's disease, these ulcerations involve the full thickness of the intestinal lining.

When the inflamed intestine heals, it may become scarred around the areas previously inflamed. This may lead to a narrowing of the bowel, or stricture, which can lead to partial or total blockage of the intestinal flow (bowel obstruction).

TREATMENT AND THERAPY

Crohn's disease is a baffling, unpredictable disease for which a truly successful treatment has not been found. Some of the medications used in treatment are corticosteroids, such as prednisone and adrenocorticotropic hormone (ACTH), and sulfasalazine-type drugs, such as Azulfidine. Both have limited benefits and some side effects. Prednisone-type drugs reduce tissue inflammation and thereby relieve symptoms such as diarrhea, rectal bleeding, abdominal pain, and fever. They may cause side effects including rounding of the face, increased facial hair, fluid retention, bone loss (osteoporosis), high blood pressure, and high blood sugar levels. These drugs also may cause mood swings. They are prescribed conservatively by most doctors. Sulfasalazine contains two active ingredients, a sulfa preparation (sulfapyridine) and an aspirin-like drug (5-aminosalicylic acid, or 5-ASA), which are bonded together. The 5-ASA medication is thought to act on the surface of the lining of the intestine, suppressing tissue inflammation.

The drug 6-mercaptopurine, or 6-MP, is an immunosuppressive, a substance that alters the body's normal immune response to a disease or antigen. Immunosuppressive drugs have been used to treat autoimmune diseases, conditions in which the body literally attacks itself, among them Crohn's disease. It is believed that these drugs can stop the mechanism that causes the body to attack itself.

Drugs can offer relief of symptoms, but no drug has yet been found to alter the long-term progression or natural course of Crohn's disease. Surgical removal of the

---

INFORMATION ON CROHN'S DISEASE

CAUSES: Infection

SYMPTOMS: Diarrhea, abdominal pain, rectal bleeding, fever, weight loss, anal sores, hemorrhoids, fissures, fistulas, abscesses, nausea, vomiting

DURATION: Chronic

TREATMENTS: Medications for symptom alleviation

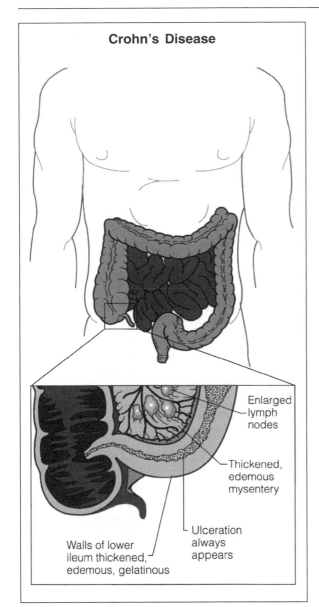

Crohn's Disease

Enlarged lymph nodes

Thickened, edemous mysentery

Ulceration always appears

Walls of lower ileum thickened, edemous, gelatinous

Crohn's disease can cause inflammation and ulceration within any region of the digestive tract, but most often in the ileum.

diseased intestine is usually reserved for cases in which medical treatment has failed. The recurrence rates of Crohn's disease following surgery are high.

PERSPECTIVE AND PROSPECTS

Unlike ulcerative colitis, which affects only the inner lining of the intestines, Crohn's disease affects the full thickness of the bowel wall. Both types of IBD occur in predominantly Western or developed countries, especially Scandinavia, England, Western Europe, Israel, and the United States. In recent years, IBD has been reported in Japan. IBD is seen rarely in Africa, most of Asia, and parts of South America. IBD seems to cluster in families, suggesting a genetic factor. Up to 20 percent of people with IBD have one or more blood relatives with the disease.

American gastroenterologist Burrill B. Crohn first identified Crohn's disease in 1932. The prognosis for sufferers was poor, and their quality of life was limited. Surgical removal of the diseased colon or small colon was the only treatment. Prednisone was the first of the above-mentioned medications to be used to treat Crohn's disease. Investigation into the causes and treatment of IBD continues in many areas, including genetic studies. Current research offers reason for optimism that the causes of IBD will be found and that a cure will follow.

—*Lisa Levin Sobczak, R.N.C.*

See also Colitis; Diarrhea and dysentery; Gastroenterology; Gastroenterology, pediatric; Gastrointestinal system; Immune system; Intestinal disorders; Intestines; Irritable bowel syndrome (IBS); Nausea and vomiting.

FOR FURTHER INFORMATION:

Brandt, Lawrence J., and Penny Steiner-Grossman, eds. *Treating IBD: A Patient's Guide to the Medical and Surgical Management of Inflammatory Bowel Disease*. Reprint. Philadelphia: Lippincott-Raven, 1996. One of the most thorough introductions to ulcerative colitis and Crohn's disease. Writing for patients, the authors, who are all medical experts, present technical information and guidelines on symptoms, drugs, surgical procedures, nutritional management, psychotherapy, and counseling.

Crohn's and Colitis Foundation of America. http://www.ccfa.org/. Provides support groups and a wide range of educational publications and programs on Crohn's and ulcerative colitis.

Kalibjian, Cliff. *Straight from the Gut: Living with Crohn's Disease and Ulcerative Colitis*. Cambridge, Mass.: O'Reilly and Associates, 2003. Shares numerous personal stories from those suffering from colitis and offers advice on all aspects of living with the disease.

Murray, Michael T. *Stomach Ailments and Digestive Disturbances: How You Can Benefit from Diet, Vitamins, Minerals, Herbs, Exercise, and Other Natural Methods*. Rocklin, Calif.: Prima, 1997. Chronic stomach ailments affect many Americans, and the number can only increase as the population ages. Murray counters that trend with practical information and sensible advice for getting well and staying well naturally.

Saibil, Fred. *Crohn's Disease and Ulcerative Colitis: Everything You Need to Know.* Rev. ed. Toronto: Firefly Books, 2003. A leading expert on IBD, Saibil covers topics such as signs and symptoms, how the gastrointestinal system works normally and how IBD affects it, procedures and instruments used to diagnose IBD, effects of diet, children and IBD, and effects on sexual activity and child-bearing.

Sklar, Jill, Manual Sklar, and Annabel Cohen. *The First Year—Crohn's Disease and Ulcerative Colitis: An Essential Guide for the Newly Diagnosed.* New York: Avalon, 2002. A unique guide for patients with specific gastrointestinal disorders, setting expectations and answering questions related to the first week of diagnosis, the first months, and the first year. Topics include treatment options, dietary choices, fertility issues, and holistic alternatives.

Steiner-Grossman, Penny, Peter A. Banks, and Daniel H. Present, eds. *The New People, Not Patients: A Source Book for Living with Inflammatory Bowel Disease.* Rev. ed. Dubuque, Iowa: Kendall/Hunt, 1997. Written to help IBD patients live with the disease, this book combines very practical information—about support groups and patients' rights, for example—with overviews of symptoms and treatments. Its main strength, however, lies in case histories of patients from different walks of life.

Zonderman, Jon, and Ronald S. Vender. *Understanding Crohn Disease and Ulcerative Colitis.* Jackson: University Press of Mississippi, 2000. Crohn's patient Zonderman and Vender, his gastroenterologist, base their presentation of the medical and psychological aspects of two inflammatory bowel diseases on solid medical evidence. They deal with related medical conditions and how Crohn's disease and ulcerative colitis can affect persons of different ages differently.

CROSSED EYES. *See* STRABISMUS.

CROUP

DISEASE/DISORDER

ALSO KNOWN AS: Viral croup, spasmodic croup, laryngotracheobronchitis

ANATOMY OR SYSTEM AFFECTED: Lungs, respiratory system, throat

SPECIALTIES AND RELATED FIELDS: Emergency medicine, otorhinolaryngology, pediatrics, preventive medicine, virology

DEFINITION: An inflammation of the larynx, throat, and upper bronchial tubes causing hoarseness, cough, and difficult breathing.

KEY TERMS:

cortisone: a steroid hormone used to reduce inflammation

epiglottis: a small piece of cartilage that covers the entry to the windpipe during swallowing

epiglottitis: a serious condition caused by a bacterial infection sometimes confused with croup

epinephrine: a hormone that helps the body manage physical stress

larynx: the voice box

stridor: the characteristic noisy, labored breathing present with croup

trachea: the windpipe

CAUSES AND SYMPTOMS

Croup is an inflammation of the larynx, trachea, and upper bronchial tubes of the lungs affecting children between the ages of six months and generally no older than five years. Two-year-olds seem to be the most commonly affected. The inflammation of the trachea causes a narrowing of the child's already small airways, making breathing difficult. Technically, croup is a syndrome, or collection of symptoms associated with several different kinds of infections. These symptoms include hoarseness, a distinctive cough most often described as "barky" and noisy, and labored breathing known as stridor.

Croup occurs in three different forms. The first, viral croup, usually begins with a cold and is most commonly caused by parainfluenza viruses. Indeed, studies indicate that the parainfluenza viruses are responsible for about 70 to 75 percent of croup cases. Viral croup is often accompanied by a low-grade fever. A second type of croup is called spasmodic croup. This condition tends to occur with changes of the weather and/or seasons, and the child does not usually run a fever. Allergies are often thought to be responsible for this kind of croup. A third, but rare, form is a bacterial infection caused by mycoplasma. This form can be very serious and is often identified by the extreme difficulty that the child experiences with breathing.

Studies indicate that attacks of croup most commonly occur in October through March and generally strike at night. In general, boys are somewhat

INFORMATION ON CROUP

CAUSES: Viral or bacterial infection, allergens, change in environment (seasonal change)
SYMPTOMS: Hoarseness, "barking" cough, difficulty breathing
DURATION: Acute
TREATMENTS: Medications (cortisone, antibiotics), humidifier; if severe, emergency care and oxygen tent

more likely to be affected by croup than are girls.

A serious, but rare, condition known as epiglottitis can sometimes be mistaken for croup. In this condition, the epiglottis, the flap that covers the windpipe during swallowing, becomes inflamed and swollen, potentially cutting off the child's air supply. The symptoms of epiglottitis are similar to those of croup, but the child's difficulty in breathing is much more severe, and the child will often run a high fever, drool, and be unable to make voiced sounds. Epiglottitis develops quickly; a child's life can be in jeopardy in only a few hours. Consequently, this condition must be treated as an emergency, requiring hospital care.

TREATMENT AND THERAPY

A number of treatments are generally used to bring relief to the child suffering from viral or spasmodic croup. The use of a cool mist humidifier can ward off an attack in the child who exhibits a tendency toward developing croup. A mild attack can also be alleviated through use of the humidifier. If the attack of croup is well under way or if it is severe, however, a cool mist humidifier may not be adequate. Many doctors recommend that after an attack of croup, a cool mist humidifier should be run in the child's room for the next three or four evenings. Another commonly used treatment is to take the child, properly dressed, outside at night. Usually the cold, damp air will soothe the child's inflamed airways.

Still another technique reported to relieve the symptoms of croup is to fill the bathroom with steam by running a hot shower. Setting the child in the steam-filled room for fifteen to twenty minutes often eases the child's breathing. The most successful use of this treatment requires that the child be held, not placed on the floor, because steam rises.

Neither cough syrups nor antibiotics are appropriate treatments for croup. Cough syrups prevent the expulsion of phlegm, while antibiotics have no effect on viral infections. Croup caused by mycoplasma, however, is treated with an antibiotic, generally erythromycin.

Pediatricians recommend that the child's doctor be called in the event of a croup attack. Serious attacks are generally treated in a hospital emergency room. There, the child may be given cortisone by injection or by mouth. In addition, hospitals can administer breathing treatments.

Bacterial croup is also treated at a hospital with antibiotics and an oxygen tent as needed. Indeed, immediate emergency room treatment is called for if there is a whistling sound in the breathing that seems to grow louder, if the child does not have enough breath to speak, or if the child is struggling to breathe.

PERSPECTIVE AND PROSPECTS

Accounts of croup can be found in medical literature dating back to the eighteenth century. Membranous croup, also known as diphtheria, was a great killer of children and adults alike in the past. Immunization made this kind of croup extremely rare, however, by the mid-twentieth century.

During the last quarter of the twentieth century, doctors continued to research the uses of corticosteroids in the treatment of croup, as well as the most effective way to deliver the drugs.

—*Diane Andrews Henningfeld, Ph.D.*

See also Bacterial infections; Bronchitis; Childhood infectious diseases; Coughing; Diphtheria; Epiglottitis; Laryngitis; Respiration; Sore throat; Viral infections; Wheezing.

FOR FURTHER INFORMATION:

American Medical Association. *American Medical Association Family Medical Guide.* 4th rev. ed. Hoboken, N.J.: John Wiley & Sons, 2004. An excellent reference for the beginner. The scientific accuracy of the text is not compromised by its accessibility.

Nathanson, Laura Walter. "Coping with Croup." *Parents* 70, no. 9 (September, 1995): 29-31. Practical advice for treating the scary-sounding cough known as croup is offered to parents. Although home remedies can help alleviate the croup, special medications allow a child to breathe easier and recover faster.

Niederman, Michael S., George A. Sarosi, and Jeffrey Glassroth. *Respiratory Infections.* 2d ed. Philadelphia: Lippincott Williams & Wilkins, 2001. Text that covers a range of respiratory problems, including croup.

Shelov, Steven P., et al. *Caring for Your Baby and Young Child: Birth to Age Five.* 4th ed. New York: Bantam Books, 2004. Offers a comprehensive discussion of illnesses that commonly affect young children.

Spock, Benjamin, and Robert Needlman. *Dr. Spock's Baby and Child Care.* 8th ed. New York: Pocket Books, 2004. For more than a half century, this book has been a virtual bible for parents seeking trustworthy information on child care. Informative, easy to use, and responsive to the changes in society, this revised and updated edition makes a classic work more essential than ever.

West, John B. *Pulmonary Pathophysiology: The Essentials.* 6th ed. Baltimore: Lippincott Williams & Wilkins, 2003. Examines lungs afflicted with obstructive, restrictive, vascular, and environmental diseases.

Woolf, Alan D., et al., eds. *The Children's Hospital Guide to Your Child's Health and Development.* Cambridge, Mass.: Perseus, 2002. An authoritative and comprehensive guide to children's health, providing a guide to every common illness or condition that affects children and a carefully designed emergency section.

CROWNS AND BRIDGES

TREATMENTS

ANATOMY OR SYSTEM AFFECTED: Gums, mouth, teeth

SPECIALTIES AND RELATED FIELDS: Dentistry

DEFINITION: Devices implanted to restore proper functioning and aesthetics of the teeth.

INDICATIONS AND PROCEDURES

With the aging process, the teeth undergo wear, increased sensitivity, decay, and in some cases, disease that may result in the loss of some or all of the teeth. This is particularly true in the elderly. Dentists can restore natural teeth that are damaged, decayed, or lost by using crowns and bridges. A crown may be constructed to restore an individual damaged tooth back to its original form and function, while a bridge may be utilized to replace one or more missing teeth. Each of these restorations is cemented onto the teeth and is referred to as fixed dentistry, in contrast to a restoration of missing teeth with a removable appliance or partial denture.

A crown, or cap, fits over a tooth. It strengthens and protects the covered tooth structure and can improve the overall appearance of the teeth. Crowns and bridges can be made from different materials, which include natural-looking porcelain, porcelain fused to a metal crown, or an all-metal crown. The patient and the dentist decide which type is the most appropriate, depending on the strength requirements and aesthetic concerns of the tooth or teeth involved. Cost will be a primary concern for many elderly.

A crown is produced using an indirect procedure. The tooth to be capped is modified by drilling and then prepared using special instruments. A copy of the prepared tooth is made by taking an impression, which is sent to a laboratory where the crown is constructed. Once the impression stage is completed, the dentist places a temporary plastic or acrylic crown on the prepared tooth to protect it and the gum tissues until the permanent crown is ready to be cemented onto the tooth.

When one or more teeth are lost, five or more other teeth may be affected. Remaining teeth may shift or tilt into the open space, changing the bite, which may result in sore jaws, gum disease, or decay. When teeth are missing and there are teeth on either side of the open space, a bridge is the best way to replace the missing teeth. Replacement teeth can be attached to two crowns constructed for the two teeth on either side of the open space.

A fixed bridge is used to replace one or several teeth. To prepare the bridge, diagnostic models are used to study the optimum way to perform the procedure. After these studies are completed, the tooth on each end of the open space is carefully reshaped, impressions are taken, and crowns are made for the end teeth so that they can serve as anchors for the bridge. While the permanent bridge is being prepared, which usually takes about two to three weeks, a temporary acrylic bridge is cemented into place. Since the bridge and attaching crowns are made as one solid piece, it is necessary to use a special type of dental floss that goes under the bridge in order to keep this area of gum tissue healthy.

—*Alvin K. Benson, Ph.D.*

See also Aging; Bone disorders; Cavities; Dental diseases; Dentistry; Dentures; Teeth.

FOR FURTHER INFORMATION:

Diamond, Richard. *Dental First Aid for Families.* Ravensdale, Wash.: Idyll Arbor, 2000.

Howe, Leslie C., et al. *Inlays, Crowns, and Bridges: A Clinical Handbook.* Edited by George F. Kantorowicz. 5th ed. Boston: Wright, 1993.

Smith, Rebecca W. *The Columbia University School of Dental and Oral Surgery's Guide to Family Dental Care*. New York: W. W. Norton, 1997.

Woodall, Irene R., ed. *Comprehensive Dental Hygiene Care*. 4th ed. St. Louis: C. V. Mosby, 1993.

CRYOSURGERY

PROCEDURE

ALSO KNOWN AS: Cryotherapy

ANATOMY OR SYSTEM AFFECTED: All

SPECIALTIES AND RELATED FIELDS: Dermatology, family medicine, general surgery, gynecology, neurology, oncology, otorhinolaryngology, plastic surgery, urology

DEFINITION: The destruction of undesired or abnormal body tissues by exposure to extreme cold.

KEY TERMS:

cryogenic agent: a substance (such as liquid nitrogen) that produces low temperatures

cryoprobe: a liquid nitrogen-cooled, probelike tool used in cryosurgery

lesion: abnormal or diseased tissue

INDICATIONS AND PROCEDURES

Cryosurgery, the therapeutic use of extreme cold, is used to remove minor skin lesions such as freckles and warts as well as cancers of the skin and other tissues. Skin heals well after cold injury, and skin pathologies were among the first lesions treated cryosurgically. Although cryosurgery is not the first treatment choice for all skin problems, it is a popular one because of the availability of liquid nitrogen, the main cryogenic agent. In addition, cryosurgery is inexpensive, compared to other procedures, and can be performed without surgical facilities. For example, family physicians and dermatologists use it to treat minor skin lesions at their offices.

Cryosurgery kills tissue via extracellular and intracellular ice. When cells freeze, extracellular ice squeezes them together and changes their extracellular/intracellular volumes. Thawing causes similar, opposite changes that break cell membranes. The rapid temperature drops used in cryosurgery produce intracellular ice, another major source of cell destruction. The result is altered solute concentrations in tissue fluid, electrolyte loss from cells, disrupted membranes, and protein inactivation and transmigration. Reversed temperature gradients cause more destruction during thawing.

Cryosurgery results in tissue hyperemia, discoloration, and ice buildup. On thawing, edema (swelling) develops, yielding necrosis (cell death) in four days. Dead tissue sloughs off in three more days. Within a month, it is replaced by granulation tissue, which yields normal tissue.

Cryosurgery uses between one and five freeze-thaw cycles (FTCs). The freeze speed is 300 degrees Celsius per minute—from 37 degrees Celsius to −196 degrees Celsius—followed by crash (about ten-second), short (one-minute), medium (about three-minute), or long (ten-minute) thaws, depending on the type of lesion treated.

For external tissue treatment, liquid nitrogen (at −196 degrees Celsius) may be applied by swab or in a spray. More often, liquid nitrogen-cooled cryoprobes are pressed on lesions. Cryoprobes are cylindrical, with flat contact surfaces. The duration of cryoprobe use depends on the lesion size and type. For example, genital warts of the cervix are treated by quick freeze, a several-minute thaw, and refreezing.

Treating cancer is more complex. In treating internal cancer, liquid nitrogen is circulated through a cryoprobe touching the lesion. Its position and cell freezing are monitored by ultrasound, which also minimizes the destruction of healthy tissue and identifies the extent of cancer death. The size of the cryoprobe depends on the size of the lesion. If a lesion is not destroyed entirely, then the number of FTCs and the treatment time can be lengthened at follow-up visits.

USES AND COMPLICATIONS

The complexity of cryosurgery varies. Cervical warts require one FTC and a cryoprobe, without any anesthetic. Because of the possibility of postoperative fainting, patients are observed for twenty minutes and should arrange for a ride home. Mild abdominal cramps or vaginal discharge may occur. The surgeon should be contacted about prolonged bleeding, infection, or cramps lasting more than twenty-four hours.

Most skin cancers, most often basal and squamous cell carcinomas, can be treated cryosurgically. Often, three to four FTCs are used. Ear, eyelid, and nose cartilage sites are good targets because scarring and necrosis of surrounding tissue are rare. Superficial basal cell carcinoma exhibits a near 100 percent cure rate, as do nose and ear lesions because these cancers rarely enter cartilage. Squamous cell carcinoma often does, however, and is harder to treat without creating scars. Cryosurgery is the treatment of choice for facial Bowen's squamous cell carcinoma, with a cure rate near 100 percent, and cancers of the cervix or penis; removing these

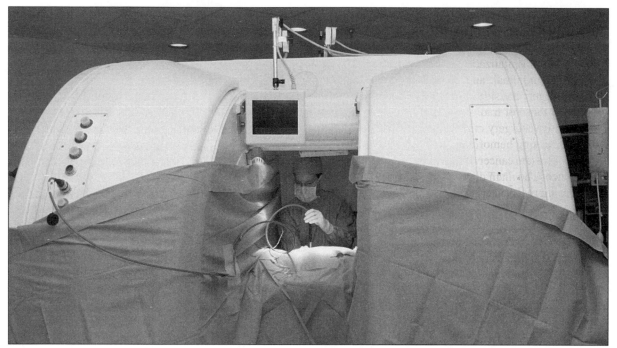

A doctor performs MRI renal cryosurgery, a procedure in which a surgical tube with a freezing tip at the end is used to destroy cancerous kidney tumors while the patient is monitored with MRI. (AP/Wide World Photos)

cancers does not leave scars. Treating lesions on the eyelids, however, may cause them to swell shut.

Cryosurgery can also be used for localized prostate cancer. Warm saline is passed through a urethral catheter to prevent freezing. Cryoprobe placement is achieved through incisions between the anus and scrotum, guided by ultrasound. As with conventional surgery, anesthesia is needed for pain. The appearance of prostate tissue changes during cryosurgery, and damage to healthy tissue can be minimized through the observation of ultrasound images. The prostate gland swells postoperatively, and a catheter in the bladder is used to prevent urination stoppage. This complication and bruises from probe insertion sites can result in hospital stays. However, cryosurgery causes less bleeding, shorter hospitalization and recovery periods, and less pain than does surgical removal of the prostate. Assurance of complete cancer destruction requires follow-up with radiation or chemotherapy.

Cryosurgery is also used to treat liver, pancreas, and breast cancers, and the applicability of cryosurgery to bone, brain, and spinal cancers is under study. In these cases, cryosurgery is part of a mixed treatment, including conventional surgery and radiation or chemotherapy. Initial reports are encouraging, but the long-term effectiveness here is unknown. When standard treatments fail or are unusable in primary or secondary liver cancer, cryosurgery may be used alone. If the surgical removal of cancer from other internal organs is impossible, then cryosurgery may be used to increase symptom-free survival time.

With all cryosurgeries, the discoloration of treated areas and minor scarring may occur. The skin can lose pigment, sweat glands, and hair follicles. Therefore, cryosurgery is less desirable for dark skin and is not suggested for lesions at sites where alopecia (hair loss) would be a problem.

Perspective and Prospects

The first use of cryosurgery was in the early twentieth century through liquid air freezing for skin cancer treatment and cosmetic surgery. In the mid-1950's, improved cryotools began the expansion of cryosurgery to its modern state. This progress was enhanced by the availability of liquid nitrogen, which enabled clinicians to work at temperatures of .196 degrees Celsius.

Cryosurgery is a standard method used in cosmetic surgery and the treatment of skin cancers and is accepted for use with other cancers, including prostate, liver, pancreatic, uterine, lung, and brain cancers. Cryosurgery is employed alone and with other treatments (such as traditional surgery), or when other methods fail. After cryosurgery, many patients regain a high quality of life and are pain-free. Moreover, they are often outpatients, spend little time under the knife, have short hospitalizations, and recuperate rapidly. Scarring is minimal, and cure rates are high.

Cryosurgery has side effects, though they are less severe than those of traditional surgery. In treatment of the liver, cryosurgery may damage bile ducts or blood vessels, causing hemorrhage or infection. In the treatment of prostate cancer, it may cause incontinence and impotence. The main disadvantage, unclear long-term value in internal cancer surgery, is sure to be addressed.

—*Sanford S. Singer, Ph.D.*

See also Cancer; Cervical procedures; Dermatology; Electrocauterization; Melanoma; Moles; Prostate cancer; Skin; Skin cancer; Skin disorders; Skin lesion removal; Tumor removal; Tumors; Warts.

FOR FURTHER INFORMATION:
Dehn, Richard W., and David P. Asprey, eds. *Clinical Procedures for Physician Assistants*. Philadelphia: W. B. Saunders, 2002. The chapter on cryosurgery provides useful information for patients and general readers.

Jackson, Arthur, Graham Colver, and Rodney Dawber. *Cutaneous Cryosurgery: Principles and Clinical Practice*. 3d ed. New York: Taylor & Francis, 2006. An illustrated handbook that provides the information needed for running a cryosurgery clinic.

Korpin, Nikolai N., ed. *Basics of Cryosurgery*. New York: Springer-Verlag, 2001. Discusses cryosurgery from cosmetic work to major surgery. Indexed, with references and illustrations.

Lask, Gary P, and Ronald L. Moy, eds. *Principles and Techniques of Cutaneous Surgery*. New York: McGraw-Hill, 1996. A classic text with a chapter on cryosurgery.

CT SCANNING. *See* COMPUTED TOMOGRAPHY (CT) SCANNING.

CULDOCENTESIS
PROCEDURE
ANATOMY OR SYSTEM AFFECTED: Abdomen, reproductive system
SPECIALTIES AND RELATED FIELDS: Gynecology, general surgery
DEFINITION: A diagnostic procedure in which fluid in the cul-de-sac of Douglas, the space behind the uterus and in front of the rectum, is removed using a needle inserted through the vagina.

INDICATIONS AND PROCEDURES
Culdocentesis is indicated in cases where a woman is suspected of having fluid in the abdomen or pelvis with an unclear cause. The patient may have an acutely painful and tender abdomen. Culdocentesis can identify the presence of fluid in the pelvis as well as distinguish whether the fluid is the result of active bleeding, infection, perforated organ, or other causes.

For culdocentesis, the patient lies on her back with her legs in stirrups, as for a pelvic examination. A speculum is inserted into the vagina to visualize the cervix, and the cervix is gently lifted with a grasping instrument. A long, thin needle is inserted through the vagina, behind the cervix, and into the cul-de-sac of Douglas. Any fluid in this cul-de-sac is aspirated, and analysis of the fluid is subsequently performed.

USES AND COMPLICATIONS
Culdocentesis is not common, as noninvasive imaging modalities such as pelvic ultrasound with vaginal transducer have replaced this procedure to evaluate fluid collections in the abdomen and pelvis. Nevertheless, culdocentesis can yield useful information regarding the nature of abdominal or pelvic fluid, and hence it can assist in diagnosis and treatment decisions. For instance, nonclotted bloody fluid can be consistent with active bleeding, such as from a ruptured ectopic pregnancy or hemorrhagic ovarian cyst. Either of these conditions may require immediate surgery to stop the bleeding. The fluid aspirated from the cul-de-sac may be bile or bowel contents, indicating perforation of the gastrointestinal tract and possible need for urgent surgery. Infected fluid suggests pelvic inflammatory disease (PID) or abscess, for which surgery may not be the first line of treatment. Nonbloody, noninfected fluid may be caused by the rupture of a benign ovarian cyst, which would not require intervention.

Complications associated with culdocentesis are very rare. They include perforation of internal organs, such as the bowel or uterus, with the needle. In almost all cases, no serious aftereffects occur from these perforations, as the needle used is thin, but there are case reports of bleeding from organ perforations that require surgical intervention. Other examples of risks involved with culdocentesis are infection and bleeding from the puncture site.

—*Anne Lynn S. Chang, M.D.*

See also Abscess drainage; Abscesses; Cyst removal; Cysts; Ectopic pregnancy; Gynecology; Invasive tests; Pelvic inflammatory disease (PID); Reproductive system; Women's health.

FOR FURTHER INFORMATION:

Doherty, Gerard M., and Lawrence W. Way, eds. *Current Surgical Diagnosis and Treatment*. 12th ed. New York: Lange Medical Books/McGraw-Hill, 2006.

Rock, John A., and Howard W. Jones III, eds. *Te Linde's Operative Gynecology*. 9th ed. Philadelphia: Lippincott Williams & Wilkins, 2003.

Stenchever, Morton A., et al. *Comprehensive Gynecology*. 4th ed. St. Louis: Mosby, 2006.

CUSHING'S SYNDROME
DISEASE/DISORDER

ANATOMY OR SYSTEM AFFECTED: Abdomen, back, blood, bones, endocrine system, glands, hair, muscles, skin

SPECIALTIES AND RELATED FIELDS: Endocrinology, family medicine, immunology, internal medicine, nutrition, radiology, urology

DEFINITION: A hormonal disorder caused primarily by chronic exposure of body tissues to excessive levels of cortisol.

CAUSES AND SYMPTOMS

Cushing's syndrome is a group of abnormalities that result from either excessive levels of hormones produced by the outer layer of the adrenal glands or from the taking of steroid hormones. The primary source of the disorder is the hormone cortisol. This condition is typically triggered by an excess production of adrenocorticotropic hormone (ACTH) from the pituitary gland. ACTH in turn stimulates the adrenal glands to produce hormones, particularly cortisol. Excessive production of ACTH may result from a pituitary gland tumor or a tumor associated with other organs or as a side effect from taking steroid hormones used to treat asthma, rheumatoid arthritis, and other serious diseases. Adrenal gland tumors also produce excess amounts of cortisol. Though extremely rare, an inherited tendency to develop endocrine gland tumors is another cause of Cushing's syndrome.

Since the hormones produced by the adrenal glands regulate processes throughout the body, excess production can cause widespread disorders. Some of the more common symptoms of Cushing's syndrome are a rounded face, a fat trunk with thin arms and legs, fat pads over the neck and shoulders, purple stretch marks on the skin, easy bruising, muscle weakness, poor wound healing, fractures in weakened bones, high blood pressure, diabetes mellitus, emotional instability, and severe fatigue. Men can experience diminished desire for sex, while women have increased hairiness, acne, and decreased or absent menstrual periods. Children are usually obese, and their growth rate is slow.

TREATMENT AND THERAPY

Cushing's syndrome is treated by restoring the hormonal balance within the body, which may take several months. If Cushing's syndrome is left untreated, it can lead to death. The disease is diagnosed through blood and urine tests to determine excess amounts of cortisol. Pituitary tumors and tumors at other locations

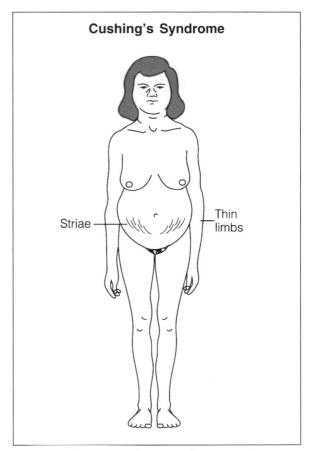

Cushing's Syndrome

Striae — Thin limbs

An adrenal disorder, Cushing's syndrome causes symptomatic fatty deposits, striae, and thin limbs and may be associated with a variety of mild to serious conditions.

INFORMATION ON CUSHING'S SYNDROME

CAUSES: Chronic exposure of body tissues to excess cortisol from overproduction by adrenal glands (tumor) or steroid use

SYMPTOMS: Rounded face, fat trunk with thin arms and legs, fat pads over neck and shoulders, purple stretch marks, easy bruising, muscle weakness, poor wound healing, fractures, high blood pressure, diabetes mellitus, emotional instability

DURATION: Chronic until treated

TREATMENTS: Restoration of hormonal balance, surgical removal of tumor, discontinuance of steroid use

in the body that have been diagnosed as producing ACTH are surgically removed, when possible, or are treated with radiation or chemotherapy. Cortisol replacement therapy is provided after surgery until cortisol production resumes. Life-long cortisol replacement therapy may be necessary. If steroids are not being used to control a life-threatening illness, they should be discontinued.

Adrenal and pituitary tumors are always surgically removed. The remaining adrenal gland, which has usually diminished in size as a result of inactivity, will return to its normal size and function. As it is doing so, steroid hormones are administered to supply the needed cortisol and then tapered off over time. Some tumors may recur after surgical excision.

PERSPECTIVE AND PROSPECTS

The first diagnosis of Cushing's syndrome was made by Dr. Harvey Cushing in 1912. In 1932, he linked the disease to an abnormality in the pituitary gland that stimulated an overproduction of cortisol from the adrenal glands. Pituitary tumors cause approximately 70 percent of the disease. Cushing's syndrome is more frequent in women than in men, with most cases occurring between the ages of twenty-five and forty-five. The disease can be very serious, possibly even fatal, unless diagnosed and treated early.

—*Alvin K. Benson, Ph.D.; updated by Sharon W. Stark, R.N., A.P.R.N., D.N.Sc.*

See also Addison's disease; Corticosteroids; Endocrine disorders; Endocrinology; Endocrinology, pediatric; Hormones; Tumors.

FOR FURTHER INFORMATION:

Endocrine and Metabolic Diseases Information Service. National Institute of Diabetes and Digestive and Kidney Diseases (NIDDK). National Institutes of Health. *Cushing's Syndrome.* http://endocrine .niddk.nih.gov/pubs/cushings/cushings.htm. Comprehensive overview of Cushing's syndrome, its diagnosis and treatment.

Fox, Stuart I. *Human Physiology.* 9th ed. New York, McGraw-Hill, 2006. Hill, 2006. A college-level human physiology textbook that is well written and richly illustrated.

Larsen, P. Reed, et al., eds. *Williams Textbook of Endocrinology.* 10th ed. Philadelphia: W. B. Saunders, 2003. Comprehensive information regarding endocrine diseases, pathophysiology, diagnoses, treatment, and prognoses

MedlincPlus. *Cushing's Syndrome.* Edited by Nikheel S. Kolatkar. http://www.nlm.nih.gov/medlineplus/ ency/article/000410.htm. General information regarding Cushing's syndrome, diagnosis, treatment, complications expectations and prevention.

CYANOSIS

DISEASE/DISORDER

ANATOMY OR SYSTEM AFFECTED: Blood, skin

SPECIALTIES AND RELATED FIELDS: Hematology, internal medicine, pulmonary medicine, toxicology

DEFINITION: Dark blue discoloration of the skin and nail beds resulting from decreases in the oxygenation of hemoglobin in the red blood cells in the arteries.

KEY TERMS:

arterial blood: blood from an artery receiving blood from the left ventricle; usually bright red

hemoglobin: the protein in red cells that combines reversibly with oxygen to form oxyhemoglobin; also referred to as reduced hemoglobin or deoxyhemoglobin

hemoglobin saturation: the portion of total hemoglobin that is combined with oxygen, usually expressed as a percentage

methemoglobin: oxidized hemoglobin, which is present normally as up to 1 percent of total hemoglobin; it does not combine reversibly rapidly with oxygen and cannot serve in oxygen transport

oxyhemoglobin: a reversibly oxygenated form of hemoglobin

sulfhemoglobin: the reaction product of hemoglobin with certain toxic agents (oxidants) *venous blood:* blood from a vein conducting blood to the right ventricle, before passage through the lungs

CAUSES AND SYMPTOMS

Cyanosis, a dark blue discoloration of the skin and nail beds, is a sign of a disorder, not a disease in itself, and it may have several causes. It is also not a symptom sensed by a patient but a physical finding. To appear, cyanosis requires a concentration in arterial blood of 4 to 5 grams per deciliter of reduced hemoglobin. Anemic patients may not show cyanosis even though their hemoglobin saturations are low. Its presence indicates one or more of the following: inadequate oxygenation of arterial blood (a decrease of oxygen saturation to 85 percent or less), the presence of a normal constituent (methemoglobin) in increased concentration, or the presence of an abnormal constituent (sulfhemoglobin).

Inadequate oxygenation of normally circulating blood. The obstruction of large airways (the tracheo-bronchial system) can occur from external compression (hanging) or the aspiration of solid or semisolid materials (foodstuffs, particularly ground meat). Laryngospasm may be a factor. The aspiration of aqueous fluids, as in drowning in freshwater, can fill the alveoli and decrease or prevent the contact of inspired air with the blood in the pulmonary capillaries. Freshwater can pass rapidly into the blood and eventually free the alveoli for gas exchanges. Drowning in seawater is usually accompanied by marked laryngospasm. If the hypertonic seawater reaches the alveoli, then water will cross from the blood into the alveoli and produce even more fluid and froth in the lungs (pulmonary edema).

The inhalation of certain toxic agents, available industrially or used in warfare, can damage the alveoli and the pulmonary capillaries and produce pulmonary edema. Typical agents are chlorine and phosgene. Smoke inhalation is another possible cause of lung damage. Pulmonary edema from cardiac failure can occur as a result of increased pressure in the alveolar capillaries. Respiratory distress syndrome, or noncardiogenic pulmonary edema, occurs probably as the end result of a variety of initiators (shock, sepsis) culminating in the production of damaging free radicals.

Pharmacologically active agents such as heroin and morphine injected intravenously, as by drug abusers, can produce fulminating pulmonary edema extremely rapidly, possibly as the result of alpha-adrenergic discharge. Substances such as ethchlorvynol (Placidyl) can also produce this condition if injected intravenously, although they may be innocuous if taken orally.

Pulmonary infections such as pneumococcal pneumonia can cause edema through the perfusion of alveoli which are filled with fluid, that is, nonventilated. This condition is essentially venous admixture, and it can occur when three or more lobes of the lungs are involved. Chronic obstructive pulmonary disease (COPD) can produce cyanosis because of destruction of lung tissue (emphysema) and because of obstruction to air movement. Oxygenation is incomplete, and cyanosis is a common feature of advanced disease.

Low oxygen concentration in ambient atmosphere occurs with ascent to high altitudes. In certain caves, oxygen may be displaced by carbon dioxide. Incorrect gas mixtures may be administered to patients under anesthesia or on artificial respiration. The oxygen of the ambient atmosphere may be decreased in closed environments such as submarines. Polycythemia (increased numbers of red blood cells per unit volume of blood) may occur as a result of chronic exposure to high altitudes or as a spontaneous problem (polycythemia vera). The oxygen content of the blood may be normal or high, but the unoxygenated portion may be increased so that a ruddy cyanosis may be present.

Admixture of venous and arterial blood flows. Patent ductus arteriosus is a heart defect that produces blue baby syndrome. It offers a classic example of the direct entry of venous blood into the arterial system, as the lungs are partially bypassed. Other cardiopulmonary abnormalities, such as right-to-left shunts, can also produce cyanosis.

Localized circulatory problems. Frostbite and Raynaud's phenomenon are examples of localized occurrence of cyanosis. In these conditions, vascular changes limit blood flow, leading to congestion and unsaturation.

Increased concentrations of methemoglobin or sulfhemoglobin. Naturally occurring methemoglobin is present at about the 1 percent level in blood. From 0.5

INFORMATION ON CYANOSIS

CAUSES: Inadequate oxygenation of hemoglobin in arterial blood from various injuries, illnesses, and disorders
SYMPTOMS: Dark blue discoloration of skin and nails
DURATION: Chronic until treated
TREATMENTS: Oxygen administration, treatment of underlying disorder

to 3 percent of the total hemoglobin is oxidized each day and returned to deoxyhemoglobin through enzymatic reductase activity. In congenital forms of methemoglobinemia, cyanosis appears when the concentration of methemoglobin approaches 10 percent of the total (about 1.4 grams per deciliter).

Acquired increased concentration can be caused by a variety of agents (such as sodium perchorate, Paraquat, nitroglycerine, inhaled butyl and isobutyl nitrites) by oxidizing hemoglobin to methemoglobin through the formation of free radicals. Nitrates, absorbed by mouth, are transformed into nitrites in the gut and also produce methemoglobin. Sulfhemoglobin can also be formed and produces cyanosis at concentrations of 0.5 gram per deciliter.

TREATMENT AND THERAPY

Treatment is directed not to the cyanosis itself but to the underlying problem. Oxygen administration is crucial in many but not all cases.

For airway obstruction, the Heimlich maneuver may be lifesaving, as may an emergency tracheostomy. Drowning requires artificial respiration, positioning of the body so that drainage of fluid from the lungs is facilitated, and administration of oxygen, if available. Full cardiopulmonary resuscitation (CPR) may be indicated. Pulmonary edema from cardiac failure or respiratory distress syndrome calls into use a variety of approaches, but oxygen is almost always provided. Artificial respiration and oxygen are usually required in heroin, morphine, and ethchlorvynol pulmonary edema. COPD and emphysema are chronic, progressive disorders in which oxygen, bronchodilators, antibiotics, steroids, and surgical interventions (lung volume reduction) may be used. In methemoglobinemia, the congenital forms may not require any treatment. If the cyanosis is the result of exposure to nitrites and other potential oxidants, then methylene blue is usually effective.

PERSPECTIVE AND PROSPECTS

Cyanosis has been recognized for centuries as a sign or indicator of an underlying problem. The focus of investigations has been on identifying these problems. The properties of the hemoglobins have been investigated by physiologists and hematologists, leading to an understanding of their structures and functions. Surgical correction of the vascular abnormalities of so-called blue babies by Alfred Blalock and Helen Taussig led to the opening of the field of cardiovascular surgery. Mo-

lecular biology has provided knowledge of the enzymatic and genetic factors involved in the development of methemoglobinemia.

—*Francis P. Chinard, M.D.*

See also Accidents; Altitude sickness; Asphyxiation; Blood and blood disorders; Blue baby syndrome; Cardiology; Cardiology, pediatric; Choking; Chronic obstructive pulmonary disease (COPD); Circulation; Congenital heart disease; Edema; Emphysema; Frostbite; Heart; Heart failure; Heimlich maneuver; Hyperbaric oxygen therapy; Lungs; Poisoning; Pneumonia; Pulmonary diseases; Pulmonary medicine; Pulmonary medicine, pediatric; Respiration; Respiratory distress syndrome; Toxicology; Vascular system.

FOR FURTHER INFORMATION:

Dickerson, Richard E., and Irving Geis. *Hemoglobin: Structure, Function, Evolution, and Pathology.* Menlo Park, Calif.: Benjamin/Cummings, 1983.

Icon Health. *Cyanosis: A Medical Dictionary, Bibliography, and Annotated Research Guide to Internet References.* San Diego, Calif.: Author, 2004.

Nagel, Ronald L., ed. *Hemoglobin Disorders: Molecular Methods and Protocols.* Totowa, N.J.: Humana Press, 2003.

Weibel, Ewald. R. *The Pathway for Oxygen: Structure and Function in the Mammalian Respiratory System.* Cambridge, Mass.: Harvard University Press, 1984.

CYST REMOVAL

PROCEDURE

ANATOMY OR SYSTEM AFFECTED: Breasts, genitals, glands, joints, reproductive system, skin

SPECIALTIES AND RELATED FIELDS: Dermatology, general surgery, gynecology, plastic surgery

DEFINITION: A surgical procedure to remove a fluid-filled nodule, performed in a physician's office or a hospital depending on the type and location of the cyst.

KEY TERMS:

aspirate: to remove a substance using suction; a cyst can be aspirated using a needle and syringe to withdraw its contents

cyst: a sac containing a fluid or semifluid substance

incision: a cut made with a scalpel during a surgical procedure

laparoscope: a small surgical tube which can be inserted through a small incision into the abdominal cavity to view and perform surgery on abdominal organs

INDICATIONS AND PROCEDURES

Many types of cysts can develop in the body. The vast majority of them are noncancerous, although in rare cases small areas of cancerous tissue may be found within a cyst. The indications and procedures for removing cysts depend on the type of cyst, its location, and whether it is causing symptoms. Examples of common types of cysts are Baker's, Bartholin's, ovarian, sebaceous, thyroglossal, and breast cysts.

Baker's cysts are small lumps that form behind the knee. Fluid-filled sacs found around joints, known as bursas, normally protect the moving joint from causing damage to overlying skin, tendons, and muscles. When the bursas behind the knee accumulate excess fluid, they can expand and form a Baker's cyst. This fluid accumulation often occurs if the knee is arthritic. Physicians usually apply pressure bandages to reduce the bursal swelling. If this does not work, then the cyst must be excised surgically.

Bartholin's gland cysts are formed when the Bartholin's glands found in the female genital area (specifically the vulva) become occluded and swollen with fluid. Infections can occur in the ducts of these glands, causing pain and scarring. Bartholin's cysts are treated with conservative measures such as warm water soaks, antibiotics, and Word's catheter placement (a catheter that continuously drains the cyst). If these methods fail, then the cyst may be incised in the operating room and then marsupialized, a procedure which sutures the inner cyst wall to the vulvar skin and keeps the cyst open and draining.

Ovarian cysts do not usually need to be removed, and many of them are physiologic and come and go with the menstrual cycle. When an ovarian cyst becomes large (greater than 6 centimeters in diameter), it may cause the ovary to twist, a condition called ovarian torsion. A twisted ovary is at risk for necrosis, since its blood supply is cut off. In this case, the ovarian cyst would need to be removed. Other reasons for removing an ovarian cyst include a cyst that is persistent and growing with time and a cyst with characteristics upon ultrasound examination that suggest malignancy.

If an ovarian cyst is thought to be noncancerous, then it can usually be removed through the abdomen using a laparoscope. The laparoscope enables visualization of the cyst, while manipulation of the ovary and cyst is accomplished through incisions and tools placed on the sides of the abdomen. The cyst is usually shelled out from the remainder of the ovary using blunt dissection, and the remaining ovary is inspected for areas of bleed-ing, which may be cauterized. Many patients do not need to be hospitalized if the surgery was straightforward. If there is a concern about cancer within an ovarian cyst, then an open abdominal surgery is indicated. In this case, the abdomen is opened surgically and the cyst is removed, along with any other abnormal-appearing tissue surrounding the cyst.

A sebaceous cyst may develop when a duct from a sebaceous gland in the skin becomes blocked and the oily fluid is unable to escape. These glands, which are associated with hair follicles, secrete sebum to lubricate the hair and skin. If the sebaceous cyst is very large or infected with bacteria, then surgical removal is usually indicated. This operation can be done in a physician's office under local anesthesia. A small incision is made in the skin, and the entire cyst is removed or drained. The complete wall of the cyst is removed in order to prevent recurrence. A few sutures are usually placed to close the wound.

Thyroglossal cysts usually arise because of a congenital defect in which the duct that connects the base of the tongue to the thyroid gland fails to disappear. If a cyst develops in this area, a noticeable swelling will occur above the thyroid cartilage (Adam's apple). This cyst nearly always becomes infected and thus should be removed surgically. This procedure involves an incision just above the thyroid cartilage and gland. The surgeon then separates surrounding tissue up to the base of the tongue to gain access to the cyst. The cyst can then be removed and the skin sutured.

Breast cysts are common and can come and go with the menstrual cycle. They are usually detected as a breast lump on physical examination. If they are persistent, then they can be visualized on ultrasound (or mammogram) to confirm that they are fluid-filled (rather than solid, which could be indicative of cancer). Breast cysts can be drained using a needle and the fluid sent for pathological analysis. If the fluid is benign, then no further procedures are indicated.

USES AND COMPLICATIONS

The uses of cyst removal in general are to relieve pain and discomfort, minimize the chance of infection, and preserve the normal anatomy and function of surrounding organs. In addition, the cyst can be sent for pathological analysis after it is removed, in order to determine if any portions suggest cancer.

Complications common to all cyst removal procedures include bleeding at the site where the cyst has been removed, damage to organ structures surrounding the cysts during the excision process, and risk of infection from the excision procedure itself, as foreign instruments are introduced into the field. Another complication is that the cysts may recur, necessitating further intervention. In addition, each type of cyst removal has its own specific risks. For instance, thyroglossal cyst removal surgery may inadvertently remove thyroid tissue, which can lead to thyroid hormone deficiency and the need for thyroid medication for replacement.

—*Matthew Berria, Ph.D.,*
and Douglas Reinhart, M.D.;
updated by Anne Lynn S. Chang, M.D.

See also Abscess drainage; Abscesses; Biopsy; Breast biopsy; Breast disorders; Breasts, female; Colon and rectal polyp removal; Colon and rectal surgery; Cysts; Dermatology; Ganglion removal; Genital disorders, female; Glands; Gynecology; Hydrocelectomy; Laparoscopy; Myomectomy; Nasal polyp removal; Reproductive system; Skin; Skin disorders; Skin lesion removal.

FOR FURTHER INFORMATION:

Doherty, Gerard M., and Lawrence W. Way, eds. *Current Surgical Diagnosis and Treatment.* 12th ed. New York: Lange Medical Books/McGraw-Hill, 2006.

Icon Health. *Ovarian Cysts: A Medical Dictionary, Bibliography, and Annotated Research Guide to Internet References.* San Diego, Calif.: Author, 2004.

Kasper, Dennis L., et al., eds. *Harrison's Principles of Internal Medicine.* 16th ed. New York: McGraw-Hill, 2005.

Tierney, Lawrence M., Stephen J. McPhee, and Maxine A. Papadakis, eds. *Current Medical Diagnosis and Treatment 2007.* New York: McGraw-Hill Medical, 2006.

CYSTIC FIBROSIS
DISEASE/DISORDER

ANATOMY OR SYSTEM AFFECTED: Chest, lungs, respiratory system, most bodily systems

SPECIALTIES AND RELATED FIELDS: Genetics, neonatology, pediatrics, pulmonary medicine

DEFINITION: A disease that affects the exocrine glands and, secondarily, most physical systems, resulting in death usually between the ages of sixteen and thirty.

KEY TERMS:

chloride transport: the movement of one of the ions found in ordinary salt across a membrane from the inside of a cell to the outside; this transport is common in human cells and is critical for many important metabolic functions

cystic fibrosis transmembrane-conductance regulator (CFTR): the protein product of the cystic fibrosis gene and a chloride transport channel

meconium ileus: the puttylike plug found in the intestines of some cystic fibrosis babies when they are born

mutation: an alteration in the deoxyribonucleic acid (DNA) sequence of a gene, which usually leads to the production of a nonfunctional enzyme or protein and thus a lack of a normal metabolic function

recessive genetic disease: a disease caused by mutated genes that must be inherited from both parents in order for that individual to show its symptoms

secretory epithelium: tissues or groups of cells that have the ability to move substances, such as chloride ions, from the inside of cells to a duct or tube

CAUSES AND SYMPTOMS

Genetic diseases are inherited, rather than caused by any specific injury or infectious agent. Thus, unlike many other types of diseases, genetic diseases range throughout a person's lifetime and often begin to exert their debilitating effects prior to birth. Since in many cases the primary defect or underlying cause of the disease is unknown, treatment is difficult or impossible and is usually restricted to treating the symptoms of the disease. Genetic diseases include sickle cell disease; thalassemia; Tay-Sachs disease; some forms of muscular dystrophy, diabetes, and hemophilia; and cystic fibrosis.

In each disease, a specific normal function is missing because of a defect in the individual's genes. Genes are sequences of deoxyribonucleic acid (DNA) contained on the chromosomes of an individual that are passed to the next generation via ova and sperm. Usually, the primary defect in a genetic disease is the inability to produce a normal enzyme, the class of proteins used to speed up, or catalyze, the chemical reactions that are necessary for cells to function. A defective gene, also called a mutation, may not allow the production of a necessary enzyme; therefore, some element of metabolism is missing from an individual with such a mutation. This lack of function leads to the symptoms associated with a genetic disease, such as the lack of insulin production in juvenile diabetes or the inability of the blood to clot in hemophilia. In the 1940's and 1950's, when the understanding of basic cellular metabolism

INFORMATION ON CYSTIC FIBROSIS

CAUSES: Genetic defect
SYMPTOMS: Severe malnutrition, production of bulky stools, chronic respiratory infections, constant coughing, compromised fertility
DURATION: Chronic and progressive
TREATMENTS: Alleviation of symptoms with dietary supplements, balanced diet, backslapping to break up mucus, antibiotics

made clear the relationship between genes, enzymes, mutant genes, and lack of enzyme function, the modern definition of genetic disease came into routine medical use.

Cystic fibrosis, one such genetic disease, has several major effects on an individual. These effects begin before birth, extend into early childhood, and become progressively more serious as the affected individual grows. The primary diagnosis for the disease is a very simple test that looks for excessive saltiness in perspiration. Although the higher-than-normal level of salt in the perspiration is, of itself, not life-threatening, the associated symptoms are. Because these other symptoms may vary from one individual to the next, the perspiration test is a very useful early diagnostic tool.

Major symptoms of cystic fibrosis include the blockage of several important internal ducts. This blockage occurs because the cystic fibrosis mutation has a critical effect on the ability of certain internal tissues called secretory epithelia to transport normal amounts of salt and water across their surfaces. These epithelia are often found in the ducts that contribute to the digestive and reproductive systems.

The blockage of ducts resulting from the production and export of overly viscous secretions reduces the delivery of digestive enzymes from the pancreas to the intestine; thus proteins in the intestine are only partly digested. Fat-emulsifying compounds, called bile salts, are often blocked as well on their route from the pancreas to the intestine, so the digestion of fats is often incomplete. These two conditions often occur prior to birth. Approximately 10 percent of newborns with cystic fibrosis have a puttylike plug of undigested material in their intestines called the meconium ileus. This plug prevents the normal movement of foods through the digestive system and can be very serious.

Because of their overall inefficiency of digestion, young children with cystic fibrosis can seem to be eating quite normally yet remain severely undernourished. They often produce bulky, foul-smelling stools as a result of the high proportion of undigested material. This symptom serves as an indicator of the progress of the disease, as such digestive problems often increase as the affected child ages.

As individuals with cystic fibrosis grow older, their respiratory problems increase because of the secretion of a thick mucus on the inner lining of the lungs. This viscous material traps white blood cells that release their contents when they rupture, which makes the mucus all the more thick and viscous. The affected individuals constantly cough in an attempt to remove this material. Of greater importance is that the mucus forms an ideal breeding ground for many types of pathogenic bacteria, and the affected individual suffers from continual respiratory infections. Male patients are almost always infertile as a result of the blockage of the ducts of the reproductive system, while female fertility is sometimes reduced as well.

Traditional treatments for cystic fibrosis have improved an individual's chance of survival and have dramatically affected the quality of life. In the 1950's, a child afflicted with cystic fibrosis usually lived only a year or two. Thus, cystic fibrosis was originally described as a children's disease and was intensively studied only by pediatricians. Today, aggressive medical intervention has changed survival rates dramatically. Affected individuals are treated by a package of therapies designed to alleviate the most severe symptoms of the disease, and taken together, they had extended the median age of survival of cystic fibrosis patients to thirty-two years by 1999. In fact, since this figure contains many individuals who were born before many of the effective treatments were developed and so did not benefit from them throughout their entire lifetimes, the true average life expectancy may be as high as forty years.

The available treatments, however, do not constitute a cure for the disease. The major roadblock to developing a cure was that the primary genetic defect remained unknown. All that was clear until the mid-1980's was that many of the secretory epithelia had a salt and water transport problem. By the late 1980's, the defect was further restricted to a problem in the transport of chloride ions, one of the two constituents of ordinary salt and a critical chemical in many important cellular processes. Because individuals who had severe forms of cystic fibrosis could still live, however, this function was deemed important but not absolutely essential for survival. Furthermore, only certain tissues and organs in the body seemed to show abnormal functions in a cystic fibrosis patient, while other organs—the heart, brain, and nerves—seemed to function normally. Thus, the defect was not uniform.

The pattern of inheritance of cystic fibrosis was relatively easy to determine. The disease acts as a recessive trait. Humans, like most animals, have two copies of each gene: one that is inherited on a chromosome from

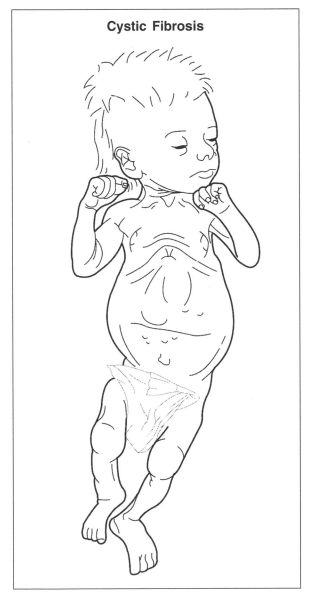

Cystic Fibrosis

Approximately 10 percent of newborns with cystic fibrosis have a puttylike plug of undigested material in their intestines called the meconium ileus, which results in emaciation with a distended abdomen.

the egg, and the other on a similar chromosome from the sperm. There is a gene in all humans that controls some normal cellular function related to the transport of chloride from the inside of a cell to the outside. If this function is missing or impaired, the individual shows the symptoms of cystic fibrosis.

A recessive trait is one that must be inherited from both the mother and the father in order to take effect. Inheriting only a single copy of the mutation from one parent does not have a deleterious effect on an individual, who would not demonstrate any of the disease symptoms. Such a person, however, is a carrier of the disease and can still pass that mutation on to his or her own children. Thus genetic diseases caused by recessive mutations, such as cystic fibrosis, can remain hidden in a family for many generations. Only when two carriers of the disease procreate are some of their children at risk. The rules of genetics, as first described by Gregor Mendel in the nineteenth century, predict that in such a marriage, approximately one in four children will have cystic fibrosis. Another one-fourth will be normal, and the remaining half will be carriers of the disease like their parents. Because the production of eggs and sperm involves a random shuffling of genes and chromosomes, however, the occurrence of normal individuals, carriers, and affected individuals cannot be predicted; only average probabilities can be discussed.

TREATMENT AND THERAPY

The treatment of cystic fibrosis typically focuses on preventing or delaying lung damage and optimizing growth and nutrition. Traditional treatments usually include dietary supplements which contain the digestive enzymes and bile salts that cannot pass through the blocked ducts; this is a daily requirement. Individuals with cystic fibrosis are also placed on special balanced diets to ensure proper nutrition despite their difficulties in digesting fats and proteins. One characteristic of cystic fibrosis treatment is the long daily ritual of back-slapping, which is designed to help break up the thick mucus in the lungs. Aggressive antibiotic therapy can keep infections of the lungs from forming or spreading. In the 1990's, an additional therapy was begun using a special enzyme which when inhaled can break down DNA in the lung mucus. Many white blood cells rupture while trapped in the thick mucus lining of the lungs, and the release of their DNA adds to the high viscosity of the mucus. Genetically engineered deoxyribonuclease (DNase), an enzyme produced from bacteria, has been found to be helpful in degrading this extra DNA, thus making it easier to break up and cough out the mucus found in the lungs of affected patients.

Another treatment approach for cystic fibrosis focused on determining the nature of the primary genetic defect. The ultimate goal was to determine which of the thousands of human genes was the one that, when defective, led to cystic fibrosis. Once accomplished, the next step would be to determine the normal function of this gene so that therapies designed to replace this function could be developed.

The classic approach to studying any genetic phenomenon involves mapping the gene. First, it must be determined which of a human's twenty-three chromosomes contains the DNA that makes up the gene. By studying the inheritance of the disease, along with other human traits, the gene was located on chromosome number 7. To localize the gene more precisely, however, modern molecular techniques had to be applied. Success came when two independent groups announced that they had identified the location of the gene in 1989. The groups were led by Lap-Chee Tsui of the Hospital for Sick Children in Toronto, Canada, and Francis Collins of the University of Michigan in Ann Arbor. The groups not only located the exact chromosomal location of the gene but also purified the gene from the vast amount of DNA in a human cell so that it could be studied in isolation. Then the structure of the normal form of the gene was compared to the DNA structure found in individuals with the disease.

DNA from more than thirty thousand individuals with cystic fibrosis was analyzed, and to the surprise of most, more than 230 differences between these defective cystic fibrosis genes and normal genes were found. Although about 70 percent of the affected individuals did have a single type of DNA difference or mutation, the other 30 percent had a tremendous variety of differences. Thus, unlike sickle cell disease, which seems to be attributable to the same defect in every affected individual, cystic fibrosis is a widely varying group of differences, which accounts for the range in severity of its symptoms. More important, this enormous diversity of defects makes developing a single, simple DNA-based screening procedure difficult. The only thing that all these individuals had in common was that, in each case, the same gene and gene product were affected.

Tsui's and Collins's groups, as well as several others, tried to determine the normal function of the protein that was coded by the cystic fibrosis gene. This protein was called cystic fibrosis transmembrane-conductance regulator (CFTR) because it was soon shown to create a channel or passage by which cells move chloride ions across their membranes. In an individual afflicted with cystic fibrosis, this channel does not work properly; both the salt and the water balance of the affected cell, and ultimately of the whole tissue, is disturbed. The thick mucus buildup in the lungs is a direct consequence of this disturbance, as is the higher-than-normal salt concentration in the patient's perspiration.

Remarkably, CFTR is an enormous protein that is embedded in the membrane of cells found in the lungs, pancreas, and the reproductive tracts. CFTR contains 1,480 amino acids linked end to end. The CFTR found in 70 percent of individuals with cystic fibrosis contains the same amino acids as normal genes, with one exception: The 508th amino acid found in a normal individual is missing. Thus, the extensive debilitating symptoms of this disease result from the mere omission of one amino acid from a long chain containing 1,479 identical ones. The other mutations affect different parts of this protein and, in all cases, reduce the ability of the CFTR protein to carry out its normal function.

In the cases of several other genetic diseases, screening programs have been developed to help patients make informed choices about having children. For Tay-Sachs disease, a fatal neurological disease found in 1 in 3,600 Ashkenazi Jews, a screening program coupled with a strong educational program combined to reduce the incidence of the disease from approximately 100 births a year in the 1970's to an average of 13 by the early 1980's. Similar screening programs have been developed for a rare genetic disease called phenylketonuria (PKU). A screening program for cystic fibrosis, however, would be much more difficult for several reasons.

First, the population at risk for cystic fibrosis is much larger; hence the costs and scope of the program would be enormous. Second, since there are many different mutations that can affect the gene responsible for causing cystic fibrosis, it may not be easy to develop a simple test which could detect this enormous variation accurately without missing affected individuals or falsely concluding that some normal individuals are affected. Finally, the symptoms shown by individuals affected with cystic fibrosis range from quite severe to nearly normal, thus making it even more difficult to provide definitive genetic counseling. For such counseling to be truly effective, large numbers of individuals from groups known to be at risk for the disease would have to undergo screening and counseling. Furthermore, a prenatal diagnostic test would need to be available to allow couples at risk to ascertain with some degree of certainty whether any particular child is going to be born with the disease. Developing these tests and coupling them with widely available, low-cost counseling remain major challenges to the medical community.

Therapies for cystic fibrosis, like those of any genetic disease, once consisted solely of ways to treat the symptoms. Since every cell in the affected individual lacked a particular metabolic function as a result of the disease, there was no easy way to replace these functions. For cystic fibrosis, this problem was exacerbated by the lack of understanding of the primary defect. The work of Tsui's and Collins's teams allowed a more direct assault on the actual defect. Gene therapy involves either replacing a defective gene with a normal one in affected cells, or adding an additional copy or copies of the normal gene to affected cells, in an attempt to restore the same functional enzymes and thus reestablish a normal metabolic process. In the case of cystic fibrosis, animal studies have shown that it is possible to produce normal lung function when either genes or genetically engineered viruses containing normal genes are sprayed into the lungs of affected animals. Yet since there is no similar direct route for getting engineered viruses or purified genes to the pancreas or reproductive system, because of their location deep within the body, other procedures will need to be developed. In the case of the lung cells, only those cells that actually receive the purified gene change, becoming normal. Since the cells lining the lung are continuously being replenished, lung gene therapy would need to be an ongoing process.

PERSPECTIVE AND PROSPECTS

Patients with the symptoms of cystic fibrosis were first described in medical records dating back to the eighteenth century. The disease was initially called muco-viscidosis and later cystic fibrosis of the pancreas. It was not clear that these symptoms were related to a single specific disease, however, until the work of Dorothy Anderson of Columbia University in the late 1930's. Anderson studied a large number of cases of persons who died with similar lung and pancreas problems. She noticed that siblings were sometimes affected and thus suspected that the disease had a genetic cause. Anderson was responsible for naming the disease on the basis of the fibrous cysts on the pancreas that she often saw in autopsies performed on affected individuals.

In the United States, cystic fibrosis is the most preva-

lent lethal genetic disease among Caucasians. Estimates vary, but most are in the range of 1 affected child in every 2,000 births. In the early 1990's, there were approximately 25,000 affected Americans and more than 50,000 affected people worldwide. The incidence of cystic fibrosis among Asian American or African American populations is considerably lower, ranging from 1 in 17,000 births for African Americans and less than 1 in 80,000 births for certain Asian American groups. What is particularly striking about this disease is that approximately 1 in 25 Caucasians is a carrier. Such individuals do not show disease symptoms but can have affected children if they procreate with another carrier.

Since this rate is so high, a premium has been placed on the development of inexpensive and accurate diagnostic procedures, which along with good genetic counseling, could greatly reduce the incidence of cystic fibrosis in the population. Yet, since carriers are perfectly normal and often do not realize that they are indeed carrying the gene, conventional genetic counseling cannot easily reduce the incidence of the mutation in human populations at risk. Only the widespread use of a DNA-based diagnostic procedure could serve to identify the large population of carriers, but even then, since three-fourths of the children of a marriage between two carriers would be normal, counseling would be fraught with severe ethical problems. Why such a deleterious gene remains in such high frequencies in the population remains a mystery.

—*Joseph G. Pelliccia, Ph.D.*

See also Birth defects; Coughing; Genetic counseling; Genetic diseases; Lungs; Respiration; Wheezing.

FOR FURTHER INFORMATION:

Cystic Fibrosis Foundation (CFF). http://www.cff.org. Web site gives comprehensive information about the disease, locations of local CFF chapters and care centers, research and clinical trials, and living with the disease.

Harris, Ann, and Maurice Super. *Cystic Fibrosis: The Facts*. 3d ed. Oxford, England: Oxford University Press, 1995. An excellent overview of the disease, its symptoms, and its treatment in a readable text.

Kepron, Wayne. *Cystic Fibrosis: Surviving Childhood, Achieving Adulthood*. Toronto: Firefly Books, 2004. A comprehensive guide that draws on current research to discuss symptoms, diagnosis, complication arising from the disease, treatments (including lung transplants), and the transition to adulthood.

Orenstein, David. *Cystic Fibrosis: A Guide for Patient and Family*. 3d ed. Philadelphia: Lippincott Williams & Wilkins, 2004. An accessible guide that examines a host of issues surrounding the disease including day-to-day concerns, physiological effects, and long-term issues.

Parker, James N., and Philip M. Parker, eds. *The Official Patient's Sourcebook on Cystic Fibrosis*. Rev. ed. San Diego, Calif.: Icon Health, 2002. Draws from public, academic, government, and peer-reviewed research to provide a wide-ranging reference about the causes, treatments, and risk factors of cystic fibrosis.

Pierce, Benjamin A. *The Family Genetic Sourcebook*. New York: John Wiley & Sons, 1990. Contains good background reading on genetics and genetic diseases. Cystic fibrosis is not the main focus of the text, but it is discussed.

Tsui, Lap-Chee. "Cystic Fibrosis, Molecular Genetics." In *The Encyclopedia of Human Biology*, edited by Renato Dulbecco. 2d ed. Vol. 2. New York: Academic Press, 1997. The pursuit of the cystic fibrosis gene is documented, along with some discussion of the function of the CFTR. Readable by someone with a strong high school science background.

U.S. Congress. Office of Technology Assessment. *Cystic Fibrosis and DNA Tests: Implications of Carrier Screening*. Washington, D.C.: Government Printing Office, 1992. An excellent overview of the scientific, ethical, social, economic, and political issues involved with screening for cystic fibrosis or for any genetic disease.

_____. *Genetic Counseling and Cystic Fibrosis Carrier Screening: Results of a Survey-Background Paper*. Washington, D.C.: Government Printing Office, 1992. A survey that looks at issues related to genetic screening for cystic fibrosis.

Yankaskas, James R., and Michael R. Knowles, eds. *Cystic Fibrosis in Adults*. Philadelphia: Lippincott-Raven, 1999. This volume covers the veritable explosion of information about cystic fibrosis in the late twentieth century, ranging from the discovery and characterization of the cystic-fibrosis transmembrane regulator (CFTR) gene and protein, to new therapeutic approaches such as anti-inflammatory, mucolytic, and inhaled antibiotic therapies.

Cystitis

Disease/disorder

Anatomy or system affected: Bladder, urinary system

Specialties and related fields: Bacteriology, gynecology, urology

Definition: An inflammation of the bladder, primarily caused by bacteria and resulting in pain, a sense of urgency to urinate, and sometimes hematuria (blood in the urine).

Key terms:

cytoscopy: a minor operation performed so that the urologist can examine the bladder

dysuria: painful urination, usually as a result of infection or an obstruction; the patient complains of a burning sensation when voiding

Escherichia coli: bacteria found in the intestines that may cause disease elsewhere

hematuria: the abnormal presence of blood in the urine

perineum: the short bridge of flesh between the anus and vagina in women and the anus and base of the penis in men

ureters: the two tubes that carry urine from the kidneys to the bladder

urethra: the tube carrying urine from the bladder to outside the body

Causes and Symptoms

The term "cystitis" is a combination of two Greek words: *kistis*, meaning hollow pouch, sac, or bladder, and *itis* meaning inflammation. Cystitis is often used generically to refer to any nonspecific inflammation of the lower urinary tract. Specifically, however, it should be used to refer to inflammation and infection of the bladder. Three true symptoms denote cystitis: dysuria, frequent urination, and hematuria. In a given year, about two million people are afflicted with cystitis; most of them are women. Fifteen percent of those affected will be struck again.

The symptoms of cystitis may appear abruptly and, often, painfully. One of the trademark symptoms signaling an onset is dysuria (burning or stinging during urination). It may precede or coincide with an overwhelming urge to urinate, and very frequently, although the amount passed may be extremely small. In addition some sufferers may experience nocturia (sleep disturbance because of a need to urinate). In many cases there may be pus in the urine. Origination of hematuria (blood in the urine), which often occurs with cystitis, may be within the bladder wall, in the urethra, or even in the upper urinary tract. These painful symptoms should be enough to spur one to seek medical attention; if left untreated, the bacteria may progress up the ureters to the kidneys, where a much more serious infection, pyelonephritis, may develop. Pyelonephritis can cause scarring of the kidney tissue and even life-threatening kidney failure. Usually kidney infections are accompanied by chills, high fever, nausea and/or vomiting, and back pain that may radiate downward.

Acute cystitis can be divided into two groups. One is when infection occurs with irregularity and with no recent history of antibiotic treatments. This type is commonly caused by the bacteria *Escherichia coli*. Types of bacteria other than *E. coli* that can cause cystitis are *Proteus*, *Klebsiella*, *Pseudomonas*, *Streptococcus*, *Enterobacter*, and, rarely, *Staphylococcus*. The second group of sufferers have undergone antibiotic treatment; those bacteria not affected by the antibiotics can cause infection. Most urinary tract infections are precipitated by the patient's own rectal flora. Once bacteria enter the bladder, whether they will cause infection depends on how many bacteria invade the bladder, how well the bacteria can adhere to the bladder wall, and how strongly the bladder can defend itself. The bladder's inherent defense system is the most important of the factors.

One of the natural defense mechanisms employed by the bladder is the flushing provided by regular urination at frequent intervals. If fluid intake is sufficient—most urologists consider this amount to be eight 8-ounce glasses daily—there will be regular and efficient emptying of the bladder, which can wash away the bacteria that have entered. This large volume of fluid also helps dilute the urine, thereby decreasing bacterial concentration. Another defense mechanism is the low pH of the bladder, which also helps control bacterial multiplication. It may be, too, that the bladder lining employs some means to repel bacteria and to inhibit their adherence to the wall. Others theorize that genetic, hormonal, and immune factors may help determine the defensive capability of the bladder.

Many women experience their first episode of cystitis as they become sexually active. So-called honeymoon cystitis, that related to sexual activity, comes about because intercourse may massage bacteria into the bladder, as can repeated thrusts of the penis, penetration of the vagina by fingers or other objects, or manual stimulation of the clitoris. Bacteria are boosted into and forced upward through the urethra. Also, a change in position—from back to front but not from front to back—may precede an attack of cystitis. When intercourse from the rear occurs, the penis may be contaminated with bacteria from the anal region, which then are transferred to the urethra. From the urethra, it is a short trip to the bladder for the bacteria. Unless they are voided upon conclusion of intercourse, they may multiply, causing inflammation and infection. Sex late in the day may be particularly hazardous if the perineal area has not been thoroughly cleansed after a bowel movement. Bathing after intercourse is too late to prevent the *E. coli* from being pushed into the urethral opening. Some instances of cystitis may be reduced if there is adequate vaginal lubrication prior to intercourse and vaginal sprays and douches are avoided.

Women who use a diaphragm as birth control are more than twice as likely to develop urinary tract infections than other sexually active women. The reason for this increased likelihood may be linked to the more alkaline vaginal environment in diaphragm users, or perhaps to the spring in the rim of the diaphragm that exerts pressure on the tissue around the urethra. Urine flow may be restricted, and the stagnant urine is a good harbor for bacterial growth.

When urine remains in the bladder for an extended period of time, its stagnation may allow for the rapid growth of bacteria, thereby leading to cystitis. Besides the use of a diaphragm, urine flow may be restricted by an enlarged prostate or pregnancy. Diabetes mellitus may also lead to cystitis, as the body's resistance to infection is lowered. Infrequent voiding for whatever reason is associated with a greater likelihood of cystitis.

Less frequently, cases have been linked to vaginitis as a result of *Monilia* or *Trichomonas*. Yeasts such as these change the pH of the vaginal fluid, which will allow and even encourage bacterial growth in the perineal region. Sometimes, it is an endless cycle: A patient takes antibiotics for cystitis, which kills her protective bacteria and allows the overgrowth of yeasts. The yeasts cause vaginitis, which may promote another

---

INFORMATION ON CYSTITIS

CAUSES: Bacterial infection
SYMPTOMS: Pain and burning upon urination, sense of urgency to urinate, sometimes blood in urine
DURATION: Acute
TREATMENTS: Antibiotics

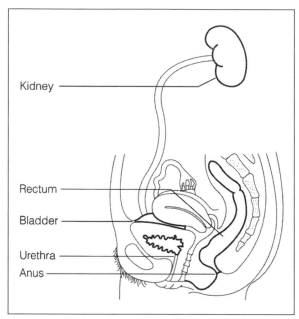

Cystitis, an inflammation of the bladder, may progress to the kidneys if left untreated.

case of cystitis, and the cycle continues. In fact, recurrent cystitis may be a result of an inappropriate course of antibiotic treatment; the antibiotic is not specific to the bacteria. More rarely, recurrent cases may be a result of constant seeding by the kidneys or a bowel fistula. The most common cause of recurrent cystitis, however, is new organisms from the rectal area that invade the perineal area. This new pool may be inadvertently changed by antibiotic treatment.

A less common but often more severe kind of cystitis is interstitial cystitis, an inflammation of the bladder caused by nonbacterial causes, such as an autoimmune or allergic response. With this type of cystitis, there may be inflammation and/or ulceration of the bladder, which may result in scarring. These problems usually cause frequent and painful urination and possible hematuria. What separates interstitial cystitis from acute cystitis is that it primarily strikes women in their early to mid-forties and that, while urine output is normal, soon after urination, the urge to void again is overwhelming. Delaying urination may cause a pink tinge to appear in the urine. This minimal bleeding is most often a result of an overly small bladder being stretched so that minute tears in the bladder wall bleed into the urine. This form is often hard to diagnose, as the symptoms may be mild or severe and may appear and disappear or be constant.

Treatment and Therapy

Medical students are typically underprepared to deal with the numerous cases of cystitis. The student is told to test urine for the presence of bacteria, prescribe a ten-day course of antibiotics, sometimes take a kidney X ray and/or perform a cytoscopy, and then perhaps prescribe more antibiotics. If the patient continues to complain, perhaps a painful dilation of the urethra or cauterizing (burning away) of the inflamed skin is performed. None of these procedures guarantees a cure.

Diagnosis of cystitis should be relatively easy; however, in a number of cases it is misdiagnosed because the doctor has failed to identify the type of bacteria, the patient's history of past cases, and possible links between cystitis and life factors (sexual activity, contraceptive method, and diet, for example). A more appropriate antibiotic given at this point might lower the risks of frequent recurrences. Diagnosis of urinary tract infection takes into account the medical history, a physical examination of the patient, and performance of special tests. The history begins with the immediate complaints of the patient and is completed with a look back at the same type of infections that the patient has had from childhood to the present. The physician should conduct urinalysis but be cognizant that, if the urine is not examined at the right time, the bacteria may not have survived and thus a false-negative reading may occur.

One special test, a cytoscopy, is used to diagnose some of the special characteristics of cystitis. These include redness of the bladder cells, enlarged capillaries with numerous small hemorrhages, and in cases of severe cystitis, swelling of bladder tissues. Swelling may be so pronounced that it partially blocks the urethral opening, making incomplete emptying of the bladder likely to occur. Pus pockets may be visible.

In a woman who first experiences cystitis when she becomes sexually active, the doctor usually instructs the patient to be alert to several details. She should wash or shower before intercourse and be warned that contraceptive method and position during intercourse may increase her chances of becoming infected. To decrease the chance of introducing the contamination of bowel flora to the urethra, wiping after urination and defecation from front to back is advised.

Children are not immune to attacks of cystitis; in fact, education at an early age may aid children in lowering their chances of developing cystitis. Some of the following may be culprits in causing cystitis and maintaining a hospitable environment for bacteria to grow:

soap or detergent that is too strong, too much fruit juice, overuse of creams and ointments, any noncotton underwear, shampoo in the bath water, bubble bath, chlorine from swimming pools, and too little fluid intake. Once children reach the teenage years, many of the above remain causes. Added to them are failure to change underwear daily, irregular periods, use of tampons, and the use of toiletries and deodorants. Careful monitoring of these conditions can greatly reduce the risk of recurrent infections.

The symptoms of cystitis are often urgent and painful enough to alert a sufferer to visit a physician as quickly as possible. Such a visit not only makes the patient feel better but also decreases the chances that the bacteria will travel toward and even into the kidney, causing pyelonephritis. Antibiotic therapy is the typical mode of treating acute or bacterial cystitis. The antibiotics chosen should reach a high concentration in theurine, should not cause the proliferation of drug-resistant bacteria, and should not kill helpful bacteria. Some antibiotics used to treat first-time sufferers of cystitis with a high success rate (80 to 100 percent) are TMP-SMX, sulfisoxazole, amoxycillin, and ampicillin. Typically, a three-day course of therapy not only will see the patient through the few days of symptoms but also will not change bowel flora significantly. When *E. coli* cause acute cystitis, there is a greater than 80 percent chance that one dose of an antibiotic such as penicillin will effectively end the bout, and again, the bowel flora will not be upset. Such antibiotics, when chosen carefully by the physician to match the bacteria, are useful in treating cystitis because they act very quickly to kill the bacteria. Sometimes, enough bacteria can be killed in one hour that the symptoms begin to abate immediately.

Yet antibiotics are not without their drawbacks: They may cause nausea, loss of appetite, dizziness, diarrhea, and fatigue and may increase the likelihood of yeast infections. The most common problem is the one posed by antibiotics that destroy all bacteria of the body. When the body's normal bacteria are gone, yeasts may proliferate in the body's warm, moist places. In one of the areas, the vagina, vaginitis causes a discharge which can seep into the urethra. The symptoms of cystitis may begin all over again.

For those suffering from recurrent cystitis, the treatment usually is a seven- to ten-day course of antibiotic treatment that will clear the urine of pus, indicating that the condition should be cured. If another bout recurs fairly soon, it is probably an indication that treatment was ended too quickly, as the infective bacteria were still present. To ensure that treatment has been effective, the urine must be checked and declared sterile.

Because cystitis is so common, and because many are frustrated by the inadequacies of treatment, self-treatment has become very popular. Self-treatment does not cure the infection but certainly makes the patient more comfortable while the doctor cultures a urine specimen, determines the type of bacteria causing the infection, and prescribes the appropriate antibiotic. Monitoring the first signs that a cystitis attack is imminent can save a victim from days of intense pain.

Those advocating home treatment do not all agree, however, on the means and methods that reduce suffering. All agree that once those first sensations are felt, the sufferer should start to drink water or water-based liquids; there is some disagreement on whether this intake should include fruit juice, especially cranberry juice. Some believe that the high acidic content of the juice may act to kill some of the bacteria, while others believe that the acid will only decrease the pH of the urine, causing more intense burnings as the acidic urine passes through the inflamed urethra. Through an increased fluid intake, more copious amounts of urine are produced. The excess urine acts to leach the bacteria from the bladder and, by diluting the urine, decreases its normal acidity. More dilute urine will relieve much of the burning discomfort during voiding. If a small amount of sodium bicarbonate is added to the water, it will aid in alkalinizing the urine. The best self-treatment is to drink one cup of water every twenty minutes for three hours; after this period, the amount can be decreased. A teaspoonful of bicarbonate every hour for three or four hours is safe (unless the person suffers from blood pressure problems or a heart condition). Additionally, the patient may wish to take a pain-killer, such as acetaminophen. If lifestyle permits, resting will enhance the cure, especially if a heating pad is used to soothe the back or stomach. After the frequent visits to the toilet, cleaning the perineal area carefully can reduce continued contamination.

Diagnosis of interstitial cystitis can only be made using a cytoscope. Since the cause is not bacterial, antibiotics are not effective in treating this type of cystitis. To enhance the healing process of an inflamed or ulcerated bladder as a result of interstitial cystitis, the bladder may be distended and the ulcers cauterized; both procedures are done under anesthesia. Corticosteroids may be prescribed to help control the inflammation.

PERSPECTIVE AND PROSPECTS

Writings throughout history indicate that people have always suffered from bladder problems, including cystitis, although the prevalence probably was not as high. The first urologists likely were the Hindus of the Vedic era, about 1500 B.C.E. They were considered experts in removing bladder stones and relieving obstructions of the urinary tract.

The recorded incidence of cystitis was possibly lower because the topic would have been taboo; women in particular would not have mentioned the problem. Couples of generations past would not have participated in intercourse as frequently; both sexes wore so many clothes and had so many children underfoot or servants around that daytime sexual activity would have been rare. Without contraception, intercourse was often for procreation; once there were several children, the couple might choose to inhabit separate bedrooms. Life spans were clearly shorter; women frequently died in childbirth. Thus, the primary causes of cystitis were not common until the twentieth century.

Those forebears did not have antibiotics, but apparently those who suffered from cystitis recovered. The treatment they did use, though, has some merit. They drank copious amounts of herb teas—chamomile, mint, and parsley. They probably added some belladonna for pain relief. All this fluid would have served to help quench the "fire." It would also have had the benefit of helping flush the bacteria from the bladder.

Infection in males is far less frequent than in females; in fact, cystitis occurs ten times more often in females than in males, and it affects about 30 percent of women at some time in their lives. Unfortunately, most urologists are better-versed in male problems. Female specialists, gynecologists, treat the reproductive system but may not have studied female urinary dysfunction. If a male suffers from urinary dysfunction, he should seek the services of a urologist. A woman who has interstitial cystitis should also see a urologist, specifically one who knows about this form of cystitis. If a female is experiencing recurrent cystitis, she is probably already seeing a gynecologist or an internist; however, if she is not getting relief, she should avail herself of a urologist, especially one specializing in female urology, if possible.

A strong social stigma is associated with bladder dysfunction, which may create an obstacle when treatment is necessary. From the time of infancy, some children are taught that anything to do with bladder or bowel function is shameful or dirty. Therefore, when dysfunction occurs, self-esteem may be decreased. As a result, the sufferer may fail to ask for help. Such a reaction must be overcome if there is to be significant progress in treating and conquering cystitis.

—*Iona C. Baldridge*

See also Antibiotics; Bacterial infections; Urethritis; Urinalysis; Urinary disorders; Urinary system; Urology; Urology, pediatric; Women's health.

FOR FURTHER INFORMATION:

Chalker, Rebecca, and Kristene E. Whitmore. *Overcoming Bladder Disorders*. New York: HarperCollins, 1990. This book was written to inform the general public about bladder disorders. It is meant to aid in diagnosis and in the selection of the right physician. Diagrams and a glossary help make this work easy to read.

Cohen, Barbara J. *Memmler's The Human Body in Health and Disease*. 10th ed. Philadelphia: Lippincott Williams & Wilkins, 2005. This textbook offers a clear presentation of how human systems maintain homeostasis through their interactions. Integral to the discussion of each system is a detailed list of the conditions that produce disease.

Gillespie, Larrian, with Sandra Blakeslee. *You Don't Have to Live with Cystitis*. New York: Avon Books, 1996. A popular work on cystitis and women's health.

Parker, James N., and Philip M. Parker, eds. *The Official Patient's Sourcebook on Urinary Tract Infection*. San Diego, Calif.: Icon Health, 2002. Draws from public, academic, government, and peer-reviewed research to provide a wide-ranging handbook for patients with recurring urinary tract infections.

Schrier, Robert W., ed. *Diseases of the Kidney and Urinary Tract*. 8th ed. Philadelphia: Wolters Kluwer Health/Lippincott Williams & Wilkins, 2007. Covers full range of the biochemical, structural, and functional correlations in the kidney, as well as hereditary diseases, urological diseases and neoplasms of the genitourinary tract, acute renal failure, nutrition, and drugs, among many additional topics.

CYSTOSCOPY

PROCEDURE

ANATOMY OR SYSTEM AFFECTED: Bladder, reproductive system, urinary system

SPECIALTIES AND RELATED FIELDS: Gynecology, urology, oncology

DEFINITION: An endoscopic procedure that utilizes a water or carbon dioxide distension system to visualize the urethra and bladder.

INDICATIONS AND PROCEDURES

Cystoscopy is indicated in patients for whom visual inspection of the urethra, bladder mucosa, and ureteral orifices is likely to yield a diagnosis. This includes patients who have hematuria (blood in the urine), incontinence, and irritative bladder symptoms for whom all obvious causes have been ruled out. In addition, patients who have undergone difficult abdominal or pelvic surgery may receive cystoscopy to verify that the bladder and the ureters, the tubes that carry urine from the kidneys to the bladder, are intact.

Cystoscopy is performed with the patient in a supine position with legs in stirrups. The cystoscope consists of a small metal tube, through which distension medium is passed. The light source, which enables visualization, also passes through this tube. The cystoscope can be attached to a video screen, or the clinician can visualize the urethral and bladder mucosas directly through the cystoscope. The cystoscope may be angled at 0 degrees, 30 degrees, or 70 degrees in order to facilitate visualization of different parts of the bladder. The procedure involves passing the cystoscope into the urethra and then the bladder under direct visualization. Cystoscopy is performed in a systematic fashion to ensure complete coverage of the urethral and bladder mucosas. Abnormal areas can be biopsied. The ureteral orifices can be visualized using the cystoscope, and the presence of urine flow from the orifices confirms patency (lack of obstruction) of the ureters.

USES AND COMPLICATIONS

Cystoscopy can be used to diagnose a variety of benign and malignant conditions of the lower urinary tract. Among the benign conditions commonly found through cystoscopy are endometriosis of the bladder, interstitial cystitis, foreign bodies, and anatomic abnormalities such as fistulas (communicating tracts between the bladder and another organ such as the bowels) or diverticula (small outpouchings of the bladder or urethra). By filling the bladder with distension fluid during cystoscopy, it is also possible to perform limited bladder function tests. Malignant conditions that may be found on cystoscopy include bladder cancers and cancers of adjacent pelvic organs, such as the cervix, which may invade the bladder.

Cystoscopy is an extremely safe procedure. Theoretical risks include the possibility of bladder injury or perforation from the cystoscope.

—*Anne Lynn S. Chang, M.D.*

See also Bladder cancer; Bladder removal; Cervical, ovarian, and uterine cancers; Cystitis; Diverticulitis and diverticulosis; Endometriosis; Endoscopy; Fistula repair; Incontinence; Invasive tests; Urethritis; Urinalysis; Urinary disorders; Urinary system; Urology; Urology, pediatric.

FOR FURTHER INFORMATION:

Doherty, Gerard M., and Lawrence W. Way, eds. *Current Surgical Diagnosis and Treatment*. 12th ed. New York: Lange Medical Books/McGraw-Hill, 2006.

Miller, Brigitte E. *An Atlas of Sigmoidoscopy and Cystoscopy*. Boca Raton, Fla.: Parthenon, 2002.

Rock, John A., and Howard W. Jones III, eds. *Te Linde's Operative Gynecology*. 9th ed. Philadelphia: Lippincott Williams & Wilkins, 2003.

Stenchever, Morton A., et al. *Comprehensive Gynecology*. 4th ed. St. Louis: Mosby, 2006.

CYSTS

DISEASE/DISORDER

ANATOMY OR SYSTEM AFFECTED: All

SPECIALTIES AND RELATED FIELDS: All

DEFINITION: A walled-off sac that is not normally found in the tissue where it occurs. To be a true cyst, a lump must have a capsule around it. Cysts usually contain a liquid or semisolid core (center) and vary in size from microscopic to very large. They may occur in any tissue of the body in a person of any age.

KEY TERMS:

asymptomatic: not causing any symptoms

benign: not malignant; noncancerous

capsule: the wall that encloses a cyst

computed tomography (CT) scan: a technique that generates detailed pictures from a series of X rays

genetic: inherited

magnetic resonance imaging (MRI): a radiologic technique that uses radio signals and magnets and a computer to produce highly detailed images of tissues

malignant: cancerous; able to spread into and destroy nearby tissues and to spread to distant areas

renal: pertaining to the kidney

sebaceous: pertaining to glands in the skin that secrete an oily substance called sebum

ultrasonography: the use of sound waves to create an image of the soft tissues of the body

INFORMATION ON CYSTS

CAUSES: Unknown; likely arises when hair follicle becomes blocked
SYMPTOMS: Lumps in skin or areas such as breast, brain, or bone; may put pressure on surrounding organs, causing pain
DURATION: Varies
TREATMENTS: Surgical drainage, sometimes antibiotics to prevent infection

CAUSES AND SYMPTOMS

Cysts can be caused by a many different processes, including infections, defects in the development of an embryo during pregnancy, various obstructions to the flow of body fluids, tumors, a number of different inflammatory conditions, and genetic diseases.

Cysts may have no symptoms at all, or they may be quite noticeable, depending on their size and location. For example, a person with a cyst in the skin or breast will most likely be able to feel the lump. On the other hand, a cyst on an internal organ may not produce any symptoms unless it becomes so large that it keeps the organ from functioning properly or presses on another organ. Many times, internal cysts are discovered by chance on an X ray, computed tomography (CT) scan, magnetic resonance imaging (MRI) scan, or ultrasound for an unrelated condition.

It is impossible to list all the different types of cysts that might form in the body, but they are usually benign. Only very rarely are cysts associated with cancer or with serious infection. Some of the common types of cysts include sebaceous cysts, which are found in the oil-secreting glands of the skin. They may become quite large and contain a foul-smelling, cheesy substance within the capsule. Breast cysts are filled with fluid and may enlarge and recede with the changing hormones of the menstrual cycle. Just before menses, breast cysts may be quite tender. Ganglion cysts occur over joints and on the tendons of the body. A chalazion, or cyst in the eyelid, is usually not painful but can be quite irritating.

Some cyst development is part of a particular disease or disorder. For example, cysts form on the ovaries in a disorder called polycystic ovary syndrome. There are also a number of different renal diseases that involve the development of cysts on the kidney.

TREATMENT AND THERAPY

The treatment for cysts depends on their size and location and whether they are causing symptoms. A small, asymptomatic cyst is often simply monitored.

When surgery is performed to remove a cyst, it is usually "shelled out" so that the entire capsule and its contents are removed. (If the capsule is left intact, then it might simply fill up again.) Depending on the location of the cyst, this may be performed in an office using local anesthesia or in the operating room of a hospital. When cancer is a possibility, the cell wall and any fluids are evaluated microscopically to determine whether any malignant cells are present.

Aspiration is another technique for treating cysts. A needle is inserted into the middle of the cyst, and any fluid is removed (aspirated) through the needle. If the cyst is deep within the body, then the aspiration may be guided by ultrasound or another radiologic technique. Aspiration may make the cyst disappear, or it may fill up again.

Some cysts are treated by incision and drainage. An opening is made in the cyst, and all the material in the core is removed. The cyst is then packed with gauze to ensure that the surgical incision does not close and allow the cyst to fill up again. The gauze is replaced periodically until healing takes place.

Ganglion cysts on tendons or joints may be successfully treated by injection with a steroid. If the cyst is part of another medical condition such as polycstic ovary syndrome, then any treatment is usually aimed at the medical condition rather than the cyst itself.

—*Rebecca Lovell Scott, Ph.D., PA-C*

See also Abscess removal; Abscesses; Acne; Bone disorders; Bones and the skeleton; Breast disorders; Breasts, female; Cyst removal; Ganglion removal; Kidney disorders; Kidneys; Ovarian cysts; Plastic surgery; Reproductive system; Skin; Skin disorders; Tendon disorders.

FOR FURTHER INFORMATION:

American Medical Association. *American Medical Association Family Medical Guide.* 4th rev. ed. Hoboken, N.J.: John Wiley & Sons, 2004.

Komaroff, Anthony, ed. *Harvard Medical School Family Health Guide.* New York: Free Press, 2005.

Stoppard, Miriam. *Family Health Guide.* New York: DK, 2004.

CYTOLOGY

SPECIALTY

ANATOMY OR SYSTEM AFFECTED: Cells, immune system

SPECIALTIES AND RELATED FIELDS: Bacteriology, hematology, histology, immunology, oncology, pathology, serology

DEFINITION: The study of the appearance of cells, usually with the aid of a microscope, in order to diagnose diseases.

KEY TERMS:

cell: a tiny baglike structure within which the basic functions of the body are carried out

chromosomes: rodlike cell parts made up of the genes that are the blueprints for every feature of the body; located in the nucleus of almost all cells

electron: a tiny particle with an electronic charge; a component of an atom

enzyme: a protein that is able to speed up a particular chemical reaction in the body

membranes: sheetlike structures that enclose each cell and separate the various organelles from one another

nucleus: the "control center" of plant and animal cells; a large spherical mass occupying up to one-third of the volume of a typical cell

organelles: specialized parts of cells

pathologist: a physician who is specially trained to use cytology and related methods to diagnose disease

protein: an abundant kind of molecule found in cells; proteins have many functions, from acting as enzymes to forming mechanical structures such as tendons and hair

SCIENCE AND PROFESSION

Cytology is the study of the appearance of cells, the fundamental units that make up all living organisms. Cells are complex structures constructed from many different subcomponents that must work together in a precisely regulated fashion. Each cell must also cooperate with neighboring cells within the organism. A cell is like a complex automobile: many separate components must be synchronized, and the cell (or car) must follow a strict order of function in order to coordinate successfully with its neighbors. Because illness results from the malfunction of cells, physicians must be able to measure key cell functions accurately. The normal and abnormal function of cells can be evaluated in many different ways; cytology is the study of cells using microscopes. A sophisticated collection of cytological techniques is available to pathologists; with

these a precise diagnosis of cellular malfunction is possible.

All cells share several basic features. They are surrounded by a membrane, a flexible, sheetlike structure which encloses the fluid contents of the cell but allows required materials to move into the cell and waste products to move out of it. The complex salty fluid contained by the membrane is the cytoplasm; the other subcomponents of the cell, called organelles, are suspended in this substance. Each cell contains a set of genes, located on chromosomes, which function as blueprints for all other structures of the cell; the genes are inherited from one's parents. In plant and animal cells, the chromosomes are contained in a prominent organelle called the nucleus, which is surrounded by its own membrane inside the cell. Cells must also have a collection of enzymes used to convert food into energy in order to power the cell. In the cells of animals and plants, these enzymes are packaged into organelles called mitochondria. Membranes, the nucleus, and the mitochondria are the most prominent parts of a cell that are visible with a microscope, but cells also contain a variety of other specialized parts that are required for them to function properly. In addition, cells can also export (secrete) a variety of materials. For example, secreted materials make up bone, cartilage, tendons, mucus, sweat, and saliva.

Despite these basic features, the different types of cells have very distinct appearances. The cells of bacteria, plants, and animals are easily distinguishable from one another using a microscope. Bacterial cells are simplified, lacking organized nuclei and mitochondria. Different kinds of bacteria can be precisely distinguished; for example, strep throat is caused by spherical bacteria that form chains, like beads of a necklace. Some dangerous bacteria can be colored with dyes that do not stain harmless bacteria. Because so many human diseases are caused by bacteria, highly accurate procedures have been developed for their identification.

The adult human body is made up of several trillion individual cells. Although much larger than bacteria, all of these are far too small to be seen with the naked eye (typically about 20 microns in diameter). Each organ of the body—the brain, liver, kidney, skin, and so on—is made up of several kinds of cells, specialized for particular functions. They must cooperate closely: Mistakes in the activities of any of these many cells can cause disease. A pathologist is able to recognize small changes in the appearance of each of many different cell types.

A few of the characteristic cell types in the human body include nerve, muscle, secretory, and epithelial cells. Nerve cells are designed to pass information throughout the nervous system. The nerve cells function much like electrical wires, so they have slender wirelike extensions that can be several feet long. Defects in the wiring circuits, for example in patients with Alzheimer's disease, can be readily detected. Muscle cells are easily identified because they are elongated cylinders packed with special fibers that cause muscular contraction. Secretory cells produce and release such substances as digestive enzymes. Such cells are often filled with membrane-bound packets of their specialized product, ready to be released from the cell. The skin and the surfaces of various internal organs are encased in a cell type called epithelium. Epithelial cells are tilelike and are often fastened tightly to neighboring epithelial cells by special kinds of connectors. Numerous other specialized cell types are found in the body as well, but these four types represent the most common cell designs.

Cells are sophisticated and delicate structures that carry out specific functions efficiently. The structure and function of normal cells are stable and predictable. If significant numbers of cells are somehow damaged, disease is the result. Such defective cells change in their appearance in characteristic ways. Therefore, cytology is an important element in the diagnosis of many

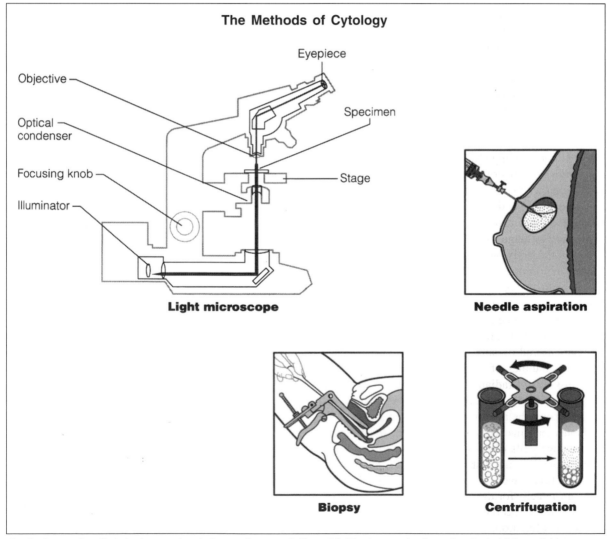

The Methods of Cytology

Eyepiece

Objective

Optical condenser

Focusing knob

Illuminator

Specimen

Stage

Light microscope

Needle aspiration

Biopsy

Centrifugation

Cytologists study cells in both normal and abnormal states. Cells and fluid to be examined may be obtained through biopsy, separated by centrifugation, and studied under a light microscope.

diseases and for monitoring the cellular response to therapy.

Many different types of stress can cause cell damage. One of the most common stresses is oxygen deprivation, known as hypoxia. Even a brief interruption of oxygen can cause irreversible damage to cells because it is needed for energy production. Since oxygen is transported in the blood, the most common cause of hypoxia is loss of blood supply, which can occur with blockage by blood clots or narrowed blood vessels and with several kinds of lung or heart problems. Carbon monoxide poisoning results from interference with the blood's ability to absorb and carry oxygen, while the poison cyanide interferes with a cell's ability to make use of oxygen.

Poisons such as cyanide can damage cells in many other ways, as can drugs. Prolonged use of barbiturates or alcohol can damage liver cells. These cells are also sensitive to common chemicals such as carbon tetrachloride, one used widely as a household cleaning agent. The liver is where foreign chemicals are changed to harmless forms, which explains why the liver cells are often damaged. Even useful chemicals, however, can cause harm to cells in some circumstances. Constant high levels of glucose, a sugar used by all cells, may overwork certain cells of the pancreas to the point where they become defective. Some foods (especially fats) and certain food additives, if they are eaten in excess, can interfere with how cells work.

Physical damage to cells—caused, for example, by blows to the body—can dislocate parts of cells, preventing their proper coordination. Extreme cold can interfere with the blood supply, causing hypoxia; extreme heat can cause cells to speed up their rate of metabolism, again exceeding the oxygen-carrying capacity of the circulatory system. The "bends," the affliction suffered by surfacing deep-sea divers, results from tiny bubbles of nitrogen that block capillaries. Various kinds of radiant energy, such as radioactivity or ultraviolet light, can damage specific chemicals of cells, causing them to malfunction. Electrical energy generates extreme local heat within the body, which can damage cells directly.

Many small living organisms can interfere with cellular function as well. Viruses are effective parasites of cells, using cells for their own survival. This relationship can result in cell death, as in poliomyelitis; in depressed cell function, as in viral hepatitis; or in abnormal cell growth, as in some cancers. Bacteria can also live as parasites, releasing toxins that interfere with cellular function in a variety of ways. Malaria is caused by a single-celled animal that damages blood cells, athlete's foot is caused by a fungus, and tiny worms called nematodes can invade cells and cause them to work improperly.

All cell types are not equally sensitive to damage by each agent. Liver cells are particularly sensitive to damage by toxic chemicals. Nerve and muscle cells are the first to be injured by hypoxia. Kidney cells are also easily damaged by loss of blood supply. Lung cells are affected by anything that is inhaled.

DIAGNOSTIC AND TREATMENT TECHNIQUES

Before cells can be successfully observed, they must be prepared through several steps. First, it is necessary to select a relatively small sample of a particular organ for closer scrutiny. Such a sample is called a biopsy when it is collected by a physician who wishes to test for a disease. The biopsy must then be preserved, or fixed, so that its parts will not deteriorate. Next, the specimen must be encased within a solid substance so that it can be handled without damage. Most often, the fixed specimen is soaked in melted paraffin, which then is allowed to solidify in a mold. For some kinds of microscopes, harder plastic materials are used. Next, the specimen must be thinly sliced so that the internal details can be seen. The delicate slices are mounted on a support, typically a thin glass slide for light microscopy. Finally, the parts of the cell must be colored, or stained. Without this coloring, the cell parts would be transparent and thus unobservable.

The basic tool of the cytologist is the light microscope. It can magnify up to about seven hundred times. Numerous sophisticated methods are used with light microscopy. Specific stains have been developed for distinguishing the different molecules that make up cells. For example, Alcian blue is a dye that stains a type of complex sugar that accumulates outside certain abnormal cells, making it easier to identify these cells. Also, specially prepared antibodies can recognize particular proteins within cells. Disease-causing proteins, including the proteins of dangerous viruses and bacteria, can be precisely identified in this way.

A major advance in cytology is the electron microscope. It forms images in essentially the same way as a light microscope does, but using electrons rather than visible light. Because of the properties of electrons, this type of microscope can magnify tens of thousands of times beyond life size. A wide range of new cell features has been revealed with the electron microscope.

The details of how genes work, how materials enter and leave cells, how energy is produced, and how molecules are synthesized have been made clearer. The steps for preparing specimens for electron microscopy are delicate, time-consuming, and demanding. Furthermore, the electron microscope itself is complex and expensive. Considerable skill is required to use it effectively. For these reasons, electron microscopy is not commonly used for routine medical diagnoses.

Cell injury causes predictable changes in cells that can be interpreted by a pathologist to suggest the underlying cause of the damage and how best to treat it. Almost all forms of reversible injury cause changes in the size and shape of cells. Cellular swelling is an obvious symptom that almost always reflects a serious underlying problem. Such cells also have a characteristic cloudy appearance. Swelling and cloudiness indicate loss of energy reserves and abnormal uptake of water into the cell through improperly functioning cell-surface membranes. An indication of serious damage is the accumulation within the cell of vacuoles—small, fluid-filled sacs that have a characteristic clear appearance when viewed through a microscope. More severe injury can cause the formation of vacuoles that contain fat, giving the cells a foamy appearance. Such damage is most often seen in cells of the heart, kidneys, and lungs. These changes appear to reflect both membrane abnormalities and the defective metabolism of fats.

Cells that are damaged beyond the point of repair will die, a process called necrosis. The two key processes in necrosis are the breakdown and mopping up of cellular contents, and large changes in structure of cellular proteins in ways that can be identified using a microscope. The most conspicuous and reliable indicators of necrosis are changes in the appearance of the nucleus, which can shrink or even break into pieces and which eventually disappears completely. Ultimately, the entire cell disappears.

Cancer provides a good illustration of how cytology is employed in the diagnosis of a specific disease. A skilled cytologist can detect cells at an early stage of cancer development and, with accuracy, can gauge how dangerous a cancer cell is or is likely to become. Cancer is a disease of abnormal growth. Cancer cells may have few abnormal features other than their improper growth; tumors made up of such cells are generally not dangerous and so are labeled benign. Malignant tumor cells, on the other hand, are highly abnormal. They can damage and invade other parts of the body, making these cells much more dangerous.

The cells of benign tumors may have nearly the same appearance as the cells of the normal tissue from which they arose. Benign cancers of skin, bone, muscle, and nerve keep the obvious structures that allow these highly specialized cell types to carry out their normal functions. Ironically, however, continued normal function can itself become a problem, because there are too many cells producing specialized products. For example, tumors in tissues that produce hormones can result in massive excesses of such hormones, causing severe imbalances in the function of the body's organs. Malignant tumor cells, on the other hand, have lost some or all of the functional and cytological features of their parent normal cells. They have a simpler and more primitive appearance, termed anaplasia by pathologists. The degree of anaplasia is one of the most reliable hallmarks of how malignant a cell has become.

Almost any part of the cell can become anaplastic. A common change is in the chromosomes of a cancer cell. The number, size, and shape of chromosomes change, and detailed analysis of these changes is often important in diagnosis, as in leukemia. Many malignant tumor cells secrete enzymes that attack surrounding connective tissue, changing its appearance in characteristic ways. Membrane systems of anaplastic cells are also abnormal, with serious consequences. The movement of materials in and out of cells becomes defective, and energy production mechanisms are upset, causing the characteristic changes in appearance described above. A general feature of tumors made up of anaplastic cells is the variability among individual cells. Some cells can appear virtually normal, while other tumor cells nearby can appear highly abnormal in several ways.

The cells of benign tumors remain where they arose. The cells of malignant tumors, however, have the ability to spread through the body (metastasize), penetrating and damaging other organs in the process. These abilities, to invade and metastasize, have serious effects on the rest of the body. Invading cells often can be identified easily with a microscope. Extensions of the tumor cells may reach into surrounding normal organ parts. Tumor cells can be observed penetrating into blood and lymph vessels and other body cavities, such as the abdominal cavity and air pockets in the lung. Small clusters of tumor cells can be found in blood and identified in distant organs. These cells can begin the process of invasion all over again, producing so-called secondary tumors in other organs. How malignant cancer cells can cause so much harm becomes clear.

PERSPECTIVE AND PROSPECTS

Of the diagnostic procedures that are available to physicians, cytologic techniques are among the most popular. Because the cells being examined are so tiny, the microscopes used must be able to magnify the cells enough to allow observation of their characteristics. Historically, the use of cytology in medical practice has closely paralleled the development of adequate microscopes and methods for preparing specimens.

Magnifying lenses by themselves lack the power required for observing cells. A microscope of adequate power must use several such lenses stacked together. The first crude microscopes with this design appeared late in the sixteenth century. During the next several hundred years, microscopes were mostly used to observe cells of plant material because the woody parts of plants can be thinly sliced and then observed directly, without the need for further preparation. The word "cell" was first employed by Robert Hooke (1635-1703) in a paper published in 1665. He observed small chambers in pieces of cork, which were where cells had been located in the living cork tree. These chambers reminded Hooke of monks' cells in a monastery, hence the name.

The great anatomist Marcello Malpighi (1628-1694) may have been the first to observe mammalian cells, within capillaries. The real giant of this era, however, was the Dutch microscopist Antoni van Leeuwenhoek (1632-1723), who greatly improved the quality of microscopes and then used them to observe single-celled animals, bacteria, sperm, and the nuclei within certain blood cells. Although most progress continued to be made with plants, numerous observations accumulated during the seventeenth and eighteenth centuries which suggested that animals are made up of tiny saclike units, and Hooke's word "cell" was applied to describe them. This concept was clearly stated in 1839 by Theodor Schwann (1810-1882); his idea that all animals are composed of cells and cellular products quickly gained acceptance. At this time, however, there was essentially no comprehension of how cells work. Without an understanding of normal cell function, cytology was still of little use in identifying and understanding disease.

During the late nineteenth and early twentieth centuries, the appearance of different cell types was carefully described. The main organelles of cells were identified, and such fundamental processes as cell division were observed and understood. At last it was possible to utilize cytology for medical purposes. The principles of medical cytology were established by the great pathologist Rudolf Virchow (1821-1902), who suggested for the first time that diseases originate from changes in specific cells of the body.

Rapid progress in cytology was made in the 1940's and 1950's, for two reasons. First, improved microscopes were developed, allowing greater accuracy in observing cell structure. The second reason—rapid progress in genetics and biochemistry—greatly increased the knowledge of how cells function and of the significance of specific changes in their appearance. Because cells are the basic units of life, scientists will continue to study them in detail, and the medical world will benefit directly from further, improved understanding in this field.

—*Howard L. Hosick, Ph.D.*

See also Bacterial infections; Bacteriology; Biopsy; Blood and blood disorders; Blood testing; Cancer; Cells; Cytopathology; Gram staining; Hematology; Hematology, pediatric; Histology; Karyotyping; Laboratory tests; Malignancy and metastasis; Microbiology; Microscopy; Oncology; Pathology; Serology; Urinalysis; Viral infections.

FOR FURTHER INFORMATION:

Kumar, Vinay, et al., eds. *Robbins Basic Pathology*. 8th ed. Philadelphia: Saunders/Elsevier, 2007. Presents a reasonably concise overview of the entire field of pathology, but the emphasis is on cytology. The chapter on disease at the cellular level is excellent and readable. The authors are unusually adept at explaining the facts in a simple and interesting way.

Taylor, Ron. *Through the Microscope*. Vol. 22 in *The World of Science*. New York: Facts On File, 1986. A fine introduction to the wonders of microscopy, recommended for all readers. In a large format with more than one hundred beautiful photographs. The clear, simple, and brief text explains how microscopes work and what is being seen. The section "Microscopes, Health, and Disease" is particularly relevant, explaining cytological detective work.

Wolfe, Stephen L. *Cell Ultrastructure*. Belmont, Calif.: Wadsworth, 1985. This book presents electron microscope photographs of the important structures of viruses, bacteria, and plant and animal cells. Included for most structures are three-dimensional drawings that are particularly useful for visualizing how cells are put together.

CYTOMEGALOVIRUS (CMV)

DISEASE/DISORDER

ANATOMY OR SYSTEM AFFECTED: Blood, brain, cells, ears, eyes, gastrointestinal system, immune system, liver, lungs

SPECIALTIES AND RELATED FIELDS: Family medicine, gastroenterology, hematology, immunology, obstetrics, pediatrics, virology

DEFINITION: A viral disease normally producing mild symptoms in healthy individuals but severe infections in the immunocompromised. Congenital infection may lead to malformations or fetal death.

KEY TERMS:

hepatitis: inflammation of the liver; usually caused by viral infections, toxic substances, or immunological disturbances

hepatosplenomegaly: enlargement of the liver and spleen such that they may be felt below the rib margins

heterophil antibodies: antibodies that are detected using antigens other than the antigens that induced them

jaundice: yellow staining of the skin, eyes, and other tissues and excretions with excess bile pigments in the blood

latency: following an acute infection by a virus, a period of dormancy from which the virus may be reactivated during times of stress or immunocompromise

microcephaly: a congenital condition involving an abnormally small head associated with an incompletely developed brain

CAUSES AND SYMPTOMS

Cytomegalovirus (CMV) is a member of the herpesvirus group that includes such viruses as the Epstein-Barr virus, which causes infectious mononucleosis, and the varicella-zoster virus, which causes chickenpox. CMV is a ubiquitous virus that is transmitted in a number of different ways. A newly infected woman may transmit the virus across the placenta to her unborn child. Infection may also occur in the birth canal or via mother's milk. Young children commonly transmit CMV by means of saliva. Sexual transmission is common in adults. Blood transfusions and organ transplants may also transmit cytomegalovirus to recipients. More than 80 percent of adults worldwide have antibodies indicating exposure to cytomegalovirus.

Congenital cytomegaloviral infection is universally common and especially prevalent in developing nations. Approximately 1 percent of live births in the United States are infected. Most congenitally infected infants exhibit no symptoms. Normal development may follow, but some infants suffer problems such as deafness, visual impairment, and/or mental retardation. Approximately 10 to 20 percent exhibit clinically obvious evidence of cytomegalic inclusion disease: hepatosplenomegaly, jaundice, microcephaly, deafness, seizures, cerebral palsy, and blood disorders such as thrombocytopenia (a decrease in platelets) and hemolytic anemia (in which red blood cells are destroyed). Giant cells having nuclei containing large inclusions are found in affected organs. Cytomegalovirus is a leading cause of mental retardation and responsible for about 10 percent of cases of microcephaly.

In immunocompetent adults and older children, cytomegalovirus can cause heterophil-negative mononucleosis, an infectious mononucleosis in which no heterophil antibodies are formed. Such antibodies are found in infectious mononucleosis caused by the Epstein-Barr virus. Heterophil-negative mononucleosis is characterized by fever, hepatitis, lethargy, and abnormal lymphocytes in blood.

Severe systemic cytomegalovirus infections are frequently seen in the immunocompromised. Transplant patients are intentionally immunosuppressed to reduce the likelihood of graft rejection, making them vulnerable to infection by cytomegalovirus either by reactivation or by acquisition of the virus from the donor organ. Resulting systemic infections are manifested in diseases such as pneumonia, hepatitis, and retinitis. In addition to these CMV diseases, acquired immunodeficiency syndrome (AIDS) patients suffer from infections of the central nervous system and gastrointestinal tract. Their blood cells may also be affected, resulting in disorders such as thrombocytopenia. AIDS patients frequently have intestinal CMV infections leading to

---

INFORMATION ON CYTOMEGALOVIRUS (CMV)

CAUSES: Viral infection spread during childbirth or through body fluid exchange

SYMPTOMS: Deafness, visual impairment, mental retardation, jaundice, microcephaly, seizures, cerebral palsy, blood disorders, infectious mononucleosis

DURATION: Varies

TREATMENTS: Antiviral drugs (ganciclovir, foscarnet)

chronic diarrhea. Cytomegalovirus retinitis in AIDS patients is particularly serious and may lead to retinal detachment and blindness. This is the most common sight-damaging opportunistic eye infection found in AIDS patients.

Treatment and Therapy

Ganciclovir, valganciclovir, foscarnet, and cidofovir are all antiviral agents which have been found useful in treating CMV infections in immunocompromised patients. Toxic properties, however, can limit their long-term administration. Ganciclovir exhibits hematopoietic toxicity; that is, it has an adverse affect on blood cells that may result in neutropenia, a decrease in the number of neutrophils in the blood. Foscarnet has more side effects than ganciclovir. It is a nephrotoxic substance, which means that it may damage the kidneys and thus cannot be used in patients with renal failure.

Valganciclovir, the oral form of ganciclovir, has been used effectively to prevent CMV infection in transplant recipients. It is administered to CMV-seronegative transplant patients receiving an organ from a CMV-seropositive donor as well as in CMV-seropositive recipients who will be undergoing immunosuppression to prevent rejection of the transplanted organ. Another material employed as a prophylaxis for bone marrow and renal transplant recipients is intravenous cytomegalovirus immune globulin.

Therapy for CMV retinitis involves intravenous treatment with either ganciclovir, foscarnet, or cidofovir plus oral probenecid or oral valganciclovir. Alternatively, an intraocular ganciclovir implant may be used along with one of the systemic treatments mentioned above. Therapy of retinitis as well as other types of CMV infection in AIDS patients should be accompanied by highly active antiretroviral therapy (HAART) to treat the human immunodeficiency virus and improve the immune function in the the the patient. Successful HAART may allow the CMV antiviral therapy to be discontinued, but the patient must be carefully monitored for relapse of the CMV infection.

Retinal detachment is another complication arising from cytomegalovirus retinitis. It may occur even in those undergoing successful antiviral treatment. Surgical intervention is required to restore functional vision in these cases.

Perspective and Prospects

The term "cytomegalia" was first used in 1921 to describe the condition of an infant with intranuclear inclusions in the lungs, kidney, and liver. This condition in an adult was first attributed to a virus of the herpes group in 1925. Twenty-five cases of apparent cytomegalic inclusion disease had been described by 1932. Cytomegalovirus was pursued and isolated in the mid-1950's by Margaret Smith in St. Louis. Around the same time, independently and serendipitously, groups in Boston and in Bethesda, Maryland, also isolated the virus.

Development of new antiviral drugs and measures to reduce the immunocompromised state should continue to progress and improve the outcomes for patients infected with CMV.

—Nancy Handshaw Clark, Ph.D.;
updated by H. Bradford Hawley, M.D.

See also Acquired immunodeficiency syndrome (AIDS); Birth defects; Eye surgery; Eyes; Hepatitis; Herpes; Immune system; Immunodeficiency disorders; Immunology; Mental retardation; Mononucleosis; Pregnancy and gestation; Stillbirth; Transplantation; Viral infections; Vision disorders.

For Further Information:

Bellenir, Karen, and Peter D. Dresser, eds. *Contagious and Noncontagious Infectious Diseases Sourcebook*. Detroit: Omnigraphics, 1997. A handy reference source on infectious diseases. Includes bibliographical references and an index.

Roizman, Bernard, ed. *Infectious Diseases in an Age of Change: The Impact of Human Ecology and Behavior on Disease Transmission*. Washington, D.C.: National Academy Press, 1995. This book reports on major infectious diseases on the rise today, such as sexually transmitted diseases, Lyme disease, human cytomegalovirus, diarrheal diseases, dengue fever, hepatitis viruses, HIV, and malaria.

Roizman, Bernard, Richard J. Whitley, and Carlos Lopez, eds. *The Human Herpesviruses*. New York: Raven Press, 1993. A helpful text discussing all aspects of the herpesvirus and offering information on vaccination against the disease. Includes bibliographical references and an index.

Scheld, W. Michael, Richard J. Whitley, and Christina M. Marra, eds. *Infections of the Central Nervous System*. 3d ed. Philadelphia: Lippincott Williams & Wilkins, 2004. This comprehensive multiauthor book covers viral infections, with six separate chapters on one herpesvirus group: herpes simplex, varicella zoster, cytomegalovirus, Epstein-Barr virus, human herpesvirus 6, and B virus.

Wagner, Edward K., and Martinez J. Hewlett. *Basic Virology*. 2d ed. Malden, Mass.: Blackwell Science, 2004. A very readable undergraduate text covering issues of virology and viral disease, properties of viruses and virus-cell interaction, working with viruses, and replication patterns of specific viruses.

CYTOPATHOLOGY

SPECIALTY

ANATOMY OR SYSTEM AFFECTED: Cells, immune system

SPECIALTIES AND RELATED FIELDS: Bacteriology, cytology, forensic pathology, hematology, histology, oncology, pathology, serology

DEFINITION: The medical field that deals with changes in cell structure or physiology as a result of injuries, infectious agents, or toxic substances.

SCIENCE AND PROFESSION

The profession of cytopathology deals with the search for lesions or abnormalities within individual cells or groups of cells. Generally speaking, a pathologist is a physician trained in pathology, the study of the nature of diseases. Observations of tissue or cell lesions are utilized in the diagnosis of disease or other agents associated with damage to cells.

Cell damage may result from endogenous phenomena, including the aging process, or from exogenous agents such as biological organisms (viruses or bacteria), chemical agents (bacterial toxins or other poisons), and physical agents (heat, cold, or electricity). For example, particular biological agents produce recognizable lesions that may be useful in the diagnosis of disease, such as the crystalline structures characteristic of certain viral infections.

The type of necrosis, or cell death, encountered is useful in diagnosing the problem. For example, certain types of enzymatic dissolution of cells, which result in areas of liquefaction, are the result of bacterial infection. Gangrenous necrosis often follows the restriction of the blood supply, because of either infection or a blood clot.

Pathologic changes within the cell can also help pinpoint the time of death. Organelles degenerate at a rate dependent on their use of oxygen. For example, mitochondria, which utilize significant amounts of oxygen, are among the first organelles to degenerate.

DIAGNOSTIC AND TREATMENT TECHNIQUES

The diagnosis and treatment of cancer are prime examples of the use of cytopathology. The extent of pleomorphism in cell size and shape, irregularity of the nucleus, and presence (or absence) of organelles all provide the basis for the choice of treatment and help determine the ultimate prognosis. Specific organelles are stained with characteristic histochemicals, followed by microscopic observation. A preponderance of large, irregularly shaped cells provides for a poorer prognosis than if cells appear more normally differentiated. The nuclei in highly malignant tumors show a greater variation in size and chromatin pattern, as compared with those of cells from benign growths. Such differences lead directly to decisions on the choice of treatment: surgical removal, chemotherapy, or radiation.

—*Richard Adler, Ph.D.*

See also Bacteriology; Biopsy; Blood and blood disorders; Blood testing; Cancer; Cells; Cytology; Gram staining; Hematology; Hematology, pediatric; Histology; Laboratory tests; Malignancy and metastasis; Microbiology; Microscopy; Oncology; Pathology; Serology; Toxicology; Tumors; Urinalysis.

FOR FURTHER INFORMATION:

Geisinger, Kim R., et al. *Modern Cytopathology*. Philadelphia: Churchill Livingstone, 2004.

Kumar, Vinay, et al., eds. *Robbins Basic Pathology*. 8th ed. Philadelphia: Saunders/Elsevier, 2007.

Lewin, Benjamin, et al., eds. *Cells*. Sudbury, Mass.: Jones and Bartlett, 2007.

Majno, Guido, and Isabelle Joris. *Cells, Tissues, and Disease: Principles of General Pathology*. 2d ed. New York: Oxford University Press, 2004.

Silverberg, Steven G., ed. *Silverberg's Principles and Practice of Surgical Pathology and Cytopathology*. 4th ed. Edinburgh, Scotland: Elsevier Churchill Livingstone, 2006.

DEAFNESS

DISEASE/DISORDER

ALSO KNOWN AS: Hearing loss, hearing impairment, presbycusis

ANATOMY OR SYSTEM AFFECTED: Ears, nervous system

SPECIALTIES AND RELATED FIELDS: Audiology, geriatrics and gerontology, speech pathology

DEFINITION: Deafness is either partial or complete loss of hearing. Hearing loss occurs most often in older adults, but people may be born deaf or become deaf at young ages.

KEY TERMS:

acquired: not present at birth; developing after birth

auditory: pertaining to hearing

cerumen: earwax produced by specialized glands to protect and lubricate the ear canal

cochlea: the organ of hearing in the inner ear that takes the vibrations from the middle ear organs and converts them into nerve impulses for the brain to interpret

congenital: present at birth

eighth cranial nerve: also known as the auditory nerve or the vestibulocochlear nerve; the nerve running between the ear and the brain, involved with hearing and balance

genetic: inherited

ossicles: the chain of tiny bones in the middle ear which carry the vibrations of the tympanic membrane to the cochlea

ototoxic: toxic or harmful to the ears

tympanic membrane: also called the eardrum; a thin membrane that separates the external or outer ear from the middle ear

CAUSES AND SYMPTOMS

To understand deafness, it is first necessary to understand how sound is heard. The sound waves produced by any noise travel through the air and are funneled down the ear canal by the external ear, which is specially shaped for this function. The sound waves then cause the tympanic membrane to vibrate, which in turn causes the chain of tiny ossicles to vibrate. This mechanical energy of vibration is then transformed by the cochlea into nerve impulses which travel along the eighth cranial nerve to the spinal cord. These impulses are transmitted to the auditory cortex (center) of the brain, where they are interpreted. The ability to hear depends on all these elements working properly.

Deafness can occur when any particular part of this hearing pathway is not functioning as it should. If the ear canal is blocked with cerumen, a foreign body, fluid, or the products of infection or inflammation, then the sound waves are unable to travel to the eardrum. If the eardrum has ruptured or if it has become stiff (sclerosed), then it cannot vibrate. If the ossicles have been damaged in any way, then they cannot vibrate. If the middle ear is filled with fluid from inflammation or infection, then the eardrum and ossicles cannot work properly. If the cochlea, auditory nerve, or both have been damaged through trauma or use of an ototoxic drug or disease, then they cannot do their job of converting vibration into nerve impulses and transmitting them to the brain. If the auditory center of the brain is damaged, then it cannot interpret the nerve impulses correctly.

Hearing loss is classified by the cause: conductive, sensory, and neural. Conductive losses are those that affect the conduction of sound waves; they involve problems with the external ear, ear canal, tympanic membrane, and ossicles. The sensory and neural causes are usually classified together as "sensorineural"; these losses affect the cochlea, auditory nerve, or auditory cortex of the brain.

The most common cause of hearing loss in children is otitis media, or middle-ear infection, which causes fluid to build up behind the tympanic membrane. It is usually reversible with time and treatment. This is a type of conductive loss, as is hearing loss attributable to cerumen impaction (excessive buildup of earwax), which can occur in both children and adults. Sensorineural losses are caused by such things as excessive noise exposure, ototoxic drugs, exposure to toxins in the environment, and diseases such as rubella (German

---

INFORMATION ON DEAFNESS

CAUSES: Aging; ear canal blockage (earwax, foreign body, fluid); ruptured or stiff eardrum; middle-ear infection; cochlea or auditory nerve damage (excessive noise exposure, ototoxic drugs, environmental toxins); genetic defect or predisposition

SYMPTOMS: Hearing loss ranging from moderate to total

DURATION: Acute, permanent, or progressive

TREATMENTS: Depends on cause; for permanent loss, hearing aids, cochlear implants, other assistive devices

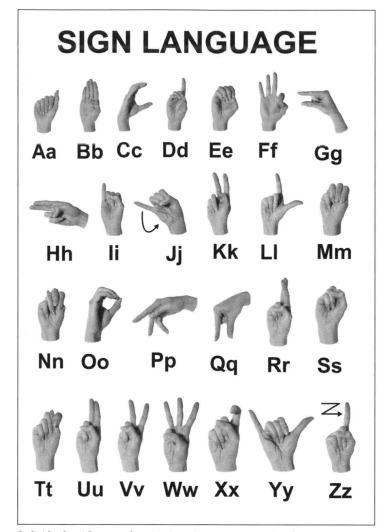

SIGN LANGUAGE

Aa Bb Cc Dd Ee Ff Gg

Hh Ii Jj Kk Ll Mm

Nn Oo Pp Qq Rr Ss

Tt Uu Vv Ww Xx Yy Zz

Individuals with severe hearing impairment may use sign language to communicate. (© Stephen Coburn/Dreamstime.com)

Likewise, deafness that occurs after birth may be either acquired or genetic. Deafness associated with exposure to loud noises is acquired, for example, while many forms of deafness that occur in older age are genetic. About one-third of people between the ages of sixty-five and seventy-five years and 40 percent of those over seventy-five have hearing loss.

TREATMENT AND THERAPY

The best treatment for deafness is prevention. Immunizations against rubella, ear protection against noise exposure, and avoidance of too much aspirin are all examples of prevention against deafness.

Once hearing impairment has occurred, determination of the cause is essential. The primary care provider, an otolaryngologist (ear, nose, and throat doctor), an audiologist (hearing specialist), and a neurologist may be involved in this assessment. Reversible causes of deafness or loss can be addressed medically or surgically, as in the removal of earwax. For nonreversible causes, hearing aids and other assistive hearing devices may be helpful. These devices have become increasingly sophisticated. Some allow the person to adjust the hearing aid to specific circumstances, while older versions amplified all sounds equally.

Cochlear implants are electronic devices that give profoundly deaf persons a sense of sound that helps them understand speech and other noises. A microphone picks up sounds, which are processed, converted to electric impulses, and sent to different areas of the auditory nerve.

In addition to these products, many new assistive devices are available to help persons with severe hearing impairment function independently. For example, special telephones, alarm clocks, and doorbells that flash a light or shake the bed in addition to ringing are readily available.

—Rebecca Lovell Scott, Ph.D., PA-C

See also Aging; Audiology; Ear infections and disorders; Ear surgery; Ears; Hearing aids; Hearing loss; Hearing tests; Neuralgia, neuritis, and neuropathy; Otorhinolaryngology; Sense organs; Speech disorders.

measles). The type of sensorineural loss that many people experience as they get older is called presbycusis, which means "a condition of elder hearing." Many people with sensorineural losses have a genetic predisposition for hearing loss.

Congenital deafness is deafness that is present at the time a baby is born. Before the widespread availability of immunization against rubella, mothers who contracted German measles during pregnancy were at great risk of having a baby with congenital deafness. In this case, the congenital deafness is acquired. Congenital deafness may also be genetic. For example, if a child inherits defective copies of the GJB2 gene from each parent, then that child will be deaf even if both parents can hear.

FOR FURTHER INFORMATION:

American Medical Association. *American Medical Association Family Medical Guide*. 4th rev. ed. Hoboken, N.J.: John Wiley & Sons, 2004.

Carmen, Richard, ed. *The Consumer Handbook on Hearing Loss and Hearing Aids: A Bridge to Healing*. 2d rev. ed. Sedona, Ariz.: Auricle Ink, 2004.

Dillon, Harvey. *Hearing Aids*. New York: Thieme, 2001.

Komaroff, Anthony, ed. *Harvard Medical School Family Health Guide*. New York: Free Press, 2005.

Romoff, Arlene. *Hear Again: Back to Life with a Cochlear Implant*. New York: League for the Hard of Hearing, 1999.

Stoppard, Miriam. *Family Health Guide*. New York: DK, 2004.

DEATH AND DYING
DISEASE/DISORDER

ANATOMY OR SYSTEM AFFECTED: Psychic-emotional system, all bodily systems

SPECIALTIES AND RELATED FIELDS: Family medicine, geriatrics and gerontology, psychology

KEY TERMS:

anticipatory depression: a depressive reaction to the awaited death of either oneself or a significant other; also called anticipatory grieving, preparatory grieving, or preparatory depression

bereavement: the general, overall process of mourning and grieving; considered to have progressive stages which include anticipation, grieving, mourning, postmourning, depression, loneliness, and reentry into society

depression: a general term covering mild states (sadness, inhibition, unhappiness, discouragement) to severe states (hopelessness, despair); typically part of normal, healthy grieving; considered the fourth stage of death and dying, between bargaining and acceptance

grief: the emotional and psychological response to loss; always painful, grieving is a type of psychological work and requires some significant duration of time

mourning: the acute phase of grief; characterized by distress, hopelessness, fear, acute loss, crying, insomnia, loss of appetite, anxiety, guilt, and restlessness

reactive depression: depression occurring as a result of overt events that have already taken place; it universally occurs in the bereaved

thanatology: the study and investigation of life-threatening actions, terminal illness, suicide, homicide, death, dying, grief, and bereavement

uncomplicated bereavement: a technical psychiatric label describing normal, average, and expectant grieving; despite an experience of great psychological pain, grieving is considered normal and healthy unless it continues much beyond one year

CAUSES AND SYMPTOMS

Medicine determines that death has occurred by assessing bodily functions in either of two areas. Persons with irreversible cessation of respiration and circulation are dead; persons with irreversible cessation of ascertainable brain functions are also dead. There are standard procedures used to diagnose death, including simple observation, brain-stem reflex studies, and the use of confirmatory testing such as electrocardiography (ECG or EKG), electroencephalography (EEG), and arterial blood gas analysis (ABG). The particular circumstances—anticipated or unanticipated, observed or unobserved, the patient's age, drug or metabolic intoxication, or suspicion of hypothermia—will favor some procedures over others, but in all cases both cessation of functions and their irreversibility are required before death can be declared.

Between 60 and 75 percent of all people die from chronic terminal conditions. Therefore, except in sudden death (as in a fatal accident) or when there is no evidence of consciousness (as in a head injury which destroys cerebral, thinking functions while leaving brain-stem, reflexive functions intact), dying is both a physical and a psychological process. In most cases, dying takes time, and the time allows patients to react to the reality of their own passing. Often, they react by becoming vigilant about bodily symptoms and any changes in them. They also anticipate changes that have yet to occur. For example, long before the terminal stages of illness become manifest, dying patients commonly fear physical pain, shortness of breath, invasive procedures, loneliness, becoming a burden to loved ones, losing decision-making authority, and facing the unknown of death itself.

As physical deterioration proceeds, all people cope by resorting to what has worked for them before: the unique means and mechanisms which have helped maintain a sense of self and personal stability. People seem to go through the process of dying much as they have gone through the process of living—with the more salient features of their personalities, whether good or bad, becoming sharper and more prominent. People seem to face death much as they have faced life.

Medicine has come to acknowledge that physicians should understand what it means to die. Indeed, while all persons should understand what their own deaths will mean, physicians must additionally understand how their dying patients find this meaning. Physicians who see death as the final calamity coming at the end of life, and thus primarily as something that only geriatric medicine has to face, are mistaken. Independent of beliefs about "life after life," the life process on this planet inexorably comes to an end for everyone, whether as a result of accident, injury, or progressive deterioration.

In 1969, psychiatrist Elisabeth Kübler-Ross published the landmark *On Death and Dying*, based on her work with two hundred terminally ill patients. Technologically driven, Western medicine had come to define its role as primarily dealing with extending life and thwarting death by defeating specific diseases. Too few physicians saw a role for themselves once the prognosis turned grave. In the decades that followed *On Death and Dying*, the profession has reaccepted that death and dying are part of life and that, while treating the dying may not mean extending the length of life, it can and should mean extending its quality.

Kübler-Ross provided a framework which explained how people cope with and adapt to the profound and terrible news that their illness is going to kill them. Although other physicians, psychologists, and thanatologists have shortened, expanded, and adapted her five stages of the dying process, neither the actual number of stages nor what they are specifically called is as important as the information and insight that any stage theory of dying yields. As with any human process, dying is complex, multifaceted, multidimensional, and polymorphic.

Well-intentioned, but misguided, professionals and family members may try to help move dying patients through each of the stages only to encounter active resentment or passive withdrawal. Patients, even dying patients, cannot be psychologically moved to where they are not ready to be. Rather than making the terminally ill die the "right" way, it is more respectful and helpful to understand any stage as a description of normal reactions to serious loss, and that these reactions normally vary among different individuals and also within the same individual over time. The reactions appear, disappear, and reappear in any order and in any combination. What the living must do is respect the unfolding of an adaptational schema which is the dying person's own. No one should presume to know how someone else should die.

COMPLICATIONS AND DISORDERS

Denial is Kübler-Ross's first stage, but it is also linked to shock and isolation. Whether the news is told outright or gradual self-realization occurs, most people react to the knowledge of their impending death with existential shock: Their whole selves recoil at the idea, and they say, in some fashion, "This cannot be happening to me. I must be dreaming." Broadly considered, denial is a complex cognitive-emotional capacity which enables temporary postponement of active, acute, but in some way detrimental, recognition of reality. In the dying process, this putting off of the truth prevents a person from being overwhelmed while promoting psychological survival. Denial plays an important stabilizing role, holding back more than could be otherwise managed while allowing the individual to marshal psychological resources and reserves. It enables patients to consider the possibility, even the inevitability, of death and then to put the consideration away so that they can pursue life in the ways that are still available. In this way, denial is truly a mechanism of defense.

Many other researchers, along with Kübler-Ross, report anger as the second stage of dying. The stage is also linked to rage, fury, envy, resentment, and loathing. When "This cannot be happening to me," becomes, "This is happening to me. There was no mistake," patients are beginning to replace denial with attempts to understand what is happening to and inside them. When they do, they often ask, "Why me?" Though logically an unanswerable question, the logic of the question is clear. People, to remain human, must try to make intelligible their experiences and reality. The asking of this question is an important feature of the way in which all dying persons adapt to and cope with the reality of death.

People react with anger when they lose something of value; they react with greater anger when something of value is taken away from them by someone or something. Rage and fury, in fact, are often more accurate descriptions of people's reactions to the loss of their own life than anger. Anger is a difficult stage for professionals and loved ones, more so when the anger and rage are displaced and projected randomly into any corner and crevice of the patient's world. An unfortunate result is that caregivers often experience the anger as personal, and the caregivers' own feelings of guilt, shame, grief, and rejection can contribute to lessening contact with the dying person, which increases his or her sense of isolation.

Bargaining is Kübler-Ross's third stage, but it is also the one about which she wrote the least and the one that other thanatologists are most likely to leave unrepresented in their own models and stages of how people cope with dying. Nevertheless, it is a common phenomenon wherein dying people fall back on their faith, belief systems, or sense of the transcendent and the spiritual and try to make a deal—with God, life, fate, a higher power, or the composite of all the randomly colliding atoms in the universe. They ask for more time to help family members reconcile or to achieve something of importance. They may ask if they can simply attend their child's wedding or graduation or if they can see their first grandchild born. Then they will be ready to die; they will go willingly. Often, they mean that they will die without fighting death, if death can only be delayed or will delay itself. Some get what they want; others do not.

At some point, when terminally ill individuals are faced with decisions about more procedures, tests, surgeries, or medications or when their thinness, weakness, or deterioration becomes impossible to ignore, the anger, rage, numbness, stoicism, and even humor will likely give way to depression, Kübler-Ross's fourth stage and the one reaction that all thanatologists include in their models of how people cope with dying.

The depression can take many forms, for indeed there are always many losses, and each loss individually or several losses collectively might need to be experienced and worked through. For example, dying parents might ask themselves who will take care of the children, get them through school, walk them down the aisle, or guide them through life. Children, even adult children who are parents themselves, may ask whether they can cope without their own parents. They wonder who will support and anchor them in times of distress, who will (or could) love, nurture, and nourish them the way that their parents did. Depression accompanies the realization that each role, each function, will never be performed again. Both the dying and those who love them mourn.

Much of the depression takes the form of anticipatory grieving, which often occurs both in the dying and in those who will be affected most by their death. It is a part of the dying process experienced by the living, both terminal and nonterminal. Patients, family, and friends can psychologically anticipate what it will be like when the death does occur and what life will, and

will not, be like afterward. The grieving begins while there is still life left to live.

Bereavement specialists generally agree that anticipatory grieving, when it occurs, seems to help people cope with what is a terrible and frightening loss. It is an adaptive psychological mechanism wherein emotional, mental, and existential stability is painfully maintained. When depression develops, not only in reaction to death but also in preparation for it, it seems to be a necessary part of how those who are left behind cope in order to survive the loss themselves. Those who advocate or advise cheering up or looking on the bright side are either unrealistic or unable to tolerate the sadness in themselves or others. The dying are in the process of losing everything and everyone they love. Cheering up does not help them; the advice to "be strong" only helps the "helpers" deny the truth of the dying experience.

Both preparatory and reactive depression are frequently accompanied by unrealistic self-recrimination, shame, and guilt in the dying person. Those who are dying may judge themselves harshly and criticize themselves for the wrongs that they committed and for the good that they did not accomplish. They may judge themselves to be unattractive, unappealing, and repulsive because of how the illness and its treatment have made them appear. These feelings and states of minds, which have nothing to do with the reality of the situation, are often amenable to the interventions of understanding and caring people. Disfigured breasts do not make a woman less a woman; the removal of the testes does not make a man less a man. Financial and other obligations can be restructured and reassigned. Being forgiven and forgiving can help finish what was left undone.

Kübler-Ross's fifth stage, acceptance, is an intellectual and emotional coming to terms with death's reality, permanence, and inevitability. Ironically, it is manifested by diminished emotionality and interests and increased fatigue and inner (many would say spiritual) self-focus. It is a time without depression or anger. Envy of the healthy, the fear of losing all, and bargaining for another day or week are also absent. This final stage is often misunderstood. Some see it either as resignation and giving up or as achieving a happy serenity. Some think that acceptance is the goal of dying well and that all people are supposed to go through this stage. None of these viewpoints is accurate. Acceptance, when it does occur, comes from within the dying person. It is marked more by an emotional void and psychological detachment from people and things once held important and necessary and by an interest in some transcendental value (for the atheist) or his or her God (for the theist). It has little to do with what others believe is important or "should" be done. It is when dying people become more intimate with themselves and appreciate their separateness from others more than at any other time.

PERSPECTIVE AND PROSPECTS

All patients die—a fact that the actual practice of clinical Western medicine has too often discounted. Dealing with death is difficult in life, and it is difficult in medicine. As the ultimate outcome of all medical interventions, however, it is unavoidable. Dealing with the dying and those who care about them is also difficult. Patients ask questions that cannot be answered; families in despair and anger seek to find cause and sometimes lay blame. It takes courage to be with individuals as they face their deaths, struggling to find meaning in the time that they have left. It takes special courage simply to witness this struggle in a profession which prides itself on how well it intervenes. Working with death also reminds professionals of their own inevitable death. Facing that fact inwardly, spiritually, and existentially also requires courage.

Cure and treatment become care and management in the dying. They should live relatively pain-free, be supported in accomplishing their goals, be respected, be involved in decision making as appropriate, be encouraged to function as fully as their illness allows, and be provided with others to whom control can comfortably and confidently be passed. The lack of a cure and the certainty of the end can intimidate health care providers, family members, and close friends. They may dread genuine encounters with those whose days are knowingly numbered. Yet the dying have the same rights to be helped as any of the living, and how a society assists them bears directly on the meaning that its members are willing to attach to their own lives.

Today, largely in response to what dying patients have told researchers, medicine recognizes its role to assist these patients in working toward an appropriate death. Caretakers must determine the optimum treatments, interventions, and conditions which will enable such a death to occur. For each terminally ill person, these should be unique and specific. Caretakers should respond to the patient's needs and priorities, at the patient's own pace and as much as possible following the patient's lead. For some dying patients, the goal is to remain as pain-free as is feasible and to feel as well

as possible. For others, finishing whatever unfinished business remains becomes the priority. Making amends, forgiving and being forgiven, resolving old conflicts, and reconciling with self and others may be the most therapeutic and healing of interventions. Those who are to be bereaved fear the death of those they love. The dying fear the separation from all they know and love, but they fear as well the loss of autonomy, letting family and friends down, the pain and invasion of further treatment, disfigurement, dementia, loneliness, the unknown, becoming a burden, and the loss of dignity.

The English writer C. S. Lewis said that bereavement is the universal and integral part of the experience of loss. It requires effort, authenticity, mental and emotional work, a willingness to be afraid, and an openness to what is happening and what is going to happen. It requires an attitude which accepts, tolerates suffering, takes respite from the reality, reinvests in whatever life remains, and moves on. The only way to cope with dying or witnessing the dying of loved ones is by grieving through the pain, fear, loneliness, and loss of meaning. This process, which researcher Stephen Levine has likened to opening the heart in hell, is a viscous morass for most, and all people need to learn their own way through it and to have that learning respected. Healing begins with the first halting, unsteady, and frightening steps of genuine grief, which sometimes occur years before the "time of death" can be recorded as a historical event and which may never completely end.

—Paul Moglia, Ph.D.

See also Acquired immunodeficiency syndrome (AIDS); Aging; Depression; Ethics; Euthanasia; Grief and guilt; Hospice; Midlife crisis; Phobias; Psychiatry; Psychiatry, child and adolescent; Psychiatry, geriatric; Stress; Sudden infant death syndrome (SIDS); Suicide; Terminally ill: Extended care.

FOR FURTHER INFORMATION:

Becker, Ernest. *The Denial of Death.* New York: Free Press, 1997. Written by an anthropologist and philosopher, this is an erudite and insightful analysis and synthesis of the role that the fear of death plays in motivating human activity, society, and individual actions. A profound work.

Cook, Alicia Skinner, and Daniel S. Dworkin. *Helping the Bereaved: Therapeutic Interventions for Children, Adolescents, and Adults.* New York: Basic Books, 1992. Although not a self-help book, this work is useful to professionals and nonprofessionals alike as a review of the state of the art in grief therapy. Practical and readable. Of special interest for those becoming involved in grief counseling.

Corr, Charles A., Clyde M. Nabe, and Donna M. Corr. *Death and Dying, Life and Living.* 5th ed. Belmont, Calif.: Wadsworth, 2005. This book provides perspective on common issues associated with death and dying for family members and others affected by life-threatening circumstances.

Forman, Walter B., et al., eds. *Hospice and Palliative Care: Concepts and Practice.* 2d ed. Sudbury, Mass.: Jones and Bartlett, 2003. A text that examines the theoretical perspectives and practical information about hospice care. Other topics include community medical care, geriatric care, nursing care, pain management, research, counseling, and hospice management.

Kübler-Ross, Elisabeth, ed. *Death: The Final Stage of Growth.* Reprint. New York: Simon & Schuster, 1997. A psychiatrist by training, Kübler-Ross brings together other researchers' views of how death provides the key to how human beings make meaning in their own personal worlds. The author addresses practical concerns over how people express grief and accept the death of those close to them, and how they might prepare for their own inevitable ends.

Kushner, Harold. *When Bad Things Happen to Good People.* 20th anniversary ed. New York: Schocken Books, 2001. The first of Rabbi Kushner's works on finding meaning in one's life, it was originally his personal response to make intelligible the death of his own child. It has become a highly regarded reference for those who struggle with the meaning of pain, suffering, and death in their lives. Highly recommended.

McFarlane, Rodger, and Philip Bashe. *The Complete Bedside Companion: No-Nonsense Advice on Caring for the Seriously Ill.* New York: Simon & Schuster, 1998. A comprehensive and practical guide to caregiving for patients with serious illnesses. The first section deals with the general needs of caring for the sick, while the second section covers specific illnesses in depth. Includes bibliographies and lists of support organizations.

DECONGESTANTS
TREATMENT

ANATOMY OR SYSTEM AFFECTED: Circulatory system, ears, nose, respiratory system, throat

SPECIALTIES AND RELATED FIELDS: Family medicine, otorhinolaryngology

DEFINITION: Oral and topical medications that are used to relieve nasal and sinus congestion and to promote the opening of collapsed Eustachian tubes.

KEY TERMS:

adjunctive: referring to the treatment of symptoms associated with a condition, not the condition itself

contraindication: a condition that makes a particular treatment not advisable; contraindications may be absolute (should never be used) or relative (should be used only with caution when the benefits outweigh the potential problems)

evidence-based medicine: a method of basing clinical medical practice decisions on systematic reviews of published medical studies

systemic: affecting the entire body; systemic treatments may be administered orally, directly into a vein, into the muscle, or through mucous membranes

topical: referring to treatments applied directly to the skin or mucous membranes that affect primarily the area in which they are applied

upper respiratory tract: the nose, sinuses, throat, ears, Eustachian tubes, and trachea

INDICATIONS AND PROCEDURES

Decongestants are used to shrink inflamed mucous membranes, promote drainage, or open collapsed Eustachian tubes. They are often used for the temporary relief of congestion caused by an upper respiratory tract infection (a cold), a sinus infection, or hay fever and other nasal allergies by promoting both nasal and sinus drainage. They are also often used as adjunctive therapy in the treatment of middle-ear infection (otitis media) in order to decrease congestion around the openings of the Eustachian tubes, and they may relieve the ear pressure, blockage, and pain experienced by some people during air travel. Careful scientific evaluation of the effectiveness of decongestants, however, has shown somewhat contradictory results.

The action of decongestants is accomplished primarily through stimulation of specific receptors in the smooth muscle of the upper respiratory tract, which in turn leads to constriction of the blood vessels and shrinkage of the mucous membranes. This improves air flow through the upper respiratory tract and relieves the sensation of stuffiness.

USES AND COMPLICATIONS

Decongestants may be applied topically, as sprays or drops, or taken by mouth. Commonly used decongestants include ephedrine, epinephrine, naphazoline, oxymetazoline, phenylephrine, pseudoephedrine, tetrahydrozoline, and xylometazoline. Some of these drugs are available over the counter and some by prescription only.

Oral preparations must be used with caution in elderly persons, children, and people with high blood pressure or other cardiac problems. If used as directed, decongestants do not usually cause excessive increases in blood pressure, overstimulate the heart, or change the distribution of blood in the circulatory system. The topical preparations are somewhat safer, because they are less likely to cause side effects, but they must also be used with caution.

The major advantage of oral decongestants is their long duration of action. Topical decongestants work more quickly but last a shorter period of time and are more likely to cause irritation of the tissues to which they are applied. If used too often or for too long a period of time (more than three to five days), nasal preparations may lead to a condition called rhinitis medicamentosa or rebound congestion, in which the congestion may be worse than before the person started using the medication.

People who take a certain type of antidepressant medication called a monoamine oxidase inhibitor (MAOI) and those with severe high blood pressure or heart disease should not take decongestants at all. People with thyroid disease, diabetes mellitus, glaucoma, or an enlarged prostate gland should take these drugs only after consulting a health care professional. Specific decongestants are contraindicated in infants and children.

People who take excessive doses of decongestants or who take them with other drugs that stimulate the central nervous system may experience insomnia, restlessness, dizziness, tremors, or nervousness. Overdose or long-term use of high doses may lead to hallucinations, convulsions, cardiovascular collapse, or even death.

PERSPECTIVE AND PROSPECTS

Although decongestants have been widely used for decades, evidence-based medicine reveals few good studies indicating that decongestants do, in fact, treat illnesses. Systematic and careful reviews of the scientific studies available in the medical literature suggest that a single dose of a decongestant may relieve the stuffiness associated with the common cold in adults, but that no evidence exists for the usefulness of repeated doses. In people with a cough, a combination decongestant-antihistamine provides some relief in adults but not in children. In children with otitis media, there is a small statistical benefit from use of a combination decongestant-antihistamine, but it is not clear that the children benefit clinically. An evidence-based medicine review suggests that they not be used in children, especially given the increased risk of side effects from these medications in this age group.

—*Rebecca Lovell Scott, Ph.D., PA-C*

See also Allergies; Antihistamines; Anti-inflammatory drugs; Common cold; Ear infections and disorders; Hay fever; Host-defense mechanisms; Immune system; Immunology; Multiple chemical sensitivity syndrome; Nasopharyngeal disorders; Otorhinolaryngology; Over-the-counter medications; Pharmacology; Pharmacy; Sinusitis; Smell.

FOR FURTHER INFORMATION:

Flynn, C. A., G. Griffin, and F. Tudiver. "Decongestants and Antihistamines for Acute Otitis Media in Children." In *The Cochrane Library, Issue 4.* Chichester, England: John Wiley & Sons, 2003.

Komaroff, Anthony, ed. *Harvard Medical School Family Health Guide.* New York: Free Press, 2005.

Lacy, Charles F., et al. *The Drug Information Handbook.* 14th ed. Hudson, Ohio: Lexi-Comp, 2006.

Schiff, Donald, and Steven Shelov, eds. *American Academy of Pediatrics Guide to Your Child's Symptoms: The Official, Complete Home Reference, Birth Through Adolescence.* New York: Villard, 1997.

Schroeder, K., and T. Fahey. "Over-the-Counter Medications for Acute Cough in Children and Adults in Ambulatory Settings." In *The Cochrane Library, Issue 4.* Chichester, England: John Wiley & Sons, 2003.

Taverner, D., L. Bickford, and M. Draper. "Nasal Decongestants for the Common Cold." In *The Cochrane Library, Issue 4.* Chichester, England: John Wiley & Sons, 2003.

DEHYDRATION
DISEASE/DISORDER

ANATOMY OR SYSTEM AFFECTED: Brain, circulatory system, cells

SPECIALTIES AND RELATED FIELDS: Exercise physiology, family medicine, sports medicine, vascular medicine

DEFINITION: Excessive loss of body water, which is often accompanied by disturbances in electrolyte balance.

KEY TERMS:

electrolytes: elements dissolved within body fluids that help regulate metabolism

plasma: the fluid portion of the blood

relative humidity: the percent moisture saturation of ambient air

CAUSES AND SYMPTOMS

The average adult's total body weight is approximately 60 percent water. Daily water requirements vary based on age, gender, level of physical activity, and climate. Dehydration, loss of 3 percent or more of body weight from the rapid loss of water, is often accompanied by the loss of essential electrolytes such as sodium, potassium, and chloride. Conditions that deplete body water faster than it is absorbed include fever-induced sweating, diarrhea, vomiting, acidosis, anorexia nervosa, bulimia, diabetes mellitus and insipidus, undernutrition, obesity, a sedentary lifestyle, and lack of acclimatization to heat stress. People exercising in hot, humid environments provide an excellent example of how dehydration develops and progresses. Symptoms of dehydration may include dry mouth, lips, and skin; decreased salivation; dizziness; weakness; constipation; and confusion.

Heat gain is higher and evaporative heat loss is lower during physical exertion in a hot environment in children as compared to adults, predisposing children to more rapid and severe dehydration. Both child and adult bodies attempt to reduce the buildup of metabolic heat through blood flow adjustments and sweat gland secretion. Flushed, red skin indicates that peripheral blood vessels have dilated, carrying blood and internal heat to the body surface for cooling. Once the heat is carried to the periphery by the bloodstream, dissipation occurs mainly by sweat evaporation. Large quantities of sweat may roll off the skin in a high humidity environment, but cooling only occurs when the sweat evaporates. Children exhibit a higher number of sweat glands per unit of body surface area than do adults, with each immature sweat gland producing about 40 percent as much sweat as an adult sweat gland. Children also gain heat from the environment faster than do adults because of their larger body surface area to body weight ratio; they dehydrate quicker as a result of lower overall fluid storage capacity. A large portion of the fluid released as sweat comes from the circulating blood plasma, making fluid consumption to rebuild blood plasma volume and to replenish lost water weight very important. Children acclimatize to a heat stress environment such as a sauna more slowly than do adults. They generally need at least six exposures before adjusting, whereas adults need only about three acclimation bouts.

The effects of dehydration are of particular concern in infants and young children, since their electrolyte balance can become precarious, leading to recommendations such as never allowing an infant to get a suntan.

TREATMENT AND THERAPY

Rapid restoration of fluid volume and electrolyte balance are primary treatment goals that may require intravenous infusion if sufficient fluid cannot be ingested orally.

"Prehydrating" the body by consuming liberal amounts of fluid before anticipated heat stress and "trickle hydrating" while losing body fluid are critical. Cool fluids of about 40 degrees Fahrenheit (about 5 degrees Celsius) empty from the gastrointestinal tract and supply the dehydrated cells quicker than warmer or colder temperature fluid. Studies of fluid absorption indicate that excessive sugar in electrolyte drinks slows water movement into the bloodstream. Children have been shown voluntarily to drink nearly twice as much when flavored fluids, as compared to plain water, are allowed.

Monitoring body weight before and after dehydration episodes and drinking enough water to regain lost weight is important. Nearly all body weight lost during exercise is attributable to water loss, not fat loss. Consuming 1 pint (473 milliliters) of fluid will replenish 1 pound (9.45 kilograms) of water weight loss. People should drink back all lost water weight even though

---

INFORMATION ON DEHYDRATION

CAUSES: Fever-induced sweating, diarrhea, vomiting, acidosis, diabetes mellitus and insipidus, anorexia nervosa, bulimia, malnutrition, obesity, sedentary lifestyle, lack of acclimatization to heat stress

SYMPTOMS: Flushed skin, dark yellow urine, cramps, and heat exhaustion or stroke, causing cool and clammy skin, low blood pressure, rapid but weak heart rate, faintness, dizziness, headaches

DURATION: Acute

TREATMENTS: Rapid restoration of fluid volume and electrolyte balance

they may not feel thirsty, as the human thirst mechanism is not a good indicator of actual need. Checking the urine is also recommended, as dark yellow urine indicates that more water consumption is needed and nearly colorless urine indicates that adequate rehydration has been achieved. Wearing light-colored, loose-fitting clothing in the heat is recommended, as rubberized or tight-weave clothing interferes with sweat evaporation and body cooling.

Other suggestions for countering dehydration include getting into good physical condition and acclimatizing to the heat. Conditioning increases the body's metabolic efficiency so that fewer of the calories burned accumulate as heat, enhances blood plasma volume to enable a larger sweat reserve, and reduces fat weight that insulates the body and retards heat dissipation. Eating a carbohydrate-enriched diet will retain water in muscle cells at a rate of nearly 3 grams of water per 1 gram of stored glycogen, whereas stored fat retains minimal water.

PERSPECTIVE AND PROSPECTS

Many episodes of dehydration can be prevented from developing into heat cramps, heat exhaustion, and heat stroke during sporting events by adhering to the aforementioned guidelines. Heat cramps, especially muscle spasms in the calves and stomach, may occur during intense sweating, with the accompanying loss of electrolytes. Mineral loss, however, is always of secondary importance to fluid loss because water provides the medium in which all cellular processes occur.

Heat exhaustion occurs when increased sweating and peripheral blood flow reduce venous return of blood to the heart, resulting in cool and clammy skin, lower-than-normal blood pressure, and a rapid but weak heart rate. Less blood is pumped to the brain, causing weakness, faintness, dizziness, headaches, and a grayish look to the face. Treatment includes lying down in a shaded, breezy place, drinking cool fluids, and removing excess clothing. Heat stroke occurs when the brain can no longer maintain thermal balance, as evidenced by the cessation of sweating, hot (sometimes white to gray) skin, rapid and full pulse, and a rise in body temperature over 104 degrees Fahrenheit leading to disorientation and unconsciousness. Heat stroke is rare but requires immediate medical attention to reduce body temperature. The body temperature should be lowered quickly by placing ice packs to the groin, neck, and under the arms. Cool sheets may be placed over and under the patient. The patient should not be al-

lowed to shiver, which increases the body temperature. Others should be alert for seizures and the possible need to perform cardiopulmonary resuscitation (CPR). The most effective treatment is prevention through proper hydration.

—Daniel G. Graetzer, Ph.D.;
updated by Amy Webb Bull, D.S.N., A.P.N.

See also Anorexia nervosa; Appetite loss; Bulimia; Cardiovascular system; Constipation; Diabetes mellitus; Diarrhea and dysentery; Dizziness and fainting; Emergency medicine; Emergency medicine, pediatric; Enterocolitis; Exercise physiology; Fever; Headaches; Heat exhaustion and heat stroke; Malnutrition; Motion sickness; Nausea and vomiting; Nutrition; Obesity; Pyloric stenosis; Seizures; Sweating; Well-baby examinations.

FOR FURTHER INFORMATION:

Brody, Jane E. "For Lifelong Gains, Just Add Water. Repeat." *The New York Times*, July 11, 2000, p. F8. The average American consumes slightly more than half the recommended amount of water per day. To avoid the symptoms of dehydration (headache, lethargy, dizziness, mental fuzziness, and loss of appetite), one should drink at least eight glasses of water per day.

McArdle, William, Frank I. Katch, and Victor L. Katch. *Exercise Physiology: Energy, Nutrition, and Human Performance*. 6th ed. Philadelphia: Lippincott Williams & Wilkins, 2007. A wide ranging text on exercise and the human body, covering topics such as nutrition, energy transfer, exercise training, systems of energy delivery and utilization, enhancement of energy capacity, the effect of environmental stress, and the effect of exercise on successful aging and disease prevention.

Sawka, Michael N., Samuel N. Cheuvront, and Robert Carter. "Human Water Needs." *Nutrition Reviews* 63, no. 6 (June, 2005): S30-S39. Provides information on daily water needs and the estimated amount of water intake required by an average adult male.

Sawka, Michael N., and Scott J. Montain. "Fluid and Electrolyte Supplementation for Exercise Heat Stress." *The American Journal of Clinical Nutrition* 72, no. 2S (August, 2000): S564-S572. During exercise in the heat, sweat output often exceeds water intake, resulting in a body water deficit (hypohydration) and electrolyte losses. Because daily water losses can be substantial, persons need to emphasize drinking during exercise as well as at meals.

Scanlon, Valerie, and Tina Sanders. *Essentials of Anatomy and Physiology*. 5th ed. Philadelphia: F. A. Davis, 2007. A text designed around three themes: the relationship between physiology and anatomy, the interrelations among the organ systems, and the relationship of each organ system to homeostasis.

Sturt, Patty Ann. "Environmental Conditions." In *Mosby's Emergency Nursing Reference*, edited by Julia Fulz and Sturt. 3d ed. St. Louis: Elsevier Mosby, 2005. A helpful resource.

DELUSIONS

DISEASE/DISORDER

ANATOMY OR SYSTEM AFFECTED: Psychic-emotional system

SPECIALTIES AND RELATED FIELDS: Psychiatry, psychology

DEFINITION: False beliefs regarding the self or persons or objects outside the self that persist despite the facts and are common in paranoia, schizophrenia, and psychotic depressed states.

CAUSES AND SYMPTOMS

Clinical delusion is defined as the presence of one or more nonbizarre false beliefs, persisting for a period of at least one month. To avoid confusion, delusions are not typically linked to the direct physiological effects of a substance or a general medical condition. Determination of "nonbizarre false beliefs" may be difficult to determine. Usually "nonbizarre" refers to situations that could occur in real life; "bizarre" refers to situations that could not occur in real life.

Life management with delusions varies. Some individuals may appear relatively unimpaired in their interpersonal and occupational roles. In others, life management issues may be so severe that isolation and withdrawal are common results. In general, however, life management functions are more likely to be adversely affected than cognitive or vocational activities.

TREATMENT AND THERAPY

Options for treatment and therapy vary depending on the severity of the delusions and the degrading effects on life management issues. Interventions vary depending on the theoretical orientation of the mental health professional combined with severity of the delusion. A thorough evaluation should begin the process. Clinical interviews should be combined with appropriate psychological testing and corroborative data collection. Therapy can vary from individual to group sessions,

---

INFORMATION ON DELUSIONS

CAUSES: Psychological disorders
SYMPTOMS: Isolation, withdrawal, impaired life management
DURATION: One month to chronic
TREATMENTS: Psychotherapy, counseling, drug therapy

"talk" therapies to pharmacological therapy, and inpatient or outpatient venues. Delusions tend to wax and wane in intensity and degrees of severity. Maintaining good general physical health is an important part of managing delusions. Maintenance of neurochemical systems, especially neurotransmitters, with vitamin-B complex foods, is an important consideration.

PERSPECTIVE AND PROSPECTS

Delusions, in and of themselves, may not prevent successful life management functioning for most individuals. When the delusion represents a life management issue as a result of a loss of contact with reality, in the client's best interest, intervention and treatment is appropriate. Although popular media and common myths present otherwise, individuals with delusions are no more dangerous and no more aggressive than the general population. While they may be the targets of ridicule, challenge, and harassment, individuals with delusions may also reorient successfully with appropriate intervention.

—*Daniel L. Yazak, D.E.D.*

See also Anxiety; Hallucinations; Paranoia; Psychiatric disorders; Psychiatry; Psychiatry, child and adolescent; Psychiatry, geriatric; Psychosis; Schizophrenia.

FOR FURTHER INFORMATION:

American Psychiatric Association. *Diagnostic and Statistical Manual of Mental Disorders: DSM-IV-TR*. 4th rev. ed. Washington, D.C.: Author, 2000.

Brems, Christiane. *Basic Skills in Psychotherapy and Counseling*. Belmont, Calif.: Brooks/Cole Thomson Learning, 2001.

Bruno, Frank J. *Psychological Symptoms*. New York: John Wiley & Sons, 1993.

Sadock, Benjamin James, and Virginia A. Sadock. *Kaplan and Sadock's Synopsis of Psychiatry: Behavioral Sciences/Clinical Psychiatry*. 9th ed. Philadelphia: Lippincott Williams & Wilkins, 2003.

Torrey, E. Fuller. *Surviving Schizophrenia: A Manual for Families, Consumers, and Providers.* 4th ed. New York: HarperCollins, 2001.

DEMENTIAS

DISEASE/DISORDER

ANATOMY OR SYSTEM AFFECTED: Brain, nervous system, psychic-emotional system

SPECIALTIES AND RELATED FIELDS: Geriatrics and gerontology, neurology, psychiatry

DEFINITION: A group of disorders involving pervasive, progressive, and irreversible decline in cognitive functioning resulting from a variety of causes; differs from mental retardation, in which the affected person never reaches an expected level of mental growth.

KEY TERMS:

basal ganglia: a collection of nerve cells deep inside the brain, below the cortex, that controls muscle tone and automatic actions such as walking

cortical dementia: dementia resulting from damage to the brain cortex, the outer layer of the brain that contains the bodies of the nerve cells

delirium: an acute condition characterized by confusion, a fluctuating level of consciousness, and visual, auditory, and even tactile hallucinations; often caused by acute disease, such as infection or intoxication

hydrocephalus: a condition resulting from the accumulation of fluid inside the brain in cavities known as ventricles; as fluid accumulates, it exerts pressure on the neighboring brain cells, which may be destroyed

subcortical dementia: dementia resulting from damage to the area of the brain below the cortex; this area contains nerve fibers that connect various parts of the brain with one another and with the basal ganglia

vascular dementia: dementia caused by repeated strokes, resulting in interference with the blood supply to parts of the brain

CAUSES AND SYMPTOMS

Dementia affects between four and five million people in the United States and is a major cause of disability in individuals over sixty. Its prevalence increases with age. Dementia is characterized by a permanent memory deficit affecting recent memory in particular and of sufficient severity to interfere with the patient's ability to take part in professional and social activities. Dementia is not part of the normal aging process. It also is not synonymous with benign senescent forgetfulness, which is more common and affects recent memory. Although the latter is a source of frustration, it does not significantly interfere with the individual's professional and social activities because it tends to affect only trivial matters (or what the individual considers trivial). Furthermore, patients with benign forgetfulness usually can remember what was forgotten by utilizing a number of strategies, such as writing lists or notes to themselves and leaving them in conspicuous places. Individuals with benign forgetfulness also are acutely aware of their memory deficit, while those with dementia, except in the early stages of the disease or for specific types of dementia, generally have no insight into their memory deficit and often blame others for their problems.

In addition to the memory deficit interfering with the patient's daily activities, patients with dementia often show evidence of impaired abstract thinking, impaired judgment, or other disturbances of higher cortical functions such as aphasia (the inability to use or comprehend language), apraxia (the inability to execute complex, coordinated movements), or agnosia (the inability to recognize familiar objects).

Dementia may result from damage to the cerebral cortex (the outer layer of the brain), as in Alzheimer's disease, or from damage to the subcortical structures (the structures below the cortex), such as white matter, the thalamus, or the basal ganglia. Although memory is impaired in both cortical and subcortical dementias, the associated features are different. In cortical dementias, for example, cognitive functions such as the ability to understand speech and to talk and the ability to perform mathematical calculations are severely impaired. In subcortical dementias, on the other hand, there is evidence of disturbances of arousal, motivation, and mood, in addition to a significant slowing of cognition and of information processing.

Alzheimer's disease, the most common cause of presenile dementia, is characterized by progressive disorientation, memory loss, speech disturbances, and personality disorders. Pick's disease is another cortical dementia, but unlike Alzheimer's disease, it is rare, tends to affect younger patients, and is more common in women. In the early stages of Pick's disease, changes in personality, absence of inhibition, inappropriate social and sexual conduct, and lack of foresight may be evident—features that are not common in Alzheimer's disease. Patients also may become euphoric or apathetic. Poverty of speech is often present and gradually progresses to mutism, although speech comprehension is usually spared. Pick's disease is characterized by cortical atrophy localized to the frontal and temporal lobes.

Vascular dementia is the second most common cause of dementia in patients over the age of sixty-five and is responsible for 8 percent to 20 percent of all dementia cases. It is caused by interference with the blood flow to the brain. Although the overall prevalence of vascular dementia is decreasing, there are some geographical variations, with the prevalence being higher in countries with a high incidence of cardiovascular and cerebrovascular diseases, such as Finland and Japan. About 20 percent of patients with dementia have both Alzheimer's disease and vascular dementia. Several types of vascular dementia have been identified.

Multiple infarct dementia (MID) is the most common type of vascular dementia. As its name implies, it is the result of multiple, discrete cerebral infarcts (strokes) that have destroyed enough brain tissue to interfere with the patient's higher mental functions. The onset of MID is usually sudden and is associated with neurological deficit, such as the paralysis or weakness of an arm or leg or the inability to speak. The disease characteristically progresses in steps: With each stroke experienced, the patient's condition suddenly deteriorates and then stabilizes or even improves slightly until another stroke occurs. In about 20 percent of patients with MID, however, the disease displays an insidious onset and causes gradual deterioration. Most patients also show evidence of arteriosclerosis and other factors predisposing them to the development of strokes, such as hypertension, cigarette smoking, high blood cholesterol, diabetes mellitus, narrowing of one or both carotid arteries, or cardiac disorders, especially atrial fibrillation (an irregular heartbeat). Somatic complaints, mood changes, depression, and nocturnal confusion tend to be more common in vascular dementias, although there is relative preservation of the patient's personality. In such cases, magnetic resonance imaging (MRI) or a computed tomography (CT) scan of the brain often shows evidence of multiple strokes.

Strokes are not always associated with clinical evidence of neurological deficits, since the stroke may affect a "silent" area of the brain or may be so small that its immediate impact is not noticeable. Nevertheless, when several of these small strokes have occurred, the resulting loss of brain tissue may interfere with the patient's cognitive functions. This is, in fact, the basis of the lacunar dementias. The infarcted tissue is absorbed into the rest of the brain, leaving a small cavity or lacuna. Brain-imaging techniques and especially MRI are useful in detecting these lacunae.

A number of neurological disorders are associated with dementia. The combination of dementia, urinary incontinence, and muscle rigidity causing difficulties in walking should raise the suspicion of hydrocephalus. In this condition, fluid accumulates inside the ventricles (cavities within the brain) and results in increased pressure on the brain cells. A CT scan demonstrates enlargement of the ventricles. Although some patients may respond well to surgical shunting of the cerebrospinal fluid, it is often difficult to identify those who will benefit from surgery. Postoperative complications are significant and include strokes and subdural hematomas.

Dementia has been linked to Parkinson's disease, a chronic, progressive neurological disorder that usually manifests itself in middle or late life. It has an insidious onset and a very slow progression rate. Although intellectual deterioration is not part of the classical features of Parkinson's disease, dementia is being recognized as a late manifestation of the disease, with as many as one-third of the patients eventually being afflicted. The dementing process also has an insidious onset and slow progression rate. Some of the medication used to treat Parkinson's disease also may induce confusion, particularly in older patients.

Subdural hematomas (collections of blood inside the brain) may lead to mental impairment and are usually precipitated by trauma to the head. Usually, the trauma is slight and the patient neither loses consciousness nor experiences any immediate significant effects. A few days or even weeks later, however, the patient may develop evidence of mental impairment. By that time, the patient and caregivers may have forgotten about the

---

INFORMATION ON DEMENTIAS

CAUSES: Aging, diseases (Alzheimer's, Pick's, Parkinson's), stroke, chronic infections, head trauma

SYMPTOMS: Impaired abstract thinking, impaired judgment, inability to use or comprehend language, inability to recognize familiar objects, inability to execute complex movements

DURATION: Chronic

TREATMENTS: None; alleviation of symptoms

slight trauma that the patient had experienced. A subdural hematoma should be suspected in the presence of a fairly sudden onset and progressing course. Headaches are common. A CT scan can reveal the presence of a hematoma. The surgical removal of the hematoma is usually associated with a good prognosis if the surgery is done in a timely manner, before irreversible brain damage occurs.

Brain tumors may lead to dementia, particularly if they are slow growing. Most tumors of this type can be diagnosed by CT scanning or MRI. Occasionally, cancer may induce dementia through an inflammation of the brain.

Many chronic infections affecting the brain can lead to dementia; they include conditions that, when treated, may reverse or prevent the progression of dementia, such as syphilis, tuberculosis, slow viruses, and some fungal and protozoal infections. Human immunodeficiency virus (HIV) infection is also a cause of dementia, and it may be suspected if the rate of progress is rapid and the patient has risk factors for the development of HIV infection. Although the dementia is part of the acquired immunodeficiency syndrome (AIDS) complex, it may occasionally be the first manifestation of the disease.

It is often difficult to differentiate depression from dementia. Nevertheless, sudden onset—especially if preceded by an emotional event, the presence of sleep disturbances, and a history of previous psychiatric illness—is suggestive of depression. The level of mental functioning of patients with depression is often inconsistent. They may, for example, be able to give clear accounts of topics that are of personal interest to them but be very vague about, and at times may not even attempt to answer, questions on topics that are of no interest to them. Variability in performance during testing is suggestive of depression, especially if it improves with positive reinforcement.

TREATMENT AND THERAPY

It is estimated that dementia affects about 1 percent of the population aged sixty to sixty-four years. By age eighty-five and higher, however, it affects anywhere from 30 to 50 percent of individuals. While different surveys may yield different results, depending on the criteria used to define dementia, it is clear that this is a significant problem.

For physicians, an important aspect of diagnosing patients with dementia is detecting potentially reversible causes which may be responsible for the impaired mental functions. A detailed history followed by a meticulous and thorough clinical examination and a few selected laboratory tests are usually sufficient to reach a diagnosis. Various investigators have estimated that reversible causes of dementia can be identified in 10 percent to 20 percent of patients with dementia. Recommended investigations include brain imaging (CT scanning or MRI), a complete blood count, and tests of erythrocyte sedimentation rate, blood glucose, serum electrolytes, serum calcium, liver function, thyroid function, and serum B_{12} and folate. Some investigators also recommend routine testing for syphilis. Other tests, such as those for the detection of HIV infection, cerebrospinal fluid examination, neuropsychological testing, drug and toxin screening, serum copper and ceruloplasmin analysis, carotid and cerebral angiography, and electroencephalography, are performed when appropriate.

It is of paramount importance for health care providers to adopt a positive attitude when managing patients with dementia. Although at present little can be done to treat and reverse dementia, it is important to identify the cause of the dementia. In some cases, it may be possible to prevent the disease from progressing. For example, if the dementia is the result of hypertension, adequate control of this condition may prevent further brain damage. Moreover, the prevalence of vascular dementia is decreasing in countries where efforts to reduce cardiovascular and cerebrovascular diseases have been successful. Similarly, if the dementia is the result of repeated emboli (blood clots reaching the brain) complicating atrial fibrillation, then anticoagulants or aspirin may be recommended.

Even after a diagnosis of dementia is made, it is important for the physician to detect the presence of other conditions that may worsen the patient's mental functions, such as the inadvertent intake of medications that may induce confusion and mental impairment. Medications with this potential are numerous and include not only those that act on the brain, such as sedatives and hypnotics, but also hypotensive agents (especially if given in large doses), diuretics, and antibiotics. Whenever the condition of a patient with dementia deteriorates, the physician meticulously reviews all the medications that the patient is taking, both medical prescriptions and medications that may have been purchased over the counter. Even if innocuous, some over-the-counter preparations may interact with other medications that the patient is taking and lead to a worsening of mental functions. Inquiries are also made into the patient's alcohol intake. The brain of an older person is much more sensitive to the effects of alcohol than that of a younger person, and some medications may interact with the alcohol to impair the patient's cognitive functions further.

Many other disease states also may worsen the patient's mental functions. For example, patients with diabetes mellitus are susceptible to developing a variety of metabolic abnormalities including a low or high blood glucose level, both of which may be associated with confusional states. Similarly, dehydration and acid-base or electrolyte disorders, which may result from prolonged vomiting or diarrhea, may also precipitate confusional states. Infections, particularly respiratory and urinary tract infections, often worsen the patient's cognitive deficit. Finally, patients with dementia may experience myocardial infarctions (heart attacks) that are not associated with any chest pain but that may manifest themselves with confusion.

The casual observer of the dementing process is often overwhelmed with concern for the patient, but it is the family that truly suffers. The patients themselves experience no physical pain or distress, and except in the very early stages of the disease, they are oblivious to their plight as a result of their loss of insight. Health care professionals therefore are alert to the stress imposed on the caregivers by dealing with loved ones with dementia. Adequate support from agencies available in the community is essential.

When a diagnosis of dementia is made, the physician discusses a number of ethical, financial, and legal issues with the family, and also the patient if it is believed that he or she can understand the implications of this discussion. Families are encouraged to make a list of all the patient's assets, including insurance policies, and to discuss this information with an attorney in order to protect the patient's and the family's assets. If the patient is still competent, it is recommended that he or she select a trusted person to have durable power of attorney. Unlike the regular power of attorney, the former does not become invalidated when the patient becomes mentally incompetent and continues to be in effect regardless of the degree of mental impairment of the person who executed it. Because durable power of attorney cannot be easily reversed once the person is incompetent, great care should be taken when selecting a person, and the specific powers granted should be clearly specified. It is also important for the patient to make his or her desires known concerning advance directives and the use of life support systems.

Courts may appoint a guardian or conservator to have charge and custody of the patient's property (including real estate and money) when no responsible family members or friends are willing or available to serve as guardian. Courts supervise the actions of the guardian, who is expected to report all the patient's income and expenditures to the court once a year. The court may also charge the guardian to ensure that the patient is adequately housed, fed, and clothed and receiving appropriate medical care.

PERSPECTIVE AND PROSPECTS

Dementia is a very serious and common condition, especially among the older population. Dementia permanently robs patients of their minds and prevents them from functioning adequately in their environment by impairing memory and interfering with the ability to make rational decisions. It therefore deprives patients of their dignity and independence.

Because dementia is mostly irreversible, cannot be adequately treated at present, and is associated with a fairly long survival period, it has a significant impact not only on the patient's life but also on the patient's family and caregivers and on society in general. The expense of long-term care for patients with dementia, whether at home or in institutions, is staggering. Every effort, therefore, is made to reach an accurate diagnosis and especially to detect any other condition that may worsen the patient's underlying dementia. Finally, health care professionals do not treat the patient in isolation but also concern themselves with the impact of the illness on the patient's caregivers and family.

Much progress has been made in defining dementia and determining its cause. Terms such as "senile dementia" are no longer in use, and even the use of the term "dementia" to diagnose a patient's condition is frowned upon because there are so many types of dementia. The recognition of the type of dementia affecting a particular patient is important because of its practical implications, both for the patient and for research into the prevention, management, and treatment of dementia. The prevalence of vascular dementia, for example, is decreasing in many countries where the prevention of cardiovascular diseases such as hypertension and arteriosclerosis has been successful.

Unfortunately, there is little that can be done to cure dementia and no effective means to regenerate nerve cells. Researchers, however, are feverishly trying to identify factors that control the growth and regeneration of nerve cells. Although no single medication is expected to be of benefit to all types of dementia, it is hoped that effective therapy for many dementias will be developed.

—Ronald C. Hamdy, M.D.,
Louis A. Cancellaro, M.D.,
and Larry Hudgins, M.D.;
updated by Nancy A. Piotrowski, Ph.D.

See also Aging; Aging: Extended care; Alzheimer's disease; Amnesia; Brain; Brain disorders; Delusions; Hallucinations; Memory loss; Parkinson's disease; Pick's disease; Psychiatric disorders; Psychiatry; Psychiatry, geriatric; Strokes.

FOR FURTHER INFORMATION:

Ballard, Clive, et al. *Dementia: Management of Behavioural and Psychological Symptoms*. New York: Oxford University Press, 2001. Details the nature of dementia symptoms, assesses their severity, and recommends a structured and sequential approach to management.

Coons, Dorothy H., ed. *Specialized Dementia Care Units*. Baltimore: Johns Hopkins University Press, 1991. A collection of articles reviewing the benefits and disadvantages of caring for patients with dementia in specialized care units. Several problems encountered when running such units are addressed.

Dana.org. http://www.dana.org/. A nonprofit organization of neuroscientists, which was formed to provide information about the personal and public benefits of brain research. The Web site is research oriented and gives excellent information and links on current brain studies, new diagnosis and treatment technology, and brain-related news stories.

Hamdy, Ronald C., et al., eds. *Alzheimer's Disease: A Handbook for Caregivers*. 3d ed. St. Louis: Mosby Year Book, 1998. A comprehensive discussion of the symptoms and characteristic features of Alzheimer's disease and other dementias. Abnormal brain structure and function in these patients are discussed, and the normal effects of aging are reviewed.

Howe, M. L., M. J. Stones, and C. J. Brainerd, eds. *Cognitive and Behavioral Performance Factors in Atypical Aging*. New York: Springer-Verlag, 1990. A review of the factors controlling behavior, test performance, and brain function in both young and older patients.

Kovach, Christine, ed. *Late-Stage Dementia Care: A Basic Guide*. Washington, D.C.: Taylor & Francis, 1997. Provides information on assessment and treatment management for individuals experiencing dementia. A valuable source for caregivers and family members of those affected.

Mace, Nancy L., and Peter V. Rabins. *The Thirty-Six-Hour Day: A Family Guide to Caring for Persons with Alzheimer Disease, Related Dementing Illnesses, and Memory Loss in Later Life*. 4th ed. Baltimore: Johns Hopkins University Press, 2006. Provides a wealth of information for families coping with Alzheimer's disease, including topics such as the evaluation of persons with dementia, hospice care, assisted living facilities and financing care, and the latest findings on eating and nutrition.

O'Brien, John, et al., eds. *Dementia*. 2d ed. New York: Oxford University Press, 2000. Text that covers advances in the research of degenerative disorders, current diagnostic criteria, rating scales, investigations, neurobiological mechanisms, therapeutic options and services, and all aspects of management, including psychosocial and psychological approaches, among other topics.

U.S. Congress. Office of Technology Assessment. *Confused Minds, Burdened Families: Finding Help for People with Alzheimer's and Other Dementias*. Washington, D.C.: Government Printing Office, 1990. A report from the Office of Technology Assessment analyzing the problems of locating and arranging services for people with dementia in the United States.

DENTAL DISEASES

DISEASE/DISORDER

ANATOMY OR SYSTEM AFFECTED: Gums, mouth, teeth

SPECIALTIES AND RELATED FIELDS: Dentistry

DEFINITION: Diseases that affect the teeth, such as dental caries, and the gums, such as gingivitis, pyorrhea, or cancer.

KEY TERMS:

dental caries: tooth decay

dentin: a hard, bonelike tissue lying beneath the tooth enamel

enamel: the hard surface covering of teeth

gingivae: the soft tissue surrounding the teeth; the gums

gingivitis: an inflammation of the gums

periodontal diseases: diseases characterized by inflammation of the gingivae

pyorrhea: the second stage of gingivitis

tooth pulp: the tissue at the center of teeth, surrounded by dentin

Vincent's infection: a bacterial infection of the gingivae, also known as trench mouth

Causes and Symptoms

Dental diseases fall into four major categories: dental caries, or tooth decay; periodontal disease, including gingivitis and pyorrhea; Vincent's infection, or trench mouth; and oral cancer. The first of these diseases was the largest contributor to tooth loss among people under thirty-five in the United States before the widespread fluoridation of drinking water was begun; it remains a major cause of tooth loss in much of the world. Periodontal disease in its two stages, gingivitis and pyorrhea, is the most widespread dental problem for people over thirty-five. Most people who suffer the loss of all of their teeth are victims of this condition. Vincent's infection, which shares many characteristics with gingivitis, is a bacterial infection. The infection flares up, is treated, and disappears, whereas gingivitis is more often a continuing condition that requires both persistent home treatment and specialized treatment. The most serious but least frequently occurring dental disease is oral cancer. It is the only dental disease commonly considered life-threatening, and there is a risk that it may spread to other parts of the body.

Dental caries occur because the food that one eats becomes trapped in the irregularities of the teeth, creating lactic acids that penetrate the enamel through holes (often microscopic) in it. Once lodged between the teeth or below the gum line, carbohydrates and starches combine with saliva to form acids that, over time, can penetrate a tooth's enamel, enter the dentin directly below it, and progressively destroy the dentin while spreading toward the tooth's center, the pulp.

This process often is not confined to a single tooth. As decay spreads, adjoining teeth may be affected. Some people have much harder tooth enamel than others. Therefore, some individuals may experience little or no decay, whereas others who follow similar diets and practice similar methods of dental hygiene may develop substantial decay.

Toothache occurs when decay eats through the dentin and enters the nerve-filled dental pulp, causing inflammation, infection, and pain. A dull, continuous ache, either mild or severe and often pulsating, may indicate that the infection has entered the jawbone beneath the tooth. An aching or sensitivity in the back teeth during chewing is sometimes a side effect of sinusitis.

INFORMATION ON DENTAL DISEASES

Causes: Tooth decay, periodontal disease (gingivitis, pyorrhea), Vincent's infection (trench mouth), oral cancer

Symptoms: Varies; may include dull, continuous ache; gum soreness, swelling, and bleeding; receding gums forming pockets for infections; bone destruction and tooth loss; fever; persistent mouth sores

Duration: Short-term to chronic

Treatments: Dependent on condition; may include medications (dextrose, antibiotics), tooth implantation, gum surgery, laser treatment, radiation, chemotherapy, surgery

---

One of dentistry's nagging problems is periodontal disease, which results from a buildup of calculus, or tartar, formed by hardened plaque. Plaque is formed when food, particularly carbohydrates and starches, interacts with the saliva that coats the teeth, creating a yellowish film. If this film is not removed, it inevitably lodges between the gums and the teeth, where, within twenty-four hours, it hardens into calculus. Dental hygienists can remove most of this calculus mechanically. If it is allowed to build up over extended periods, however, the calculus will irritate the gums, causing the soreness, swelling, and bleeding that signal gum infection. Eventually, this infection becomes entrenched and difficult to treat.

Periodontists can control but not cure most periodontal disease. In its early manifestations, periodontal disease results in gingivitis, marked by inflammation and bleeding. Untreated, it progresses to pyorrhea, which is characterized by gums that recede from the teeth and form pockets in which infections flourish. As pyorrhea advances, the bone that underlies the teeth and holds them in place is compromised and ultimately destroyed, causing looseness and eventual tooth loss.

Vincent's infection (trench mouth) is communicable through kissing or sharing eating utensils. Although it is sometimes mistaken for gingivitis, Vincent's infection has one distinguishing characteristic that gingivitis does not have: It is accompanied by a fever stemming from sustained bacterial infection, which also causes extremely foul breath. Vincent's infection is curable through proper treatment. It is unlikely to recur unless one is again exposed to the infection.

Oral cancer is the most serious of oral diseases. It often spreads quickly, destroying the tissues of the mouth during its ravaging advance. It not only threatens its original site but also can spread to other areas of the body and to vital organs. Fortunately, oral cancer is uncommon. Nevertheless, dentists look vigilantly for signs of it when they perform mouth examinations because early detection is vital to successful treatment, containment, and cure. People who have persistent mouth sores that do not heal may be experiencing the early manifestations of oral cancer and should see their dentists or physicians immediately.

Two other dental conditions afflict many people: malocclusion and toothache. Malocclusion occurs when, for a variety of reasons, the teeth are out of alignment. People with malocclusion are prime candidates for dental caries and periodontal disease, largely because their teeth are difficult to reach and hard to clean. Malocclusion may also cause one or more teeth to strike the teeth above or below them, causing injury to teeth and possibly fracturing them.

TREATMENT AND THERAPY

Modern dentistry has succeeded in controlling most dental diseases. In the United States, dental caries have been almost eliminated in the young, for example, by the addition of fluoride to most water systems. Used over time, fluoride strengthens the teeth by increasing the hardness of the enamel, making it resistant to the acids that form in the mouth and cause decay.

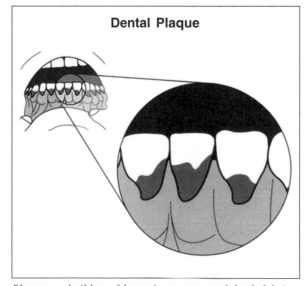

Dental Plaque

Plaque—a buildup of bacteria, mucus, and food debris— leads to dental caries (tooth decay) if not regularly removed by brushing, flossing, and professional tooth cleaning.

Since the 1950's, many American children have been reared on fluoridated water. Those whose water supply is not fluoridated have usually had their teeth treated with fluoride by their dentists. Many have brushed their teeth regularly with fluoridated toothpaste, which offers considerable protection from dental caries. From the 1950's to the 1990's, fluoride reduced dental decay in Americans under the age of twenty-one by more than 70 percent.

Current research into ways of preventing dental decay centers on several projects of the National Institute of Dental Research. Researchers for this organization discovered in the mid-1960's that a substance found in the mouth's streptococcal bacteria creates dextran. Dextran enables bacteria to cling to the surface of the teeth and invade them with the lactic acid that they generate. Researchers ultimately discovered dextrase, an enzyme effective in dissolving dextran. Strides are being made to use dextrase in toothpaste or mouthwash in order to reduce or eliminate the effects of dextran.

Some people's teeth seem to be impervious to tooth decay. It has been determined that such people have a common substance in their blood that protects their teeth from dental caries. Attempts are being made to identify and isolate this substance and to make it generally available to the public and to dentists in an applicable form. Some dentists coat the teeth with a durable plastic substance to make them resistant to penetration by the acids that cause dental decay, creating a hard protective coating above the enamel and making it difficult for food to lodge between the teeth or in irregularities in the teeth.

Because malocclusion can lead to tooth decay, dentists have become increasingly aware of the need to replace lost teeth so that the alignment of the remaining teeth will not be disturbed. Tooth implantation, a process by which a tooth, either artificial or natural, is anchored directly and permanently in the gum, solves many dental problems that in the past were addressed by attaching artificial teeth to existing ones beside them. In situations where malocclusion is caused by malformations, the use of orthodontic braces results in a more regular alignment.

Nutrition has come to the forefront of recent research in dental health. A lack of calciferol, a form of vitamin D_2, may result in dental abnormalities, including malocclusion. Among substantial numbers of hospital patients who suffer from nutritional problems, the earliest symptoms occur in the soft tissue of the mouth.

Brushing the teeth after meals and before bed controls plaque, as does regular flossing. Such daily attention must be supplemented by twice-yearly cleaning, performed by a dentist or dental hygienist, and by annual or biennial whole-mouth X rays to reveal incipient decay. Various mouthwashes also contain substances that control decay.

People who cannot brush after every meal should use a mouthwash or rinse the mouth out with water after eating, then brush as soon as they can. Special attention must be given to the back surfaces of the lower front teeth because the salivary glands are located there. This area is a breeding ground for the bacteria that cause the formation of lactic acid. Routine home care of this kind, particularly daily flossing, will help prevent both tooth decay and periodontal disease, and can also reverse some of the inroads that periodontal disease has made. When gingivitis advances to pyorrhea, however, dental surgery may be indicated.

The major villain in both gingivitis and pyorrhea is tartar, or calculus, which is produced when plaque hardens. When tartar accumulates beneath the gums, it causes an irritation that can lead to infection. Sometimes, this infection moves to other parts of the body, causing joint problems and other difficulties.

People can control plaque by practicing daily dental hygiene at home. They must also have accumulated tartar regularly scraped away or removed by ultrasound in the dentist's office. Malocclusions and defects in the production of saliva can be corrected by dentists and can greatly reduce the progress of periodontal disease.

When gum surgery is advised for the removal of the deep gum pockets that occur with pyorrhea, further surgery can usually be avoided by regular home care. Meanwhile, researchers are trying to develop a vaccine to immunize its recipients against the bacteria that cause tooth decay. Other decay-inhibiting agents are being studied closely with the expectation that they may in time be added to common foods and beverages.

Vincent's infection is successfully treated with antibiotics, accompanied by a prescribed course of dental hygiene that is begun in the dentist's office and continues at home on a daily basis. Some patients have found a peroxide mouthwash helpful in treating this disease.

Oral cancer, when it is discovered by a dentist, is usually referred immediately to the patient's family physician, who then refers the case to an oncologist. Laser treatment and radiation are used in controlling this sort of cancer, as are chemotherapy and surgery. The most important element in cancer treatment is time. It is essential, therefore, that specialized treat-

ment be initiated as soon as oral cancer is discovered or suspected. In cases of oral cancer, a delay of even days can affect outcomes negatively.

The most immediate treatments for toothache range from the application of cold compresses to the taking of aspirin or some other analgesic every few hours. If the decayed part of the tooth is visible and reachable, sometimes applying a mixture of oil of cloves and benzocaine to the decayed area with a small swab soothes the pain. These treatments, however, offer only temporary relief.

Dentists resist treating toothache by removing the tooth, although removal offers an immediate solution to the problem. In some cases, dentists can drill out the decay and fill the tooth with silver amalgam, gold, or plastic. Quite often, by the time a tooth begins to ache, the pulp and dentin have been ravaged by decay. The best solution is endodontistry, or root canal, which will preserve the tooth but may necessitate the attachment of a crown.

PERSPECTIVE AND PROSPECTS

Great strides have been made in the United States in preventing and treating dental disease, as researchers have reached deeper understandings of the root causes of such disease. Dentistry has become increasingly less painful through the use of anesthetics and high-speed, water-cooled drills. The public at large has grown aware of the close relationship between dental health and general health. People are unwilling to accept tooth loss as a natural consequence of aging. They have also begun to realize that orthodontistry is more than a cosmetic procedure. Rather, it is a necessary procedure for correcting misalignments of the teeth that can result in difficulty if uncorrected.

National attention has been given to preventing tooth decay through the fluoridation of water supplies and, although some groups still fight fluoridation, it is for most Americans an accepted fact of modern life. Fluoridation, more than any other factor, has changed the emphasis in dentistry from preventing and treating dental caries to more sophisticated pursuits such as orthodontistry, endodontistry, and periodontistry. The establishment of the National Institute for Dental Research by Congress in 1948 has, more than any other single factor, stimulated dental research in the United States.

Advances in preventing and treating dental disease are constantly being made. Through genetic engineering, it is almost inevitable that substances will soon be available to increase an individual's resistance to tooth decay. Nevertheless, controlling the buildup of calculus, the major factor in periodontal disease, will probably remain the responsibility of individuals through daily home care and twice-yearly visits to their dentists.

—*R. Baird Shuman, Ph.D.*

See also Canker sores; Cavities; Crowns and bridges; Dentistry; Dentistry, pediatric; Dentures; Endodontic disease; Fluoride treatments; Fracture repair; Gingivitis; Gum disease; Jaw wiring; Orthodontics; Periodontal surgery; Periodontitis; Root canal treatment; Teeth; Teething; Tooth extraction; Toothache; Wisdom teeth.

FOR FURTHER INFORMATION:

Anderson, Pauline C., and Alice E. Pendleton. *The Dental Assistant*. 7th ed. Albany, N.Y.: Thomson Delmar Learning, 2000. Designed as a textbook for dental hygienists, this popular volume is particularly clear in its discussion of periodontal disease and dental caries. Although it is not directed specifically to laypersons, the book is easily accessible to nonspecialized readers.

Diamond, Richard. *Dental First Aid for Families*. Ravensdale, Wash.: Idyll Arbor, 2000. Retired dentist Diamond discusses what to do when a dental problem arises and an immediate visit to the dentist is impossible. His practical, easy-to-understand advice is built on just enough basic science to put dental problems in context.

Fairpo, Jenifer E. H., and C. Gavin Fairpo. *Heinemann Dental Dictionary*. 4th ed. Boston: Butterworth-Heinemann, 1998. This is the fourth edition of a dictionary of dental and medical terms that includes several quick-reference charts on anatomy, abbreviations, and journals. The purpose is to provide a reference for dental students and other professional and nonprofessional people associated with the science and practice of dentistry.

Foster, Malcolm S. *Protecting Our Children's Teeth: A Guide to Quality Dental Care from Infancy Through Age Twelve*. Cambridge, Mass.: Perseus, 1992. This book, meant for parents, is clear and easy to understand. The illustrations are useful. A good starting point.

Gluck, George M., and William M. Morganstein. *Jong's Community Dental Health*. 5th ed. St. Louis: Mosby, 2003. Explores the role of dentistry in public health, examining such topics as dental care delivery, demographic shifts and dental health, distribution of dental disease and prevention, and research in dental public health.

Langlais, Robert P., and Craig S. Miller. *Color Atlas of Common Oral Diseases*. 3d ed. Philadelphia: Lippincott Williams & Wilkins, 2003. Provides six hundred color photographs of the most commonly seen oral problems accompanied by descriptive text for each condition.

Newman, Michael G., Henry H. Takei, and Perry R. Klokkevold, eds. *Carranza's Clinical Periodontology*. 10th ed. St. Louis: Saunders Elsevier, 2006. Explores the clinical aspects of modern periodontology and its relationships with anatomy, physiology, etiology, and pathology.

Ring, Malvin E. *Dentistry: An Illustrated History*. New York: Abrams, 1985. Ring's coverage of dentistry is broad and accurate. The illustrations are particularly useful in helping readers understand dental diseases. An excellent starting point for those unfamiliar with the topic.

Woodall, Irene R., ed. *Comprehensive Dental Hygiene Care*. 4th ed. St. Louis: C. V. Mosby, 1993. This illustrated text addresses topics in dental hygiene and prophylaxis.

DENTISTRY

SPECIALTY

ANATOMY OR SYSTEM AFFECTED: Gums, mouth, teeth

SPECIALTIES AND RELATED FIELDS: Anesthesiology, orthodontics

DEFINITION: The field of health involving the diagnosis and treatment of diseases of the teeth and related tissues in the oral cavity.

KEY TERMS:

dental caries: the scientific term for tooth decay

dentist: a doctor with specialized training to diagnose and treat diseases of the teeth and oral tissues

endodontics: the dental specialty that treats diseases of infected pulp tissue

oral surgery: the dental specialty that surgically removes diseased teeth and oral tissues and treats fractures of the jawbone

orthodontics: the dental specialty that treats malocclusions or improperly aligned teeth by straightening the teeth in the jaws

pedodontics: the dental specialty that treats children

periodontics: the dental specialty that treats the diseases of the supporting tissues of the teeth *prosthodontics:* the dental specialty that restores missing teeth with fixed or removable dentures

SCIENCE AND PROFESSION

The practice of dentistry is a highly specialized area of medicine that treats the diseases of the teeth and their surrounding tissues in the oral cavity. Dental education normally takes four years to complete, with predental training preceding it. Prior to entering a dental school, students are usually required to have a bachelor's degree from a college or university. This degree should have major emphasis in biology or chemistry. Predental courses are concentrated in both inorganic and organic chemistry. The biology courses can cover such subjects as comparative anatomy, histology, physiology, and microbiology. Other courses that can help students to prepare for both dental school and the future practice of dentistry are English, speech skills, economics, physics, computer technology, and subjects, such as sculpture, that teach spatial relationships. Upon entering dental school, students are faced with two distinct parts of their education: didactics and techniques.

The didactic courses offered in dental schools are required to achieve knowledge of the human body, most particularly the head and neck. Some of the courses required are human anatomy (including dissection of a human cadaver), physiology, biochemistry, microbiology, general and oral histology and pathology, dental anatomy, pharmacology, anesthesiology, and radiology. One course specific to dental school is occlusion, which emphasizes the structure of the temporomandibular joint and its accompanying neurology and musculature.

In addition, students must know the properties of the materials used in the practice of dentistry. The physical properties of metals, acrylic plastics, gypsum plasters, impression materials, porcelains, glass ionomers, dental composites, sealant resins, and other substances must be thoroughly understood to determine the proper restorations for diseased tissues in the mouth. Knowledge of resistance to wear by chewing forces, thermal conductivity, and corrosion and staining by mouth fluids and foods is important. Information concerning the materials used in dental treatment in terms of resistance to recurrent decay, possible toxicity, or irritation to the hard and soft tissues of the oral cavity is also necessary.

The technical phase of dental education addresses the practical use of this didactic knowledge in treating diseases of the mouth. Students are trained to operate on diseased teeth and to prepare the teeth to receive restorations that will function as biomechanical prostheses in, or adjacent to, living tissue. An understanding of anatomy, physiology, and pathology is necessary for successful restoration of the teeth. During this course of study, students are required to construct fillings, cast-gold crowns and inlays, fixed and removable dentures, porcelain crowns and inlays, and other restorations on mannequins, plastic models, or extracted teeth. These activities are undertaken prior to working on patients. Through practice and repetition of these techniques, dental students soon become aware of the importance of mastering this phase of the education prior to their application in a clinical environment.

The clinical phase of dental education integrates the didactic and technical instruction that has taken place throughout the first years of professional study. Students learn to treat patients under the close supervision of their instructors. The treatment of patients in all the specialties of dentistry is required of students before they receive the degree for general dentistry. Some students may opt for extra training in one of several specialties. In order to become a specialist, postgraduate education is required. This education commonly encompasses two years of study but is sometimes longer.

Upon graduation, students receive their professional degrees. Before they can legally practice dentistry in the United States, however, they must successfully pass an examination offered by the board of dental examiners in their chosen state. National exams in didactics are offered during dental school, and most states accept them as part of their state examination. The technical portion of the exam may only be taken after the student has received a doctorate. The emphasis regarding techniques may vary from state to state. Many states allow reciprocity, which means that a student who has passed the examination in one state may become licensed to practice in another. In states that do not accept reciprocity, the student must pass the practical examination of that state prior to obtaining a license. There have been attempts to make reciprocity universal among all states, but several states insist on governing the quality of their dental health care.

Dental education can be quite expensive. After a dentist receives a license to practice, the cost of equipping an office must also be borne. A dental office must have dental chairs, office and reception room furniture, a dental laboratory, a sterilizing room, X-ray units, instruments, and various supplies. Because of these expenses, new dentists often initially practice as an associate or partner of an established dentist, as an employee of a dental clinic, in the military or Public Health Service, or in state institutions. Some dentists enjoy the academic atmosphere of dental schools and return to become part-time or full-time educators.

DIAGNOSTIC AND TREATMENT TECHNIQUES

The practice of dentistry is quite different in modern times compared to the past. While some techniques and materials are still in use, there have been improvements in materials and instruments because of expanded knowledge in many scientific fields. This knowledge has increased to such an extent that dentistry has divided into several specialties. While the general dentist uses all disciplines of dentistry to treat patients, complex problems often require referral and the expertise of a specialist.

The general dentist is involved primarily in the treatment of caries or tooth decay and the replacement of missing teeth. Bacterial acids that dissolve the enamel and dentin of teeth cause caries. A diseased or damaged tooth must be prepared mechanically by the removal of the decayed material using a dental drill and tough, sharp bits called burs. The amount of damage and the position of the tooth in the mouth determine the type of restoration. In the posterior or back teeth, initial cavities may be restored with silver amalgam or bonded composite resins. In addition to removing the decayed tooth structure, the dentist must take into consideration the closeness of the dental pulp, the chewing forces of the opposing teeth, and the aesthetics of the finished restoration. In the anterior or front teeth, aesthetic restorative materials are used to fill small cavities. In this case also, the size and position of the defect determine the choice of restorative material.

When the amount of tooth destruction caused by decay becomes too large for conservative filling materials, the remaining tooth structure must be reinforced by the use of cast metal or porcelain restorations. The tooth is prepared for the specific restoration, and accurate impressions are taken of the prepared teeth. The crown or inlay is fabricated on hard plaster models reproduced from the impressions and then cemented into place on the tooth. This process is also used for fixed partial dentures, or bridges, which are used to replace one or more missing teeth. Two or more teeth are prepared on either end of the space of missing teeth to support the span. The bridge is constructed with metal and porcelain as a single unit. It is then cemented on the prepared abutment teeth.

The health of the supporting tissues of the teeth, the periodontium, is necessary for the long-term retention of any mechanical restoration. When teeth become loose in the jaws because of periodontal disease, or pyorrhea, the restoration of these teeth often depends on the treatment by a periodontist, the specialist in this field. Periodontists treat the diseased tissues by scraping off harmful deposits on the roots of the teeth and by removing the diseased soft tissue and bone through curettage, surgery, or both techniques. At present, there is no means to regenerate or regrow bone lost by periodontal disease. Some newer techniques of grafting the patient's bone with sterile freeze-dried bone, implanting stainless steel pins, or using other artificial materials show great promise.

If the tooth decay reaches the dental pulp and infects it, there are two choices of treatment: removal of the tooth or endodontic therapy, commonly known as root canal treatment. If the tooth is well supported by a healthy periodontium, it is better to save the tooth by endodontics. The basic procedure of a root canal is to enter the tooth through the chewing surface on teeth toward the rear of the mouth or the inside surface or lingual aspect of teeth in the front of the mouth. Files, reamers, and broaches to the tip of the root remove diseased or decaying (necrotic) material of the dental pulp. The now-empty canal is filled by cementing a point that fits into it. Although the tooth is now nonvital, meaning that it has lost its blood supply and nerve, it can remain in the mouth for many years and provide good service.

The maintenance of the health of the primary dentition, or baby teeth, is very important. These deciduous teeth, although lost during childhood and adolescence, are important not only to the dental health of the child but to the permanent teeth as well. The deciduous teeth act as guides and spacers for the correct placement of adult teeth when they erupt. A pediodontist, who specializes in the practice of dentistry for children, must have a good knowledge of the specific mechanics of children's mouths in treating primary teeth. This specialist must also have a thorough foundation in the treatment of congenital diseases. The pediodontist prepares the way for dental treatment by an adult dentist and often assists an orthodontist by doing some preliminary straightening of teeth.

An orthodontist treats malocclusions, or ill-fitting teeth (so-called bad bites) with mechanical appliances that reposition the teeth into an occlusion that is closer to ideal. These appliances, known commonly as braces, move the teeth through the bone of the jaws until the

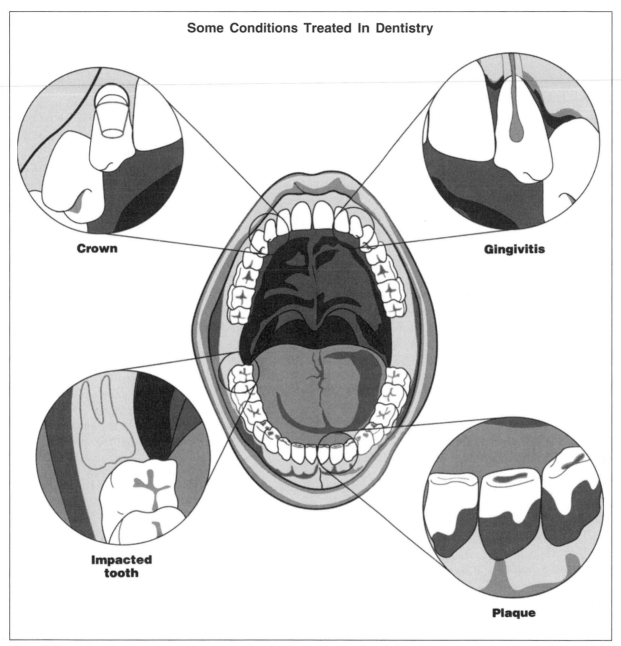

Some Conditions Treated In Dentistry

Crown

Gingivitis

Impacted tooth

Plaque

Care of the teeth and supporting structures may involve the treatment of such dental diseases as gingivitis (infection of the gums), the removal of dental plaque (hard deposits on the teeth), the surgical excision of impacted molars (teeth trapped beneath the gums), and the fitting of a crown (an artificial covering for a tooth) following root canal treatment.

opposing teeth occlude in a balanced bite. The side benefit of this treatment is that the teeth become properly positioned for an attractive smile.

Sometimes the teeth or their supporting tissues become so diseased that there is no alternative but to remove them. A general dentist often does routine extractions of these diseased teeth. If the patient has com-

plications beyond the training of a general dentist or is medically compromised by systemic illness, an oral surgeon, with specialized training, is typically consulted. This specialist not only removes teeth under difficult conditions but also is trained to remove tumors of the oral cavity, treat fractures of the jaws, and perform the surgical placement of dental implants.

Although the total loss of teeth is becoming rarer, there are still many patients who are without teeth. Often, they have been wearing complete, removable dentures that, over a period of time, have caused the loss or resorption of underlying bone. Prosthodontists are specialists trained to construct fixed and removable dentures for difficult cases. The increased success of titanium implants in the jaws and the appliances connected to them have aided prosthodontists in treating the complex cases. They also construct appliances to replace tissues and structures lost from cancer surgery of the oral cavity and congenital deformities such as cleft palate.

Perspective and Prospects

In the past, dentistry only treated pain caused by a diseased tooth; the usual mode of treatment was extraction. Today, the prevention of disease, the retention of teeth, and the restoration of the dentition are the treatment goals of dentists.

The development of composite resins has successfully addressed many aesthetic problems associated with restorations. Although metal fillings of silver amalgam (actually a mixture of silver, lead, and a small amount of mercury) and cast-gold restorations are often the treatments of choice, the display of metal is offensive to some patients. Plastic composite materials that are chemically bonded to the enamel and dentin of teeth are more aesthetically pleasing than metals. They have also shown great promise for longevity. There is still some concern about the resistance of these materials to chewing forces and leakage of the bonding to the tooth, but the techniques and materials are improving.

Dental porcelains improved greatly in the last half of the twentieth century. Although porcelain fused to metal crowns is often the material of choice, in certain cases crowns, inlays, and fixed bridges of a newer type of porcelain are being used. Thin veneers of porcelain are also used to restore front teeth that are congenitally or chemically stained. The result is cosmetically more appealing. Through a similar bonding process of composites, these veneers on the front surfaces of the teeth offer maximum aesthetics with minimum destruction of tooth structure.

While implantation of metals into the jawbones to support dentures and other prosthetic appliances is not new, the recent use of titanium implants and precision techniques promises long-term retention. Special drills are used to prepare the implant site, and titanium cylinders are either threaded into the bone or pushed into the jaw. The implant is covered by the gum tissue and allowed to heal for six to eight months, so that the process of osseointegration (joining of bone and metal) can occur. The bone will actually fuse to the pure metal, anchoring the implant for an eventual prosthetic appliance.

Laser technology is an exciting field that may have some applications in dentistry. Lasers have been used in gum surgery. Some theorists believe that if the enamel surface of the teeth were to be fused, it would be highly resistant to decay. The heat generated by lasers is a concern, but steps are being taken to control this problem. One of the most promising uses of lasers is in the specialty of endodontics. A thin laser fiber-optic probe advanced down the root canal, preparing and sterilizing the canal prior to filling, vaporizes diseased or degenerating pulp.

Computer science is also being integrated into the treatment phase of dentistry. For example, after scanning a patient's mouth, projected results of treatment can be displayed on a computer screen. In addition, restorations can be developed using the concept of computer-aided design/computer-aided manufacturing (CAD/CAM). A computer scans a prepared tooth for a crown or inlay. The restoration is then designed for a three-dimensional model on the screen. After the model restoration has been chosen, the computer transfers the data to a computer-activated milling machine in the dental laboratory, and a restoration is reproduced in a ceramic or composite resin material in the designed image. The restoration is then cemented into the prepared tooth.

Such improvements in techniques and materials have advanced dentistry into a new era in providing treatment for patients. The basic fundamentals of treatment of the teeth and their surrounding tissues must be maintained, however, in view of the peculiar anatomy and physiology of the teeth.

The above discussion reflects the state of dentistry in North America and Western Europe. In other parts of the world, resources are not available for such advanced techniques. In these countries, teeth are still more likely to be extracted than restored. Prosthetic devices are less common, and many chemical treatments are simply not available. The underlying reason is lack of money.

—William D. Stark, D.D.S.; updated by
L. Fleming Fallon, Jr., M.D., Ph.D., M.P.H.
See also Anesthesia; Anesthesiology; Canker sores; Cavities; Crowns and bridges; Dental diseases; Den-

tistry, pediatric; Dentures; Endodontic disease; Fluoride treatments; Fracture repair; Gastrointestinal system; Gingivitis; Gum disease; Halitosis; Head and neck disorders; Jaw wiring; Orthodontics; Periodontal surgery; Periodontitis; Root canal treatment; Teeth; Teething; Temporomandibular joint (TMJ) syndrome; Tooth extraction; Toothache; Wisdom teeth.

FOR FURTHER INFORMATION:

Foster, Malcolm S. *Protecting Our Children's Teeth: A Guide to Quality Dental Care from Infancy Through Age Twelve*. Cambridge, Mass.: Perseus, 1992. This book is written for parents and other interested readers. It gives insights and suggestions for promoting general dental health.

Gluck, George M., and William M. Morganstein. *Jong's Community Dental Health*. 5th ed. St. Louis: Mosby, 2003. Explores the role of dentistry in public health, examining such topics as dental care delivery, demographic shifts and dental health, distribution of dental disease and prevention, and research in dental public health.

Kendall, Bonnie L. *Opportunities in Dental Care Careers*. Revised by Blythe Camenson. Lincolnwood, Ill.: VGM Career Horizons, 2000. This text provides guidance for students interested in the field of dentistry. It provides information about careers in all allied dentistry fields. Admission requirements for different careers and the names of professional schools that can supply the training are listed.

Moss, Stephen J. *Growing Up Cavity Free: A Parent's Guide to Prevention*. New York: Edition Q, 1994. This rather brief book is written in easy-to-understand language. There are standard suggestions for preventing dental problems.

Parker, James N., and Philip M. Parker, eds. *The Official Patient's Sourcebook on Gingivitis*. San Diego, Calif.: Icon Health, 2002. Draws from public, academic, government, and peer-reviewed research to provide a wide-ranging handbook for patients with gingivitis.

_____. *The Official Patient's Sourcebook on Periodontitis*. San Diego, Calif.: Icon Health, 2002. Draws from public, academic, government, and peer-reviewed research to provide a wide-ranging handbook for patients with periodontitis.

Ring, Malvin E. *Dentistry: An Illustrated History*. New York: Abrams, 1985. Ring's coverage of dentistry is broad and accurate. The illustrations are particularly useful in helping readers understand dental diseases. An excellent starting point for those unfamiliar with the topic.

Smith, Rebecca W. *The Columbia University School of Dental and Oral Surgery's Guide to Family Dental Care*. New York: W. W. Norton, 1997. This classic text provides easy-to-understand explanations of all common dental problems and procedures and many less common procedures. The text is written for the general reader.

DENTISTRY, PEDIATRIC
SPECIALTY

ANATOMY OR SYSTEM AFFECTED: Gums, mouth, teeth
SPECIALTIES AND RELATED FIELDS: Orthodontics
DEFINITION: The specialty that addresses all aspects of dental treatment needed by children from infancy to age eighteen.

KEY TERMS:

caries: tooth decay or cavities

deciduous teeth: the temporary teeth that normally appear between eight months and two years and that begin to fall out after the child turns six or seven; also called baby teeth

endodontist: a dentist whose specialty is the treatment of disorders of the dental pulp

orthodontist: a dentist whose specialty is straightening teeth

pedodontist: a dentist whose specialty is the treatment of children's teeth from infancy to late adolescence

permanent teeth: the teeth that appear between age seven and adolescence

sealant: a substance used to seal the chewing surfaces of teeth and prevent the development of caries

wisdom teeth: the permanent teeth that may appear between late adolescence and early adulthood

SCIENCE AND PROFESSION

Dental education normally takes four years to complete. Courses offered at dental schools teach knowledge of anatomy, particularly the head and neck. Students must also learn the properties of materials—such as metals, acrylic plastics, porcelains, and sealant resins—used in dentistry. Prior to working on patients, students are trained to operate on diseased teeth using mannequins, plastic models, or extracted teeth. Then they treat patients under the close supervision of instructors. Students must treat patients in all specialties of dentistry before they can receive a degree in general dentistry. Postgraduate education is required to become a specialist in pediatric dentistry.

General dental care for children may be given by a family dentist or by a pedodontist. Pedodontists are dentists specializing in the practice of dentistry for children. They must understand the specific mechanics of children's anatomy and have a thorough foundation in the treatment of congenital diseases. Many pedodontists also assist orthodontists by doing some preliminary straightening of teeth.

Diagnostic and Treatment Techniques

In the second half of the twentieth century, dentists did an excellent job of educating parents and children about the importance of regular dental care. It is now generally understood that regular dental care from early childhood through adolescence is essential for the proper development of children. The dentist will also take advantage of each visit to discuss with parents and children proper techniques for brushing and flossing. If good habits are developed at an early age, serious dental problems can be reduced in the future.

Many parents do not understand the central importance of deciduous teeth, or baby teeth. These teeth appear in infants between eight months and two years and begin to fall out when children are about six or seven. By the age of two, most children have twenty deciduous teeth. If baby teeth are extracted too early, the other teeth will move, which will create orthodontic problems.

Dentists recommend that every child be examined by the age of three. If cavities or other problems are discovered, the affected teeth should be treated and saved. Fillings and even steel crowns are often required.

Since permanent teeth are located below baby teeth, abscesses in baby teeth can spread below the gums and damage permanent teeth. If X rays reveal that there are no permanent teeth to replace baby teeth, the dentist will make every effort to preserve baby teeth for as long as possible. Frequently, a dentist will have to explain to parents that paying for fillings or crowns now will save a much larger amount of money in the future by shortening the period of time required for orthodontics.

As the permanent teeth begin to break through and replace baby teeth, the dentist may discover that there are too many teeth or not enough teeth. Extra teeth,

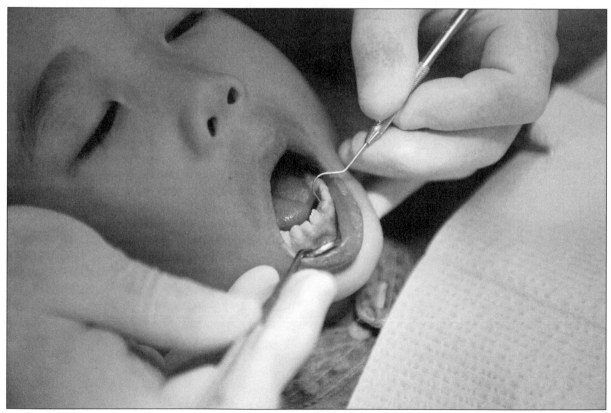

A dentist checks a child's teeth. Proper dental care is important for both deciduous and permanent teeth. (PhotoDisc)

called supernumerary teeth, must be extracted because they occupy space needed for the proper alignment of permanent teeth.

It is not uncommon for children's teeth to be injured as a result of accidents. In such cases, a dentist may refer the child to an endodontist, who will perform a root canal to repair damaged dental pulp. After the root canal has been completed, the family dentist or pedodontist will put a crown on the affected tooth.

A major expense for parents is orthodontics, but straightening teeth is not purely cosmetic. If there is a significant overbite, the child may develop speech problems that will not disappear until the malocclusion, or improper positioning of teeth, is eliminated. If a pedodontist or family dentist concludes that braces are needed to straighten a child's teeth, the child will be referred to an orthodontist, who will examine the child, take X rays, determine whether the child is ready for braces, and decide how to straighten the teeth and, if necessary, realign the jaws. Orthodontic treatment often lasts two to three years. Parents are usually asked to make a large initial payment and monthly payments thereafter. This expense can be significant if parents have two or more children in braces at the same time. Parents often consult several orthodontists in order to compare prices.

Orthodontists must motivate children to cooperate with their instructions in using bands as directed and brushing their teeth carefully. Both orthodontists and pedodontists or family dentists must remind children that it is easy for tooth decay to take place under braces.

As children become adolescents, other dental problems may occur, including tooth decay. Pedodontists often perform fluoride treatments, and they may apply sealants to the surface of the teeth. Frequently, oral surgery is performed on older adolescents or young adults to extract wisdom teeth that are impacted, or trapped within the gums.

PERSPECTIVE AND PROSPECTS

The quality of pediatric dental care available in economically advanced countries is excellent. Nevertheless, the cost of dental care concerns many parents, who wonder how they can afford to spend thousands of dollars for orthodontics and hundreds of dollars for a single crown or root canal. Dental insurance has become readily available in the United States, and most other countries have state-supported medical insurance programs that also cover dental treatment. Developing countries often have great difficulty paying for quality dental care. Efforts have been made to ensure that some of the international aid sent from developed to developing countries is used to improve dental care.

—Edmund J. Campion, Ph.D.

See also Dental diseases; Dentistry; Fluoride treatments; Orthodontics; Teeth; Teething; Thumb sucking; Wisdom teeth.

FOR FURTHER INFORMATION:

Foster, Malcolm S. *Protecting Our Children's Teeth: A Guide to Quality Dental Care from Infancy Through Age Twelve.* Cambridge, Mass.: Perseus, 1992.

Moss, Stephen J. *Growing Up Cavity Free: A Parent's Guide to Prevention.* New York: Edition Q, 1994.

Schou, Lone, and Anthony S. Blinkhorn, eds. *Oral Health Promotion.* New York: Oxford University Press, 1993.

Taintor, Jerry F., and Mary Jane Taintor. *The Complete Guide to Better Dental Care.* Reprint. New York: Checkmark Books, 1999.

DENTURES

TREATMENT

ANATOMY OR SYSTEM AFFECTED: Gums, mouth, teeth

SPECIALTIES AND RELATED FIELDS: Dentistry

DEFINITION: Removable artificial teeth worn to replace missing or diseased teeth, thus restoring both facial appearance and the ability to speak clearly and chew food by maintaining the shape of the jaw

INDICATIONS AND PROCEDURES

With the aging process, disease of the teeth and surrounding tissues often increases, leading to the eventual loss of some or all the teeth. When teeth are missing, the remaining teeth can change position, drifting into the surrounding space. Teeth that are out of position can damage tissues in the mouth. It is also more difficult to clean thoroughly between crooked teeth, resulting in an increased risk of tooth decay, gum disease, and additional loss of teeth. The solution is to replace the missing teeth with a denture. In 1999, more than thirty-two million Americans were wearing some type of denture, and the majority were over fifty-five years of age.

When a large number of teeth are missing, and a sufficient number of adjacent teeth are not present to support a bridge, or fixed partial denture, a removable partial denture is the solution. It consists of replacement teeth attached to pink or gum-colored plastic bases, which are connected by a metal framework. This prosthetic device is usually secured by clasping it to several of the remaining teeth. The clasps are typically made out of gold or a cobalt-steel alloy. Although more costly, precision attachments are nearly invisible and generally more aesthetically pleasing than metal clasps. Crowns on the adjacent natural teeth may improve the fit of a removable partial denture, and they are usually required with precision attachments.

When all the teeth need replacement, a full denture is constructed. It is usually made of acrylic, occasionally reinforced with metal. Full dentures replace all the teeth in either jaw and are generally held in place by suction created between saliva and the soft tissues of the mouth. A temporary soft liner can be placed in a new or old denture to help improve the health of the gum tissues by absorbing some of the pressures of mastication and providing maximum retention by fitting around undercuts in the bone and gums.

USES AND COMPLICATIONS

A common misconception is that when all the teeth are extracted and replaced by full dentures, all teeth problems cease. In fact, properly fitted full dentures at best are only about 25 to 35 percent as efficient as natural teeth. Many elderly have little trouble adjusting, but some find it difficult to adapt to and learn to use dentures properly. Furthermore, the tissues of the mouth undergo constant changes, which may result in loose or bad-fitting dentures, which may cause damage to the mouth tissues. Consequently, a person who wears dentures should continue to see a dentist for regular annual checkups.

Full and partial dentures are removable and must be taken out frequently and cleansed. In addition, the supporting soft tissues of the mouth need thorough cleansing with a soft mouth brush two to three times daily. It typically takes a few weeks to get used to inserting, wearing, eating with, removing, and maintaining dentures. Careful attention to all the instructions given by the dentist is vital.

—*Alvin K. Benson, Ph.D.*

See also Aging; Bone disorders; Cavities; Crowns and bridges; Dental diseases; Dentistry; Otorhinolaryngology; Periodontitis; Teeth; Tooth extraction.

FOR FURTHER INFORMATION:

Devlin, Hugh. *Complete Dentures: A Clinical Manual for the General Dental Practitioner.* New York: Springer, 2002.
Schillingburg, Warren, et al. *Fundamentals of Fixed Prosthodontics.* 3d ed. Chicago: Quintessence, 1997.
Smith, Rebecca W. *The Columbia University School of Dental and Oral Surgery's Guide to Family Dental Care.* New York: W. W. Norton, 1997.
Woodforde, John. *The Strange Story of False Teeth.* New York: Universe Books, 1983.

DEPRESSION
DISEASE/DISORDER

ANATOMY OR SYSTEM AFFECTED: Brain, heart, musculoskeletal system, psychic-emotional system

SPECIALTIES AND RELATED FIELDS: Family medicine, geriatrics and gerontology, psychiatry, psychology

DEFINITION: One of the most common psychiatric disorders to occur in most lifetimes, caused by biological, psychological, social, and/or environmental factors.

KEY TERMS:

bipolar disorders: mood disorders characterized by symptoms of mania and symptoms of depression

cyclothymia: a mood disorder characterized by fewer and less intense symptoms of elevated mood and depressed mood than bipolar disorders

dysthymia: a mood disorder characterized by symptoms similar to depression that are fewer in number but last for a much longer period of time

electroconvulsive therapy (ECT): the use of electric shocks to induce seizure in depressed patients as a form of treatment

major depressive disorder: a pattern of major depressive episodes that form an identified psychiatric disorder

major depressive episode: a syndrome of symptoms characterized by depressed mood; required for the diagnosis of some mood disorders

manic episode: a syndrome of symptoms characterized by elevated, expansive, or irritable mood; required for the diagnosis of some mood disorders

psychopharmacology: the drug treatment of psychiatric disorders

psychosurgery: the surgical removal or destruction of part of the brain of depressed patients as a form of treatment

psychotherapy: the "talk" therapies that target the emotional, social, and other contributors to and consequences of depression

seasonal affective disorder (SAD): a mood disorder associated with the winter season, when the amount of daylight hours is reduced

CAUSES AND SYMPTOMS

The word "depression" is used to describe many different things. For some, it defines a fleeting mood, for others an outward physical appearance of sadness, and for others a diagnosable clinical disorder. In any year, more than twenty million American adults suffer from a clinically diagnosed depression, a mood disorder that often affects personal, vocational, social, and health functioning. The *Diagnostic and Statistical Manual of Mental Disorders: DSM-IV-TR* (4th rev. ed., 2000) of the American Psychiatric Association delineates a number of mood disorders that include clinical depression, known as major depression.

A major depressive episode is a syndrome of symptoms, present during a two-week period and representing a change from previous functioning. The symptoms include at least five of the following: depressed or irritable mood, diminished interest in previously pleasurable activities, significant weight loss or weight gain, insomnia or hypersomnia, physical excitation or slowness, loss of energy, feelings of worthlessness or guilt, indecisiveness or a diminished ability to concentrate, and recurrent thoughts of death. The clinical depression cannot be initiated or maintained by another illness or condition, and it cannot be a normal reaction to the death of a loved one (some symptoms of depression are a normal part of the grief reaction).

In major depressive disorder, the patient experiences a major depressive episode and does not have a history of mania or hypomania. Major depressive disorder is often first recognized in the patient's late twenties, while a major depressive episode can occur at any age, including infancy. Women are twice as likely to suffer from the disorder than are men.

There are several potential causes of major depressive disorder. Genetic studies suggest a familial link with higher rates of clinical depression in first-degree relatives. There also appears to be a relationship between clinical depression and levels of the brain's neurochemicals, specifically dopamine, norepinephrine, and serotonin, as well as hormones. It is important to keep in mind, however, that anywhere from 15 to 40 percent of adults will experience depression in their lifetimes. Furthermore, not everyone has a biological cause for this depression. Common causes of clinical depression also include psychosocial stressors such as

the death of a loved one, financial stress, loss of a job, interpersonal problems, or world events. It is unclear, however, why some people respond to a specific psychosocial stressor with a clinical depression and others do not. Finally, certain prescription medications have been noted to cause or be related to clinical depression. These drugs include muscle relaxants, heart medications, hypertensive medications, ulcer medications, oral contraceptives, painkillers, narcotics, and steroids. Thus there are many causes of clinical depression, and no single cause is sufficient to explain all clinical depressions.

Another category of depressive disorder is bipolar disorders. Bipolar disorders occur in about 1 percent of the population as a whole. In persons over the age of eighteen, about two to three persons out of one hundred are diagnosed. Bipolar I disorder is characterized by one or more manic episodes along with persisting symptoms of depression. A manic episode is defined as a distinct period of abnormally and persistently elevated, expansive, or irritable mood. Three of the following symptoms must occur during the period of mood disturbance: inflated self-esteem, decreased need for sleep, unusual talkativeness or pressure to keep talking, racing thoughts, distractibility, excessive goal-oriented activities (especially in work, school, or social areas), and reckless activities with a high potential for negative consequences (such as buying sprees or risky business ventures). For a diagnosis of bipolar disorder, the symptoms must be sufficiently severe to cause impairment in functioning and/or concern regarding the person's danger to himself/herself or to

---

INFORMATION ON DEPRESSION

CAUSES: Genetic factors, psychosocial stressors, neurochemical dysfunction, certain medications

SYMPTOMS: Irritable mood, diminished interest in previously pleasurable activities, significant weight loss or gain, insomnia or hypersomnia, physical excitation or slowness, loss of energy, feelings of worthlessness or guilt, indecisiveness, recurrent thoughts of death

DURATION: Ranges from short-term to chronic

TREATMENTS: Drug therapy, individual and group psychotherapy, light therapy, electroconvulsive therapy

others, must not be superimposed on another psychotic disorder, and must not be initiated or maintained by another illness or condition. Bipolar II disorder is characterized by symptoms of a history of a major depressive episode and symptoms of hypomania.

Cyclothymia is another cyclic mood disorder related to depression. It involves symptoms of both depression and mania. However, the manic symptoms are without marked social or occupational impairment and are known as hypomanic episodes. Similarly, the symptoms of major depressive episodes do not meet the clinical criteria (less than five of the nine symptoms described above), but the symptoms must be present for at least two years. Cyclothymia cannot be superimposed on another psychotic disorder and cannot be initiated or maintained by another illness or condition. This mood disorder is a particularly persistent and chronic disorder with an identified familial pattern.

Dysthymia is another chronic mood disorder affecting approximately 6 percent of the population in a lifetime. Dysthymia is characterized by at least a two-year history of depressed mood and at least two of the following symptoms: poor appetite, insomnia or hypersomnia, low energy or fatigue, low self-esteem, poor concentration or decision making, or feelings of hopelessness. There cannot be evidence of a major depressive episode during the first two years of the dysthymia or a history of manic episodes or hypomanic episodes. The individual cannot be without the symptoms for more than two months at a time, the disorder cannot be superimposed on another psychotic disorder, and it cannot be initiated or maintained by another illness or condition. Dysthymia is more common in adult females, equally common in both sexes of children, and with a greater prevalence in families. The causes of dysthymia are believed to be similar to those listed for major depressive disorder, but the disorder is less well understood than is depression.

A final variant of clinical depression is known as seasonal affective disorder. Patients with this illness demonstrate a pattern of clinical depression during the winter, when there is a reduction in the amount of daylight hours. For these patients, the reduction in available light is thought to be the cause of the depression.

Treatment and Therapy

Crucial to the choice of treatment for clinical depression is determining the variant of depression being experienced. Each of the diagnostic categories has associated treatment approaches that are more effective for a particular diagnosis. Multiple assessment techniques are available to the health care professional to determine the type of clinical depression. The most valid and reliable is the clinical interview. The health care provider may conduct either an informal interview or a structured, formal clinical interview assessing the symptoms that would confirm the diagnosis of clinical depression. If the patient meets the criteria set forth in the DSM-IV, then the patient is considered for depression treatments. Patients who meet many but not all diagnostic criteria are sometimes diagnosed with a "subclinical" depression. These patients might also be considered appropriate for the treatment of depression, at the discretion of their health care providers.

Another assessment technique is the "paper-and-pencil" measure, or depression questionnaire. A variety of questionnaires have proven useful in confirming the diagnosis of clinical depression. Questionnaires such as the Beck Depression Inventory, Hamilton Depression Rating Scale, Zung Self-Rating Depression Scale, and the Center for Epidemiologic Studies Depression Scale are used to identify persons with clinical depression and to document changes with treatment. This technique is often used as an adjunct to the clinical interview and rarely stands alone as the definitive assessment approach to diagnosing clinical depression.

Laboratory tests, most notably the dexamethasone suppression test, have also been used in the diagnosis of depression. The dexamethasone suppression test involves injecting a steroid (dexamethasone) into the patient and measuring the production levels of another steroid (cortisol) in response. Studies have demonstrated, however, that certain severely depressed patients do not reveal the suppression of cortisol production that would be expected following the administration of dexamethasone. The test has also failed to identify some patients who were depressed and has mistakenly identified others as depressed. Research continues to determine the efficacy of other laboratory measures of brain activity to include computed tomography (CT) scanning, positron emission tomography (PET) scanning, and magnetic resonance imaging (MRI). At this time, laboratory tests are not a reliable diagnostic strategy for depression.

Once a clinical depression (or a subclinical depression) is identified, several types of treatment options are available. These options are dependent on the subtype and severity of the depression. They include psychopharmacology (drug therapy), individual and group psychotherapy, light therapy, family therapy, electroconvulsive therapy (ECT), and other less traditional treatments. These treatment options can be provided to the patient as part of an outpatient program or, in certain severe cases of clinical depression in which the person is a danger to himself/herself or others, as part of a hospitalization.

Clinical depression often affects the patient physically, emotionally, and socially. Therefore, prior to beginning any treatment with a clinically depressed individual, the health care provider will attempt to develop an open and communicative relationship with the patient. This relationship will allow the health care provider to provide patient education on the illness and to solicit the collaboration of the patient in treatment. Supportiveness, understanding, and collaboration are all necessary components of any treatment approach.

Three primary types of medications are used in the treatment of clinical depression: cyclic antidepressants, monoamine oxidase inhibitors (MAOIs), and lithium salts. These medications are considered equally effective in decreasing the symptoms of depression, which begin to resolve in three to four weeks after initiating treatment. The health care professional will select an antidepressant based on side effects, dosing convenience (once daily versus three times a day), and cost.

The cyclic antidepressants are the largest class of antidepressant medications. As the name implies, the chemical makeup of the medication contains chemical rings, or "cycles." There are unicyclic (buproprion and fluoxetine, or Prozac), bicyclic (sertraline and trazodone), tricyclic (amitriptyline, desipramine, and nortriptyline), and tetracyclic (maprotiline) antidepressants. These antidepressants function to either block the reuptake of neurotransmitters by the neurons, allowing more of the neurotransmitter to be available at a receptor site, or increase the amount of neurotransmitter produced. The side effects associated with the cyclic antidepressants—dry mouth, blurred vision, constipation, urinary difficulties, palpitations, and sleep disturbance—vary and can be quite problematic. Some of these antidepressants have deadly toxic effects at high levels, so they are not prescribed to patients who are at risk of suicide. The newer drugs are more specific in terms of the drug action. For instance, fluoxetine is a selective serotonin reuptake inhibitor (SSRI) and works specifically on the neurotransmitter serotonin. Similarly, buproprion is a norepinephrine and dopamine reuptake inhibitor (NDRI) and works specifically on the neurotransmitters norepinephrine and dopamine. More specific drugs generally create fewer side effects.

Fewer side effects can be associated with greater medication compliance, potentially making these drugs a more effective treatment.

Monoamine oxidase inhibitors (isocarboxazid, phenelzine, and tranylcypromine) are the second class of antidepressants. They function by slowing the production of the enzyme monoamine oxidase. This enzyme is responsible for breaking down the neurotransmitters norepinephrine and serotonin, which are believed to be responsible for depression. By slowing the decomposition of these transmitters, more of them are available to the receptors for a longer period of time. Restlessness, dizziness, weight gain, insomnia, and sexual dysfunction are common side effects of the MAOIs. MAOIs are most notable because of the dangerous adverse reaction (severely high blood pressure) that can occur if the patient consumes large quantities of foods high in tyramine (such as aged cheeses, fermented sausages, red wine, foods with a heavy yeast content, and pickled fish). Because of this potentially dangerous reaction, MAOIs are not usually the first choice of medication and are more commonly reserved for depressed patients who do not respond to the cyclic antidepressants.

A third class of medication used in the treatment of mood disorders are mood stabilizers, the most notable being lithium carbonate, which is used primarily for bipolar disorder. Lithium is a chemical salt that is believed to effect mood stabilization by influencing the production, storage, release, and reuptake of certain neurotransmitters. It is particularly useful in stabilizing and preventing manic episodes and preventing depressive episodes in patients with bipolar disorder.

Psychotherapy refers to a number of different treatment techniques used to deal with the psychosocial contributors and consequences of clinical depression. Psychotherapy is a common supplement to drug therapy. In psychotherapy, the patients develop knowledge and insight into the causes and treatment for their clinical depression. In cognitive psychotherapy, symptom relief comes from assisting patients in modifying maladaptive, irrational, or automatic beliefs that can lead to clinical depression. In behavioral psychotherapy, patients modify their environment such that social or personal rewards are more forthcoming. This process might involve being more assertive, reducing isolation by becoming more socially active, increasing physical activities or exercise, or learning relaxation techniques. Research on the effectiveness of these and other psychotherapy techniques indicates that psychotherapy is as effective as certain antidepressants for many patients and, in combination with certain medications, is more effective than either treatment alone.

Electroconvulsive (or "shock") therapy is the single most effective treatment for severe and persistent depression. If the clinically depressed patient fails to respond to medications or psychotherapy and the depression is life-threatening, electroconvulsive therapy is considered. It is also considered if the patient cannot physically tolerate antidepressants, as with elders who have other medical conditions. This therapy involves inducing a seizure in the patient by administering an electrical current to specific parts of the brain. The therapy has become quite sophisticated and much safer than it was in the mid-1900's, and it involves fewer risks to the patient. Patients undergo several treatments over a period of time, such as a week, and show marked treatment benefit. Some temporary memory impairment is a common side effect of this treatment. In the past, however, more memory impairment, of lasting duration for some, was more common.

A special treatment used for individuals with seasonal affective disorder is light therapy, or phototherapy. Light therapy involves exposing patients to bright light for a period of time each day during seasons of the year when there is decreased light. This may be done as a preventive measure and also during depressive episodes. The manner in which this treatment approach modifies the depression is unclear and awaits further research, but some believe it affects the internal clock of the body, or circadian rhythm. Studies of the effectiveness of light therapy have been mixed, but interest in this promising treatment is strong, as it may prove useful for working with nonseasonal mood disorders as well. It should be noted, however, that light therapy does have some risks associated with it. Caution must be used to protect the eyes and use the light as directed. Additionally, the intensity of light must be correct so as to achieve therapeutic effects and not cause other problems. Finally, some individuals can experience manic episodes if they are exposed to too much light, so caution must be exercised in terms of the length of time for light exposure treatment sessions.

Psychosurgery, the final treatment option, is quite rare. It refers to surgical removal or destruction of certain portions of the brain believed to be responsible for causing severe depression. Psychosurgery is used only after all treatment options have failed and the clinical depression is life-threatening. Approximately 50 percent of patients who undergo psychosurgery benefit from the procedure.

Perspective and Prospects

Depression, or the more historical term "melancholy," has had a history predating modern medicine. Writings from the time of the ancient Greek physician Hippocrates refer to patients with a symptom complex similar to the present-day definition of clinical depression.

The rates of clinical depression have increased since the early twentieth century, while the age of onset of clinical depression has decreased. Women appear to be at least twice as likely as men to suffer from clinical depression, and people who are happily married have a lower risk for clinical depression than those who are separated, divorced, or dissatisfied in their marital relationship. These data, along with recurrence rates of 50 to 70 percent, indicate the importance of this psychiatric disorder.

While most psychiatric disorders are nonfatal, clinical depression can lead to death. About 60 percent of individuals who commit suicide have a mood disorder such as depression at the time. In a lifetime, however, only about 7 percent of men and 1 percent of women with lifetime histories of depression will commit suicide. Though these numbers are very high, what this means is that not everyone who is depressed will commit suicide. In fact, many receive help and recover from this illness. There are, however, other costs of clinical depression. In the United States, billions of dollars are spent on clinical depression, divided among the following areas: treatment, suicide, and absenteeism (the largest). Clinical depression obviously has a significant economic impact on a society.

The future of clinical depression lies in early identification and treatment. Identification will involve two areas. The first is improving the social awareness of mental health issues to include clinical depression. By eliminating the negative social stigma associated with mental illness and mental health treatment, there will be an increased level of the reporting of depression symptoms and thereby an improved opportunity for early intervention, preventing the progression of the disorder to the point of suicide. The second approach to identification involves the development of reliable assessment strategies for clinical depression. Data suggest that the majority of those who commit suicide see a physician within thirty days of the suicide. The field will continue to strive to identify biological markers and other methods to predict and/or identify clinical depression more accurately. Treatment advances will focus on further development of pharmacological strategies and drugs with more specific actions and fewer side effects. Adjuncts to traditional drug therapies need continued development and refinement to maximize the success of integrated treatments.

—Oliver Oyama, Ph.D.;
updated by Nancy A. Piotrowski, Ph.D.

See also Antidepressants; Anxiety; Bipolar disorders; Brain; Death and dying; Dementias; Eating disorders; Emotions, biochemical causes and effects of; Geriatrics and gerontology; Grief and guilt; Hypochondriasis; Light therapy; Midlife crisis; Neurology; Neurology, pediatric; Neurosis; Neurosurgery; Obsessive-compulsive disorder; Panic attacks; Paranoia; Pharmacology; Phobias; Postpartum depression; Post-traumatic stress disorder; Psychiatric disorders; Psychiatry; Psychiatry, child and adolescent; Psychiatry, geriatric; Psychoanalysis; Psychosomatic disorders; Seasonal affective disorder; Shock therapy; Stress; Suicide.

FOR FURTHER INFORMATION:

American Psychiatric Association. *Diagnostic and Statistical Manual of Mental Disorders: DSM-IV-TR*. Rev. 4th ed. Washington, D.C.: Author, 2000. This reference book lists the clinical criteria for psychiatric disorders, including mood disorders.

DePaulo, J. Raymond, Jr., and Leslie Ann Horvitz. *Understanding Depression: What We Know and What You Can Do About It.* New York: Wiley, 2003. A leading expert on depression examines the disease's nature, causes, effects, and treatments.

Depression and Bipolar Support Alliance. http://www .dbsalliance.org/. Offers information on mood disorders, support groups, referrals for mental health professionals, research links, and discussion forums.

Jones, Steven. *Coping with Bipolar Disorder: A Guide to Living with Manic Depression.* Oxford, England: Oneworld, 2002. A handbook for living with bipolar disorder, outlining causes, symptoms, and treatments, giving case studies, and listing support organizations and Internet groups.

Koplewicz, Harold S. *More than Moody: Recognizing and Treating Adolescent Depression.* New York: Penguin, 2002. A leading clinician and researcher helps parents distinguish between normal teenage angst and depression, examining the warning signs, risk factors, and key behaviors, as well as treatment options.

DERMATITIS

DISEASE/DISORDER

ALSO KNOWN AS: Eczema

ANATOMY OR SYSTEM AFFECTED: Hair, skin

SPECIALTIES AND RELATED FIELDS: Dermatology

DEFINITION: A wide range of skin disorders, some the result of allergy, some caused by contact with a skin irritant, and some attributable to other causes.

KEY TERMS:

allergen: a substance that excites an immunologic response; also called an antigen

crusting: the appearance of slightly elevated skin lesions made up of dried serum, blood, or pus; they can be brown, red, black, tan, or yellowish

immunoglobulin E (IgE): ordinarily, a relatively rare antibody; in patients with atopic dermatitis, levels can be significantly higher than in the general population

lesion: any pathologic change in tissue

scaling: a buildup of hard, horny skin cells

secondary infection: a bacterial, viral, or other infection that results from or follows another disease

wheal: a small swelling in the skin

CAUSES AND SYMPTOMS

The term "dermatitis" does not refer to a single skin disease, but rather to a wide range of disorders. "Dermatitis" is often used interchangeably with "eczema." The two most common dermatitides are atopic (allergic) dermatitis, in which the individual appears to inherit a predilection for the disease, and contact dermatitis, in which the individual's skin reacts immediately on contact with a substance, or develops sensitivity to it.

Atopic dermatitis often occurs in individuals with a personal or family history of allergy, such as hay fever or asthma. Thirty to 50 percent of children with atopic dermatitis develop asthma or hay fever, a rate that is three to five times higher than for the general population. These people often have high serum levels of a certain antibody, immunoglobulin E (IgE), which may be associated with their skin's tendency to break out, although a specific antigen-antibody reaction has not been demonstrated.

There are many distinct characteristics of atopic dermatitis, some of which depend on the age of the patient. The disease usually starts early in childhood. It is often first discovered in infants in the first months of life when redness and weeping, crusted lesions appear mostly on the face, although the scalp, arms, and legs may also be affected. There is intense itching. Papules

INFORMATION ON DERMATITIS

CAUSES: Allergies, infection, contact irritation, altered immune system

SYMPTOMS: Dry and itchy skin, rashes, inflammation, pain

DURATION: Short-term to chronic

TREATMENTS: Topical corticosteroids or antihistamines, antibiotics, dietary changes, and specialized lotions, soaps, or shampoos

(pimples), vesicles (small, blisterlike lesions filled with fluid), edema (swelling), serous exudation (discharge of fluid), and scaly crusts may be seen. At one year of age, oval, scaly lesions appear on the arms, legs, face, and torso. In older children and adults, the lesions are usually localized in the crook of the elbow and the back of the knees, and the face and neck may be involved. The course of the disease is variable. It usually subsides by the third or fourth year of life, but periodic outbreaks may occur throughout childhood, adolescence, and adulthood. In 75 percent of cases, atopic dermatitis improves between the ages of ten and fourteen. Cases persisting past the patient's middle twenties, or beginning then, are the most difficult to treat.

Dryness and itching are always present in atopic dermatitis. People with atopic dermatitis seem to lose skin moisture more readily than average people: Rather than soft, pliable skin, they develop dry, rough, sensitive skin that is particularly prone to chapping and splitting. The skin becomes itchy, and the individual's tendency to scratch significantly aggravates the condition in what is called the "itch-scratch-itch" cycle or the "scratch-rash-itch" cycle: The individual scratches to relieve the itching, which causes a rash, which in turn causes increased itching, which invites increased scratching and increased irritation. After years of itching and scratching, the skin of older children and adults with atopic dermatitis develops red, lichenified (rough, thickened) patches in the crook of the arm and behind the knees, as well as on the eyelids, neck, and wrists.

Constant chafing of the affected area invites bacterial infection and lymphadenitis (inflammation of lymph nodes). Furthermore, patients with atopic dermatitis seem to have altered immune systems. They appear to be more susceptible than others to skin infections, warts, and contagious skin diseases. *Staphylococcus aureus* and certain streptococci are common infecting bacteria in these patients. Pyoderma is often seen as a result of bacterial infection in atopic dermatitis. This condition features redness, oozing, scaling, and crusting, as well as the formation of small pustules (pus-filled pimples).

Patients with atopic dermatitis are also particularly sensitive to herpes simplex and vaccinia viruses. Exposure to either could cause a severe skin disease called Kaposi's varicelliform eruption. Vaccinia virus (the agent that causes cowpox) is used in the preparation of smallpox vaccine. Therefore, patients with atopic dermatitis must not be vaccinated against smallpox. Furthermore, they must be isolated from patients with active herpes simplex and those recently vaccinated against smallpox.

Patients with atopic dermatitis may also develop contact dermatitis, which can greatly exacerbate their condition. They are also sensitive to a wide range of allergens, which can bring on outbreaks, as well as to low humidity (such as in centrally heated houses in winter), which would contribute to dry skin. They may not be able to tolerate woolen clothing.

A condition called keratosis pilaris often develops in the presence of atopic dermatitis. It is not seen in young infants, but it does appear in childhood. Hair follicles on the torso, buttocks, arms, and legs become plugged with horny matter and protrude above the skin, giving the appearance of goose bumps or "chicken skin." The palms of the hands of patients with atopic dermatitis have significantly more fine lines than those of average people. In many patients, there is a tiny "pleat" under the eyes. They are often prone to cold hands and may have pallor, seen as a blanching of the skin around the nose, mouth, and ears.

When ordinary skin is lightly rubbed with a pointed object, almost immediately there is a red line, followed by a red flare, and finally, a wheal or slight elevation of the skin along the line. In patients with atopic dermatitis, however, there is a completely different reaction: The red line appears, but almost instantly it becomes white. The flare and the wheal do not appear.

About 4 to 12 percent of patients with atopic dermatitis develop cataracts at an early age. Normally, cataracts do not appear until the fifties and sixties; those with atopic dermatitis may develop them in their twenties. These cataracts usually affect both eyes simultaneously and develop quickly.

Psychologically, children with atopic dermatitis often show distinct personality characteristics. They are reported to be bright, aggressive, energetic, and prone to fits of anger. Children with severe, unmanageable cases of atopic dermatitis may become selfish and domineering, and some go on to develop significant personality disorders.

It is not known exactly what happens to cause the itching and dry skin that are the fundamental signs of atopic dermatitis and the root of many of its complications. Various theories suggest various origins. It is by definition an allergic disorder, but the allergens that are specifically involved and how they produce the signs of atopic dermatitis are unknown. One of the most interesting theories involves the antibody IgE. Theoretically, the union of IgE with an antigen causes certain cells to release pharmacologic mediators, such as histamine, bradykinin, and slow-reacting substance (SRS-A), that cause itching and thus begin the cycle of scratching and irritation characteristic of atopic dermatitis. The fact that patients with atopic dermatitis have higher than normal levels of IgE, and that there is a relationship between IgE levels and the severity of atopic dermatitis, seems to lend support to this theory.

Contact dermatitis could resemble atopic dermatitis at certain stages, but the dry skin of atopic dermatitis may not be seen. Contact dermatitis is usually characterized by a rash consisting of small bumps, itchiness, blisters, and general swelling. It occurs when the skin has been exposed to a substance to which the body is sensitive or allergic. If the contact dermatitis is caused by direct irritation by a caustic substance, it is called irritant contact dermatitis. The causative agents are primary irritants that cause inflammation at first contact. Some obvious irritants are acids, alkalis, and other harsh chemicals or substances. An example is fiberglass dermatitis, in which fine glass particles from fiberglass fabrics or insulation enter the skin and cause redness and inflammation.

If the dermatitis is caused by allergic sensitivity to a substance, it is called allergic contact dermatitis. In this case, it may take hours, days, weeks, or years for the patient to develop sensitivity to the point where exposure to these substances causes allergic contact dermatitis. These agents include soaps, acetone, skin creams, cosmetics, poison ivy, and poison sumac.

Allergic contact dermatitis comprises the largest variety of contact dermatitides, many of them named for the allergens that cause them. Hence, there is pollen dermatitis; plant and flower dermatitis, such as poison ivy or poison oak; clothing dermatitis; shoe, and even sandal strap, dermatitis; metal and metal salt dermatitis; cosmetic dermatitis; and adhesive tape dermatitis, among others. They all have one thing in common: The skin is exposed to an allergen from any of these sources and becomes so sensitive to it that further exposure causes a rash, itching, and blistering.

The development of sensitivity to an allergen is an immunological response to exposure to that substance. With many allergens, the first contact elicits no immediate immunological reaction. Sensitivity develops after the allergen has been presented to the T lymphocytes that mediate the immune response.

Because it often takes a long time to develop sensitivity, patients are surprised to discover that they have become allergic to substances that they have been using for years. For example, a patient who has been applying a topical medication to treat a skin condition may one day find that the medication causes an outbreak of dermatitis. Ironically, some of the ingredients in medications commonly used to treat skin conditions are among the major allergens that cause allergic contact dermatitis. These include antibiotics, antihistamines, topical anesthetics, and antiseptics, as well as the inactive ingredients used in formulating the medications, such as stabilizers.

Other substances to which the patient may develop sensitivity include the chemicals used in making fabric for clothing, tanning chemicals used in making leather, dyes, and ingredients in cosmetics. Many patients develop sensitivity to allergens found in the workplace. The list of potential allergens in the industrial setting is virtually endless. It includes solvents, petroleum products, chemicals commonly used in manufacturing processes, and coal tar derivatives.

In some cases, the allergen requires sunlight or other forms of light to precipitate an outbreak of contact dermatitis. This is called photoallergic contact dermatitis, and it may be caused by such agents as aftershave lotions, sunscreens, topical sulfonamides, and other preparations applied to the skin. Another light reaction, termed phototoxic contact dermatitis, can be caused by exposure to sunlight after exposure to perfumes, coal tar, certain medications, and various chemicals.

A different form of dermatitis involves the sebaceous glands, which secrete sebum, a fatty substance that lubricates the skin and helps retain moisture. Sebaceous dermatitis is usually seen in areas of the body with high concentrations of sebaceous glands, such as on the scalp or face, behind the ears, on the chest, and in areas where skin rubs against skin, such as the buttocks and the groin. It is seen most often in infants and adolescents, although it may persist into adulthood or start at that time.

In infants, sebaceous dermatitis can begin within the first month of life and appears as a thick, yellow, crusted lesion on the scalp called cradle cap. There can be yellow scaling behind the ears and red pimples on the face. Diaper rash may be persistent in these infants. In older children, the lesion may appear as thick, yellow plaques in the scalp. When sebaceous dermatitis begins in adulthood, it starts slowly, and usually its only manifestation is scaling on the scalp (dandruff). In severe cases, yellowish-red scaling pimples develop along the hairline and on the face and chest. Its cause is unknown, but a yeast commonly found in the hair follicles, *Pityrosporum ovale*, may be involved.

There are many other kinds of dermatitis. Diaper dermatitis, or diaper rash, is a complex skin disorder that involves irritation of the skin by urine and feces, irritation by constant rubbing, and secondary infection by *Candida albicans*. Nummular dermatitis (from *nummus*, meaning coin) is characterized by crusting, scaly, disc-shaped papules and vesicles filled with fluid and often pus. Pityriasis alba is a common dermatitis with pale, scaly patches. In lichen simplex chronicus, there is intense itching, with lesions caused by, and perpetuated by, scratching and rubbing. Stasis dermatitis occurs at the ankles; brown discoloration, swelling, scaling, and varicose veins are common. Hyperimmunoglobulin E (Hyper IgE) syndrome is characterized by extremely high IgE levels, ten to one hundred times higher than normal, and a family history of allergy; the patient has frequent skin infections, suppurative (pus-forming) lymphadenitis, pustules, plaques, and abscesses. Pompholyx occurs on the hands and soles of the feet; there is excessive sweating, with eruptions of deep vesicles accompanied by burning or itching.

Friction can also cause dermatitis. In intertrigo, the friction of skin rubbing against skin causes inflammation that can become infected. In frictional lichenoid dermatitis, or sandbox dermatitis, it is thought that the abrasive action of sand or other gritty material on the skin causes the characteristic lesions. Winter eczema seems to be caused by the skin-drying effects of low humidity as well as by harsh soaps and overfrequent bathing; dry skin and itching are common. The acrodermatitis diseases (from *acro*, meaning the extremities) may be limited to the hands and feet, or, like acrodermatitis enteropathica, may erupt in other parts of the body, such as around the mouth and on the buttocks. In fixed-drug eruption, lesions appear in direct response to the administration of a drug; the lesions are generally in the same parts of the body, but they may spread. Swimmer's itch is a parasitic infection from an organism that lives in fresh water lakes and ponds, while seabather's eruption seems to be caused by a similar saltwater organism.

Treatment and Therapy

Many dermatitides resemble one another, and it is important for a physician to identify the patient's complaint precisely in order to treat it effectively. Therefore, the physician will confirm the identity of the condition through a process known as differential diagnosis. This method allows him or her to rule out all similar conditions, pinpoint the exact nature of the patient's problem, and develop a therapeutic regimen to treat it.

In treating atopic dermatitis, one of the first goals is to relieve dryness and itching. The patient is cautioned not to bathe excessively because this dries the skin. Lotions are used to lubricate the skin and retain moisture. The patient is advised not to scratch, because this could break the skin and invite infection. The patient is advised to avoid any known offending agents and not to apply any medication to the skin without the doctor's knowledge.

Wet compresses can bring relief to patients with atopic dermatitis. Topical corticosteroids are used to help resolve acute flare-ups, but only for short-term therapy, because their prolonged use might produce undesirable side effects. Oral antihistamines are often given to relieve itching and to help the patient sleep. Diet may play a role in atopic dermatitis in infants: Some pediatric dermatologists and other physicians recommend elimination of milk, eggs, tomatoes, citrus fruits, wheat products, chocolate, spices, fish, and nuts from the diets of these patients. Soft cotton clothing is recommended, as is the avoidance of pets or fuzzy toys that might be allergenic. For secondary infections that arise from atopic dermatitis, the physician prescribes appropriate antibiotic therapy.

In primary irritant contact dermatitis, the offending agent is eliminated or avoided. In allergic contact dermatitis, one of the main goals is to discover the offending agent so that the patient can avoid contact with it. Sometimes this information can be elicited from the patient interview, and sometimes it is necessary to conduct a series of patch tests. In this procedure, known allergens are applied to the skin of the patient to find those that cause irritation. Avoidance of the offending agent can cause the patient some difficulty if the agent happens to be something that is found everywhere. An example is the metal nickel, which is in coins, jewelry, and hundreds of other objects. Patients who insist on wearing nickel-plated jewelry are advised to paint it with clear nail polish periodically to avoid contact of the metal with the skin. Similarly, many other allergens are in common use. Patients are advised to read cosmetic labels and food and medical ingredients lists in order to avoid contact with agents to which they are sensitive.

Because there is such a wide range of allergic contact dermatitides, treatment of the flare-ups varies considerably. Topical and oral steroids are used, as well as antihistamines. Sometimes the physician finds it necessary to drain large blisters and apply drying agents to weeping lesions. Sometimes the condition calls for wet compresses to relieve itching and soothe the patient. Specialized lotions, soaps, and shampoos are also used, some to treat dryness and others, as in the case of sebaceous dermatitis, to remove scales and to relieve oiliness.

Other treatments depend on the type of dermatitis from which the patient suffers. Patients with photoallergic or phototoxic dermatitis are advised to avoid light. Acrodermatitis enteropathica is caused by a zinc deficiency; in addition to palliative therapy to relieve the symptoms, these patients are given zinc sulfate, which results in complete remission of the disease. As with atopic dermatitis, bacterial infections occurring as a result of a flare-up of allergic contact dermatitis are treated with appropriate antibiotic therapy.

PERSPECTIVE AND PROSPECTS

The skin is the largest organ of the human body, and it is subject to an extraordinary range and number of diseases, with atopic dermatitis and contact dermatitis among the most common. They may afflict patients of all ages, but they are particularly prevalent in children. Many of the dermatitides start in the first weeks of life and continue through childhood. In many cases, the disease is resolved by the time that the child reaches adolescence, but in some it continues into adulthood.

In spite of the fact that disorders of the skin are readily apparent, an understanding of them has been imperfect throughout history. For example, the allergic nature of many of the dermatitides was not explained until the twentieth century. In addition, because their symptoms are similar to one another and to diseases that are not properly classified as dermatitides, there has been much confusion in identifying them. It has

been suggested that many of the biblical lepers were in fact suffering only from a form of dermatitis. With prolonged exposure, however, they probably contracted leprosy in time.

The dermatitides are often highly complex diseases, involving genetic, allergic, metabolic, and immune and infective factors, among many others. They are not usually life-threatening, but they take an enormous toll in pain, discomfort, and disfigurement, with an equal toll in psychological distress that can be suffered by patients.

Understanding of these disorders improves constantly, and with understanding comes new methods of treating them. Nevertheless, progress will probably be limited. There is the possibility that patients can be desensitized to allow them to tolerate the allergens that bring about their eruptions, as many hay fever sufferers have been desensitized against the pollens and dusts that trigger their allergy. It is unlikely, however, that there will ever be vaccines to immunize against this group of diseases, nor can many of them be cured, except in the sense that the discomfort that they bring can be treated and the agents that cause them can be avoided.

—*C. Richard Falcon*

See also Acne; Allergies; Blisters; Dermatology; Dermatology, pediatric; Dermatopathology; Diaper rash; Eczema; Hives; Itching; Multiple chemical sensitivity syndrome; Poisonous plants; Psoriasis; Rashes; Rosacea; Scabies; Skin; Skin disorders.

FOR FURTHER INFORMATION:

Adelman, Daniel C., et al., eds. *Manual of Allergy and Immunology.* 4th ed. Philadelphia: Lippincott Williams & Wilkins, 2002. Examines research developments and the clinical diagnosis and treatment of allergies and immune disorders. Topics include asthma, disorders of the skin, diseases of the lung, anaphlaxism, insect allergies, drug allergies, rheumatic diseases, transplantation immunology, and immunization.

American Academy of Dermatology. http://www.aad .org/. The site's "Public Resources" section has good information about dermatitis, as well as coverage of other dermatological disorders.

Litin, Scott C., ed. *Mayo Clinic Family Health Book.* 3d ed. New York: HarperResource, 2003. An excellent general reference for the layperson, with good coverage of the dermatological diseases.

Middlemiss, Prisca. *What's That Rash? How to Identify*

and Treat Childhood Rashes. London: Hamlyn, 2002. A comprehensive guide to the identification and treatment of childhood rashes.

Parker, James N., and Philip M. Parker, eds. *The Official Patient's Sourcebook on Atopic Dermatitis*. San Diego, Calif.: Icon Health, 2002. Draws from public, academic, government, and peer-reviewed research to provide a wide-ranging handbook for patients with dermatitis.

Rietschel, Robert L., and Joseph F. Fowler, eds. *Fisher's Contact Dermatitis*. 5th ed. Philadelphia: Lippincott Williams & Wilkins, 2001. An encyclopedic reference on contact dermatitis. Offers extensive lists of causative agents.

Titman, Penny. *Understanding Childhood Eczema*. New York: Wiley, 2003. Discusses the physical and emotional toll of eczema on young patients and provides practical advice for choosing and managing different treatments.

Weston, William L., et al. *Color Textbook of Pediatric Dermatology*. 3d ed. New York: Elsevier, 2002. Clinical textbook that covers a range of disorders, including drug reactions, hair disorders, nail disorders, and sun sensitivity. Clinical features, differential diagnosis, pathogenesis, treatment, and patient education are discussed.

Williams, Hywel C., ed. *Atopic Dermatitis: The Epidemiology, Causes, and Prevention of Atopic Eczema*. New York: Cambridge University Press, 2000. Provides a comprehensive review of this increasingly common disorder. Discusses the distribution, frequency, and underlying causes of atopic dermatitis.

DERMATOLOGY

SPECIALTY

ANATOMY OR SYSTEM AFFECTED: Hair, immune system, nails, skin

SPECIALTIES AND RELATED FIELDS: Cytology, histology, immunology, oncology, public health

DEFINITION: The study of a variety of irritations or lesions affecting one of several layers of the skin.

KEY TERMS:

allergens: foreign substances in the surrounding environment that may cause an allergic response, such as a skin reaction

dermatitis: a general term for nonspecific skin irritations that may be caused by bacteria, viruses, or fungi

keratin: a fibrous molecule essential to the tissue structure of hair, nails, or the skin

melanin: a polymer made up of several compounds (including the amino acid tyrosine) that causes pigmentation in the skin, hair, and eyes

SCIENCE AND PROFESSION

Dermatology is the subfield of medicine that deals with diseases of the skin. Some disorders affecting the hair and fingernails may also fall under this category.

Dermatological study requires attention to three distinct layers of the skin, each of which can be affected differently by different disorders. The deepest layer is the subcutaneous tissue where fat is formed and stored. It is also here that the deeper hair follicles and sweat glands originate. Blood vessels and nerves pass from this layer to the dermis. The dermis is mainly connective tissue that contains the oil-producing, or sebaceous, glands and shorter hair follicles. On the surface of the skin is the epidermis, which is itself multilayered. The innermost basal layer is made up of specialized keratin- and melanin-forming cells, whereas the outermost, horny cell layer consists of keratinized dead cells.

The diagnosis of apparent skin disease requires dermatologists to determine whether symptomatic sores, or lesions, are primary (the original symptoms of suspected disease) or secondary (such as infection or irritation caused by scratching which may overshadow the original disorder). Dermatologists are trained to recognize categories of lesions and to determine whether they represent actual diseases or relatively common disorders characteristic of age, or even genetic predispositions. The most common categories of lesions include vesicles, bullae, and crusts; scaling; keratosis; lichenification; pustules; atrophy; and tumors.

Vesicles and bullae are bubblelike eruptions filled with clear serous fluid. As primary lesions, they are often the symptoms of diseases such as chickenpox and herpes zoster. Crusts are formed by tissue fluid that remains in a dried form after the rupture of microscopic vesicles.

Scaling is noticeably different from crusting. These flakes on the surface of the skin may represent a subsiding stage of earlier inflammation. Scaling may be a secondary lesion associated with psoriasis. Keratoses are rough lesions that show strongly adherent (not loose) flaking. Lichenification involves a thickening of the epidermis, with a more pronounced visibility of lined patterns on the skin surface. Pustules are lesions filled with pus, which serves as a growth medium for microorganisms. Atrophy always involves shrinkage of skin

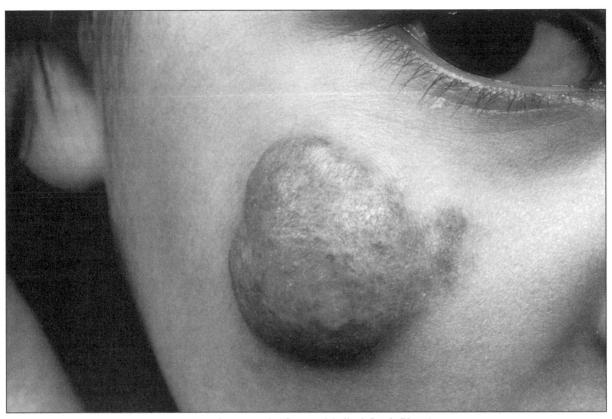

A strawberry mark. (Custom Medical Stock Photo)

tissues, creating in some cases visible depressions in the area of the lesion. The last category of primary lesions, tumors, may be found either on the surface of or underneath the skin. Tumorous growths can signal a condition as benign as seborrheic keratosis (the appearance of thick scales in isolated spots, particularly as age advances) or as serious as one of several forms of skin cancer.

Secondary lesions appear as the primary, or causal, skin disorder progresses, creating different symptoms in the secondary stage. Examples of secondary lesions include scales (dandruff and psoriasis), crusts (impetigo), ulcers (advanced syphilis), and scarring, the growth of connective tissue that actually replaces damaged tissues following burns or other traumatic injuries.

In addition to these general categories of lesions associated with dermatological diseases, a number of localized problems in blood flow—called vascular nevoid lesions, or birthmarks—may be visible at or soon after birth. Dermatologists assume that some of these lesions may be caused by genetic factors. The most common vascular nevi categories are nevus

flammeus (port-wine stain), a purple discoloring of the skin resulting from dilated dermal vessels, and capillary hemangioma (strawberry mark), which begins as a bruiselike lesion but soon grows into a protruding mass. Unlike port-wine stains, which remain throughout the individual's lifetime unless they are removed through laser surgery, strawberry marks will usually subside and disappear on their own, leaving at most visible puckering of the skin. Unless there are complications (such as ulceration), treatment is usually simple, consisting of the application of elastic bandages to maintain constant pressure, thus reducing the distortion caused by the rapid expansion of skin tissue in a localized area.

Probably the most commonly recognized dermatological disorder, acne, usually occurs among adolescents and young adults. Although this problem is likely to occur as part of the normal process of maturation, lack of proper care of acne may cause complications and lifelong scarring. Acne, as with equally common cases of seborrheic dermatitis (or dandruff, a subcategory of psoriasis), afflicts those areas of the body where oil gland secretions are plentiful and where many forms of bacteria are present on the skin (mainly the face, neck, and upper trunk). The points of lesion for acne are always specific: the hair follicles that are so numerous in these areas of the body. Two phenomena, so-called blackheads and the pimples associated with acne, occur when the normal draining of follicle secretions is blocked in a sac called a comedo. Blackheads occur when the residue trapped in the comedo—keratin, sebum, and various microorganisms—becomes chemically oxidized. When conditions associated with acne appear, an increase in bacterial growth within the comedones produces characteristic pimples which, if traumatized by scratching or picking, may burst, leading to the possibility of further infection. There is no way to prevent acne from appearing, but dermatological therapy to soothe the effects of advanced cases may be recommended.

Another relatively benign but persistently insoluble dermatological problem, the appearance of warts, occurs most often among the middle-aged or older segment of the adult population. Modern dermatological research dating from the 1960's has determined that warts are associated with particular viral strains (papillomaviruses). At least four subtypes have been associated with the appearance of warts on the human body. Warts may vary greatly in appearance—from plantar warts, which grow well below the skin surface and exhibit a drier consistency, to plane warts, which are even with the skin surface, to a very visible brownish and moist lump, which is often found on the face or hands. All warts are localized viral infections that destroy the normal skin tissue in the area of infection. Despite their common occurrence—dermatologists experience a high rate of patient demand for their removal—warts have always carried a certain social stigma. As viruses, they may be transferred to others through contact, particularly if the lesion is an open one.

The term "seborrheic dermatitis" can refer to the recurrent and common problem of dandruff (redness and scaling mainly in skin areas where body hair is present). Like acne, seborrheic dermatitis is more a condition resulting from secretion imbalances and chemical reactions affecting the skin than an actual disease. Dermatological complications arise when excessive scratching of sensitive areas causes secondary lesions to form.

Beyond these categories of common skin disorders are far more serious diseases that require professional dermatological treatment. For example, psoriasis, although varying in possible locations all over the body (including the hands and feet), seems to share symptoms with seborrheic dermatitis, specifically the flaking away of dry skin. What begins as limited patches of flaking, usually on elbows or in the armpits, however, may spread rapidly and have traumatic effects. Dermatologists usually associate psoriasis with stress and anxiety. When irritations are limited in scope, treatment through topical medications—most containing coal tar, sulfur, salicylic acid, or ammoniated mercury solutions—may be successful. Advanced cases may demand systemic treatment with more sophisticated drugs.

Herpes simplex is another common viral infection which leads directly to surface lesions that may be communicable, in this case cold sores. As with warts, folk knowledge has it that improper hygienic practices lead to the much more virulent eruptions associated with herpes simplex. Medical observations have shown, however, that various factors may unleash a dermatological reaction from latent viral sources in an individual. A herpes simplex reaction to increased levels of exposure to sunlight is a good example. On the other hand, many cases of herpes simplex occur in both the male and female genital areas. Although these eruptions are not necessarily connected with much more serious sexually transmitted diseases, their communicability is clearly associated with levels of hygiene in intimate sexual contact. Whatever the cause of herpes simplex, its highly contagious nature may demand dermatological attention to avoid more serious complications. Any occurrence of herpes simplex inflammation near a vital organ, for example, must be treated immediately to prevent the spread of viral infection, particularly in the area surrounding the eyes.

Herpes zoster, commonly referred to as shingles, is thought to be a recurrence in the adult years of a common viral infection that most people experience at an earlier age: chickenpox. The persistence of the symptoms of shingles among adults, however, is not comparable to the mild effect of the virus during childhood. The appearance of painful lesions, usually but not always in the trunk area, may come after a short period of tingling. Although inflammation may pass, many elderly patients, especially those suffering from systemic diseases such as diabetes mellitus, are plagued by continuous long-term discomfort. In addition to discomfort, there may be (as in herpes simplex) a danger of complications if the area of inflammation is close to vulnerable tissues or key organs, such as the eyes or ears. In cases where lesions may affect the eyes, dermatologists must go beyond topical treatment to enhance the healing process. Additional emergency therapy may include systemic steroid treatment, the intravenous administration of corticotropin, or oral doses of prednisone.

DIAGNOSTIC AND TREATMENT TECHNIQUES

The diagnosis of specific dermatoses, or potentially serious skin diseases, may or may not require cutaneous biopsies; because their symptoms are not shared by other diseases, a diagnosis can often be made by observation alone. Less easily recognized problems include lichen planus, an uncommon chronic pruritic disease; such potentially dangerous bullous diseases as pemphigus vulgaris, which is characterized by flat-topped papules on the wrists and legs that resemble poison ivy reactions; and skin cancer. Such conditions usually require biopsy to ensure that a mistaken diagnosis does not lead to the wrong treatment. Several methods of biopsy are employed, according to the nature of the lesion under examination. For example, the cutaneous punch technique, which utilizes a special surgical tool that penetrates to about 4 millimeters, may not be appropriate if the lesion is close to the surface. In this case, either curettage (scraping) or shave biopsy (cutting a layer corresponding to the thickness of the lesion) may be used in combination with the cutaneous punch method.

The total number of dermatoses that can be diagnosed is far too great for review here. The conditions that are most commonly treated, however, range from mildly serious but clearly irritating lesions such as acne or warts to much more serious phenomena such as psoriasis and lupus erythematosus. Several early and potentially dangerous conditions, especially basal cell carcinoma, may deteriorate into fatal skin cancers.

Dermatologists classify serious skin diseases under several key divisions. Pruritic dermatoses are characterized by itching. Vascular dermatoses, including several categories of urticaria, are all characterized by sudden outbreaks of papules—some temporary in their irritation and therefore merely disorders, as with hives as a reaction to poison ivy or medicines such as penicillin, and others more serious, such as swelling of the glottis, which may accompany angioneurotic edema. Papulosquamous dermatoses include psoriasis and lichen planus, both localized irritations that involve redness and flaking. In addition to these categories of dermatoses, a wide variety of common dermatologic viruses demand special medical attention because they are socially communicable. These include herpes simplex and herpes zoster. Other serious viruses affecting the skin, such as smallpox and measles, have been controlled by preventive vaccinations. Impetigo, once common during childhood in certain environments, is a bacterial infection, not a viral one. One formerly lethal sexually transmitted disease is syphilis, a form of spirochetal infection. Although far from eradicated, syphilis has been treatable through the use of benzathine penicillin since the mid-twentieth century.

The most serious challenge to dermatologists is the early diagnosis and treatment of skin cancer. The most common forms of skin cancer are basal cell epithelioma, which originates in the epidermis, often as a result of excessive exposure to the sun, and squamous cell carcinoma, which may affect the epidermis or mucosal surfaces (the inside of the mouth or throat). Early diagnosis of both types is essential to prevent metastasis (spreading). The most dangerous skin cancer is malignant melanoma, which may reveal itself through changes in size or color of a body mark such as a mole. This cancer can metastasize very rapidly and endanger the life of the patient.

Possible treatments for different types of skin disease vary considerably. Surgical operations, although certainly not unknown, tend to be associated with more extreme disorders, most notably skin cancer. In such cases, it is usually not the dermatologist but a specialized surgeon who performs the procedure.

The most common treatments used by dermatologists involve the application of various pharmaceutical preparations directly to the surface of the skin. For the treatment of common skin disorders, dermatologists may choose between a variety of medications.

The effect of antipruritic agents (menthol, phenol, camphor, or coal tar solutions) is to reduce itching. Keratoplastic agents (salicylic acid) and keratolytic agents (stronger doses of salicylic acid, resorcinol, or sulfur) affect the relative thickness or softness of the horny layer of the skin. They are associated with the treatment of diseases or disorders characterized by flaking.

Antieczematous agents, including coal tar solutions and hydrocortisone, halt oozing from vesicular lesions. By far the most commonly used drugs in dermatology are antiseptics which, according to their classification, control or kill bacteria, fungi, and viruses. Antibacterial agents that have been widely used for many years include iodochlorhydroxyquin and ammoniated mercury. Ointments to combat viral infections are much less common on the pharmaceutical market, but the recently developed drug acyclovir has been marketed under the name Zovirax.

These and many other topical applications may be only the first steps, however, in soothing the irritating side effects of more serious or chronically persistent dermatological diseases. Doctors may turn to more active therapies to treat specific ailments, beginning with the general category of electrosurgery, of which there are five specialized subtreatments: electrodesiccation, or the drying of tissues; electrocoagulation, which involves more intense heat; electrocautery, the actual burning of tissues; electrolysis, which produces the cauterization of lesions by chemical reaction; and electrosection, or the removal of tissues by cutting, achieved by the focus of electrical currents produced by various forms of vacuum tubes. By the 1990's, rapid progress in laser beam technology—particularly the carbon dioxide laser, which is a beam of infrared electromagnetic energy with an almost infinitesimal wavelength of 10,600 nanometers—began to replace some of these time-tested methods in cases in which electrosurgery had been commonplace for almost half a century.

Other modes of treatment that penetrate the subsurface layers of the skin include radiation therapy and cryosurgery, which is the immediate freezing of tissues by application of agents such as solid carbon dioxide (−78.5 degrees Celsius) or liquid nitrogen (−195.8 degrees Celsius). These methods are used to treat conditions ranging from psoriasis and pruritic dermatoses to skin cancer.

PERSPECTIVE AND PROSPECTS

One common feature—visible body surface symptoms—means that the medical identification and attempted treatment of human skin diseases can be traced to almost all cultures in all historical periods. An outstanding example of ancient peoples' concerns for eruptions on the skin can be found in the Old Testament or Talmud in Leviticus. In the Scripture, however, as well as in many medieval texts, one sees that a variety of skin diseases tended to be classified as leprosy. The physical location of skin lesions often determined the results of very general attempts at diagnosis.

It was not until the last quarter of the eighteenth century that Viennese physicians ushered in what could be called the first phase of scientific study of the skin and its disorders, or dermatology. This early Viennese school insisted on the study of the morphological nature of the lesions. Until this time, physicians had grouped skin diseases according to their appearance in different places on the body. By the mid-nineteenth century another Austrian, Ferdinand von Hebra, made considerable progress in classifying skin diseases.

Because so many lesions of the skin could potentially lead to diagnoses of sexually transmitted diseases, early generations of dermatologists concentrated most of their emphasis in this area. Discovery of a treatment for syphilis in the early twentieth century freed researchers to diversify their physiological investigations, opening the field to broader applications of biochemistry for treatment of different skin conditions, a field developed by the American doctor Stephen Rothman in the 1930's. Some categories, such as fungal diseases, were brought under control by treatments that were developed fairly quickly. By the second half of the century, dermatologists could alleviate most of the complications caused by psoriasis. Then, during the last quarter of the twentieth century, impressive advances in the discovery and patenting of sophisticated drugs brought most of the major dermatological diseases, including those caused in large part by nervous stress, under general control.

Although the treatment of life-threatening diseases, particularly skin cancers, continues to fall short of guaranteed cures, early recognition of their symptoms has steadily increased patients' chances for survival.

—*Byron D. Cannon, Ph.D.*

See also Abscess drainage; Abscesses; Acne; Age spots; Albinos; Athlete's foot; Biopsy; Birthmarks; Blisters; Boils; Bruises; Burns and scalds; Cancer; Carcinoma; Chickenpox; Cryosurgery; Cyst removal; Cysts; Dermatitis; Dermatology, pediatric; Dermatopathology; Diaper rash; Eczema; Electrocauterization; Fifth disease; Fungal infections; Glands; Grafts and grafting; Hair; Hair loss and baldness; Hair transplantation; Hand-foot-and-mouth disease; Healing; Histology; Hives; Human papillomavirus (HPV); Itching; Impetigo; Lice, mites, and ticks; Melanoma; Moles; Multiple chemical sensitivity syndrome; Nail removal; Necrotizing fasciitis; Neurofibromatosis; Pigmentation; Plastic surgery; Poisonous plants; Psoriasis; Rashes; Ringworm; Rosacea; Scabies; Sense organs; Skin; Skin cancer; Skin disorders; Skin lesion removal; Styes; Sunburn; Systemic lupus erythematosus (SLE); Tattoo removal; Tattoos and body piercing; Touch; Warts.

FOR FURTHER INFORMATION:

Braverman, Irwin M. *Skin Signs of Systemic Disease.* 3d ed. Philadelphia: W. B. Saunders, 1998. This book deals with the side effects of chronic diseases such as lymphomas and leukemia that may, at certain stages, be diagnosed through dermatological analysis.

Ceaser, Jennifer. *Everything You Need to Know About Acne.* Rev. ed. New York: Rosen, 2003. Covers the different forms of acne, their causes, and treatment forms in an approachable manner.

Hall, John C. *Sauer's Manual of Skin Diseases.* 9th ed. Philadelphia: Lippincott Williams & Wilkins, 2006. This very detailed and frequently updated text is among the most widely used in medical schools. Part of its organization consists of "reminder boxes" to emphasize salient points for diagnosis and therapy.

Jacknin, Jeanette. *Smart Medicine for Your Skin.* New York: Putnam, 2001. An accessible guide to skin care, written in an A-to-Z format. Explores both alternative and conventional therapies for everything from common acne to diminishing wrinkles.

Monk, B. E., R. A. C. Graham-Brown, and I. Sarkany, eds. *Skin Disorders in the Elderly.* Boston: Blackwell Scientific, 1988. As the title suggests, this collection of studies deals with typical skin problems among the elderly, many of which stem from infections elsewhere in the body.

Turkington, Carol, and Jeffrey S. Dover. *The Encyclopedia of Skin and Skin Disorders.* New York: Facts On File, 2002. More than one thousand entries on skin-related topics, including diseases, treatments, resources and organizations, skin cancer, acne treatment, FDA approvals of new treatments, and remedies for wrinkled skin.

Weedon, David. *Skin Pathology.* 2d ed. New York: Churchill Livingstone, 2002. Text with extensive photographs, covering tissue reaction patterns; the epidermis, dermis, and subcutis; the skin in systemic and miscellaneous diseases; infections and infestations; and tumors, among other topics.

DERMATOLOGY, PEDIATRIC
SPECIALTY

ANATOMY OR SYSTEM AFFECTED: Skin

SPECIALTIES AND RELATED FIELDS: Oncology, pediatrics, plastic surgery

DEFINITION: The medical specialty that deals with the diagnosis and treatment of diseases and disorders of the skin that occur in infants and children.

KEY TERMS:

congenital: existing or present at birth; usually also existing before birth

dermatitis: an inflammation of the skin

dermatosis: a condition of the skin; any skin disease not characterized by inflammation

skin biopsy: a small sample of skin removed for laboratory evaluation to help establish a diagnosis

systemic: affecting the entire body

topical treatment: a treatment that is placed on the skin itself

SCIENCE AND PROFESSION

A pediatric dermatologist is a skin doctor who has specialized training in the diagnosis and treatment of childhood skin disorders. The full course of training requires a medical degree followed by specialized residency training, usually at a large teaching hospital. Skin problems account for nearly one-third of all children's doctor visits. Most skin problems, however, are diagnosed in the primary care setting, by a pediatrician, family physician, physician assistant, or nurse practitioner. Primary care clinicians typically refer children with those conditions most difficult to diagnose or treat to the pediatric dermatologist. In addition, many general dermatologists also diagnose and treat children with skin problems.

The skin is the largest organ of the body and serves many functions. It is the body's first line of defense against infection, harmful substances, and radiation. It regulates body temperature. It conserves body fluids and also serves as a barrier to water. It helps in the production of vitamin D. The skin is also important in helping individuals sense the environment around them through special receptors for touch, heat, pain, and vibration. Any or all of these functions of the skin can be disrupted by the diseases and disorders that are diagnosed and treated by the pediatric dermatologist.

Children have some skin problems that are unique to childhood and share some skin problems with adults. For example, people of almost any age can have a condition called seborrheic dermatitis. Yet, each age group from infancy through adolescence has its own characteristic skin conditions or problems. For example, newborns may have salmon patches (commonly known as "stork bites"), infants may have diaper rash, and adolescents may have acne. Some childhood diseases, such as chickenpox, are found mostly in toddlers and school-age children. Likewise, some skin conditions, such as seborrheic keratoses, are found primarily in adults.

Changes in the skin may represent diseases and disorders of the skin itself, as in diaper dermatitis (diaper rash) or sunburn. Skin changes may also reflect a systemic disease or disorder, as in the rash associated with scarlet fever. Some skin lesions are markers for serious underlying conditions, either congenital or acquired. For example, a condition called neurofibromatosis may be signaled by the presence of multiple café-au-lait spots on the trunk. Thus, the pediatric dermatologist must be knowledgeable not only about the skin but also about all systemic diseases that produce skin changes.

DIAGNOSTIC AND TREATMENT TECHNIQUES

Most diagnoses relating to the skin are based on the appearance of the lesion itself. Lesions may be flat or raised, wet or dry, scattered or clustered, tender or nontender. They may have characteristic colors. They may be on the skin surface or extend beneath it. Typically, skin lesions are described according to their location on the body, their configuration, color, any changes that may have occurred as the result of secondary infection or scratching, and what the individual lesion itself looks like. In general, the pediatric dermatologist will inspect the skin of the entire body, even though only a small area may seem to be involved. In addition, the dermatologist will obtain a history related to the skin lesion: how long it has been there, whether it comes and goes, any changes that have taken place, what the patient or parents have used to treat the problem, allergies, and other symptoms such as pain or itching.

Usually, a thorough history and physical examination are sufficient to make the diagnosis of skin problems; however, the pediatric dermatologist may need to perform certain diagnostic or confirmatory tests. These tests may include a culture if a skin lesion is thought to be the result of an infection by a virus or bacterium. The dermatologist may gently scrape a lesion (particularly when a fungus is suspected) and examine the scrapings under a microscope. Certain dermatoses require the performance of a skin biopsy. In some cases, dermatologists punch out a small part of the skin lesion; in other cases, they cut out the entire lesion and a certain amount of surrounding tissue.

Treatments used by pediatric dermatologists may be topical, systemic, or surgical. Diaper dermatitis, for example, is usually treated with a topical cream or ointment aimed at killing the fungus that causes it. Impetigo, a bacterial infection of the skin, is usually treated with systemic antibiotics. Many kinds of skin lesions are treated with steroid creams, gels, or ointments. The dermatologist may surgically remove a mole with changes suspicious of skin cancer or use a laser to remove a birthmark.

PERSPECTIVE AND PROSPECTS

In the United States, many pediatric dermatologists (or general dermatologists with an interest in children's problems) belong to the Society for Pediatric Dermatology. The purpose of this group, formed in 1975, is to promote, develop, and advance education and research on skin conditions in children and to improve care. The group meets twice a year to present the latest advances in this field. The American Academy of Dermatology, while not specifically devoted to children's dermatology, also educates physicians about childhood problems. Another organization devoted specifically to children's skin problems is the International Society of Pediatric Dermatology.

—*Rebecca Lovell Scott, Ph.D., PA-C*

See also Acne; Albinos; Allergies; Birthmarks; Blisters; Boils; Bruises; Burns and scalds; Chickenpox; Childhood infectious diseases; Cradle cap; Dermatitis; Diaper rash; Fifth disease; Frostbite; Fungal infections; Hand-foot-and-mouth disease; Hives; Impetigo; Itching; Lice, mites, and ticks; Measles; Moles; Neurofibromatosis; Pityriasis alba; Pityriasis rosea; Plastic surgery; Poisonous plants; Psoriasis; Rashes; Ringworm; Roseola; Rubella; Scabies; Scarlet fever; Skin; Skin disorders; Styes; Sunburn; Tattoo removal; Tattoos and body piercing; Warts.

FOR FURTHER INFORMATION:

American Medical Association. *American Medical Association Family Medical Guide*. 4th rev. ed. Hoboken, N.J.: John Wiley & Sons, 2004. An excellent reference for the beginner. The scientific accuracy of the text is not compromised by its accessibility.

Beers, Mark H., et al., eds. *The Merck Manual of Medical Information, Second Home Edition*. Whitehouse Station, N.J.: Merck Research Laboratories, 2003. A team of nearly two hundred experts, consultants, and authors has assembled a body of information so vast that listing select items fails to do it justice.

Middlemiss, Prisca. *What's That Rash? How to Identify and Treat Childhood Rashes*. London: Hamlyn, 2002. A comprehensive guide to the identification and treatment of childhood rashes.

Schmitt, Barton D. *Your Child's Health: The Parents'*

One-Stop Reference Guide to Symptoms, Emergencies, Common Illnesses, Behavior Problems, Healthy Development. Rev. ed. New York: Bantam Books, 2005. Written for parents in a format that takes the guesswork out of when to call your health provider. This book covers almost any situation a parent could encounter. An essential resource.

Thompson, June. *Spots, Birthmarks, and Rashes: The Complete Guide to Caring for Your Child's Skin.* Toronto: Firefly Books, 2003. Guide for identifying and treating skin disorders with special attention to birthmarks and growths. Text accompanied by clear, color photographs.

Titman, Penny. *Understanding Childhood Eczema.* New York: Wiley, 2003. Discusses the physical and emotional toll of eczema on young patients and provides practical advice for choosing and managing different treatments.

Weston, William L., et al. *Color Textbook of Pediatric Dermatology.* 3d ed. New York: Elsevier, 2002. Clinical textbook that covers a range of disorders, including drug reactions, hair disorders, nail disorders, and sun sensitivity. Clinical features, differential diagnosis, pathogenesis, treatment, and patient education are discussed.

Woolf, Alan D., et al., eds. *The Children's Hospital Guide to Your Child's Health and Development.* Cambridge, Mass.: Perseus, 2002. An authoritative and comprehensive guide to children's health, providing a guide to every common illness or condition that affects children and a carefully designed emergency section.

DERMATOPATHOLOGY

SPECIALTY

ANATOMY OR SYSTEM AFFECTED: Immune system, skin

SPECIALTIES AND RELATED FIELDS: Cytology, dermatology, forensic medicine, histology, immunology, oncology, pathology

DEFINITION: The study of the causes and characteristics of diseases or changes involving the skin.

KEY TERMS:

basal cells: cells at the base of the epidermis that migrate upward and become the principal source of epidermal tissue

dermatoses: disorders of the skin

dermis: the layer of skin just below the surface, in which is found blood and lymphatic vessels, sebaceous (oil) glands, and nerves; also called the corium

epidermis: the outer layer of the skin, consisting of a dead superficial layer and an underlying cellular section

SCIENCE AND PROFESSION

Dermatopathology is the medical specialty that utilizes external clinical features of the body's surface, as well as histological changes that are observed microscopically, to define diseases of the skin. The dermatopathologist is a physician who has specialized in pathology, the clinical study of disease, and/or in histology, the microscopic study of cells and tissues. Although the specific clinical field of this specialty involves the skin, the practitioner has also received broader training in pathology.

The skin is the tough, cutaneous layer that covers the entire surface of the body. In addition to the epidermal tissue of the surface, the skin contains an extensive network of underlying structures, including lymphatic vessels, nerves and nerve endings, and hair follicles. The dead cells on the surface of the epidermis continually slough off, to be replaced by dividing cells from the underlying basal layers. As these cells proceed to the surface, they mature and die, forming the outer layer of the skin.

When a disease or condition of the skin is being diagnosed, the initial observations are often carried out by a general practitioner or dermatologist. This person will make a gross observation; if warranted, biopsies or samples of the lesion may then be provided to the dermatopathologist for examination. The most common forms of skin lesions are those associated with allergies, such as contact dermatitis associated with exposure to plant oils (poison ivy) or chemicals (antibiotics). More serious dermatologic diseases may also require diagnosis. Specific types of disease are often represented by specific kinds of lesions; these may include a variety of forms of skin cancers, lesions associated with bacterial or viral infections (such as impetigo or herpes simplex), and autoimmune disorders (such as lupus). The dermatopathologist may also be concerned with diseases of underlying tissue, such as lymphoid cancers or lesions penetrating into mucous membranes.

The dermatopathologist is involved in the diagnosis of the problem but generally is not involved with specific forms of treatment. Nevertheless, his or her recommendations may certainly influence any decisions. The major role of the dermatopathologist is observation; this may then be followed by an interpretation of results, including a possible prognosis or outcome.

DIAGNOSTIC AND TREATMENT TECHNIQUES

The clinical examination of skin lesions initially falls within the realm of the dermatologist. If the gross observations are insufficient to warrant diagnosis, however, a sample of the lesion can be sent to the dermatopathologist for further examination. In addition to the tissue sample, information on the age, sex, and skin color of the patient should be included, along with any history of the suspected condition.

If the lesion is superficial, as in dermatoses such as warts or even certain types of cancer, a superficial shave biopsy is sufficient for examination. If the lesion involves an infiltrating tumor, inflammation, or possible metabolic problems, a deeper section of tissue is necessary. The specimen is immediately placed in a fixative solution such as formalin, in order to prevent deterioration.

The dermatopathologist initially embeds the sample in paraffin, which can be sectioned into thin slices after hardening. The tissue is stained, most commonly with hematoxylin and eosin (H & E), and observed microscopically.

Anything about the cells that is out of the ordinary may be helpful in the diagnosis of the problem. For example, in the case of basal cell carcinoma, the cells may be abnormally shaped, with enlarged nuclei. They may also be observed infiltrating other layers of tissue. With contact dermatitis, the lesion is characterized by infiltration of large numbers of white blood cells, particularly lymphocytes, with their easily observed large nuclei. Edema, the abnormal accumulation of fluid, is also common with these types of lesions.

The presence of bacteria, as with boils or impetigo, warrants the use of antibiotics, unlike other inflammatory lesions. In this matter, the dermatopathology of the sample can determine the appropriate form of treatment.

While dermatopathology is primarily observational, recommendations regarding treatment may be made by its practitioners. For example, the study of a sample for the type and extent of cancer may lead to a recommendation concerning how extensive the surgical removal of the tumor should be.

PERSPECTIVE AND PROSPECTS

The use of the physical appearance of the skin as a means of diagnosis represents one of the earliest attempts to understand disease. With the microscopic examination of tissue, first performed during the nineteenth century, it became possible to match the presence of histological lesions to specific diseases and to differentiate these diseases from one another.

The field of dermatopathology was greatly refined during the twentieth century. The development of differential and immunological staining methods allowed for a greater understanding of the roles played by the wide variety of cells in the body. For example, the dendritic cells of the skin were found to have a critical function in the immune responses which begin at that level.

In many Western countries, there was a significant shift during the twentieth century in the types of skin disease most commonly seen, mostly reflecting changes in lifestyle. The prevalence of malignant melanomas and basal cell carcinomas became much higher as a result of increased exposure to sun during leisure hours. The recognition of such problems has become an important aspect of the training of clinicians less specialized than dermatopathologists, such as family physicians.

—*Richard Adler, Ph.D.*

See also Autoimmune disorders; Bacterial infections; Biopsy; Cancer; Carcinoma; Cytopathology; Dermatitis; Dermatology; Edema; Electrocauterization; Grafts and grafting; Herpes; Histology; Human papillomavirus (HPV); Melanoma; Microscopy; Oncology; Pathology; Pigmentation; Plastic surgery; Skin; Skin cancer; Skin disorders; Skin lesion removal; Systemic lupus erythematosus (SLE); Viral infections; Warts.

FOR FURTHER INFORMATION:

Caputo, Ruggero, and Carlo Gemetti. *Pediatric Dermatology and Dermatopathology: A Concise Atlas*. Washington, D.C.: Taylor & Francis, 2002. Reviews childhood dermatologic diseases in alphabetical order with a brief description and photos of clinical and pathological features.

McKee, Phillip. *A Concise Atlas of Dermatopathology*. New York: Gower Medical, 1993. This atlas of skin problems discusses histopathology, among other topics. Includes an index.

Mehregan, Amir H., et al. *Pinkus' Guide to Dermatohistopathology*. 6th ed. Norwalk, Conn.: Appleton & Lange, 1995. The sixth edition of a diagnostic reference to dermal pathology, for dermatology residents and practitioners. References extensively updated. Abundant halftone illustrations.

Tierney, Lawrence M., Stephen J. McPhee, and Maxine A. Papadakis, eds. *Current Medical Diagnosis and Treatment 2007*. New York: McGraw-Hill

Medical, 2006. This text, updated yearly, is the point of reference for physicians and other health care practitioners. It incorporates each year's biomedical research discoveries that have immediate, relevant, and applicable use for the patient.

Weedon, David. *Skin Pathology.* 2d ed. New York: Churchill Livingstone, 2002. Text with extensive photographs, covering tissue reaction patterns; the epidermis, dermis, and subcutis; the skin in systemic and miscellaneous diseases; infections and infestations; and tumors, among other topics.

Developmental stages
Development

Anatomy or system affected: Brain, nervous system, psychic-emotional system

Specialties and related fields: Neurology, psychiatry, psychology

Definition: The growth and changes that occur over time in children's mental and physical processes as they develop from birth to adulthood.

Key terms:

attachment: special relationship of mutual closeness established between an infant and a caregiver; based on consistent caring, it confers an anticipation of security in relationships

concrete operations stage: Jean Piaget's cognitive stage in which concrete, easily visualized objects can be grouped together, combined, and transformed in equivalent ways; "concrete" contrasts with "formal" operations, which involve abstract and hypothetical transformations

initiative versus guilt: Erik Erikson's characterization for the young child's imaginative exploration of wishes and impulses in fantasy and dramatic play, restrained by emerging pangs of conscience

mental operations: comprehension of the reversibility of such events as regrouping objects into different categories or transferring a fixed quantity of a substance into containers of different shapes

preoperational stage: Piaget's transitional stage of young childhood in which absent objects can be remembered from mental representations but cannot be grouped or logically manipulated

sensorimotor stage: Piaget's stage in infancy in which objects can be recognized by appropriate habitual reactions to them

stage: a period in a progressive, invariant sequence of events when specified cognitive and motivational events are programmed to occur

Physical and Psychological Factors

The development of the human being from the infant to the child to the adolescent to the adult is a story of increasing physical, cognitive, social, and emotional adequacy in coping with environmental demands. Major observers of human development have added a key corollary concerning the nature and pace of this development: It occurs in stages.

Development in stages implies several features about the process. The first implication is that developmental changes are not simply quantitative but also qualitative, changes not only in degree but also in kind. With advancement to another stage, perceptions, thoughts, motives, and social interactions are fundamentally altered. A second implication is that development is uneven in its pace—sometimes flowing and sometimes ebbing, sometimes fast and sometimes slow and steady in apparent equilibrium. A third implication is that the order of the stages is invariant: One always moves from lower to higher stages. No individual skips stages; each subsequent stage is a necessary antecedent to the more mature or advanced stages to come. The invariant sequence is preordained by the biological maturation of neurological systems and by the necessary requirements of human societies.

Descriptions of development in terms of stages are found in the writings of many psychologists, especially cognitive psychologists, who are interested in age-related changes in thinking styles, and psychoanalytic psychologists, influenced by Sigmund Freud, who concern themselves with changes in the growing child's emotional involvements. The most significant, influential, and comprehensive of stage descriptions of development are those of two seminal scientists, Jean Piaget (1896-1980) and Erik Erikson (1902-1994).

Piaget, a cognitive developmental psychologist, outlined a series of shifts in children's cognition, their ways of thinking about and interpreting the world. They include the sensorimotor stage in infancy, the preoperational stage beginning in toddlerhood, the intuitive preoperational substage of the preschool child, the concrete operations stage of the school-age child, and the formal operations stage beginning in adolescence.

Erikson, who updated psychoanalytic theory, outlined a series of age-related shifts in motives and ways of relating to others, each one related to a psychosocial crisis. These psychosocial stages include an infancy stage of trust versus mistrust, a toddlerhood stage of autonomy versus shame and doubt, a preschool childhood stage of initiative versus guilt, a school-age stage of competence versus inferiority, and an adolescent stage of identity versus role diffusion.

The approaches of Piaget and Erikson originated independently, each emphasizing different aspects of development. The stages that they describe, however, should be viewed as complementary. Since the social changes result in large part from shifts in the child's thinking, the psychosocial stages of Erikson closely parallel the cognitive stages outlined by Piaget.

In infancy, a period lasting from birth to about eighteen months, sensorimotor cognitive development is initiated by rapid brain development. During the first six months of life, the nerve cells in the forebrain that control coordinated movements, refined sensory discriminations, speech, and intellect increase greatly in number and size and develop a rich network of connections. This neural growth makes possible dramatic progress in the child's ability to discriminate relevant objects and to coordinate precise movements of arms, legs, and fingers in relating to these objects. The infant who was capable of only a few reflexes at birth by six months can grasp a dangling object. The infant who was born with very poor visual acuity by six months can recognize detailed patterns in toys and faces. The infant shows recognition and knowledge of an object by relating to it repeatedly with the same pattern of movements. During the first few months of life, the infant has very limited ability to recall objects when they are not directly seen or heard and, in fact, will fail to look for a toy when it is not in view. Sensorimotor integrations, therefore, form the infant's principal method of representing reality. Only gradually does attention span increase and does the infant acquire the capacity to think about missing objects. The capacity to keep out-of-sight objects in mind, the gradual appreciation of object permanence, is a key achievement of the sensorimotor stage.

The corresponding psychosocial stage of infancy is built around the establishment of trust, some sort of sustaining faith in the stability of the world and the security of human relationships. Crucial to the establishing of this trust is the stability of the infant's relationship with a primary caregiver, most commonly a mother. Babies begin to pay special attention to the caregiver on a schedule determined by their cognitive development. The primary caregiving adult is among the first significant objects identified by the infant. Indeed, it appears that infants are wired to be especially responsive to a human caregiver. Infants of only two or

three months of age find the human face the most interesting object and will focus on faces and facelike designs in preference to almost any other stimulus object. By the age of six months, infants clearly recognize the caregiver as special but for some time cannot appreciate that the caregiver continues to exist during absences. Thus, conspicuous anxiety sometimes occurs when the caregiver leaves.

It is little wonder that an infant perceives the caregiver as special. The human caregiver is wonderfully reinforcing to the infant. Relief from all kinds of pain, smiling responses to infantile smiles, vocal responses to infant babbling, soft and warm cuddling contact, and games all offer to the infant what is most craved. By six to nine months of age, the baby seems dependent on the caregiver for a basic feeling of security. Until the age of two or three, most infants seem more secure when their mother or primary caregiver is physically present. The relationship between the quality and warmth of infant-mother interactions and the infant's feelings of security has been supported by voluminous research on mother-infant attachment.

By about age two, neural and physical developments make possible the advance to more adaptive styles of cognitive interpretations. Piaget characterized the cognitive stage of toddlerhood as preoperational. Brain centers important for language and movement continue to develop rapidly. Now the child can deal cognitively with reality in a new way, by representing out-of-sight and distant objects and events by words, images, and symbols. The child can also imitate the actions of people not present. Thinking during this stage remains limited. The child cannot yet hold several thoughts simultaneously in mind and manipulate them—that is, perform mental operations. This stage is, therefore, "preoperational."

Erikson described the psychosocial crisis of toddlerhood as autonomy versus shame and doubt. This crisis results in part from the child's cognitive growth. The preoperational child has acquired an increasing ability to appreciate the temporary nature of a caregiver's absence and to move about independently. The toddler can now assert autonomy and often does so emphatically. Resistance to parental demands is possible, and the toddler seems to delight in such resistance. "No" becomes a favorite word. Since this period corresponds to the time when children are toilet trained, parent-child tugs-of-war often involve issues of bowel control and cleanliness. The beginning of shame, the humiliation that comes from overextending freedom foolishly and making mistakes, begins to serve as a self-imposed check on this autonomy.

Piaget characterized the thinking of three-, four-, and five-year-olds as "intuitive." This thinking is still preoperational. Children can represent to themselves all sorts of objects but cannot keep these objects in the focus of attention long enough to classify them or consider how these objects could be regrouped or transformed. If six tin soldiers are stretched into three groups of two, the preschool child assumes that there are now more than before. Thinking is egocentric because children lack the ability to put themselves in the perspective of others while keeping their own perspective. Yet preschool children make all sorts of intuitive attempts to fit remembered events and scenes into underlying plots or themes. Fanciful attempts to understand events often result in misconstruing the nature of things. Children at this stage are easily misled by appearances. A man in a tiger suit could become a tiger; a boy who wears a dress could become a girl and grow up to be a mother. Appearance becomes reality.

Erikson characterized the corresponding psychosocial stage of the preschool child as involving the crisis of initiative versus guilt. The child's new initiative is expressed in playful exploration of fanciful possibilities. Children can pretend and transform themselves in play as never before and never again. From dramatic play, the child's conceptions of the many possibilities of the world of bigger people are enacted. The earlier psychoanalyst, Freud, focused particularly on how children experience their first sexual urges at this time of life and sometimes weave into their ruminations fantastic themes of possession of the opposite-sex parent and jealous triumph over the same-sex parent. To Erikson, such themes are merely examples of the many playful fantasies essential to later, more realistic involvements.

Piaget characterized the cognitive stage of the school-age child as the concrete operations stage. The child is capable of mental operations. The school-age child can focus on several incidents, objects, or events simultaneously. Now it is obvious that six tin soldiers sorted into three pairs of two could easily be transformed back into a single group of six. Regardless of grouping, the total quantity is the same. The formerly egocentric child becomes cognitively capable of empathetic role taking, of assuming the perspective of another person while keeping the perspective of the self in mind. In making ethical choices, the child can now appreciate the impact of alternative possibilities on particular people in particular situations. The harshness of absolute dictates is softened by empathetic understanding of others.

Erikson characterized the psychosocial crisis of the school-age child as one of competence versus inferiority. Now is the time for children to acquire the many verbal, computational, and social skills that are required for adequate adulthood. Learning experiences are structured and planned, and performances are evaluated. Newly empathetic children are only too aware of how their skill levels are perceived by others. Adequacy is being assessed. The schoolchild must not only be good but also be good at something.

The cognitive stage of the adolescent was described by Piaget as formal operational. The dramatic physical changes that signal sexual maturity are accompanied by less obvious neural changes, especially a fine tuning of the frontal lobes of the brain, the brain's organizing, sequencing, executive center. Cognitively, the adolescent becomes capable of dealing with formal operations. Unlike concrete operations, which can be visualized, formal operations include abstract possibilities that are purely hypothetical, abstract strategies useful in ordering a sequence of investigations, and "as if" or "let us suppose" propositions.

Erikson's corresponding psychosocial crisis of adolescence was that of identity versus role diffusion. The many physical and mental changes and the impending necessity of finding occupational, social, marital, religious, and political roles in the adult world impel a concern with the question, "Who am I?" To interact as an adult, one must know what one likes and loathes, what one values and despises, and what one can do well, poorly, and not at all. Most adolescents succeed in finding themselves—some by adopting the identity of family and parents, some after a soul-searching struggle.

DISORDERS AND EFFECTS

Stage theories define success as advancement through the series of stages to maturity. Psychosocially, each successful advance yields a virtue that makes life endurable: hope, will, purpose, competence, and finally fidelity to one's own true self. As a final reward for normal developmental success, one can enjoy the benefits of adulthood: intimacy, or the sharing of one's identity with another, and generativity, or the contribution of one's own gifts to the benefit of the next generation and to the collective progress of humankind. Cognitively, maturity means the capacity for formal operational thought. Hypothetical thinking of this type is basic to most fields of higher learning, to the sciences, to philosophy, and even to the comprehension of such abstract moral principles as justice.

Advancement to each subsequent stage of cognitive development is dependent on both neurological maturation and a culture that presents appropriate problems. Adults who fail to attain concrete operational thought are considered mentally retarded. A failure in neurological maturation is a frequent cause. Failures to attain formal operational thought, on the other hand, are not unusual among normal adults. Cultural experience must nourish advancement to formal operational thinking within a domain of inquiry by the provision of moderately novel and challenging but not overwhelming tasks. When people are not confronted with such complex problems within some domain, then abstract, formal operational thought fails to occur. Abstract ethical reasoning is a case in point. Cross-cultural studies suggest that concepts of justice that involve the application of abstract rules are rare in cultures where people seldom confront questions of ethical complexity.

Psychosocial pathology is evidenced by development arrested in one of the immature stages of psychosocial development. It results from a social environment that fails to foster growth or exaggerates the particular apprehensions that are most acute in one of the developmental stages.

The development of trust in infancy requires a loving, available, and sensitive caretaker. If the infant's caretaker is unavailable, missing, neglectful, or abusive, the pathology of mistrust develops. The world is perceived as unstable. Close personal relationships are viewed as unreliable, fickle, and possibly malicious. Later, closeness in relationships may be rejected. Confident exploration of the possibilities of life may never be attempted.

Similarly, the apprehensions of each subsequent psychosocial stage can be exaggerated to the point of pathology. The toddler, shamed out of troublesome expressions of autonomy, may compensate for doubts with the rigidly excessive controls of the compulsive lifestyle. The preschool child can become so overwhelmed with guilt over playful fantasies, particularly sexual and aggressively tinged fantasies, that adult possibilities become severely restricted. The school-age child can become so wounded by humiliations in a harshly competitive school environment that the child becomes beaten down into enduring feelings of inferiority. An adolescent may so fear the risks of exploring the possibilities of life that future adulthood becomes a shallow diffusion of roles, a yielding to social pressures and whims unguided by any knowledge of who one really is.

The successful confrontation of the tasks of adulthood—finding a partner to share intimacy and caring for the next generation—are most easily attainable for adults who have overcome each of these earlier developmental hurdles.

Perspective and Prospects

Stage theories of development are found as early as 1900 in the work of American psychologist James Mark Baldwin and in Freud's psychoanalysis. Baldwin, much influenced by Charles Darwin's theory of evolution by natural selection, hypothesized that the infant emerges from a sensorimotor stage of infancy to a symbolic mode of thinking, an advancement yielding enormous evolutionary advantages. Freud, the Viennese psychoanalyst, based his conception of emotional development on what he called psychosexual stages. Progression occurs from an oral period of infancy, when sensory pleasure is concentrated on the mouth region, to an anal stage of toddlerhood, when anal pleasures and the control of such pleasures become of concern. When sexual pleasure shifts to the genital region in the three-year-old, the love of the opposite-sex parent becomes sexually tinged, and the child becomes jealous of the same-sex parent. Working through these so-called Oedipal fantasies was, to Freud, crucial to the formation of personality.

Neither Baldwin nor Freud and his followers were the sort of rigorous scientists most respected by scientific psychology in the mid-twentieth century. Far more influential in American psychology between 1920 to about 1960 were behavioral conceptions of the developmental process as steady, incremental growth. To behaviorists such as B. F. Skinner, becoming an adult was conceived as a process of continuously being reinforced for learning progressively more adequate responses.

The stage approaches of Piaget and Erikson were introduced to most American psychologists in 1950, the year that both Piaget's *Psychology of Intelligence* and Erikson's *Childhood and Society* were published in English. Piaget's description of cognitive stages was much more complete than Baldwin's earlier account and was much better supported by clever behavioral observations. Erikson's thesis of psychosocial stages incorporated most of Freud's observations about stages. Erikson treated the social environmental pressures intrinsic to each stage as events of primary importance and shifts in the locus of bodily pleasures as secondary.

By the 1970's, Piaget's and Erikson's accounts of stages were awarded an important place in most developmental texts. This influence occurred for several reasons. First, researchable hypotheses were derived, and most of this research was supportive. Cross-cultural comparisons suggested that these stages could be found in a similar sequence in differing cultures. Second, the theses of Piaget and Erikson were mutually supportive. The stage-related cognitive changes, in fact, would seem to explain the corresponding psychosocial concerns. Finally, these approaches generated productive spinoffs in related theory and research. In 1969, basing his work on the cognitive changes outlined by Piaget, Lawrence Kohlberg elaborated a stage sequence of progressively more adequate methods of moral reasoning. In 1978, basing her work on Erikson's hypotheses about trust, Mary Ainsworth began a productive research program on the antecedents and consequents of stable and unstable mother-infant attachment styles.

The most recent challenges to cognitive and psychosocial stage theory arise from the alternative perspectives of biopsychology and information-processing theory. Some psychologists argue that biologically rooted temperament, rather than the social environment, affects both styles of attachment and identity formation. Not only do babies respond to caregivers, but caregivers respond to babies as well. A baby who begins with a shy, passive temperament may be more susceptible to an avoidant attachment style and more likely to elicit detached, unresponsive caregiver behavior. Temperament, it is maintained, is more important than psychosocial environment.

Information processing theorists have challenged the discontinuity implied by stage concepts. They suggest that the appearance of global transformations in the structure of thought may be an illusion. Development is a continuous growth of efficiency in processing and problem solving. The growing child combines an expanding number of ideas, increases the level and speed of processing by increments, and learns more effective problem-solving strategies. To select particular points in this continuous development and call them "stages," they argue, is purely arbitrary.

The final research to settle the question of the ultimate nature of stages has not been performed. A psychosocial stage theorist can acknowledge the role of temperament but still maintain that loving, trust-creating environments are also significant in encouraging the child to apply temperamental potential in positive social directions rather than in angry antagonism or frightened withdrawal. At the very least, Piagetian and Eriksonian stage concepts have the practical usefulness of highlighting significant developmental events and interpersonal reactions to these events. The warmth of caregivers for infants, the later tolerance of children's struggles to become themselves, and environments that present challenging problems appropriate to the child's developmental level are vital to emotional and intellectual growth.

For some purposes, it may be instructive to break the achievement of cognitive and emotional growth into increments that can be seen as if under a microscope. For other purposes, it is instructive to go up for an aerial view to gain perspective on the nature and direction of such achievements. The aerial view is the contribution of stage theories of development.

—Thomas E. DeWolfe, Ph.D.

See also Bed-wetting; Bonding; Cognitive development; Motor skill development; Puberty and adolescence; Reflexes, primitive; Separation anxiety; Soiling; Speech disorders; Teething; Thumb sucking; Toilet training; Weaning.

For Further Information:

Berk, Laura E. *Child Development*. 7th ed. Boston: Pearson/Allyn and Bacon, 2006. A text that reviews theory and research in child development, cognitive and language development, personality and social development, and the foundations and contexts of development.

Feldman, Robert S. *Development Across the Life Span*. 4th ed. Upper Saddle River, N.J.: Pearson/Prentice Hall, 2006. Traces the physical, cognitive, and social and personality development of one's life span, focusing on basic theories, research findings, and current applications of theory.

Ginsburg, Herbert, and Sylvia Opper. *Piaget's Theory of Intellectual Development*. 3d ed. Englewood Cliffs, N.J.: Prentice Hall, 1988. A detailed, book-length elaboration of Jean Piaget's stage theory of cognitive development.

Hall, Calvin S., Gardner Lindzey, and John B. Campbell. *Theories of Personality*. 4th ed. New York: John Wiley & Sons, 1998. Chapter 5, "Current Psychoanalytic Theory," describes Erikson's psychosocial stages and current research inspired by this theory. Chapter 2 describes Sigmund Freud's earlier psychosexual stages.

Karen, Robert. "Becoming Attached." *Atlantic Monthly* 265, no. 2 (February, 1990): 35-70. A thorough, fair, and readable account of the research on attachment and its relationship to trust in people.

Miller, Patricia H. *Theories of Developmental Psychology*. 4th ed. New York: Worth, 2002. A comparative analysis of developmental theories. Piaget's cognitive stage theory and Freud's and Erikson's psychoanalytic theories are described and compared with other developmental approaches.

Nathanson, Laura Walther. *The Portable Pediatrician: A Practicing Pediatrician's Guide to Your Child's Growth, Development, Health, and Behavior from Birth to Age Five*. 2d ed. New York: HarperCollins, 2002. An engaging, easy-to-read guide for parents to assess their child's development, medical symptoms, and behavioral problems.

Parke, Ross D., et al., eds. *A Century of Developmental Psychology*. Washington, D.C.: American Psychological Association, 1994. Contains material on the early approaches of James Mark Baldwin and a review of attachment theory and research.

Sternberg, Robert J. *Psychology: In Search of the Human Mind*. 3d ed. Fort Worth, Tex.: Harcourt College, 2001. As in most other texts in introductory psychology, the stage theories of Erik Erikson and Jean Piaget are described in the chapter on human development. A good discussion of the concept of developmental stages.

Diabetes mellitus
Disease/disorder

Anatomy or system affected: Abdomen, blood vessels, circulatory system, endocrine system, eyes, gastrointestinal system, glands, heart, kidneys, nervous system, pancreas

Specialties and related fields: Endocrinology, family medicine, genetics, internal medicine, nephrology, neurology, pediatrics, vascular medicine

Definition: A hormonal disorder in which the pancreas is not able to produce sufficient insulin to process and maintain proper blood sugar levels, insulin resistence, or both; if left untreated, it leads to secondary complications such as blindness, cardiovascular disease, dementia, kidney disease, and eventually death.

Key terms:

beta cells: the insulin-producing cells located at the core of the islets of Langerhans in the pancreas; the

alpha, or glucagon-producing, cells form an outer coat

cross-linking: a chemical reaction, triggered by the binding of glucose to tissue proteins, that results in the attachment of one protein to another and the loss of elasticity in aging tissues

glucosuria: a condition in which the concentration of blood glucose exceeds the ability of the kidney to reabsorb it; as a result, glucose spills into the urine, taking with it body water and electrolytes

hyperglycemia: excessive levels of glucose in the circulating blood

insulin-dependent diabetes mellitus (IDDM): Type I diabetes, a state of absolute insulin deficiency in which the body does not produce sufficient insulin to move glucose into the cells

insulin resistance: a lack of insulin action; a reduction in the effectiveness of insulin to lower blood glucose concentrations; characteristic of Type II diabetes

insulitis: the selective destruction of the insulin-producing beta cells in Type I diabetes

islets of Langerhans: clusters of cells scattered throughout the pancreas; they produce three hormones involved in sugar metabolism: insulin, glucagon, and somatostatin

ketoacidosis: high levels of ketones in the blood that result from a lack of circulating insulin

non-insulin-dependent diabetes mellitus (NIDDM): Type II diabetes, which is the state of a relative insulin deficiency; although insulin is released, its target cells do not adequately respond to it by taking up blood glucose

Causes and Symptoms

Diabetes mellitus is by far the most common of all endocrine (hormonal) disorders. The word "diabetes" is derived from the Greek word for "siphon" or "running through," a reference to the potentially large urine volume that can accompany the condition. *Mellitus*, the Latin word for "honey," was added when physicians began to make the diagnosis of diabetes mellitus based on the sweet taste of the patient's urine. The disease has been depicted as a state of starvation in the midst of plenty. Although there is plenty of sugar in the blood, without insulin it does not reach the cells that need it for energy. Glucose, the simplest form of sugar, is the primary source of energy for many vital functions. Deprived of glucose, cells starve and tissues begin to degenerate. The unused glucose builds up in the bloodstream, which leads to a series of secondary complications.

The most common symptoms of diabetes mellitus are related to hyperglycemia, glycosuria, and ketoacidosis. The acute symptoms of diabetes mellitus are all attributable to inadequate insulin action. The immediate consequence of an insulin insufficiency is a marked decrease in the ability of both muscle and adipose (fat) tissue to remove glucose from the blood. In the presence of inadequate insulin action, a second problem manifests itself. People with diabetes continue to make the hormone glucagon. Glucagon, which raises the level of blood sugar, can be considered insulin's biological opposite. Like insulin, glucagon is released from the pancreatic islets. The release of glucagon is normally inhibited by insulin; therefore, in the absence of insulin, glucagon action elevates concentrations of glucose. For this reason, diabetes may be considered a "two-hormone disease." With a reduction in the conversion of glucose into its storage forms of glycogen in liver and muscle tissue and lipids in adipose cells, concentrations of glucose in the blood steadily increase (hyperglycemia). When the amount of glucose in the blood exceeds the capacity of the kidney to reabsorb this nutrient, glucose begins to spill into the urine (glucosuria). Glucose in the urine then drags additional body water along with it so that the volume of urine dramatically increases. In the absence of adequate fluid intake, the loss of body water and accompanying electrolytes (sodium) leads to dehydration and, ultimately, death caused by the failure of the peripheral circulatory system.

Insulin deficiency also results in a decrease in the synthesis of triglycerides (storage forms of fatty acids) and stimulates the breakdown of fats in adipose tissue. Although glucose cannot enter the cells and be used as an energy source, the body can use its supply of lipids from the fat cells as an alternate source of energy. Fatty acids increase in the blood, causing hyperlipidemia. With large amounts of circulating free fatty acids available for processing by the liver, the production and release of ketone bodies (breakdown products of fatty acids) into the circulation are accelerated, causing both ketonemia and an increase in the acidity of the blood. Since the ketone levels soon also exceed the capacity of the kidney to reabsorb them, ketone bodies soon appear in the urine (ketonuria).

Insulin deficiency and glucagon excess also cause pronounced effects on protein metabolism and result in an overall increase in the breakdown of proteins and a

---

INFORMATION ON DIABETES MELLITUS

CAUSES: Genetic and environmental factors
SYMPTOMS: Large urine output, excessive thirst, dehydration, low blood pressure, weight loss despite increased appetite, fatigue, nausea, vomiting, blurred vision
DURATION: Chronic
TREATMENTS: Insulin or oral hypoglycemic drugs, lifestyle changes (diet modification and exercise)

---

reduction in the uptake of amino acid precursors into muscle protein. This leads to the wasting and weakening of skeletal muscles and, in children who are diabetics, results in a reduction in overall growth. Unfortunately, the increased level of amino acids in the blood provides an additional source of material for glucose production (gluconeogenesis) by the liver. All these acute metabolic changes in carbohydrates, lipids, and protein metabolism can be prevented or reversed by the administration of insulin.

There are three distinct types of diabetes mellitus. Type I, or insulin-dependent diabetes mellitus (IDDM), is an absolute deficiency of insulin that accounts for approximately 10 percent of all cases of diabetes. Until the discovery of insulin, people stricken with Type I diabetes faced certain death within about a year of diagnosis. In Type II or non-insulin-dependent diabetes mellitus (NIDDM), insulin secretion may be normal or even increased, but the target cells for insulin are less responsive than normal (insulin resistance); therefore, insulin is not as effective in lowering blood glucose concentrations. Although either type can be manifested at any age, Type I diabetes has a greater prevalence in children, whereas the incidence of Type II diabetes increases markedly after the age of forty and is the most common type of diabetes. Genetic and environmental factors are important in the expression of both of these types of diabetes mellitus. The third type is gestational diabetes, which is characterized by high blood glucose during pregnancy in a person who did not previously have diabetes.

Type I diabetes is an autoimmune process that involves the selective destruction of the insulin-producing beta cells in the islets of Langerhans (insulitis). The triggering event that initiates this process in genetically susceptible persons is linked to environmental factors that result from an infection, a virus, or, more likely, the presence of toxins in the diet. The body's own T lymphocytes progressively attack the beta cells but leave the other hormone-producing cell types intact. T lymphocytes are white blood cells that normally attack virus-invaded cells and cancer cells. For up to ten years, there remains a sufficient number of insulin-producing cells to respond effectively to a glucose load, but when approximately 80 percent of the beta cells are destroyed, there is insufficient insulin release in response to a meal and the deadly spiral of the consequences of diabetes mellitus is triggered. Insulin injection can halt this lethal process and prevent it from recurring but cannot mimic the normal pattern of insulin release from the pancreas. It is interesting that not everyone who has insulitis actually progresses to experience overt symptoms of the disease, although it is known that the incidence of Type I diabetes around the world is on the increase.

Type II diabetes is normally associated with obesity and lack of exercise as well as with genetic predisposition. Recently, with the reported increased rates of obesity and inactivity in children, there has also been an increase of Type II diabetes at younger and younger ages. Family studies have shown that as many as 25 to 35 percent of persons with Type II diabetes have a sibling or parent with the disease. The risk of diabetes doubles if both parents are affected. Native Americans and other ethnic minorities have a higher incidence of Type II diabetes in youth than do Caucasians. Even in adults, the prevalence of this type of diabetes is higher in minority groups, such as Hispanics, Native Americans, and African Americans, than it is in Caucasians.

Because there is a reduction in the sensitivity of the target cells to insulin, people with Type II diabetes must secrete more insulin to maintain blood glucose at normal levels. Because insulin is a storage, or anabolic, hormone, this increased secretion further contributes to obesity. In response to the elevated insulin concentrations, the number of insulin receptors on the target cell gradually decreases, which triggers an even greater secretion of insulin. In this way, the excess glucose is stored despite the decreased availability of insulin binding sites on the cell. Over time, the demands for insulin eventually exceed even the reserve capacity of the "genetically weakened" beta cells, and symptoms of insulin deficiency develop as the plasma glucose concentrations remain high for increasingly longer periods of time. Because the symptoms of Type II diabetes are usually less severe than those of Type I diabetes, many persons have the disease but remain unaware of it. Unfortunately, once the diagnosis of diabetes is made in these individuals, they also exhibit symptoms of long-term complications that include atherosclerosis and nerve damage. Hence, Type II diabetes has been called the "silent killer."

Gestational diabetes develops during pregnancy in a person who did not have diabetes before becoming pregnant. It occurs in approximately 7 percent of all pregnancies. Women with gestational diabetes have an increased risk of developing diabetes after pregnancy. Children of women with gestational diabetes have a higher risk of obesity, glucose intolerance, and diabetes in adolescence.

Prediabetes is a condition in which individuals have blood glucose levels that are high, but not high enough to be diagnosed with Type II diabetes; they are at higher risk to develop diabetes in the future.

Treatment and Therapy

Insulin is the only treatment available for Type I diabetes, and in many cases it is used to treat individuals with Type II diabetes. Insulin is available in many formulations, which differ in respect to the time of onset of action, activity, and duration of action. Insulin preparations are classified as fast-acting, intermediate-acting, and long-acting; the effects of fast-acting insulin last for thirty minutes to twenty-four hours, while those of

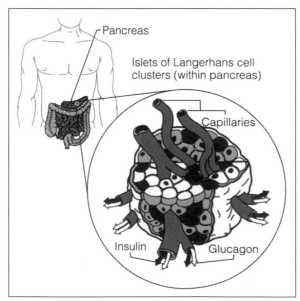

Location of the pancreas, with a section showing the specialized cells (islets of Langerhans) that produce the sugar-metabolizing hormones.

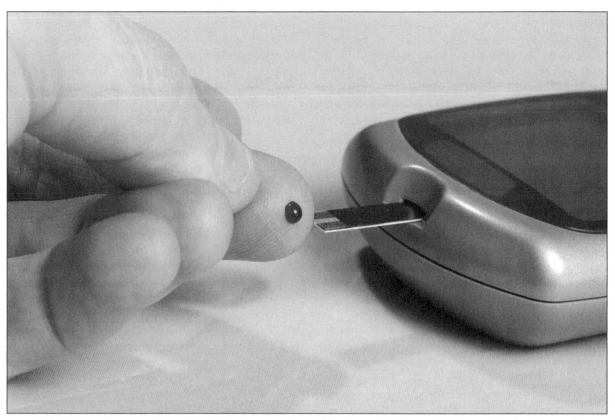

A diabetic performs a glucose level check using a finger blood test. (© Eugene Bochkarev/iStockphoto.com)

long-acting preparations last from four to thirty-six hours. Some of the factors that affect the rate of insulin absorption include the site of injection, the patient's age and health status, and the patient's level of physical activity. For a person with diabetes, however, insulin is a reprieve, not a cure. In 2006, the Food and Drug Administration (FDA) approved the use of inhaled insulin for individuals eighteen years or older. It is absorbed into the bloodstream via the lungs. Studies have shown promise in its effectiveness in controlling blood glucose.

Because of the complications that arise from chronic exposure to glucose, it is recommended that glucose concentrations in the blood be maintained as close to physiologically normal levels as possible. For this reason, it is preferable to administer multiple doses of insulin during the day. By monitoring plasma glucose concentrations, the diabetic person can adjust the dosage of insulin administered and thus mimic normal concentrations of glucose relatively closely. Basal concentrations of plasma insulin can also be maintained throughout the day by means of electromechanical insulin delivery systems. Whether internal or external,

such insulin pumps can be programmed to deliver a constant infusion of insulin at a rate designed to meet minimum requirements. The infusion can then be supplemented by a bolus injection prior to a meal. Increasingly sophisticated systems automatically monitor blood glucose concentrations and adjust the delivery rate of insulin accordingly. These alternative delivery systems are intended to prevent the development of long-term tissue complications.

There are a number of chronic complications that account for the shorter life expectancy of diabetic persons. These include atherosclerotic changes throughout the entire vascular system. The thickening of basement membranes that surround the capillaries can affect their ability to exchange nutrients. Cardiovascular lesions are the most common cause of premature death in diabetic persons. Kidney disease, which is commonly found in longtime diabetics, can ultimately lead to kidney failure. For these persons, expensive medical care, including dialysis and the possibility of a kidney transplant, overshadows their lives. Diabetes is the leading cause of new blindness in the United States. Delayed gastric emptying (gastroparesis) occurs when the stomach takes too long to empty its contents; it results from damage to the vagus nerve from long-term exposure to high glucose levels. In addition, diabetes leads to a gradual decline in the ability of nerves to conduct sensory information to the brain. For example, the feet of some diabetics feel more like stumps of wood than living tissue. Consequently, weight is not distributed properly; in concert with the reduction in blood flow, this problem can lead to pressure ulcers. If not properly cared for, areas of the foot can develop gangrene, which may then lead to amputation of the foot. Finally, in male patients, there are problems with reproductive function that generally result in impotence.

IN THE NEWS: INCREASE IN TYPE II DIABETES IN ADULTS AND CHILDREN

There is no doubt that the United States, as well as many other countries around the world, is affected by an "obesity epidemic." Poor eating habits and sedentary lifestyles are causing higher rates of obesity across all age groups and ethnic backgrounds. Approximately 30 percent of adults in the United States are obese. The rate of obesity in children aged two to five and aged twelve to nineteen has tripled since the mid-1970's. In children aged six to eleven, this rate has quadrupled from 4 to an alarming 19 percent.

Type II diabetes is occurring with increasing frequency in children, adolescents, and adults. The number of people with diabetes has doubled since the mid-1980's, and Type II diabetes accounts for 90 to 95 percent of these cases. The Centers for Disease Control and Prevention estimates that 8 to 43 percent of new cases of diabetes in children are Type II diabetes. These young people are usually overweight or obese, have a family history of diabetes, have signs of insulin resistance such as acanthosis nigricans, are members of an ethnic group with a high risk of Type II diabetes, and are more often girls than boys.

This increase has many causes. The serving sizes of foods sold in stores and restaurants have increased. In many neighborhoods, there are more fast food restaurants than grocery stores. Approximately 30 percent of all calories consumed by Americans are in the form of sodas and fruit-flavored drinks. Teenagers drink more soda than milk, and about half of children aged six to eleven drink soda daily. Less than 25 percent of Americans eat five or more servings of fruit and vegetables daily. To compound the problem, more than 30 percent of high school students do not exercise regularly and more than half of adults do not get enough physical activity.

This epidemic can be stopped in a number of ways. Healthier eating habits and regular physical activity can decrease rates of obesity, diabetes, and many other chronic diseases. Breast-feeding is associated with lower rates of obesity in children. Parents can advocate for regular physical activity in schools and healthy snacks and drinks in vending machines. Limiting television viewing and computer time, encouraging physical activity at home, and providing healthy meals and smaller portions can all contribute to controlling the "obesity epidemic" in children.

—Julie M. Slocum, R.N., M.S., C.D.E.

The mechanism responsible for the development of these long-term complications of diabetes is genetic in origin and dependent on the amount of time the tissues are exposed to the elevated plasma glucose concentrations. What, then, is the link between glucose concentrations and diabetic complications?

As an animal ages, most of its cells become less efficient in replacing damaged material, while its tissues lose their elasticity and gradually stiffen. For example, the lungs and heart muscle expand less successfully, blood vessels become increasingly rigid, and ligaments begin to tighten. These apparently diverse age-related changes are accelerated in diabetes, and the causative agent is glucose. Glucose becomes chemically attached to proteins and deoxyribonucleic acid (DNA) in the body without the aid of enzymes to speed the reaction along. What is important is the duration of exposure to the elevated glucose concentrations. Once glucose is bound to tissue proteins, a series of chemical reactions is triggered that, over the passage of months and years, can result in the formation and eventual accumulation of cross-links between adjacent proteins. The higher glucose concentrations in diabetics accelerate this process, and the effects become evident in specific tissues throughout the body.

Understanding the chemical basis of protein cross-linking in diabetes has permitted the development and study of compounds that can intervene in this process. Certain compounds, when added to the diet, can limit the glucose-induced cross-linking of proteins by preventing their formation. One of the best-studied compounds, aminoguanidine, can help prevent the cross-linking of collagen; this fact is shown in a decrease in the accumulation of trapped lipoproteins on artery walls. Aminoguanidine also prevents thickening of the capillary basement membrane in the kidney. Aminoguanidine acts by blocking glucose's ability to react with neighboring proteins. Vitamins C and B_6 are also effective in reducing cross-linking. All these substances may be considered antiaging compounds.

Alternatively, transplantation of the entire pancreas is an effective means of achieving an insulin-independent state in persons with Type I diabetes mellitus. Both the technical problems of pancreas transplantation and the possible rejection of the foreign tissue, however, have limited this procedure as a treatment for diabetes. Diabetes is usually manageable; therefore, a pancreas transplant is not necessarily lifesaving. Some limited success in treating diabetes has been achieved by transplanting only the insulin-producing islet cells from the pancreas or grafts from fetal pancreas tissue. It may one day be possible to use genetic engineering to permit cells of the liver to self-regulate glucose concentrations by synthesizing and releasing their own insulin into the blood.

Some of the less severe forms of Type II diabetes mellitus can be controlled by the use of oral hypoglycemic agents that bring about a reduction in blood glucose. These drugs can be taken orally to drive the beta cells to release even more insulin than usual. These drugs also increase the ability of insulin to act on the target cells, which ultimately reduces the insulin requirement. The use of these agents remains controversial, because they overwork the already strained beta cells. If a diabetic person is reliant on these drugs for extended periods of time, the insulin cells could "burn out" and completely lose their ability to synthesize insulin. In this situation, the previously non-insulin-dependent person would have to be placed on insulin therapy for life. Other hypoglycemic agents lower blood glucose by decreasing hepatic glucose output, reducing insulin resistance, and delaying the absorption of glucose from the gastrointestinal tract.

If obesity is a factor in the expression of Type II diabetes, as it is in most cases, the best therapy is a combination of a reduction of calorie intake and an increase in activity. More than any other disease, Type II diabetes is related to lifestyle. It is often the case that people prefer having an injection or taking a pill to improving their quality of life by changing their diet and level of activity. Attention to diet and exercise results in a dramatic decrease in the need for drug therapy in nine out of ten diabetics. In some cases, the loss of only a small percentage of body weight results in an increased sensitivity to insulin. Exercise is particularly helpful in the management of both types of diabetes, because working muscle does not require insulin to metabolize glucose. Thus, exercising muscles take up and use some of the excess glucose in the blood, which reduces the overall need for insulin. Permanent weight reduction and exercise also help to prevent long-term complications and permit a healthier and more active lifestyle.

Perspective and Prospects

Diabetes mellitus is a disease of ancient origin. The first written reference to diabetes, which was discovered in the tomb of Thebes in Egypt (1500 B.C.E.), described an illness associated with the passage of vast quantities of sweet urine and an excessive thirst.

The study of diabetes owes much to the Franco-Prussian War. In 1870, during the siege of Paris, it was noted by French physicians that the widespread famine in the besieged city had a curative influence on diabetic patients. Their glycosuria decreased or disappeared. These observations supported the view of clinicians at the time who had previously prescribed periods of fasting and increased muscular work for the treatment of the overweight diabetic individual.

It was Oscar Minkowski of Germany who, in 1889, accidentally traced the origin of diabetes to the pancreas. Following the complete removal of the pancreas from a dog, Minkowski's technician noted the animal's subsequent copious urine production. Acting on the basis of a hunch, Minkowski tested the urine and determined that its sugar content was greater than 10 percent.

In 1921, Frederick Banting and Charles Best, at the University of Toronto, successfully extracted the antidiabetic substance "insulin" using a cold alcohol-hydrochloric acid mixture to inactivate the harsh digestive enzymes of the pancreas. Using this substance, they first controlled the disease in a depancreatized dog and then, a few months later, successfully treated the first human diabetic patient. The clinical application of a discovery normally takes a long time, but in this case a mere twenty weeks had passed between the first injection of insulin into the diabetic dog and the first trial with a diabetic human. Three years later, in 1923,

Banting and Best were awarded the Nobel Prize in Physiology or Medicine for their remarkable achievement.

Although insulin, when combined with an appropriate diet and exercise, alleviates the symptoms of diabetes to such an extent that a diabetic can lead an essentially normal life, insulin therapy is not a cure. The complications that arise in diabetics are typical of those found in the general population except that they happen much earlier in the diabetic. With regard to these glucose-induced complications, it was first postulated in 1908 that sugars could react with proteins. In 1912, Louis Camille Maillard further characterized this reaction at the Sorbonne and realized that the consequences of this reaction were relevant to diabetics. Maillard suggested that sugars were destroying the body's amino acids, which then led to increased excretion in diabetics. It was not until the mid-1970's, however, that Anthony Cerami in New York introduced the concept of the nonenzymatic attachment of glucose to protein and recognized its potential role in diabetic complications. A decade later, this development led to the discovery of aminoguanidine, the first compound to limit the cross-linking of tissue proteins and thus delay the development of certain diabetic complications.

In 1974, Josiah Brown published the first report showing that diabetes could be reversed by transplanting fetal pancreatic tissue. By the mid-1980's, procedures had been devised for the isolation of massive numbers of human islets that could then be transplanted into diabetics. For persons with diabetes, both procedures represent more than a treatment; they may offer a cure for the disease.

By the turn of the twenty-first century, a rise in the prevalence of Type II diabetes in both developing and developed countries was noticed. In the United States, it is estimated that at least 16 million people have diabetes, and the number is expected to rise to 22 million by the year 2025. Although the incidence of Type II diabetes generally increases with age, there has been a dramatic rise in this type of diabetes in young adults: The largest increase is in the thirteen-to-thirty-nine-year-old age bracket, which saw a 70 percent increase between 1990 and 1998. Another 12 million adults have impaired fasting glucose tolerance, meaning they will develop diabetes if they do not address the problem quickly. Obesity is clearly linked to the increase of Type II diabetes. The growing sedentary lifestyle and increase in energy-dense food intake in the United States are significant risk factors. The Centers for Dis-

ease Control reported that obesity more than doubled in the United States from 15 percent in 1980 to 31 percent in 2000. In the twenty-to-seventy-four age bracket, 65 percent of adults were overweight or obese in 1999-2000.

—Hillar Klandorf, Ph.D.; updated by
Sharon W. Stark, R.N., A.P.R.N., D.N.Sc.

See also Blindness; Endocrine disorders; Endocrinology; Endocrinology, pediatric; Eye infections and disorders; Gangrene; Gastroenterology; Gastroenterology, pediatric; Gastrointestinal system; Gestational diabetes; Glands; Heart attack; Hormones; Hyperadiposis; Hypoglycemia; Insulin resistance syndrome; Internal medicine; Metabolic disorders; Metabolic syndrome; Obesity; Pancreas; Pancreatitis.

FOR FURTHER INFORMATION:

American Diabetes Association. "Gestational Diabetes." *Diabetes Care* 26 (2003): S103-S105. Discussion of gestational diabetes risk factors, diagnosis, and treatment.

_____. http://www.diabetes.org/homepage.jsp. Gives comprehensive information on both Type I and Type II diabetes and current research and scientific findings, provides community forums and news stories, and helps decipher health insurance issues, among other features.

American Diabetes Association Complete Guide to Diabetes. 4th ed. Alexandria, Va.: American Diabetes Association, 2005. A comprehensive consumer guide for all issues surrounding diabetes.

Becker, Gretchen. *The First Year—Type II Diabetes: An Essential Guide for the Newly Diagnosed.* New York: Avalon, 2001. A unique guide for patients with Type II diabetes, setting expectations and answering questions related to the first week of diagnosis, the first months, and the first year. Topics include treatment options, dietary choices, and holistic alternatives.

Biermann, June, and Barbara Toohey. *The Diabetic's Book: All Your Questions Answered.* 4th ed. New York: G. P. Putnam's Sons, 1993. This extremely helpful book deals with both Type I and Type II diabetes. It is filled with useful information to help patients live a more healthful and satisfying life and contains answers to 130 frequently asked questions about the disease, including lifestyle, diet, and therapy.

Centers for Disease Control and Prevention. *Diabetes and Me.* http://www.cdc.gov/diabetes/consumer/

index.htm. Concise overview of diabetes—its diagnosis, treatment, and prevention.

Children with Diabetes. http://www.childrenwithdiabetes.com/index_cwd.htm. Site provides information that helps children with diabetes and their families learn about diabetes, meet people with diabetes, and help others with diabetes.

Jovanovic-Peterson, Lois, Charles M. Peterson, and Morton B. Stori. *A Touch of Diabetes*. 3d ed. Minneapolis: Chronimed, 1998. A straightforward guide for people with Type II diabetes. Provides useful information on the disease and suggestions of how to change eating habits and monitor one's lifestyle.

Larsen, P. Reed, et al., eds. *Williams Textbook of Endocrinology*. 10th ed. Philadelphia: W. B. Saunders, 2003. Comprehensive information regarding endocrine diseases, pathophysiology, diagnoses, treatment, and prognoses.

MedlinePlus. *Diabetes*. http://www.nlm.nih.gov/medlineplus/diabetes.html. A Web site dedicated to the description, causes, symptoms, treatments, and support related to diabetes and diabetic care.

National Diabetes Information Clearinghouse (NDIC). National Institute of Diabetes and Digestive and Kidney Diseases (NIDDK). National Institutes of Health. *Diabetes*. http://diabetes.niddk.nih.gov/dm/pubs/overview/index.htm. Good discussion of diabetes, diagnosis, treatment, future directions in treatment, and points to remember.

Powers, Margaret A., ed. *Handbook of Diabetes Medical Nutrition Therapy*. Rev. ed. Gaithersburg, Md.: Aspen, 1996. A comprehensive book written by dietitians for persons interested in the nutritional treatment of diabetes; blends new scientific knowledge and thought with recent advances in clinical practice.

DIALYSIS

PROCEDURE

ANATOMY OR SYSTEM AFFECTED: Abdomen, blood, circulatory system, kidneys, urinary system

SPECIALTIES AND RELATED FIELDS: Biotechnology, hematology, internal medicine, nephrology, serology, urology

DEFINITION: The artificial replacement of renal (kidney) function, which involves the removal of toxins in the blood by selective diffusion through a semipermeable membrane.

KEY TERMS:

hemodialysis: the removal of toxins from blood through the process of dialysis

osmosis: the diffusion of molecules through a semipermeable membrane until there is an equal concentration on either side of the membrane

peritoneal dialysis: the removal of toxins from blood by dialysis in the peritoneal cavity

peritoneum: the membrane lining the walls of the abdominal cavity and enclosing the viscera

INDICATIONS AND PROCEDURES

The two major functions of the kidneys are to produce urine, thereby excreting toxic substances and maintaining an optimal concentration of solutes in the blood, and to produce and secrete hormones that regulate blood flow, blood production, calcium and bone metabolism, and vascular tone. These functions can be impaired or even completely halted by kidney failure that may or may not be related to diseases such as hepatitis and diabetes. The kidney is the only human organ with a function—that is, the excretion of toxic substances from the blood—that can be artificially replaced on a reliable and chronic basis. Although dialysis cannot duplicate the intricate processes of normal renal function, it is possible to provide patients with a tolerable level of life.

If a solute is added to a container of water, it will be distributed at uniform concentration through the water. This process is called diffusion and results from random movement of the solute molecules in the solvent; it can be seen as a chemical mixing of the solution. The mixing will ensure an even distribution of solute molecules throughout the solution. The time required for complete mixing depends on factors such as the nature of the solute, its molecular size, the temperature of the solution, and the size of the container. The process of dialysis is based on the diffusion of solute molecules (urea and other substances) from the blood or fluids of a patient to a sterile solution called dialysate. The artificial kidney or dialysis system is designed to provide controllable osmosis, or the transfer of solutes and water across a semipermeable membrane separating streams of blood (contaminated as a result of renal failure) and dialysate (a sterile solution). For solutes such as urea, the outflowing blood concentration is high, while the concentration in the inflowing dialysate is usually zero. The result is a concentration gradient that guarantees osmosis of urea molecules from the blood to the dialysate solution. The same process will take place for other toxins present in the blood but absent from the dialysate solution.

There are two types of clinical dialysis, hemodialysis and peritoneal dialysis. In hemodialysis, the device utilized is called a dialyzer. The three basic structural elements of all dialyzers are the blood compartment, the membrane, and the dialysate compartment. In a perfect dialyzer, diffusion equilibrium would result in the blood and dialysate streams during passage through the device, and virtually all the urea and toxins contained in the inflowing blood stream would be transferred to the dialysate stream. This level of efficiency is not achieved, however, and for maximum efficiency, dialysate flow rate should be from two to two and one-half times the actual blood flow rate.

Several fundamental material and design requirements must be met in the construction of efficient dialyzers suitable for clinical use. First, the surfaces in contact with blood and the flow geometry must not induce the formation of blood clots. The materials used must be nontoxic and free of leachable toxic substances. The ratio of membrane surface area to contained volume must be high to ensure maximum transference of substances, and the resistance to blood flow must be low and predictable.

There are three basic designs for a dialyzer: the coil, parallel plate, and hollow fiber configurations. The coil dialyzer was the earliest design. In it, the blood compartment consisted of one or two membrane tubes placed between support screens and then wound with the screens around a plastic core. This resulted in a coiled tubular membrane laminated between support screens, which was then enclosed in a rigid cylindrical case. This design had serious performance limitations, such as a high hydraulic resistance to blood flow and an increase in contained blood volume as blood flow through the device was increased.

The coil design has all but been replaced by more efficient devices. In the parallel plate dialyzer, sheets of membrane are mounted on a plastic support screen and then stacked in multiple layers, allowing for multiple parallel blood and dialysate flow channels. The original design had problems with membrane stretching and nonuniform channel performance. In order to minimize these problems, smaller plates and better membrane supports have been developed. The hollow fiber dialyzer is the most effective design for providing low volume and high efficiency together with modest resistance to flow. Developed in the 1970's, the membrane is composed of tiny cellulose or synthetic hollow fibers about the size of a human hair. Between seven thousand and twenty-five thousand of those fibers are enclosed in a cylindrical jacket, with the blood inlet and outlet at

the top and bottom of the cylinder and the dialysate inlet and outlet being simply expanded sections of the jacket itself. This is the most commonly used geometry for hemodialysis. Extreme care must be taken to ensure that all the extra fluids that might have entered the blood during dialysis are removed. Ultrafiltration refers to the removal of water from the blood after dialysis and is a critical component of the dialysis process.

The delivery system of a dialyzer provides on-line proportioning of water with dialysate concentrate and monitors the dialysate for temperature, composition, and blood leaks. It also controls the ultrafiltration rate and regulates the dialysate flow. Normally included in the system are a blood pump, blood pressure and air monitors, and an anticoagulant pump.

The composition of the dialysate is designed to approximate the normal electrolyte concentration found in plasma and extracellular water; it contains calcium, magnesium, sodium and potassium chloride, sodium acetate, sodium carbonate, and lactic acid, kept at a pH of 7.4. The water used in this preparation is purified, heated to between 35 and 37 degrees Celsius, and deaerated to prevent air embolism. An anticoagulant must be added in the process to prevent the formation of blood clots. Heparin is the most commonly used anticoagulant, mainly because its effect is immediate, is easily measured, and can be almost immediately terminated by adding protamine. In addition, because of its high molecular weight and substantial protein binding, it is not dialyzable and will not be lost from the blood in the process.

Several types of polymers are commonly employed for the manufacture of the membranes utilized in hemodialysis. Cellulosic membranes, or membranes generated from the plant product cellulose, are the most commonly used polymers. (Cellophane was originally used, and later cuprophan and hemophan were introduced.) Noncellulosic artificial membranes made from synthetic polymers such as polycarbonate and polyamide are also used.

The development of efficient and more permeable synthetic membranes and ultrafiltration control delivery systems has reduced treatment time to two or three hours. Dialysis remains a potentially lethal procedure, and careful monitoring of equipment and solutions is necessary. For example, the dialysate must be monitored for hypertonic or hypotonic conditions that can result in hemolysis and death, and the flow from the dialyzer outlet back to the patient must have, among other things, an air bubble detector and filters to remove clots.

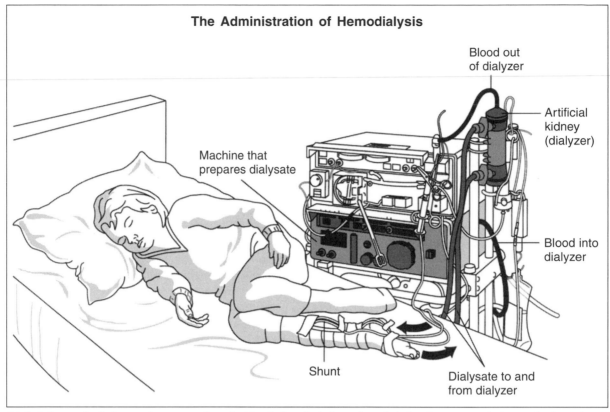

The Administration of Hemodialysis

Blood out of dialyzer

Artificial kidney (dialyzer)

Machine that prepares dialysate

Blood into dialyzer

Shunt

Dialysate to and from dialyzer

Dialysis is a method of removing wastes from the blood when the kidneys have failed to do so. Hemodialysis, which employs a machine that acts as an artificial kidney, is performed in a hospital or a local dialysis center in a session lasting two to six hours in which the blood is filtered to eliminate wastes, toxins, and excess fluid.

Peritoneal dialysis involves the transfer of solutes and water from the peritoneal capillary blood to the dialysate in the peritoneal cavity and the absorption of glucose and other solutes from the peritoneal fluid into the blood. The physiology of this process is less understood than that of hemodialysis. The process involves the introduction in the peritoneal cavity of a certain volume of dialysate and its removal after the dialysis process is complete. The main type of procedure is chronic intermittent peritoneal dialysis (CIPD). This process is performed three to seven times per week and takes from eight to twelve hours. It is mostly done overnight, when a pump introduces the dialysate to the peritoneal cavity and gravity removes it. Two systems are commonly used for this purpose: One is the reverse osmosis machine, which provides continuous flow through the night in a fast manner, while the other system utilizes a cycler for the cycling of the dialysate during the night. Cyclers are semiautomated systems with simple operation and a low initial expense that provide basically trouble-free performance but are expensive in the long

run because they use premixed dialysates and many disposable components. Chronic ambulatory peritoneal dialysis (CAPD) is the most versatile and manageable of the techniques. In this case, the inflow and outflow of dialysate is done manually by gravity. With about 2 liters of dialysate used per exchange, it normally takes ten minutes for inflow and fifteen to twenty minutes for outflow. There are an average of four exchanges per day and one overnight. This is an easy, safe, and effective method of dialysis. A variation of CAPD is continuous cycling peritoneal dialysis (CCPD), introduced in 1980. It basically reverses the CAPD cycle: Cyclers are used during the night to achieve three to four exchanges, and there is a long period without exchange during the day. This minimizes the inconvenience of scheduling exchanges during the day, and many patients can alternate between the two methods without experiencing problems.

For peritoneal dialysis, the dialysate includes dextrose, lactate, sodium, calcium, and magnesium salts. An anticoagulant such as heparin can be added when needed, such as if blood is seen in the peritoneal fluid. Other substances—such as insulin for both diabetic and nondiabetic patients, antibiotics if there is peritonitis, and bicarbonate to prevent abdominal discomfort—can also be added without major complications.

Peritoneal dialysis may be a better choice than hemodialysis for certain patients when factors such as coronary artery disease, diabetes mellitus, age, or severe hemodialysis-related symptoms are present. It is also the choice for patients whose residence is remote from a dialysis center, who wish to travel frequently, or who live alone.

USES AND COMPLICATIONS

Hemodialysis is used in acute and chronic renal failure patients. Some individuals, however, do not tolerate hemodialysis well, such as children, infants, geriatric patients, diabetics, and victims of traumatic injuries. Therefore, the selection of patients for this procedure must be closely monitored. The process also can be used for treatment of drug overdose (since drugs can be removed from the blood during the dialysis procedure) and hypercalcemia, an excess of calcium.

For many years, peritoneal dialysis was reserved for the treatment of acute renal failure (ARF) or for those patients awaiting transplantation or the availability of hemodialysis. Although it is used principally for the treatment of patients with end-stage renal disease, it remains a valuable tool in the management of ARF because of its simplicity and widespread availability. Essentially, it can be provided in any hospital by most internists or surgeons without the need for specially trained nephrology personnel. It also avoids the need for systematic anticoagulation, making it a good choice for patients in the immediate postoperative period with severe trauma, intracerebral hemorrhage, or hypocoagulable states. It is most suitable for the treatment of patients with an unstable cardiovascular system and for pediatric or elderly patients. It could be impossible to use, however, in postsurgical patients with many abdominal drains, with hernias, or with severe gastroesophageal reflux.

For many years, peritoneal dialysis was not used for patients with CRF (chronic renal failure) because of the problems involved in the maintenance of permanent peritoneal access, the inconvenience of manual dialysate exchanges, the high rate of peritonitis observed in these patients, and the rapid progress made in hemodialysis in the early 1960's. The advent of a safe, permanent peritoneal catheter in the late 1960's and the simultaneous development of automated reverse osmosis peritoneal delivery systems created new interest in the technique and resulted in safer, more effective systems. Peritoneal dialysis can also be used or is recommended in the following cases: for diabetic patients, since it provides a continuous source of insulin and also has the advantage of providing blood pressure control; for edema patients, since the process is useful in the treatment of intractable edema states such as congestive heart failure; and for pancreatitis patients or individuals who suffer from the release of pancreatic enzymes into the abdominal cavity and their subsequent absorption into the circulation. For the latter, the removal of the enzymes through peritoneal dialysis may prevent the necrotic process. Individuals exhibiting hypothermia as a consequence of accidental exposure, cold water immersion, central nervous system disorders, intoxication, or burns can be treated by performing peritoneal dialysis with dialysate solutions between 40 and 45 degrees Celsius. This will bring the body back to 34 degrees Celsius (a stable temperature) in a few hours, and, if the cause of the hypothermia is intoxication, the drugs causing the condition can be removed at the same time.

PERSPECTIVE AND PROSPECTS

As early as the 1600's, the relationship between blood and various diseases was known. At that time, however, great difficulties existed in the transport and study of blood. By the 1800's, the techniques for entering the blood vessels had been refined. The dangers of air embolization (air entering the patient) and clotting were well recognized. Prior to 1850, there was no treatment for patients with renal failure, but crude methods such as applying heat, immersing in warm baths, bloodletting, or administering diaphoretic (perspiration-inducing) mixtures of nitric acid in alcohol and wine were commonly used. (In fact, diaphoretic mixtures and bloodletting for renal failure were used as late as the 1950's.)

In 1854, Thomas Graham, a Scottish chemist, presented a paper on osmotic force, which was the first reference to the process of separating a substance using a semipermeable membrane. His definitions and experimental proofs of the laws of diffusion and osmosis form the foundation upon which dialysis is based. Between 1872 and 1900, the control of membrane manufacture and the dialysis of animal blood were critical developments. One of the key turning points in the development of dialysis occurred in 1913, when John Jacob

Abel, using anticoagulants, created the first extracorporeal device that could be used to diffuse a substance from blood and developed methods to quantify this diffusion. World War I brought the development of the first plate dialyzer, by Heinrich Necheles, a German-born physician. It included an air bubble trap, continuous blood flow, and an entry port for a saline solution to be used as dialysate; it was only used for animals. George Haas must be credited as the first to perform dialysis on a uremic human, in October, 1924. He used heparin, an anticoagulant discovered by William H. Howell and Luther E. Holt, two Americans. Haas had all the pieces together: a dialyzer with a large surface area, a workable membrane, a blood pump, and an anticoagulant.

The emergence of manufactured membranes in the 1930's (such as cellophane, which allows small molecules to pass through it) was crucial in the development of the technique. The lifesaving potential of an artificial kidney was shown by Willem Kolff, a physician from the Netherlands, who saved a patient from coma. His classic work *New Ways of Treating Uraemia*, published in 1947, laid out the principles that are still used and was the first manual for the treatment of patients undergoing hemodialysis. In the United States, the first clinical dialysis was performed on January 26, 1948, at Mt. Sinai Hospital in New York City, by physicians Irving Kroop and Alfred Fishman. The number of groups developing artificial kidney devices and programs between 1945 and 1950 was large. The first complete artificial kidney system commercially available came into existence in 1956, and the first home patient was treated in 1964 by Belding Scribner, from the University of Washington.

Soon the dialyzing fluid delivery systems became smaller and easier to use, the designs were simplified and made more compact, and a better understanding of the physiology of the patient was obtained. Calcium depletion, bone disease, neuropathy, dietary management, and anemia were being looked at closely in order to determine better how much dialysis was required for effective treatment. The late 1960's brought the miniaturization of the systems, in-home care, and lower prices. In fact, in 1973, legislation was enacted in the United States that provided payment through the Social Security system for the care of dialysis patients.

In the latter part of the 1970's, a shift to totally automated systems and an emphasis on negative-pressure dialysis had major impacts, resulting in a move from coil to hollow-fiber dialyzers. Some patients, however, such as diabetics, children, and older patients, did not tolerate hemodialysis well. Therefore, a closer look was taken at peritoneal and automated peritoneal dialysis delivery systems. The earliest reference to peritoneal diffusion was in 1876, and in 1895 it was formally presented as an alternative to remove toxins from the bloodstream. Nevertheless, peritoneal dialysis lay dormant until the 1940's. The basic procedure of using solutions and instilling them into the peritoneal cavity in order to reduce the toxin levels in the blood was first used in 1945 by a group of physicians in Beth Israel Hospital in Boston. The full implications of its use came in the late 1970's, with the development of reverse osmosis technology and the introduction of continuous ambulatory peritoneal dialysis. In the 1980's, the introduction of continuous intermittent peritoneal dialysis gave patients yet another treatment option.

One of the main goals of the medical community and industry is to provide the quality of care that will minimize the burden of those afflicted with renal disease. The main goal, however, remains to obtain the necessary knowledge to understand the causes of progressive renal failure and then prevent, control, or eliminate the consequences of renal disease.

—Maria Pacheco, Ph.D.

See also Blood and blood disorders; Circulation; Diabetes mellitus; Edema; Heart failure; Hematology; Hematology, pediatric; Hemolytic uremic syndrome; Hepatitis; Hyperthermia and hypothermia; Kidney cancer; Kidney disorders; Kidney transplantation; Kidneys; Nephrectomy; Nephritis; Nephrology; Nephrology, pediatric; Pancreatitis; Polycystic kidney disease; Renal failure.

For Further Information:

Cameron, J. Stewart. *History of the Treatment of Renal Failure by Dialysis*. New York: Oxford University Press, 2002. Traces the history of dialysis, including discussions of the concepts of diffusion and anticoagulation, early attempts of dialysis in animals and humans, and recent developments in the field.

Cogan, Martin G., and Patricia Schoenfeld, eds. *Introduction to Dialysis*. 2d ed. New York: Churchill Livingstone, 1991. An excellent and thorough presentation of the topic. Somewhat technical, however, since it includes derivations for the equations governing the different parts of the process. A good reference work for those interested in the theoretical and practical aspects of the dialysis process.

Fine, Leonard W., Herbert Beall, and John Stuehr.

Chemistry for Engineers and Scientists. Fort Worth, Tex.: Saunders College, 2000. A good chemistry book that explains the chemical and physical bases of diffusion and dialysis in a nontechnical presentation.

Nissenson, Allen R., and Richard N. Fine, eds. *Clinical Dialysis*. 4th ed. New York: McGraw-Hill Medical, 2005. A compilation of works by various authorities in the field of dialysis. Contains an excellent presentation of the development of the technique and of its many aspects and applications.

_____. *Dialysis Therapy*. 3d ed. Philadelphia: Hanley and Belfus, 2002. A compilation of works dealing with the theory, applications, advantages, and complications of dialysis. The reader will need some background in the area to make the best use of the book.

Voet, Donald, and Judith G. Voet. *Biochemistry*. 3d ed. Hoboken, N.J.: John Wiley & Sons, 2004. A good book to use for the description and explanation of the chemical processes taking place in the kidney and other areas of the body.

Diaper rash

Disease/disorder

Anatomy or system affected: Anus, skin

Specialties and related fields: Family medicine, pediatrics

Definition: A skin condition characterized by irritation in the diaper area which can vary from slight redness to severe inflammation with sores or blisters.

Key terms:

rash: the breaking out of spots or patches on the skin

sensitive skin: skin that is easily irritated

Causes and Symptoms

Nearly all babies have diaper rash at some time during their infancy. Whether cloth diapers or disposable diapers are used does not affect whether the baby will have this rash. Diaper rash is less likely to occur, however, in very young infants who are fed breast milk than it is in babies who are bottle-fed. Breast milk is more completely digested by the baby than is formula or cow's milk. Thus, babies who are breast-fed produce less waste material than do babies who are bottle-fed, providing fewer opportunities for fecal material to irritate the baby's diaper area.

When a baby starts on solids or juices, occasional diaper rash is likely to occur. Sometimes when new foods are fed to the baby, the baby's body may not be able to digest the food completely; enzymes in the food can cause diaper rash. These enzymes can break down a baby's skin, causing irritation and even sores. Acid in foods and juices can also cause irritation; a bright red scald around the urethral opening or on the buttocks can result when the baby cannot digest the acid in such foods as tomatoes or orange juice.

Interaction between the baby's urine and bacteria on the baby's skin produces ammonia. Ammonia can be caustic to the diaper area, causing burns. Prolonged wetness can cause the rash to form bumps, which then become white-headed pimples and even weeping areas. These white-headed, weeping pimples are likely to appear if a baby sleeps in a wet diaper for ten to twelve hours or if a baby has a cold, sore throat, or ear infection.

Another cause of diaper rash is yeast infections, such as candidiasis. A rash from a yeast infection is fiery red and bumpy; it may have scaly edges. The rash caused by candidiasis may appear when a baby has been ill, since some antibiotics taken for certain illnesses may destroy the bacteria that control the growth of yeast in the body.

Babies are likely to get diaper rash when they have had diarrhea or an illness. Diarrhea burn is indicated by a bright red burn encircling the baby's anus after a bout with diarrhea. Streptococcal bacteria may also produce diaper rash; often, diaper rash caused by strep infection will appear after other members of the family have been infected. This rash will be bright red, with swollen areas near the rectum. There may also be slits in the skin.

There are also inorganic causes of diaper rash. A diaper that fits too snugly may cause a rash. Usually, such a rash is shiny and red but not sore. Sensitive skin may also develop a rash when exposed to fabric softeners, detergents, and various toiletries. Such rashes are often tiny red blisters. If the baby wears cloth diapers, a rash can occur if the diaper has been washed in a detergent that contains an enzyme or bleach. The plastic in some disposable diapers can also cause red patches.

Treatment and Therapy

When diaper rash develops, particularly a rash that appears to be a burn, the baby's diet should be examined to determine if certain foods are contributing to the rash. Highly acidic foods such as orange juice and tomatoes can cause scalding burns. Mixing water with

INFORMATION ON DIAPER RASH

CAUSES: Yeast infections, food irritants, antibiotics, streptococcal bacteria
SYMPTOMS: Pain, inflammation, red prick marks or radiating redness
DURATION: Short-term
TREATMENTS: Use of protective ointment, dietary change, allowing diaper area to dry completely before diapering, frequent diapering, administration of antifungal agents (nystatin)

acidic juices will help reduce the likelihood of rash formation.

The best way to eliminate diaper rash is to keep a baby clean and dry. Caregivers should remove wet or soiled diapers as soon as they are aware of them. The baby should be washed with warm water and dried off at each diaper change. If there is a rash, the baby should be allowed, whenever possible, to lie for an hour with the diaper area uncovered. If air is allowed to move around the diaper area, it is less likely that a rash will form, and if one does occur, it is more likely that the rash will heal. Therefore, the baby's diapers should not be fastened too tightly to the skin.

If the baby's diaper rash is caused by a yeast infection, then a prescription medication such as nystatin will be needed to clear up the problem. Severe diaper rash caused by prolonged wetness can sometimes be controlled by using extra-absorbency disposable diapers. A doctor may recommend 1 percent hydrocortisone ointment for such a rash, but caregivers should be careful when using hydrocortisone creams, since they can affect the baby's own production of cortisone.

If the diaper rash appears to be a result of irritation from detergents used in washing cloth diapers, then the diapers should be washed in milder detergents. Drying diapers in a very hot dryer or in the sunshine will kill organisms that can cause rashes. If all else fails, boiling diapers for a half hour or more will destroy most bacteria.

Diaper rash can be prevented by coating the diaper area with a protective ointment such as petroleum jelly. If a diaper rash does develop, the ointment can prevent further spread of the rash. Care must be taken, however, because medicated ointments can prevent the stay-dry liner of disposable diapers from drawing moisture away from the body, making the rash worse.

A physician should be consulted for a diaper rash that resembles a chemical burn, develops blisters, or becomes infected. Impetigo, which must be treated by a doctor, is a fairly common complication of diaper rash. This communicable infection is characterized by blisters that itch, break, ooze, and crust over.

PERSPECTIVE AND PROSPECTS

Undoubtedly, diaper rash has been around since babies began to wear diapers. It can be largely prevented through vigilant caregivers who make sure that diapers are changed as soon as they become soiled or wet. Nevertheless, when new foods are introduced, a baby is sick, or sensitive skin comes in contact with irritants such as detergents, it is likely that diaper rash will occur.

—Annita Marie Ward, Ed.D.

See also Allergies; Bacterial infections; Breastfeeding; Burns and scalds; Dermatology, pediatric; Fungal infections; Impetigo; Nutrition; Pediatrics; Rashes; Skin; Skin disorders.

FOR FURTHER INFORMATION:

Illingworth, Ronald S. *The Normal Child: Some Problems of the Early Years and Their Treatment.* 10th ed. Edinburgh, Scotland: Churchill Livingstone, 1991. Although intended as a text for pediatric students, the approach and style make this book equally useful for parents who are unafraid of occasional medical terminology.

Jones, Sandy. *Crying Baby, Sleepless Nights: Why Your Baby Is Crying and What You Can Do About It.* Rev. ed. Boston: Harvard Common Press, 1992. Writing with empathy for parents and infants alike, Jones helps parents identify the source of their baby's distress. She covers basic soothing techniques, infants' sleep-wake patterns, feeding problems, the colic-allergy connection, and colic drugs.

Kemper, Kathi J. *The Holistic Pediatrician: A Pediatrician's Comprehensive Guide to Safe and Effective Therapies for the Twenty-five Most Common Ailments of Infants, Children, and Adolescents.* 2d ed. New York: HarperCollins, 2002. Integrates mainstream and alternative medicine to aid parents in dealing with the most common childhood health problems such as diaper rash, ear infections, and allergies.

Leach, Penelope. *Your Baby and Child: From Birth to Age Five.* 3d ed. New York: Alfred A. Knopf, 1997. Each developmental stage—newborn, settled baby, older baby, toddler, and young child—is discussed in terms of feeding, teeth and teething, growing, excreting, crying, sleeping, playing, and everyday care.

Sullivan, Michele G. "Diaper Rash: Common, Yet Poorly Understood." *Pediatric News* 38, no. 9 (September 1, 2004): 43. Discusses the etiology of and treatment options for diaper rash.

Woolf, Alan D., et al., eds. *The Children's Hospital Guide to Your Child's Health and Development.* Cambridge, Mass.: Perseus, 2002. An authoritative and comprehensive guide to children's health, providing a guide to every common illness or condition that affects children and a carefully designed emergency section.

Diarrhea and dysentery

Disease/disorder

Anatomy or system affected: Abdomen, gastrointestinal system, intestines

Specialties and related fields: Family medicine, gastroenterology, internal medicine, pediatrics, public health

Definition: Intestinal disorders that may indicate minor emotional distress or a variety of diseases, some serious; diarrhea is loose, watery, copious bowel movements, whereas dysentery is an intestinal infection characterized by severe diarrhea.

Key terms:

electrolytes: inorganic ions dissolved in body water, including sodium, potassium, calcium, magnesium, chloride, phosphate, bicarbonate, and sulphate

functional disease: a derangement in the way that normal anatomy operates

gastroenterology: the medical subspecialty devoted to care of the digestive tract and related organs

intestines: the tube connecting the stomach and anus in which nutrients are absorbed from food; divided into the small intestine and the colon, or large intestine

mucosa: the semipermeable layers of cells lining the gut, through which fluid and nutrients are absorbed

organic disease: disease resulting from an identifiable cause, such as an enzyme deficiency, growth, hole, or organism

pathogen: an organism that causes disease

peristalsis: the wavelike muscular contractions that move food and waste products through the intestines; problems with peristalsis are called motility disorders

stool: the waste products expelled from the anus during defecation

---

Information on Diarrhea and Dysentery

Causes: Bacterial, viral, or parasitic infection; laxative abuse; hormones; inflammatory bowel disease

Symptoms: Dehydration, weakness, malnutrition, nausea, bleeding, fever, bloating, persistent intestinal pain

Duration: Acute to chronic

Treatments: Oral rehydration, antibiotics if needed

Causes and Symptoms

A symptom of various diseases rather than a disease in itself, diarrhea is so difficult to define and can result from so many disparate causes that it is sometimes called the gastroenterologist's nightmare. Dysentery (bloody diarrhea), a more threatening symptom, presents even further complexity.

Uncontrolled, some forms of diarrhea result in dehydration, weakness, and malnutrition and quickly turn deadly. Diarrhea is implicated in more infant deaths worldwide than any other affliction. Even in mild forms, it produces so much distress in victims and has inspired so many remedies that its psychological and economic toll is monumental.

Common medical definitions of diarrhea seek to bring diagnostic precision to a nebulous complaint and to distinguish between acute and chronic forms and between organic and functional causes. For example, *The Merck Manual of Diagnosis and Therapy* (17th ed., 1999), a widely respected reference for physicians, associates diarrhea with increased amount and fluidity of fecal matter and frequent defecation relative to a person's usual pattern, emphasizing the importance of volume (more than 300 grams of stool daily, of which 60 to 90 percent is water) in the definition. The key phrase here is "relative to a usual pattern": Because quantity, frequency, and firmness of bowel movements vary greatly among healthy people, a more precise generalization is difficult to make. Yet some specialists demand greater specificity from the definition. For example, W. Grant Thompson, a professor of medicine and popular author on the digestive tract, proposed the operational definition of "loose or watery stools more than 75 percent of the time" in *Gut Reactions* (1989). Acute diarrhea seldom lasts more than five days, although acute dysentery may continue up to ten days;

most causes are infections, that is, resulting from the presence of microorganisms (viruses, bacteria, or parasites). Physicians differ over how long the symptoms must persist before a condition is identified as chronic diarrhea, proposing from two weeks to three months; impaired functioning of the intestinal tract (functional diarrhea) is usually responsible, although persistent malfunctions may originate from pathogens that in most cases provoke only acute diarrhea.

In a single day, water intake, saliva, gastric juice, bile, pancreatic juices, and electrolyte secretions in the upper small intestine produce about 9 to 10 liters of fluid in the average person. About 1 to 2 liters of this amount empty into the colon, and 100 to 150 milligrams are excreted in the stool; the rest is absorbed through the intestinal mucosa. If for any reason more fluid enters the colon than it can absorb, diarrhea results. Schemes classifying diarrhea according to the biochemical mechanisms causing it vary considerably, although all authorities agree on three broad types of malfunction.

The first is secretory diarrhea. The intestines, especially the small intestine, normally add water and electrolytes—principally sodium, potassium, chloride, and bicarbonate—into the nutrient load during the biochemical reactions of digestion. In a healthy person, more fluid is absorbed than is secreted. Many agents and conditions can reverse this ratio and stimulate the mucosa to exude more water than can be absorbed: toxin-producing bacteria; various organic chemicals, including caffeine and some laxatives; acids; hormones; some cancers; and inflammatory diseases of the bowel. Large stool volume (more than 1 liter a day), with little or no decrease during fasting and with normal sodium and potassium content in the body fluid, characterizes secretory diarrhea.

Second, the nutrient load in the gut may include substances that exert osmotic force but cannot be absorbed, causing osmotic diarrhea. Some laxatives (especially those containing magnesium), an inability to absorb the lactose in dairy products or the artificial sweeteners in diet foods, and enzyme deficiencies are

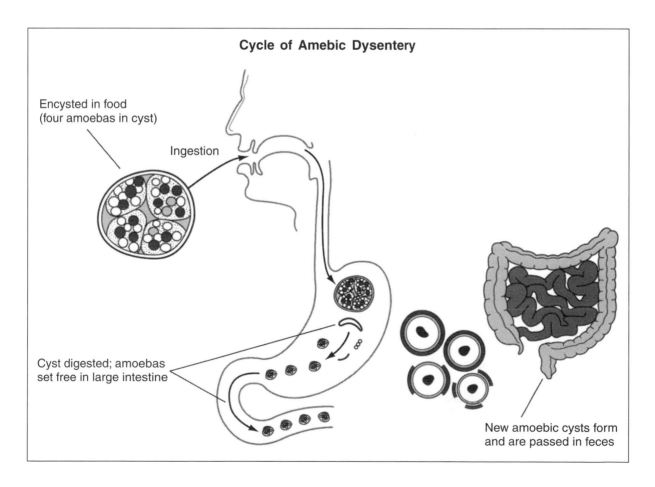

Cycle of Amebic Dysentery

Encysted in food
(four amoebas in cyst)

Ingestion

Cyst digested; amoebas
set free in large intestine

New amoebic cysts form
and are passed in feces

the principal causes. Stool volume tends to be less than 1 liter a day and decreases during fasting, and the sodium and potassium content of stool water is low.

Third, motility disorders occur when peristalsis, the natural wavelike contractions of the bowel wall that move waste matter toward the rectum for defecation, becomes deranged. Some drugs, irritable bowel syndrome (IBS), hyperthyroidism, and gut nerve damage (as from diabetes mellitus) may have this effect. Fluid passes through the intestines too quickly or in an uncoordinated fashion, and too little is removed from the waste matter.

These mechanisms do not conform exactly with popular names for diarrhea. For example, travelers' diarrhea, the most infamous, comprises a diverse group of microorganism infections that come from drinking polluted water or eating tainted foods. When a person is not a native to an area, and so has little or no resistance to locally abundant pathogens, these pathogens can radically alter the balance of intestinal flora or attack the mucosa, increasing secretion and disrupting absorption and motility. Similarly, terms such as "Montezuma's revenge," "the backdoor trots," and "beaver fever" can refer to a variety of organic diseases, although the last commonly refers to *Giardia lamblia* infection.

Dysentery occurs with infectious diarrhea, most commonly from bacteria and amoebas, such as *Shigella*, *Salmonella*, and *Escherichia coli* (*E. coli*), and with inflammatory diseases of the bowel, such as colitis and Crohn's disease. Any pathogen that injures and inflames the bowel wall, ulcerating the mucosa, may cause blood and pus to ooze into the feces. To the greatest threat from diarrhea—dehydration—dysentery often adds fever, chills, cramping, blood loss, and nausea, and in extreme cases delirium, convulsions, and coma.

Although most diarrheas result from physiological mechanisms, one relatively rare form of chronic diarrhea ultimately has a psychological origin: laxative abuse. Physicians consider this curious phenomenon a specialized manifestation of Münchausen syndrome, named after the German soldier Baron Münchausen (1720-1797), who was famous for his wild tales of military exploits and injuries in battles. In order to be admitted to hospitals, patients mutilate themselves in such a way that the injuries mimic acute, dramatic, and convincing symptoms of serious physiological diseases. Laxative abusers secretly dose themselves with nonprescription laxatives and suffer continual diarrhea, weight loss, and weakness. When they present themselves to physicians, they lie about taking laxatives, which makes a correct diagnosis extremely difficult; even when confronted with irrefutable evidence of the abuse, they deny it and persist in taking the laxatives.

TREATMENT AND THERAPY

Almost everyone, at one time or another, produces stools that seem somehow unusual; if the bowel movement comes swiftly and is preceded by intestinal cramps and if the stool has anything from a watery to an oatmeal-like consistency, victims are likely to believe that they have diarrhea. Such episodes seldom indicate anything except perhaps a dietary excess or a temporary motility disturbance. Normal bowel movement returns on its own, and no medical treatment is called for. When loose feces are uncontrollable, even explosive, however, and other symptoms coexist, such as nausea, bleeding, fever, bloating, and persistent intestinal pain, the distress may indicate serious illness.

Because so many organic and functional diseases can lead to diarrhea, physicians follow carefully designed algorithms when treating patients. Essentially, such an algorithm seeks to eliminate possibilities systematically. Step by step, physicians interview patients, conduct physical examinations, and, when called for, perform tests that gradually narrow the range of possible causes until one seems most likely. Only then can the physician decide upon an effective therapy. This painstaking approach is necessary because treatments for some mechanisms of diarrhea prove useless against or worsen other mechanisms. If the underlying disease is complex or uncommon, the process can be long and frustrating.

One treatment, however, always precedes a complete investigation. Because dehydration is the most immediately serious effect of diarrhea, the physician first tries to prevent or reduce dehydration in a patient through oral rehydration; that is, the patient is given fluids with electrolytes to drink. Often, mineral water or fruit juice with soda crackers is sufficient to restore fluid balance.

If the diarrhea lasts fewer than three days and no other serious symptoms accompany it, the physician is unlikely to recommend treatment other than oral rehydration because whatever caused the upset is already resolving itself. If the diarrhea is persistent, however, the physician queries the patient about his or her recent experience, which is called "taking a history." Fever, tenesmus (the urgent need to defecate without the ability to do so satisfactorily), blood in the stool, and abdominal pain will suggest that a pathogen has in-

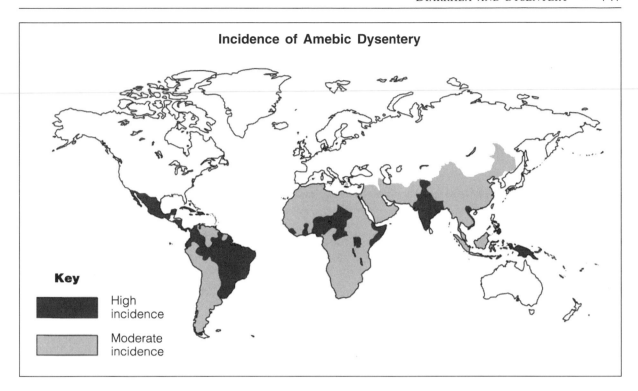

Incidence of Amebic Dysentery

Key

High incidence

Moderate incidence

fected the patient. If the patient has recently eaten seafood, traveled abroad, suffered an immune system disorder, or engaged in sexual activity without the protection of condoms, the physician has reason to suspect that viruses, bacteria, or parasites are responsible.

At that point, a stool sample is taken. If few or no white cells turn up in the stool, then the diarrhea has not caused inflammation. Several common bacteria and parasites, usually contracted during travel, induce diarrhea without inflammation, most notably some types of *E. coli*, cryptosporidium, rotavirus, Norwalk virus, and *Giardia lamblia*. Further tests, such as the culturing and staining of stool samples and electron microscopy of stool or bowel wall tissue, will distinguish between bacterial and parasite infection. Most noninflammatory bacterial diarrheas are allowed to run their course without drug therapy; only the effects of the diarrhea (especially dehydration) are treated. If the agent responsible is a parasite, the patient is given specific antiparasite medications.

The presence of white cells in the stool is evidence of inflammatory diarrhea, and the physician considers a completely separate group of microorganisms, especially *Shigella*, *Salmonella*, amoebas, and various forms of *E. coli*. Because the inflammation may cause bleeding and pockets of pus, which in turn can lead to anemia and fever, inflammatory diarrhea often requires

aggressive treatment. Cell cultures help identify the specific microorganism involved, and that identification enables the physician to select the proper antibiotic to kill the infecting agents.

If cell cultures, microscopic examination of stool samples, biopsies, or staining fails to identify a microorganism (and some, like the parasite *Giardia lamblia*, are difficult to spot), the physician suspects that the diarrhea derives from a source other than an infectious agent. IBS, a chronic and relapsing disorder, may be making its first appearance. Overuse of antibiotics, antacids, or laxatives is frequently the cause, in which case the cure is simple: Elimination of the drugs clears up the symptom.

When neither drugs nor IBS is responsible, the physician looks for other diseases, organic or functional; these can range from the readily identifiable to the obscure, and they are often chronic. Chemical tests, for example, can show that a patient has enzyme deficiencies that produce intolerance to types of food, such as dairy products, or conditions resulting from malfunctioning organs, such as hyperthyroidism and pancreatic insufficiency. Looking through an endoscope, a long flexible fiber-optic tube, the physician can locate diarrhea-causing tumors or the abrasions and inflammation typical of colitis and Crohn's disease. Yet neither tests nor direct examination may pin down the dysfunction. For example, diarrhea figures prominently among a group of symptoms, probably derived from assorted dysfunctions, that characterize IBS; this mild functional disease is estimated to afflict between 10 and 20 percent of Americans.

Cancers, Crohn's disease, and some forms of colitis can be alleviated with surgery, although in the case of Crohn's disease the relief from diarrhea may be only temporary. The surgery itself, however, may impair bowel function, worsening diarrhea rather than stopping it. Food intolerances are managed by removing the offending food from the patient's diet; similarly, some types of colitis and IBS sometimes improve after the physician and patient experiment with altering the patient's diet. Medications are available that supplement or counteract the biochemical imbalances created by malfunctioning organs, such as treatment for hyperthyroidism. Yet, in many cases, the disease must simply be endured and the diarrhea can only be palliated with bulking agents, which often contain aluminum and bismuth, or opiates, such as morphine and codeine, which slow peristalsis.

The surest protection from diarrhea of all types is a balanced, moderate, pathogen-free diet, although diet alone seldom prevents organic diseases. When dietary control is difficult, such as when a person travels and especially when the itinerary includes underdeveloped countries, other measures may help. Bacterial infection accounts for 80 percent of cases of travelers' diarrhea, so some physicians recommend regular doses of antibiotics or a bismuth subsalicylate preparation (such as Pepto Bismol) to kill off the pathogens before they can cause trouble. Such prophylactic treatment is controversial because the drugs, taken over long periods, can have serious side effects, including rashes, tinnitus (ringing in the ear), sensitivity to sunlight, and shock. Also, preventive doses of drugs may give travelers a false sense of security so that they fail to exercise caution in eating foreign foods. Also, widespread use of antibiotics for this purpose fosters the emergence of bacteria that are resistant to them, ultimately making the treatment of disease more difficult.

PERSPECTIVE AND PROSPECTS

In effect, diarrhea is an urgent message from the body that something is wrong. Although it is often difficult for a physician to interpret, persistent diarrhea sends a signal that cannot be ignored without endangering the patient. Similarly, when significant numbers of people in an area suffer diarrhea, the disease is an urgent social

and political message to local governments: Public health is endangered and steps must be taken to improve living conditions.

Although some endemic diarrheal diseases do exist in wealthy industrialized countries such as the United States, most severe, long-lasting plagues of diarrhea occur in impoverished nations that have inadequate sanitation systems and poor standards for food handling. Most viral, bacterial, and parasitic diarrheas are transmitted by food and water. Any food can harbor bacteria after being grown in or washed with infected water. Meat is especially vulnerable during slaughtering, but refrigerating, drying, salting, fermenting, freezing, or irradiating it prevents the bacteria from proliferating to numbers that cause illness. If the food is stored in a warm place, as is often the case in countries lacking the resources for refrigeration or other safe storage techniques, the diarrhea-causing organisms can spoil the food in hours. Spoiled food becomes a particular nuisance when served at restaurants or by street vendors, because great numbers and varieties of people are infected.

Organisms that cause many forms of diarrhea travel in human excrement. When an infected person defecates, the organism-rich stool enters the sewer system, and if that system is not well designed, the infected excrement may leak into the local water supply, spreading the infection when the water is drunk or used to wash food. Furthermore, infected persons, if they fail to wash themselves well, may have traces of excrement on their hands, and when they touch food during its preparation or touch other people directly, the organism can find a new host.

In 1989, the World Health Organization (WHO) issued ten rules for safe food preparation in an attempt to improve food handling practices worldwide and combat diarrheal diseases. The effort, it was hoped, would reduce infant mortality in developing countries, since diarrheal dehydration kills children younger than two years of age at rates disproportionate to other age groups. WHO advises food handlers to choose foods that are already processed, to cook foods thoroughly, to serve cooked foods immediately, to store foods carefully, to reheat foods thoroughly, to prevent raw and cooked foods from touching, to wash their hands repeatedly, to clean all kitchen surfaces meticulously, to protect foods from insects and rodents, and to use pure water.

Eliminating endemic infectious diarrheal diseases would improve general health significantly throughout the world, since diarrhea is one of the most incapacitating of afflictions even in its mild forms. International travel would also become safer; of the estimated 300 million people who cross national borders yearly, 20 to 50 percent contract diarrheal illnesses. Noninfectious diarrhea from chronic functional diseases will remain a knotty problem, but it is rare in comparison to acute infectious diarrhea and cannot be transmitted, so has little or no effect on public health.

—Roger Smith, Ph.D.

See also Abdominal disorders; Bacterial infections; Colitis; Colon cancer; Crohn's disease; Digestion; *E. coli* infection; Food poisoning; Gastroenterology; Gastroenterology, pediatric; Gastrointestinal disorders; Gastrointestinal system; Incontinence; Indigestion; Intestinal disorders; Intestines; Irritable bowel syndrome (IBS); Lactose intolerance; Noroviruses; Over-the-counter medications; Rotavirus; Viral infections.

FOR FURTHER INFORMATION:

Biddle, Wayne. *A Field Guide to Germs.* 2d ed. New York: Anchor Books, 2002. This comprehensive book is easily accessible to the nonspecialist and includes a discussion of nearly every virus, bacterium, and fungus known to cause human and nonhuman animal disease. The history of the microbe and the treatment of diseases are included.

DuPont, Herbert L., and Charles D. Ericsson. "Drug Therapy: Prevention and Treatment of Traveler's Diarrhea." *The New England Journal of Medicine* 328 (June 24, 1993): 1821-1826. This article, a periodic update on the subject from the Center for Infectious Diseases, is a review of existing knowledge. It should be basic reading for international travelers, or anyone who wants an accurate overview of travelers' diarrhea.

Gracey, Michael, ed. *Diarrhea.* Boca Raton, Fla.: CRC Press, 1991. The fourteen essays in this collection cover major types of acute and chronic diarrhea in depth. Although written by academic physicians, the essays are accessible to readers with a basic knowledge of physiology, and the clarity and wealth of information make the book a valuable resource.

Janowitz, Henry D. *Your Gut Feelings: A Complete Guide to Living Better with Intestinal Problems.* Rev. ed. New York: Oxford University Press, 1994. An eminent gastroenterologist and popular writer on intestinal subjects, Janowitz writes plainly and offers much helpful advice. His section on travelers' diarrhea is particularly valuable.

Parker, James N., and Philip M. Parker, eds. *The Official Patient's Sourcebook on Diarrhea.* San Diego, Calif.: Icon Health, 2002. Draws from public, academic, government, and peer-reviewed research to provide a wide-ranging handbook for patients with diarrhea.

Peikin, Steven R. *Gastrointestinal Health.* Rev. ed. New York: HarperCollins, 1999. Examines a range of gastrointestinal ailments in depth, including diarrhea and colitis, and offers tips for managing them via diet, stress management, and drugs.

Saibil, Fred. *Crohn's Disease and Ulcerative Colitis: Everything You Need to Know.* Rev. ed. Toronto: Firefly Books, 2003. A leading expert on inflammatory bowel disease (IBD), Saibil covers topics such as signs and symptoms, how the gastrointestinal system works normally and how IBD affects it, procedures and instruments used to diagnose IBD, effects of diet, and children and IBD.

Scarpignato, Carmelo, and P. Rampal, eds. *Traveler's Diarrhea: Recent Advances.* New York: S. Karger, 1995. The authors discuss the latest methods in the prevention, control, and treatment of diarrhea.

Thompson, W. Grant. *Gut Reactions: Understanding Symptoms of the Digestive Tract.* New York: Plenum Press, 1989. With much charm, Grant writes for the general reader, laying out the essential information that patients need in order to comprehend most gastrointestinal ailments. His chapter on diarrhea addresses only the functional diseases.

DIET. *See* NUTRITION.

DIETARY DEFICIENCIES. *See* MALNUTRITION; NUTRITION; VITAMINS AND MINERALS.

DiGEORGE SYNDROME
DISEASE/DISORDER

ALSO KNOWN AS: Chromosome 22 interstitial deletion, 22q11.2 deletion syndrome

ANATOMY OR SYSTEM AFFECTED: Glands, heart, immune system, lymphatic system, mouth

SPECIALTIES AND RELATED FIELDS: Cardiology, genetics, immunology, pediatrics, plastic surgery

DEFINITION: A pediatric syndrome caused by a missing piece of chromosome 22 and characterized by congenital heart defects, the absence or hypoplasia of the thymus and parathyroid glands, cleft palate, and dysmorphic facial features.

Causes and Symptoms

Chromosomes possess two parts. The upper arms are called "p" arms and the lower arms are called "q" arms. Patients with DiGeorge syndrome are missing a tiny interstitial piece inside the long arm of chromosome 22. The specific region inside the long "q" arm is labeled 11.2. Thus, DiGeorge syndrome is also referred to as 22q11.2 deletion syndrome or chromosome 22 interstitial deletion.

Most microdeletions such as these cannot be observed under a microscope because they are so tiny. A molecular cytogenetic test known as fluorescence in situ hybridization (FISH) is used. It includes the use of deoxyribonucleic acid (DNA) probes made from the DiGeorge chromosomal region (DGCR). A green fluorescent probe is used to identify chromosome 22, while a red probe is specific to the DGCR. In DiGeorge syndrome, one of the chromosomes will lack the red fluorescence.

About 93 percent of patients have a spontaneous (de novo) deletion of a 22q11.2, and 7 percent have inherited the deletion from a parent. The very high de novo rate indicates that the deletion recurs with a high frequency as a result of new mutations occurring in the population. This deletion is inherited in an autosomal dominant manner. The offspring of persons with the deletion have a 50 percent chance of inheriting it. This interstitial deletion encompasses about 3 million base pairs of DNA in the majority of patients. About 90 percent of patients have the same 3 million base pair deletion, while 10 percent have a 1.5 million base pair deletion. Therefore, the deletion is large enough to contain nearly one hundred genes.

DiGeorge syndrome is initiated by defective embryonic development of the third and fourth pharyngeal pouches during the fifth week of development. These pouches normally become the thymus and the parathyroid glands. In the absence of a thymus, T lymphocyte maturation is stopped at the pre-cell stage. DiGeorge syndrome is one of the most severe forms of deficient T-cell immunity. Children with DiGeorge syndrome develop recurrent viral infections and have abnormal cellular immunity, as characterized by severely reduced or absent T lymphocytes. They also have defects in T cell-dependent antibody production. A spectrum of abnormal phenotypes may develop. These defects arise from the absence of key genes that are not available for normal development when a 22q microdeletion is present. Infants with this disease may suffer from congenital heart disease of various types, palatal abnormalities (such as cleft palate), and learning difficulties.

Treatment and Therapy

Children with a 22q11.2 deletion may exhibit a wide spectrum of problems and much variation in the severity of symptoms. A patient with DiGeorge syndrome may have several organs or systems affected. DiGeorge syndrome may result in problems in different body systems, such as the heart or palate, and in cognition, such as learning style. Consequently, a multidisciplinary approach is needed for management of a specific patient.

In the neonatal period, the following clinical and laboratory studies are pursued. The serum is tested for calcium; a low concentration points to the need for supplementation. The lymphocytes are measured; a low absolute count means referral to an immunologist, who will look at T and B cell subsets. A renal ultrasound examination should be performed because of the high incidence of structural renal abnormalities. A chest X ray is needed to identify thoracic vertebral anomalies. A cardiac evaluation is recommended for all patients with DiGeorge syndrome because possible malformations may include tetralogy of Fallot, ventricular septal defect, interrupted aortic arch, or truncus arteriosus. Pediatric cardiologists are necessary for the treatment and therapy that is needed. An endocrinologist could follow up possible growth hormone deficiencies. Since there is a high incidence of speech and language delay, speech therapy and early educational intervention are highly recommended. All children with the 22q deletion should be seen by a cleft palate team to diagnose problems and schedule surgery if necessary.

Other medical needs of children are met through evaluation by a feeding specialist, especially in the

---

INFORMATION ON DiGeorge Syndrome

Causes: Chromosomal abnormality resulting in absence of thymus and parathyroid glands

Symptoms: Recurrent viral infections, reduced or absent T lymphocytes, defects in antibody production, congenital heart disease, cleft palate, learning difficulties

Duration: Lifelong

Treatments: Growth hormone, speech therapy, surgery to correct heart defects and cleft palate

newborn period; a neurologist, for possible seizure disorders or problems with balance; a urologist, for possible kidney problems; and an otorhinolaryngologist (ear, nose, and throat doctor) for problems in this region.

PERSPECTIVE AND PROSPECTS

DiGeorge syndrome is relatively frequent, occurring with a frequency of 1 in 4,000 live births. Therefore, this disorder is a significant health concern in the general population. Since the phenotype associated with it is broad and variable, many types of clinical and laboratory specialists are needed. The medical geneticist is the most likely person to have an overview of the diagnosis. A yearly genetics evaluation is beneficial in answering questions. Parents should be tested to determine their chromosomal status. Genetic counseling could provide individuals and families with information on the nature, inheritance, and implications of DiGeorge syndrome to help them make informed medical and personal decisions. Current and future research using model organisms may help to explain the problems of phenotypic variability in DiGeorge syndrome.

—*Phillip A. Farber, Ph.D.*

See also Birth defects; Cleft lip and palate; Congenital heart disease; Genetic counseling; Genetic diseases; Genetics and inheritance; Immune system; Immunodeficiency disorders; Lymphatic system.

FOR FURTHER INFORMATION:

Emanuel, Beverly S., et al. "The 22q11.2 Deletion Syndrome." *Advances in Pediatrics* 48 (2001): 33-73.

King, Richard A., Jerome I. Rotter, and Arno G. Motulsky, eds. *The Genetic Basis of Common Diseases*. 2d ed. New York: Oxford University Press, 2002.

Maroni, Gustavo. *Molecular and Genetic Analysis of Human Traits*. Malden, Mass.: Blackwell Scientific, 2001.

Rimoin, David L., et al., eds. *Emery and Rimoin's Principles and Practice of Medical Genetics*. 5th ed. New York: Churchill Livingstone, 2006.

Stocker, J. Thomas, and Louis P. Dehner, eds. *Pediatric Pathology*. 2d ed. Philadelphia: Lippincott Williams & Wilkins, 2001.

Turnpenny, Peter, and Sian Ellard. *Emery's Elements of Medical Genetics*. 12th ed. New York: Elsevier Churchill Livingstone, 2005.

DIGESTION

BIOLOGY

ANATOMY OR SYSTEM AFFECTED: Abdomen, gastrointestinal system, intestines, pancreas, stomach

SPECIALTIES AND RELATED FIELDS: Biochemistry, family medicine, gastroenterology, internal medicine, nutrition, pharmacology

DEFINITION: The chemical breakdown of food materials in the stomach and small intestine and the absorption into the bloodstream of essential nutrients through the intestinal walls.

KEY TERMS:

amino acids: the product of proteins broken down by digestive enzymes; essential for the building of tissue throughout the body

cecum: the dividing passageway between the small intestine and the large intestine, or colon

chyme: partially broken down food materials that pass from the stomach into the small intestine

dyspepsia: a general term applied to several forms of indigestion

villi: fingerlike projections on the intestinal lining that absorb essential body nutrients after enzymes break down chyme

STRUCTURE AND FUNCTIONS

In the most general terms, digestion is a multiple-stage process that begins by breaking down foodstuffs taken in by an organism. Some specialists consider that the actual process of digestion occurs after this breaking-down stage, when essential nutritional elements are absorbed into the body. Even after division of the digestive process into two main functions, there remains a third, by-product stage: disposal by the body of waste material in the form of urine and feces.

Several different vital organs, all contained in the abdominal cavity, contribute either directly or indirectly to the digestive process at each successive stage. Certain imbalances in the functioning of any one, or a combination of, these organs can lead to what is commonly called indigestion. Chronic imbalances in the functioning of any of the key digestive organs—the stomach, small intestine, large intestine (or colon), liver, gallbladder, and pancreas—may indicate symptoms of diseases that are far more serious than mere indigestion.

In a very broad sense, the process of digestion begins even before food that has been chewed and swallowed passes into the stomach. In fact, while chewing is underway, a first stage of glandular activity—the release of saliva by the salivary glands into the food being chewed (a process referred to as intraluminal digestion)—provides a natural lubricant to help propel masticated material down the esophagus. Although the esophagus does not perform a digestive function, its muscular contractions, which are necessary for swallowing, are like a preliminary stage to the muscular operation that begins in the stomach.

The human stomach has two main sections: the baglike upper portion, or fundus, and the lower part, which is twice as large as the fundus, called the antrum. The function of the fundus is essentially to receive and hold foods that reach the stomach via the esophagus, allowing intermittent delivery into the antrum. Here two dynamic elements of the breaking-down process occur, one physical, the other chemical. The muscular tissue surrounding the antrum acts to churn the partially liquefied food in the lower stomach, while a series of what are commonly called gastric juices flow into the mixture held by the stomach.

The most active element that is secreted from special parietal cells in the mucous membranes lining the stomach is hydrochloric acid. The possibility of damage to the stomach lining is minimized (but not removed entirely) first by the chemical reaction between the acid and the mildly alkaline chewed food and second by the presence of other gastric juices in the antrum. Primary among these is the enzyme pepsin, which is secreted by a different set of specialized cells in the gastric lining. Secretions of both hydrochloric acid and pepsin become mixed and interact chemically with food materials, while the antrum itself moves in rhythmic pulses caused by muscular contractions (peristalsis). One of the key functions of pepsin during this stage is to break down protein molecules into shorter molecular strings of less complicated amino acids, which eventually serve as building material for many body tissues.

At a certain point, food materials are sufficiently reduced to pass beyond the antrum into the duodenum, the first section of the small intestine, where a different stage in the digestive process takes place. At this juncture, the partially broken-down food material is referred to as chyme. The transfer of food from one digestive organ to another is actually monitored by a special autonomic nerve, called the vagus nerve, which originates in the medulla at the head of the spinal cord. Although the vagus nerve innervates a number of vital zones in the abdominal cavity, its function here is quite specific: It adjusts the intensity of muscular movement in the stomach wall and thus limits the amount of food passing into the small intestine.

The exact amount of food that is allowed to enter the intestinal tract represents only part of the essential question of balance between agents contributing to the digestive process. The presence of a now slightly acidic food-gastric juice mixture in the duodenum sparks what is called an enterogastric reflex. Two hormones, secretin and cholecystokinin, begin to flow from the mucous membranes of the duodenum. These hormones serve to limit the acidic strength of stomach secretions and trigger reactions in the liver, gallbladder, and pancreas—other key organs that contribute to digestion as the chyme passes through the intestines.

While in the compact, coiled mass of the small intestine (compared to the thicker, but much shorter, colon, or large intestine), food materials, especially proteins, are broken down into one of twenty possible amino acid components by the chemical action of two pancreatic enzymes, trypsinogen and chymotrypsinogen, and two enzymes produced in the intestinal walls themselves, aminopeptidase and dipeptidase. It is interesting to note that the body, which is itself in large part constructed of protein material, has its own mechanism to prevent protein-splitting enzymes from devouring the very organs that produce them. Thus, when they leave the pancreas, both trypsinogen and chymotrypsinogen are inactive compounds. They become active "protein-breakers" only when joined by another enzyme—enterokinase—which is secreted from cells in the wall of the small intestine itself.

Other nutritional components contained in chyme interact chemically with other specialized enzymes that are secreted into the small intestine. Carbohydrate molecules, especially starch, begin to break down when exposed to the enzyme amylase in saliva. This process is intensified greatly when pancreatic amylase flows into the small intestine and mixes with the chyme. The products created when carbohydrates break down are simple sugars, including disaccharides and monosaccharides, especially maltose. As these sugars are all broken down into monosaccharides, a final process that occurs in the wall of the small intestine itself (which contains more specialized enzymes such as maltase, sucrase, and lactase), they become the most rapidly assimilated body nutrients.

The process needed to break down fats is more complicated, since fats are water insoluble and enter the intestine in the form of enzyme-resistant globules. Before the fat-splitting enzyme lipase can be chemically active, bile, a fluid produced by the liver and stored in the gallbladder, must be present. Bile serves to dissolve fat globules into tiny droplets that can be broken down for absorption, like all other nutritive elements, into the body via the epithelial lining of the intestinal wall. Such absorption is locally specialized. Iron and calcium pass through the epithelial lining of the duodenum. Protein, fat, sugars, and vitamins pass through the lining of the jejunum, or middle small intestine. Finally, salt, vitamin B_{12}, and bile salts pass through the lining of the lower small intestine, or ileum.

It is this stage that many scientists consider to be the true process of digestion. Absorption occurs through enterocytes, which are specialized cells located on the surface of the epithelium. The surface of the epithelium is increased substantially by the existence of fingerlike projections called villi. These tiny protrusions are surrounded by the fluid elements of chemically altered food. Specialized enterocyte cells selectively absorb these elements into the capillaries that are inside each of the hundreds of thousands of villi. From the capillaries, the nutrients enter the blood and are carried by the portal vein to the liver. This organ carries out the essential chemical processes that prepare fats, carbohydrates, and proteins for their eventual delivery, through the main bloodstream, to various parts of the body.

Elements that are left after the enzymes in the small intestine have done their work are essentially waste material, or feces. These pass from the small intestine to the large intestine, or colon, through a dividing passageway called the cecum. The disposal of waste materials may or may not be considered to be technically part of the main digestive process.

After essential amounts of water and certain salts are absorbed into the body through the walls of the colon, the remaining waste material is expulsed from the bowels through the rectum and anus. If any prior stage in the digestive process is incomplete or if chemical imbalances have occurred, the first symptoms of indigestion may manifest themselves as bowel movement irregularities.

DISORDERS AND DISEASES

Malfunctions in any of the delicate processes that make up digestion can produce symptoms that range from what is commonly called simple indigestion to potentially serious diseases of the gastrointestinal tract. Functional indigestion, or dyspepsia, is one of the most common sources of physical discomfort experienced not only by human beings but by most animals as well. Generally speaking, dyspepsias are not the result of organic disease, but rather of a temporary imbalance in one of the functions described above. There are many possible causes of such an imbalance, including nervous stress and changes in the nature and content of foods eaten.

The most common causes of dyspepsia and their symptoms, although serious enough in chronic cases to require expert medical attention, are far less dangerous than diseases afflicting one of the digestive organs. Such diseases include gallstones, pancreatitis, peptic ulcers (in which excessive acid causes lesions in the stomach wall), and, most serious of all, cancers afflicting any of the abdominal organs.

Dyspepsia may stem from either physical or chemical causes. On the physical side, it is clear that an important part of the digestive process depends on muscular or nerve-related impulses that move partially digested food through the gastrointestinal tract. When, for reasons that are not yet fully understood, the organism fails to coordinate such physical reactions, spasms may occur at several points from the esophagus through to the colon. If extensive, such muscular contractions can create abdominal pains that are symptomatic of at least one category of functional indigestion.

Problems of motility, or physical movement of food materials through the digestive tract, may also cause one common discomfort associated with indigestion: heartburn. This condition occurs when the system fails to move adequate quantities of the mixture of food and gastric juices, including hydrochloric acid, from the stomach into the duodenum. The resultant backup of food forces part of the acidic liquid mass into the esophagus, causing instant discomfort.

Insufficient motility may also cause delays in the movement of feces through the colon, resulting in constipation. Just as the vagus nerve monitors the muscular movements that are necessary to move food from the stomach to the small intestine, an essential gastrocolic reflex, tied to the organism's nervous system, is needed to ensure a constant rhythm in the movement of feces into the rectum for elimination. If this function is delayed (as a result of nervous stress in some individuals, or because of the dilated physical state of the colon in aged persons), food residues become too tightly compressed in the bowels. As the colon continues to carry out its normal last-stage digestive function of reabsorbing essential water from waste material before it is eliminated, the feces become drier and even more compacted, making defecation difficult and sometimes painful.

Most other imbalances in digestive functions are

chemical in nature. Highly spiced or unfamiliar foods frequently upset the balance in the body's chemical digestion. Symptoms may appear either in the abdomen itself (in particular, a bloated stomach accompanied by what is commonly called gas, a symptom of chemical disharmony in the digestive process) or in the stool. If the chemical breakdown of chyme is incomplete because of an imbalance in the proportion (either excessive or inadequate) of enzymes secreted into the stomach or intestines, the normal process of absorption will not take place, creating one of a number of symptoms of indigestion.

The most common symptom of indigestion is diarrhea, which can result from a variety of causes. Because movement in the bowels is affected by different nerve signals, some diarrhea attacks may be linked to nonchemical reactions, such as extreme nervousness. Relaxation of the sphincter, however, as well as the rise in the contractile pressure of the lower colon that precedes defecation (the gastroileal reflex), is also affected by the presence of gastrointestinal hormones, particularly gastrin itself. An imbalance in the amount of concentration of such components in the gastrointestinal tract (attributable to incomplete digestive chemistry) tends to relax the bowels to such a degree that elimination cannot be prevented except through determined mental resistance. It is important to note that if diarrhea continues for an extended time, its effect on the body is not simply the loss of essential body nutrients that pass through the bowels without being fully digested; the inability of the colon to reabsorb into the body an adequate proportion of the water content from the feces can lead to dehydration of the organism, especially in infants.

In most areas of the world, there is widespread consensus that treatment of indigestion is a matter of taking over-the-counter drugs whose function is to right the imbalance in some of the chemical processes described above. In theory as well as in practice, such treatments do work, since the basic chemical imbalance, if it is has not extended beyond the point of indigestion (in the case of peptic ulcers, for example), is fairly easily diagnosed, even by pharmacists. Increasingly, however, the public is becoming aware that digestion can be aided, and indigestion avoided, by paying closer attention to dietary habits, particularly the importance of increasing fiber intake to facilitate the digestive process. Critical advances are also being made in knowledge of the potentially harmful effects on digestion of chemical additives to processed foods.

PERSPECTIVE AND PROSPECTS

Historical traces of the medical observation of indigestion, as well as the prescription of remedies, can be found as far back as ancient Egypt. A famous medical text from about 1600 B.C.E. known as the Ebers Papyrus contains suggested remedies (mainly herbal drugs) for digestive ailments, as well as instructions for the use of suppositories to loosen the lower bowel. For centuries, however, such practical advice for treating indigestion was never accompanied by an adequate theoretical conception of the digestion function itself.

In the medieval Western world, many erroneous guidelines for understanding the digestive process were handed down from the works of Galen of Pergamum (129-c. 199 C.E.). Galen taught that food material passed from the intestines to the liver, where it was transformed into blood. At this point, a vital life-giving spirit, or "pneuma," gave the blood power to drive the body. Similar misconceptions would continue until, following the work of William Harvey (1578-1657), medical science gained more accurate knowledge of the circulatory function of the bloodstream. By the eighteenth century, rapid advances had been made in studies of the function of the stomach and intestines, notably by the French naturalist René de Réaumur (1683-1757), who demonstrated that food is broken down by gastric juices in the stomach, and by the Italian physiologist Lazzaro Spallanzani (1729-1799), who discovered that the stomach itself is the source of gastric juices.

It was an American army surgeon, William Beaumont (1785-1853), who wrote what became, until well into the twentieth century, the most complete medical guide to digestive functions. Beaumont carried out direct clinical observations of the actions of gastric juices in humans. He also observed the way in which the anticipation of eating can spark not only the secretion of such fluids but also the muscular stimuli that promote motility in the digestive process. Soon after Beaumont's findings were published, the German physiologist Theodor Schwann (1810-1882) first isolated pepsin. Others would show that a variety of enzymes in the gastrointestinal tract are secreted by different organs in the abdomen, notably the pancreas.

—Byron D. Cannon, Ph.D.

See also Acid-base chemistry; Acid reflux disease; Celiac sprue; Colitis; Constipation; Crohn's disease; Diarrhea and dysentery; Enzymes; Food biochemistry; Food poisoning; Gastroenterology; Gastroenterology, pediatric; Gastrointestinal disorders; Gastrointestinal system; Heartburn; Hirschsprung's disease; Indigestion; Intestines; Irritable bowel syndrome (IBS); Malabsorption; Metabolism; Nutrition; Over-the-counter medications; Peristalsis; Supplements; Ulcer surgery; Ulcers; Vagotomy; Vitamins and minerals.

For Further Information:

Bonci, Leslie. *American Dietetic Association Guide to Better Digestion.* New York: Wiley, 2003. A user-friendly guide to help analyze one's eating habits, map out a dietary plan to manage and reduce the uncomfortable symptoms of digestive disorders, and find practical recommendations for implementing lifestyle changes.

Jackson, Gordon, and Philip Whitfield. *Digestion: Fueling the System.* New York: Torstar Books, 1984. This compact and excellently illustrated volume is designed for the informed layperson.

Janowitz, Henry D. *Indigestion: Living Better with Upper Intestinal Problems from Heartburn to Ulcers and Gallstones.* New York: Oxford University Press, 1994. Deals with common problems of indigestion and includes medical approaches to the treatment of chronic cases.

Johnson, Leonard R., ed. *Gastrointestinal Physiology.* 7th ed. Philadelphia: Mosby Elsevier, 2007. This book contains a variety of different "self-contained" specialized topics dealt with by experts. Offers the excellent chapters "Gastric Motility" and "Pancreatic Secretion."

Magee, Donal F., and Arthur F. Dalley. *Digestion and the Structure and Function of the Gut.* Basel, Switzerland: S. Karger, 1986. This textbook is part of a continuing education publication series. Although it covers all topics with full technical detail, it is easily understood by a well-informed reader.

Mayo Clinic. *Mayo Clinic on Digestive Health: Enjoy Better Digestion with Answers to More than Twelve Common Conditions.* 2d ed. Rochester, Minn.: Author, 2004. Reviews the causes and treatments of common digestive conditions.

Scanlon, Valerie, and Tina Sanders. *Essentials of Anatomy and Physiology.* 5th ed. Philadelphia: F. A. Davis, 2007. A text designed around three themes: the relationship between physiology and anatomy, the interrelations among the organ systems, and the relationship of each organ system to homeostasis.

Diphtheria
Disease/disorder

Anatomy or system affected: Heart, nervous system, throat

Specialties and related fields: Bacteriology, cardiology, epidemiology, family medicine, microbiology, pediatrics, toxicology

Definition: An acute, contagious disease found primarily in children, associated with toxin production by the bacterium *Corynebacterium diphtheriae*.

Causes and Symptoms

The etiological agent of diphtheria, *Corynebacterium diphtheriae*, is found in some individuals as an inhabitant of the nasopharynx (nose and throat). Its symptoms are associated with the production of a toxin. Only those strains of the organism carrying a bacteriophage in a lysogenic state produce the toxin. Spread of diphtheria is generally person to person through respiratory secretions or through contaminated environmental surfaces.

Following an incubation period of several days to a week, symptoms often have a sudden onset and typically include a sore throat, malaise, and a mild fever. The disease is further characterized by an exudative, pseudomembrane formation on the mucous surface of the throat, which results from replication of the organism in the pharynx or surrounding areas. The pseudomembrane can become quite thick and may cause respiratory stress through obstruction of the breathing passages. Toxin is secreted into the bloodstream, where its presence can result in damage to the heart, nervous system, or other organs. Diagnosis is based upon a combination of symptoms, as well as isolation of the organism in a throat culture.

A less common form of diphtheria may be observed on skin surfaces. It contains bacteria that can be spread

---

Information on Diphtheria

Causes: Toxin production by bacteria

Symptoms: Sore throat, malaise, mild fever, pseudomembrane formation in throat; when systemic, damage to heart, nervous system, or other organs

Duration: Acute

Treatments: Antibiotics (penicillin, erythromycin), antitoxin

through contaminated environmental surfaces. Infection generally occurs through small cuts in the skin. Cutaneous diphtheria is characterized by an ulcer that heals slowly. If the organism is a strain that produces toxin, then systemic damage may result.

TREATMENT AND THERAPY

Most diphtheria infections respond to antibiotics, either a single dose of penicillin or a seven-day or ten-day course of erythromycin. Since symptoms are associated with toxin production, the administration of antitoxin is critical to early treatment. Once toxin has been incorporated into the target, cell death is irreversible. Antibiotic treatment, however, does result in the elimination of the organism and the termination of further toxin production.

Vaccination with diphtheria toxoid, an inactivated form of the toxin, has proven effective in immunization against the disease. Prophylaxis is generally started early in childhood as part of the trivalent DPT (diphtheria, pertussis, tetanus) series. Boosters are recommended at ten-year intervals.

PERSPECTIVE AND PROSPECTS

Introduction of the diphtheria vaccine in the first decades of the twentieth century served to reduce significantly the incidence of the disease in the West. The use of antibiotic therapy further reduced the fatality rate associated with this disease, which ranged from 30 to 50 percent at its peak. On average, fewer than ten cases per year are now observed in the United States, generally associated with asymptomatic carriers. Diphtheria still exists as a childhood scourge, however, in much of the Third World.

—*Richard Adler, Ph.D.*

See also Antibiotics; Bacterial infections; Bacteriology; Childhood infectious diseases; Immunization and vaccination; Sore throat.

FOR FURTHER INFORMATION:

Forbes, Betty, Daniel F. Sahm, and Alice S. Weissfeld. *Bailey and Scott's Diagnostic Microbiology.* 11th ed. St. Louis: Mosby, 2002.

Grob, Gerald N. *The Deadly Truth: A History of Disease in America.* Cambridge, Mass.: Harvard University Press, 2002.

Parker, James N., and Philip M. Parker, eds. *The Official Patient's Sourcebook on Diphtheria.* San Diego, Calif.: Icon Health, 2002.

DISEASE

DISEASE/DISORDER

ANATOMY OR SYSTEM AFFECTED: All

SPECIALTIES AND RELATED FIELDS: All

DEFINITION: A morbid (pathological) process with a characteristic set of symptoms that may affect the entire body or any of its parts; the cause, pathology, and course of a disease may be known or unknown.

KEY TERMS:

diagnosis: the art of distinguishing one disease from another

lesion: any pathologic or traumatic discontinuity of tissue or loss of function of a body part

pathology: the study of the essential nature of disease, especially as it relates to the structural and functional changes that are caused by that disease

prognosis: a forecast regarding the probable cause and result of an attack of disease

syndrome: a congregation of a set of signs and symptoms that characterize a particular disease process, but without a specific etiology or a constant lesion

TYPES OF DISEASE

It is difficult to answer the question "What is disease?" To the patient, disease means discomfort and disharmony with the environment. To the treating physician or surgeon, it means a set of signs and symptoms. To the pathologist, it means one or more structural changes in body tissues, called lesions, which may be viewed with or without the aid of magnifying lenses.

The study of lesions, which are the essential expression of disease, forms part of the modern science of pathology. Pathology had its beginnings in the morgue and the autopsy room, where investigations into the cause of death led to the appreciation of "morbid anatomy"—at first by gross (naked-eye) examination and later microscopically. Much later, the investigation of disease moved from the cold autopsy room to the patient's bedside, from the dead body to the living body, on which laboratory tests and biopsies are performed for the purpose of establishing a diagnosis and addressing proper treatment.

Diagnosis is the art of determining not only the character of the lesion but also its etiology, or cause. Because so much of this diagnostic work is done in laboratories, the term "laboratory medicine" has gained in popularity. The explosion in high technology has expanded the field of laboratory medicine tremendously. The diagnostic laboratory today is highly automated and sophisticated, containing a team of laboratory technologists and scientific researchers rather than a single pathologist.

The lesions laid bare by the pathologist usually bear an obvious relation to the symptoms, as in the gross lesions of acute appendicitis, the microscopic lesions in poliomyelitis, or even the chromosomal lesions in genetically inherited conditions such as Down syndrome. Yet there may be lesions without symptoms, as in early cancer or "silent" diseases such as tuberculosis. There may also be symptoms without obvious lesions, as in the so-called psychosomatic diseases, functional disorders, and psychiatric illnesses. It is likely that future research will reveal the presence of "biochemical lesions" in these cases. The presence of lesions distinguishes organic disease, in which there are gross or microscopic pathologic changes in an organ, from functional disease, in which there is a disturbance of function without a corresponding obvious organic lesion. Although most diagnoses consist largely of naming the lesion (such as cancer of the lung or a tooth abscess), diseases should truly be considered in the light of disordered function rather than altered structure. Scientists are searching beyond the presence of obvious lesions in tissues and cells to the submicroscopic, molecular, and biochemical alterations affecting the chemistry of cells.

Not every disease has a specific etiology. A syndrome is a complex of signs and symptoms with no specific etiology or constant lesion. It results from interference at some point with a chain of body processes, causing impairment of body function in one or more systems. With a syndrome, a specific biochemical molecular derangement caused by yet undiscovered agents is usually found. An example is acquired immunodeficiency syndrome (AIDS), for which a specific human immunodeficiency virus (HIV) agent is now accepted as the etiologic agent.

Some diseases have an acute (sudden) onset and run a relatively short course, as with acute tonsillitis (strep throat) or the common cold. Others run a long, protracted course, as with tuberculosis and rheumatoid arthritis; these are called chronic illnesses. The healthy body is in a natural state of readiness to combat disease, and thus there is a natural tendency to recover from disease. This is especially true in acute illness, in which inflammation tends to heal with full resolution of structure and function. Sometimes, however, healing does not occur and the disease overwhelms the body and leads to death. Therefore, a patient with acute pneumonia may have a full recovery, with complete healing and resolution of structure and function, or may die. The outcome of disease can vary between the extremes of full recovery or death and can run a chronic, protracted course eventually leading to severe loss of function. This outcome is the prognosis, a forecast of what may be expected to happen. The accurate diagnosis of disease is essential for its treatment and prognosis.

There are four aspects to the study of disease. The first is etiology or cause; for example, the common cold virus causes the common cold. The second is pathogenesis, or course; it refers to the sequence of events in the body that occurs in response to injury and the method of the lesion's production and development. The relation of an etiologic agent to disease, of cause to effect, is not always as simple a matter as it is in most acute illnesses; for example, a herpesvirus causes the development of fever blisters. In many illnesses, indeed in most chronic illnesses, the concept of one agent causing one disease is an oversimplification. In tuberculosis, for example, the causative agent is a characteristic slender microbe called tubercle bacillus (*Mycobacterium tuberculosis*). Many people may be exposed to and inhale the tuberculosis bacteria, but only a few will get the disease; also, the bacteria may lurk in the body for years and become clinically active only as a result of an unrelated, stressful situation that alters the body's immunity, such as prolonged strain, malnutrition, or another infection. In investigating the causation and pathogenesis of disease, several factors—such as heredity, sex, environment, nutrition, immunity, and age—must be considered. That is why there is no simple answer to the questions, "Does cigarette smoking cause cancer?" or "Does a cholesterol-rich diet cause hardening of the blood vessels (atherosclerosis)?" The third aspect to the study of disease relates to morphologic and structural changes associated with the functional alterations in cells and tissues that are characteristic of the disease. These are the gross and microscopic findings that allow the pathologist to establish a diagnosis. The fourth aspect to disease study is the evaluation of functional abnormalities and their clinical significance; the nature of the morphologic changes and their distribution in different organs or tissues influence normal function and determine the clinical features, signs and symptoms, and course and outcome (prognosis) of disease.

All forms of tissue injury start with molecular and structural changes in cells. Cells are the smallest living units of tissues and organs. Along with their substructural components, they are the seat of disease. Cellular pathology is the study of disease as it relates to the origins, molecular mechanisms, and structural changes of cell injury.

The normal cell is similar to a factory. It is confined to a fairly narrow range of function and structure, dictated by its genetic code, the constraints of neighboring cells, the availability of and access to nutrition, and the disposal of its waste products. It is said to be in a "steady state," able to handle normal physiologic demands and to respond by adapting to other excessive or strenuous demands (such as the muscle enlargement seen in bodybuilders) to achieve a new equilibrium with a sustained workload. This type of adaptive response is called hypertrophy. Conversely, atrophy is an adaptive response to decreased demand, with a resulting diminished size and function.

If the limits of these adaptive responses are exceeded, or if no adaptive response is possible, a sequence of events follows which results in cell injury. Cell injury is reversible up to a certain point, but if the stimulus persists or is severe, then the cell suffers irreversible injury and eventual death. For example, if the blood supply to the heart muscle is cut off for only a few minutes and then restored, the heart muscle cells will experience injury but can recover and function normally. If the blood flow is not restored until one hour later, however, the cells will die.

Whether specific types of stress induce an adaptive response, a reversible injury, or cell death depends on the nature and severity of the stress and on other inherent, variable qualities of the cell itself. The causes of cell injury are many and range from obvious physical trauma, as in automobile accidents, to a subtle, genetic lack of enzymes or hormones, as in diabetes mellitus. Broadly speaking, the causes of cell injury and death can be grouped into the following categories: hypoxia, or a decrease in the delivery of available oxygen; physical agents, as with mechanical and thermal injuries; chemical poisons, such as carbon monoxide and alcohol, tobacco, and other addictive drugs; infectious agents, such as viruses and bacteria; immunological and allergic reactions, as in patients with certain sensitivities; genetic defects, as with sickle cell disease; and nutritional imbalances, such as severe malnutrition and vitamin deficiencies or nutritional excesses predisposing a patient to heart disease and atherosclerosis.

CAUSES OF DISEASE

By far the most common cause of disease is infection, especially by bacteria. Certain lowly forms of animal life known as animal parasites may also live in the body and produce disease; parasitic diseases are common in poor societies and countries. Finally, there are viruses, forms of living matter so minute that they cannot be seen with the most powerful light microscope; they are visible, however, with the electron microscope. Viruses, as agents of disease, have attracted much attention for their role in many diseases, including cancer.

Bacteria, or germs, can be divided into three morphologic groups: cocci, which are round; bacilli, which are rod-shaped; and spirilla or spirochetes, which are spiral-shaped, like a corkscrew. Bacteria produce disease either by their presence in tissues or by their production of toxins (poisons). They cause inflammation and either act on surrounding tissues, as in an abscess, or are carried by the bloodstream to other distant organs. Strep throat is an example of a local infection by cocci—in this case, streptococci. Some dysenteries and travelers' diarrheas are caused by coliform bacilli. Syphilis is an example of a disease caused by a spirochete. The great epidemics of history, such as bubonic plague and cholera, have been caused by bacteria, as are tuberculosis, leprosy, typhoid, gas gangrene, and many others. Bacterial infections are treatable with antibiotics, such as penicillin.

Viruses, on the other hand, are not affected by antibiotics; they infect the cell itself and live within it, and are therefore protected. Viruses cause a wide variety of diseases. Some are short-lived and run a few days' course, such as many childhood diseases, the measles, and the common cold. Others can cause serious body impairment, such as poliomyelitis and AIDS. Still others are probably involved in causing cancer and such diseases as multiple sclerosis.

Of the many physical agents causing injury, trauma is the most obvious; others relate to external temperatures, ones that are either too high or too low. A high temperature may produce local injury, such as a burn, or general disease, such as heat stroke. Heat stroke results from prolonged direct exposure to the sun (sunstroke) or from very high temperatures, so that the heat-regulating mechanism of the body becomes paralyzed. The internal body temperature shoots up to alarming heights; collapse, coma, and even death may result. Low temperatures can cause local frostbite or general hypothermia, which can also lead to death.

Other forms of physical agents causing injury are radiation and atmospheric pressure. Increased atmospheric pressure is best illustrated by the "bends," a decompression sickness which can affect deep sea divers.

The pressure of the water causes inert gases, such as nitrogen, to be dissolved in the blood plasma. If the diver passes too rapidly from a high to a normal atmospheric pressure, the excessive nitrogen is released, forming gas bubbles in the blood. These tiny bubbles can cause the blockage of small vessels of the brain and result in brain damage. The same problem can occur in high-altitude aviators unless the airplane is pressurized.

The study of chemical poisoning, or toxicology, as a cause of disease is a large and specialized field. Poisons may be introduced into the body by accident (especially in young children), in the course of suicide or homicide, and, most important, as industrial pollution. Lead poisoning is a danger because of the use of lead in paints and soldering. Acids and carbon monoxide are emitted into the atmosphere by industry, and various chemicals are dumped into the ground and water. Such environmental damage will eventually affect plants, livestock, and humans.

Hypoxia (lack of oxygen) is probably the most common cause of cell injury, and it may also be the ultimate mechanism of cell death by a wide variety of physical, biological, and chemical agents. Loss of adequate blood and oxygen supply to a body part, such as a leg, is called ischemia. (This is a local loss of blood, in contrast to anemia, which is a general condition of poor oxygen-carrying capacity affecting the entire body.) If the blood loss is very severe, the result is hypoxia or anoxia. This condition may also result from narrowing of the blood vessels, called atherosclerosis. If this narrowing occurs in the artery of the leg, as may be seen in patients with advanced diabetes, then the tissues of the foot will eventually die, a condition known as gangrene. An even more critical example of ischemia is blockage of the coronary arteries of the heart, resulting in a myocardial infarction (heart attack), with damage to the heart muscle. Similarly, severe blockage of arteries to the brain can cause a stroke.

Nutritional diseases can be caused either by an excessive intake and storage of foodstuffs, as in extreme obesity, or by a deficiency. Obesity is a complex condition, often associated with hereditary tendencies and hormonal imbalances. The deficiency conditions are many. Starvation and malnutrition can occur because of intestinal illnesses that prevent the delivery of food to the blood (malabsorption) or because of debilitating diseases such as advanced cancer. Even more important than general malnutrition as a cause of disease is a deficiency of essential nutrients such as minerals, vitamins, and other trace elements. Iron deficiency causes anemia, and calcium deficiency causes osteoporosis (bone fragility). Vitamin deficiencies are also numerous, and deficiency of the trace element iodine causes a thyroid condition called goiter.

Genetic defects as a cause of cellular injury and disease are of major interest to many biologists. The genetic injury may be as gross as the congenital malformations seen in patients with Down syndrome or as subtle as molecular alterations in the coding of the hemoglobin molecule that causes sickle cell disease.

Cellular injuries and diseases can be induced by immune mechanisms. The anaphylactic reaction to a foreign protein, such as a bee sting or drug, can actually cause death. In the so-called autoimmune diseases, such as lupus erythematosus, the immune system turns against the cellular components of the very body that it is supposed to protect.

Finally, neoplastic diseases, or cancer, are presently of unknown etiology. Some are innocuous growths, while others are highly lethal. Diagnosing cancer and determining its precise nature can be an elaborate, and elusive, process. The methods involve clinical observations and laboratory tests; a biopsy of the involved organ may be taken and analyzed.

PERSPECTIVE AND PROSPECTS

It is sometimes said that the nature of disease is changing, that one hears more often of people dying of heart failure and cancer than was once the case. This does not mean that these diseases have actually become more common, although more people do die from them. This increase is attributable to a longer life span and vastly improved diagnostic methods.

For primitive humans, there were no diseases, only patients stricken by evil; therefore, magic was the plausible recourse. Magic entails recognition of the principle of causality—that, given the same predisposing conditions, the same results will follow. In a profound sense, magic is early science. In ancient Egypt, the priests assumed the role of healers. Unlike magic, religion springs from a different source. Here the system is based on the achievement of results against, or in spite of, a regular sequence of events. Religion heals with miracles and antinaturals that require the violation of causality. The purely religious concept of disease, as an expression of the wrath of gods, became embodied in many religious traditions.

The ancient Greeks are credited with attempts at introducing reason to the study of disease by asking questions about the nature of things and considering the notion of health as a harmony, as the adjustment of such opposites as high and low, hot and cold, dry and moist. Disease, therefore, was a disharmony of the four elements that make up life: earth, air, fire, and water. This concept was refined by Galen in the second century and became dogma throughout the Dark Ages until the Renaissance, when the seat of disease was finally assigned to organs within the body itself through autopsy studies. Much later, in the nineteenth century, the principles espoused by French physiologist Claude Bernard were introduced, whereby disease was considered not a thing but a process that distorts normal physiologic and anatomic features. The nineteenth century German pathologist Rudolf Virchow emphasized the same principle—that disease is an alteration of life's processes—by championing the concept of cellular pathology, identifying the cell as the smallest unit of life and as the seat of disease.

As new diseases are discovered and old medical mysteries are deciphered, as promising new medicinal drugs and vaccines are tested and public health programs implemented, the age-old goal of medicine as a healing art seems to be closer at hand.

—Victor H. Nassar, M.D.

See also Centers for Disease Control and Prevention (CDC); Childhood infectious diseases; Dental diseases; Environmental diseases; Gallbladder diseases; Genetic diseases; Infection; Insect-borne diseases; Motor neuron diseases; National Institutes of Health (NIH); Parasitic diseases; Pathology; Prion diseases; Protozoan diseases; Pulmonary diseases; Sexually transmitted diseases (STDs); Zoonoses; *specific diseases*.

FOR FURTHER INFORMATION:

Biddle, Wayne. *A Field Guide to Germs.* 2d ed. New York: Anchor Books, 2002. This comprehensive book is easily accessible to the nonspecialist and includes a discussion of nearly every virus, bacterium, and fungus known to cause human and nonhuman animal disease. The history of the microbe and the treatment of diseases are included.

Boyd, William. *Boyd's Introduction to the Study of Disease.* 11th ed. Philadelphia: Lea & Febiger, 1992. A textbook for students in the medical and allied health sciences. The text and illustrations emphasize the view of disease as a disturbed functional alteration.

Frank, Steven A. *Immunology and Evolution of Infectious Disease.* Princeton, N.J.: Princeton University Press, 2002. Blends research from molecular biology, immunology, pathogen biology, and population dynamics to discuss how and why parasites vary to escape recognition by the immune system, vaccine design, and the control of epidemics.

Grist, Norman R., et al. *Diseases of Infection: An Illustrated Textbook.* 2d ed. New York: Oxford University Press, 1992. An informative survey of communicable diseases. Contains copious illustrations.

Kumar, Vinay, Abul K. Abbas, and Nelson Fausto, eds. *Robbins and Cotran Pathologic Basis of Disease.* 7th ed. Philadelphia: Elsevier Saunders, 2005. The standard textbook on disease for medical students.

McCance, Kathryn L., and Sue M. Huether. *Pathophysiology: The Biologic Basis for Disease in Adults and Children.* 5th ed. St. Louis: Elsevier Mosby, 2006. A text that explores the myriad cellular and genetic causes of disease. Topics include cell injury, immunity, inflammation and wound healing, coping and illness, and ontogenesis.

Shaw, Michael, ed. *Everything You Need to Know About Diseases.* Springhouse, Pa.: Springhouse Press, 1996. This well-illustrated consumer reference, compiled by more than one hundred doctors and medical experts, describes five hundred illnesses and conditions, their causes, symptoms, diagnosis, treatment, and prevention. A valuable reference book for everyone interested in health and disease.

Strauss, James, and Ellen Strauss. *Viruses and Human Disease.* San Diego, Calif.: Academic Press, 2001. An undergraduate text that examines virology from a human disease perspective.

DISK REMOVAL

PROCEDURE

ANATOMY OR SYSTEM AFFECTED: Back, bones, nervous system, spine

SPECIALTIES AND RELATED FIELDS: General surgery, neurology, orthopedics, physical therapy

DEFINITION: A surgical procedure used to remove intervertebral disks that are compressing nerves that enter and exit the spinal cord.

KEY TERMS:

cervical vertebrae: the first seven bones of the spinal column, located in the neck

disk prolapse: the protrusion (herniation) of intervertebral disk material, which may press on spinal nerves

intervertebral disks: flattened disks of fibrocartilage

that separate the vertebrae and allow cushioned flexibility of the spinal column

lumbar vertebrae: the five bones of the spinal column
in the lower back, which experience the greatest
stress in the spine

spinal cord: a column of nervous tissue housed in the
vertebral column which carries messages to and
from the brain

INDICATIONS AND PROCEDURES

A relatively common disorder which causes lower back
and sometimes leg pain is the herniation or prolapse of
an intervertebral disk in the lower back. These disks are
made of cartilage and serve to separate the bones that
make up the vertebral column. The spinal cord is located within the bony structure of the vertebrae and
has nerves which enter and exit between these bones.
These sensory and motor nerves must pass alongside
the intervertebral disks. When a disk's jellylike center bulges out through a weakened area of the firmer
outer core, the disk is said to be herniated or prolapsed.
This may compress the spinal cord or the nerve roots
and yield such symptoms as interference with muscle
strength or pain and numbness of the lower back and
leg.

More than 90 percent of disk prolapses occur in the
lumbar region of the back, but they may also occur in
the cervical vertebrae. Occasionally, disk herniation is
caused by improper lifting of heavy objects, sudden
twisting of the spinal column, or trauma to the back or
neck. More typically, however, a prolapsed disk develops gradually as the patient ages and the intervertebral
disks degenerate.

In order to diagnose a prolapsed disk, a physician
will likely want to visualize the vertebrae and spinal
cord using X rays, computed tomography (CT) scans,
or magnetic resonance imaging (MRI). Once diagnosed, most cases can be treated with analgesics, muscle relaxants (such as cyclobenzaprine and metho-
carbamol), and physical therapy. If the symptoms recur,
however, it may be necessary to have the protruding
portion of the disk or the whole disk surgically removed. This procedure usually requires that the patient
have general anesthesia and remain hospitalized for
several days.

For a lumbar procedure, the patient is anesthetized
and placed on the operating room table in a modified
kneeling position, with the abdomen suspended and the
legs placed over the end of the table. The lower back is
then prepared for a sterile procedure, and the surgeon

makes an incision in the middle of the back along the
spine. The surrounding tissues are retracted, and the
vertebrae are exposed. At this time, the surgeon must
make a careful dissection of the tissues in order to identify the affected nerves and intervertebral disk. Once
the prolapsed disk is found, the physician will cut away
the fragment of the disk impinging on the nerve. It is
important that all free fragments be removed, as these
could cause symptoms at a later time. Often, the surgeon must remove some of the vertebrae to gain access
to the disk. This is known as a laminectomy.

USES AND COMPLICATIONS

Because the vertebral column houses the spinal cord,
any surgical manipulation of this area must be ap-
proached with extreme caution. Very large arteries (the
aorta) and veins (the vena cava) lie adjacent to the spinal column, and accidental cuts can lead to rapid blood
loss. The spinal cord is surrounded by a covering called
the meninges, which helps to protect the cord and
which contains the cerebral spinal fluid. Trauma to the
meninges may cause the fluid to leak out or lead to
meningitis (inflammation of the meninges). One surgical approach to reduce the adverse affects of a lesion on
the meninges is to use some of the patient's fat to pack
the leak and help prevent scarring. Patients with operative trauma to the meninges may complain of headache, which usually decreases in severity as the lesion
heals.

Other complications that may arise include infections in approximately 3 percent of patients, thromboembolism in less than 1 percent, and death in about one
patient per 1,000. One study reports an overall complication rate of 4 percent. Unfortunately, one of the major
long-term complications reported in the study involved
a worsening of symptoms after surgery.

PERSPECTIVE AND PROSPECTS

Even with some potential complications, disk removal
typically has a favorable outcome, although this varies
somewhat depending on the patient, the treatment
method, and what the patient and physician consider "a
good result." Typically, favorable outcomes range
from 50 to 95 percent. The number of patients who
need a second operation ranges from 4 to 25 percent.

Health care professionals are beginning to emphasize the importance of prevention of back pain. Educating patients on proper lifting techniques, such as
bending the legs rather than the back and avoiding
twisting, will reduce the potential for damage to the

intervertebral disks. Individuals who are overweight are also at risk for developing lower back pain because of the added stress to the lumbar spine, as well as because of their relatively weak abdominal muscles. The abdominal muscles are important in stabilizing and supporting the lower back. Exercises which help strengthen these muscles are recommended for a weight-reducing exercise and diet program. Patients who must sit for long periods of time are also at risk for lower back pain. These people should take several quick breaks to stand and stretch, which reduces the constant stress on the lumbar spine.

—*Matthew Berria, Ph.D.,*
and Douglas Reinhart, M.D.

See also Back pain; Bone disorders; Bones and the skeleton; Braces, orthopedic; Laminectomy and spinal fusion; Meningitis; Orthopedic surgery; Orthopedics; Slipped disk; Spinal cord disorders; Spine, vertebrae, and disks.

For Further Information:

Aminoff, Michael J. "Nervous System." In *Current Medical Diagnosis and Treatment 2004*, edited by Lawrence M. Tierney, Jr., Stephen J. McPhee, and Maxine A. Papadakis. 43d ed. New York: McGraw-Hill, 2003. A chapter in a text which is the point of reference for physicians and other health care practitioners. It incorporates each year's biomedical research discoveries that have immediate, relevant, and applicable use for the patient.

Bradford, David S., and Thomas A. Zdeblick, eds. *The Spine*. 2d ed. Philadelphia: Lippincott Williams & Wilkins, 2004. Discusses surgical methods and options for the treatment of the spine. Includes bibliographical references and an index.

Canale, S. Terry, ed. *Campbell's Operative Orthopaedics*. 10th ed. 4 vols. St. Louis: Mosby, 2003. The section "The Spine" contains an essay, "Lower Back Pain and Disorders of Intervertebral Discs," which discusses such topics as microsurgery, nontraumatic bone and joint disorders, arthrodesis, arthroplasty, and congenital anomalies.

Filler, Aaron G. *Do You Really Need Back Surgery? A Surgeon's Guide to Back and Neck Pain and How to Choose Your Treatment*. Rev. ed. New York: Oxford University Press, 2007. A good review of diagnosis and treatment options.

Haldeman, Scott, William H. Kirkaldy-Willis, and Thomas N. Bernard, Jr. *Atlas of Back Pain*. Boca Raton, Fla.: Parthenon, 2002. A clinical text that ex-

plains how to determine the underlying causes of back conditions and describes the various treatment options available.

Leikin, Jerrold B., and Martin S. Lipsky, eds. *American Medical Association Complete Medical Encyclopedia*. New York: Random House Reference, 2003. A concise presentation of numerous medical terms and illnesses. A good general reference.

Dislocation. *See* Fracture and dislocation.

Disseminated intravascular coagulation (DIC)

Disease/disorder

Also known as: Consumption coagulopathy

Anatomy or system affected: Blood, blood vessels, circulatory system, immune system

Specialties and related fields: Hematology, internal medicine, neonatology, obstetrics, oncology

Definition: A hemorrhagic disorder that occurs as a complication of several different disease states and results from abnormally initiated and accelerated blood clotting.

Key terms:

acute DIC: a disorder of the blood-clotting mechanism that develops within hours of an initial attack on an underlying body system

chronic DIC: a disorder of the blood-clotting mechanism that persists in a suppressed state until a coagulation disorder worsens

coagulation: the process of blood clot formation

coagulation cascade: the series of steps starting with the activation of the intrinsic or extrinsic pathways of coagulation and proceeding through the common pathway of coagulation leading to the formation of fibrin clots

ecchymosis: bleeding into the skin, subcutaneous tissue, or mucous membranes, resulting in bruising

hemostasis: the stopping of blood flow through the blood vessels, usually as a result of blood clotting

petechiae: round pinpoint hemorrhages in the skin

platelets: cells, found in the blood of all mammals, that are involved in the coagulation of blood and the contraction of blood clots

thrombocytopenia: a markedly decreased number of platelets in the blood

thromboembolism: the obstruction of a blood vessel with a clot that has broken loose from its site of origin

CAUSES AND SYMPTOMS

Disseminated intravascular coagulation (DIC) is a disorder that occurs as a life-threatening complication of many different conditions. It is most commonly seen as a complication of bacterial, fungal, parasitic, or viral infections; inflammatory bowel disease; pregnancy; cancer; surgery; major trauma; burns; heat stroke; shock; transplant rejection; toxicity resulting from recreational drug use; or snakebite. It can occur as either an acute or a chronic condition, depending on the underlying cause.

In both forms, DIC involves the systemic activation of the hemostasis system. In its acute form, DIC involves hemorrhaging, the development of ecchymoses, bleeding of the mucosa, and depletion or absence of platelets and clotting factors in the blood. In the most severe cases, it is accompanied by extensive consumption of the proteins involved in coagulation, significant deposits of fibrin in the vasculature and organs, and bleeding that may lead to organ failure and death. In its chronic form, it is more subtle and usually includes thromboembolism along with activation of the coagulation system.

In acute DIC, the introduction of tissue factors into the circulation (from injury, surgery, or tissue necrosis), stagnant blood flow (from shock or cardiac arrest), or the presence of infectious agents leads to systemic activation of the coagulation system. A massive clotting cascade is triggered and leads to the formation of blood clots, possibly compromising the blood supply to major organs, and simultaneously to the exhaustion of platelets and coagulation factors, resulting in hemorrhaging.

Thus, DIC occurs when endothelial cells or monocytes are damaged by toxic substances. When these cells are injured, they release tissue factor on the surface of the cell, which in turn triggers the hemostasis system, activating a coagulation cascade. Thrombin accumulates rapidly, and fibrin is produced in large quantities and is deposited in the microvasculature, leading to blood clots throughout the capillary system. This clot formation leads rapidly to the depletion of platelets and coagulation factors throughout the body. Simultaneously, thrombin activates fibrinolytic pathways that release anticoagulants and dissolve the clots by turning them into fibrin split products, further contributing to uncontrollable bleeding.

In chronic DIC, these events occur more slowly, allowing compensation to take place.

The diagnosis of DIC is based on clinical signs and laboratory findings. In acute DIC, the symptoms include multiple bleeding sites, the development of petechiae on the skin, ecchymoses of the skin and mucous membranes, visceral hemorrhaging, and the development of ischemic tissue. In chronic DIC, symptoms will include deep vein or arterial thrombosis or embolism, superficial venous thrombosis (especially in the absence of varicose veins), multiple and simultaneous thrombus sites, or serial thrombotic episodes. Laboratory findings indicative of DIC are decreased platelet count, prolonged prothrombin time (PT), activated partial thromboplastin time (APTT), and thrombin time along with decreased fibrinogen levels and increased fibrin-fibrinogen degradation product (FDP) levels. Peripheral smears will show the presence of schistocytes (fragments of red blood cells).

TREATMENT AND THERAPY

The treatment of either the acute or the chronic form of DIC is based on the etiology and pathophysiology of the underlying clinical condition. Aside from the treatment of the underlying disorder, acute DIC requires aggressive treatment of the bleeding through the use of anticoagulants (such as heparin or antithrombin III) and antifibrinolytics (Amicar or Cykokapron), as well as the administration of blood products, including fresh frozen plasma, cryoprecipitate, red blood cells, and platelets. The prognosis is determined by the underly-

---

INFORMATION ON DISSEMINATED INTRAVASCULAR COAGULATION (DIC)

CAUSES: Accelerated blood clotting that may be complication of bacterial, fungal, parasitic, or viral infections; inflammatory bowel disease; pregnancy; cancer; surgery; major trauma; burns; heat stroke; shock; transplant rejection; drug use; snakebite

SYMPTOMS: Hemorrhaging, bruising, bleeding of mucosa, depletion or absence of platelets and clotting factors in blood

DURATION: Acute or chronic, depending on cause

TREATMENTS: Dependent on underlying condition; anticoagulants (heparin, antithrombin III), antifibrinolytics (Amicar, Cykokapron), blood products (fresh frozen plasma, cryoprecipitate, red blood cells, platelets)

ing condition that led to DIC, as well as the severity of the DIC. Follow-up care for those who survive is provided by a primary physician, for the underlying disorder, and by a hematologist.

PERSPECTIVE AND PROSPECTS

It is unclear when disseminated intravascular coagulation was first mentioned in the medical literature. Historically, it has always been considered a secondary disease (resulting as a consequence of some underlying disorder). Thus, DIC has always referred to the secondary activation of the coagulation system as a result of an underlying problem. It occurs with equal frequency in males and females and does not appear to be age-related. Approximately 20,000 cases per year were diagnosed in the United States during the mid-1990's.

While DIC is generally categorized, treated, and evaluated based on the pathophysiology of the underlying disorder, Rodger L. Bick has proposed a DIC scoring system to assess the severity of the coagulation disorder, as well as the effectiveness of the treatment modalities. New treatment modalities, such as the use of recombinant activated protein C, are being investigated in large multicenter clinical trials.

—Robin Kamienny Montvilo, Ph.D.

See also Bleeding; Blood and blood disorders; Circulation; Hematology; Hematology, pediatric; Ischemia; Thrombosis and thrombus.

FOR FURTHER INFORMATION:

Bick, Rodger L. "Disseminated Intravascular Coagulation: Objective Criteria for Diagnosis and Management." *Medical Clinics of North America* 78 (1994): 511-543.

Kasper, Dennis L., et al., eds. *Harrison's Principles of Internal Medicine.* 16th ed. New York: McGraw-Hill, 2005.

Lichtman, Marshall A., et al., eds. *Williams Hematology.* 7th ed. New York: McGraw-Hill, 2006.

DIVERTICULITIS AND DIVERTICULOSIS
DISEASE/DISORDER

ANATOMY OR SYSTEM AFFECTED: Abdomen, gastrointestinal system, intestines

SPECIALTIES AND RELATED FIELDS: Gastroenterology, internal medicine, proctology

DEFINITION: Diverticulosis is a disease involving multiple outpouchings, or diverticuli, of the wall of the colon; these diverticuli may become inflamed, leading to the painful condition called diverticulitis.

KEY TERMS:

colon: the portion of the large intestine excluding the cecum and rectum; it includes the ascending, transverse, descending, and sigmoid colon

dietary fiber: indigestible plant substances that humans eat; fiber may be soluble, meaning that it dissolves in water, or insoluble, meaning that it does not dissolve in water

hernia: the bulging out of part or all of an organ through the wall of the cavity that usually contains it

infection: multiplication of disease-causing microorganisms in the body; the body normally also contains microorganisms that do not cause disease

inflammation: a tissue response to injury involving local reactions that attempt to destroy the injurious material and begin healing

lumen: the channel within a hollow or tubular organ

mucosa: the inner lining of the digestive tract; in the colon, the major function of the mucosal cells is to reabsorb liquid from feces, creating a semisolid material

perforation: an abnormal opening, such as a hole in the wall of the colon

peritoneal cavity: the cavity in the abdomen and pelvis that contains the internal organs

prevalence: the frequency of disease cases in a population, often expressed as a fraction (such as cases per 100,000)

CAUSES AND SYMPTOMS

Diverticulosis is an acquired condition of the colon that involves a few to hundreds of blueberry-sized outpouchings of its wall, called diverticuli. Diverticular disease is usually manifested by the presence of multiple diverticuli that are at risk of causing abdominal pain, inflammation, or bleeding.

Although the wall of the colon is thin, microscopically it has four layers. The innermost layer is called the mucosa. Its main function is to absorb fluids from the substance entering the colon, turning it into a semisolid material called feces. Outside the mucosa is the submucosa, a layer which contains blood vessels as well as nerve cells that control the functions of mucosal cells. Outside the submucosa is the muscularis, which contains muscle cells that are able to contract, pushing feces along the colon and eventually out through the rectum. Outside the muscularis is the serosa, which forms a wrap around the colon and helps prevent infections in this organ from spreading beyond its walls.

The definition of a diverticulum, taken from *Sted-*

INFORMATION ON DIVERTICULITIS AND DIVERTICULOSIS

CAUSES: Aging, low-fiber diet
SYMPTOMS: Abdominal pain; rectal bleeding; sudden urge to defecate followed by passage of red blood, clots, or maroon-colored stool; sometimes fever
DURATION: Chronic, with acute episodes
TREATMENTS: Increased dietary fiber, intravenous fluids, antispasmodic drugs, antibiotics, blood transfusions, surgery

man's *Medical Dictionary* (27th ed., 2000), is "a pouch or sac opening from a tubular or saccular organ, such as the gut or bladder." The diverticuli that form in the colon are not true diverticuli, in that the entire wall is not present in the outpouching. If examined microscopically, only the mucosal and submucosal layers pouch out through weakened areas in the muscularis layer. If examined by the naked eye, however, it appears as if the entire wall of the colon is involved in the tiny outpouching. The mucosa bulges out in the part of the colonic wall that is weakened: This is where arteries penetrate through clefts in the muscularis.

The large intestine begins with the cecum, which is connected to the small intestine. The cecum is a pouch leading to the colon, whose components are the ascending, transverse, descending, and sigmoid colon. The sigmoid colon leads to the rectum, which is connected to the outside of the body by the anal canal. Although diverticuli can appear at a variety of locations in the gastrointestinal (GI) tract, they are usually located in the colon, most commonly in the sigmoid colon.

The most common form of diverticulosis is called spastic colon diverticulosis, which is a condition involving diverticuli in the sigmoid colon whose lumen is abnormally narrowed. Since the circumference of the colon normally alternately narrows and widens along its length, muscle contractions may result in local occlusions of the lumen at the narrowed sections. Occlusion may cause the lumen of the colon to become multiple, separate chambers. When this happens, the pressure within the chambers can increase to the point where the mucosa herniates out through small clefts in the muscularis, creating diverticuli.

Most people with diverticulosis never notice it. When abdominal pain related to painful diverticular disease develops, it is felt in the lower abdomen and

may last for hours or days. Eating usually makes it worse, whereas passing gas or having a bowel movement may relieve it.

Besides causing abdominal pain, diverticuli may cause rectal bleeding, which may vary from mild to life-threatening. Usually, there is a sudden urge to defecate followed by passage of red blood, clots, or maroon-colored stool. If the stool is black, the bleeding is probably from the upper GI tract.

Since the colon may be studded with multiple diverticuli, and the bleeding may stop by the time of evaluation, it is often difficult to tell which one bled. Diverticulosis is most common in elderly people, who may have other conditions of the colon that are associated with bleeding. Therefore, it is often impossible to confirm that the cause of bleeding was diverticular disease—even if the colon is lined with hundreds of diverticuli.

What is most important is to establish what part of the GI tract is bleeding. To find out if the bleeding could have come from the upper GI tract, a tube is passed through the nose into the stomach, and the contents are aspirated. If blood is not present, this suggests lower GI bleeding. In addition, the esophagus, stomach, and upper small intestine can be visualized with a flexible, snakelike instrument called an endoscope to exclude a source such as a bleeding ulcer.

It is more difficult to examine the lower GI tract. The simplest procedure is anoscopy, by which the physician can examine the inside of the anal canal for hemorrhoids. Proctosigmoidoscopy, a procedure similar to endoscopy, offers a view of the rectum and part of the sigmoid colon. It may reveal diverticuli or other lesions such as a bleeding growth called a polyp.

Angiography is a test done in the radiology department; it involves injecting dye into the vessels that lead to the colon. If there is active bleeding, it can help localize the source. Even if the bleeding has stopped, this procedure can sometimes identify abnormal blood vessel formations suggestive of cancer or a blood vessel abnormality called angiodysplasia. Colonoscopy is most easily performed after bleeding has stopped. It requires cleaning out the contents of the colon and then inserting a long, flexible instrument called a colonoscope all the way to the cecum. The entire lining of the colon can be visualized while withdrawing the colonoscope.

About 15 percent of people with diverticulosis suffer from one or more episodes of diverticulitis, which is an inflammatory condition that may progress to an infection. Initially, feces may become trapped and inspissated (thickened) in a diverticulum, irritating it and leading to inflammation. Inflammation is a tissue response to injury which involves local reactions that attempt to destroy the injurious material and begin the healing process. It is usually the first step in the body's attempt to prevent infection and involves the migration of white blood cells out of blood vessels and into tissues, where they begin to fight off bacteria. The white blood cells release enzymes that cause tissue destruction. Because it is thin, the wall of the diverticulum may develop a tiny perforation.

Feces are made up of waste material and bacteria that normally do not cause problems when confined within the lumen of the colon. When a diverticulum perforates, however, they travel outside the colon and into other regions such as the peritoneal cavity, causing an infection. This infection along the outside of the colon is often limited, because many adjacent structures are able to wall off the bacteria, limiting their ability to extend through the peritoneal cavity. Although they become sealed off, they often form a pus-filled lesion called an abscess.

Fever and abdominal pain are the most common symptoms of diverticulitis. The fever may be high and associated with shaking chills. The pain is often sudden in onset, is often continuous, and may radiate from the left lower abdomen to the back. Laboratory findings usually include an elevated white blood cell count, a nonspecific finding that occurs with a variety of infections.

Radiographic studies are helpful for diagnosing and assessing the severity of diverticulitis. For example, a computed tomography (CT) scan can detect diverticuli or a thickening of the bowel wall associated with diverticulitis and can help assess whether abscesses are present.

TREATMENT AND THERAPY

There are two treatment goals in treating uncomplicated, painful diverticular disease: prevention of further development of diverticuli and pain relief. It is important to understand that the pressure that is able to develop inside the lumen of the colon is inversely related to the radius of the lumen. Therefore, if the lumen's radius can be increased, the pressures within the lumen will lessen, theoretically decreasing the chance of diverticuli formation. One key to increasing the radius of the lumen of the colon is to increase the bulk of the stool by the addition of dietary fiber.

A Western diet tends to be high in fiber-free animal foods and to lose much of its fiber during processing. This low-fiber diet may contribute to diverticulosis, which is prevalent in countries that have low-fiber diets. The typical American diet contains an average of 12 grams of fiber per day, whereas diets from Africa and India contain from 40 to 150 grams of fiber per day. A high-fiber diet can increase stool bulk by 40 to 100 percent. Fiber adds bulk to the stool because it acts like a sponge, retaining water that would normally be reabsorbed by the colonic mucosa. Fiber also increases stool bulk because 50 to 70 percent of the fiber is degraded by the bacteria in the colon and the products of degradation attract water by a process called osmosis.

The main fibers that increase stool bulk are the water-insoluble fibers, such as cellulose, hemicellulose, and lignin; they are derived from plants such as vegetables and whole grain cereals. Diets high in these fibers have been shown to decrease the intraluminal

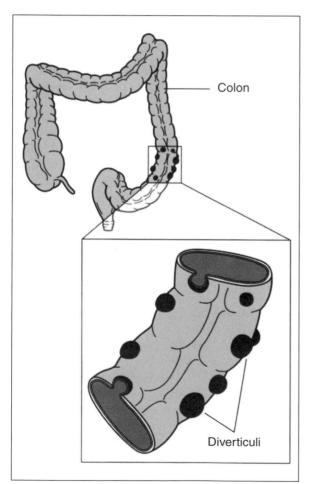

Diverticulosis occurs when multiple diverticuli (outpouchings) appear on the colon wall.

pressure in the sigmoid colon, as well as to relieve the pain associated with uncomplicated diverticular disease. The best results have been with the addition of 10 to 25 grams per day of coarse, unprocessed wheat bran to various liquid and semisolid foods. The sudden addition of large amounts of bran to one's diet, however, may cause bloating. Commercial preparations such as methylcellulose may be better tolerated during the first few weeks of therapy; their use may then be tapered off as bran is added to the diet. There are also various antispasmodic drugs available for inhibiting the muscle spasms of the colon, but many of those used in the United States are not very effective for decreasing symptoms.

For diverticular bleeding, the most effective therapy is patience. Most episodes stop on their own, and conservative treatments such as maintaining the patient's blood volume with intravenous fluids and possibly performing blood transfusions are all that is necessary. In those patients with continued active bleeding and in whom the source of the bleeding can be identified with angiography, a drug called vasopressin may be administered into the artery over several hours. This causes constriction of the vessel and stops bleeding most of the time. Once the vasopressin is stopped, however, patients may resume bleeding.

If vasopressin fails, surgery may be necessary. Surgery is most often successful if the bleeding site has been well localized before the operation. In that case, only the involved segment of the colon needs to be removed. If the bleeding site cannot be identified, it may be necessary to remove a majority of the colon; this procedure is associated with a higher rate of postoperative complications.

Diverticulitis that warrants hospitalization is initially treated with intravenous antibiotics for seven to ten days. Antibiotics help prevent 70 to 85 percent of patients from needing surgery. Most of those who respond to antibiotics will not have future attacks severe enough to warrant hospitalization.

Other measures may be necessary for the care of someone with diverticulitis, because the inflammation around the colon may be associated with problems such as narrowing of the bowel lumen to the point where it causes a partial or complete colonic obstruction. In this case, nothing should be given by mouth, and a tube should be passed through the nose into the stomach in order to suck out air and the stomach contents. This suction helps to reduce the amount of material that can pass through the colon and worsen the

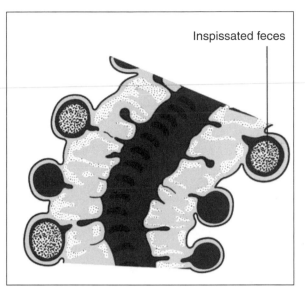

Diverticulitis begins when fecal material invades diverticuli and thickens (inspissated feces); when a diverticulum perforates, bacteria travel outside the colon into other regions and cause serious symptoms, including lower abdominal pain, fever, chills, and abscesses.

dilation of the colon that occurs proximal to the obstruction.

If the fever persists for more than a few days, the diverticulitis may be associated with complications. One complication is the formation of a large abscess outside the colon, which may be detected by a CT scan. An abscess has a rim around it that makes it difficult for antibiotics to penetrate the liquid center. If it does not go away despite antibiotic therapy, surgery may be necessary. If the abscess is small, it is possible to remove the involved segment of bowel and reattach the two free ends. If the abscess is very large, it may be necessary first to drain the abscess and then to cut across the colon proximal to the diseased segment, attaching the free end of the proximal segment to the abdominal wall, a procedure called a diverting colostomy. Later, the diseased segment of colon can be removed, and the remaining two free ends of colon can be joined. Another option is to drain the abscess with the aid of visual guidance by the CT scan and then operate on the colon. Draining the abscess in this manner helps get the infection under control before surgery is performed. Other indications for surgery in diverticulitis include complications such as a persistent bowel obstruction. In this case, it is often necessary to use a two-stage approach rather than to cure the problem in one operation.

Another complication of diverticulitis is a generalized infection of the peritoneal cavity, called peritonitis. Surgery for peritonitis involves removing the leaking segment of bowel and attaching the remaining two free ends of the colon to the abdominal wall. In addition, the peritoneal cavity is rinsed with a sterile solution in an attempt to clean out the contaminating materials.

Diverticulitis may also be complicated by the presence of a perforation of a diverticulum leading to a fistula, an abnormally existing channel connecting two hollow organs. When there is a fistula between the colon and the bladder, stool can travel into the bladder. The bacteria in the stool can cause severe, recurrent urinary tract infections. Another symptom is that bowel gas gets into the bladder; when the patient urinates, there is an intermittent stream because of colonic gas being passed along with the urine. When a fistula exists, it is necessary to remove the diseased segment of colon, the fistula tract, and a small portion of the bladder where the tract entered it.

Even if a patient with diverticulitis seems to improve and is able to return home from the hospital without needing surgery, there is still a chance that surgery will be necessary in the future. Surgery may be needed if the patient continues to have repeated, severe attacks of diverticulitis, or when a fistula between the colon and bladder causes recurring urinary tract infections. Another reason for surgery is persistent partial colonic obstruction and no possibility of inspecting the narrowed region of colon to exclude a constricting cancerous lesion as the cause of the obstruction.

Perspective and Prospects

Diverticuli are quite common in the United States and other developed countries that tend to eat processed, low-fiber foods. In the United States, for example, diverticulosis is uncommon before the age of forty but is seen in 30 to 50 percent of elderly people at autopsy. Of those with diverticuli, only about one-fifth suffer any symptoms. Although members of ethnic groups who live in underdeveloped countries and eat a high-fiber diet tend to have a low prevalence of diverticulosis, their risk of developing this disease increases within ten years of moving to more developed countries.

Before 1900, the presence of colonic diverticuli in the United States was considered a curiosity, whereas now it is found in one-third to one-half of all autopsies of people over the age of sixty. There are a few possible explanations for why this increasing prevalence is seen.

First, the change in the American diet probably plays a large part in the pathogenesis of diverticular disease.

Fiber consumption may have fallen off by as much as 30 percent during the twentieth century. Many people in the United States eat foods such as quick-cooking rice, highly processed cereals, and processed flour, all of which contain less fiber than their unprocessed counterparts. In addition, the population tends to eat more fats and proteins and less carbohydrates. Many fibers are from food sources rich in carbohydrates and are carbohydrates themselves.

The increasing prevalence of diverticular disease may also be attributable to the changing survival pattern. In 1900, the average life expectancy in the United States was forty-nine; in 1983, it was seventy-one years for men and seventy-eight years for women. The proportion of people over sixty-five has risen: It was 4.1 percent in 1900 and increased to 11.6 percent in 1986. Thus, the American population is not only growing but also getting older. Since diverticulosis is seen in increasing frequencies with aging, it is understandable that more of it was seen in the late twentieth century than during the early 1900's.

Most poor people in the world live largely on plant foods rich in fiber, being largely dependent on cereal grains such as wheat, rice, and corn for both their calorie and their protein sources. Although one can look at the amount of fiber in the diet of rural Africans and compare it to that in the United States, there may be other differences in lifestyles that contribute to the higher prevalence of diverticular disease in the United States. Living in rural Africa, without traffic jams and the fast pace of developed countries, may cause people to have less stressful lives, and the lower stress is associated with fewer muscle spasms in the colon. Since it has been documented that stress can increase colonic contractions, and stress may worsen another disorder of the colon involving muscle spasm called irritable bowel syndrome (IBS), one might postulate that the stress of Western society contributes to the spasms in the sigmoid colon that may lead to diverticular disease.

Another reason for the increase in the prevalence of diverticular disease could be improvements in detection. Now it is detected not only at autopsy but also by barium enema, during sigmoidoscopy, and during surgery. Thus, there are more opportunities for discovering diverticulosis.

—Marc H. Walters, M.D.

See also Colon and rectal polyp removal; Colon and rectal surgery; Colon cancer; Colon therapy; Colonoscopy and sigmoidoscopy; Constipation; Digestion; Gastroenterology; Gastroenterology, pediatric; Gastrointestinal disorders; Gastrointestinal system; Intestinal disorders; Intestines; Irritable bowel syndrome (IBS); Nutrition; Peritonitis.

FOR FURTHER INFORMATION:

Achkar, Edgar, Richard G. Farmer, and Bertram Fleshler, eds. *Clinical Gastroenterology.* 2d ed. Philadelphia: Lea & Febiger, 1992. This book is written by gastroenterologists from the Cleveland Clinic. Contains excellent chapters on abdominal pain, gastrointestinal bleeding, and diverticular disease. Less detailed but more readable than Marvin Sleisenger and John Fordtran's textbook.

Feldman, Mark, Lawrence S. Friedman, and Lawrence J. Brandt, eds. *Sleisenger and Fordtran's Gastrointestinal and Liver Disease: Pathophysiology, Diagnosis, Management.* 8th ed. 2 vols. Philadelphia: W. B. Saunders, 2006. This text is the best comprehensive textbook on gastrointestinal diseases and physiology. Contains excellent information on diverticular disease.

Ganong, William F. *Review of Medical Physiology.* 22d ed. New York: Lange Medical Books/McGraw-Hill Medical, 2005. This classic book has a nice section emphasizing normal gastrointestinal physiology which would provide a solid background for understanding diverticulosis.

Kapadia, Cyrus R., James M. Crawford, and Caroline Taylor. *An Atlas of Gastroenterology: A Guide to Diagnosis and Differential Diagnosis.* Boca Raton, Fla.: Pantheon, 2003. Provides a fully illustrated, nonspecialist understanding of myriad gastrointestinal diseases, including heartburn, dyspepsia, diarrhea, irritable bowel syndrome, and pancreatitis. Includes bibliographic references and index.

Kumar, Vinay, et al., eds. *Robbins Basic Pathology.* 8th ed. Philadelphia: Saunders/Elsevier, 2007. An introductory pathology textbook. Less detailed than texts used by physicians, but still contains useful information on diverticular disease.

Peikin, Steven R. *Gastrointestinal Health.* Rev. ed. New York: HarperCollins, 1999. Discusses a range of gastrointestinal disorders, including diverticulosis, IBS, and ulcers.

Tortora, Gerard J., and Bryan Derrickson. *Principles of Anatomy and Physiology.* 11th ed. Hoboken, N.J.: John Wiley & Sons, 2006. An outstanding textbook of human anatomy and physiology, and a good first text to consult before reading more advanced gastroenterology texts and journal articles.

DIZZINESS AND FAINTING
DISEASE/DISORDER

ANATOMY OR SYSTEM AFFECTED: Blood vessels, brain, circulatory system, head, nervous system, psychic-emotional system

SPECIALTIES AND RELATED FIELDS: Cardiology, emergency medicine, family medicine, internal medicine, neurology

DEFINITION: Dizziness is a feeling of light-headedness and unsteadiness, sometimes accompanied by a feeling of spinning or other spatial motion; fainting is a loss of consciousness as a result of insufficient amounts of blood reaching the brain. Both are symptoms of many conditions, which may be harmless or serious.

KEY TERMS:

cardiac output: the amount of blood that the heart can pump per unit of time (usually per minute); if the brain does not receive enough of the cardiac output, the person becomes dizzy and may faint

dizziness: a sensation of whirling, with difficulty balancing

fainting: a weak feeling followed by a loss of consciousness, usually due to a lack of blood flow to the brain; also called syncope

hypertension: a condition in which the patient's blood pressure is higher than that demanded by the body

hypotension: decrease in blood pressure to the point that insufficient blood flow causes symptoms

vasoconstriction: a reduction in the diameter of arteries, which increases the amount of work required for the heart to move blood

vasodilation: an increase in the diameter of arteries, which decreases the amount of work required for the heart to move blood

venous return: the amount of blood returning to the heart; one factor that determines the amount of blood the heart can pump out

vertigo: a sensation of moving in space or having objects move about when the patient is stationary, the most common symptom of which is dizziness; vertigo results from a disturbance in the organs of equilibrium

CAUSES AND SYMPTOMS

In humans, several mechanisms have evolved by which adequate blood flow to organs is maintained. Without a constant blood supply, the body's tissues would die from a lack of essential nutrients and oxygen. In particular, the brain and heart are very sensitive to changes in their blood supply as they, more than any other organs, must receive oxygen and nutrients at all times. If they do not, their cells will die and cannot be replaced.

While the heart supplies most of the force needed to propel the blood throughout the body, tissues rely on changes in the size of arteries to redirect blood flow to where it is needed most. For example, after a large meal the blood vessels that lead to the gastrointestinal tract enlarge (vasodilate) so that more blood can be present to collect the nutrients from the meal. At the same time, the blood vessels that supply muscles decrease in diameter (vasoconstrict) and effectively shunt the blood toward the stomach and intestines. On the other hand, during exercise, the blood vessels that supply the muscles dilate and the ones leading to the intestinal tract vasoconstrict. This mechanism allows the cardiovascular system to supply the most blood to the most active tissues.

The brain is somewhat special in that the body tries to maintain a nearly constant blood flow to it. Located in the walls of the carotid arteries, which carry blood to the brain, are specialized sensory cells that have the ability to detect changes in blood pressure. These cells are known as baroreceptors. If the blood pressure going to the brain is too low, the baroreceptors send an impulse to the brain, which in turn speeds up the heart rate and causes a generalized vasoconstriction. This reflex response raises the body's blood pressure, reestablishing adequate blood flow to the brain. If the baroreceptors detect too high a blood pressure, they send a signal to the brain, which in turn slows the heart rate and causes the arteries of the body to dilate. These reflexes prevent large fluctuations in blood flow to the brain and other tissues.

Most people have experienced a dizzy feeling or maybe even a fainting response when they have stood up too quickly from a prone position. The ability of the baroreceptors to maintain relatively constant arterial pressure is extremely important when a person stands after having been lying down. Immediately upon standing, the pressure in the carotid arteries falls, and a reduction of this pressure can cause dizziness or even fainting. Fortunately, the falling pressure at the baroreceptors elicits an immediate reflex, resulting in a more rapid heart rate and vasoconstriction, minimizing the decrease in blood flow to the brain.

Blood pressure is not the only factor that is essential in maintaining tissue viability. The accumulation of waste products and a lack of essential nutrients and gases can also have a profound effect on how much

---

INFORMATION ON DIZZINESS AND FAINTING

CAUSES: Environmental factors, dehydration, postural hypotension, inner ear infection, brain stem disorders, brain tumors, blood flow deficiency disorders

SYMPTOMS: Light-headedness, unsteadiness, feeling of spinning or other spatial motion, nausea, vomiting

DURATION: Usually temporary

TREATMENTS: Deep breathing, rest, adequate blood flow to brain, drug therapy, rehydration

---

blood flows through a particular tissue and how quickly. In a region of the carotid arteries near the baroreceptors are chemoreceptors. Chemoreceptors detect the concentration of the essential gas oxygen and the concentration of the gaseous waste product carbon dioxide. When carbon dioxide concentrations increase and oxygen concentrations decrease, the chemoreceptors stimulate regions in the brain to increase the heart rate and blood pressure in an attempt to supply the tissues with more oxygen and flush away the excess carbon dioxide. If the chemoreceptors detect high levels of oxygen and low levels of carbon dioxide, an impulse is transmitted to the brain, which in turn slows the heart rate and decreases the blood pressure.

Normally, most of the blood flow to the brain is controlled by the baroreceptor and chemoreceptor reflexes. However, the brain has a backup system. If blood flow decreases enough to cause a deficiency of nutrients and oxygen and an accumulation of waste products, special nerve cells respond directly to the lack of adequate energy sources and become strongly excited. When this occurs, the heart is stimulated and blood pressure rises.

Dizziness is a sensation of light-headedness often accompanied by a sensation of spinning (vertigo). Occasionally, a person experiencing dizziness will feel nauseated and may even vomit. Most attacks of dizziness are harmless, resulting from a brief reduction in blood flow to the brain. There are several causes of dizziness, and each alters blood flow to the brain for a slightly different reason.

A person rising rapidly from a sitting or lying position may become dizzy. This is known as postural hypotension, which is caused by a relatively slow reflexive response to the reduced blood pressure in the arteries providing blood to the brain. Rising requires increased blood pressure to supply the brain with adequate amounts of blood. Postural hypotension is more common in the elderly and in individuals prescribed antihypertensive medicines (drugs used to lower high blood pressure).

If the patient experiences vertigo with dizziness, the condition is usually caused by a disorder of the inner ear equilibrium system. Two disorders of the inner ear that can cause dizziness are labyrinthitis and Ménière's disease. Labyrinthitis, inflammation of the fluid-filled canals of the inner ear, is usually caused by a virus. Since these canals are involved in maintaining equilibrium, when they become infected and inflamed, one experiences the symptom of dizziness. Ménière's disease is a degenerative disorder of the ear in which the patient experiences not only dizziness but also progressive hearing loss.

Some brain-stem disorders also cause dizziness. The brain stem houses the vestibulocochlear nerve, which transmits messages from the ear to several other parts of the nervous system. Any disorder that alters the functions of this nerve will result in dizziness and vertigo. Meningitis (inflammation of the coverings of the brain and spinal cord), brain tumors, and blood-flow deficiency disorders such as atherosclerosis may affect the function of the vestibulocochlear nerve.

Syncope (fainting) is often preceded by dizziness. Syncope is the temporary loss of consciousness as a result of an inadequate blood flow to the brain. In addition to losing consciousness, the patient may be pale and sweaty. The most common cause of syncope is a vasovagal attack, in which an overstimulation of the vagus nerve slows the heart. Often vasovagal syncope results from severe pain, stress, or fear. For example, people may faint when hearing bad news or at the sight of blood. More commonly, individuals who have received a painful injury will faint. Rarely, vasovagal syncope may be caused by prolonged coughing, straining to defecate or urinate, pregnancy, or forcing expiration. Standing still for long periods of time or standing up rapidly after lying or sitting can cause fainting. With the exception of vasovagal syncope, all the causes of syncope are attributable to inadequate blood returning to the heart. If blood pools in the lower extremities, there is a reduced amount available for the heart to pump to the brain. In vasovagal syncope and some disorders of heart rhythm such as Adams-Stokes syndrome, it is the heart itself that does not force enough blood toward the brain.

TREATMENT AND THERAPY

Short periods of dizziness usually subside after a few minutes. Deep breathing and rest will usually relieve the symptom. Prolonged episodes of dizziness and vertigo should be brought to the attention of a physician.

Recovery from fainting likewise will occur when adequate blood flow to the brain is reestablished. This happens within minutes because falling to the ground places the head at the same level as the heart and helps return the blood from the legs. If a person does not regain consciousness within a few minutes, a physician or emergency medical team should be notified.

The most common cause of syncope is decreased cerebral blood flow resulting from limitation of cardiac output. When the heart rate falls below its normal seventy-five beats per minute to approximately thirty-five beats per minute, the patient usually becomes dizzy and faints. Although slow heart rates can occur in any age group, they are most often found in elderly people who have other heart conditions. Drug-induced syncope can also occur. Drugs for congestive heart failure (digoxin) or antihypertensive medications that slow the heart rate (propranolol, metoprolol) may reduce blood flow to the brain sufficiently to cause dizziness and fainting.

Exertional syncope occurs when individuals perform some physical activity to which they are not accustomed. These physical efforts demand more work from the cardiovascular system, and in patients with some obstruction of the arteries which leave the heart, the cardiovascular system is overstressed. This defect, combined with the vasodilation in the blood vessels that provide blood to the working muscles, reduces the amount of blood available for use by the brain. If the person also hyperventilates during exercise, he or she will effectively reduce the amount of carbon dioxide in the blood and rid the cardiovascular system of this normal stimulus for increasing heart rate and blood flow to the brain. Some persons also hold their breath during periods of high exertion. For example, people attempting to lift something very heavy often take a deep breath just prior to exerting and then hold their breath when they lift the object. This practice, known as the Valsalva maneuver, increases the pressure within the chest cavity, which in turn reduces the amount of blood returning to the heart. A decrease in blood returning to the heart (venous return) causes a decrease in the availability of blood to be pumped out of the heart and reduces cardiac output. The reduction in cardiac output decreases the amount of blood flowing to the brain and initiates a fainting response. It is interesting to note that humans also use the Valsalva maneuver when defecating or urinating, particularly when they strain. These acts can also lead to exertional syncope.

In order for a physician to diagnose and treat dizziness and fainting accurately, he or she must take an accurate medical history, paying particular attention to cardiovascular and neurological problems. In addition to experiencing episodes of dizziness and fainting, patients often have a weak pulse, low blood pressure (hypotension), sweating, and shallow breathing. Heart rate and blood pressure are monitored while the patient assumes different positions. The clinician also listens to the heart and carotid arteries to determine whether there are any problems with these tissues, such as a heart valve problem or atherosclerosis of the carotid arteries. An electrocardiogram (ECG or EKG) can detect abnormal heart rates and rhythms that may reduce cardiac output. Laboratory tests are used to determine whether the patient has low blood sugar (hypoglycemia), too little blood volume (hypovolemia), too few red blood cells (anemia), or abnormal blood gases suggesting a lung disorder. Finally, if the physician suspects a neurological problem such as a seizure disorder, he or she may run an electroencephalogram (EEG) to record brain activity.

Treatment for any of these underlying disorders may cure the dizziness and fainting episodes. In patients with postural hypotension, merely being aware of the condition will allow them to change their behavior to lessen the chances of becoming dizzy and fainting. These patients should not make any sudden changes in posture that could precipitate an attack. Often, this means simply slowing down their movements and learning to assume a horizontal position if they feel dizzy. Patients also can learn to contract their leg muscles and not hold their breath when rising. This increases the amount of blood available for the heart to pump toward the brain. If these techniques do not provide an adequate solution for postural hypotension, then a physician can prescribe drugs, such as ephedrine, which increase blood pressure.

Heart rhythm disturbances that cause an abnormally fast or slow heart rate can be corrected with drug therapy such as quinidine or disopyramide (if the rate is too rapid) or a pacemaker (if the rate is too slow). It is interesting to note that even too fast a heart rate can cause dizziness and fainting. In patients with this type of arrhythmia, the heart beats at such a rapid rate that it can-

not efficiently fill with blood before the next contraction. Therefore, less blood is pumped with each beat.

Other treatments for dizziness and fainting may include correcting the levels of certain blood elements. Patients with hypoglycemia often feel dizzy. The brain and spinal cord require glucose as their energy source. In fact, the brain and spinal cord have a very limited ability to utilize other substrates such as fat or protein for energy. Because of this, patients often feel lightheaded when there are inadequate levels of glucose in the blood. Patients can correct this condition by eating more frequent meals, and if necessary, physicians can administer drugs such as epinephrine or glucagon. These agents liberate glucose from storage sites in the liver.

Individuals with a low blood volume are often dehydrated and upon becoming rehydrated no longer have dizziness or fainting episodes. If dehydration is not corrected and becomes worse, the patient can go into shock, a state of inadequate blood flow to tissues that will result in death if left untreated. In addition to being dizzy or fainting, the patient is often cold to the touch and has a rapid heart rate, low blood pressure, bluish skin, and rapid breathing. These patients are treated by emergency medical personnel, who keep the individual warm, elevate the legs, and infuse fluid into a vein. Drugs may be used to help bring blood pressure back to normal. The cause of the shock should be identified and corrected.

PERSPECTIVE AND PROSPECTS

As humans evolved, they assumed an upright posture. This was advantageous because it allows for the use of the front limbs for other things besides locomotion. Unlike most four-legged animals, however, humans have their brains above their hearts and must continually force blood uphill to reach this vital tissue. This adaptation to the upright posture is a continuing physiological problem because the cardiovascular system must counteract the forces of gravity to provide the brain with blood. If this does not occur, the individual becomes dizzy and faints.

Another significant problem that humans face is adaptation to brain blood flow during exercise. The amount of blood flowing to a tissue is usually proportional to the metabolic demand of the tissue. At rest, various organs throughout the body receive a certain amount of the cardiac output. For example, blood flow to abdominal organs such as the spleen and the kidneys requires about 43 percent of the total blood volume.

The total flow to the brain is estimated to be only 13 percent, and the skin and skeletal muscles require 21 percent and 9 percent, respectively. Other areas such as the gastrointestinal tract and heart receive the remaining 14 percent. During exercise, the skeletal muscles may receive up to 80 percent of the cardiac output while the rest of the organs are perfused at a much reduced rate.

Most data indicate that the brain receives only 3 percent of the total cardiac output during heavy exercise. Even though there is a large change in the redistribution of cardiac output, physiologists do not know the absolute amount of blood reaching the brain or the mechanism for the change in the perfusion rate.

With strenuous aerobic exercise such as jogging, there is an increase in cardiac output. During strenuous anaerobic exercise such as weight lifting, however, there may be a decrease in cardiac output, attributable to the Valsalva maneuver. Therefore, it has been difficult to predict accurately, using available techniques, the volume of blood reaching this critical tissue.

—Matthew Berria, Ph.D.

See also Anxiety; Balance disorders; Brain; Brain disorders; Ear infections and disorders; Ears; Exercise physiology; Headaches; Huntington's disease; Hypotension; Ménière's disease; Meningitis; Migraine headaches; Multiple chemical sensitivity syndrome; Narcolepsy; Nausea and vomiting; Nervous system; Neuralgia, neuritis, and neuropathy; Neurology; Neurology, pediatric; Palpitations; Unconsciousness.

FOR FURTHER INFORMATION:

Babikian, Viken K., and Lawrence R. Wechsler, eds. *Transcranial Doppler Ultrasonography.* 2d ed. Boston: Butterworth-Heinemann, 1999. Describes a noninvasive way to measure blood flow to the brain using ultrasound techniques. The authors provide information on how drugs such as anesthetics alter this blood flow.

Brandt, Thomas. *Vertigo: Its Multisensory Syndromes.* 2d ed. New York: Springer, 2003. Uses an interdisciplinary approach in its discussion of clinical symptoms; central vestibular, nerve, and labyrinthine disorders; hereditary factors; and epilepsy, among other topics.

Furman, Joseph M., and Stephen P. Cass. *Vestibular Disorders: A Case-Study Approach.* New York: Oxford University Press, 2003. A text that examines case studies to elucidate the causes of vestibular disorders. History, physical examination, laboratory testing, differential diagnosis, and treatment are discussed.

Geelen, G., and J. E. Greenleaf. "Orthostasis: Exercise and Exercise Training." *Exercise and Sport Sciences Reviews* 21 (1993): 201-230. Provides an excellent, complete discussion of the relationship between exercise and dizziness and fainting. These authors describe the current theories on blood flow regulation to the brain in athletes.

Guyton, Arthur C. *Human Physiology and Mechanisms of Disease.* 6th ed. Philadelphia: W. B. Saunders, 1997. This textbook introduces human physiology and basic pathology for individuals without an extensive background in medicine. Guyton offers several chapters on blood pressure regulation in humans and gives brief explanations as to what happens when blood pressure is not adequately regulated.

Leikin, Jerrold B., and Martin S. Lipsky, eds. *American Medical Association Complete Medical Encyclopedia.* New York: Random House Reference, 2003. This encyclopedia lists in alphabetical order medical terms, diseases, and medical procedures. It does an excellent job of explaining rather complex medical subjects for the nonprofessional audience. In the sections on dizziness and fainting, flow charts detail the appropriate first aid treatments.

DNA AND RNA

BIOLOGY

ANATOMY OR SYSTEM AFFECTED: Cells

SPECIALTIES AND RELATED FIELDS: Genetics

DEFINITION: Molecules that store coded genetic information and express this information as functional proteins; deoxyribonucleic acid (DNA) is a long, thin, double-stranded fibrous molecule which holds coded information that determines the type, amount, and timing of protein production, while ribonucleic acid (RNA) is a long, single-stranded molecule that amplifies, transports, and expresses this coded information.

KEY TERMS:

genetic disease: a disease state that exists because of a decrease in or the absence of normal protein activity as the result of an alteration in the information carried in the DNA

mutation: an alteration in the information stored in DNA that may lead to an alteration in the structure of proteins produced from this information

replication: the process by which the DNA of a cell is duplicated so that the information stored there can be passed on to new cells after cell division

transcription: the process by which the information stored in DNA is copied into the structure of RNA for transport to the cytoplasm

translation: the process by which the copied information in RNA is utilized in the production of a protein

STRUCTURE AND FUNCTIONS

Each human being is a biologically unique individual. That uniqueness has its basis in one's cellular makeup. Appearance derives from the arrangement of cells during fetal development, size depends on the cells' ability to grow and divide, and the function of organs depends on the biochemical function of the individual cells that constitute each organ. The functions of cells depend on

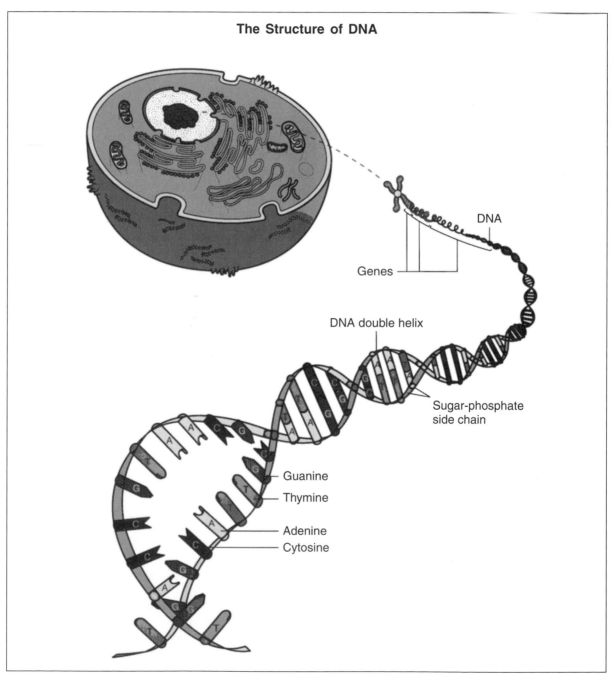

The Structure of DNA

DNA

Genes

DNA double helix

Sugar-phosphate side chain

Guanine

Thymine

Adenine

Cytosine

the types and amounts of the different proteins that they synthesize. The substance that holds the information that determines the structure of proteins, when they should be produced, and in what amounts is deoxyribonucleic acid (DNA).

DNA is the molecule of heredity, and as a child receives half of his or her DNA from each biological parent, each individual is the product of a mixture of information. Therefore, while children resemble their parents, they are unique. Each cell in an individual's body (except for the sex cells) has a complete set of genetic information contained in the chromosomes of the cell's nucleus. Human cells have forty-six chromosomes (twenty-three pairs). Each chromosome is a single piece of DNA associated with many types of proteins. The major function of DNA is to store, in a stable manner, the information that is the "blueprint" for all physiological aspects of an individual. Stability is one of the key attributes of DNA. An information storage molecule is of little use if it can be altered or damaged easily. Another key characteristic of DNA is its ability to be replicated. When a cell divides, the information in the DNA must be replicated so that each of the two new cells can have a complete set.

Stability, the ability to be replicated, and the ability to store vast amounts of coded information have their basis in the structure of DNA. DNA is a long, incredibly thin fiber. The chromosomes in some cells would be as long as a foot or more if they were fully extended. The shape of the DNA molecule can be imagined as a long ladder whose rails are chains of two alternating molecules: deoxyribose (a sugar) and phosphate (an acid containing phosphorus and oxygen). The steps of the ladder are made of pairs of organic bases, of which there are four types: adenine (A), guanine (G), thymine (T), and cytosine (C). Adenine always pairs up with thymine to form a step in the ladder (A-T), and guanine always pairs with cytosine (C-G). This complementarity of base-pairing is the basis for DNA replication and for transferring information from DNA out of the nucleus and into the cytoplasm. Finally, the whole DNA molecule is twisted into a stable right-handed spiral, or helix. Because there is no restriction on the sequence in which the base pairs appear along the molecule, the bases have the potential to be used as a four-letter alphabet that can encode information into "words" of varying lengths, called genes. Each information sequence, or gene, holds the information needed to synthesize a linear chain of amino acids, which are the building blocks of proteins. The informa-

tion encoded in the base sequences of DNA determines the quantities and composition of all proteins made in the cell.

Under certain conditions, DNA can be separated lengthwise into two halves, or denatured, by breaking the base pairs so that one of each pair remains attached to one sugar-phosphate chain and the other base remains attached to the other sugar-phosphate chain. Because this forms two strands of DNA, whole DNA is usually referred to as being double-stranded. Such separation rarely happens by accident because of the extreme length of DNA. If any area becomes denatured, the rest of the base pairs hold the molecule together. In addition, an area of denaturation will automatically try to renature, since complementary bases have a natural attraction for each other. As stable as these traits make it, DNA must be capable of being duplicated so that each newly divided cell has a complete copy of the stored information. DNA is replicated by breaking the base pairs, separating the DNA into two halves, and building a new half onto each of the old halves. This is possible because the complementarity rule (A pairs with T, and C pairs with G) allows each half of a denatured DNA molecule to hold the information needed to construct a new second half. This is accomplished by special sets of proteins that separate the old DNA as they move along the molecule and build new DNA in their wake.

All the information needed to produce proteins is located in the DNA within the nucleus of the cell, but all protein synthesis occurs outside the nucleus in the cytoplasm. An information transfer molecule is required to copy or transcribe information from the genes of the DNA and carry it to the cytoplasm, where large globular protein complexes called ribosomes take the information and translate it into the amino acid structure of specific proteins. This information transfer molecule is ribonucleic acid (RNA). Many RNA copies can be made for any single piece of information on the DNA and used as a template to synthesize many proteins. In this way, the information in DNA is also amplified by RNA. RNA also participates in the synthesis of proteins from the genetic information. RNA resembles one half of a DNA molecule and is usually referred to as being single-stranded. It consists of a single chain of alternating sugars and phosphates with a single organic base attached to each sugar. The sugar in this case is ribose, similar to deoxyribose, and the bases are identical to those in DNA with the exception of thymine, which is replaced by a very similar base called uracil (U).

There are three major types of RNA. Messenger RNA (mRNA) is responsible for the transfer of information from the DNA sequences in the nucleus to the ribosomes in the cytoplasm. Ribosomal RNA (rRNA) interacts with dozens of proteins to form the ribosome. It aids in the interaction between mRNA and the ribosome. Transfer RNA (tRNA) is a group of small RNAs that helps translate the information coded in the mRNA into the structure of specific proteins. They carry the amino acids to the ribosome and match the correct amino acid to its corresponding sequence of bases in the mRNA.

The first step in producing a specific protein is the accurate copying or transcription of information in a gene into information on a piece of mRNA. There are specific sets of proteins that separate the double-stranded DNA in the immediate vicinity of a gene into two single-stranded portions and then, using the DNA as a template, build a piece of mRNA that is a complementary copy of the information in the gene. This is possible because RNA also uses organic bases in its structure. The A, C, G, and T of the single-stranded portion of DNA form base pairs with the U, G, C, and A of the mRNA, respectively. The complementary copy of mRNA, when complete, falls away from the DNA and moves to the cytoplasm of the cell.

In the cytoplasm, the mRNA binds to a ribosome. As the ribosome moves down the length of the mRNA, the tRNAs interact with both the ribosome and the mRNA in order to match the proper amino acid (carried by the tRNAs) to the proper sequence of bases in the mRNA. The order of amino acids in the protein is thus determined by the order of bases in the DNA. Achieving the correct order of amino acids is critical for the correct functioning of the protein. The order of amino acids in the chain determines the way in which it interacts with itself and folds into a three-dimensional structure. The function of all proteins depends on their assuming the correct shape for interaction with other molecules. Therefore, the sequence of bases in the DNA ultimately determines the shape and function of proteins.

DISORDERS AND DISEASES

When the normal structure of DNA is altered (a process called a mutation), the number of proteins produced and/or the functions of proteins may be affected. At one extreme, a mutation may cause no problem at all to the person involved. At the other extreme, it may cause devastating damage to the person and result in genetic disease or cancer.

Mutations are changes in the normal sequence of bases in the DNA that carry the information to build a protein or that regulate the amount of protein to be produced. There are different types of mutations, such as the alteration of one base into another, the deletion of one or many bases, or the insertion of bases that were not in the sequence previously. Mutations can have many different causes, such as ultraviolet rays, X rays, mutagenic chemicals, invading viruses, or even heat. Sometimes mutations are caused by mistakes made during the process of DNA replication or cell division. Cells have several systems that constantly repair mutations, but occasionally some of these alterations slip by and become permanent.

Mutations may affect protein structure in several ways. The protein may be too short or too long, with amino acids missing or new ones added. It might have new amino acids substituting for the correct ones. Sometimes as small a change as one amino acid can have noticeable effects. In any of these cases, changes in the amino acid sequence of a protein may drastically affect the way the protein interacts with itself and folds itself into a three-dimensional structure. If a protein does not assume the correct three-dimensional structure, its function may be impaired. It is important to note that how severely a protein's function is affected by a mutation depends on which amino acids are involved. Some amino acids are more important than others in maintaining a protein's shape and function. A change in amino acid sequence may have virtually no effect on a protein or it may destroy that protein's ability to function.

If a mutation occurs that affects the regulation of a particular protein, that gene may be perfectly normal and the protein may be fully functional, but it may exist in the cell in an improper amount—too much, too little, or even none at all. It is important to note that the overproduction of a protein, as well as its underproduction or absence, can be harmful to the cell or to the person in general. The genetic disease known as Down syndrome, for example, is the result of the overproduction of many proteins at the same time.

The term "genetic disease" is used for a heritable disease that can be passed from parent to child. The mutation responsible for the disease is contributed by the parents to the affected child via the sperm or the egg or (as is usually the case) both. The parents are, for the most part, quite unaffected. Because all creatures more complex than bacteria have at least two copies of all their genes, a person may carry a mutated gene and be perfectly healthy because the other normal gene compensates by producing adequate amounts of normal protein. If two individuals carrying the same mutated gene produce a child, that child has a chance of obtaining two mutant genes—one from each parent. Every cell in that child's body carries the error with no normal genes to compensate, and every cell that would normally use that gene must produce an abnormal protein or abnormal amounts of that protein. The medical consequences vary, depending on which gene is affected and which protein is altered. The following are two specific examples of genetic diseases in which the connection between specific mutations and the disease states are well documented.

Sickle cell disease is a genetic disease that results from an error in the gene that carries the information for the protein beta globin. Beta globin is one of the building blocks of hemoglobin, the molecule that binds to and carries oxygen in the red blood cells. The error or mutation is a surprisingly small one and serves to illustrate the fact that the replacement of even a single amino acid can change the chemical nature and function of a protein. Normal beta globin has a glutamic acid as the sixth amino acid in the protein chain. The mutation of a single base in the DNA

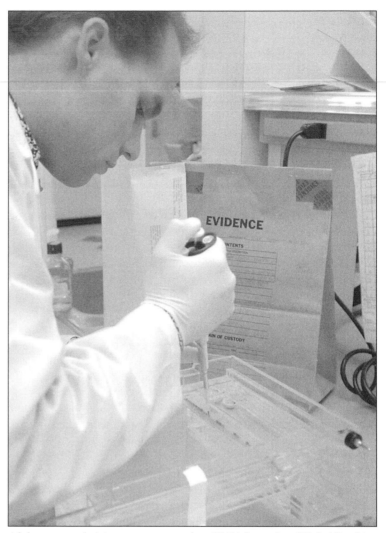

A laboratory technician prepares samples of DNA for testing. (Digital Stock)

changes the coded information such that the amino acid valine replaces glutamic acid as the sixth position in the protein chain. This single alteration causes the hemoglobin in the red blood cell to crystallize under conditions of low oxygen concentration. As the crystals grow, they twist and deform the normally flexible and disk-shaped red blood cells into rigid sickle shapes. These affected cells lose their capacity to bind and hold oxygen, thereby causing anemia, and their new structure can cause blockages in small capillaries of the circulatory system, causing pain and widespread organ damage. There is no safe and effective treatment or cure for this condition.

Phenylketonuria (PKU) is caused by a mutation in the gene that controls the synthesis of the protein phenylalanine hydroxylase (PAH). There are several mu-

tations of the PAH gene that can lead to a drastic decrease in PAH activity (by greater than 1 percent of normal activity). Some are changes in one base that lead to the replacement of a single amino acid for another. For example, one of the most common mutations in the PAH gene is the alteration of a C to a T that results in amino acid number 408 changing from an arginine to a tryptophan. Some mutations are deletions of whole sequences of bases in the gene. One such deletion removes the tail end of the gene. In any case, the amino acid structure of PAH is altered significantly enough to remove its ability to function. Without this protein, the amino acid phenylalanine cannot be converted into tyrosine, another useful amino acid. The problem is not a shortage of tyrosine, since there is plenty in most foods, but rather an accumulation of undesirable products that form as the unused phenylalanine begins to break down. Since developing brain cells are particularly sensitive to these products, the condition can cause mental retardation unless treated immediately after birth. While there is no cure, the disease is easily diagnosed and treatment is simple. The patient must stay on a diet in which phenylalanine is restricted. Food products that contain the artificial sweetener aspartame (NutraSweet) must have warnings to PKU patients printed on them since phenylalanine is a major component of aspartame.

PERSPECTIVE AND PROSPECTS

Genetics is a young science whose starting point is traditionally considered to be 1866, the year in which Gregor Mendel published his work on hereditary patterns in pea plants. While he knew nothing of DNA or its structure, Mendel showed mathematically that discrete units of inheritance, which are now called genes, existed as pairs in an organism and that different combinations of these units determined that organism's characteristics. Unfortunately, Mendel's work was ahead of its time and thus ignored until rediscovered by several researchers simultaneously in 1900.

DNA itself was discovered in 1869 by Friedrich Miescher, who extracted it from cell nuclei but did not realize its importance as the carrier of hereditary information. Chromosomes were first seen in the 1870's as threadlike structures in the nucleus, and because of the precise way they are replicated and equally parceled out to newly divided cells, August Weismann and Theodor Boveri, in the 1880's, postulated that chromosomes were the carriers of inheritance.

In 1900, Hugo de Vries, Karl Correns, and Erich Tschermak von Seysenegg—all plant biologists who were working on patterns of inheritance—independently rediscovered Mendel's work. De Vries had in the meantime discovered mutation around 1890 as a source of hereditary variation, but he did not postulate a mechanism. Mendel's theories and the then-current knowledge of chromosomes merged perfectly. Mendel's units of inheritance were thought somehow to be carried on the chromosomes. Pairs of chromosomes would carry Mendel's pairs of hereditary units which, in 1909, were dubbed "genes."

At that point, genes were still a theoretical concept and had not been proved to be carried on the chromosomes. In 1909, Thomas Hunt Morgan began the work that would provide that proof and allow the mapping of specific genes to specific areas of a chromosome. The

nature of a gene, or how it expressed itself, was still a mystery. In 1941, George Beadle and Edward Tatum proved that genes regulated the production of proteins, but the nature of genes was still in debate. There were two candidates for the chemical substance of genes; one was protein and the other was the deceptively simple DNA. In 1944, Oswald Avery proved in experiments with pure DNA that DNA was indeed the molecule of inheritance. In 1953, James D. Watson and Francis Crick, using the work of Rosalind Franklin, elucidated the chemical structure of the double helix, and soon after, Matthew Meselson and Franklin Stahl proved that DNA replicated itself. By the end of the 1950's, RNA was being implicated in protein synthesis, and much of the mechanism of translation was postulated by Marshall Nirenberg and Johann Matthaei in 1961.

The concept of heritable genetic disease is also a relatively recent one. The first direct evidence that a mutation can result in the production of an altered protein came in 1949 with studies on sickle cell disease. Since then, thousands of genetic diseases have been characterized. The advent of recombinant DNA technology in the 1970's, which allows the direct manipulation of DNA, has increased the knowledge of these diseases manyfold, as well as demonstrating the genetic influences in maladies such as cancer and behavioral disorders. This technology has led to vastly improved diagnostic methods and therapies while pointing the way toward potential cures.

—*Robert D. Meyer, Ph.D.*

See also Bioinformatics; Cells; Gene therapy; Genetic counseling; Genetic diseases; Genetic engineering; Genetics and inheritance; Genomics; Karyotyping; Mutation; Proteomics.

FOR FURTHER INFORMATION:

Campbell, Neil A., et al. *Biology: Concepts and Connections.* 5th ed. San Francisco: Pearson/Benjamin Cummings, 2006. This classic introductory textbook provides an excellent discussion of essential biological structures and mechanisms. Its extensive and detailed illustrations help to make even difficult concepts accessible to the nonspecialist. Of particular interest are the chapters constituting the unit titled "The Gene."

Drlica, Karl. *Understanding DNA and Gene Cloning: A Guide for the Curious.* 4th ed. Hoboken, N.J.: Wiley, 2004. This book for the uninitiated explains the basic principles of genetic mechanisms without requiring knowledge of chemistry. The first third is especially good on the fundamentals, but the remainder may be too deep for some readers.

Frank-Kamenetskii, Maxim D. *Unraveling DNA: The Most Important Molecule of Life*. Translated by Lev Liapin. Rev. ed. Reading, Mass.: Addison-Wesley, 1997. This very readable book provides an excellent history of the discovery of DNA. Also describes the nature of DNA and discusses genetic engineering and the ethical questions that surround its use.

Glick, Bernard, and Jack Pasternak. *Molecular Biotechnology: Principles and Applications of Recombinant DNA*. 3d ed. Washington, D.C.: ASM Press, 2003. Explores the scientific principles of recombinant DNA technology and its wide-ranging use in industry, agriculture, and the pharmaceutical and biomedical sectors.

Gonick, Larry, and Mark Wheelis. *The Cartoon Guide to Genetics*. Rev. ed. HarperPerennial, 1991. An effective mixture of humor and fact makes this book a nonthreatening reference on genetics for nonscientists. Presented using historical context, it covers DNA and RNA structure and function and much more.

Gribbin, John. *In Search of the Double Helix*. New York: Bantam Books, 1985. Gribbin is a renowned science writer who is capable of explaining complex subjects in a way that anyone can understand. In this book, he goes from Charles Darwin's theories to quantum mechanics in his rendition of the history of the discovery of DNA. Very readable.

Hofstadter, Douglas R. "The Genetic Code: Arbitrary?" In *Metamagical Themas: Questing for the Essence of Mind and Pattern*. New York: Basic Books, 1985. While only a thirty-page chapter in a large book, this piece by Hofstadter is an excellent and thought-provoking explanation of transcription and translation written for the nonscientist.

Miklos, David A., Greg A. Freyer, and David A. Crotty. *DNA Science: A First Course in DNA Technology*. 2d ed. Cold Springs Harbor, N.Y.: Cold Springs Harbor Press, 2002. Text that combines an introductory discussion of the principles of genetics, DNA structure and function, and methods for analyzing DNA with twelve laboratory experiments that illustrate the basic techniques of DNA restriction, transformation, isolation, and analysis.

Nicholl, Desmond S. T. *Introduction to Genetic Engineering*. 2d ed. New York: Cambridge University Press, 2002. A valuable textbook for the nonspecialist and anyone interested in genetic engineering. It provides an excellent foundation in molecular biology and builds on that foundation to show how organisms can be genetically engineered.

Watson, James D., and Andrew Berry. *DNA: The Secret of Life*. New York: Knopf, 2003. Nobel Prize-winning scientist Watson guides readers through the rapid advances in genetic technology and what these advances mean for modern life. Covers all aspects of the genome in a readable fashion.

DOMESTIC VIOLENCE

DISEASE/DISORDER

ANATOMY OR SYSTEM AFFECTED: Psychic-emotional system, all bodily systems

SPECIALTIES AND RELATED FIELDS: Emergency medicine, family medicine, geriatrics and gerontology, internal medicine, pediatrics, psychiatry, psychology, public health

DEFINITION: Assaultive behavior intended to punish, dominate, or control another in an intimate family relationship; physicians are often best able to identify situations of domestic violence and assist victims to implement preventive interventions.

KEY TERMS:

cycle of violence: a repeating pattern of violence characterized by increasing tension, culminating in violent action, and followed by remorse

family violence: violence against a family member, typically to assert domination, control actions, or punish, which occurs as a pattern of behavior, not as a single, isolated act; also called battering, marital violence, domestic violence, relationship violence, child abuse, or elder abuse

funneling: an interviewing technique for assessing violence in a patient's relationship, beginning with broad questions of relationship conflict and gradually narrowing to focus on specific violent actions

hands-off violence: indirect attacks meant to terrorize or control a victim; may include property or pet destruction, threats, intimidating behavior, verbal abuse, stalking, and monitoring

hands-on violence: direct attacks upon the victim's body, including physical and sexual violence; comprises a continuum of acts ranging from seemingly minor to obviously severe

lethality: the potential, given the particular dynamics of violence in a relationship, for one or both partners to be killed

safety planning: the development of a specific set of actions and strategies to enable a victim either to avoid violence altogether or, once violence has begun, to escape and minimize damage and injury

CAUSES AND SYMPTOMS

Domestic or family violence is the intentional use of violence against a family member. The purpose of the violence is to assert domination, to control the victim's actions, or to punish the victim for some actions. Family violence generally occurs as a pattern of behavior over time rather than as a single, isolated act.

Forms of family violence include child physical abuse, child sexual abuse, spousal or partner abuse, and elder abuse. These forms of violence are related, in that they occur within the context of the family unit. Therefore, the victims and perpetrators know one another, are related to one another, may live together, and may love one another. These various forms of violence also differ insofar as victims may be children, adults, or frail, elderly adults. The needs of victims differ with age and independence, but there are also many similarities between the different types of violence. One such similarity is the relationship between the offender and the victim. Specifically, victims of abuse are always less powerful than abusers. Power includes the ability to exert physical and psychological control over situations. For example, a child abuser has the ability to lock a child in a bathroom or to abandon him or her in a remote area in order to control access to authorities. A spouse abuser has the ability to physically injure a spouse, disconnect the phone, and keep the victim from leaving for help. An elder abuser can exert similar control. Such differences in power between victims and offenders are seen as a primary cause of abuse; that is, people batter others because they can.

Families that are violent are often isolated. The members usually keep to themselves and have few or no friends or relatives with whom they are involved, even if they live in a city. This social isolation prevents victims from seeking help from others and allows the abuser to establish rules for the relationship without answering to anyone for these actions. Abuse continues and worsens because the violence occurs in private, with few consequences for the abuser.

Victims of all forms of family violence share common experiences. In addition to physical violence, victims are also attacked psychologically, being told they are worthless and responsible for the abuse that they receive. Because they are socially isolated, victims do not

have an opportunity to take social roles where they can experience success, recognition, or love. As a result, victims often have low self-esteem and truly believe that they cause the violence. Without the experience of being worthwhile, victims often become severely depressed and anxious, and they experience more stress-related illnesses such as headaches, fatigue, or gastrointestinal problems.

Child and partner abuse are linked in several ways. About half of the men who batter their wives also batter their children. Further, women who are battered are more likely to abuse their children than are nonbattered women. Even if a child of a spouse-abusing father is not battered, living in a violent home and observing the father's violence has negative effects. Such children often experience low self-esteem, aggression toward other children, and school problems. Moreover, abused children are more likely to commit violent offenses as adults. Children, especially males, who have observed violence between parents are at increased risk of assaulting their partners as adults. Adult sexual offenders have an increased likelihood of having been sexually abused as children. Yet, while these and other problems are reported more frequently by adults who were abused as children than by adults who were not, many former victims do not become violent. The most common outcomes of childhood abuse in adults are emotional problems. Although much less is known about the relationship between child abuse and future elder abuse, many elder abusers did suffer abuse as children. While most people who have been abused do not themselves become abusers, this intergenerational effect remains a cause for concern.

In its various forms, family violence is a public health epidemic in the United States. Once thought to be rare, family violence occurs with high frequency in the general population. Although exact figures are lacking and domestic violence tends to be underreported, it is estimated that each year 1.9 million children are physically abused, 250,000 children are sexually molested, 1.6 million women are assaulted by their male partners, and between 500,000 and 2.5 million elders are abused. Rates of violence directed toward unmarried heterosexual women, married heterosexual women, and members of homosexual male and female couples tend to be similar. No one is immune: Victims come from all social classes, races, and religions. Partner violence directed toward heterosexual men, however, is rare and usually occurs in relationships in which the male hits first.

Because family violence is so pervasive, physicians encounter many victims. One out of every three to five women visiting emergency rooms is seeking medical care for injuries related to partner violence. In primary care clinics, including family medicine, internal medicine, and obstetrics and gynecology, one out of every four female patients reports violence in the past year, and two out of five report violence at some time in their lives. It is therefore reasonable to expect all physicians and other health care professionals working in primary care and emergency rooms to provide services for victims of family violence.

Family violence typically consists of a pattern of behavior occurring over time and involving both hands-on and hands-off violence. Hands-on violence consists of direct attacks against the victim's body. Such acts range from pushing, shoving, and restraining to slapping, punching, kicking, clubbing, choking, burning, stabbing, or shooting. Hands-on violence also includes sexual assault, ranging from forced fondling of breasts, buttocks, and genitals; to forced touching of the abuser; to forced intercourse with the abuser or with other people.

Hands-off violence includes physical violence that is not directed at the victim's body but is intended to display destructive power and assert domination and control. Examples include breaking through windows or locked doors, punching holes through walls, smashing objects, destroying personal property, and harming or killing pet animals. The victim is often blamed for this destruction and forced to clean up the mess. Hands-off violence also includes psychological control, coercion, and terror. This includes name calling, threats of violence or abandonment, gestures suggesting the possibility of violence, monitoring of the victim's whereabouts, controlling of resources (such as money, transportation, and property), forced viewing of pornography, sexual exposure, or threatening to contest child custody. These psychological tactics may occur simultaneously with physical assaults or may occur separately. Whatever the pattern of psychological and physical tactics, abusers exert extreme control over their partners.

Neglect—the failure of one person to provide for the basic needs of another dependent person—is another form of hands-off abuse. Neglect may involve failure to provide food, clothing, health care, or shelter. Children, older adults, and developmentally delayed or physically handicapped people are particularly vulnerable to neglect.

Family violence differs in two respects from violence directed at strangers. First, the offender and victim are related and may love each other, live together, share property, have children, and share friends and relatives. Hence, unlike victims of stranger violence, victims of family violence cannot quickly or easily sever ties with or avoid seeing their assailants. Second, family violence often increases slowly in intensity, progressing until victims feel immobilized, unworthy, and responsible for the violence that is directed toward them. Victims may also feel substantial and well-grounded fear about leaving their abusers or seeking legal help, because they have been threatened or assaulted in the past and may encounter significant difficulty obtaining help to escape. In the case of children, the frail and elderly, or people with disabilities, dependency upon the caregiver and cognitive limitations make escape from an abuser difficult. Remaining in the relationship increases the risk of continued victimization. Understanding this unique context of the violent family can help physicians and other health care providers understand why battered victims often have difficulty admitting abuse or leaving the abuser.

Family violence follows a characteristic cycle. This cycle of violence begins with escalating tension and anger in the abuser. Victims describe a feeling of "walking on eggs." Next comes an outburst of violence. Outbursts of violence sometimes coincide with episodes of alcohol and drug abuse. Following the outburst, the abuser may feel remorse and expect forgiveness. The abuser often demands reconciliation, including sexual interaction. After a period of calm, the abuser again becomes increasingly tense and angry. This cycle generally repeats, with violence becoming increasingly severe. In partner abuse, victims are at greatest risk when there is a transition in the relationship such as pregnancy, divorce, or separation. In the case of elder abuse, risk increases as the elder becomes increasingly dependent on the primary caregiver, who may be inexperienced or unwilling to provide needed assistance. Without active intervention, the abuser rarely stops spontaneously and often becomes more violent.

TREATMENT AND THERAPY

Physicians play an important role in stopping family violence by first identifying people who are victims of violence, then taking steps to intervene and help. Physicians use different techniques with each age group because children, adults, and older adults each have special needs and varying abilities to help themselves.

This section will first consider the physician's role with children and will then examine the physician's role with adults and older adults.

Because children do not usually tell a physician directly if they are being abused physically or sexually, physicians use several strategies to identify child and adolescent victims. Physicians screen for abuse during regular checkups by asking children if anyone has hurt them, touched them in private places, or scared them. To accomplish this screening with five-year-old patients having routine checkups, physicians may teach their young patients about private areas of the body; let them know that they can tell a parent, teacher, or doctor if anyone ever touches them in private places; and ask the patients if anyone has ever touched them in a way that they did not like. For fifteen-year-old patients, physicians may screen potential victims by providing information on sexual abuse and date rape, then asking the patients whether they have ever experienced either.

A second strategy that physicians use to identify children who are victims of family violence is to remain alert for general signs of distress that may indicate a child or youth lives in a violent situation. General signs of distress in children, which may be caused by family violence or by other stressors, include depression, anxiety, low self-esteem, hyperactivity, disruptive behaviors, aggressiveness toward other children, and lack of friends.

In addition to general signs of distress, there are certain specific signs and symptoms of physical and sexual abuse in children which indicate that the child has probably been exposed to violence. For example, a bruise that looks like a handprint, belt mark, or rope burn would indicate abuse. X rays can show a history of broken bones that are suspicious. Intentional burns from hot water, fire, or cigarettes often have a characteristic pattern. Sexually transmitted diseases in the genital, anal, or oral cavity of a child who is aged fourteen or under would suggest sexual abuse.

A physician observing specific signs of abuse or violence in a child, or even suspecting physical or sexual abuse, has an ethical and legal obligation to provide this information to state child protective services. Every state has laws that require physicians to report suspected child abuse. Physicians do not need to find proof of abuse before filing a report. In fact, the physician should never attempt to prove abuse or interview the child in detail because this can interfere with interviews conducted by experts in law, psychology, and the medicine of child abuse. When children are in immediate

danger, they may be hospitalized so that they may receive a thorough medical and psychological evaluation while also being removed from the dangerous situation. In addition to filing a report, the physician records all observations in the child's medical file. This record includes anything that the child or parents said, drawings or photographs of the injury, the physician's professional opinion regarding exposure to violence, and a description of the child abuse report.

The physician's final step is to offer support to the child's family. Families of child victims often have multiple problems, including violence between adults, drug and alcohol abuse, economic problems, and social isolation. Appropriate interventions for promoting safety include foster care for children, court-ordered counseling for one or both parents, and in-home education in parenting skills. The physician's goal, however, is to maintain a nonjudgmental manner while encouraging parental involvement.

Physicians also play a key role in helping victims of partner violence. Like children and adolescents, adult victims will usually not disclose violence; therefore, physicians should screen for partner violence and ask about partner violence whenever they notice specific signs of abuse or general signs of distress. Physicians screen for current and past violence during routine patient visits, such as during initial appointments; school, athletic, and work physicals; premarital exams; obstetrical visits; and regular checkups. General signs of distress include depression, anxiety disorders, low self-esteem, suicidal ideation, drug and alcohol abuse, stress illnesses (headache, stomach problems, chronic pain), or patient comments about a partner being jealous, angry, controlling, or irritable. Specific signs of violence include physical injury consistent with assault, including that requiring emergency treatment.

When a victim reports partner violence, there are several steps that a physician can take to help. Communicating belief and support is the first step. Sometimes abuse is extreme and patient reports may seem incredible. The physician validates the victim's experience by expressing belief in the story and exonerating the patient of blame. The physician can begin this process by making eye contact and telling the victim, "You have a right to be safe and respected" and "No one should be treated this way."

Another step is helping the patient assess danger. This is done by asking about types and severity of violent acts, duration and frequency of violence, and injuries received. Specific factors that seem to increase the risk of death in violent relationships include the abuser's use of drugs and alcohol, threats to kill the victim, and the victim's suicidal ideation or attempts. Finally, the physician should ask if the victim feels safe returning home. With this information, the physician can help the patient assess lethal potential and begin to make appropriate safety plans.

Another step is helping the patient identify resources and make a safety plan. The physician begins this process by simply expressing concern for the victim's safety and providing information about local resources such as mandatory arrest laws, legal advocacy services, and shelters. For patients planning to return to an abusive relationship, the physician should encourage a detailed safety plan by helping the patient identify safe havens with family members, friends, or a shelter; assess escape routes from the residence; make specific plans for dangerous situations or when violence recurs; and gather copies of important papers, money, and extra clothing in a safe place in or out of the home against the event of a quick exit. Before the patient leaves, the physician should give the patient a follow-up appointment within two weeks. This provides the victim with a specific, known resource. Follow-up visits should continue until the victim has developed other supportive resources.

The physician's final step is documentation in the patient's medical file. This written note includes the victim's report of violence, the physician's own observations of injuries and behavior, assessment of danger, safety planning, and follow-up. This record can be helpful in the event of criminal or civil action taken by the victim against the offender. The medical file and all communications with the patient are kept strictly confidential. Confronting the offender about the abuse can place the victim at risk of further, more severe violence. Improper disclosure can also result in loss of the patient's trust, precluding further opportunities for help.

There are several things that a physician should never do when working with a patient-victim. The physician should not encourage a patient to leave a violent relationship as a first or primary choice. Leaving an abuser is the most dangerous time for victims and should be attempted only with adequate planning and resources. The physician should not recommend couples counseling. Couples counseling endangers victims by raising the victim's expectation that issues can be discussed safely. The abuser often batters the victim after disclosure of sensitive information. Finally, the physician should not overlook violence if the violence

appears to be "minor." Seemingly minor acts of aggression can be highly injurious.

Physicians also play an important role in helping adults who are older, developmentally delayed, or physically disabled. People in all three groups experience a high rate of family violence. Each group presents unique challenges for the physician. One common element among all three groups is that the victims may be somewhat dependent upon other adults to meet their basic needs. Because of this dependence, abuse may sometimes take the form of failing to provide basic needs such as adequate food or medical care. In many states, adults who are developmentally delayed are covered by mandatory child abuse reporting laws.

The signs and symptoms of the abuse of elders are similar to those of the other forms of family violence. These include physical injuries consistent with assault, signs of distress, and neglect, including self-neglect. Elder abuse victims are often reluctant to reveal abuse because of fear of retaliation, abandonment, or institutionalization. Therefore, a key to intervention is coordinating with appropriate social service and allied health agencies to support an elder adequately, either at home or in a care center. Such agencies include aging councils, visiting nurses, home health aides, and respite or adult day care centers. Counseling and assistance for caregivers are also important parts of intervention.

Many states require physicians to report suspected elder abuse. Because many elder abuse victims are mentally competent, however, it is important that they be made part of the decision-making and reporting process. Such collaboration puts needed control in the elder's hands and therefore facilitates healing. Many other aspects of intervention described for partner abuse apply to working with elders, including providing emotional support, assessing danger, safety planning, and documentation.

In addition to helping the victims of acute, ongoing family violence, physicians have an important role to play in helping survivors of past family violence. People who have survived family violence may continue to experience negative effects similar to those experienced by acute victims. Physicians can identify survivors of family violence by screening for past violence during routine exams. A careful history can determine whether the patient has been suffering medical or psychological problems related to the violence. Finally, the physician should identify local resources for the patient, including a mutual help group and a therapist.

Physicians can also help prevent family violence.

One avenue of prevention is through education of patients by discussing partner violence with patients at key life transitions, such as during adolescence when youths begin dating, prior to marriage, during pregnancy, and during divorce or separation. A second avenue of prevention is making medical clinic waiting rooms and examination rooms into education centers by displaying educational posters and providing pamphlets.

PERSPECTIVE AND PROSPECTS

Despite its frequency, family violence has not always been viewed as a problem. In the 1800's, it was legal in the United States for a man to beat his wife, or for parents to use brutal physical punishment with children. Although the formation of the New York Society for the Prevention of Cruelty to Children in 1874 signaled rising concern about child maltreatment, the extent of the problem was underestimated. As recently as 1960, family violence was viewed as a rare, aberrant phenomenon, and women who were victims of violence were often seen as partially responsible because of "masochistic tendencies." Several factors combined to turn the tide during the next thirty years. Medical research published in the early 1960's began documenting the severity of the problem of child abuse. By 1968, every state in the United States had passed a law requiring that physicians report suspected child abuse, and many states had established child protective services to investigate and protect vulnerable children.

Progress in the battle against partner violence was slower. The battered women's movement brought new attention and a feminist understanding to the widespread and serious nature of partner violence. This growing awareness provided the impetus, during the 1970's and 1980's, for reform in the criminal justice system, scientific research, continued growth of women's shelters, and the development of treatment programs for offenders.

The medical profession's response to partner abuse followed these changes. In 1986, Surgeon General C. Everett Koop declared family violence to be a public health problem and called upon physicians to learn to identify and intervene with victims. In 1992, the American Medical Association (AMA) echoed the surgeon general and stated that physicians have an ethical obligation to identify and assist victims of partner violence, and it established standards and protocols for identifying and helping victims of family violence. Because partner and elder abuse have been recognized only recently by the medical community, many physicians are just beginning to learn about their essential role.

Family violence has at various times been considered as a social problem, a legal problem, a political problem, and a medical problem. Because of this shifting understanding and because of the grassroots political origins of the child and partner violence movements, some may question why physicians should be involved. There are three compelling reasons.

First, there is a medical need: Family violence is one of the most common causes of injury, illness, and death for women and children. Victims seeking treatment for acute injuries make up a sizable portion of emergency room visits. Even in outpatient clinics, women report high rates of recent and ongoing violence and injury from partners. In addition to physical injuries, many victims experience stress-related medical problems for which they seek medical care. Among obstetrical patients who are battered, there is a risk of injury to both the woman and her unborn child. Hence, physicians working in clinics and emergency rooms will see many people who are victims.

Second, physicians have a stake in breaking the cycle of violence because they are interested in injury prevention and health promotion. When a physician treats a child or adult victim for physical or psychological injury but does not identify root causes, the victim will return to a dangerous situation. Prevention of future injury requires proper diagnosis of root causes, rather than mere treatment of symptoms.

Third, physicians have a stake in treatment of partner violence because it is a professional and ethical obligation. Two principles of medical ethics apply. First, a physician's actions should benefit the patient. Physicians can benefit patients who are suffering the effects of family violence only if they correctly recognize the root cause and intervene in a sensitive and professional manner. Physicians should also "do no harm." A physician who fails to recognize and treat partner violence will harm the patient by providing inappropriate advice and treatment.

—L. Kevin Hamberger, Ph.D.,
and Bruce Ambuel, Ph.D.

See also Addiction; Alcoholism; Bipolar disorders; Depression; Ethics; Intoxication; Münchausen syndrome by proxy; Paranoia; Psychiatric disorders; Psychiatry; Psychiatry, child and adolescent; Psychiatry, geriatric; Psychoanalysis; Psychosis; Schizophrenia; Stress.

For Further Information:

Bancroft, Lundy, and Jay G. Silverman. *The Batterer as Parent: Addressing the Impact of Domestic Violence on Family Dynamics*. Thousand Oaks, Calif.: Sage Publications, 2002. Examines how partner abuse affects each relationship in a family and explains how children's emotional recovery is inextricably linked to the healing and empowerment of their mothers.

Barnett, Ola, Cindy L. Miller-Perrin, and Robin D. Perrin. *Family Violence Across the Lifespan: An Introduction*. 2d ed. Thousand Oaks, Calif.: Sage Publications, 2005. Provides information about the different ways that domestic violence, and the warning signs associated with it, may be recognized at various stages in the life spans of individuals and families.

Dutton, Donald G. *The Abusive Personality: Violence and Control in Intimate Relationships*. Rev. ed. New York: The Guilford Press, 2003. Dutton, a psychologist, began as a disciple of social learning theory and eventually came to understand that theory alone was inadequate to explain the multifaceted origins of spousal abuse.

Island, David, and Patrick Letellier. *Men Who Beat the Men Who Love Them: Battered Gay Men and Domestic Violence*. New York: Haworth Press, 1991. The first published book that tackles the issue of gay male partner violence. The authors write in a lively, straightforward manner that is easy to understand. Proposes novel ways of thinking about partner violence.

Kakar, Suman. *Domestic Abuse*. San Francisco: Austin & Infield, 2002. Offers theoretical and analytical explanations for domestic violence and includes detailed discussion of violence against children, youth, and the elderly.

Levine, Murray, and Adeline Levine. *Helping Children: A Social History*. New York: Oxford University Press, 1992. The Levines provide an excellent history of child maltreatment in the United States, as well as the various legal, social, and medical strategies that have been used to help abused children.

National Coalition Against Domestic Violence. http://www.ncadv.org/. A site that defines domestic violence and offers information on community responses, getting help, and public policy.

Raphael, Jody. *Saving Bernice: Battered Women, Welfare, and Poverty*. Boston: Northeastern University Press, 2000. Raphael uses the case study of one welfare mother and survivor of domestic violence to exemplify the broader issues connecting domestic violence and poverty. In interviews taped during 1995-1999, Bernice, a mother of two and on welfare for eight years, recounts the trauma of abuse, harassment, and stalking by her former partner.

Wilson, K. J. *When Violence Begins at Home: A Comprehensive Guide to Understanding and Ending Domestic Violence*. Alameda, Calif.: Hunter House, 1997. Wilson seeks to share her wealth of knowledge stemming from experience as the current training director at the Austin Center for Battered Women, as an educator, and as a survivor of domestic abuse.

Down syndrome
Disease/disorder

Anatomy or system affected: Brain, nervous system, psychic-emotional system

Specialties and related fields: Embryology, genetics, obstetrics, pediatrics

Definition: A congenital abnormality characterized by moderate to severe mental retardation and a distinctive physical appearance caused by a chromosomal aberration, the result of either an error during embryonic cell division or the inheritance of defective chromosomal material.

Key terms:

chromosomes: small, threadlike bodies containing the genes that are microscopically visible during cell division

gametes: the egg and sperm cells that unite to form the fertilized egg (zygote) in reproduction

gene: a segment of the DNA strand containing instructions for the production of a protein

homologous chromosomes: chromosome pairs of the same size and centromere position that possess genes for the same traits; one homologous chromosome is inherited from the father and the other from the mother

meiosis: the type of cell division that produces the cells of reproduction, which contain one-half of the chromosome number found in the original cell before division

mitosis: the type of cell division that occurs in nonsex cells, which conserves chromosome number by equal allocation to each of the newly formed cells

translocation: an aberration in chromosome structure resulting from the attachment of chromosomal material to a nonhomologous chromosome

Causes and Symptoms

Down syndrome is an example of a genetic disorder, that is, a disorder arising from an abnormality in an individual's genetic material. Down syndrome results from an incorrect transfer of genetic material in the formation of cells. Genetic information is contained in large "library" molecules of deoxyribonucleic acid (DNA). DNA molecules are formed by joining together units called nucleotides which come in four different varieties: adenosine, thymine, cytosine, and guanine (identified by their initials A, T, C, and G). These nucleotides store hereditary information by forming "words" with this four-letter alphabet. In a gene, a section of DNA which contains the chemical message controlling an inherited trait, three consecutive nucleotides combine to specify a particular amino acid. This word order forms the "sentences" of a recipe telling cells how to construct proteins, such as those coloring the hair and eyes, from amino acids.

In living systems, tissue growth occurs through cell division processes in which an original cell divides to form two cells containing duplicate genetic material. Just before a cell divides, the DNA organizes itself into distinct, compact bundles called chromosomes. Normal human cells, diploid cells, contain twenty-three pairs (or a total of forty-six) of these chromosomes. Each pair is a set of homologues containing genes for the same traits. These chromosomes are composed of two DNA strands, chromatids, joined at a constricted region known as the centromere. The bundle is similar in shape to the letter X. The arms are the parts above and below the constriction, which may be centered or offset toward one end (giving arms of equal or different lengths, respectively). During mitosis, the division of nonsex cells, the chromatids separate at the centromere, forming two sets of single-stranded chromosomes, which migrate to opposite ends of the cell. The cell then splits into two genetically equivalent cells,

each containing twenty-three single-stranded chromosomes that will duplicate to form the original number of forty-six chromosomes.

In sexual reproduction, haploid egg and sperm cells, each containing twenty-three single-stranded chromosomes, unite in fertilization to produce a zygote cell with forty-six chromosomes. Haploid cells are created through a different, two-step cell division process termed meiosis. Meiosis begins when the homologues in a diploid cell pair up at the equator of the cell. The attractions between the members of each pair then break, allowing the homologues to migrate to opposite ends of the cell, each twin to a different pole, without splitting at the centromere. The parent cell then divides once to give two cells containing twenty-three double-stranded chromosomes, and then divides again through the process of mitosis to form cells that contain only twenty-three single-stranded chromosomes. Thus, each cell contains half of the original chromosomes.

Although cell division is normally a precise process, occasionally an error called nondisjunction occurs when a chromosome either fails to separate or fails to migrate to the proper pole. In meiosis, the failure to move to the proper pole results in the formation of one gamete having twenty-four chromosomes and one having twenty-two chromosomes. Upon fertilization, zygotes of forty-seven or forty-five chromosomes are produced, and the developing embryo must function with either extra or missing genes. Since every chromosome contains a multitude of genes, problems result from the absence or excess of proteins produced. In fact, the embryos formed from most nondisjunctional fertilizations die at an early stage in development and are spontaneously aborted. Occasionally, nondisjunction occurs in mitosis, when a chromosome migrates before the chromatids separate, yielding one cell with an extra copy of the chromosome and no copy in the other cell.

Down syndrome is also termed trisomy 21 because it most commonly results from the presence of an extra copy of the smallest human chromosome, chromosome 21. Actually, it is not the entire extra chromosome 21 that is responsible, but rather a small segment of the long arm of this chromosome. Only two other trisomies occur with any significant frequency: trisomy 13 (Patau's syndrome) and trisomy 18 (Edwards' syndrome). Both of these disorders are accompanied by multiple severe malformations, resulting in death within a few months of birth. Most incidences of Down syndrome are a consequence of a nondisjunction dur-

---

Information on Down Syndrome

Causes: Genetic defect
Symptoms: Mental retardation, characteristic facial appearance, lack of muscle tone, increased risk for heart malformations, increased disease susceptibility
Duration: Lifelong
Treatments: None

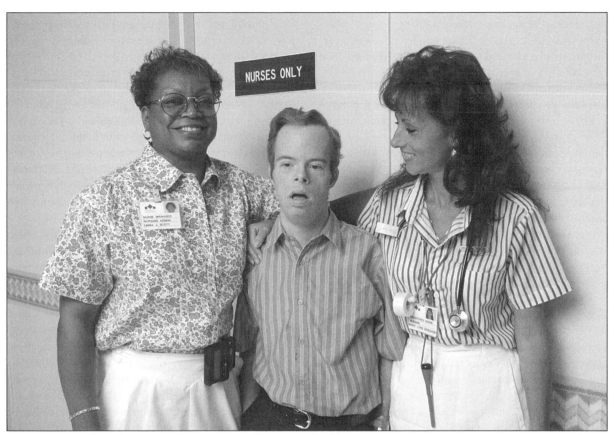

Nurses and other health care professionals can offer both medical and emotional support to people with Down syndrome. (PhotoDisc)

ing meiosis. In about 75 percent of these cases, the extra chromosome is present in the egg. About 1 percent of Down syndrome cases occur after the fertilization of normal gametes from a mitosis nondisjunction, producing a mosaic in which some of the embryo's cells are normal and some exhibit trisomy. The degree of mosaicism and its location will determine the physiological consequences of the nondisjunction. Although mosaic individuals range from apparent normality to completely affected, typically the disorder is less severe.

In about 4 percent of all Down syndrome cases, the individual possesses not an entire third copy of chromosome 21 but rather extra chromosome 21 material, which has been incorporated via a translocation into a nonhomologous chromosome. In translocation, pieces of arms are swapped between two nonrelated chromosomes, forming "hybrid" chromosomes. The most common translocation associated with Down syndrome is that between the long arm (Down gene area) of chromosome 21 and an end of chromosome 14. The

individual in whom the translocation has occurred shows no evidence of the aberration, since the normal complement of genetic material is still present, only at different chromosomal locations. The difficulty arises when this individual forms gametes. A mother who possesses the 21/14 translocation, for example, has one normal 21, one normal 14, and the hybrid chromosomes. She is a genetic carrier for the disorder, because she can pass it on to her offspring even though she is clinically normal. This mother could produce three types of viable gametes: one containing the normal 14 and 21; one containing both translocations, which would result in clinical normality; and one containing the normal 21 and the translocated 14 having the long arm of 21. If each gamete were fertilized by normal sperm, two apparently normal embryos and one partial trisomy 21 Down syndrome embryo would result. Down syndrome that results from the passing on of translocations is termed familial Down syndrome and is an inherited disorder.

The presence of an extra copy of the long arm of

chromosome 21 causes defects in many tissues and organs. One major effect of Down syndrome is mental retardation. The intelligence quotients (IQs) of affected individuals are typically in the range of 40-50. The IQ varies with age, being higher in childhood than in adolescence or adult life. The disorder is often accompanied by physical traits such as short stature, stubby fingers and toes, protruding tongue, and an unusual pattern of hand creases. Perhaps the most recognized physical feature is the distinctive slanting of the eyes, caused by a vertical fold (epicanthal fold) of skin near the nasal bridge which pulls and tilts the eyes slightly toward the nostrils. For normal Caucasians, the eye runs parallel to the skin fold below the eyebrow; for Asians, this skin fold covers a major portion of the upper eyelid. In contrast, the epicanthal fold in trisomy 21 does not cover a major part of the upper eyelid.

It should be noted that not all defects associated with Down syndrome are found in every affected individual. About 40 percent of Down syndrome patients have congenital heart defects, while about 10 percent have intestinal blockages. Affected individuals are prone to respiratory infections and contract leukemia at a rate twenty times that of the general population. Although Down syndrome children develop the same types of leukemia in the same proportions as other children, the survival rates of the two groups are markedly different. While the survival rate for patients without Down syndrome after ten years is about 30 percent, survival beyond five years is negligible in those with Down syndrome. It appears that the extra copy of chromosome 21 not only increases the risk of contracting the cancer but also exerts a decisive influence on the disease's outcome. Reproductively, males are sterile while some females are fertile. Although many Down syndrome infants die in the first year of life, the average life expectancy is about fifty years. This reduced life expectancy results from defects in the immune system, causing a high susceptibility to infectious disease. Many individuals with Down syndrome develop an Alzheimer's-like condition later in life.

TREATMENT AND THERAPY

Trisomy 21 is one of the most common human chromosomal aberrations, occurring in about 0.5 percent of all conceptions and in one out of every seven hundred to eight hundred live births. About 15 percent of the patients institutionalized for mental deficiency suffer from Down syndrome.

Even before the chromosomal basis for the disorder was determined, the frequency of Down syndrome births was correlated with increased maternal age. For mothers at age twenty, the incidence of Down syndrome is about 0.05 percent, which increases to 0.9 percent by age thirty-five and 3 percent at age forty-five. Studies comparing the chromosomes of the affected offspring with those of both parents have shown that the nondisjunction event is maternal about 75 percent of the time. This maternal age effect is thought to result from the different manner in which the male and female gametes are produced. Gamete production in the male is a continual, lifelong process, while it is a one-time event in females.

Formation of the female's gametes begins early in embryonic life, somewhere between the eighth and twentieth weeks. During this time, cells in the developing ovary divide rapidly by mitosis, forming cells called primary oocytes. These cells then begin meiosis by pairing up the homologues. The process is interrupted at this point, and the cells are held in a state of suspended animation until needed in reproduction, when they are triggered to complete their division and form eggs. It appears that the frequency of nondisjunction events increases with the length of the storage period. Studies have demonstrated that cells in a state of meiosis are particularly sensitive to environmental influences such as viruses, X rays, and cytotoxic chemicals. It is possible that environmental influences may play a role in nondisjunction events. Up to age thirty-two, males contribute an extra chromosome 21 as often as do females. Beyond this age, there is a rapid increase in nondisjunctional eggs, while the number of nondisjunctional sperm remains constant. Where the maternal age effect is minimal, mosaicism may be an important source of the trisomy. An apparently normal mother who possesses undetected mosaicism can produce trisomy offspring if gametes with an extra chromosome are produced. In some instances, characteristics such as abnormal fingerprint patterns have been observed in the mothers and their Down syndrome offspring.

Techniques such as amniocentesis, chorionic villus sampling, and alpha-fetoprotein screening are available for prenatal diagnosis of Down syndrome in fetuses. Amniocentesis, the most widely used technique for prenatal diagnosis, is generally performed between the fourteenth and sixteenth weeks of pregnancy. In this technique, about one ounce of fluid is removed from the amniotic cavity surrounding the fetus by a needle inserted through the mother's abdomen. Although some testing can be done directly on the fluid (such as the assay for spina bifida), more information is obtained from the cells shed from the fetus that accompany the fluid. The mixture obtained in the amniocentesis is spun in a centrifuge to separate the fluid from the fetal cells. Unfortunately, the chromosome analysis for Down syndrome cannot be conducted directly on the amount of cellular material obtained. Although the majority of the cells collected are nonviable, some will grow in culture. These cells are allowed to grow and multiply in culture for two to four weeks, and then the chromosomes undergo karyotyping, which will detect both trisomy 21 and translocational aberration.

In karyotyping, the chromosomes are spread on a microscope slide, stained, and photographed. Each type of chromosome gives a unique, observable banding pattern when stained, which allows it to be identified. The chromosomes are then cut out of the photograph and arranged in homologous pairs, in numerical order. Trisomy 21 is easily observed, since three copies of chromosome 21 are present, while the translocation shows up as an abnormal banding pattern. Termination of the pregnancy in the wake of an unfavorable amniocentesis diagnosis is complicated, because the fetus at this point is usually about eighteen to twenty weeks old, and elective abortions are normally performed between the sixth and twelfth weeks of pregnancy. Earlier sampling of the amniotic fluid is not possible because of the small amount of fluid present.

An alternate testing procedure called chorionic villus sampling became available in the mid-1980's. In this procedure, a chromosomal analysis is conducted on a piece of placental tissue that is obtained either vaginally or through the abdomen during the eighth to eleventh week of pregnancy. The advantages of this procedure are that it can be done much earlier in the pregnancy and that enough tissue can be collected to conduct the chromosome analysis immediately, without the cell culture step. Consequently, diagnosis can be completed during the first trimester of the pregnancy, making therapeutic abortion an option for the parents. Chorionic villus sampling does have some negative aspects. One disadvantage is the slightly higher incidence of test-induced miscarriage as compared to amniocentesis—around 1 percent (versus less than 0.5 percent). Also, because tissue of both the mother and the fetus are obtained in the sampling process, they must be carefully separated, complicating the analysis. Occasionally, chromosomal abnormalities are observed in the tested tissue that are not present in the fetus itself.

Prenatal maternal alpha-fetoprotein testing has also been used to diagnose Down syndrome. Abnormal levels of a substance called maternal alpha-fetoprotein are often associated with chromosomal disorders. Several research studies have described a high correlation between low levels of maternal alpha-fetoprotein and the occurrence of trisomy 21 in the fetus. By correlating alpha-fetoprotein levels, the age of the mother, and specific female hormone levels, between 60 percent and 80 percent of fetuses with Down syndrome can be detected. Although techniques allow Down syndrome to be detected readily in a fetus, there is no effective intrauterine therapy available to correct the abnormality.

The care of a Down syndrome child presents many challenges for the family unit. Until the 1970's, most of these children spent their lives in institutions. With the increased support services available, however, it is now common for such children to remain in the family environment. Although many Down syndrome children have happy dispositions, a significant number have behavioral problems that can consume the energies of the parents, to the detriment of other children. Rearing a Down syndrome child often places a large financial burden on the family: Such children are, for example, susceptible to illness; they also have special educational needs. Since Down syndrome children are often conceived late in the parents' reproductive period, the parents may not be able to continue to care for these children throughout their offspring's adult years. This is problematic because many Down syndrome individuals do not possess sufficient mental skills to earn a living or to manage their affairs without supervision.

All women in their mid-thirties have an increased risk of producing a Down syndrome infant. Since the resultant trisomy 21 is not of a hereditary nature, the abnormality can be detected only by the prenatal screening, which is recommended for all pregnancies of women older than age thirty-four.

For parents who have produced a Down syndrome child, genetic counseling can be beneficial in determining their risk factor for future pregnancies. The genetic counselor determines the specific chromosomal aberration that occurred utilizing chromosome studies of the parents and affected child, along with additional information provided by the family history. If the cause was nondisjunction and the mother is young, the recurrence risk is much less than 1 percent; for mothers over the age of thirty-four, it is about 5 percent. If the cause was translocational, the Down syndrome is hereditary and risk is greater—statistically, a one-in-three chance. In addition, there is a one-in-three chance that clinically normal offspring will be carriers of the syndrome, producing it in the next generation. It is suggested that couples who come from families having a history of spontaneous abortions, which often result from lethal chromosomal aberrations, and/or incidence of Down syndrome, undergo chromosomal screening to detect the presence of a Down syndrome translocation.

PERSPECTIVE AND PROSPECTS

English physician John L. H. Down is credited with the first clinical description of Down syndrome, in 1886. Since the distinctive epicanthic fold gave Down children an appearance that John Down associated with Asians, he called the condition "mongolism"—an unfortunate term implying that those affected with the condition are throwbacks to a more "primitive" racial group. Today, the inappropriate term has been replaced with the name Down syndrome.

A French physician, Jérôme Lejeune, suspected that Down syndrome had a genetic basis and began to study the condition in 1953. A comparison of the fingerprints and palm prints of affected individuals with those of unaffected individuals showed a high frequency of abnormalities in the prints of those with Down syndrome. These prints appear very early in development and serve as a record of events that take place early in embryogenesis. The extent of the changes in print patterns led Lejeune to the conclusion that the condition was not a result of the action of one or two genes but rather of many genes or even an entire chromosome. Upon microscopic examination, he observed that Down syndrome children possess forty-seven chromosomes instead of the forty-six chromosomes found in normal children. In 1959, Lejeune published his findings, showing that Down syndrome is caused by the presence of the extra chromosome which was later identified as a copy of chromosome 21. This first observation of a human chromosomal abnormality marked a turning point in the study of human genetics. It demonstrated that genetic defects not only were caused by mutations of single genes but also could be associated with changes in chromosome number. Although the presence of an extra chromosome allows varying degrees of development to occur, most of these abnormalities result in fetal death, with only a few resulting in live birth. Down syndrome is unusual in that the affected individual often survives into adulthood.

—*Arlene R. Courtney, Ph.D.*

See also Amniocentesis; Birth defects; Chorionic villus sampling; DNA and RNA; Genetic diseases; Genetics and inheritance; Leukemia; Mental retardation; Mutation.

FOR FURTHER INFORMATION:

Cohen, William, Lynn Nadel, and Myra E. Madnick, eds. *Down Syndrome: Visions for the Twenty-first Century.* New York: Wiley-Liss, 2002. Reviews the medical and research advances in the clinical, educational, developmental, psychosocial, and vocational aspects of Down syndrome.

Hassold, Terry J., and David Patterson, eds. *Down Syndrome: A Promising Future, Together.* New York: Wiley-Liss, 1999. Discusses clinical, educational, developmental, psychosocial, and vocational issues relevant to people with Down syndrome.

Miller, Jon F., Mark Leddy, and Lewis A. Leavitt, eds. *Improving the Communication of People with Down Syndrome.* Baltimore: Paul H. Brookes, 1999. Discusses how to assess and treat speech, language, and communication problems in children and adults with Down syndrome.

Moore, Keith L., and T. V. N. Persaud. *The Developing Human.* 7th ed. Philadelphia: W. B. Saunders, 2003. An outstanding textbook on human embryonic development, with specific information about the causes of congenital malformations and common defects occurring in each of the body's systems.

National Down Syndrome Society. http://www.ndss .org/. An excellent organization that focuses on research, advocacy, and education. The Web site promotes virtual communities and provides up-to-date information about upcoming events.

Pueschel, Siegfried M. *A Parent's Guide to Down Syndrome.* 2d ed. Baltimore: Paul H. Brookes, 2000. An informative guide highlighting the important developmental stages in the life of a child with Down syndrome.

_____, ed. *Adults with Down Syndrome.* Baltimore: Paul H. Brookes, 2006. Discusses health care and medical issues, psychiatric disorders, sexuality, education and employment, and community involvement.

Rondal, Jean A., et al., eds. *Down's Syndrome: Psychological, Psychobiological, and Socioeducational Perspectives.* San Diego, Calif.: Singular, 1996. An academic text on issues surrounding Down syndrome. Includes references and an index.

DROWNING

DISEASE/DISORDER

ANATOMY OR SYSTEM AFFECTED: Brain, circulatory system, heart, kidneys, lungs, nervous system, respiratory system, stomach, throat

SPECIALTIES AND RELATED FIELDS: Critical care, emergency medicine, environmental health, nursing, pulmonary medicine

DEFINITION: A drowning victim dies by suffocation from submersion in a liquid medium, usually water.

KEY TERMS:

alveolar ventilation: the volume of air that ventilates all the perfused alveoli; the normal average is four to five liters per minute

asphyxia: cessation of breathing

bradycardia: a heart rate below sixty beats per minute

glottis: the opening to the larynx

hypertonic fluid: a solution that increases the degree of osmotic pressure on a semipermeable membrane

hypothermia: an abnormal and dangerous condition in which the temperature of the body is below 95 degrees Fahrenheit; usually caused by prolonged exposure to cold

hypoxia: inadequate oxygen at the cellular level

intrapulmonary shunting: a condition of perfusion without ventilation

laryngospasm: spasm of the larynx

CAUSES AND SYMPTOMS

Drowning is the leading cause of accidental death in the United States. The victim dies by suffocation from submersion in a liquid medium. Although suffocation most commonly results from aspiration of fresh or salt water into the lungs, about 10 percent to 20 percent of victims experience laryngospasm with subsequent glottic closure followed by asphyxiation. Near-drowning is defined as recovery after submersion. Victims are typically children or adolescents. Males more often engage in risk-taking behavior and have a significantly greater incidence of drowning and near-drowning than do females.

Victims of near-drowning, if rescued and resuscitated quickly enough, may fully recover. In many instances, however, near-drowning victims are left with mild to severe neurologic effects. Even if the victim has been submerged in water for some time, vigorous attempts at resuscitation are indicated because of documented recovery following such incidents.

Boating and swimming accidents account for the largest number of drownings in the adult population, and many are alcohol-related. Factors that influence the extent of damage in near-drowning include the length of time submerged, the temperature of the water, and the victim's resistance to asphyxia and anoxia (oxygen deprivation). Recovery may be more successful if the victim drowns in cold water, because the induced hypothermia lowers the body's metabolic demands and, therefore, oxygen needs. Extremely cold water may decrease the victim's core body temperature so rapidly that death from hypothermia may actually occur before drowning.

Generally, there is an inverse relation between the victim's age and the victim's resistance to asphyxia and anoxia. The younger the victim, the greater the resistance. The resistance is especially strong in very young victims, usually under two or three years of age, because of the diving reflex triggered in young children when the face is immersed in very cold water. Blood is shunted to the vital organs, especially the brain and heart. Hypothermia offers some protection to the hypoxic brain by reducing the cerebral metabolic rate. Although the victim suffers severe bradycardia, the remaining oxygen supply is concentrated in the heart and brain. The diving reflex is generally not a factor in adult drownings.

Approximately 10 percent of drowning victims develop laryngospasm concurrently with the first gulp of water and thus do not aspirate (swallow) fluid. Even in the majority of victims who do aspirate, the amount of fluid aspirated is small. In the past, salt water and freshwater drowning were differentiated. These differences are of little clinical significance in humans, primarily

---

INFORMATION ON DROWNING

CAUSES: Submersion in a liquid medium, resulting in aspiration or asphyxiation

SYMPTOMS: Slow heart rate, hypoxemia, ineffective circulation, cardiac arrest, brain injury, brain death; following near-drowning, may include acute respiratory failure, cerebral and pulmonary edema, shock acidosis, electrolyte imbalance, stupor, coma, cardiac arrest

DURATION: Acute and often fatal; possible permanent effects for near-drowning

TREATMENTS: For near-drowning, cardiopulmonary resuscitation (CPR), intubation, mechanical ventilation, stomach decompression, sometimes induced coma and hypothermia

because so little fluid is aspirated. In both cases, drowning quickly diminishes perfusion to the alveoli, interfering with ventilation and soon leading to hypoxemia, ineffective circulation, cardiac arrest, brain injury, and brain death.

When water is aspirated into the lungs, the composition of the water is a key factor in the pathophysiology of the near-drowning event. Aspiration of freshwater causes surfactant to wash out of the lungs. Surfactant reduces surface tension within the alveoli, increases lung compliance and alveolar radius, and decreases the work of breathing. Loss of surfactant from freshwater aspiration destabilizes the alveoli and leads to increased airway resistance. Conversely, salt water—a hypertonic fluid—creates an osmotic gradient that draws protein-rich fluid from the vascular space into the alveoli. The consequences of both types of aspiration include impaired alveolar ventilation and resultant intrapulmonary shunting, which further compound the hypoxic state.

When submersion is brief, the near-drowning victim may spontaneously regain consciousness or may recover quickly following rescue. Even when victims have not aspirated fluid, they should be hospitalized for observation because respiratory symptoms may not develop for twelve to twenty-four hours. Victims who have been submerged for longer periods may show varying degrees of recovery following resuscitation. Manifestations may include acute respiratory failure, pulmonary edema, shock acidosis, electrolyte imbalance, stupor, coma, and cardiac arrest. Damage causes cerebral edema (brain swelling) and may lead to increased intracranial pressure. Care for the patient who has suffered brain damage involves careful and frequent assessment of the patient's neurologic status, including vital signs, pupil reaction, and reflexes.

TREATMENT AND THERAPY

Immediate care should focus on a safe rescue of the victim. Once rescuers gain access to the victim, priorities include safe removal from the water, while maintaining spine stabilization with a board or flotation device, and initiating airway clearance and ventilatory support measures. If hypothermia is a concern, then gentle handling of the victim is essential to prevent ventricular fibrillation. Abdominal thrusts should only be delivered if airway obstruction is suspected. Once the victim is safely removed from the water, airway and cardiopulmonary support interventions begin. Emergency care involves cardiopulmonary resuscitation (CPR), intubation, and mechanical ventilation with 100 percent oxygen.

In the clinical setting, stomach decompression using a tube down the nose or mouth is indicated to prevent the aspiration of gastric contents and to improve breathing.

Patients who experience near-drowning require complex care to support their body systems. The full spectrum of critical care technology may be needed to manage the physiological problems and effects associated with near-drowning, including lung infection, acute respiratory distress syndrome, and central nervous system impairment. Metabolic acidosis results from severe hypoxia. Arterial blood gases must be monitored frequently, and sodium bicarbonate is usually administered to correct the acidosis. Coma may be induced with barbiturates and a state of hypothermia maintained for several days following the near-drowning. These interventions reduce the metabolic and oxygen demands of the brain. Diuretics are prescribed to treat pulmonary and cerebral edema. Fluid therapy must be monitored carefully to prevent fluid overload and promote adequate renal function.

PERSPECTIVE AND PROSPECTS

Drowning is the second leading cause of preventable death in children according to the American Academy of Pediatrics. New drowning prevention recommendations warn parents to be certain that everyone caring for a child understands the need for constant supervision around water and other liquids.

—*Jane C. Norman, Ph.D., R.N.*

See also Accidents; Asphyxiation; Brain damage; Cardiopulmonary resuscitation (CPR); Choking; Critical care; Critical care, pediatric; Emergency medicine; Emergency medicine, pediatric; Hyperbaric oxygen therapy; Lungs; Pulmonary medicine; Pulmonary medicine, pediatric; Respiration; Resuscitation; Unconsciousness.

FOR FURTHER INFORMATION:

Black, Joyce M., and Jane H. Hawks, eds. *Medical-Surgical Nursing: Clinical Management for Positive Outcomes.* 7th ed. St. Louis: Elsevier Saunders, 2005.

Lewis, Sharon M., et al., eds. *Medical-Surgical Nursing: Assessment and Management of Clinical Problems.* 6th ed. St. Louis: Mosby, 2004.

Smeltzer, Suzanne C., and Brenda G. Bare, eds. *Brunner and Suddarth's Textbook of Medical-Surgical Nursing.* 10th ed. St. Louis: Mosby, 2004.

DRUG ADDICTION. *See* ADDICTION.

DRUG RESISTANCE

DISEASE/DISORDER

ANATOMY OR SYSTEM AFFECTED: All

SPECIALTIES AND RELATED FIELDS: Bacteriology, microbiology, pharmacology, public health, virology

DEFINITION: The ability of a pathogen, formerly susceptible to a particular medication, to change in such a way that it is no longer affected by it.

KEY TERMS:

antibiotic: a substance that kills or prevents the growth of a pathogen

bacteria: microscopic single-celled organisms

bacterial chromosome: a circular cell component in bacteria that contains deoxyribonucleic acid (DNA)

bacteriophage: a virus that attaches itself to bacteria

conjugation: the direct exchange of genetic material between bacteria

nosocomial infection: a disease or organism that is acquired in a hospital

pathogen: a living organism that causes disease

plasmids: circular pieces of DNA within bacteria; these are much smaller than bacterial chromosomes

transduction: the indirect transfer of genetic material between bacteria by a bacteriophage

transposons: pieces of DNA that can be transferred between plasmids and chromosomes

virus: a microscopic organism consisting of DNA or ribonucleic acid (RNA) within a protein coating

CAUSES AND SYMPTOMS

Drug resistance occurs whenever pathogens—disease-causing organisms such as bacteria, viruses, or fungi—that have been successfully eradicated with a chemical agent develop the ability to resist that agent. The most clinically important form of drug resistance is the ability of bacteria to develop resistance to antibiotics.

An antibiotic attacks a bacterial cell by interfering with a vital biochemical process needed by the organism. Antibiotics generally are engineered to kill bacteria, while leaving body cells unharmed. This bacteria-specific approach creates a safe way of killing pathogens with strong chemicals, while keeping the affected person safe from harm.

Bacteria can develop resistance to an antibiotic in several ways, but the spread of that resistance may be blamed on one primary phenomenon related to evolution: selection. Selection is the "weeding out" of individuals in a population, leaving a smaller number of "tougher" individuals. If environmental pressure (such as an antibiotic treatment) is placed on any population of organisms, the only individuals that will survive and reproduce are those resistant to that pressure.

Resistance to a particular antibiotic arises in a bacterial cell by random genetic mutation. Because a particular cell is genetically altered and survives the antibiotic treatment that destroys other bacteria of the same kind, it is able to survive, unlike its susceptible relatives. The small, resistant population that is left grows rapidly and cannot be halted.

Even if an antibiotic is completely successful in eradicating a particular type of bacteria, problems with drug resistance can still arise. The human body contains billions of bacteria of many different kinds. These bacteria fill large and small environmental niches in the microflora that human beings carry in and on their bodies. When one or more of these susceptible bacteria types are eliminated by an antibiotic, their niches are left empty. This leaves room for the resistant bacteria that are left to multiply in greater numbers. This is not generally a problem because most of the resistant bacteria are harmless, but even if they are, they may have the ability to genetically transfer antibiotic resistance to pathogenic bacteria.

Use of multiple antibiotics or broad spectrum antibiotics that attack many kinds of bacteria can cause other problems. By eliminating a large number of the bacteria normally present and emptying essentially all the environmental niches, powerful antibiotics encourage the growth of fungi such as *Candida albicans*. Fungal infections are not affected by bacterial antibiotics and require special antifungal drugs.

The ability to resist a particular antibiotic is encoded as genetic information in deoxyribonucleic acid (DNA) molecules. Bacterial DNA is located in a special bacterial chromosome found in the cytoplasm of a bacterial cell. Additionally, bacterial DNA may be found on small, circular fragments of DNA called plasmids. These plasmids are separate from the bacterial chromosome and carry special information needed for the bacteria to survive under adverse environmental conditions. Plasmids carry "mating" genes, which allow the bacteria to transfer a plasmid from one bacteria to another. They also carry genes that make a bacteria resistant to a particular antibiotic. Consequently, plasmids are of particular importance because they allow antibiotic resistance to be transferred between bacteria.

Two bacterial cells may exchange plasmids by direct contact in a process known as conjugation. Not all plasmids can be exchanged in this way, but the genetic information that encodes for resistance may be transferred from a plasmid that cannot be exchanged to one that can. This occurs when a small piece of DNA known as a transposon breaks away from one plasmid and attaches itself to another. A transposon may also break away from a bacterial chromosome and attach itself elsewhere on the chromosome or onto a plasmid.

Antibiotic resistance may also be transferred between bacteria indirectly by a bacteriophage in transduction. A bacteriophage is a virus that attaches itself to a bacterial cell. The virus sometimes incorporates DNA from the invaded bacterial cell into its own DNA. The virus may then transfer this DNA to the next bacterial cell to which it attaches. In this way, it can transfer drug resistance between bacteria that are unable to undergo conjugation.

The various ways in which genetic information can be exchanged between bacteria may result in organisms with resistance to multiple drugs. Some bacteria are known to be resistant to at least ten different antibiotics. They carry a series of genes on their plasmids able to make enzymes that can degrade and destroy antibiotics. For example, bacteria able to resist penicillin treatments carry an enzyme called penicillinase that destroys penicillin, thus protecting the bacteria.

An important factor in the emergence of antibiotic resistance is the misuse of antibiotics. For example, antibiotics have no effect on viruses but are often used against viral illnesses. A study published in 1997 revealed that at least half of all patients in the United States who visited doctors' offices with colds, upper respiratory tract infections, and bronchitis received antibiotics, even though 90 percent of these illnesses are caused by viruses. The same study showed that almost a third of all antibiotic prescriptions written in doctors' offices were used for these kinds of illnesses. Similar problems are also seen in hospitals. It is also important to remember that misuse can include underutilizing prescribed drugs, such as may stem from poor patient compliance with medical directions. If patients do not take their medications as directed, typically until the whole course of antibiotics has been consumed, then it may encourage the development of drug resistance, as the antibiotics did not have the opportunity to exert their full effect on the bacteria causing the problem. The bacteria that survive the partial course may be more likely to be resistant to that drug, making future administrations less effective.

This misuse of antibiotics has been one of the strongest forces pushing selection of antibiotic-resistant bacteria—but this is not only because of its use in humans. Specifically, even if doctors stopped overprescribing antibiotics today, other factors are at work. In 2000, an estimated fifty million pounds of antibiotics were used in the United States; half that amount was used for veterinary and agricultural purposes. Antibiotics are administered in huge doses to farm animals to keep them healthy and allow them to grow larger. These drugs are even being used in the petroleum industry for cleaning pipelines. The World Health Organization (WHO) noted a sharp decrease in the incidence of antibiotic-resistant bacterial strains in Denmark after antibiotic use was all but eliminated from livestock in 1998.

A final factor in the increase in antibiotic resistance is the use and overuse of substandard and counterfeit antimicrobial agents in developing countries. In Nigeria, for example, WHO estimates that there are twenty thousand unlicensed medical stands scattered throughout the country. These street vendors do not require prescriptions to dose patients. Additionally, the common use of antibiotics in developing nations to "sterilize" households risks the development of cross-resistant bacterial strains.

Several public health concerns have arisen as a result of drug resistance. One of the earliest problems occurred in Japan in 1955, when an outbreak of dysentery was caused by bacteria resistant to four antibiotics. For the last fifty years multiple antibiotic resistance has emerged in bacteria causing pneumonia, gonorrhea, meningitis, and other serious illnesses.

In the 1980's, drug-resistant tuberculosis emerged as a public health concern. In 1991, in New York City, for example, 33 percent of all tuberculosis infections were resistant to at least one drug, and 19 percent were resistant to both of the most effective drugs used to treat the disease. Because of resistance, many tuberculosis patients now require treatment with four drugs for several months. Some patients are required to be directly observed by a health care worker every time they take a dose of medication to ensure compliance. The use of multiple drugs and the need for increased numbers of health care workers greatly increase the cost of treating tuberculosis.

A new challenge appeared in 1997, when patients in Japan and the United States developed infections caused by bacteria known as *Staphylococcus aureus*. This bacteria is an ordinarily harmless organism found on human skin, but it can cause potentially fatal infections when it enters the bloodstream. The most pathogenic strain is known as the multiresistant *Staphylococcus aureus* (MRSA). Since 1997, vancomycin-resistant *Staphylococcus aureus* (VRSA) has emerged, causing major public health problems.

TREATMENT AND THERAPY

The antibiotic vancomycin is one of a small group of "glycopeptide" antibiotics. At one time, its administration was considered a last resort. Vancomycin is toxic to humans in the wrong dosage, so it must be dispensed carefully by a physician. The drug eradicates bacteria by inhibiting the synthesis of their outer protective wall. Without this outer cell wall, bacteria become sensitive to minor environmental changes and die. Vancomycin has been a valuable antibiotic because it is so important in the fight against bacteria that are resistant to penicillin. The VRSA-type bacteria have nullified this valuable antibiotic and made it much less useful.

The most common sites for MRSA and VRSA invasion and growth are wounds, the nasal cavities, and surgical incisions. Both these strains generally arise as nosocomial infections, that is, infections contracted in a hospital.

The *Enterococcus* bacteria are the second most common nosocomial infection found in hospitals. These bacteria often give rise to infections in the urinary tracts of patients, but they are also the cause of meningitis, septicemia, and endocarditis. Most frequently, *Enterococcus* is found in children, the elderly, HIV-infected individuals, or the immunologically compromised, whose immune systems are not fully functioning. *Enterococcus* bacteria are now resistant to vancomycin. This means that vancomycin-resistant *Enterococcus* (VRE) can spread vancomycin resistance to other organisms, producing major medical problems.

Another problem bacteria is pneumococcus. This bacterial species was once completely sensitive to penicillin, but now, according to bacteriologist Perry Dickinson, up to 55 percent of the pneumococcal strains are penicillin-resistant. The group most at risk for infection with the drug-resistant *Streptococcus pneumoniae* (DRSP) is children age six or younger. Adult pneumococcal strains seem not to be as generally antibiotic resistant. The resistant strains are becoming quite a serious threat among children, but pneumococcus is still vancomycin-sensitive and amoxicillin is still effective at high dosages.

One of the most promising new superdrugs, line-zolid (Zyvox), developed to combat antibiotic resistance, falls into a new category of antibiotics called oxazolidinones. These drugs act at an early stage in the synthesis of protein by bacteria. Without protein production, bacteria cannot multiply, and they die. The antibiotic linezolid acts strongly against many bacteria, including MRSA, VRSA, VRE, and penicillin-resistant pneumococci. In hospital trials involving patients with MRSA infections, linezolid produced clinical success in more than 83 percent of the patients. The drug can be taken orally or injected, making it quite versatile. Robert Moellering of Harvard University Medical School suggests that this versatility is convenient for patients because they can complete their therapy at home. This drug has also been shown to have few side effects.

A whole series of promising new antibiotics are presently being examined by the Food and Drug Administration (FDA) for use against the variously resistant superbugs. GlaxoWellcome has at least three new antibiotics that are effective against VRE, MRSA, and VRSA infections. These include Sanfetrinem, GV143253, and Grepafloxacin. The company Microcide, Incorporated, has recently developed MC02479, a cephalosporin-type antibiotic that works in a fashion similar to penicillin and is strongly active against VRE, MRSA, and VRSA. As long as these drugs and others like them are used and prescribed responsibly, they may offer a therapeutic benefit for decades to come.

It is important to remember, however, that drug resistance is not simply about fixing problems with antibiotics. Though this is a large concern, similar concerns exist with respect to other pathogens, such as viruses and fungi. With viruses, there are concerns about global pandemics, such as those caused by influenza strains, particularly avian influenza (bird flu). With fungi, there are concerns because of the damage that they can do to individuals with compromised immune systems.

PERSPECTIVE AND PROSPECTS

Several different strategies have been suggested for handling the problem of drug resistance. In general, these strategies involve educating the public and health care workers; monitoring antibiotic, antiviral, and antifungal use; and promoting research into methods to deal with resistant pathogens.

The general public should be aware of the proper use of these medicines as well. Many patients expect to be given antibiotics for illnesses that do not respond to them, such as viral infections. Similarly, they may pressure physicians into prescribing antiviral or antifungal medications even when physicians are aware that these drugs are useless. Patients must learn to understand the difference between a bacterial and a viral infection and how each is treated. Patients must also be educated not to use another person's medicines or an old supply of medicines that they have saved from previous illnesses. Finally, patients must learn to take the entire course of medicines. Often, patients who begin to feel better may fail to take the entire amount prescribed. This leads to an increased risk of drug-resistant infection if they do not completely eliminate the original infection.

All health care workers should be aware of the importance of avoiding the spread of resistant pathogens from one patient to another. In the late 1990's, about two million Americans per year acquired nosocomial infections. These infections were responsible for about eighty thousand deaths per year. The most important factors in reducing the rate of nosocomial infections are frequent and thorough hand washing, glove changes, and disinfectant applications.

Children should be immunized at a young age against pneumococcal infections. Children who are immunized do not get the infections; hence, no antibiotics are needed, and no extra antibiotics enter into the general population. Additionally, children who are ill should be kept home from day care centers. Day care centers are becoming dangerous incubators, where disease may potentially run rampant. In these places, children spread bacterial infections among themselves, often amplifying pathogenicity and drug resistance. This can be avoided by isolating sick children at home.

Physicians need to be aware of the proper ways to use antibiotics. Microbiologists have suggested better instruction in antibiotic use in medical schools, more continuing education on the subject for practicing physicians, and the development of computer programs to aid physicians in selecting antibiotics. Some have suggested that all physicians prescribing antibiotics in hospitals be required to consult with physicians who specialize in infectious diseases. Standardized order forms that include guidelines for proper use of each antibiotic have also been proposed. Additionally, doctors who have been thoroughly educated must learn not to accede to patient demands for antibiotics, and they must defer antibiotic use in self-limiting infections that will heal on their own. They must also avoid prescribing antibiotics over the phone.

Unfortunately, overall antibiotic prescription rates still seem to be rising, despite warnings of increased antimicrobial resistance. Since 1992, yearly prescriptions have increased by more than thirty million. The most commonly prescribed antibiotic has been amoxicillin, which represents more than 25 percent of the total prescriptions. Erythromycin use has fallen to less than 7 percent, while penicillin and tetracycline use have fallen as well. The new broad-spectrum antibiotics called macrolides have replaced these drugs and make up more than 10 percent of antibiotic use. Despite the overall increases, the proportion of antibiotic prescriptions for the common cold has decreased to 40 percent from a high of 52 percent in 1994.

Researchers agree that monitoring antibiotic use is critical in fighting drug resistance. A study published in 1997 demonstrated the effectiveness of education and monitoring in reducing resistance. Physicians in Finland were educated in the proper use of the antibiotic erythromycin, and use of the drug was monitored. In 1992, 16.5 percent of bacteria known as group A *Streptococci* were resistant to erythromycin. In 1996, only 8.6 percent were resistant. Some experts have proposed using computers to share information about antibiotic use and resistance among as many health care facilities as possible.

Faster development of new antibiotics for use on multiply resistant bacteria is another improvement. Researchers stress, however, that these new antibiotics must be used only when necessary, in order to avoid promoting resistance to them. Consequently, linezolid and other new antibiotics are being used sparingly.

Other methods have been proposed for minimizing antibiotic resistance. Because patients often expect or demand prescriptions when they visit physicians, some experts have suggested that the physician write a lifestyle prescription when drug use is not appropriate. Such a prescription would explain why antibiotics should not be used in a particular situation and would give the patient specific instructions on how to treat the illness without them.

Eliminating the routine use of antibiotics in farm animals would be of great help. As the Danish study suggests, the risk of resistant bacterial strains in livestock could be reduced, making human lives safer as well.

International concerns over antibiotic resistance are at such a height that in 2000, eight international medical societies gathered to spend a full day discussing the problem. They called this event Global Resistance Day, and the medical professionals discussed the dilemma and solutions for global antibiotic resistance.

—Rose Secrest; James J. Campanella, Ph.D.;
updated by Nancy A. Piotrowski, Ph.D.

See also Antibiotics; Bacterial infections; Bacteriology; Epidemiology; Fungal infections; Hospitals; Iatrogenic disorders; Infection; Microbiology; Mutation; Pharmacology; Pharmacy; Viral infections.

FOR FURTHER INFORMATION:

Harrison, Polly F., et al., eds. *Antimicrobial Resistance: Issues and Options*. Washington, D.C.: National Academy Press, 1998. An excellent, up-to-date text describing the problems that society faces with antibiotic resistance, and possible solutions.

Levy, Stuart B. *The Antibiotic Paradox: How the Misuse of Antibiotics Destroys Their Curative Powers*. Cambridge, Mass.: Perseus, 2002. A leading researcher in molecular biology explores a modern-day massive evolutionary change in bacteria due to misuse of antibiotics. He argues that a buildup of new antibiotic-resistant bacteria in individuals and in the environment is leading medicine into a dangerous territory where "miracle" drugs may be obsolete.

McLean, Angela, et al., eds. *SARS: A Case Study in Emerging Infections*. New York: Oxford University Press, 2005. Describes the emergence of severe acute respiratory syndrome (SARS) and how it affected perceptions of global travel and public health.

Murray, Barbara E. "Can Antibiotic Resistance Be Controlled?" *New England Journal of Medicine* 330, no. 17 (April 28, 1994): 1229-1230. An editorial that outlines the future consequences of increasing drug resistance and offers several suggestions for fighting it.

Rosen, Barry P., and Shahriar Mobashery, eds. *Resolving the Antibiotic Paradox: Progress in Understanding Drug Resistance and Development of New Antibiotics*. New York: Plenum, 1998. A more technical book than some others. It addresses the issue of bacterial resistance, highlighting both conventional and new drug discovery approaches.

Shnayerson, Michael, and Mark J. Plotkin. *The Killers Within: The Deadly Rise of Drug Resistant Bacteria*. New York: Little, Brown, 2002. Traces the evolution of drug-resistant bacteria and how physicians are trying to combat it.

Smaglik, Paul. "Proliferation of Pills." *Science News* 151, no. 20 (May 17, 1997): 310-311. An account of the frequent misuse of antibiotics, with opinions from several experts.

Walsh, Christopher. *Antibiotics: Actions, Origins, Resistance*. Washington, D.C.: ASM Press, 2003. Examines such topics as how antibiotics block specific proteins, how the molecular structure of drugs enables such activity, the development of bacterial resistance, and the molecular logic of antibiotic biosynthesis.

DRUG THERAPY. *See* **ANTIBIOTICS; ANTIDEPRESSANTS; ANTIHISTAMINES; ANTI-INFLAMMATORY DRUGS; APHRODISIACS; CHEMOTHERAPY; DECONGESTANTS; NARCOTICS; OVER-THE-COUNTER MEDICATIONS; STEROIDS.**

DWARFISM
DISEASE/DISORDER

ANATOMY OR SYSTEM AFFECTED: Back, bones, brain, endocrine system, glands, hips, legs, musculoskeletal system, nervous system, respiratory system

SPECIALTIES AND RELATED FIELDS: Endocrinology, genetics, orthopedics, pediatrics

DEFINITION: Underdevelopment of the body, most often caused by a variety of genetic or endocrinological dysfunctions and resulting in either proportionate or disproportionate development, sometimes accompanied by other physical abnormalities and/or mental deficiencies.

KEY TERMS:

amino acid: the building blocks of protein

autosomal: refers to all chromosomes except the X and Y chromosomes (sex chromosomes) that determine body traits

cleft palate: a gap in the roof of the mouth, sometimes present at birth and frequently combined with harelip

collagen: protein material of which the white fibers of the connective tissue of the body are composed

hypoglycemia: low blood sugar

laminae: arches of the vertebral bones

spondylosis: a condition characterized by restriction of movement of the vertebral bones; occurs naturally as a child grows

stenosis: any narrowing of a passage or orifice of the body

CAUSES AND SYMPTOMS

A person of unusually small stature is generally termed a "dwarf." Dwarfism in humans may be caused by a number of conditions that occur either before birth or in early childhood. When short stature is the only observable feature, growth—though abnormal relative to height—is proportionate. Short stature is nearly always blamed on endocrinological dysfunction, but few cases are actually the result of endocrinopathy. If shortness is caused by endocrinopathy, it is often attributable to a deficiency in one or two glands: the pituitary gland (which produces growth hormone) and the thyroid gland. Those who are unusually short but have no other obvious disease are divided into two categories: those who were afflicted prenatally and those who were afflicted postnatally. Many of those born "growth-retarded" are actually the result of chromosomal aberrations and skeletal abnormalities; other events that may cause prenatal growth retardation might include magnesium deficiency (which would prohibit ribosome synthesis and, in turn, halt protein synthesis) or a uterus that is too small. Postnatal growth retardation may be caused by heredity if both parents are short; there is no skeletal abnormality at fault. Other short-statured children may simply mature at a much slower rate, yet grow normally. Typically, one of the parents may have had a late onset of puberty; such children may reach normal height in their late teens.

Unusually short-statured males are those who are shorter than five feet tall; in females, fifty-eight inches and below is short-statured. Children are classified as dwarfs if their height is below the third percentile for their age. When this is the case, doctors will look primarily to four major causes of dwarfism: an underactive or inactive pituitary gland, achondroplasia (failure of normal development in cartilage), emotional or nutritional deprivation, or Turner syndrome (the possession of a single, X, chromosome). If the answer is not found in one of these alternatives, then it may be found in rarer causes, either genetically based or disease-induced.

Growth hormone, also called somatotropin, determines a person's height. Growth hormone does not affect brain growth but may influence the brain's functions. In addition, it may enhance the growth of nerves radiating from the brain so that they can reach their targets. Growth hormone elevates the appetite, increases metabolic rate, maintains the immune system, and works in coordination with other hormones to regulate carbohydrate, protein, lipid, nucleic acid, water, and electrolyte metabolism. Target areas for growth hormone include cell membranes, as well as other cell organelles, in bone, cartilage, bone marrow, adipose tissue, and the liver, kidney, heart, pancreas, mammary glands, ovaries, testes, thymus gland, and hypothalamus. Fetuses not producing growth hormone still grow

---

Information on Dwarfism

Causes: Genetic or endocrinological dysfunctions
Symptoms: Short stature, higher-than-average body fat, high forehead, wrinkled skin, high-pitched voice, episodic hypoglycemia during childhood, late onset of puberty
Duration: Lifelong
Treatments: Growth hormone

---

normally until birth; they may even weigh more than average at birth. These babies may thrive at first, but if no growth hormone is administered, they will be "miniature" adults with a maximum height of two and a half feet. Other telltale physical attributes include higher-than-average body fat, a high forehead, wrinkled skin, and a high-pitched voice. During childhood, there may be episodic hypoglycemia attacks. If the endocrine system is functioning properly, puberty may be delayed but still will occur. Complete reproductive maturity will be reached, and there is great likelihood that the afflicted person will develop his or her complete intellectual potential. When it is inherited, growth hormone deficiency occurs as an autosomal recessive trait. Yet the genetic basis for growth hormone deficiency may not simply be caused by a gene. The condition could, in theory, be the result of a structural defect in the pituitary gland or the hypothalamus, or in the secretory mechanisms of growth hormone itself. Prenatal factors that contribute to growth retardation include toxemia, kidney and heart disease, rubella, maternal malnutrition, maternal age, small uterus, and environmental influences such as alcohol and drug use.

Prenatal thyroid dysfunction that goes untreated results in cretinism. Cretins do not undergo nervous, skeletal, or reproductive maturation; they may not grow over thirty inches tall. Before two months of age, treatment can cause a complete reversal of symptoms. Delayed treatment, however, cannot reverse brain damage, although growth and reproductive organs can be dramatically affected.

Achondroplasia is the most common form of short-limb dwarfism. It is inherited as an autosomal dominant form of dwarfism. Only when one dominant gene is inherited is achondroplasia expressed; when an offspring inherits the dominant gene from both parents, the condition is lethal. Incidence of achondroplasia increases with parental age and is more closely related to the father's age. Mutations may account for a majority of cases of achondroplasia, since in only 15 to 20 percent of cases is there an afflicted parent. Achondroplasia results from abnormal embryonic development that affects bone growth; metaphyseal development is prevented, which means that cartilaginous bone growth is impaired. This impairment is accompanied by unusually small laminae of the spine, resulting in spinal stenosis. The spinal cord may become compressed during the normal process of spondylosis. These individuals may experience slowly progressing spastic weakness of the legs as a result of the spinal cord compression. The torso may be normal, but the head will be disproportionately large and the limbs may be dwarfed and curved. In addition, there will be a prominent forehead and a depressed nasal bridge. A shallow thoracic cage and pelvic tilt may cause a protuberant abdomen. Bowlegs are caused by overly long fibulae. Many infants so affected are stillborn. Those surviving to adulthood are typically three feet to five feet tall and have unusual muscular strength; reproductive and mental development are not affected, and neither is longevity.

Marasmus, severe emaciation resulting from malnutrition prenatally or in early infancy, may be considered a form of dwarfism. It is caused by extremely low caloric and protein intake, which causes a wasting of body tissues. Usually marasmus is found in babies either weaned very early or never breast-fed. All growth is retarded, including head circumference. If the area housing the brain fails to grow, then it cannot house a normal-sized brain, and some degree of retardation will occur. Not only is growth stunted, but such infants will be apathetic and hyperirritable as well. As they lie in bed, they are completely unresponsive to their environment and are irritable when moved or handled. Although the symptoms are treatable and may disappear, the growth failure is permanent.

Occasionally, dwarfism may be induced by emotional starvation. This type of child abuse causes extreme growth retardation, inhibition of skeletal growth, and delayed psychomotor development. Fortunately, it can be reversed by social and dietary changes. These children are extremely small but perfectly proportioned; however, they have distended abdomens.

The height achieved in females with Turner syndrome is typically between four and a half and five feet. Turner syndrome results when an egg has no X chromosome and is fertilized by an X-bearing sperm. The offspring are females with only one X; their ovaries never develop and are unable to function. These individuals cannot undergo puberty; physical manifestations of Turner syndrome include short stature, stocky build, and a webbed neck.

Another cause of short stature may be as a consequence of chronic disease. Children suffering from chronic renal (kidney) failure nearly always experience growth retardation because of hormonal, metabolic, and nutritional abnormalities, effects seen in 35 to 65 percent of children with renal failure. The failure to grow occurs more often in children with congenital renal disease than in those with acquired renal disease.

With congenital heart disease, several factors may prohibit growth. Growth failure may be a direct result of the disease or an indirect result of other problems associated with heart disease. These babies experience stress, with periods of cardiac failure, and either caloric or protein deficiency. These inadequacies grossly slow the multiplication of cells and hence growth. If surgery corrects the condition, some catching up can be expected, but normal growth is dependent on how much time has elapsed without treatment.

TREATMENT AND THERAPY

In the United States population in 1992, there were roughly five million people of short stature, with 40 percent of this number under the age of twenty-one. The more a child is below the average stature, the greater is the likelihood of determining the cause. A child who is short-statured should be evaluated so that if an endocrine disorder is the root, the child can be treated. Time is an important consideration with hypothyroidism especially, since the longer it goes untreated, the more likely it is that mental development will be arrested.

Children born with congenital growth hormone deficiency are sometimes small for their gestational age; however, the majority of growth hormone-deficient children acquire the disorder after birth. The first year or two, the children grow normally; then growth dramatically decreases. Diagnosis of growth hormone deficiency requires numerous tests and sampling. If bone age appears the same as the child's age, then growth hormone deficiency can be eliminated. A test for normal growth hormone secretion is done by measuring a blood sample for growth hormone twenty minutes after exercise in a fasting child. If this test shows a hormone deficiency, then growth hormone therapy may help the child overcome the obstacles of being labeled "short."

At first, growth hormone was harvested from human pituitary glands after persons' deaths. This process was so expensive, however, that few children with hormone deficiency could be treated. Even worse, some of those who did get this treatment were inadvertently infected with a slow-acting virus that proved fatal. In the mid-1980's, it was found that some men who had received human growth hormone died at an early age of a neurological disorder called Creutzfeldt-Jakob disease (CJD). These men were found to have been given the disease via a growth hormone that had been obtained from pituitary glands during autopsies. Once the relationship was determined, more victims were traced. CJD is a nervous disorder caused by a slow-acting, viruslike particle. Its symptoms include difficulty in balance while walking, loss of muscular control, slurred speech, impairment of vision, and other muscular disorders including spasticity and rigidity. Behavioral changes and mental incapacities may also occur (memory loss, confusion, dementia). The symptoms appear, progress rapidly over the next months, and usually cause death in less than a year. There is no treatment or cure.

These unfortunate circumstances led to the development of a synthetic growth hormone. It is made by encoding bacterial deoxyribonucleic acid (DNA) with the sequence of human growth hormone; the bacteria used are those that grow normally in the human intestinal tract. The bacteria synthesize human growth hormone using the preprogrammed human sequence of DNA; it is then purified so that no bacteria remain in the hormone that is used for treatment. The Food and Drug Administration (FDA) approved the biosynthetic hormone in 1985. The sole difference between the synthetic and the naturally produced growth hormone was one amino acid; in 1987, a new synthetic form without the extra amino acid became available. This synthetic hormone works exactly as natural growth hormone does. Moreover, it does not carry the danger of contamination attributed to human growth hormone. In most cases, the patient's immune system fails to interfere with the synthetic growth hormone's effectiveness. In fact, no major health-threatening side effects have surfaced in using artificial growth hormone. In 1992, more than 150,000 growth hormone-deficient children in the United States were receiving growth hormone therapy.

Those children suffering from various forms of chondrodystrophies (cartilage disorders), such as achondroplasia, are diagnosed by using skeletal measurements, clinical manifestations, X rays, laboratory study and analysis of cartilage, and observed abnormalities of the body's proteins, such as collagen and cell membranes. In chondrodystrophies, skeletal growth is disproportionate, with shortened limbs more common than a shortened trunk. If visual examination is not confirmation enough, the diagnosis may be assured through X rays. Although histological studies do not necessarily enhance diagnosis, making an analysis of the patient's cartilage may lead to a better understanding of the disease. Biochemical studies of abnormal proteins in chondrodystrophies actually have little diagnostic value, but they too may lead to better understanding. Because achondroplasia is genetically inherited, prevention of the affliction involves genetic counseling before conception.

A child so affected may be treated symptomatically; surgery on the fibulae to correct bowlegs may be desirable, either for cosmetic reasons or for functional reasons. Laminectomies or skull surgery may be indicated for neurological problems. Orthodontic surgery may be necessary to correct malocclusions and other dental deformities. If hearing loss occurs because of recurrent ear infections, then corrective surgery may be necessary. Achondroplasiacs generally enjoy a normal life span, barring complications.

Other chondrodystrophies that cause dwarfism may have more severe symptoms than achondroplasia. Cockayne syndrome, a type of progeria, is the sudden onset of premature old age in extremely young children. It is the result of inheritance of an autosomal recessive gene. Physical signs of the disease begin after a normal first year of life. In the second year, growth begins to falter, and psychomotor development becomes abnormal. As time passes, dwarfism, and sometimes mental retardation, becomes evident. Other observable characteristics that develop are a shrunken face with sunken eyes and a thin nose, optic degeneration, cavities of the teeth, a photosensitive skin rash that produces scarring, disproportionately long limbs with large hands and feet, and hair loss. The life span for children with this disease is very short.

Another chondrodystrophy inherited through autosomal recessive genes is thanotophoric dwarfism. All known cases have died during the first four weeks of life as a result of respiratory distress; most are stillborn. Postnatal death occurs as a result of an extremely small thoracic cage with only eleven pairs of ribs present. Other physical characteristics of the disease are that the infant has a large skull relative to its face, which is often elongated with a prominent forehead. The eyes are widely spaced, and there is a broad, flat nasal bridge. Frequently, cleft palate is present. The ears are low-set and poorly formed, and the neck is short and fleshy. The limbs, particularly the legs, are bowed; clubfoot is common, as are dislocated hip joints.

A small percentage of short-statured individuals may be unusually short because of social and psychological factors. This condition is called psychosocial dwarfism. This type of nongrowth is secondary to emotional deprivation and is representative of a type of child abuse. The behavior of such children is characterized by apathy and inadequate interpersonal relationships, with retarded motor and language development. They generally do not gain weight in spite of their extraordinary appetite and excessive thirst; such a child may steal and hoard food yet have the distended abdomen of a starving child. Diagnosis generally identifies a growth hormone deficiency, and when these children are moved to stimulating and accepting environments, their behavior becomes more normal. Their caloric intake decreases as their growth hormone secretion becomes normal, and their growth undergoes a dramatic catch-up.

Perspective and Prospects

Dwarfism is certainly not a new phenomenon. Two well-known Egyptian deities, Bes and Ptah, are represented as dwarfs. At one time, short-statured individuals were attractions in the royal courts. Jeffery Hudson, a favorite of Charles I of England, is said to have been only eighteen inches high at the age of thirty, and Bébé, the celebrated dwarf in the court of Stanisław I of Poland, was thirty-three inches tall. More recently, perfectly proportioned dwarfs have made a living by working in circuses and sideshows. It is likely that the best known of these individuals was P. T. Barnum's General Tom Thumb (Charles Stratton), who at age twenty-five was thirty-one inches tall.

Today, because of the negative consequences of being short-statured, counseling should begin early. Counseling would be preceded by a physical examination to determine the nature of the affliction. If it is ascertained that the short stature cannot be treated, both patient and parents should be informed of the nature of the disease. The patient should be assured that intelligence will not be affected, even if the head is somewhat large. Ear infections are common, and the child should be closely watched to avoid hearing loss. Normal fertility is the rule, but giving birth will necessitate a cesarean section. These characteristics of a majority of dwarfism cases should assure families that, as the child matures, he or she will not be limited physically or mentally. The problems that the patients may face usually deal with social and emotional consequences. Short-statured children will usually be thought younger than their age; finding appropriate clothes and shoes may be difficult. Children are often cruel, and as afflicted individuals are highly noticeable, they may be the butt of jokes and teasing and will experience discrimination on many fronts. Seeking affiliation with support groups may aid in coping with the difficulties that a short-statured person will undoubtedly meet. Additionally, counseling for children and parents of dwarf children should be provided to assist in coping with their anomalies and to facilitate positive outcomes.

The rate at which those diagnosed with dwarfism develop psychologically is directly related to two components: if their parents treat them according to their age rather than their size, and if they can cope with the notoriety that their size brings them. It is common for such children to lag in development; personality traits often exhibited with delayed maturation are withdrawal, inhibition, dissociation, and learning problems. There have been no observed tendencies toward aggression or acting out. Inhibition and withdrawal are likely if affected children are appalled by their notoriety; if they use it to measure popularity, they may act the clown to minimize their size difference.

—Iona C. Baldridge; updated by Sharon W. Stark, R.N., A.P.R.N., D.N.Sc.

See also Congenital heart disease; Cornelia de Lange syndrome; Endocrine disorders; Endocrinology; Endocrinology, pediatric; Gigantism; Growth; Hormones; Metabolic disorders; Rubinstein-Taybi syndrome.

For Further Information:

Adelson, B., and J. Hall. *Dwarfism: Medical and Psychological Aspects of Profound Short Stature.* Baltimore: Johns Hopkins University Press, 2005. Overview of problems related to dwarfism and medical progress in treatment.

Brooks, S. J., and Robert S. Bar. *Early Diagnosis and Treatment of Endocrine Disorders.* Totowa, N.J.: Humana Press, 2003. Reviews the early signs and symptoms of common endocrine diseases, surveys the clinical testing needed for a diagnosis, and presents recommendations for therapy.

Healthline. *Dwarfism.* http://www.healthline.com/search?q1=dwarfism. Compilation of various types of dwarfism, definitions, causes, and treatments.

Juul, Anders, and Jens O. L. Jorgensen, eds. *Growth Hormone in Adults: Physiological and Clinical As-*

pects. 2d ed. New York: Cambridge University Press, 2000. This book examines the use of somatotropin on adults to treat dwarfism.

Kelly, Thaddeus E. *Clinical Genetics and Genetic Counseling*. 2d ed. Chicago: Year Book Medical, 1986. This text of genetic disorders and their treatment was written to aid medical students and physicians. Aside from the sometimes difficult medical terminology, the case illustrations and discussions of genetic counseling are interesting.

Larsen, P. Reed, et al., eds. *Williams Textbook of Endocrinology*. 10th ed. Philadelphia: W. B. Saunders, 2003. Comprehensive information regarding endocrine diseases, pathophysiology, diagnoses, treatment, and prognoses.

Little People of America. http://www.lpaonline.org/. A nonprofit organization that provides support and information to people of short stature and their families. Web site offers a research library, FAQs, chat rooms, and information on local chapters.

MedlinePlus. *Dwarfism*. http://www.nlm.nih.gov/medlineplus/dwarfism.html. This Web site offers an overview of dwarfism and resources from which to obtain additional information.

Morgan, Brian L. G., and Roberta Morgan. *Hormones: How They Affect Behavior, Metabolism, Growth, Development, and Relationships*. Los Angeles: Price, Stern, Sloan, 1989. A book written for use by the general reader as a resource on hormones and their roles in the human body. Very readable, it also contains sections about hormonal diseases and includes a bibliography.

Shaw, Michael, ed. *Everything You Need to Know About Diseases*. Springhouse, Pa.: Springhouse Press, 1996. This well-illustrated consumer reference, compiled by more than one hundred doctors and medical experts, describes five hundred illnesses and conditions, as well as their causes, symptoms, diagnosis, treatment, and prevention. Of particular interest is chapter 21, "Genetic Disorders."

DYSENTERY. *See* DIARRHEA AND DYSENTERY.

DYSLEXIA
DISEASE/DISORDER

ANATOMY OR SYSTEM AFFECTED: Brain, ears, eyes, nervous system, psychic-emotional system

SPECIALTIES AND RELATED FIELDS: Audiology, neurology, psychology, speech pathology

DEFINITION: Severe reading disability in children with average to above-average intelligence.

KEY TERMS:

auditory dyslexia: the inability to perceive individual sounds that are associated with written language

cognitive: relating to the mental process by which knowledge is acquired

computed tomography (CT) scan: a detailed X-ray picture that identifies abnormalities of fine tissue structure

dysgraphia: illegible handwriting resulting from impaired hand-eye coordination

electroencephalogram: a graphic record of the brain's electrical activity

imprinting: training that overcomes reading problems by use of repeated, exaggerated language drills

kinesthetic: related to sensation of body position, presence, or movement, resulting mostly from the stimulation of sensory nerves in muscles, tendons, and joints

phonetics: the science of speech sounds; also called phonology

visual dyslexia: the inability to translate observed written or printed language into meaningful terms

CAUSES AND SYMPTOMS

Nearly 25 percent of the individuals in the United States and in many other industrialized societies who otherwise possess at least average intelligence cannot read well. Many such people are viewed as suffering from a neurological disorder called dyslexia. This term was first introduced by the German ophthalmologist Rudolf Berlin in the nineteenth century. Berlin defined it as designating all those individuals who possessed average or above-average intelligence quotients (IQs) but who could not read adequately because of their inability to process language symbols. At the same time as Berlin and later, others reported on dyslexic children. These children saw everything perfectly well but acted as if they were blind to all written language. For example, they could see a bird flying but were unable to identify the written word "bird" seen in a sentence.

The problem involved in dyslexia has been defined and redefined many times since its introduction. The modern definition of the disorder, which is close to Berlin's definition, is based on long-term, extensive studies of dyslexic children. These studies have identified dyslexia as a complex syndrome composed of a large number of associated behavioral dysfunctions

INFORMATION ON DYSLEXIA

CAUSES: Unknown; possibly neurological disorder from accident, disease, or hereditary faults in body biochemistry; dormant, immature, or undeveloped learning centers in the brain

SYMPTOMS: Poor written schoolwork, easy distractibility, clumsiness, poor coordination, poor spatial orientation, confused writing and/or spelling, poor left-right orientation

DURATION: Often long term

TREATMENTS: Medication, patterning, teaching of specific reading skills and repeated language drills (imprinting)

that are related to visual-motor brain immaturity and/or brain dysfunction. These problems include a poor memory for details, easy distractibility, poor motor skills, visual letter and word reversal, and the inability to distinguish between important elements of the spoken language.

Understanding dyslexia in order to correct this reading disability is crucial and difficult. To learn to read well, an individual must acquire many basic cognitive and linguistic skills. First, it is necessary to pay close attention, to concentrate, to follow directions, and to understand the language spoken in daily life. Next, one must develop an auditory and visual memory, strong sequencing ability, solid word decoding skills, the ability to carry out structural-contextual language analysis, the capability to interpret the written language, a solid vocabulary which expands as quickly as is needed, and speed in scanning and interpreting written language. These skills are taught in good developmental reading programs, but some or all are found to be deficient in dyslexic individuals.

Two basic explanations have evolved for dyslexia. Many physicians propose that it is caused by brain damage or brain dysfunction. Evolution of the problem is attributed to accident, disease, and/or hereditary faults in body biochemistry. Here, the diagnosis of dyslexia is made by the use of electroencephalograms (EEGs), computed tomography (CT) scans, and related neurological technology. After such evaluation is complete, medication is often used to diminish hyperactivity and nervousness, and a group of physical training procedures called patterning is used to counter the neurological defects in the dyslexic individual.

In contrast, many special educators and other re-

searchers believe that the problem of dyslexia is one of dormant, immature, or undeveloped learning centers in the brain. Many proponents of this concept strongly encourage the correction of dyslexic problems by the teaching of specific reading skills. While such experts agree that the use of medication can be of great value, they attempt to cure dyslexia mostly through a process called imprinting. This technique essentially trains dyslexic individuals and corrects their problems via the use of exaggerated, repeated language drills.

Another interesting point of view, expressed by some experts, is the idea that dyslexia may be the fault of the written languages of the Western world. For example, Rudolf F. Wagner notes that Japanese children exhibit an incidence of dyslexia that is less than 1 percent. The explanation for this, say Wagner and others, is that unlike Japanese, the languages of Western countries require both reading from left to right and phonetic word attack. These characteristics—absent in Japanese—may make the Western languages either much harder to learn or much less suitable for learning.

A number of experts propose three types of dyslexia. The most common type and the one most often identified as dyslexia is called visual dyslexia, the lack of ability to translate the observed written or printed language into meaningful terms. The major difficulty is that afflicted people see certain words or letters backward or upside down. The resultant problem is that—to the visual dyslexic—any written sentence is a jumble of many letters whose accurate translation may require five or more times as much effort as is needed by an unafflicted person. The other two problems viewed as dyslexia are auditory dyslexia and dysgraphia. Auditory dyslexia is the inability to perceive individual sounds of spoken language. Despite having normal hearing, auditory dyslexics are deaf to the differences between certain vowel and/or consonant sounds, and what they cannot hear they cannot write. Dysgraphia is the inability to write legibly. The basis for this problem is a lack of the hand-eye coordination that is required to write clearly.

Many children who suffer from visual dyslexia also exhibit elements of auditory dyslexia. This complicates the issue of teaching many dyslexic students because only one type of dyslexic symptom can be treated at a time. Also, dyslexia appears to be a sex-linked disorder, being much more common in boys than in girls. Estimates vary between three and seven times as many boys having dyslexia as girls.

TREATMENT AND THERAPY

The early diagnosis and treatment of dyslexia is essential to its eventual correction. Many experts agree that if a treatment begins before the third grade, there is an 80 percent probability that the dyslexia can be corrected. If the disorder remains undetected until the fifth grade, however, success at treating dyslexia is cut in half. If treatment does not begin until the seventh grade, the probability of successful treatment drops below 5 percent.

The preliminary identification of a dyslexic child can be made from symptoms that include poor written schoolwork, easy distractibility, clumsiness, poor co-ordination, poor spatial orientation, confused writing and/or spelling, and poor left-right orientation. Because numerous nondyslexic children also show many of these symptoms, a second step is required for such identification: the use of written tests designed to identify dyslexics. These tests include the Peabody Individual Achievement Test, the Halstead-Reitan Neuropsychological Test Battery, and the SOYBAR Criterion Tests.

Electroencephalograms and CT scans are often performed in the hope of pinning down concrete brain abnormalities in dyslexic patients. There is considerable disagreement, however, over the value of these techniques, beyond finding evidence of tumors or severe brain damage—both of which may indicate that the condition observed is not dyslexia. Most researchers agree that children who seem to be dyslexic but who lack tumors or damage are no more likely to have EEG or CT scan abnormalities than nondyslexics. An interesting adjunct to EEG use is a technique called brain electrical activity mapping (BEAM). BEAM converts an EEG into a brain map. Viewed by some workers in the area as a valuable technique, BEAM is contested by many others.

Once conclusive identification of a dyslexic child has been made, it becomes possible to begin corrective treatment. Such treatment is usually the preserve of special education programs. These programs are carried out by the special education teacher in school resource rooms. They also involve special classes limited to children with reading disabilities and schools that specialize in treating learning disabilities.

An often-cited method used is that of Grace Fernald, which utilizes kinesthetic imprinting, based on combined language experience and tactile stimulation. In this popular method or adaptations of it, a dyslexic child learns to read in the following way. First, the child tells a spontaneous story to the teacher, who transcribes it. Next, each word that is unrecognizable to the child is written down by the teacher, and the child traces its letters repeatedly until he or she can write the word without using the model. Each word learned becomes part of the child's word file. A large number of stories are handled this way. Though the method is quite slow, many reports praise its results. Nevertheless, no formal studies of its effectiveness have been made.

A second common teaching technique used by special educators is the Orton-Gillingham-Stillman method, which was developed in a collaboration between two teachers and a pediatric neurologist, Samuel T. Orton. The method evolved from Orton's conceptualization of language as developing from a sequence of processes in the nervous system that ends in its unilateral control by the left cerebral hemisphere. He proposed that dyslexia arises from conflicts between this cerebral hemisphere and the right cerebral hemisphere, which is usually involved in the handling of nonverbal, pictorial, and spatial stimuli.

Consequently, the corrective method that is used is a multisensory and kinesthetic approach, like that of Fernald. It begins, however, with the teaching of individual letters and phonemes. Then, it progresses to dealing with syllables, words, and sentences. Children taught by this method are drilled systematically, to imprint them with a mastery of phonics and the sounding out of unknown written words. They are encouraged to

Dyslexia may make it difficult to distinguish letters and words that are mirror images of each other, thus making it difficult for an otherwise intelligent child to learn to read.

learn how the elements of written language look, how they sound, how it feels to pronounce them, and how it feels to write them down. Although the Orton-Gillingham-Stillman method is as laborious as that of Fernald, it is widely used and appears to be successful.

Another treatment aspect that merits discussion is the use of therapeutic drugs in the handling of dyslexia. Most physicians and educators propose the use of these drugs as a useful adjunct to the special education training of those dyslexic children who are restless and easily distracted and who have low morale because of continued embarrassment in school in front of their peers. The drugs that are utilized most often are amphetamine, Dexedrine, and methylphenidate (Ritalin).

These stimulants, given at appropriate dose levels, will lengthen the time period during which certain dyslexic children function well in the classroom and can also produce feelings of self-confidence. Side effects of their overuse, however, include loss of appetite, nausea, nervousness, and sleeplessness. Furthermore, there is also the potential problem of drug abuse. When they are administered carefully and under close medical supervision, however, the benefits of these drugs far outweigh any possible risks.

A proponent of an entirely medical treatment of dyslexia is psychiatrist Harold N. Levinson. He proposes that the root of dyslexia is in inner ear dysfunction and that it can be treated with the judicious application of proper medications. Levinson's treatment includes amphetamines, antihistamines, drugs used against motion sickness, vitamins, health food components, and nutrients mixed in the proper combination for each patient. He asserts that he has cured more than ten thousand dyslexics and documents many cases. Critics of Levinson's work pose several questions, including whether the studies reported were well controlled and whether the patients treated were actually dyslexics. A major basis for the latter criticism is Levinson's statement that many of his cured patients were described to him as outstanding students. The contention is that dyslexic students are never outstanding students and cannot work at expected age levels.

An important aspect of dyslexia treatment is parental support of these children. Such emotional support helps dyslexics to cope with their problems and with the judgment of their peers. Useful aspects of this support include a positive attitude toward an afflicted child, appropriate home help that complements efforts at school, encouragement and praise for achievements, lack of recrimination when repeated mistakes are made, and positive interaction with special education teachers.

PERSPECTIVE AND PROSPECTS

The identification of dyslexia by German physician Rudolf Berlin and England's W. A. Morgan began the efforts to solve this unfortunate disorder. In 1917, Scottish eye surgeon James Hinshelwood published a book on dyslexia, which he viewed as being a hereditary problem, and the phenomenon became much better known to many physicians.

Attempts at educating dyslexics were highly individualized until the endeavors of Orton and his co-workers and of Fernald led to more standardized and widely used methods. These procedures, their adaptations, and several others not mentioned here had become the standard treatments for dyslexia by the late twentieth century.

Interestingly, many famous people—including Hans Christian Andersen, Winston Churchill, Albert Einstein, General George Patton, and Woodrow Wilson—had symptoms of dyslexia, which they subsequently overcame. This was fortunate for them, because adults who remain dyslexic are very often at a great disadvantage. In many cases in modern society, such people are among the functionally illiterate and the poor. Job opportunities open to dyslexics of otherwise adequate intelligence are quite limited.

Furthermore, with the development of a more complete understanding of the brain and its many functions, better counseling facilities, and the conceptualization and actualization of both parent-child and parent-counselor interactions, the probability of success in dyslexic training has improved greatly. Moreover, while environmental and socioeconomic factors contribute relatively little to the occurrence of dyslexia, they strongly affect the outcome of its treatment.

The endeavors of special education have so far made the greatest inroads in the treatment of dyslexia. It is hoped that many more advances in the area will be made as the science of the mind grows and diversifies, and the contributions of psychologists, physicians, physiologists, and special educators mesh even more effectively. Perhaps BEAM or the therapeutic methodology suggested by Levinson may provide or contribute to definitive understanding of and treatment of dyslexia.

—Sanford S. Singer, Ph.D.
See also Learning disabilities.

FOR FURTHER INFORMATION:

Huston, Anne Marshall. *Understanding Dyslexia: A Practical Approach for Parents and Teachers.* Rev. ed. Lanham, Md.: Madison Books, 1992. Explains dyslexia, describes its three main types, identifies causes and treatments, and covers useful teaching techniques. A bibliography, a useful glossary, appendices, and teaching materials are valuable additions.

International Dyslexia Association. http://www.inter dys.org/index.jsp. Web site includes a bookstore and information on new assistive technology. Site is divided into sections for children, teens, college students, adults, educators, and parents.

Jordan, Dale R. *Overcoming Dyslexia in Children, Adolescents, and Adults.* 3d ed. Austin, Tex.: Pro-Ed, 2002. Examines the role of genetics and brain development in relation to learning disabilities and explains the perceptual and emotional nature of dyslexia. Eight "success stories," strategies for improving academic performance and social skills, and assessment checklists are included.

Levinson, Harold N. *Smart but Feeling Dumb: The Challenging New Research on Dyslexia—and How It May Help You.* Rev. ed. New York: Warner Books, 2003. Argues that the basis of dyslexia and other disorders is an inner ear dysfunction that can be cured with judicious application of the correct medications. Also discusses adults and families with dyslexia, speech disorders, and attention deficit disorders.

Reid, Gavin, and Jane Kirk. *Dyslexia in Adults: Education and Employment.* New York: John Wiley & Sons, 2001. Offers a comprehensive guide for professionals to working with adults with dyslexia in the learning and working environment.

Snowling, Margaret. *Dyslexia: A Cognitive Developmental Perspective.* 2d ed. New York: Basil Blackwell, 2000. Covers aspects of dyslexia, including its identification, associated cognitive defects, the basis for language skill development, and the importance of phonetics.

Wolraich, Mark L., ed. *Disorders of Development and Learning: A Practical Guide to Assessment and Management.* 3d ed. Hamilton, Ont.: BC Decker, 2003. Summarizes salient facts about learning disorders, including etiology, assessment, management, and outcome.

DYSMENORRHEA

DISEASE/DISORDER

ANATOMY OR SYSTEM AFFECTED: Reproductive system, uterus

SPECIALTIES AND RELATED FIELDS: Gynecology

DEFINITION: A common menstrual disorder characterized by painful menstrual flow that is more severe than the usual cramps experienced by women with menstruation.

CAUSES AND SYMPTOMS

Dysmenorrhea is classified into primary and secondary dysmenorrhea. In primary dysmenorrhea, no organic cause of the menstrual pain is found, although multiple theories exist in the medical literature as to why pain occurs. Dysmenorrhea is associated with a number of psychological symptoms, including depression, irritability, and insomnia, although it is not clear whether these psychological symptoms are causes or effects.

Secondary dysmenorrhea is painful menstruation that occurs in the setting of known pelvic disease, such as endometriosis, adenomyosis, infection such as endometritis or pelvic inflammatory disease (PID), or anatomic abnormalities such as uterine fibroids or developmental abnormalities of the uterus, cervix, or vagina.

The symptoms of dysmenorrhea involve dull lower abdominal pain or cramping at the midline. The discomfort may radiate to the lower back or thighs. It can be associated with a number of other symptoms, most commonly nausea and vomiting or fatigue. Dysmenorrhea can occur up to one to two days before the onset

---

INFORMATION ON DYSMENORRHEA

CAUSES: Primary type unknown but associated with psychological symptoms (depression, irritability, insomnia); secondary type caused by pelvic disease (endometriosis or adenomyosis), infection (endometritis or pelvic inflammatory disease), or anatomic abnormalities (uterine fibroids or developmental abnormalities of uterus, cervix, or vagina)

SYMPTOMS: Dull lower abdominal pain or cramping radiating to lower back or thighs; associated with nausea, vomiting, fatigue

DURATION: Two or three days

TREATMENTS: Hormones, prostaglandin synthetase inhibitors, treatment of underlying condition

of menstrual flow and usually lasts for forty-eight to seventy-two hours. The most severe pain usually occurs on the first day of menstrual flow.

TREATMENT AND THERAPY

Treatment is recommended if dysmenorrhea interferes with activities of daily living. The two most common treatments are hormones and prostaglandin synthetase inhibitors. In women who do not desire pregnancy, oral contraceptive pills are an effective method of controlling dysmenorrhea, as they can reduce the volume of blood flow and the number of menstrual periods a woman has, if the pills are taken in continuous fashion.

In women nearing the menopause, hormones that artificially induce the menopause can serve as a bridge until natural menopause occurs. In women with primary dysmenorrhea whose symptoms do not improve after six to twelve months of medical treatment, laparoscopy may be considered to search for organic causes of pain.

In secondary dysmenorrhea, the treatment of any underlying pelvic disease may ameliorate the symptoms. For instance, any anatomic abnormalities may be amenable to surgery. Endometriosis may be treated with hormones or removal procedures.

Pain from either primary or secondary amenorrhea is often responsive to prostaglandin synthetase inhibitors, such as ibuprofen. These drugs decrease the levels of prostaglandins (which cause uterine cramping) in the menstrual blood. Patients with psychological symptoms accompanying their dysmenorrhea may benefit from psychological counseling and therapy. In cases of dysmenorrhea that resist standard treatment, a number of alternate treatments have been tried, with varying levels of success. They include nonspecific analgesics (such as opioids), acupuncture, and even surgical procedures such as presacral neurectomy, the interruption of the nerves going to the uterus.

—*Anne Lynn S. Chang, M.D.*

See also Endometriosis; Gynecology; Hormones; Menstruation; Pain; Pain management; Pelvic inflammatory disease (PID); Premenstrual syndrome (PMS); Reproductive system; Women's health.

FOR FURTHER INFORMATION:

Golub, Sharon. *Periods: From Menarche to Menopause.* Newbury Park, Calif.: Sage Publications, 1992.

Kasper, Dennis L., et al., eds. *Harrison's Principles of Internal Medicine.* 16th ed. New York: McGraw-Hill, 2005.

Minkin, Mary Jane, and Carol V. Wright. *The Yale Guide to Women's Reproductive Health: From Menarche to Menopause.* New Haven, Conn.: Yale University Press, 2003.

Stenchever, Morton A., et al. *Comprehensive Gynecology.* 4th ed. St. Louis: Mosby, 2006.

Tierney, Lawrence M., Stephen J. McPhee, and Maxine A. Papadakis, eds. *Current Medical Diagnosis and Treatment 2007.* New York: McGraw-Hill Medical, 2006.

DYSPHASIA. *See* APHASIA AND DYSPHASIA.

E. COLI INFECTION

DISEASE/DISORDER

ANATOMY OR SYSTEM AFFECTED: Blood, cells, gastrointestinal system, immune system, intestines, nervous system, urinary system

SPECIALTIES AND RELATED FIELDS: Bacteriology, cytology, epidemiology, gastroenterology, internal medicine, microbiology, neonatology, nephrology, public health, urology

DEFINITION: Infection with a rod-shaped, anaerobic, self-propelling bacterium of the family Enterobacteriaceae. It normally inhabits mammal intestines without ill effect, but some strains can cause life-threatening illness.

KEY TERMS:

intestines: the bowel, a two-part tube (the small intestine and the large intestine, or colon) connecting the stomach and anus; it absorbs nutrients from food

mucosa: a mucus-secreting membrane lining the bowel wall

strain: a subgroup in a species

toxin: a substance, usually a protein made by a cell, that causes injury

CAUSES AND SYMPTOMS

Escherichia coli (*E. coli*), the organism most often used for experiments in microbiology, is the best understood type of cell. These bacteria dwell in large numbers in the colons of mammals and constitute a major part of normal feces. More than 250 strains of *E. coli* are known, nearly all harmless to humans, although some may sicken other mammals. Scientists classify those strains that are toxic to humans according to the manner in which they cause disease (pathogenesis). People infected with the bacteria do not always develop symptoms.

Enterotoxigenic *E. coli* (ETEC) strains are the most common source of "travelers' diarrhea" in the United States and Europe. They colonize the small intestine and make it secrete fluid rather than absorb fluid. The result may be watery diarrhea. The afflicted person does not have a fever or inflammation of the bowel wall, which is not damaged by the bacteria.

Enteropathogenic *E. coli* (EPEC) strains attack the lower section of the small intestine, the ileum. Binding tightly to the mucosa cells, they damage the bowel wall. The infected person may feel cramps and have bloody diarrhea (dysentery).

Enterohemorrhagic *E. coli* (EHEC) strains can inflame the colon, damaging the mucosa and causing bleeding and severe cramps, a condition known as hemorrhagic colitis. In some cases, toxins absorbed through the bowel wall enter the bloodstream and travel to the kidneys. There, the glomeruli are attacked and red blood cells are destroyed, a condition called hemolytic uremic syndrome (HUS). The infected person will have difficulty urinating, and the urine will contain blood products such as hemoglobin. Fever may ensue, and the kidneys may fail, potentially a fatal condition. A related condition, thrombotic thrombocytopenic purpura, in which platelets and red blood cells are destroyed, produces high fever, vomiting, cramps, and damage to one or more organs. Untreated, it is almost always fatal.

Enteroinvasive *E. coli* (EIEC) strains penetrate the mucosa of the colon. The result is intense inflammation and moderate dysentery. A related set of strains afflict infants less than six months of age; the diarrhea may persist for weeks, and the resulting malnutrition and dehydration can be fatal. These strains are rare in the United States.

E. coli strains that enter the bloodstream can cause inflammation when they lodge and multiply in a localized part of the body: meningitis in the spine, prostatitis in the prostate gland, or cystitis in the bladder. After infection, people with depressed immune systems, such as those with acquired immunodeficiency syndrome (AIDS), may develop septicemia—blood poisoning throughout the body that can harm organs and cause sudden fevers, vomiting, skin eruptions, diarrhea, and, if persistent, death.

TREATMENT AND THERAPY

There is no specific treatment for *E. coli* infection. Medical research recommends managing the symptoms and providing supportive therapy while waiting for the body's immune system to clear the disease on its own. Thus, doctors seek to reduce fever, stop diarrhea, and ensure that the patient gets nourishment and enough fluid to prevent dehydration. Bed rest is often necessary in moderate and severe cases.

If the infection leads to a secondary disease, such as HUS, then doctors treat symptoms vigorously. Dialysis can support patients during kidney failure. Infusions of plasma can amend anemia from blood loss. A variety of medications can be taken to reduce the inflammation in such disorders as meningitis and prostatitis.

Most studies do not recommend antibiotics for killing *E. coli* bacteria. Clinical trials have not shown that such treatments help the patient. On the contrary, antibacterial medications appear to increase the patient's chance of developing a secondary condition, particularly HUS. Use of antidiarrheal drugs may also foster HUS.

PERSPECTIVES AND PROSPECTS

German biochemist Theodor Escherich (1857-1911) first isolated *Escherichia coli* in 1884; the species is named after him. The bacteria were best known as the "laboratory rats" of microbiologists until several outbreaks of the O157:H7 EHEC strain attracted public attention in the 1990's. *E. coli* bacteria spread most often from food or beverages contaminated by feces of cattle and humans. Hamburger was the usual culprit, although deer jerky, unpasteurized apple juice, milk, and bean sprouts have also been linked to outbreaks. Many secondary infections arose in people who had contact with those infected from foods. Dozens died, nearly all of them children or the elderly.

Proper food handling is the best defense against *E. coli*: Making sure that foods and liquids do not touch feces prevents the bacteria from spreading. If they do spread, the bacteria are relatively easy to kill. Pasteurization cleanses liquids; thorough cooking purifies meats and vegetables.

Studies in the mid-1990's found, unexpectedly, that some strains of *E. coli*—O157:H7, for example— mutate at an extremely high rate. Most mutations are harmless, but the chance of a new toxic variety is appreciable. Additionally, some types of *E. coli* have shown increasing resistance to antibiotics; however, epidemiologists deny that an *E. coli* strain such as O157:H7 could be an epidemic-causing "superbug." *E. coli* of all types cause less sickness in the United States than *Campylobacter*, *Salmonella*, and *Shigella* bacteria.

—*Roger Smith, Ph.D.*

See also Antibiotics; Bacterial infections; Bacteriology; Centers for Disease Control and Prevention (CDC); Colitis; Diarrhea and dysentery; Drug resistance; Food poisoning; Gastroenterology; Gastroenterology, pediatric; Gastrointestinal disorders; Gastrointestinal system; Hemolytic uremic syndrome; Infection; Intestinal disorders; Intestines; Meningitis; Microbiology; Mutation; Renal failure.

FOR FURTHER INFORMATION:

Biddle, Wayne. *A Field Guide to Germs*. 2d ed. New York: Anchor Books, 2002. This comprehensive book is easily accessible to the nonspecialist and includes a discussion of nearly every virus, bacterium, and fungus known to cause human and nonhuman animal disease. The history of the microbe and the treatment of diseases are included.

Dixon, Bernard. *Power Unseen: How Microbes Rule the World*. New York: W. H. Freeman, 1994. This book portrays the many, diverse, and often unexpected activities of microbes through a series of seventy-five vignettes, each focusing on one particular organism and its characteristic behavior. Dixon leaves the reader in no doubt that microbes, not macrobes, rule the world.

Donnenberg, Michael S., ed. *"Escherichia coli": Virulence Mechanisms of a Versatile Pathogen*. Boston: Academic Press, 2002. Provides a comprehensive analysis of the biology and molecular mechanisms that enable these organisms to cause human disease.

Lederberg, Joshua, ed. *Encyclopedia of Microbiology*. 2d ed. San Diego, Calif.: Academic Press, 2000. This encyclopedic reference source covers all aspects of microbiology. Includes bibliographical references and an index.

Parker, James N., and Philip M. Parker, eds. *The Official Patient's Sourcebook on E. Coli*. San Diego, Calif.: Icon Health, 2002. Draws from public, academic, government, and peer-reviewed research to provide a wide-ranging handbook for patients with *E. coli*.

Snyder, Larry, and Wendy Champness. *Molecular Genetics of Bacteria*. 3d ed. Washington, D.C.: ASM Press, 2003. A text that introduces the field of bacterial molecular genetics and describes the mechanisms of mutations and gene exchange in bacteria and phages. Concentrates specifically on the bacterium *E. coli* while using examples from other bacteria as appropriate.

Wilson, Michael, Brian Henderson, and Rod McNab.

Bacterial Virulence Mechanisms. New York: Cambridge University Press, 2002. Basing their discussion on research advances in microbiology, molecular biology, and cell biology, the authors describe the interactions that exist between bacteria and human cells both in health and during infection.

EAR INFECTIONS AND DISORDERS
DISEASE/DISORDER

ANATOMY OR SYSTEM AFFECTED: Ears

SPECIALTIES AND RELATED FIELDS: Audiology, neurology, otorhinolaryngology

DEFINITION: Infections or disorders of the outer, middle, or inner ear, which may result in hearing impairment or loss.

KEY TERMS:

conductive loss: a hearing loss caused by an outer-ear or middle-ear problem which results in reduced transmission of sound

frequency: the number of vibrations per second of a source of sound, measured in hertz; correlates with perceived pitch

intensity of sound: the physical phenomenon that correlates approximately with perceived loudness; measured in decibels

otitis: any inflammation of the outer or middle ear

sensorineural loss: a hearing loss caused by a problem in the inner ear; this impairment is caused by a hair cell or nerve problem and is usually not amenable to surgical correction

CAUSES AND SYMPTOMS

The hearing mechanism, one of the most intricate and delicate structures of the human body, consists of three sections: the outer ear, the middle ear, and the inner ear. The outer ear converts sound waves into the mechanical motion of the eardrum (tympanic membrane), and the middle ear transmits this mechanical motion to the inner ear, where it is transformed into nerve impulses sent to the brain.

The outer ear consists of the visible portion, the ear canal, and the eardrum. The middle ear is a small chamber containing three tiny bones—the auditory ossicles, termed malleus (hammer), incus (anvil), and stapes (stirrup)—which transmit the vibrations of the eardrum (attached to the hammer) into the inner ear. The chamber is connected to the back of the throat by the Eustachian tube, which allows equalization with the external air pressure. The inner ear, or cochlea, is a fluid-filled cavity containing the complex structure necessary to

convert the mechanical vibrations of the cochlear fluid into nerve pulses. The cochlea, shaped something like a snail's shell, is divided lengthwise by a slightly flexible partition into upper and lower chambers. The upper chamber begins at the oval window, to which the stirrup is attached. When the oval window is pushed or pulled by the stirrup, vibrations of the eardrum are transformed into cochlear fluid vibrations.

The lower surface of the cochlear partition, the basilar membrane, is set into vibration by the pressure difference between the fluids of the upper and lower ducts. Lying on the basilar membrane is the organ of Corti, containing tens of thousands of hair cells attached to the nerve transmission lines leading to the brain. When the basilar membrane vibrates, the cilia of these cells are bent, stimulating them to produce electrochemical impulses. These impulses travel along the auditory nerve to the brain, where they are interpreted as sound.

Although well protected against normal environmental exposure, the ear, because of its delicate nature, is subject to various infections and disorders. These disorders, which usually lead to some hearing loss, can occur in any of the three parts of the ear.

The ear canal can be blocked by a buildup of waxy secretions or by infection. Although earwax serves the useful purpose of trapping foreign particles that might otherwise be deposited on the eardrum, if the canal becomes clogged with an excess of wax, less sound will reach the eardrum, and hearing will be impaired.

Swimmer's ear, or otitis externa, is an inflammation caused by contaminated water which has not been completely drained from the ear canal. A moist condition in a region with little light favors fungal growth. Symptoms of swimmer's ear include an itchy and tender ear canal and a small amount of foul-smelling drainage. If

---

**INFORMATION ON
EAR INFECTIONS AND DISORDERS**

CAUSES: Infection, buildup of earwax, fluid retention, injury, fungal growth, allergies, exposure to loud noise, sudden change in air pressure, certain drugs

SYMPTOMS: Hearing impairment or loss, itchiness, pain, inflammation, discharge, tinnitus

DURATION: Temporary to chronic

TREATMENTS: Wide ranging; can include flushing ear with a warm solution under pressure, antibiotics, surgery

the canal is allowed to become clogged by the concomitant swelling, hearing will be noticeably impaired.

A perforated eardrum may result from a sharp blow to the side of the head, an infection, the insertion of objects into the ear, or a sudden change in air pressure (such as a nearby explosion). Small perforations are usually self-healing, but larger tears require medical treatment.

Inflammation of the middle ear, acute otitis media, is one of the most common ear infections, especially among children. Infection usually spreads from the throat to the middle ear through the Eustachian tube. Children are particularly susceptible to this problem because their short Eustachian tubes afford bacteria in the throat easy access to the middle ear. When the middle ear becomes infected, pus begins to accumulate, forcing the eardrum outward. This pressure stretches the auditory ossicles to their limit and tenses the ligaments so that vibration conduction is severely impaired. Untreated, this condition may eventually rupture the eardrum or permanently damage the ossicular chain. Furthermore, the pus from the infection may invade nearby structures, including the facial nerve, mastoid bones, the inner ear, or even the brain. The most common symptom of otitis is a sudden severe pain and an impairment of hearing resulting from the reduced mobility of the eardrum and the ossicles.

Secretory otitis media is caused by occlusion of the Eustachian tube as a result of conditions such as a head cold, diseased tonsils and adenoids, sinusitis, improper blowing of the nose, or riding in unpressurized airplanes. People with allergic nasal blockage are particularly prone to this condition. The blocked Eustachian tube causes the middle-ear cavity to fill with a pale yellow, noninfected discharge which exerts pressure on the eardrum, causing pain and impairment of hearing. Eventually, the middle-ear cavity is completely filled with fluid instead of air, impeding the movement of the ossicles and causing hearing impairment.

A mild, temporary hearing impairment resulting from airplane flights is termed aero-otitis media. This disorder results when a head cold or allergic reaction does not permit the Eustachian tube to equalize the air pressure in the middle ear with atmospheric pressure when a rapid change in altitude occurs. As the pressure outside the eardrum becomes greater than the pressure within, the membrane is forced inward, while the opening of the tube into the upper part of the throat is closed by the increased pressure. Symptoms are a severe sense of pressure in the ear, pain, and hearing impairment.

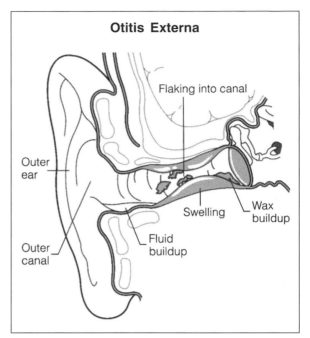

Otitis externa (swimmers' ear) results when the outer ear is inflamed by contaminated water that has not been completely drained from the ear canal.

Although the pressure difference may cause the eardrum to rupture, more often the pain continues until the middle ear fills with fluid or the tube opens to equalize pressure.

Chronic otitis media may result from inadequate drainage of pus during the acute form of this disease or from a permanent eardrum perforation that allows dust, water, and bacteria easy access to the middle-ear cavity. The main symptoms of this disease are fluids discharging from the outer ear and hearing loss. Perforations of the eardrum result in hearing loss because of the reduced vibrating surface and a buildup of fibrous tissue which further induces conductive losses. In some cases, an infection may heal but still cause hearing loss by immobilizing the ossicles. There are two distinct types of chronic otitis, one relatively harmless and the other quite dangerous. An odorless, stringy discharge from the mucous membrane lining the middle ear characterizes the harmless type. The dangerous type is characterized by a foul-smelling discharge coming from a bone-invading process beneath the mucous lining. If neglected, this process can lead to serious complications, such as meningitis, paralysis of the facial nerve, or complete sensorineural deafness.

The ossicles may be disrupted by infection or by a jarring blow to the head. Most often, a separation of the linkage occurs at the weakest point, where the anvil joins the stirrup. A partial separation results in a mild hearing loss, while complete separation causes severe hearing impairment.

Disablement of the mechanical linkage of the middle ear may also occur if the stirrup becomes calcified, a condition termed otosclerosis. The normal bone is resorbed and replaced by very irregular, often richly vascularized bone. The increased stiffness of the stirrup produces conductive hearing loss. In extreme cases, the stirrup becomes completely immobile and must be surgically removed. Although the exact cause of this disease is unknown, it seems to be hereditary. About half of the cases occur in families in which one or more relatives have the same condition, and it occurs more frequently in females than in males. There is also some evidence that the condition may be triggered by a lack of fluoride in drinking water and that increasing the intake of fluoride may retard the calcification process.

Tinnitus is characterized by ringing, hissing, or clicking noises in the ear that seem to come and go spontaneously without any sound stimulus. While technically tinnitus is not a disease of the ear, it is a common symptom of various ear problems. Possible

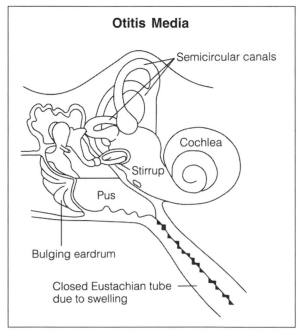

Otitis Media

Semicircular canals

Cochlea

Stirrup

Pus

Bulging eardrum

Closed Eustachian tube due to swelling

Otitis media occurs when infection spreads from the throat to the middle ear via the Eustachian tube; it is a serious condition which, left untreated, may lead to permanent ear damage and even infection of the brain.

causes of tinnitus are earwax lodged against the eardrum, a perforated or inflamed eardrum, otosclerosis, high aspirin dosage, or excessive use of the telephone. Tinnitus is most serious when caused by an inner-ear problem or by exposure to very intense sounds, and it often accompanies hearing loss at high frequencies.

Ménière's disease is caused by production of excess cochlear fluid, which increases the pressure in the cochlea. This condition may be precipitated by allergy, infection, kidney disease, or any number of other causes, including severe stress. The increased pressure is exerted on the walls of the semicircular canals, as well as on the cochlear partition. The excess pressure in the semicircular canals (the organs of balance) is interpreted by the brain as a rapid spinning motion, and the victim experiences abrupt attacks of vertigo and nausea. The excess pressure in the cochlear partition has the same effect as a very loud sound and rapidly destroys hair cells. A single attack causes a noticeable hearing loss and could result in total deafness without prompt treatment.

Of all ear diseases, damage to the hair cells in the cochlea causes the most serious impairment. Cilia may be destroyed by high fevers or from a sudden or prolonged exposure to intensely loud sounds. Problems include destroyed or missing hair cells, hair cells which fire spontaneously, and damaged hair cells that require unusually strong stimuli to excite them. At the present time, there is no means of repairing damaged cilia or of replacing those which have been lost.

Viral nerve deafness is a result of a viral infection in one or both ears. The mumps virus is one of the most common causes of severe nerve damage, with the measles and influenza viruses as secondary causes.

Ototoxic (ear-poisoning) drugs can cause temporary or permanent hearing impairment by damaging auditory nerve tissues, although susceptibility is highly individualistic. A temporary decrease of hearing (in addition to tinnitus) accompanies the ingestion of large quantities of aspirin or quinine. Certain antibiotics, such as those of the mycin family, may also create permanent damage to the auditory nerves.

Repeated exposure to loud noise (in excess of 90 decibels) will cause a gradual deterioration of hearing by destroying cilia. The extent of damage, however, depends on the loudness and the duration of the sound. Rock bands often exceed 110 decibels; farm machinery averages 100 decibels.

Presbycusis (hearing loss with age) is the inability to hear high-frequency sounds because of the increasing deterioration of the hair cells. By age thirty, a perceptible high-frequency hearing loss is present. This deterioration progresses into old age, often resulting in severe impairment. The problem is accelerated by frequent unprotected exposure to noisy environments. The extent of damage depends on the frequency, intensity, and duration of exposure, as well as on the individual's predisposition to hearing loss.

Treatment and Therapy

The simplest ear problems to treat are a buildup of earwax, swimmer's ear, and a perforated eardrum. A large accumulation of wax in the ear canal is best removed by having a medical professional flush the ear with a warm solution under pressure. One should never attempt to remove wax plugs with a sharp instrument. A small accumulation of earwax may be softened by a few drops of baby oil left in the ear overnight, then washed out with warm water and a soft rubber ear syringe. Swimmer's ear can usually be prevented by thoroughly draining the ears after swimming. The disease can be treated by an application of antibiotic eardrops after the ear canal has been thoroughly cleaned. A small perforation of the eardrum will usually heal itself. Larger tears, however, require an operation, tympanoplasty, that grafts a piece of skin over the perforation.

Fortunately, the bacteria that usually cause acute otitis respond quickly to antibiotics. Although antibiotics may relieve the symptoms, complications can arise unless the pus is thoroughly drained. The two-part treatment—draining the fluid from the middle ear and antibiotic therapy—resolves the acute otitis infection within a week. Secretory otitis is cured by finding and removing the cause of the occluded Eustachian tube. The serous fluid is then removed by means of an aspirating needle or by an incision in the eardrum so as to inflate the tube by forcing air through it. In some cases, a tiny polyethylene tube is inserted through the eardrum to aid in reestablishing normal ventilation. If the Eustachian tube remains inadequate, a small plastic grommet may be inserted. The improvement in hearing is often immediate and dramatic. The pain and hearing loss of aero-otitis is usually temporary and disappears of its own accord. If, during or immediately after flight, yawning or swallowing does not allow the Eustachian tube to open and equalize the pressure, medicine or surgical puncture of the eardrum may be required. The harmless form of chronic otitis is treated with applied medications to kill the bacteria and to dry the chronic drainage. The eardrum perforation may then be closed

to restore the functioning of the ear and to recover hearing. The more dangerous chronic form of this disease does not respond well to antibacterial agents, but careful X-ray examination allows diagnosis and surgical removal of the bone-eroding cyst.

Ossicular interruption can be surgically treated to restore the conductive link by repositioning the separated bones. This relatively simple operation has a very high success rate. Otosclerosis is treated by operating on the stirrup in one of several ways. The stirrup can be mechanically freed by fracturing the calcified foot plate, or by fracturing the foot plate and one of the arms. Although this operation is usually successful, recalcification often occurs. Alternatively, the stirrup can be completely removed and replaced by a prosthesis of wire or silicon, yielding excellent and permanent results.

Since tinnitus has many possible, and often not readily identifiable, causes, only about 10 percent of the cases are treated successfully. The tinnitus masker has been invented to help sufferers live with this annoyance. The masker, a noise generator similar in appearance to a hearing aid, produces a constant, gentle humming sound which masks the tinnitus.

Ménière's disease, usually treated by drugs and a restricted diet, may also require surgical correction to relieve the excess pressure in severe cases. If this procedure is unsuccessful, the nerves of the inner ear may be cut. In drastic cases, the entire inner ear may be removed.

Presently there is no cure for damaged hair cells; the only treatment is to use a hearing aid. It is more advantageous to take preventive measures, such as reducing noise at the source, replacing noisy equipment with quieter models, or using ear protection devices. Recreational exposure to loud music should be severely curtailed, if not completely eliminated.

Perspective and Prospects

For many centuries, treatment of the ear was associated with that of the eye. In the nineteenth century, the development of the laryngoscope (to examine the larynx) and the otoscope (to examine the ears) enabled doctors to examine and treat disorders such as croup, sore throat, and draining ears, which eventually led to the control of these diseases. As an offshoot of the medical advances made possible by these technological devices, the connection between the ear and throat became known, and otologists became associated with laryngologists.

The study of ear diseases did not develop scientifically until the early nineteenth century, when Jean-Marc-Gaspard Itard and Prosper Ménière made systematic investigations of ear physiology and disease. In 1853, William R. Wilde of Dublin published the first scientific treatise on ear diseases and treatments, setting the field on a firm scientific foundation. Meanwhile, the scientific investigation of the diseased larynx was aided by the laryngoscope, invented in 1855 by Manuel Garcia, a Spanish singing teacher who used his invention as a teaching aid. During the late nineteenth century, this instrument was adopted for detailed studies of larynx pathology by Ludwig Türck and Jan Czermak, who also adapted this instrument to investigate the nasal cavity, which established the link between laryngology and rhinology. Friedrich Voltolini, one of Czermak's assistants, further modified the instrument so that it could be used in conjunction with the otoscope. In 1921, Carl Nylen pioneered the use of a high-powered binocular microscope to perform ear surgery. The operating microscope opened the way for delicate operations on the tiny bones of the middle ear. With the founding of the American Board of Otology in 1924, otology (later otolaryngology) became the second medical specialty to be formally established in North America.

Prior to World War II, the leading cause of deafness was the various forms of ear infection. Advances in technology and medicine have now brought ear infections under control. Today the leading type of hearing loss in industrialized countries is conductive loss, which occurs in those who are genetically predisposed to such loss and who have had lifetime exposure to noise and excessively loud sounds. In the future, ear protection devices and reasonable precautions against extensive exposure to loud sounds should reduce the incidence of hearing loss to even lower levels.

—George R. Plitnik, Ph.D.

See also Altitude sickness; Audiology; Balance disorders; Deafness; Decongestants; Ear surgery; Ears; Hearing loss; Hearing tests; Ménière's disease; Motion sickness; Myringotomy; Nasopharyngeal disorders; Neurology; Neurology, pediatric; Otoplasty; Otorhinolaryngology; Sense organs; Sinusitis; Speech disorders; Tonsillitis.

FOR FURTHER INFORMATION:

Canalis, Rinaldo, and Paul R. Lambert, eds. *The Ear: Comprehensive Otology*. Philadelphia: Lippincott Williams & Wilkins, 2000. A text covering all aspects of otology.

Dugan, Marcia B. *Living with Hearing Loss*. Washington, D.C.: Gallaudet University Press, 2003. Offers a range of practical advice for those with hearing loss, including strategies for dealing with everyday situations and emergencies, speechreading (lipreading), oral interpreters, and assertive communication.

Ferrari, Mario. *PDxMD Ear, Nose, and Throat Disorders*. New York: Elsevier, 2002. A clinical yet accessible reference text that provides a comprehensive list of disorders, with a summary of the condition, background, diagnosis, treatment, outcomes, prevention, and resources.

Friedman, Ellen M., and James M. Barassi. *My Ear Hurts! A Complete Guide to Understanding and Treating Your Child's Ear Infections*. New York: Simon & Schuster, 2001. Reviews current research on ear infections and reviews a range of treatment approaches from both conventional and alternative medicine.

Greene, Alan R. *The Parent's Complete Guide to Ear Infections*. Reprint. Allentown, Pa.: People's Medical Society, 1999. Every parent who has ever had a child with recurrent otitis will appreciate this book. It explains the anatomy of normal ears, causes of infections, prevention, symptoms, evaluation, initial and ongoing treatment, antibiotics, the pros and cons of surgical intervention, hearing loss, tubes, and complications.

Jerger, James, ed. *Hearing Disorders in Adults: Current Trends*. San Diego, Calif.: College-Hill Press, 1984. A reliable and readable introductory treatise on common hearing disorders.

Kemper, Kathi J. *The Holistic Pediatrician: A Pediatrician's Comprehensive Guide to Safe and Effective Therapies for the Twenty-five Most Common Ailments of Infants, Children, and Adolescents*. New York: HarperCollins, 2002. Integrates mainstream and alternative medicine to aid parents in dealing with the most common childhood health problems such as diaper rash, ear infections, and allergies.

"Lack of Consensus About Surgery for Ear Infections." *Health News* 18, no. 3 (June/July, 2000): 11. Children who suffer from recurrent otitis media, or ear infections, may be candidates for a surgical procedure called "myringotomy," which involves the insertion of tiny tubes into the ear drums. The goal of the surgery is to prevent future infections and reduce the chances of hearing loss.

Pender, Daniel J. *Practical Otology*. Philadelphia: J. B. Lippincott, 1992. A well-illustrated text on diseases of the ear and their surgical correction.

Roland, Peter S., Bradley F. Marple, and William L. Meyerhoff, eds. *Hearing Loss*. New York: Thieme, 1997. Provides information on hearing disorders and discusses the anatomy and physiology of the ear.

EAR, NOSE, AND THROAT MEDICINE. *See* OTORHINOLARYNGOLOGY.

EAR SURGERY

PROCEDURE

ANATOMY OR SYSTEM AFFECTED: Bones, ears, musculoskeletal system, nervous system

SPECIALTIES AND RELATED FIELDS: Audiology, general surgery, otorhinolaryngology, speech pathology

DEFINITION: An invasive procedure to correct structural problems of the ear that produce some degree of hearing loss.

KEY TERMS:

cochlea: a structure in the inner ear that receives sound vibrations from the ossicles and transmits them to the auditory nerve

myringotomy: incision of the tympanic membrane used to drain fluid and reduce middle-ear pressure

ossicles: tiny bones located between the eardrum and the cochlea

otosclerosis: a condition in which the stapes becomes progressively more rigid, and hearing loss results

stapedectomy: a surgical procedure in which the stapes is replaced with an artificial substitute

stapes: the ossicle that makes contact with the cochlea

tympanic membrane: the eardrum, which separates the external ear canal from the middle ear and ossicles and which transmits sound vibration to the ossicles

tympanoplasty: a surgical procedure to repair the tympanic membrane

INDICATIONS AND PROCEDURES

Humans are able to detect sound because of the interaction between the ears and the brain. When sound waves strike the tympanic membrane (eardrum), it vibrates. The movement of the tympanic membrane then causes the movement of the ossicles, the three tiny bones within the middle ear (malleus, incus, and stapes). These moving bones transfer the vibrations to the cochlea of the inner ear, which stimulates the auditory nerve and eventually the brain.

Hearing problems may result when any part of the ear is damaged. Hearing difficulties can be categorized into two main areas: conductive and sensorineural hearing loss. In conductive hearing loss, the ear loses its ability to transmit sound from the external ear to the cochlea. Common causes include earwax buildup in the outer ear canal; otosclerosis, in which the stapes loses mobility and cannot stimulate the cochlea effectively; and otitis media, in which the middle ear becomes infected and a sticky fluid is produced which causes the ossicles to become inflexible. Otitis media is the most common cause of conductive hearing loss and typically occurs in children. If antibiotics such as amoxicillin or ampicillin fail to clear the ear of infection, surgery may be required. Sensorineural hearing loss results from damage to the cochlea or auditory nerve. Common causes include loud noises, rubella (a type of viral infection) during embryonic development, and certain drugs such as gentamicin and streptomycin. Occasionally, a tumor (neuroma) of the auditory nerve may cause sensorineural hearing loss.

Myringotomy is a surgical procedure in which an incision is made in the tympanic membrane to allow drainage of fluid (effusion) from the middle ear to the external ear canal. The surgeon usually performs this operation to treat recurrent otitis media, a condition in which pressure builds in the middle ear and pushes outward on the tympanic membrane. The patient, usually a child, is given general anesthesia. An incision is made in the eardrum so that a small tube can be inserted to allow continuous drainage of the pus. The tube usually falls out in a few months, and the tympanic membrane heals rapidly.

Otosclerosis, the overgrowth of bone that impedes the movement of the stapes, can be treated by stapedectomy (surgical removal of the stapes). General anesthesia is used to prevent pain or movement when an incision is made in the ear canal and the tympanic membrane is folded to access the ossicles. The stapes can then be removed and a metal or plastic prosthesis inserted in its place. The eardrum is then repaired.

Tympanoplasty is an operation to repair the tympanic membrane or ossicles. Sudden pressure changes in an airplane or during deep-sea diving may perforate the tympanic membrane (barotrauma) and require tympanoplasty. The procedure is similar to stapedectomy. With the patient under general anesthesia, an incision is made next to the eardrum to provide access to the tympanic membrane and ossicles. The tympanic membrane may need to be repaired if the perforated eardrum does not heal on its own. An operating microscope is employed for optimal visualization of the middle ear. If the tympanoplasty involves the ossicles, microsurgical instruments are used to reposition, repair, or replace the damaged bones. They are then reset in their natural positions, and the eardrum is repaired.

Auditory neuromas are benign tumors of the supporting cells surrounding the auditory nerve. Although rare, these tumors can cause deafness. Once neuromas are confirmed by computed tomography (CT) scanning, surgical removal is necessary. With the patient under general anesthesia, the surgeon must make a hole in the skull and attempt to remove the tumor carefully without damaging the auditory nerve or adjacent nerves.

Uses and Complications

More than 90 percent of the patients undergoing stapedectomy experience improved hearing. Approximately 1 percent, however, show deterioration of hearing or total hearing loss postoperatively. For this reason, most surgeons perform stapedectomy on one ear at a time.

Occasionally, the surgical removal of auditory neuromas causes total deafness because of damage to the auditory nerve itself. In rare cases, damage to nearby nerves may cause weakness and/or numbness in that part of the face. Depending on the extent of nerve damage, the symptoms may or may not lessen with time.

Perspective and Prospects

Improvements in technology promise new methods of treating hearing loss. For example, cochlear implants have been developed for the treatment of total sensorineural hearing loss. These implants are surgically inserted into the inner ear. Electrodes in the cochlea receive sound signals transmitted to them from a miniature receiver implanted behind the skin of the ear. Directly over the implant, the patient wears an external transmitter which is connected to a sound processor and microphone. As the microphone picks up sound, the sound is eventually conducted to the electrodes within the cochlea.

—*Matthew Berria, Ph.D.,*
and Douglas Reinhart, M.D.

See also Audiology; Deafness; Ear infections and disorders; Ears; Hearing loss; Ménière's disease; Myringotomy; Neurology; Neurology, pediatric; Otoplasty; Otorhinolaryngology; Plastic surgery; Sense organs.

For Further Information:

Brunicardi, F. Charles, et al., eds. *Schwartz's Principles of Surgery*. 8th ed. New York: McGraw-Hill, 2005. A standard textbook on the topic. Intended for practicing surgeons, but valuable to general readers for its details.

Ferrari, Mario. *PDxMD Ear, Nose, and Throat Disorders*. New York: Elsevier, 2002. A clinical yet accessible reference text that provides a comprehensive list of disorders, with a summary of the condition, background, diagnosis, treatment, outcomes, prevention, and resources.

Leikin, Jerrold B., and Martin S. Lipsky, eds. *American Medical Association Complete Medical Encyclopedia*. New York: Random House Reference, 2003. A concise presentation of numerous medical terms and illnesses. A good general reference.

Nadol, Joseph B., Jr., and Michael J. McKenna. *Surgery of the Ear and Temporal Bone*. 2d ed. Philadelphia: Lippincott Williams & Wilkins, 2005. Written by specialists at the Massachusetts Eye and Ear Infirmary, details surgical techniques that have been found reproducible and effective, as well as surgical decision making, including discussions of indications, contraindications, complications, and therapeutic alternatives.

Pender, Daniel J. *Practical Otology*. Philadelphia: J. B. Lippincott, 1992. A well-illustrated text on diseases of the ear and their surgical correction.

Tierney, Lawrence M., Stephen J. McPhee, and Maxine A. Papadakis, eds. *Current Medical Diagnosis and Treatment 2007*. New York: McGraw-Hill Medical, 2006. The point of reference for physicians and other health care practitioners. It incorporates each year's biomedical research discoveries that have immediate, relevant, and applicable use for the patient.

Ears

Anatomy

Anatomy or system affected: Bones, musculoskeletal system, nervous system

Specialties and related fields: Audiology, neurology, otorhinolaryngology, speech pathology

Definition: The organs responsible for both hearing and balance.

Key terms:

auditory nerve: the nerve that conducts impulses originating in hair cells of cochlea to the brain for processing as the sensation of sound

cochlea: the fluid-filled coil of the inner ear containing hair cells that change vibrations in the fluid into nerve impulses

eardrum: the membrane separating the outer ear canal from the middle ear that changes sound waves into movements of the ossicles; also called the tympanic membrane

Eustachian tube: the tube connecting the middle ear to the back of the throat; air exchange through this tube equalizes air pressure in the middle ear with the outside air pressure

inner ear: an organ that includes the cochlea (for detection of sound) and the labyrinth (for detection of movement)

labyrinth: a structure consisting of three fluid-filled, semicircular canals at right angles to one another in the inner ear; they monitor the position and movement of the head

middle ear: the air-filled cavity in which vibrations are transmitted from the eardrum to the inner ear via the ossicles

ossicles: three small bones in the middle ear that transmit vibrations from the eardrum to the fluid of the inner ear

otoscope: an instrument for viewing the ear canal and the eardrum

outer ear: the visible, fleshy part of the ear and the ear canal; transmits sound waves to the eardrum

tympanic membrane: another term for the eardrum

STRUCTURE AND FUNCTIONS

The ear is composed of three parts: the outer ear, the middle ear, and the inner ear. All three parts are involved in hearing, while only the inner ear is involved in balance.

Sound can be thought of as pressure waves that travel through the air. These waves are collected by the fleshy part of the outer ear and are funneled down the ear canal to the eardrum. The eardrum, being a thin membrane, vibrates as it is hit by the sound waves. Attached to the eardrum is the first of the ossicles (the hammer or malleus), which moves when the eardrum moves. The second ossicle (the anvil or incus) is attached to the first, and the third to the second. Therefore, as the first bone moves, the others move also. The base of the third bone (the stirrup or stapes) is in contact with the oval window at the beginning of the inner ear. Movement of the oval window sets up vibrations in the fluid of the cochlea. These vibrations are detected by hair cells. Depending on their position in the cochlea,

the hair cells are sensitive to being moved by vibrations of different frequencies. When the hair of a hair cell is bent by the fluid, an impulse is generated. The impulses are transmitted to the brain via the auditory nerve. The nerve impulses are processed in the brain, and the result is the sensation of sound, in particular the sense of pitch. Thus the three parts of the ear turn sound waves into "sound" by changing air vibrations into eardrum vibrations, then ossicle movement, then fluid vibrations, and finally nerve impulses.

DISORDERS AND DISEASES

Each of the three parts of the ear can be affected by diseases that can lead to temporary or, in some cases, permanent hearing loss. Damage to the eardrum, ossicles, or any part of the ear before the cochlea results in conductive hearing loss, as these structures conduct the sound or vibrations. Damage to the hair cells or to the auditory nerve results in sensorineural hearing loss. Sound may be conducted normally but cannot be detected by the hair cells or transmitted as nerve impulses to the brain.

Disorders of the outer ear include cauliflower ear, blockage by earwax, otitis externa, and tumors. Cauliflower ear is a severe hematoma (bruise) to the outer ear. In some cases, the blood trapped beneath the skin does not resorb and instead turns into fibrous tissue that may become cartilaginous or even bonelike.

Earwax is secreted by the cells in the lining of the ear canal. Its function is to protect the eardrum from dust and dirt, and it normally works its way to the outer opening of the ear. The amount secreted varies from person to person. In some people, or in people who are continually exposed to dusty environments, excessive amounts of wax may be secreted and may block the ear canal sufficiently to interfere with its transmission of sound waves to the eardrum.

Otitis externa can take two forms, either localized or generalized. The localized form, a boil or abscess, is a bacterial infection that results from breaks in the lining of the ear canal and is often caused by attempts to scratch an itch in the ear or to remove wax. The generalized form can be a bacterial or fungal infection, known as otomycosis. Generalized otitis externa is also called swimmer's ear because it often results from swimming in polluted waters or from chronic moisture in the ear canal.

Tumors of the ear can be benign (noncancerous) or malignant (cancerous) growths of either the soft tissues or the underlying bone. Bony growths, or osteomas, can

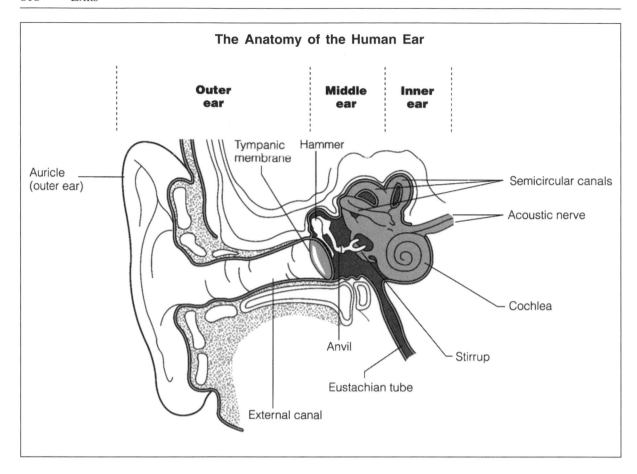

The Anatomy of the Human Ear

Outer ear   **Middle ear**   **Inner ear**

Tympanic membrane   Hammer

Auricle (outer ear)

Semicircular canals

Acoustic nerve

Cochlea

Anvil

Stirrup

Eustachian tube

External canal

cause sufficient blockage, by themselves or by leading to the buildup of earwax, to result in hearing loss.

The middle ear consists of the eardrum, three small bones called the ossicles, and the Eustachian tube. The bones of the middle ear move in an air-filled cavity. Air pressure within this cavity is normally the same as the outside air pressure because air is exchanged between the middle ear and the outside world via the Eustachian tube. When this tube swells and closes, as it often does with a head cold, one experiences a stuffy feeling, decreased hearing, mild pain, and sometimes ringing in the ears (tinnitus) or dizziness. The middle ear is susceptible to infection, such as otitis media, because bacteria and viruses can sometimes enter via the Eustachian tube. Young children are especially prone to middle-ear infections because a child's Eustachian tubes are shorter and more directly in line with the back of the throat than those of adults. Untreated ear infections can sometimes spread into the surrounding bone (mastoiditis) or into the brain (meningitis).

Fluid in the middle ear during an ear infection interferes with the free movement of the ossicles, causing

hearing loss that, although significant while it lasts, is temporary. In other instances, there is the prolonged presence of clear fluid in the middle ear, resulting from a combination of infection or allergy and Eustachian tube dysfunction, which itself can result from swelling caused by allergy. This condition, known as "glue ear" or persistent middle-ear effusion, can last long enough to cause detrimental effects on speech, particularly in young children. Middle-ear infections can sometimes become chronic, as in chronic otitis media; permanent damage to the hearing can result from the ossicles being dissolved away by the pus from these chronic infections.

During a middle-ear infection, fluid can build up and increase pressure within the middle-ear cavity sufficiently to rupture (perforate) the eardrum. Very loud noises are another form of increased pressure, in this case from the outside. If a loud noise is very sudden, such as an explosion or gunshot, then pressure cannot be equalized fast enough and the eardrum can rupture. Scuba diving without clearing one's ears (that is, getting the Eustachian tube to open and allow airflow) can also result in ruptured eardrums. Other causes of ruptured eardrums include puncture by a sharp object inserted into the ear canal to remove wax or relieve itching, a blow to the ear, or a fractured skull. Some hearing is lost when the eardrum is ruptured, but if the damage is not too severe, the eardrum heals itself and hearing returns.

The middle ear does not always fill with fluid if the Eustachian tube is blocked. In some instances, the middle-ear cavity remains filled with trapped air. This trapped air is taken up by the cells lining the middle-ear cavity, decreasing the air pressure inside the middle ear and allowing the eardrum to push inward. Cells that are constantly shed from the eardrum collect in this pocket and form a ball that can become infected. This infected ball, or cholesteatoma, produces pus, which can erode the ossicles. If left untreated, the erosion can continue through the roof of the middle-ear cavity (causing brain abscesses or meningitis) or through the walls (causing abscesses behind the ear). The symptoms of a cholesteatoma go beyond the symptoms of an earache to include headache, dizziness, and weakness of the facial muscles.

Permanent conductive hearing loss can also result from calcification of the ossicles, a condition called osteosclerosis. Abnormal spongy bone can form at the base of the stirrup bone, interfering with its normal movement against the oval window. Hearing loss caused by osteosclerosis occurs gradually over ten to fifteen years, although it may be accelerated in women by pregnancy. There is a hereditary component.

The inner ear begins at the oval window, which separates the air-filled cavity at the middle ear from the fluid-filled cavities of the inner ear. The inner ear consists of the cochlea, which is involved in hearing, and the labyrinth, which maintains balance.

Disorders of the cochlea result in permanent sensorineural hearing loss. Hair cells can be damaged by the high fever accompanying some diseases such as meningitis. They may also be damaged by some drugs. The largest, and most preventable, sources of damage to the hair cells are occupational and recreational exposure to loud sounds, particularly if they are prolonged. In some occupations, the hearing loss from working without ear protection may be confined to certain frequencies of sounds, while other occupations lead to general loss at all sound frequencies. Prolonged exposure to overamplified music will likewise cause permanent hearing loss at all frequencies. This is more severe and has much earlier onset than presbycusis—the progressive loss of hearing, particularly in the high frequencies, that occurs with normal aging.

The labyrinth is the part of the ear that maintains one's balance; therefore the major system of disorders of the labyrinth is vertigo (dizziness). Labyrinthitis is an infection, generally viral, of the labyrinth. The vertigo can be severe but is temporary.

With Ménière's disease, there is an increase in the volume of fluid in the labyrinth and a corresponding increase in internal pressure, which distorts or ruptures the membrane lining. The symptoms, which include vertigo, noises in the ear, and muffled or distorted hearing especially of low tones, flare up in attacks that may last from a few hours to several days. The frequency of these attacks varies from one individual to another, with some people having episodes every few weeks and others having them every few years. This condition, which may be accompanied by migraine headaches, usually clears spontaneously but in some people may result in deafness.

DIAGNOSTIC AND TREATMENT TECHNIQUES

The most common ear disorders, outer-ear or middle-ear infections, are diagnosed visually with an otoscope. This handheld instrument is a very bright light with a removable tip. Tips of different sizes can be attached so that the doctor can look into ear canals of various sizes. Infections or obstructions in the outer ear are readily visible. Middle-ear infections can often be discerned by the appearance of the eardrum, which may appear red and inflamed. Fluid in the middle ear can sometimes be seen through the eardrum, or its presence can be surmised if the eardrum is bulging toward the ear canal. In other cases, the eardrum will be seen to be retracted or bulging inward toward the middle-ear cavity. Holes in the eardrum can also be seen, as can scars from previous ruptures that have since healed.

Impedance testing may be used in addition to the otoscope for diagnosis of middle-ear problems. Impedance testing is based on the fact that, when sound waves hit the eardrum, some of the energy is transmitted as vibrations of the drum, while some of the energy is reflected. If the eardrum is stretched tight by fluid pushing against it or by being retracted, it will be less mobile and will reflect more sound waves than a normal eardrum. In the simplest form, the mobility of the eardrum is tested with a small air tube and bulb attached to an otoscope. The doctor gently squeezes a puff of air into the ear canal while watching through the otoscope to see how well the eardrum moves.

A far more quantitative version of impedance testing can be done in cases of suspected hearing loss. This type of impedance testing is generally administered by an audiologist, a professional trained in administering and interpreting hearing tests. The ear canal is blocked with an earplug containing a transmitter and receiver. The transmitter releases sound of known frequency and intensity into the ear canal while also changing the pressure in the ear canal by pumping air into it. The receiver then measures the amount of energy reflected back. The machine analyzes the efficiency of reflection at various pressures and prints out a graph. By comparison of the graph to that from an eardrum with normal mobility, conclusions can be drawn about the degree of immobility and, consequently, about the stage of the middle-ear infection. Many pediatricians or family physicians have handheld versions of this instrument, which resembles an otoscope but is capable of transmitting sound and measuring reflected sound intensity.

When an ear infection has been diagnosed, the treatment is generally with antibiotics. For outer-ear infections, drops containing antibiotic or antifungal agents are prescribed. For middle-ear infections, antibiotics are prescribed that can be taken by mouth. The patient is rechecked in about three weeks to ensure that the ear has healed.

In some cases, the ear does not heal, or the fluid in the middle ear does not go away. This can occur if a new infection starts before the ear is fully recovered or if the infecting microorganisms are resistant to the antibiotic used for treatment. In cases of chronic or repeated otitis media, a surgical procedure called a myringotomy can be performed in which a small slit is made in the eardrum to release fluid from the middle ear. Often, a small tube is inserted into the slit. These ear tubes, or tympanostomy tubes, keep the middle ear ventilated, allowing it to dry and heal. In most cases, these tubes are spontaneously pushed out by the eardrum as healing takes place, usually within three to six months. Patients must be cautious to keep water out of their ears while the tubes are in place.

A permanently damaged eardrum—from an explosion, for example—can be replaced by a graft. This procedure is called tympanoplasty, and the tissue used for the graft is generally taken from a vein from the same person. If the ossicles are damaged, they too can be replaced, in this case by metal copies of the bones. For example, when otosclerosis has damaged the stapes (stirrup) bone, hearing can often be restored by replacing it with a metal substitute.

Tumors, osteomas in the ear canal, or cholesteatomas on the eardrum may need to be removed surgically. Surgery may also be needed if infections have spread into the surrounding bone. Bone infections or abnormalities of the inner ear are diagnosed by X rays or by computed tomography (CT) scans.

For some persons who have complete sensorineural hearing loss, some awareness of sound can be restored with a cochlear implant. This electronic device is surgically implanted and takes the place of the nonexistent hair cells in detecting sound and generating nerve impulses.

Problems of balance may sometimes be treated successfully with drugs to limit the swelling in the labyrinth. Ringing in the ears (tinnitus) is usually resolved when the underlying condition is resolved. In some cases, tinnitus is caused by drugs (large doses of aspirin, for example) and will cease when the drugs are stopped.

Doctors who specialize in diagnosis and treatment of disorders of the ear and who do these surgeries are called otorhinolaryngologists (ear, nose, and throat doctors). They are medical doctors who have several years of training beyond medical school in surgery and in problems of the ear, nose, and throat.

PERSPECTIVE AND PROSPECTS

The basic anatomy of the ear has been known for some time. Bartolommeo Eustachio (1520-1574), an Italian anatomist, first described the Eustachian tube as well as a number of the nerves and muscles involved in the functioning of the ear. An understanding of how the ear functions to discriminate the pitch of sounds, however, was not arrived at until the twentieth century. Georg von Békésy won the Nobel Prize in Physiology or Medicine in 1961 for his work on the acoustics of the ear and how it functions to analyze sounds of varying frequencies (pitch).

Treatment of diseases of the ear has been radically changed by the advent of antibiotics. Older texts describe rupture of the eardrum by middle-ear fluid as a desired outcome of middle-ear infection, one which would ensure that the infection drained and healed, rather than becoming chronic.

Chronic ear infections used to be associated with diseases such as tuberculosis, measles, and syphilis, which themselves became far less common with the widespread use of antibiotics or vaccines. In the past, chronic ear infections were much more likely to result in mastoiditis, or infection of the air spaces of the mastoid bone, requiring surgical removal of the infected portions of the mastoid bone.

Adenoids and tonsils were frequently removed from patients with recurrent ear infections, as these were thought to be the source of the reinfection. It is now known that these tissues are involved in the formation of immunity to infectious bacteria and viruses. Their removal is not advocated in most circumstances— except, for example, when they are large enough to block the opening of the Eustachian tube.

Reconstructive surgery began in the 1950's with the development by Samuel Rosen and others of the operation to free up the calcified stapes bone in cases of otosclerosis. Today virtually all the components of the middle ear can be replaced.

While ear infections used to be much more dangerous, perhaps there is an equal danger today of taking threats to the ears too lightly. Chronic ear infections can still cause permanent hearing loss and even become life-threatening infections if left untreated. Damage involving the inner ear remains untreatable, as do many cases of tinnitus and loss of balance. Because the largest source of inner ear damage is prolonged exposure to noise, the prevention of damage is far more effective than treatment.

—*Pamela J. Baker, Ph.D.*

See also Altitude sickness; Anatomy; Audiology; Balance disorders; Biophysics; Deafness; Dyslexia; Ear infections and disorders; Ear surgery; Hearing loss; Hearing tests; Ménière's disease; Motion sickness; Myringotomy; Nervous system; Neurology; Neurology, pediatric; Otoplasty; Otorhinolaryngology; Plastic surgery; Sense organs; Speech disorders; Systems and organs.

FOR FURTHER INFORMATION:

Gelfand, Stanley A. *Essentials of Audiology*. 2d ed. New York: Thieme, 2001. Undergraduate text covering a wide range of relevant topics, including acoustics, anatomy and physiology, sound perception, auditory disorders, and the nature of hearing impairment.

Katz, Jack, ed. *Handbook of Clinical Audiology*. 5th ed. Philadelphia: Lippincott Williams & Wilkins, 2002. Text that examines advances in the scientific, clinical, and philosophical understanding of audiology. Sections of the book cover behavioral tests, physiologic tests, special populations, and the management of hearing disorders.

Leikin, Jerrold B., and Martin S. Lipsky, eds. *American Medical Association Complete Medical Encyclopedia*. New York: Random House Reference, 2003. Includes a nondetailed, readable description of the anatomy of the ear and a complete listing of common ailments, each with a section on treatment that includes "self-help" and "professional help." Good illustrations and some photographs are provided.

Mendel, Lisa Lucks, Jeffrey L. Danhauer, and Sadanand Singh. *Singular's Illustrated Dictionary of Audiology*. San Diego, Calif.: Singular, 1999. A comprehensive reference guide to the field that includes numerous photographs, charts, and diagrams. Appendixes cover acronyms, illustrations, topic categories, and physical quantities.

Nettina, Sandra M., ed. *The Lippincott Manual of Nursing Practice*. 8th ed. Philadelphia: Lippincott Williams & Wilkins, 2006. Presents hearing problems and other problems of the ear, each in outline form, with sections including clinical manifestations, management, and patient education. Contains an extensive bibliography.

Pender, Daniel J. *Practical Otology*. Philadelphia: J. B. Lippincott, 1992. A well-illustrated text on diseases of the ear and their surgical correction.

Zuckerman, Barry S., and Pamela A. M. Zuckerman. *Child Health: A Pediatrician's Guide for Parents*. New York: Hearst Books, 1986. A very readable description of the ear ailments and treatments most common to children. Includes sections on swimmer's ear, otitis media, glue ear, ear tubes, hearing tests, and other topics.

EATING DISORDERS
DISEASE/DISORDER

ANATOMY OR SYSTEM AFFECTED: Abdomen, bones, gastrointestinal system, intestines, mouth, psychic-emotional system, reproductive system, stomach, teeth, throat

SPECIALTIES AND RELATED FIELDS: Dentistry, family medicine, pediatrics, psychiatry, psychology

DEFINITION: A group of conditions characterized by disordered eating patterns, preoccupation with body size and weight, and distorted body image. Eating disorders can cause serious medical complications and even death. The causes of eating disorders are complex and involve biological, psychological, and societal factors.

KEY TERMS:

amenorrhea: the absence of menstruation

antidepressant: medication used to treat depression

cardiomyopathy: disease of the heart muscle

diuretic: an agent that promotes the secretion of urine

fast: to abstain from food

laxative: an agent that promotes evacuation of the bowel

osteopenia: reduced bone mass

osteoporosis: demineralization of the bone

neurotransmitters: chemicals in the brain that stimulate activity

pharmacotherapy: the treatment of disease with medication

satiety: the state of feeling full or fed and free from hunger

serotonin: the neurotransmitter associated with pain perception, sleep, impulsivity, and aggression; implicated in disorders associated with anxiety, depression, and migraines

CAUSES AND SYMPTOMS

Identified eating disorders include anorexia nervosa, bulimia nervosa, and binge-eating disorder. These disorders are not always distinct, and many individuals exhibit symptoms of more than one. Their prevalence has increased during the past several decades. Anorexia nervosa and bulimia nervosa predominantly affect adolescent and young adult females. However, they can also occur in males and the elderly, and binge-eating disorder occurs more frequently in males. Approximately 4 percent of females have eating disorders, although the number of those who do not meet the full criteria for diagnosing any specific disorder is much higher. There is an approximately 9 to 1 ratio of females to males with eating disorders. The incidence of eating disorders in males is rising, however, and they

---

INFORMATION ON EATING DISORDERS

CAUSES: Psychological disorder

SYMPTOMS: Intense preoccupation with food and weight, disordered eating; may include ingestion of laxatives, depression and suicidal feelings, nutritional deficiencies, dehydration, hormonal changes, gastrointestinal problems, changes in metabolism, heart disorders, persistent sore throat, teeth and gum damage

DURATION: Chronic

TREATMENTS: Psychotherapy, nutritional counseling, medication

---

are most commonly associated with sports (such as wrestling), bodybuilding, and the performing arts (such as dance). The disorders can be chronic and recur across the life span of an individual. Recognition of eating disorders in the elderly has increased, as have the negative health affects of the conditions on this population.

Anorexia nervosa is characterized by refusal to maintain normal body weight (less than 85 percent of expected weight), extreme fear of becoming fat, and relentless pursuit of thinness. Individuals with anorexia nervosa have a distorted perception of body weight and size and consider themselves to be overweight even when the opposite is true. Their view of themselves is heavily dependent on factors such as their level of adherence to a restrictive diet or the fit of their clothes. They often deny the negative aspects of low weight even in the face of serious health problems.

Two types of anorexia nervosa have been identified: the restricting type, involving dieting, fasting, or skipping meals, but not bingeing/purging; and the binge-eating/purging type, involving binge eating and purging (self-induced vomiting or misusing laxatives, enemas, or diuretics). The latter type is primarily distinguished from bulimia nervosa by refusal to maintain 85 percent of normal body weight. Dieting regimens may be severe, with intake reduced to between 300 and 600 kilocalories (Calories) per day and strict habits regarding food selection and eating.

Individuals with anorexia nervosa commonly display a set of personality and behavioral characteristics including being goal driven, perfectionistic, and overtly competent at school or work. Underlying these tendencies is often a lack of confidence and low sense of self-worth. As dieting increases, individuals may become depressed and fatigued, causing school or work to suffer and further eroding self-perception. Rigid "all or nothing" thinking influences the severity of dieting. Thus, anorexic people might believe that if they permit themselves even one lapse in dieting, then they will become obese. As starvation develops, focus on food and weight increases, and behaviors such as hoarding food, gazing in mirrors, or seeking reassurance about appearance may be observed. Significant energy is expended to keep secret the severity of weight loss efforts. Consequently, exercise may be conducted privately, family meals and public eating avoided, or food disposed of surreptitiously. In some cases, anorexia nervosa is not discovered until after a health problem has developed consequent to malnutrition.

A number of serious health problems stemming from starvation and malnutrition are seen in people with anorexia nervosa. Among the most serious are those associated with cardiac functioning, including cardiomyopathy, arrhythmias, and altered heart rates. In rare cases, sudden death can occur as a result of irregular heart muscle contractions. Other health problems caused by anorexia nervosa involve the gastrointestinal system (bloating and constipation), the reproductive system (amenorrhea, hormonal abnormalities, and infertility), and the skeletal system (osteoporosis and osteopenia). Additional complications include lowered metabolism, cold intolerance, weakness, loss of muscle mass, low body temperature, and growth suppression. While elderly individuals with anorexia nervosa may not exhibit a drive for thinness, behaviors such as food refusal, the hoarding or hiding of food, and distorted body image are often observed. The health effects of anorexia nervosa in this population are significant and worsen coexisting illnesses, sometimes hastening death. A very serious condition known as the "female athlete triad" is a combination of factors involving athletic training: disordered eating, amenorrhea, and osteoporosis. Permanent damage to bone strength can result from this condition. Despite the numerous medical problems caused by anorexia nervosa, many with the disorder appear superficially healthy even after significant weight loss.

Bulimia nervosa is characterized by recurrent episodes of binge eating followed by purging or other inappropriate efforts to avoid weight gain. The episodes are accompanied by feelings of being out of control and subsequent self-disgust, guilt, and depression. Bingeing involves eating over a limited period of time an amount of food that is markedly larger than most people would under similar circumstances. Caloric intake during binges may range from 2,000 to 10,000. Social interruption, fear of discovery, or physical discomfort (nausea or abdominal pain) typically terminates the binge episode. The binge-purge cycle may occur several times per day, with considerable effort directed toward keeping the episodes secret. Typically, bulimics recognize that their behavior is abnormal and desire to change (as opposed to those with anorexia nervosa). The disorder is divided into two types. The purging type involves self-induced vomiting or laxative, diuretic, or enema misuse as methods to avoid weight gain. The nonpurging type involves fasting or excessive exercise to prevent weight gain.

Self-induced vomiting is the most frequent method of purging and is typically accomplished by initiating the gag reflex by placing fingers down the throat. Over time, many bulimics are able to vomit reflexively without the need to use their fingers. Though employed less frequently as the sole methods of purging, laxatives, enemas, and rarely diuretics may be used in conjunction with vomiting. Abuse of laxatives is more common among the elderly.

Individuals with nonpurging bulimia nervosa, especially males, engage in hours of exercise every day or fast following bingeing. Typically, the fast is broken by another binge episode and the cycle continues.

Those with bulimia nervosa place strong emphasis on appearance, and their mood and view of themselves are highly dependent on their weight and body shape. Most are at a normal weight, but some are underweight or overweight. Often bulimia nervosa is initiated by a restrictive diet that appears to cause many of the unusual behaviors and thinking patterns associated with anorexia nervosa, such as secretive behavior, food hoarding, and extreme focus on food and eating. There may be signs of depression and anxiety as well as compulsive behavior. As opposed to anorexia nervosa, those with bulimia nervosa are more likely to be interested in social relations and to worry more about how others perceive them. Some engage in impulsive behaviors such as substance abuse or shoplifting.

Serious medical complications can result from bulimia nervosa. Chronic vomiting or laxative abuse and consequent loss of body fluids may cause dizziness, cardiac abnormalities, dehydration, and weakness. Tooth decay caused by repeated exposure to gastric acids from vomiting may occur. Erosion or tearing of the esophagus can result from chronic vomiting. Bingeing is associated with a variety of gastrointestinal disturbances including bloating, diarrhea, and constipation.

Binge-eating disorder is a relatively newly identified condition, and less is known about it. The disorder is similar to bulimia nervosa but does not involve efforts to avoid weight gain (such as purging). Individuals with the disorder regularly engage in binges lasting up to several hours, during which from 2,000 to 10,000 Calories may be consumed. Eating during binges is typically at a rapid pace and continues in spite of feeling discomfort or pain. Bingeing may occur when an individual is not very hungry, after attempting to keep a strict diet, or as a means to reduce stress. It is usually done in private and kept secret. Feeling out of control during binges is common, followed by feelings of self-disgust and shame. Preoccupation with food and unusual food-related behaviors (such as hiding food) are common. Individuals with binge-eating disorder are typically overweight and unhappy with their body shape and size. General mood and self-perception may be dependent on their weight and size. Depression and anxiety are common coexisting conditions. Distorted body image is less likely than with anorexia nervosa and bulimia nervosa. The health problems related to obesity are seen in those with binge-eating disorder. They include high blood pressure, diabetes, high cho-lesterol, and heart disease. Gastrointestinal problems may also result from bingeing.

The precise causes of eating disorders are unknown; however, a number of factors involving biological, psychological, and social variables have been identi-fied as contributing to the conditions. The primary bio-logical influences on all eating disorders are related to hunger and starvation. Research indicates that in healthy individuals, severe dieting produces moodiness, irritability, depression, food obsessions, social isola-tion, and apathy. These symptoms are also found in eating disorders and become more pronounced as starvation emerges. Thus, an-orexia nervosa, bulimia nervosa, or binge-eating disorder may de-velop after food deprivation has occurred as a result of purposeful dieting in order to lose weight or enhance athletic performance, or consequent to food restriction re-sulting from illness (especially in the elderly) or stress. Hunger re-sulting from restrictive dieting is the major stimulus for bingeing. Because a majority of those who diet do not develop eating disor-ders, there is likely some as yet unidentified biological or genetic predisposition in some individu-als. Biological abnormalities as-sociated with the hypothalamus and thyroid gland have been iden-tified in some individuals with anorexia nervosa, while other re-search points to neurochemical or hormonal imbalances. In the elderly, medications, coexisting health problems, and even poorly fitting dentures may initiate re-stricted eating, leading to an-orexia nervosa. Irregular levels of the neurotransmitter serotonin may influence bingeing in bu-limia nervosa and binge-eating disorder since it is associated with triggering signals of satiety to the brain. Knowledge of the causes of binge-eating disorder is lim-ited; however, as with bulimia

---

IN THE NEWS:
GENETIC LINKS TO EATING DISORDERS

A study published in the April, 2003, volume of the *International Journal of Eating Disorders* revealed substantial heritability for obe-sity and moderate heritability for binge eating among 2,163 female twins. The study also showed that obesity and binge eating share a moderate genetic correlation. Another study published in the same vol-ume demonstrated that some genetic influences may be activated dur-ing puberty, suggesting that age-related development may be an impor-tant factor to consider in the study of eating disorders. This study used 530 twins who were eleven years of age and 602 twins who were seven-teen years of age from the Minnesota Twins Family Study. The genetic contribution was zero in the eleven-year-olds but 55 percent in the seventeen-year-olds. The correlation of developmental stage with eat-ing disorders was also highlighted in a 2001 issue of *Aging and Mental Health*, which reported on anorexia and the elderly.

The February, 2003, issue of *Clinical Psychology Review* presented a review of relevant literature suggesting that disorders such as an-orexia nervosa and bulimia nervosa may also share relationships with other conditions that have genetic contributions. For instance, both dis-orders may be associated with depression, and anorexia has been asso-ciated with obsessive-compulsive disorder.

Similarly, a study of 256 female twins reported in a 2002 issue of *Journal of Abnormal Psychology* suggested that eating disorders might be related to inherited personality characteristics. In this study, the re-sults indicated that phenotypic associations between the Multidimen-sional Personality Questionnaire and the Eating Disorders Inventory were more likely to be genetic; however, their shared genetic variance was limited. Thus, personality may play a role in the expression of eat-ing disorders, but this role may be limited.

Together, these studies suggest that genetics and environment play roles in the development of various eating disorders. They also suggest that more than one mechanism may account for these contributions re-lated to factors such as psychiatric conditions (depression or anxiety), personality factors, and even age-related development.

—Nancy A. Piotrowski, Ph.D.

nervosa, there often is a history of being overweight or obese prior to developing the disorder.

A number of psychological factors have been identified as causing eating disorders. Most of these are not mutually exclusive, and none has been universally accepted as the primary causative factor for the conditions. Factors proposed to account for anorexia nervosa include phobic responses to food and weight gain, conflicted feelings over adolescent development and sexual maturity, and reactions to feelings of personal ineffectiveness by "controlling" hunger and the body. Faulty thinking, known as cognitive distortions, may cause misperceptions in body image and undue emphasis on the importance of appearance. Powerful needs to demonstrate self-discipline and to develop feelings of uniqueness and independence may also contribute to anorexia nervosa. Individuals with bulimia nervosa often exhibit mood fluctuations as well as impulsive behaviors. Bulimia nervosa is thought by some to be a variant of obsessive-compulsive disorder (OCD) in which bingeing results from irresistible urges to eat and purging is engaged in to alleviate overwhelming anxiety. Fewer psychological causes have been identified in binge-eating disorder. Some research suggests that characteristics seen in bulimia nervosa such as impulsivity and mood changes are also associated with this disorder. Depression, especially in the elderly population, appears to play a role in all eating disorders. Middle-aged and elderly individuals may employ behaviors such as extreme dieting, bingeing, and purging to reduce anxiety or to exert control in their lives.

Societal factors appear to also contribute to eating disorders. Popular media increasingly promotes physical appearance, and thinness is held up as the ideal body type. Since the 1950's, there have been steady decreases in the weights of influential persons such as actors, fashion models, and musicians. Many popular role models for females and males are underweight. Significant social approval is often associated with weight loss and disapproval with weight gain. Thus, females and males may feel pressured to attain an unhealthy weight or unrealistic body shape. A number of Internet sites are devoted to promoting anorexia nervosa and bulimia nervosa as a means of personal choice and self-expression and minimizing the medical and psychological damage caused by these disorders. No reliable family characteristics have been conclusively associated with eating disorders; however, some families appear to have higher than usual levels of depression, difficulties in communication, conflict, and focus on weight and appearance.

TREATMENT AND THERAPY

Treatment of eating disorders incorporates medical, behavioral, and psychological interventions. Typically, those with anorexia nervosa believe that their diet is justified, and resistance to treatment is the norm. Males may be especially resistant. Weight restoration is the central focus of initial treatment. Hospitalization is recommended for persons with more serious medical complications or who have less than 75 percent of expected weight. During hospitalization, daily monitoring of weight and caloric intake occurs, as well as any other necessary medical management. Behavioral therapy is employed to facilitate eating habits, and privileges such as social activity or family visits are made dependent upon increased eating and daily weight gains. Individual and family therapy are introduced as malnutrition eases and irritability, depression, and preoccupation with diet diminishes. Lengths of hospital stays vary from weeks to months depending on severity of illness and treatment progress.

Outpatient treatment may be recommended with individuals who have less severe medical complications, who are motivated to cooperate with treatment, and who have families that can independently monitor diet and health status. Weight restoration is facilitated by supervision of caloric intake and regular measurements as well as behavioral therapy techniques. Individual therapy focuses on altering cognitive distortions and assumptions about diet, weight, and body image and developing more effective means of dealing with stress. Family therapy aims to improve communication patterns, eating habits, and supportive behaviors.

No medications have been identified as effective agents in treating the core symptoms of anorexia nervosa. Medications that promote hunger may be used during the initial stages of treatment to facilitate eating. Also, medications to treat coexisting conditions such as depression and anxiety are often employed in the treatment regimen.

Most patients with bulimia nervosa do not require hospitalization unless medical complications are severe. Outpatient treatment involves individual psychotherapy, family therapy, and pharmacotherapy. Individual psychotherapy addresses cognitive distortions involving appearance and body image as well as behaviors, thoughts, and emotions that lead to binge episodes. Skills for problem solving and stress reduction are also taught. Treatment methods used for obsessive-compulsive disorder may also be employed, involving exposure to stimuli that usually trigger binge-purge behaviors while preventing them from occurring. Family therapy for bulimia nervosa aims at strengthening support and communication and developing healthy eating habits. With adolescents, impulsive behaviors associated with bulimia nervosa may be addressed by helping parents develop more effective methods of discipline and behavior management.

Antidepressant medications that regulate the neurotransmitter serotonin have been found to reduce bingeing, improve mood, and lesson preoccupation with weight and size. These same medications are useful in treating depression and anxiety, which are also commonly seen in those with bulimia nervosa.

Treatment of binge-eating disorder is similar to that of bulimia nervosa. Psychotherapy aims toward identifying and altering behaviors and feelings that lead to bingeing and developing effective methods of dealing with stress. Group therapy and weight loss programs with medical management may also be utilized. Antidepressants have also been found effective with binge-eating disorder.

PERSPECTIVE AND PROSPECTS

Behaviors associated with eating disorders have been identified in the earliest writings of Western civilization, including those by the ancient Greeks and early Christians. Formal identification of eating disorders as medical illnesses occurred in the nineteenth century when case studies were first recorded. Treatment methods at that time were limited and often involved "mental hygiene" measures such as rest, fresh air, and cold or hot baths.

In the early to mid-twentieth century, psychological theories influenced by Sigmund Freud, an Austrian psychiatrist, dominated treatment methods for eating disorders. These conditions were viewed as resulting from early childhood experiences that caused problems with psychological and sexual development. Treatment involved psychoanalysis, a form of psychotherapy, often lasting several years. Limited evidence for the success of this approach caused its decline in use.

More recent and successful treatment approaches involve cognitive and behavioral therapy that aims to alter thinking and behavior contributing to eating disorders. Medications have increasingly been used in treating eating disorders since the 1980's. Identifying biological causes of the conditions and refining pharmacotherapy may offer the best hope for improving treatment in the future.

Eating disorders were once thought to occur exclusively among young Caucasian females from middle- and upper-class families. Consequently, research into the disorders has historically focused on this population. Increased awareness of the illnesses has revealed that they occur in all socioeconomic classes and races, as well as in males and the elderly. Additional research into these groups is needed.

Awareness of eating disorders and their dangers has expanded among the general public since the 1970's. Nevertheless, rates of these disorders are rising. The media publicizes celebrities' struggles with these conditions, which may glamorize the illnesses even when negative aspects are reported. Establishing healthy eating habits and identifying potential problems early constitute the current focus of prevention efforts in medicine and education.

—*Paul F. Bell, Ph.D.*

See also Addiction; Amenorrhea; Anorexia nervosa; Anxiety; Appetite loss; Bariatric surgery; Bulimia; Depression; Hyperadiposis; Malnutrition; Nutrition; Obesity; Obesity, childhood; Obsessive-compulsive disorder; Psychiatric disorders; Psychiatry; Psychiatry, child and adolescent; Puberty and adolescence; Sports medicine; Stress; Vitamins and minerals; Weight loss and gain; Weight loss medications; Women's health.

FOR FURTHER INFORMATION:

American Psychiatric Association. *Diagnostic and Statistical Manual of Mental Disorders: DSM-IV-TR*. 4th rev. ed. Washington, D.C.: Author, 2000. A manual used by most mental health professionals to diagnose patients. It details the diagnostic criteria for mental health disorders, including eating disorders, identified by the American Psychiatric Association.

Duyff, Roberta Larson, ed. *365 Days of Healthy Eating from the American Dietetic Association*. Hoboken, N.J.: John Wiley & Sons, 2003. A guide for developing healthy eating habits. Provides practical recommendations for making good food choices, as well as preparation suggestions and recipes that promote healthy nutrition. Offers strategies for incorporating exercise and health-promoting activity into daily living.

National Association of Anorexia Nervosa and Associated Disorders. http://www.anad.org/site/anadweb/. A site that provides hotline counseling, a national network of free support groups, referrals to health care professionals, and education and prevention programs to promote self-acceptance and healthy lifestyles.

Parker, James M., and Philip M. Parker, eds. *The 2002 Official Patient's Sourcebook on Binge Eating Disorder.* San Diego, Calif.: Icon Health, 2002. Draws from public, academic, government, and peer-reviewed research to provide a wide-ranging handbook for patients with this eating disorder.

Paterson, Anna. *Fit to Die: Men and Eating Disorders.* London: Sage Publications, 2004. This book examines the causes and effects of eating disorders in men. Issues are explored such as how depression, self-esteem, and the drive for fitness contribute to disordered eating and disturbed body image. It offers advice and hope for those experiencing the illnesses.

Sackler, Ira M., and Marc A. Zimmer. *Dying to Be Thin: Understanding and Defeating Anorexia Nervosa and Bulimia—A Practical, Lifesaving Guide.* New York: Warner Books, 1987. Includes case histories of individuals suffering from eating disorders, with accounts from patients, family members, and treatment professionals. The causes and symptoms of eating disorders are reviewed, and treatment options and resources are presented. Information included can be helpful to those who are concerned about eating disorders for themselves or loved ones.

Thompson, Ron A., and Roberta Trattner Sherman. *Helping Athletes with Eating Disorders.* Champaign, Ill.: Human Kinetics. 1993. This book examines the connection between sports and eating disorders and the characteristics of athletes that put them at risk. The effects of eating disorders on performance and methods for coaches to approach athletes with eating disorders are detailed.

EBOLA VIRUS
DISEASE/DISORDER

ANATOMY OR SYSTEM AFFECTED: Blood, circulatory system, gastrointestinal system, muscles, skin

SPECIALTIES AND RELATED FIELDS: Epidemiology, public health, virology

DEFINITION: A virus responsible for a severe and often fatal hemorrhagic fever.

KEY TERMS:

Filoviridae: the family to which the Ebola virus belongs

maculopapular rash: a discolored skin rash observed in patients with Ebola fever.

INFORMATION ON EBOLA VIRUS

CAUSES: Viral infection

SYMPTOMS: Severe blood clotting and hemorrhaging, fever, lethargy, appetite loss, headaches, muscle aches, skin rash

DURATION: Acute

TREATMENTS: None

CAUSES AND SYMPTOMS

The Ebola virus is named after the Ebola River in northern Zaire, Africa, where it was first detected in 1976, when hundreds of deaths were recorded there as well as in neighboring Sudan. Three subtypes of the virus cause human disease: Ebola-Zaire, Ebola-Sudan, and Ebola-Ivory Coast. A fatal disease among cynomolgus laboratory monkeys that were imported from the Philippines to Texas in 1996 was caused by Ebola-Reston, a fourth subtype of the virus that causes disease in non-human primates, but not in humans. An equally devastating outbreak among humans took place again in early 1995 in Kirkwit, 500 kilometers east of Kinshasha, Zaire; the disease claimed the lives of 244 patients out of 315 reported cases, a 77 percent fatality rate. It is interesting to note that the epidemic ended within a few months, as suddenly as it began; this puzzled scientists, who are still unaware of the causes and nature of this so-called hot virus. Despite the dreadful speed with which the disease killed its victims, scientists were happy that they contained it with a relatively small number of fatalities. Outbreaks in Africa have continued to occur; a recent outbreak in Sudan resulted in twenty cases with five deaths. Recently obtained historical documentation suggests the possibility that the Athenian plague at the beginning of the Peloponnesian War around 430 B.C.E. could be attributed to the Ebola virus.

The Ebola virus appears to have an incubation period of two to twenty-one days, after which time the impact is devastating. The patient develops appetite loss, increasing fever, headaches, and muscle aches. The next stage involves disseminated intravascular coagulation (DIC), a condition characterized by both blood clots and hemorrhaging. The clots usually form in vital internal organs such as the liver, spleen, and brain, with subsequent collapse of the neighboring capillaries. Other symptoms include vomiting, diarrhea with blood and mucus, and conjunctivitis. An unusual type of skin irritation known as maculopapular rash first appears in the trunk and quickly covers the rest of the body. The final stages of the disease involve a spontaneous hemorrhaging from all body outlets, coupled with shock and kidney failure and often death within eight to seventeen days.

TREATMENT AND THERAPY

The Ebola virus is classified as a ribonucleic acid (RNA) virus and is closely related to the Marburg virus, first discovered in 1967. The Marburg and the Ebola viruses are the only two members of the Filoviridae family, which was first established in 1987. Electron microscope studies show the Ebola virus as long filaments, 650 to 14,000 nanometers in length, that are often either branched or intertwined. Its virus part, known as the virion, contains one single noninfectious minus-strand RNA molecule and an endogenous RNA polymerase. The lipoprotein envelope contains a single glycoprotein, which behaves as the type-specific antigen. Spikes are approximately 7 nanometers in length, are spaced at approximately 10-nanometer intervals, and are visible on the virion surface. It is believed that once in the body, the virus produces proteins that suppress the organism's immune system, thus allowing its uninhibited reproduction. In 2002, researchers announced a new discovery about how Ebola makes entry into and subverts human cells. Findings show that the virus targets a "lipid raft," tiny fat platforms that float atop the membranes of human cells. These rafts act as gateways for the virus, the assembly platform for making new virus particles, and the exit point where new particles bud. This research is a significant step toward one day creating drugs that would stop viruses from replicating.

The Ebola virus can be transmitted through contact with body fluids, such as blood, semen, mucus, saliva, and even urine and feces. It is thought that the first person in an outbreak acquires the virus through contact with an infected animal, including carcasses of dead animals.

The level of infectivity of the Ebola virus is quite stable at room temperature. Its inactivation is accomplished via ultraviolet or gamma irradiation, 1 percent formalin, beta propiolactone, and an exposure to phenolic disinfectants and lipid solvents, such as deoxycholase and ether. The virus isolation is usually achieved from acute-phase serum of appropriate cell cultures, such as the Ebola-Sudan virus MA-104 cells from a fetal rhesus monkey kidney cell line. Satis-

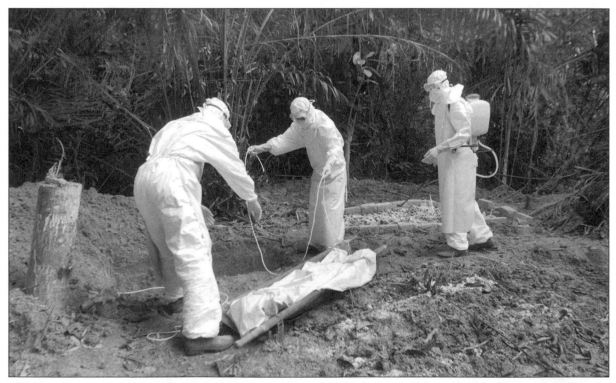

Workers wear protective clothing when burying a young victim of the Ebola virus in Gabon in 2001. (AP/Wide World Photos)

factory results have been accomplished using tissues obtained from the liver, spleen, lymph nodes, kidneys, and heart during autopsy. The virus isolation from brain and other nervous tissues, however, has been rather unsuccessful so far. Neutralization tests have been inconsistent for all filoviruses. Ebola strains, however, show cross-reactions in tests of immunofluorescence assays.

There appears to be no known or standard treatment for Ebola fever. No chemotherapeutic or immunization strategies are available, and no antiviral drug has been shown to provide positive results, even under in vitro conditions. Human interferon, human convalescent plasma, and anticoagulation therapy have been used with unconvincing results.

At this stage, therapy involves sustaining the desired fluid and electrolyte balance by the frequent administration of fluids. Bleeding may be fought off with blood and plasma transfusion. Sanitary conditions to avoid further contact with the disease are required. Proper decontamination of medical equipment, isolation of the patients from the rest of the community, and prompt disposal of infected tissues, blood, and even corpses limit the spread of the disease.

IN THE NEWS:
CONGO OUTBREAK OF EBOLA IN 2003

In December, 2002, reports that gorillas and chimpanzees were dying in remote forests within the northern region of the Republic of Congo alarmed Congolese authorities. In January, 2003, word spread of a possible outbreak of Ebola virus in the country's Cuvette-Ouest district. At that point in time, twelve people had died of apparent hemorrhagic fever in the town of Kelle, and four more persons had died at Mbomo. The previous year, in the same area, a similar episode had resulted in the deaths of forty-three people in the Republic of Congo and fifty-three residents of neighboring Gabon.

At the peak of the epidemic, most of the population of Kelle fled into the forest in the attempt to hide from the deadly virus. Volunteers from the Congolese Red Cross, clad in protective suits, cared for the sick and the elderly who were left behind. Few villagers believed that the epidemic was a natural disease brought about by eating infected primate meat—rather, they suspected witchcraft. Four teachers, accused of causing the outbreak, were reportedly killed by a mob.

Medical teams from the United Nations World Health Organization (WHO), the Red Cross, and Médecins Sans Frontières set up makeshift hospital wards in the affected area. The United States Centers for Disease Control (CDC) sent an expert epidemiologist. The European Commission's Humanitarian Aid Office appropriated 500,000 euros to support the relief work.

Aid workers began a public awareness campaign to halt the spread of the disease. The WHO held meetings with local leaders to assure them they could limit the outbreak by avoiding primate meat and by not touching the bodies of those sick with the disease. Heads of families were urged to refrain from washing deceased family members, a ritual required by traditional burial practices.

By late April, the epidemic appeared to be under control, and people began to return to their homes. Fears that the returning villagers might start a new series of infections after eating the meat of dead gorillas while hiding in the forest proved unfounded. Out of 144 reported cases, the disease claimed 126 lives, a death rate approaching 90 percent.

—*Milton Berman, Ph.D.*

PERSPECTIVE AND PROSPECTS

The puzzling characteristics of the Ebola virus are the location of its primary natural reservoir, its sudden eruption and the unknown reason for its quick end, and the unusual discovery of the virus in the organs of people who have survived it.

In the past, experimental work on the virus has been slow because of its high pathogenicity. The progress of recombinant deoxyribonucleic acid (DNA) technology has shed the first light on the molecular structure of this virus. It is hoped that further work using this technique

as well as the results of viruses of lower pathogenicity (such as the Reston virus) will provide the desired information on replication and virus-host interactions. Finally, the improvement of the various diagnostic tools will allow more accurate virus identification and assessment of transmission modes.

In 1995, the World Health Organization (WHO) investigators and epidemiologists captured about three thousand birds, rodents, and other animals and insects that are suspected of spreading the disease in order to investigate the source of the virus. The results, how-

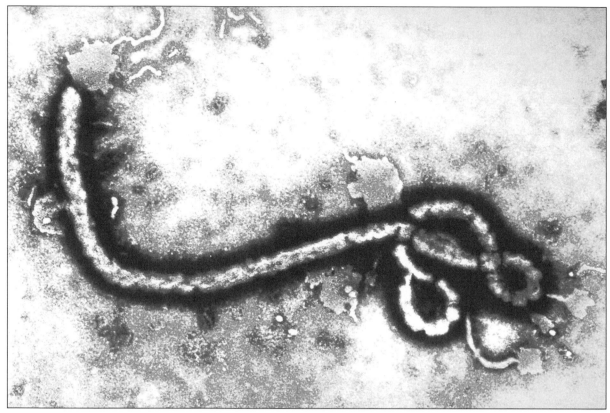

An enlarged view of the Ebola virus that causes African hemorrhagic fever. (Digital Stock)

ever, were obscure and inconclusive, and the main facts about the disease are still a mystery, with the exception of the established link between primates and Ebola virus infection in humans. This conclusion was reached after the fatal infection of a French researcher in Ivory Coast who performed an autopsy on a chimpanzee that had died from a disease with the same symptoms as Ebola fever. Yet, the human outbreaks in Zaire and the Sudan have not been traced to monkeys. As long as these puzzling questions linger, the disease should be contained, with particular emphasis on the improvement of sanitary conditions and the control of body fluid contact.

—*Soraya Ghayourmanesh, Ph.D.;*
updated by H. Bradford Hawley, M.D.
See also Bleeding; Centers for Disease Control and Prevention (CDC); Epidemiology; Marburg virus; Tropical medicine; Viral infections; Zoonoses.

FOR FURTHER INFORMATION:

Balter, Michael. "On the Trail of Ebola and Marburg Viruses." *Science* 290, no. 5493 (November 3, 2000): 923-925. Researchers are making headway on understanding hemorrhagic fever viruses. Perplexing to researchers is how Marburg and Ebola viruses cause such devastating symptoms as shock and massive bleeding.

Biddle, Wayne. *A Field Guide to Germs.* 2d ed. New York: Anchor Books, 2002. This comprehensive book is easily accessible to the nonspecialist and includes a discussion of nearly every virus, bacterium, and fungus known to cause human and nonhuman animal disease. The history of the microbe and the treatment of diseases are included.

Dyer, Nicole. "Killers Without Cures." *Science World* 57, no. 3 (October 2, 2000): 8-12. In the last thirty years, more than fifty lethal viruses once found only in animals have infected humans. A look at how virus hunters on a 1995 mission worked to stop a deadly outbreak of the Ebola virus in the Congo.

Jaax, Nancy. *Lethal Viruses, Ebola, and the Hot Zone: Worldwide Transmission of Fatal Viruses.* Lincoln: University of Nebraska Foundation, 1996. This text is based on a forum on world issues sponsored by the Cooper Foundation and the University of Nebraska at Lincoln. Illustrated.

Jahrling, Peter B., et al. "Filoviruses and Arenaviruses." In *Manual of Clinical Microbiology*, edited by Patrick R. Murray et al. 8th ed. Washington, D.C.: American Society of Microbiology, 2003. A chapter in a text devoted to medical and diagnostic microbiology. Includes bibliographical references and an index.

McGraw-Hill Encyclopedia of Science and Technology. 10th ed. 20 vols. New York: McGraw-Hill, 2007. A complete reference for the nonspecialist that offers thousands of articles written by world-renowned scientists and engineers. It includes many new and revised articles and extensive cross-references and bibliographies and is fully illustrated.

Peters, C. J., and J. W. LeDuc. "An Introduction to Ebola: The Virus and the Disease." *The Journal of Infectious Diseases* 179, supp. 1 (1999): ix-xvi. This paper is sponsored by the World Health Organization and the Centers for Disease Control and Prevention. Includes bibliographical references.

Strauss, James, and Ellen Strauss. *Viruses and Human Disease*. San Diego, Calif.: Academic Press, 2001. An undergraduate text that examines virology from a human disease perspective.

ECG OR EKG. *See* ELECTROCARDIOGRAPHY (ECG OR EKG).

ECHOCARDIOGRAPHY

PROCEDURE

ALSO KNOWN AS: Cardiac ultrasound, 2-D echo, stress echo

ANATOMY OR SYSTEM AFFECTED: Circulatory system, heart

SPECIALTIES AND RELATED FIELDS: Cardiology, critical care, emergency medicine, family medicine, internal medicine

DEFINITION: A diagnostic technique that uses ultrasound to display anatomical and physiological characteristics of the heart and related structures.

KEY TERMS:

stress echocardiography: echocardiography procedure performed while the heart is stressed, either with medications or by exercising on a treadmill

transducer: the tip of the ultrasound probe

transesophageal echocardiography: the method of performing echocardiography with the ultrasound probe inserted via the esophagus (food pipe)

transthoracic echocardiography: the routine method of performing echocardiography by placing the ultrasound probe on the chest

INDICATIONS AND PROCEDURES

Echocardiography is a technique that uses ultrasound waves to detect the structures of the heart. The most common indication for echocardiography is to evaluate chamber size, thickness of the heart muscle, valve abnormalities, and the flow of blood through the heart. The procedure is usually performed to evaluate the functioning of the heart in a patient with heart failure and can detect any damage to the heart muscles after a heart attack. In addition, valvular abnormalities of any of the four heart valves, such as thickening or leakage, can be detected. Other indications include evaluation of congenital or birth defects of the heart and fluid collection in the sac covering the heart (pericardial effusion). The use of a color Doppler further helps in assessing the velocity of blood flow through the heart.

Transthoracic echocardiography (TTE) is a simple outpatient, noninvasive procedure. While undergoing echocardiography, the patient lies down on his or her back and turns a little toward to the left so that the heart can be better visualized. The area on the left side of chest is wiped dry (no shaving is necessary), and a gel is applied over the skin for better conduction of the ultrasound waves. The operator then applies the transducer or the ultrasound probe over the chest, and two-dimensional images of the heart are seen on the attached monitor. Multiple still and motion pictures of the heart are recorded, which are then read by a cardiologist. The procedure takes about thirty minutes, and the patient is able to go home immediately after the procedure.

Special types of echocardiography include transesophageal echocardiography (TEE) and stress echocardiography. In TEE, the ultrasound probe is mounted on an endoscope and introduced into the esophagus. The structures at the back of the heart and valves are better visualized with this procedure. Stress echocardiography includes performing echocardiography while the patient is undergoing a stress test (while exercising on a treadmill or after medications such as dobutamine have been given). Both these procedures take a longer time and require experienced operators. Patients may be observed for a few hours after the procedure.

USES AND COMPLICATIONS

Echocardiography helps in identifying congenital heart defects such as tetralogy of Fallot, atrial and ventricular septal defects, valvular abnormalities such as stenosis (narrowing) or regurgitation (leaking) of the four heart valves, the functioning of the heart muscle after a heart attack, the collection of fluid in the sac covering the heart, the rupture of heart muscle, and the progression of heart failure.

Different modes of echocardiography are used in clinical practice. The most common is two-dimensional echocardiography (2-D echo), as described above, which detects cardiac structure and function and displays results in two dimensions. A newer, more expensive three-dimensional echocardiography is gaining popularity, as it displays the findings in a three-dimensional form and localizes specific lesions more accurately. Stress echocardiography is used to detect areas in the heart that have a reduced blood flow, especially during exercise or stress. This enables cardiologists to locate the diseased artery and correct it by stenting or by surgery. TEE specifically looks for blood clots in one of the heart chambers called the left atrium and also looks closely at infections of the valves (endocarditis).

TTE is a safe procedure without any known complications. Patients undergoing TEE or stress echocardiography are carefully screened before undergoing the procedure. Rare complications of stress echocardiography are chest pain and heart attack in patients with very poor circulation to the heart, and this procedure should not be performed in persons with ongoing heart attack symptoms. TEE rarely can cause rupture of the esophagus because of the invasive nature of the procedure. Occasionally, aspiration of food contents into the lungs can occur, and hence patients are required to have an empty stomach before the procedure. If complications do occur, then patients are hospitalized and treated appropriately.

PERSPECTIVES AND PROSPECTS

The term "echo' was first coined by the Roman architect Vesuvius during the rule of the Roman Empire. Karl Dussik first used ultrasound in medicine to outline the ventricles of the brain. The first use of ultrasound to examine the heart was by W. D. Keidel in the 1940's. Clinical echocardiography was initiated by Helmut Hertz and Inge Edler of Sweden using a commercial ultrasonoscope to examine the heart. Though echocardiography was introduced in the United States by John J. Wild, H. D. Crawford, and John Reid in 1960's, most of the credit for its further development and popularity goes to Harvey Feigenbaum at Indiana University.

Echocardiography is a great tool for assessing cardiac function. Recent echocardiography machines are portable and allow physicians to do bedside evaluation of the heart. Newer models are handheld, further enhancing ease of use. A role for echocardiography has been proposed in other systemic diseases such as diabetes, hypertension, pregnancy, kidney disease, and thyroid disease and also in the screening of athletes. Echocardiography is a cost-effective, versatile procedure that has a significant role in clinical medicine.

—*Venkat Raghavan Tirumala, M.D., M.H.A., M.S.*

See also Angiography; Arrhythmias; Arteriosclerosis; Cardiac rehabilitation; Cardiology; Cardiology, pediatric; Circulation; Congenital heart disease; Electrocardiography (ECG or EKG); Endocarditis; Exercise physiology; Heart attack; Heart disease; Heart failure; Hypertension; Imaging and radiology; Magnetic resonance imaging (MRI); Mitral valve prolapse; Noninvasive tests; Pacemaker implantation; Palpitations; Sports medicine; Ultrasonography; Vascular medicine; Vascular system.

FOR FURTHER INFORMATION:

Feigenbaum, Harvey, William F. Armstrong, and Thomas Ryan. *Feigenbaum's Echocardiography.* 6th ed. Philadelphia: Lippincott Williams & Wilkins, 2005. An interesting read authored by the "father of echocardiography" in the United States.

Kasper, Dennis L., et al., eds. *Harrison's Principles of Internal Medicine.* 16th ed. New York: McGraw-Hill, 2005. A textbook of medicine that includes an in-depth description of echocardiography.

Tierney, Lawrence M., Stephen J. McPhee, and Maxine A. Papadakis, eds. *Current Medical Diagnosis and Treatment 2007.* New York: McGraw-Hill Medical, 2006. An annually updated resource for medical topics.

ECLAMPSIA. *See* PREECLAMPSIA AND ECLAMPSIA.

ECTOPIC PREGNANCY
DISEASE/DISORDER
ALSO KNOWN AS: Tubal pregnancy

ANATOMY OR SYSTEM AFFECTED: Reproductive system

SPECIALTIES AND RELATED FIELDS: Embryology, gynecology

DEFINITION: The implantation of an embryo outside the uterine endometrium, most commonly in the Fallopian tube.

INFORMATION ON ECTOPIC PREGNANCY

CAUSES: Unknown; factors may include previous pelvic inflammatory disease, IUD use, tubal ligation, endometriosis, multiple abortions, pelvic adhesions

SYMPTOMS: Similar to those of early pregnancy, followed by spotting, cramping, abdominal pain (especially on one side); if Fallopian tube ruptures, bleeding and severe pain

DURATION: Acute

TREATMENTS: Only in early cases, methotrexate to end pregnancy; usually surgical removal of embryo and Fallopian tube

CAUSES AND SYMPTOMS

Although ectopic pregnancies can occur without any known cause, several factors increase a woman's risk. Studies have shown an increase in ectopic pregnancies in women with previous pelvic inflammatory disease (PID). An increase in such pregnancies is also seen in women who were using intrauterine devices (IUDs), especially those containing progesterone, at the time of conception and in women who had tubal ligations and other surgeries of the Fallopian tubes. Endometriosis, multiple induced abortions, and pelvic adhesions also may increase a woman's chance of ectopic pregnancy. In general, women whose Fallopian tubes are damaged for any reason have a higher risk. The risk is heightened because damage slows the progress of the developing embryo through the tube, allowing the embryo to be mature enough to implant itself before reaching the uterus. Another factor that may increase the chances of ectopic pregnancy is smoking. Nicotine slows the movement of cilia in the Fallopian tubes, thus slowing the progress of the embryo.

The symptoms of an early ectopic pregnancy are similar to those of any early pregnancy, except that spotting, cramping, and pain, especially on only one side of the abdomen, may occur as the embryo grows. Hormone levels mimic early pregnancy but usually do not rise as high as in a normal intrauterine implantation. If the tube ruptures, then bleeding and severe pain may occur.

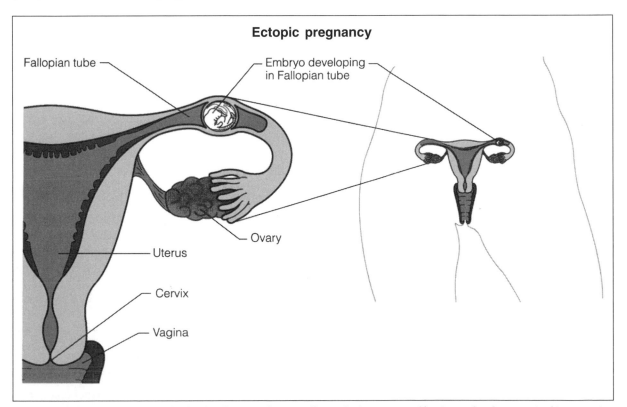

Ectopic pregnancy

Ectopic pregnancy results when the fertilized egg implants itself outside the uterus and begins to develop; surgical intervention is usually required.

TREATMENT AND THERAPY

If a tubal ectopic pregnancy is diagnosed early enough, methotrexate, a chemical that attacks quickly growing cells, may be administered. The drug causes the death of the embryo and flushes the material from the tube. Surgical removal is the most common treatment. The Fallopian tube may be split to remove the embryo, or all or part of the tube may be removed. Methotrexate may be administered to remove any remaining tissues from the pregnancy. Since there is no known way to implant the removed embryo in the uterus, surgical removal also results in the death of the embryo.

—*Richard W. Cheney, Jr., Ph.D.*

See also Conception; Contraception; Genital disorders, female; Miscarriage; Obstetrics; Pregnancy and gestation; Women's health.

FOR FURTHER INFORMATION:

Carson, Sandra Ann, ed. *Ectopic Pregnancy*. Philadelphia: Lippincott-Raven, 1999.

Hey, Valerie, et al., eds. *Hidden Loss: Miscarriage and Ectopic Pregnancy*. 2d ed. London: Women's Press, 1997.

Leach, Richard E., and Steven J. Ory, eds. *Management of Ectopic Pregnancy*. Malden, Mass.: Blackwell Science, 2000.

Stabile, Isabel. *Ectopic Pregnancy: Diagnosis and Management*. New York: Cambridge University Press, 1996.

ECZEMA

DISEASE/DISORDER

ALSO KNOWN AS: Dermatitis

ANATOMY OR SYSTEM AFFECTED: Skin

SPECIALTIES AND RELATED FIELDS: Dermatology, pediatrics

DEFINITION: An inflammation of the skin.

CAUSES AND SYMPTOMS

The term "eczema" refers to a noncontagious inflammation of the skin. Several types of eczema exist, resulting in a range of symptoms that vary in appearance, duration, and severity. The common characteristic, however, is red, dry, and itchy skin. Other symptoms may include scaling, thickening, or cracking of the skin, leading to infections and severe discomfort.

Atopic dermatitis, the most common form of eczema, is characterized by itchy and cracked skin of the cheeks, arms, and legs. The onset of this chronic type of eczema occurs most often during infancy or childhood,

---

INFORMATION ON ECZEMA

CAUSES: Genetic sensitivity to irritants (soaps, detergents, rough clothes), allergens (certain foods, pollen, animal dander), and climate or temperature changes

SYMPTOMS: Red, dry, and itchy skin; scaling, thickening, or cracking of skin

DURATION: Often chronic

TREATMENTS: Minimal exposure to irritants, drugs (corticosteroid creams and ointments, antihistamines, antibiotics); in severe cases, oral corticosteroids or phototherapy

---

although symptoms may continue into adulthood. The cause of atopic dermatitis is thought to be a hereditary predisposition to skin sensitivities to various environmental factors. These factors include irritants such as soaps, detergents, and rough clothes; allergens such as certain foods, pollen, or animal dander; and changes in climate or temperature. Other forms of eczema, such as contact dermatitis, have similar environmental causes. Seborrheic eczema, nummular eczema, and dishydrotic eczema may result from a combination of several possible causes. Emotional factors, such as stress or frustration, may aggravate the symptoms.

The diagnosis of eczema requires a careful and detailed observation of symptoms. Family and personal medical histories are often useful to determine the presence of allergies or exposure to allergens or irritants. Dermatologists may also use skin biopsies or blood tests to determine a tendency toward elevated allergic or immune response.

TREATMENT AND THERAPY

The treatment of eczema involves minimizing exposure to possible causes while at the same time managing symptoms to maintain a high quality of life. Identifying known allergens and irritants specific to the individual is an important first step. Lifestyle changes aimed at avoiding exposure to these possible causes can lower the frequency and duration of symptoms dramatically. Proper skin care to avoid excessive drying of the skin, including the use of moisturizers or creams and minimizing exposure to water, may also help reduce skin irritation. Avoiding scratching of existing irritations and eliminating sources of emotional stress are other ways that patients can lessen the severity of their symptoms. Dermatologists may prescribe additional treatments, such as corticosteroid creams and ointments, antihistamines, or antibiotics. In more severe cases, systemic corticosteroid treatments or phototherapy, the use of ultraviolet (UV) light, may be tried.

The approval of a new type of treatment for eczema called topical immunomodulators has changed the way eczema is treated in recent years. This new class of drug counteracts the inflammation of the skin without interfering in the body's normal immune response. This treatment has been successful in preventing and even eliminating symptoms of eczema.

—Paul J. Frisch

See also Allergies; Dermatitis; Dermatology; Dermatology, pediatric; Itching; Rashes; Skin; Skin disorders; Wiskott-Aldrich syndrome.

FOR FURTHER INFORMATION:

Fry, Lionel. *An Atlas of Atopic Eczema*. New York: Parthenon, 2004.

National Eczema Society. http://www.eczema.org/.

Rakel, Robert E., and Edward T. Bope, eds. *Conn's Current Therapy 2007*. Philadelphia: W. B. Saunders, 2006.

Ring, J., B. Przybilla, and T. Ruzicka, eds. *Handbook of Atopic Eczema*. 2d ed. New York: Springer, 2006.

Turkington, Carol A., and Jeffrey S. Dover. *Skin Deep: An A-Z of Skin Disorders, Treatments, and Health.* Updated ed. New York: Facts On File, 1998.

Westcott, Patsy. *Eczema: Recipes and Advice to Provide Relief.* New York: Welcome Rain, 2000.

EDEMA

DISEASE/DISORDER

ANATOMY OR SYSTEM AFFECTED: Blood vessels, circulatory system, liver, lungs, lymphatic system, respiratory system, skin

SPECIALTIES AND RELATED FIELDS: Internal medicine, nephrology, pulmonary medicine

DEFINITION: Accumulation of fluid in body tissues that may indicate a variety of diseases, including cardiovascular, kidney, liver, and medication problems.

KEY TERMS:

extracellular fluid: the fluid outside cells; includes the fluid within the vascular system and the lymphatic system and the fluid surrounding individual cells

hydrostatic pressure: the physical pressure on a fluid, such as blood; it tends to push fluids across membranes toward areas of lower pressure

interstitial fluid: the fluid between the vascular system and cells; nutrients from the vascular compartment must diffuse across the interstitial compartment to enter the cells

intracellular fluid: the fluid within cells

intravascular fluid: the fluid carried within the blood vessels; it is in a constant state of motion because of the pumping action of the heart

osmotic pressure: the ability of a concentrated fluid on one side of a membrane to draw water away from a less concentrated fluid on the other side

PROCESS AND EFFECTS

Edema is not a disease, but a condition that may be caused by a number of diseases. It signals a breakdown in the body's fluid-regulating mechanisms. The body's water can be envisioned as divided into three compartments: the intracellular compartment, the interstitial compartment, and the vascular compartment. The intracellular compartment consists of the fluid contained within the individual cells. The vascular compartment consists of all the water that is contained within the heart, the arteries, the capillaries, and the veins. The last compartment, and in many ways the most important for a discussion of edema, is called the interstitial compartment. This compartment includes all the water not contained in either the cells or the blood vessels. The interstitial compartment contains all the fluids between the intracellular compartment and the vascular compartment and the fluid in the lymphatic system. The sizes of these compartments are approximately as follows: intracellular fluid at 66 percent, interstitial fluid at 25 percent, and the vascular fluid at only 8 percent of the total body water.

When the interstitial compartment becomes overloaded with fluid, edema develops. To understand the physiology of edema formation, it may be helpful to follow a molecule of water as it travels through the various compartments, beginning when the molecule enters the aorta soon after leaving the heart. The blood has just been ejected from the heart under high pressure, and it speedily begins its trip through the body. It passes from the great vessel, the aorta, into smaller and smaller arteries that divide and spread throughout the body. At each branching, the pressure and speed of the water molecule decrease. Finally, the molecule enters a capillary, a vessel so small that red blood cells must flow in a single file. The wall of this vessel is composed only of the membrane of a single capillary cell. There are small passages between adjacent capillary cells leading to the interstitial compartment, but they are normally closed.

The hydrostatic pressure on the water molecule is much lower than when it was racing through the aorta, but it is still higher than that of the surrounding interstitial compartment. At the arterial end of the capillary, the blood pressure is sufficient to overcome the barrier of the capillary cell's membrane. A fair number of water and other molecules are pushed through the membrane into the interstitial compartment.

In the interstitial compartment, the water molecule is essentially under no pressure, and it floats amid glucose molecules, oxygen molecules, and many other compounds. Glucose and oxygen molecules enter the cells, and when the water molecule is close to a glucose molecule it is taken inside a cell with that molecule. The water molecule is eventually expelled by the cell, which has produced extra water from the metabolic process.

Back in the interstitial compartment, the molecule floats with a very subtle flow toward the venous end of the capillary. This occurs because, as the arterial end of the capillary pushes out water molecules, it loses hydrostatic pressure, eventually equaling the pressure of the interstitial compartment. Once the pressure equalizes, another phenomenon that has been thus far overshadowed by the hydrostatic pressure takes over—osmotic pressure. Osmotic pressure is the force exercised by a concentrated fluid that is separated by a membrane from a less concentrated fluid. It draws water molecules across the membrane from the less concentrated side. The more concentrated the fluid, the greater is the drawing power. The ratio of nonwater molecules to water molecules determines concentration.

The fluid that stays within the capillary remains more concentrated than the interstitial fluid for two rea-sons. First, the plasma proteins in the vascular compartment are too large to be forced across the capillary membrane; albumin is one such protein. These proteins stay within the vascular compartment and maintain a relatively concentrated state, compared to the interstitial compartment. At the same time, the concentration of the fluid in the interstitial compartment is being lowered constantly by the cellular compartment's actions. Cells remove molecules of substances such as glucose to metabolize, and afterward they release water—a by-product of the metabolic process. Both processes conspire to lower the total concentration of the interstitial compartment. The net result of this process is that water molecules return to the capillaries at the venous end because of osmotic pressure.

The water molecule is caught by this force and is returned to the vascular compartment. Back in the capillary, the molecule's journey is not yet complete. Now in a tiny vein, it moves along with blood. On the venous side of the circulatory system, the process of branching is reversed, and small veins join to form increasingly larger ones. The water molecule rides along in these progressively larger veins. The pressure surrounding the molecule is still low, but it is now higher than the pressure at the venous end of the capillary. One may wonder how this is possible if the venous pressure at the beginning of the venous system is essentially zero, and there is only one pump, the heart, in the body. As the molecule flows through the various veins, it occasionally passes one-way valves that allow blood to flow only toward the heart. The action of these valves, combined with muscular contractions from activities such as walking or tapping the foot, force blood toward the heart. Without these valves, it would be impossible for the venous blood to flow against gravity and return to the heart; the blood would simply sit at the lowest point in the body. Fortunately, these valves and contractions move the molecule against gravity, returning it to the heart to begin a new cycle.

In certain disease states, there is marked capillary dilation and excessive capillary permeability, and excessive amounts of fluid are allowed to leave the intravascular compartment. The fluid accumulates in the interstitial space. When capillary permeability is increased, plasma proteins also tend to leave the vascular space, reducing the intravascular compartment's osmotic pressure while increasing the interstitial compartment's osmotic pressure. As a result, the rate of return of fluid from the interstitial compartment to the vascular com-

---

INFORMATION ON EDEMA

CAUSES: Wide ranging; includes disease, heart failure, deep vein thrombosis, inadequate blood levels of albumin

SYMPTOMS: Varies; may include accumulated fluid, shortness of breath, pain and tenderness, impacted mobility

DURATION: Acute to chronic

TREATMENTS: Dependent on cause; may include frequent elevation of feet to heart level, support stockings, avoidance of prolonged standing or sitting, dietary changes, medications (*e.g.*, diuretics)

partment is lowered, thus increasing the interstitial fluid levels.

Another route of return of interstitial fluid to the circulation is via the lymphatic system. The lymphatic system is similar to the venous system, but it carries no red blood cells. It runs through the lymph nodes, carrying some of the interstitial fluid that has not been able to return to the vascular compartment at the capillary level. If lymphatic vessels become obstructed, water in the interstitial compartment accumulates, and edema may result.

CAUSES AND SYMPTOMS

Heart failure is a major cause of edema. When the right ventricle of the heart fails, it cannot cope with all the venous blood returning to the heart. As a consequence, the veins become distended, the interstitial compartment is overloaded, and edema occurs. If the patient with heart failure is mostly upright, the edema collects in the legs; if the patient has been lying in bed for some time, the edema tends to accumulate in the lower back. Other clinical signs of right heart failure include distended neck veins, an enlarged and tender liver, and a "galloping" sound on listening to the heart with a stethoscope.

When the left ventricle of the heart fails, the congestion affects the pulmonary veins instead of the neck and leg veins. Fluid accumulates in the same fashion within the interstitial compartment of the lungs; this condition is termed pulmonary edema. Patients develop shortness of breath with minimal activity, upon lying down, and periodically through the night. They may need to sleep on several pillows to minimize this symptom. This condition can usually be diagnosed by listening to the lungs and heart through a stethoscope and by taking an X ray of the chest.

Deep vein thrombosis is another common cause of edema of the lower limbs. When a thrombus (a blood clot inside a blood vessel) develops in a large vein of the legs, the patient usually complains of pain and tenderness of the affected leg. There is usually redness and edema as well. If the thrombus affects a small vein, it may not be noticed. The diagnosis can be made by several specialized tests, such as ultrasound testing and/or impedance plethysmography. Other tests may be needed to make the diagnosis, such as injecting radiographic dye in a vein in the foot and then taking X rays to determine whether the flow in the veins has been obstructed, or using radioactive agents that bind to the clot. Risks for developing venous thrombosis include immobility

(even for relatively short periods of time such as a long car or plane ride), injury, a personal or family history of venous thrombosis, the use of birth control pills, and certain types of cancer. Elderly patients are at particular risk because of relative immobility and an increased frequency of minor trauma to the legs.

When repeated or large thrombi develop, the veins deep inside the thigh (the deep venous system) become blocked, and blood flow shifts toward the superficial veins. The deep veins are surrounded by muscular tissue, and venous flow is assisted by muscular contractions of the leg (the muscular pump), but the superficial veins are surrounded only by skin and subcutaneous tissue and cannot take advantage of the muscular pump. As a consequence, the superficial veins become distended and visible as varicose veins.

When vein blockage occurs, the valves inside become damaged. Hydrostatic pressure of the venous system below the blockage then rises. The venous end of the capillary is normally where the osmotic pressure of the vascular compartment pulls water from the interstitial compartment back into the vascular compartment. In a situation of increased hydrostatic pressure, however, this process is slowed or stopped. As a result, fluid accumulates in the interstitial space, leading to the formation of edema.

A dangerous complication of deep vein thrombosis occurs when part of a thrombus breaks off, enters the circulation, and reaches the lung; this is called a pulmonary embolus. It blocks the flow of blood to the lung, impairing oxygenation. Small emboli may have little or no effect on the patient, while larger emboli may cause severe shortness of breath, chest pain, or even death.

Another potential cause of edema is the presence of a mass in the pelvis or abdomen compressing the large veins passing through the area and interfering with the venous return from the lower limbs to the heart. The resulting venous congestion leads to edema of the lower limbs. The edema may affect either one or both legs, depending on the size and location of the mass. This diagnosis can usually be established by a thorough clinical examination, including rectal and vaginal examinations and X-ray studies.

Postural (or gravitational) edema of the lower limbs is the most common type of edema affecting older people; it is more pronounced toward the end of the day. It can be differentiated from the edema resulting from heart failure by the lack of signs associated with heart failure and by the presence of diseases restricting the patient's degree of mobility. These diseases include

Parkinson's disease, osteoarthritis, strokes, and muscle weakness. Postural edema of the lower limbs results from a combination of factors, the most important being diminished mobility. If a person stands or sits for prolonged periods of time without moving, the muscular pump becomes ineffective. Venous compression also plays an important role in the development of this type of edema. It will occur when the veins in the thigh are compressed between the weight of the body and the surface on which the patient sits, or when the edge of a reclining chair compresses the veins in the calves. Other factors that aggravate postural edema include varicose veins, venous thrombi, heart failure, some types of medication, and low blood albumin levels.

Albumin is formed in the liver from dietary protein. It is essential to maintaining adequate osmotic pressure inside the blood vessels and ensuring the return of fluid from the interstitial space to the vascular compartment. When edema is caused by inadequate blood levels of albumin, it tends to be quite extensive. The patient's entire body and even face are often affected. There are several reasons that the liver may be unable to produce the necessary amount of albumin, including malnutrition, liver impairment, the aging process, and excessive protein loss.

In cases of malnutrition, the liver does not receive a sufficient quantity of raw material from the diet to produce albumin; this occurs when the patient does not ingest enough protein. Healthy adults need at least 0.5 gram of protein for each pound of their body weight. Two groups of people are particularly susceptible to becoming malnourished: the poor and the elderly. Infants and children of poor families who cannot afford to prepare nutritious meals often suffer from malnutrition. The elderly, especially men living on their own, are also vulnerable, regardless of their income.

A liver damaged by excessive and prolonged consumption of alcohol, diseases, or the intake of some types of medication or other chemical toxins will be unable to manufacture albumin at the rate necessary to maintain a normal concentration in the blood. Clinically, the patient shows other evidence of liver impairment in addition to edema. For example, fluid may also accumulate in the abdominal cavity, a condition known as ascites. The diagnosis of liver damage is made by clinical examination and supporting laboratory investigations. The livers of older people, even in the absence of disease, are often less efficient at producing albumin.

The albumin also can be deficient if an excessive amount of albumin is lost from the body. This condition may occur in certain types of diseases affecting the kidneys or the gastrointestinal tract. An excessive amount of protein also may be lost if a patient has large, oozing pressure ulcers, extensive burns, or chronic lung conditions that produce large amounts of sputum.

Patients with strokes and paralysis sometimes develop edema of the paralyzed limb. The mechanism of edema formation in these patients is not entirely understood. It probably results from a combination of an impairment of the nerves controlling the dilation and a constriction of the blood vessels in the affected limb, along with postural and gravitational factors.

Severe allergic states, toxic states, or local inflammation are associated with increased capillary permeability that results in edema. The amount of fluid flowing out to the capillaries far exceeds the amount that can be returned to the capillaries at the venous end. A number of medications, including steroids, estrogens, some arthritis medications, a few blood pressure medications, and certain antibiotics, can induce edema by promoting the retention of fluid. Salt intake tends to cause retention of fluid as well. Obstruction of the lymphatic system often leads to accumulation of fluid in the interstitial compartment. Obstruction can occur in certain types of cancer, after radiation treatment, and in certain parasitic infestations.

Treatment and Therapy

The management of edema depends on the specific reason for its presence. To determine the cause of edema, a thorough history, including current medications, dietary habits, and activity level, is of prime importance. Performing a detailed physical examination is also a vital step. It is frequently necessary to obtain laboratory, ultrasound, and/or X-ray studies before a final diagnosis is made. Once a treatable cause is found, then therapy aimed at the cause should be instituted.

If no treatable, specific disease is responsible for the edema, conservative treatment aimed at reducing the edema to manageable levels without inducing side effects should be initiated. Frequent elevation of the feet to the level of the heart, support stockings, and an avoidance of prolonged standing or sitting are the first steps. If support stockings are ineffective or are too uncomfortable, then custom-made, fitted stockings are available. A low-salt diet is important in the management of edema because a high salt intake worsens the fluid retention. If all these measures fail, then diuretics in small doses may be useful.

Diuretics work by increasing the amount of urine produced. Urine is made of fluids removed from the vascular compartment by the kidneys. The vascular compartment then replenishes itself by drawing water from the interstitial compartment. This reduction in the amount of interstitial fluid improves the edema. There are various types of diuretics, which differ in their potency, duration of action, and side effects. Potential side effects include dizziness, fatigue, sodium and potassium deficiency, excessively low blood pressure, dehydration, sexual dysfunction, the worsening of a diabetic's blood sugar control, increased uric acid levels, and increased blood cholesterol levels. Although diuretics are a convenient and effective means of treating simple edema, it is important to keep in mind that the cure should not be worse than the disease. When the potential side effects of diuretic therapy are compared to the almost total lack of complications of conservative treatment, one can see that mild edema which is not secondary to significant disease is best managed conservatively. Edema caused by more serious diseases, however, calls for more intensive measures.

PERSPECTIVE AND PROSPECTS

The prevalence of edema could decrease as people become more health-conscious and medical progress is made. Nutritious diets, avoidance of excessive salt, and an increased awareness of the dangers of excessive alcohol intake and of the benefits of regular physical exercise all contribute to decreasing the incidence of edema. Improved methods for the early detection, prevention, and management of diseases that may ultimately result in edema could also significantly reduce the scope of the problem. It is also expected that safer and more convenient methods of treating edema will become available.

—*Ronald C. Hamdy, M.D., Mark R. Doman, M.D., and Katherine Hoffman Doman*

See also Arteriosclerosis; Circulation; Elephantiasis; Embolism; Heart; Heart disease; Heart failure; Kidney disorders; Kidneys; Kwashiorkor; Liver; Liver disorders; Lungs; Malnutrition; Nutrition; Phlebitis; Pulmonary diseases; Pulmonary medicine; Pulmonary medicine, pediatric; Respiration; Thrombosis and thrombus; Varicose vein removal; Varicose veins; Vascular medicine; Vascular system; Venous insufficiency.

FOR FURTHER INFORMATION:

Andreoli, Thomas E., et al., eds. *Cecil Essentials of Medicine.* 6th ed. Philadelphia: W. B. Saunders, 2004. A good introductory text to internal medicine that can also be easily understood by nonscientists.

Guyton, Arthur C., and John E. Hall. *Human Physiology and Mechanisms of Disease.* 6th ed. Philadelphia: W. B. Saunders, 1997. The standard reference text in human physiology. A background in basic physiology is helpful in understanding this work.

Hosenpud, Jeffrey D., and Barry H. Greenberg, eds. *Congestive Heart Failure.* 3d ed. Philadelphia: Lippincott Williams & Wilkins, 2007. A thorough treatise on the subject of heart failure. The authors discuss the circulatory system in states of both health and disease and the drug treatment for heart failure.

Marieb, Elaine N., and Katja Hoehn. *Human Anatomy and Physiology.* 7th ed. San Francisco: Pearson Benjamin Cummings, 2007. Details the interrelationships of body organ systems, homeostasis, and how structure and function complement one another.

EDUCATION, MEDICAL
HEALTH CARE SYSTEM

DEFINITION: In the United States, the educational process that leads to obtaining and maintaining a state license to practice medicine, a process which generally involves obtaining two academic degrees and one or more medical certifications; the entire medical education takes a minimum of eleven years beyond high school.

KEY TERMS:

continuing medical education (CME): medical lectures given by hospitals, medical societies, specialists, and conferences that, in the United States, must be approved to meet the requirements for CME credits

generalist: a medical practitioner who belongs to one of the three largest specialties of medicine—family medicine, internal medicine, and pediatrics; sometimes, practitioners of obstetrics/gynecology (OB/GYN) and general surgery are considered to be generalists

internship: the first year of supervised, postgraduate training after receiving a Doctor of Medicine (M.D.) or Doctor of Osteopathy (D.O.) degree, which allows individuals to practice clinical medicine with a limited license; for M.D.'s, this is called year one of residency, and for D.O.'s this is called year one of internship

residency: a course of postgraduate medical education undertaken after receiving an M.D. or D.O. degree and leading to certification in a generalist or specialist branch of medicine

specialist: referring to specialties of medicine not categorized as generalist

STRUCTURE AND CURRICULUM

During the course of the twentieth century, the medical education system in the United States developed from a one-year or two-year program to the present requirement of eleven or more years of formal education and training after completion of secondary school.

College or university. A person who wishes to be licensed as a physician by one of the fifty states usually begins by completing a bachelor's degree at an accredited college or university. This is, by far, the norm, although it is not an absolute requirement. Some colleges and universities offer a premedical undergraduate program that emphasizes biology, chemistry, and other courses in scientific disciplines. In the past, medical schools preferred graduates of these premedical programs over those with liberal arts or science degrees. Today, many medical schools seek more well rounded students who have degrees in liberal arts disciplines. This change has been made in response to societal pressures to graduate more physicians who have a humanistic approach to medical practice. An effort has also been made to provide educational opportunities for members of disadvantaged and minority groups. Therefore, any person with a good grade point average may consider applying to medical school regardless of the type or the nature of the bachelor-level education.

Preparation. The first choice that an individual must make when considering a career as a physician is, "What type of medical school do I wish to attend?" In the United States, two medical degrees are granted: Doctor of Medicine (M.D.) and Doctor of Osteopathy (D.O.). M.D.'s are occasionally referred to as allopathic physicians to distinguish them from osteopathic physicians. Historically, allopathic education stressed the importance of disease in causing illness. Laboratory tests and the prescription of medications are generally used in diagnosis and treatment. Osteopathic education historically looked to the musculoskeletal system with respect to health and illness. This distinction is largely a historical remnant. The curricula of both M.D. and D.O. schools are nearly identical. Both types of physicians train in the same residencies, and both receive the same license to practice medicine and surgery.

Medical school (preclinical). The first two years of medical school are generally devoted to the study of academic medicine. This period is known as preclini-

cal education. These years stress the need to master material from basic sciences and to understand the scientific method of research. Courses such as anatomy, biochemistry, histology, immunology, microbiology, neurology, pathology, and physiology are taught. Achievement is marked by success in test taking through memorization, the analysis of detailed information, and the integration of new material. Actual contact with practicing physicians and their patients is not stressed. As a result, this phase is sometimes criticized for teaching medical knowledge that is separated from medical practice. Some medical schools are adjusting the curriculum in the preclinical years to reduce this dichotomy. At the end of the second year, students must pass the first component of the examination to obtain licensure.

Medical school (clinical). The second two years of medical education stress the clinical knowledge needed to become a physician. Classroom education is concerned with physical diagnosis, the identification of diseases, treatments, and associated procedures and techniques. Medical schools require students to observe physicians practicing medicine with patients in both hospital and office settings. Opportunities are available for students to spend time away from their medical school learning about various specialties. The standard curriculum requires all students to study internal medicine, surgery, pediatrics, obstetrics and gynecology, and psychiatry. Other specialties are studied on an elective basis. For example, a medical student may spend a month observing family physicians working in hospitals and their offices and receive a grade for that month. In this manner, students gain some experience by direct exposure to several medical specialties. At the end of the fourth year, students must pass the second component of the examination to obtain licensure.

It has been suggested that general medical education should include as part of the core curriculum courses in bioethics, communication, and the legal issues that affect the practice of medicine. Components of such courses would include informed consent and refusal of treatment; the ethical limits of paternalism, truthtelling, trust, confidentiality, and communication; medical research; human reproduction and the status of the embryo; issues regarding children; issues surrounding genetics, mental health, and reproduction; special duties involving death and dying; and prolonging life. Medical education in Great Britain includes such courses. In the United States, however, those courses are not a mandatory part of the curriculum in all but a very few medical schools. It is only through continuing education and individual cases that physicians and other health care providers are exposed to these problems. Humanities courses are also part of the undergraduate medical curriculum in Great Britain because it is believed that art, drama, and literature, for example, are means by which people express their joy and sorrow through human creativity. These subjects are not required in the United States curriculum.

Internship. In the past, many generalist physicians, after one year of internship, entered private practice. Today, the year of internship is completed under close medical supervision. This prepares a new physician for more independent practice. All new physicians complete their first year of internship in a residency program before receiving a full medical license in the second year of residency. Physicians who receive their medical education outside the United States must pass the same test as American medical students before being eligible to complete residency training. Some internships are spent rotating through the areas of medicine, surgery, pediatrics, and obstetrics before entering specialized training in areas such as radiology, dermatology, and some surgical specialties. During the first year of residency, a physician has a limited license to practice medicine. Upon completion of the internship or first-year residency and successful passage of the third portion of the standard licensure examination, a physician is granted a full license to practice medicine and surgery.

Residency. The three generalist areas in which resident physicians learn clinical medicine, also known as primary care specialties, are family medicine, internal medicine, and pediatrics. Family medicine treats the whole family throughout life, internal medicine treats adults, and pediatrics treats children and teenagers. The end of childhood and the beginning of adulthood are not clearly defined, and there is some overlap. Most pediatricians will treat patients up to the age of twenty-two, when they typically complete college. The lowest age for patients of internists is usually sixteen. The

THE REQUIREMENTS FOR FULLY LICENSED PHYSICIANS		
Place or Event	*Degree or Program*	*Years*
College or University	B.A. or B.S.	4
Medical School	Preclinical	2
Medical School	Clinical	2
Graduation	D.O. or M.D.	-
Internship or Residency	D.O. or M.D. Limited License	1
Residency (1st)	Generalist or Specialist	2-5
Residency (2d/3d)	Subspecialist (Optional)	0-5
Continuing Education	CME (150 credits)	every 3
	TOTAL	11-19+

many specialist areas of medicine are concerned with specific organ systems, disease processes, or prevention. For example, a psychiatrist has a residency in the area of mental illness, while an emergency room (ER) physician has a residency in the practice of medicine in the ER.

Residency education is the time when a physician who has been graduated from medical school first becomes responsible for patient care, under both direct and indirect supervision. Resident physicians are often referred to as "house officers" or "house staff." Residency teaches and evaluates the skill of a new physician in applying the knowledge gained in medical school to clinical practice. Residency programs are usually three to five years in length. After each year, the resident is given more independence of practice and more responsibility to supervise newer physicians. Upon completion of a residency program, a physician becomes eligible for certification by one of the generalist or specialist boards of medicine. Most boards require one or two years of independent practice before allowing candidates to seek board certification. A physician must take and pass yet another examination concerning knowledge related to the specialty area for which certification is desired. Many board certifications must be renewed periodically (every five to seven years) as a condition of retaining board-certified status.

Second residency (subspecialization). Some physicians choose to complete additional training in their medical specialties. This subspecialty medical education is usually called a fellowship. For example, a general surgeon may complete a multiyear residency in cardiac surgery, or a psychiatrist may complete a subspecialty residency in children's mental illness. Some highly subspecialized physicians need seven to ten years after medical school to complete their subspecialty training. An example of this level of specialization is forensic pathology, which requires residency training in pathology and fellowships in forensic and chemical pathology. Pediatric neurosurgery is another example.

Continuing medical education. All states require that physicians complete a certain number of continuing medical education (CME) credits in order to maintain their medical licensure. A common requirement is 150 CME credits over three years. Some specialties also require national examinations for recertification in the specialty. For physicians in the United States, medical education is an exercise in lifelong learning.

ISSUES AND PHILOSOPHIES

American medical education is undergoing one of the greatest challenges in its history. Medical schools are being asked to teach physicians how to be effective and efficient caregivers to all persons. The corporate system of medical care demands medical care that is effective, cost-conscious or economically efficient, and delivered in a positive and caring manner. Health maintenance organizations (HMOs), preferred provider organizations (PPOs), and other organizational alliances of physicians expect the medical educational system to teach these values and skills.

The national government adds one more criterion: Physicians must be able to do the above for all citizens. In a pluralistic and democratic society, a physician must acknowledge various social, ethnic, cultural, and regional needs. Medical educators must train socially conscious physicians. Physicians must be available to practice in either rural or inner-city areas. They must be able to treat various populations, such as African Americans and Native Americans, for their specific needs. Physicians are being asked to be cognizant of and caring toward all Americans.

The medical philosophy that allows for an increase of psychological skills and social awareness in medical education is called the biopsychosocial model. As the label indicates, it conceptualizes a medical education system which teaches physicians solid medical knowledge ("bio"), an improved ability to relate to patients ("psycho"), and an awareness of different social systems and cultural attitudes as they affect medical care ("social"). The biopsychosocial model of care is a proposed revision of what the medical education system should teach physicians. It may be the medical school curriculum of the future.

PERSPECTIVE AND PROSPECTS

The history of American medical education can be understood as falling into five periods of development. Each period stressed a certain philosophy and direction unique to its times. The current philosophy of medical education has aspects of all five periods, affecting how and what physicians are taught.

The British period (1750-1815). American medical education was established on the British model. The emphasis in British medical education was on developing a physician's medical knowledge through direct observation of patient care in clinical settings. There were few formal centers for medical training. They functioned to instruct teaching physicians and to transmit new medical knowledge. In America, there were only six medical schools. Most medical education was clinical and taught by older physicians to younger physicians in office settings. There were no formal educational requirements. Most physicians could read and write, possessing the equivalent of only two or three years of formal education.

The French period (1815-1865). French physicians, who developed the skills of classification, influenced American medical education through methods of diagnosis and the use of hospitals. In the United States, many hospitals were built, and there was a significant expansion in the number of medical schools. Large groups of patients were admitted to hospitals and grouped on wards by diagnosis. The hospital-office model of medical education began to develop.

The German period (1865-1915). Laboratory methods and germ theory were introduced into medical education from Germany. Some medical schools began to educate physicians in the laboratory approach to medicine. Office practice was less important in medical education. The period of formal education was still relatively brief, often less than two years in total length. At the end of the German period, many medical schools that were not teaching laboratory methods were closed.

The American period (1915-1965). American medical education embraced a scientific approach, first detailed by Abraham Flexner in *Medical Education in the United States and Canada*, published in 1910 in a report on reforming American medical education. Physician-scientists were to be educated by quality medical schools to provide clinical medicine according to the scientific method. This model was successfully introduced into American medical education. It was considered the norm until the concerns of corporate interests and government interests became vital.

The corporate period (1965-   ). Medicare and Medicaid programs were created and supported by the national government in order to provide quality medical care to all Americans. Corporate interests require that medical education be effective in controlling health costs to industry. Many of the current challenges facing medical education revolve around teaching physicians the two concerns of access and cost-effectiveness.

In the early 1990's, the Council on Graduate Medical Education (COGME) suggested that certain humanistic and corporate medical education goals be reached by the year 2000. At least 50 percent of residency graduates should enter practice as generalist physicians. The number of underrepresented minority students should be doubled. Shortages of physicians in rural and urban areas should be eliminated. The purpose of these goals was to avoid a severe physician shortage for some populations, areas of specialty, and geographic centers. With a system of managed medical care in place, COGME projected a shortage of 35,000 generalist physicians and a surplus of 115,000 specialist physicians by the year 2000. COGME released a report in 1999 that noted the rate of growth in the physician supply had moderated slightly but still was likely to lead to a surplus of physicians, and that the number of generalist physicians was increasing.

In 1990, fewer than one-third of all American physicians practiced primary care. It appears that in the future, the trend toward specialization will be reversed. Those who plan, those who pay, and those who orga-

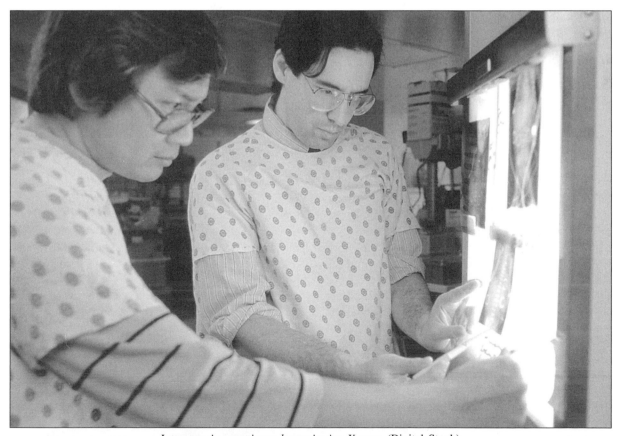

Interns gain experience by reviewing X rays. (Digital Stock)

nize the various systems to deliver medical care in the United States no longer believe that so many specialty-trained physicians will be needed. Yet, the demand by Americans for specialized health care services has not diminished. A clash between recipients and providers appears to be inevitable. The next decades in American medicine are likely to be turbulent, as various stakeholders struggle to redefine the American system of health care.

There is an acknowledged maldistribution of physicians. Most prefer to practice in suburban and medical center settings, leaving significant numbers of Americans without easy access to adequate health care. Many planners also believe that the promised efficiency of managed care will result in a decreased need for physicians. In the mid-1990's, state legislatures began to reduce the amounts of support for medical education, effectively forcing medical schools to reduce the number of physicians that they graduate. The final outcomes of these policy changes are unclear. The results of this trend, however, will be felt by American society for decades.

Women in medicine. Despite a long history of discrimination against women in medicine, women have actually practiced the profession for many centuries. In ancient Egypt, in the time of Moses, and throughout the nineteenth century and the reign of King Henry V of England, female physicians were active. Opportunities for female physicians were scarce, however, and admissions to "regular" medical schools were an anomaly.

In the United States, three medical schools were opened specifically for female applicants in 1864: in Boston, Cincinnati, and Philadelphia. Medical societies refused admission to women, however, and it was difficult for women to obtain academic positions outside a women's medical school. By 1870, women represented only 0.8 percent of physicians in the United States. By 1900, 6 percent of all physicians were women. By 1940, the percentage of women in medicine declined to 4.4 percent, and it did not reach 6 percent again until 1950. A major surge in female admissions occurred in the 1970's, when the percentage of women in medicine reached 8.9 percent. Overall, by 1997 women represented 22 percent of physicians. They are, however, an increasing proportion of the profession, constituting close to half of all medical students in the early twenty-first century. Despite the relative paucity of their numbers as physicians, women occupy the majority position as workers in the health care sector generally (85 percent).

Discrimination is present in medical schools and workplaces, and sexual harassment exists within the medical sector, a disproportionate amount of which is directed toward women. Some patients also discriminate, preferring not to deal with female physicians. Research during the 1970's revealed that patients often felt that women physicians lacked competency and experience, but as more women entered the profession, patients' attitudes toward female physicians became more positive. Overall, female physicians have a greater percentage of female patients than do male physicians. They are more likely to discuss psychological and sexual issues with their patients and to bring a sense of participation to the physician-patient relationship, relative to male physicians. Data suggest that there is greater disclosure in the same-sex doctor-patient relationship.

Women in medicine have also had to combat sexual stereotyping. The characteristics of leaders—assertion, capability, and decisiveness—when applied to women become negative attributes—pushiness, lack of femininity, and aggression. Sociologists have reported that women and men think differently and approach situations from different perspectives. Consequently, many people believe that women bring the positive traits of humanism and caring to the practice of medicine. In 2000, it was predicted that in the future male physicians will use high-tech medicine while female physicians will practice hands-on medicine.

Female physicians also experience many stresses in their professional lives. They advance more slowly in their careers and earn less money than do male physicians. One study reported that almost 65 percent of female family practitioners felt overwhelmed at least once a week. Women reportedly complain of less support from their employers and their families than do their male counterparts, and they rely more heavily on their spouses for support. A common solution to stress management has been avoidance; that is, some female physicians back off from ambition. Others, in contrast, play a domestic role while simultaneously pursuing a career. The latter group experiences extreme strain, fatigue, anxiety, and resentment about work overload with little time to accomplish their tasks. Statistics in 1999 demonstrated that about 90 percent of married female physicians have a spouse who also is a professional, and half of these marry another physician.

Techniques for reducing strain when combining roles of marriage and motherhood with medicine include role cycling (prioritizing one or another role at different times); changed expectations (developing a flexible attitude toward daily problems); decreased confrontations with social norms (reducing conflict by seeking out friends with similar backgrounds, thus reaching one's own comfort level); hiring help for child care, housework, and other chores; and concentrating one's life within a small geographic area. Relaxation techniques such as meditation and biofeedback, support groups, coaches, and professional counseling are helpful means to assist female physicians in stress reduction and coping.

—Gerald T. Terlep, Ph.D.;
L. Fleming Fallon, Jr., M.D., Ph.D., M.P.H.;
updated by Marcia J. Weiss, M.A., J.D.

See also American Medical Association (AMA); Ethics; Hippocratic oath; Nursing; Osteopathic medicine; *specific specialties.*

FOR FURTHER INFORMATION:

Birenbaum, Aaron. *Wounded Profession: American Medicine Enters the Age of Managed Care.* Westport, Conn.: Greenwood Press, 2002. Traces the evolution of health care in the United States during the 1990's and examines the rising costs, consumer backlash, and new legislation.

Bowman, Marjorie A., and Deborah I. Allen. *Stress and Women Physicians.* 2d ed. New York: Springer-Verlag, 1990. Discusses professional qualities of practicing women physicians.

Bowman, Marjorie A., Erica Frank, and Deborah I. Allen. *Women in Medicine: Career and Life Management.* New York: Springer-Verlag, 2002. An honest discussion of the challenges facing women physicians. Includes cases, appendixes, resource lists, organizations, and Web site addresses. An updated version of *Stress and Women Physicians.*

Brown, Stanford J. *Getting into Medical School.* 9th ed. Hauppauge, N.Y.: Barron's, 2001. Advice on recommended undergraduate courses, taking the Medical College Admission Test (MCAT), applying to medical school, getting through the personal interview, and alternatives for students who have been rejected. Directory of American medical schools included.

Ludmerer, Kenneth M. *Time to Heal: American Medical Education from the Turn of the Century to the Managed Care Era.* New York: Oxford University Press, 2000. Ludmerer looks at the future of medicine in America and reveals some very disturbing trends in managed care, education, and research funding. Contains a wealth of factual details and insightful questions.

Rivo, Marc L., et al. "Defining the Generalist Physician's Training." *Journal of the American Medical Association* 271 (May 18, 1994): 1499-1504. Rivo presents a clear, fact-filled article on major current issues in medical education. The article is accessible to the general reader. It also contains charts and references for further research.

Starr, Paul. "The Framework of Health Care Reform." *New England Journal of Medicine* 330, no. 15 (April 14, 1994): 1086-1088. This article reviews several proposals for health care reform. The author has provided commentary on the American health care system for many years.

Zebala, John A., Daniel B. Jones, and Stephanie B. Jones. *Medical School Admissions: The Insider's Guide.* 5th rev. ed. Memphis: Mustang, 2000. Written by medical students for medical students, gives practical advice on admission tasks such as the preparation of an effective application, improving scores on the MCAT, and writing a compelling personal essay.

EEG. *See* ELECTROENCEPHALOGRAPHY (EEG).

ELECTRICAL SHOCK
DISEASE/DISORDER

ANATOMY OR SYSTEM AFFECTED: Heart, nervous system, skin

SPECIALTIES AND RELATED FIELDS: Critical care, emergency medicine, neurology

DEFINITION: The physical effect of an electrical current entering the body and the resulting damage.

CAUSES AND SYMPTOMS

Electric shock ranges from a harmless jolt of static electricity to a power line's lethal discharge. The severity of the shock depends on the current flowing through the body, and the current is determined by the skin's electrical resistance. Dry skin has a very high resistance; thus, 110 volts produces a small, harmless current. The resistance for perspiring hands, however, is lower by a factor of 100, resulting in potentially fatal currents. Currents traveling between bodily extremities are particularly dangerous because of their proximity to the heart.

Electric shock causes injury or death in one of three ways: paralysis of the breathing center in the brain, paralysis of the heart, or ventricular fibrillation (extremely rapid and uncontrolled twitching of the heart muscle).

The threshold of feeling (the minimum current de-

INFORMATION ON ELECTRICAL SHOCK

CAUSES: Electrical current entering the body
SYMPTOMS: Unconsciousness, moderate to severe pain, ventricular fibrillation, burning or charring of skin
DURATION: Acute
TREATMENTS: Resuscitation, emergency care

tectable) ranges from 0.5 to 1.0 milliamperes. Currents up to 5.0 milliamperes, the maximum harmless current, are not hazardous, unless they trigger an accident by involuntary reaction. Currents in this range create a tingling sensation. The minimum current that causes muscular paralysis occurs between 10 and 15 milliamperes. Currents of this magnitude cause a painful jolt. Above 18 milliamperes, the current contracts chest muscles, and breathing ceases. Unconsciousness and death follow within minutes unless the current is interrupted and respiration resumed. A short exposure to currents of 50 milliamperes causes severe pain, possible fainting, and complete exhaustion, while currents in the 100- to 300-milliampere range produce ventricular fibrillation, which is fatal unless quickly corrected. During ventricular fibrillation, the heart stops its rhythmic pumping and flutters uselessly. Since blood stops flowing, the victim dies from oxygen deprivation in the brain in a matter of minutes. This is the most common cause of death for victims of electric shock.

Relatively high currents (above 300 milliamperes) may produce ventricular paralysis, deep burns in the body's tissue, or irreversible damage to the central nervous system. Victims are more likely to survive a large but brief current, even through smaller, sustained currents are usually lethal. Burning or charring of the skin at the point of contact may be a contributing factor to the delayed death that often follows severe electric shock. Very high voltage discharges of short duration, such as a lightning strike, tend to disrupt the body's nervous impulses, but victims may survive. On the other hand, any electric current large enough to raise body temperature significantly produces immediate death.

TREATMENT AND THERAPY

Before medical treatment can be applied, the current must be stopped or the shock victim must be separated from the current source without being touched. Nonconducting materials such as dry, heavy blankets or pieces of wood can be used for this purpose. If the victim is not breathing, artificial respiration immediately applied provides adequate short-term life support, though the victim may become stiff or rigid in reaction to the shock. Victims of electric shock may suffer from severe burns and permanent aftereffects, including eye cataracts, angina, or disorders of the nervous system.

Electric shock can usually be prevented by strictly adhering to safety guidelines and using commonsense precautions. Careful inspection of appliances and tools, compliance with manufacturers' safety standards, and the avoidance of unnecessary risks greatly reduce the chance of an electric shock. Electrical appliances or tools should never be used when standing in water or on damp ground, and dry gloves, shoes, and floors provide considerable protection against dangerous shocks from 110-volt circuits.

Electrical safety is also provided by isolation, guarding, insulation, grounding, and ground-fault interrupters. Isolation means that high-voltage wires strung overhead are not within reach, while guarding provides a barrier around high voltage devices, such as those found in television sets.

Old wire insulation may become brittle with age and develop small cracks. Defective wires are hazardous and should be replaced immediately. Most modern power tools are double-insulated; the motor is insulated from the plastic insulating frame. These devices do not require grounding, as no exposed metal parts become electrically live if the wire insulation fails.

In a home, grounding is accomplished by a third wire in outlets, connected through a grounding circuit to a water pipe. If an appliance plug has a third prong, it will ground the frame to the grounding circuit. In the event of a short circuit, the grounding circuit provides a low resistance path, resulting in a current surge which trips the circuit breaker.

In some instances the current may be inadequate to trip a circuit breaker (which usually requires 15 or 20 amperes), but current in excess of 10 milliamperes could still be lethal to humans. A ground-fault interrupter ensures nearly complete protection by detecting leakage currents as small as 5 milliamperes and breaking the circuit. This relatively inexpensive device operates very rapidly and provides an extremely high degree of safety against electrocution in the household. Many localities now have codes which require the installation of ground-fault interrupters in bathrooms, kitchens, and other areas where water is used.

—George R. Plitnik, Ph.D.

See also Burns and scalds; Cardiac arrest; Critical care; Critical care, pediatric; Emergency medicine; Resuscitation; Shock; Unconsciousness.

FOR FURTHER INFORMATION:

Atkinson, William. "Electric Injuries Can Be Worse than They Seem." *Electric World* 214, no. 1 (January/February, 2000): 33-36. Whether an electrical shock initially seems serious or mild, it is always a cause for concern. Aspects of electrical shock injuries are explored.

Bridges, J. E., et al., eds. *International Symposium on Electrical Shock Safety Criteria*. New York: Pergamon Press, 1985. The summary of a symposium covering the physiological effects of shock, bioelectrical conditions, and safety measures.

Hewitt, Paul G. *Conceptual Physics*. 10th ed. San Francisco: Pearson Addison Wesley, 2006. Comprehensive coverage of physics for the layperson, which includes detailed discussions of the laws of electricity and electrical devices.

Hogan, David E., and Jonathan L. Burstein. *Disaster Medicine*. Philadelphia: Lippincott Williams & Wilkins, 2002. Examines a wide range of relevant topics including natural, industrial, transportation, and conflict-related disasters; and infectious diseases, winter storms, fires, and mass burns.

Liu, Lynda. "Pullout Emergency Guide: Electric Shock." *Parents* 75, no. 1 (January, 2000): 65-66. A pull-out emergency guide for the prevention and treatment of electrical shock in children. Household hazards and electricity dos and don'ts are among the tips offered.

U.S. Department of Labor. Occupational Safety and Health Administration. *Controlling Electrical Hazards*. Rev. ed. Washington, D.C.: Author, 2002. A report which identifies common electrical hazards and discusses their prevention.

ELECTROCARDIOGRAPHY (ECG OR EKG)

PROCEDURE

ANATOMY OR SYSTEM AFFECTED: Chest, circulatory system, heart

SPECIALTIES AND RELATED FIELDS: Biotechnology, cardiology, critical care, emergency medicine, exercise physiology, preventive medicine

DEFINITION: A noninvasive procedure that provides insight into the rate, rhythm, and general health of the heart.

KEY TERMS:

ECG waves: the repeated deflections of an electrocardiogram; one complete wave consists of a P wave, followed by a QRS complex, and then a T wave and represents one complete cardiac cycle, or heartbeat

electrocardiogram (ECG or EKG): a record of the waves produced by the rhythmically changing electrical conduction within the heart; often recorded by a strip chart recorder

INDICATIONS AND PROCEDURES

Electrocardiography is a useful medical diagnostic and evaluative procedure that reveals much information about the function or malfunction of a person's heart. ECG is a noninvasive, easy-to-use, and economical tool that is an essential part of diagnosing chest pain. It serves an important role in both cardiology and emergency medicine. ECG is also commonly used in preventive medicine to monitor heart health. For this purpose, ECG is frequently used in a format known as a stress test. Athletes often have ECG analysis performed as a part of their training and cardiovascular conditioning.

In a stress test, a person is studied for regularity of rhythm, rate, and unimpeded flow of electrical conduction within the heart. ECG recordings are first made while the person is at rest, then during light exercise, and, finally, if healthy enough, during rigorous exercise. Such exercise causes the heart to work harder and allows a physician to determine whether a person has a heart that beats with a regular, repetitive rhythm and at an appropriate pace for the level of rest or exercise. The stress of exercise can also help in assessing whether the heart muscle masses contract in the proper sequence: atrial contraction followed by ventricular contraction. An irregularity of electrical conduction, poor muscle contraction, dead regions of heart tissue (from a recent or old heart attack), and other maladies can be revealed.

In order to obtain an electrocardiogram, small metallic contact points are taped to the patient's skin via an electrically conductive adhesive or gel. The electric impulses travel across the skin to these contact points; from there, leads (plastic-coated wires) are attached to the recording device so that a complete circuit is made. Either a monitor screen or a strip chart recorder traces the electrical impulses. The waves are plotted in units of millivolts (on the y-axis) versus time in units of seconds (on the x-axis).

A twelve-lead ECG has replaced the original four-lead type. A twelve-lead ECG allows the physician to

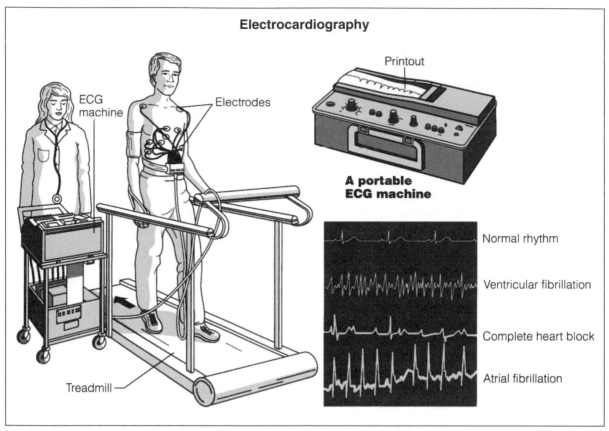

Electrocardiography

Printout

A portable ECG machine

ECG machine

Electrodes

Treadmill

Normal rhythm

Ventricular fibrillation

Complete heart block

Atrial fibrillation

The electrical activity of the heart can be measured with an electrocardiograph (ECG or EKG) machine; characteristic patterns can be used to diagnose arrhythmias (irregular heartbeats). The patient may also be asked to walk on a treadmill while the heart is monitored in order to gauge its function during exercise.

explore the performance of the heart from twelve different orientations, or angles, so that much more of the heart mass can be evaluated. Ten electrodes are placed on the body as follows: one on the right leg, which serves as the ground electrode; one on each of the other extremities; and six on the precordium, which is the area around the sternum and on the left chest wall (over the heart). The leads are explored in different combinations.

USES AND COMPLICATIONS

Healthy people, including athletes or certain members of the armed services, may take stress tests in order to have their health and cardiovascular conditioning monitored during training. Some professionals are required to take stress tests on a regular basis, such as commercial airline pilots and astronauts. In addition, people who have a family history of cardiovascular disease, or who are concerned about their heart health for other reasons, may have a stress test performed to find early warning signs and allow intervention before a crisis oc-

curs. Finally, it should be noted that some insurance companies require stress tests of their applicants in order to determine insurability before issuing or rejecting a policy.

Treatment for chest pain is highly dependent on the electrical patterns seen on the ECG. Drugs may be administered or withheld depending on the shape or duration reported for the P wave, QRS complex, and T-wave patterns. Left-sided versus right-sided heart disease can be discerned from the traces, and infarction (heart attack) can be distinguished from angina. Although the waves in the electrocardiogram for an infarcted or anginal heart are abnormal, the patterns become abnormal in a predictable, and therefore diagnostic, manner.

Diagnostic patterns can also be seen for arrhythmias (unusual and abnormal beating patterns), such as ectopic foci, in which some part of the heart other than the sinoatrial (S-A) node (the natural pacemaker) is abnormally in control of determining when the heart contracts, or heart block, whereby electrical conduction is interrupted.

ECG is routinely used to keep close tabs on heart patients and in the postsurgery monitoring of patients who have had open heart or thoracic surgery. Certain kinds of neonatal or infant malformations or malfunctions may also be evaluated with ECG.

Because ECG is a superficial and noninvasive technique, there are no real risks associated with having this procedure performed.

PERSPECTIVE AND PROSPECTS

Electrocardiography was once a wet, messy, and awkward procedure to perform: A patient dangled one arm in a huge jar filled with a conducting salt solution and placed the left leg in another saline-filled container. Changing the leads to include other limbs required the patient to take a good amount of soaking. Although it was a clumsy procedure, the basic premise of ECG remains unchanged: The heart exhibits regular patterns of electrical activity that can be useful diagnostically.

Recent advances in electrocardiography have involved the use of multiple electrode systems along with computers and recorders that allow rapid and simultaneous multiple-lead input and output. In addition, modern electronic instrumentation allows continuous ECG monitoring so that patients in intensive care units, coronary care units, or emergency rooms can be assessed on a second-by-second basis when seconds count. Undoubtedly, the ECG systems available today, coupled with thoughtful and informed interpretation by medical doctors and emergency medical technicians (EMTs), are responsible for saving many lives.

—Mary C. Fields, M.D.

See also Angina; Arrhythmias; Biofeedback; Cardiac arrest; Cardiology; Cardiology, pediatric; Cardiopulmonary resuscitation (CPR); Critical care; Critical care, pediatric; Echocardiography; Emergency medicine; Emergency medicine, pediatric; Exercise physiology; Heart; Heart attack; Paramedics; Stress; Stress reduction.

FOR FURTHER INFORMATION:

Brady, William, John Camm, and June Edhouse. *ABC of Clinical Electrocardiography*. Malden, Mass.: Blackwell Science, 2002. A quick-reference text showing a wide range of electrocardiogram patterns seen in clinical practice.

Conover, Mary Boudreau. *Understanding Electrocardiography*. 8th ed. St. Louis: Mosby, 2003. This standard text is divided into four sections: introduction to the 12-lead electrocardiogram, arrhythmia recognition, abnormal 12-lead electrocardiograms, and special diagnostic and therapeutic procedures.

Phibbs, Brendan. *The Human Heart: A Complete Text on Function and Disease*. 5th ed. St. Louis: G. W. Manning, 1992. Designed for the general reader, this resource discusses cardiology. Includes bibliographical references and an index.

Surawicz, Borys, and Timothy K. Knilans. *Chou's Electrocardiography in Clinical Practice: Adult and Pediatric*. 5th ed. Philadelphia: W. B. Saunders, 2001. Explores the values and limitations of the electrocardiogram and covers such topics as pericarditis and cardiac surgery, atrial and atrioventricular rhythms, ventricular arrhythmias, and effects of drugs on the ECG.

Thaler, Malcom S. *The Only EKG Book You'll Ever Need*. 5th ed. Philadelphia: Lippincott Williams & Wilkins, 2006. Many EKG texts delve heavily into the physics and myocardial electrophysiology associated with EKGs and overwhelm and confuse the early learner. This book avoids lengthy discussions of theory and uses wide spacing, open pages, simple text, and diagrams to allow for speedier mastery of the basics.

Wellens, Hein J. J., and Mary Conover. *The ECG in Emergency Decision Making*. 2d ed. St. Louis: Saunders Elsevier, 2006. This resource offers guidance for the professional regarding the diagnosis of heart disease in an emergency setting.

Wiederhold, Richard. *Electrocardiography: The Monitoring and Diagnostic Leads*. Philadelphia: W. B. Saunders, 1999. This textbook is intended to be a primary or introductory text to the field of electrocardiography (ECG) for students in the health care professions or clinicians who are not cardiologists.

ELECTROCAUTERIZATION

PROCEDURE

ANATOMY OR SYSTEM AFFECTED: Blood vessels, cells, circulatory system, joints, ligaments, muscles, skin, uterus

SPECIALTIES AND RELATED FIELDS: Cardiology, critical care, dermatology, emergency medicine, family medicine, general surgery, gynecology, internal medicine, vascular medicine

DEFINITION: The surgical control of bleeding from small blood vessels or the removal of unwanted tissue using a controlled electric current.

INDICATIONS AND PROCEDURES

Electrocauterization is a procedure used in many surgical operations. As a surgeon's scalpel penetrates layers of skin and tissue, numerous tiny blood vessels are cut open. To stop the associated bleeding, an assisting surgeon can seal these vessels immediately using an electrical instrument to burn just enough of the tissue to produce a tiny scar. Electrocauterization is also used to destroy unwanted tissue, such as skin lesions.

Prior to any surgery involving electrocautery, local anesthesia is applied by injection. Electrocauterization is carried out with a small needle probe that is heated with an electrical current. Enough current is applied to heat the probe to temperatures at which blood will coagulate. To prevent electrical shock, a grounding pad is placed on the patient and a small electrode is attached to the skin near the surgery site to direct any excess current away from the body. Depending on the surgery site and the size and shape of unwanted tissue, the cautery pattern may be circular, dotted, or linear. In some applications, a temperature sensor near the electrical probe allows a microprocessor-based control unit to regulate the delivered electrical power as a function of tissue temperature.

USES AND COMPLICATIONS

Electrocauterization is commonly used to destroy unwanted tissue. It has been applied to remove growths in the nasal passage, noncancerous polyps in the colon, canker sores, and lesions on or around the skin, muscles, ligaments, blood vessels, joints, and bones. It is used to stop bleeding during surgery and also when biopsies are performed. It has been used in women to remove abnormal tissue from the cervix and to stop abnormal bleeding from the uterus that is not caused by menstruation.

The healing time after electrocauterization procedures is usually two to three weeks. After electrocautery, a patient may experience pain, swelling, redness, drainage, bleeding, bruising, scarring, or itching at or around the surgery site. Headache, muscle aches, dizziness, fever, tiredness, and a general ill feeling may also occur following electrocauterization. The most serious complication can be the onset of infection. Antibiotics are typically administered if this occurs. Acetaminophen is used to diminish pain.

Excessive electrocautery can produce superficial to deep burns, which can be treated with cold packs. Electrocauterization of the cervix may lead to the misinterpretation of future Pap smear tests. When electrocau-

terization is performed multiple times to stop the occurrence of frequent nosebleeds, scar tissue can build up in the nose, leading to increased nosebleeds because of the lack of elasticity of scar tissue.

—Alvin K. Benson, Ph.D.

See also Biopsy; Canker sores; Cervical procedures; Colon and rectal polyp removal; Cryotherapy and cryosurgery; Dermatology; Dermatopathology; Genital disorders, female; Healing; Laser use in surgery; Nosebleeds; Skin; Skin disorders; Skin lesion removal; Surgery, general; Surgical procedures; Tumor removal; Tumors.

FOR FURTHER INFORMATION:

Bland, Kirby I., ed. *The Practice of General Surgery.* Philadelphia: W. B. Saunders, 2002.

Brunicardi, F. Charles, et al., eds. *Schwartz's Manual of Surgery.* 8th ed. New York: McGraw-Hill Medical, 2006.

Morreale, Barbara, David L. Roseman, and Albert K. Straus. *Inside General Surgery: An Illustrated Guide.* New Brunswick, N.J.: Johnson & Johnson, 1991.

Pollack, Sheldon V. *Electrosurgery of the Skin.* New York: Churchill Livingstone, 1991.

ELECTROENCEPHALOGRAPHY (EEG)

PROCEDURE

ANATOMY OR SYSTEM AFFECTED: Brain, head, nervous system, psychic-emotional system

SPECIALTIES AND RELATED FIELDS: Biotechnology, critical care, emergency medicine, neurology, pathology, psychiatry, psychology, speech pathology

DEFINITION: The tracing of the electrical potentials produced by brain cells on a graphic chart, as detected by electrodes placed on the scalp.

KEY TERMS:

brain stem: the medulla oblongata, pons, and mesencephalon portions of the brain, which perform motor, sensory, and reflex functions and contain the corticospinal and reticulospinal tracts

cerebrum: the largest and uppermost section of the brain, which integrates memory, speech, writing, and emotional responses

epilepsy: uncontrollable excessive activity in either all or part of the central nervous system

lesion: a visible local tissue abnormality such as a wound, sore, rash, or boil which can be benign, cancerous, gross, occult, or primary

neurological: dealing with the nervous system and its disorders *seizure:* a sudden, violent, and involuntary contraction of a group of muscles; may be paroxysmal and episodic

INDICATIONS AND PROCEDURES

Clinical electroencephalography (EEG) uses from eight to sixteen pairs of electrodes called derivations. The "international 10-20" system of electrode placement provides coverage of the scalp at standard locations denoted by the letters *F* (frontal), *C* (central), *P* (parietal), *T* (temporal), and *O* (occipital). Subscripts of odd for left-sided placement, even for right-sided placements, and *z* for midline placement further define electrode location. During the procedure, the patient remains quiet, with eyes closed, and refrains from talking or moving. In some circumstances, however, prescribed activities such as hyperventilation may be requested. An EEG test is used to diagnose seizure disorders, brain-stem disorders, focal lesions, and impaired consciousness.

Electrical potentials caused by normal brain activity have atypical amplitudes of 30 to 100 millivolts and irregular, wavelike variations in time. The main generators of the EEG are probably postsynaptic potentials, with the largest contribution arising from pyramidal cells in the third cortical layer. The ongoing rhythms on an EEG background recording are classified according to the frequencies that they produce as delta (less than 3.5 hertz), theta (4.0 to 7.5 hertz), alpha (8.0 to 13.0 hertz), and beta (greater than 13.5 hertz). In awake but relaxed normal adults, the background consists primarily of alpha activity in occipital and parietal areas and beta activity in central and frontal areas. Variations in this activity can occur as a function of behavioral state and aging. Alpha waves disappear during sleep and are replaced by synchronous beta waves of higher frequency but lower voltage. Theta waves can occur during emotional stress, particularly during extreme disappointment and frustration. Delta waves occur in deep sleep and infancy and with serious organic brain disease.

USES AND COMPLICATIONS

During neurosurgery, electrodes can be applied directly to the surface of the brain (intracranial EEG) or placed within brain tissue (depth EEG) to detect lesions or tumors. Electrical activity of the cerebrum is detected through the skull in the same way that the electrical activity originating in the heart is detected by an electrocardiogram (ECG or EKG) through the chest

wall. The amplitude of the EEG, however, is much smaller than that of the ECG because the EEG is generated by cells that are not synchronously activated and are not geometrically aligned, whereas the ECG is generated by cells that are synchronously activated and aligned. Variations in brain wave activity correlate with neurological conditions such as epilepsy, abnormal psychopathological states, and level of consciousness such as during different stages of sleep.

The two general categories of EEG abnormalities are alterations in background activity and paroxysmal activity. An EEG background with global abnormalities indicates diffuse brain dysfunction associated with developmental delay, metabolic disturbances, infections, and degenerative diseases. EEG background abnormalities are generally not specific enough to establish a diagnosis—for example, the "burst-suppression" pattern may indicate severe anoxic brain injury as well as a coma induced by barbiturates. Some disorders do have

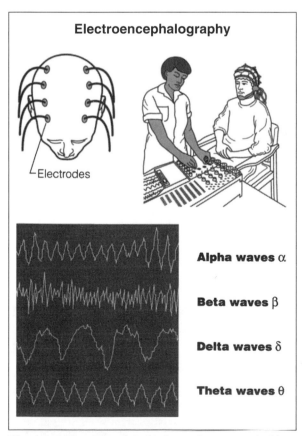

The electrical activity of the brain can be measured with an electroencephalograph (EEG) machine; characteristic patterns can be used to diagnose some brain disorders and to determine levels of consciousness.

characteristic EEG features: An excess of beta activity suggests intoxication, whereas triphasic slow waves are typical of metabolic encephalopathies, particularly as a result of hepatic or renal dysfunction. Psychiatric illness is generally not associated with prominent EEG changes. Therefore, a normal EEG helps to distinguish psychogenic unresponsiveness from neurologic disease. EEG silence is an adjunctive test in the determination of brain death, but it is not a definitive one because it may be produced by reversible conditions such as hypothermia. Focal or lateralized EEG abnormalities in the background imply similarly localized disturbances in brain function and thus suggest the presence of lesions.

Paroxysmal EEG activity consisting of spikes and sharp waves reflects the pathologic synchronization of neurons. The location and character of paroxysmal activity in epileptic patients help clarify the disorder, guide rational anticonvulsant therapy, and assist in determining a prognosis. The diagnostic value of an EEG is often enhanced by activation procedures, such as hyperventilation, photic (light) stimulation, and prolonged ambulatory monitoring, or by using special recording sites, such as nasopharyngeal leads, anterior temporal leads, and surgically placed subdural and depth electrodes. During a seizure, paroxysmal EEG activity replaces normal background activity and becomes continuous and rhythmic. In partial seizures, paroxysmal activity begins in one brain region and spreads to uninvolved regions.

PERSPECTIVE AND PROSPECTS

One of the most important uses of EEGs has been to diagnose certain types of epilepsy and to pinpoint the area in the brain causing the disturbance. Epilepsy is characterized by uncontrollable excessive activity in either all or part of the central nervous system and is classified into three types: grand mal epilepsy, petit mal epilepsy, and focal epilepsy. Additionally, EEGs are often used to localize tumors or other space-occupying lesions in the brain. Such abnormalities may be so large as to cause a complete or partial block in electrical activity in a certain portion of the cerebral cortex, resulting in reduced voltage. More frequently, however, a tumor compresses the surrounding nervous tissue and thereby causes abnormal electrical excitation in these areas.

Some researchers predict new uses of EEG technology in the future, although many of these applications appear dubious. Attempts to interpret thought patterns so that an EEG could serve as a lie detector or measurement of intellectual ability, for example, have proven unsuccessful.

—*Daniel G. Graetzer, Ph.D.*

See also Brain; Brain damage; Brain disorders; Brain tumors; Critical care; Critical care, pediatric; Emergency medicine; Epilepsy; Headaches; Neuroimaging; Neurology; Neurology, pediatric; Neurosurgery; Positron emission tomography (PET) scanning; Seizures; Tumor removal; Tumors.

FOR FURTHER INFORMATION:

Daube, Jasper R., ed. *Clinical Neurophysiology*. 2d ed. New York: Oxford University Press, 2002. Covers the basics of clinical neurophysiology, considers the assessment of disease by anatomical system, and explains how clinical neurophysiologic techniques are used in the clinical assessment of diseases of the nervous system. Electroencephalography is covered extensively.

Ebersole, John S., and Timothy A. Pedley, eds. *Current Practice of Clinical Electroencephalography*. 3d ed. Philadelphia: Lippincott Williams & Wilkins, 2002. The thoroughly revised and greatly expanded third edition of this classic work covers the full range of applications of EEG and evoked potentials in current clinical practice. The most advanced instrumentation and techniques and their use in evaluating various disorders are discussed by more than twenty of the foremost authorities in the field.

Evans, James R., and Andrew Abarbanel, eds. *Introduction to Quantitative EEG and Neurofeedback*. San Diego, Calif.: Academic Press, 1999. The stated purpose of this text is to provide "an overview of the basics of QEEG and neurofeedback in one source."

Hayakawa, Fumio, et al. "Determination of Timing of Brain Injury in Preterm Infants with Periventricular Leukomalacia with Serial Neonatal Electroencephalography." *Pediatrics* 104, no. 5 (November, 1999): 1077-1081. The authors determine the timing of brain injury in infants with periventricular leukomalacia with serial encephalography recordings during the neonatal period.

Powledge, Tabitha M. "Unlocking the Secrets of the Brain: Part II." *Bioscience* 47, no. 7 (July/August, 1997): 403-408. In the second article in a two-part series, Powledge discusses positron emission tomography (PET) scanning, electroencephalography, magnetoencephalography, and other imaging techniques that help provide an understanding of the brain.

Ricker, Joseph H., and Ross D. Zafonte. "Functional Neuroimaging and Quantitative Electroencephalography in Adult Traumatic Head Injury: Clinical Applications and Interpretive Cautions." *The Journal of Head Trauma Rehabilitation* 15, no. 2 (April, 2000): 859. This article provides an overview of the use of procedures such as positron emission tomography, single photon emission computed tomography, and quantitative electroencephalography in adults.

ELECTROLYTES. *See* FLUIDS AND ELECTROLYTES.

ELEPHANTIASIS
DISEASE/DISORDER

ALSO KNOWN AS: Bancroft's filariasis
ANATOMY OR SYSTEM AFFECTED: Lymphatic system
SPECIALTIES AND RELATED FIELDS: Environmental health, epidemiology, public health
DEFINITION: A grossly disfiguring disease caused by a roundworm parasite; it is the advanced stage of the disease Bancroft's filariasis, contracted through roundworms.

KEY TERMS:
acute disease: a disease in which symptoms develop rapidly and which runs its course quickly
chronic disease: a disease that develops more slowly than an acute disease and persists for a long time
host: any organism on or in which another organism (called a parasite) lives, usually for the purpose of nourishment or protection
inflammation: a response of the body to tissue damage caused by injury or infection and characterized by redness, pain, heat, and swelling
lymph nodes: globular structures located along the routes of the lymphatic vessels that filter microorganisms from the lymph
lymphatic system: a body system consisting of lymphatic vessels and lymph nodes that transports lymph through body tissues and organs; closely associated with the cardiovascular system
lymphatic vessels: vessels that form a system for returning lymph to the bloodstream
parasite: an organism that lives on or within another organism, called the host, from which it derives sustenance or protection at the host's expense

CAUSES AND SYMPTOMS
Elephantiasis is characterized by gross enlargement of a body part caused by the accumulation of fluid and connective tissue. It most frequently affects the legs, but may also occur in the arms, breasts, scrotum, vulva, or any other body part. The disease starts with the slight enlargement of one leg or arm (or other body part). The limb increases in size with recurrent attacks of fever. Gradually, the affected part swells, and the swelling, which is soft at first, becomes hard following the growth of connective tissue in the area. In addition, the skin over the swollen area changes so that it becomes coarse and thickened, looking almost like elephant hide. The elephant-like skin, along with the enlarged body parts, gave the disease the name "elephantiasis."

Elephantiasis is found worldwide, mostly in the tropics and subtropics. Most cases of elephantiasis are a result of infection with a parasitic worm called *Wuchereria bancrofti* (*W. bancrofti*). *W. bancrofti* belongs to a group of worms called filaria, or roundworms, and infection with a filarial worm is called filariasis. Filariasis caused by *W. bancrofti* is the most common and widespread type of human filarial infection and is often called Bancroft's filariasis. Elephantiasis is the advanced, chronic stage of Bancroft's filariasis, and only a small percentage of persons with Bancroft's filariasis will develop elephantiasis. During Bancroft's filariasis, adult forms of *W. bancrofti* live inside the human lymphatic system, and it is the person's reaction to the presence of the worm that causes the symptoms of the disease. The worm's life cycle is important in understanding how the disease is transmitted from one person to another, how the symptoms develop, and how to prevent and reduce the incidence of the disease.

The adult worms live in human lymphatic vessels and lymph nodes and measure about 4 centimeters in length for the male and 9 centimeters in length for the female. Both are threadlike and about 0.3 millimeter in diameter. After mating, the female releases large num-

---

INFORMATION ON ELEPHANTIASIS

CAUSES: Infection from roundworm parasite
SYMPTOMS: Recurrent fever, inflammation of lymph vessels, swollen and painful lymph nodes, possible gross enlargement of body part
DURATION: Acute to chronic
TREATMENTS: Bed rest, supportive measures (*e.g.*, hot and cold compresses to reduce swelling), drug diethylcarbamazine (DEC)

bers of embryos or microfilariae (microscopic round-worms), which are more than one hundred times smaller in length and ten times thinner than their parents. They make their way from the lymphatic system into the bloodstream, where they can circulate for two years or longer. Interestingly, most strains of microfilariae (all except those found in the South Pacific Islands) exhibit a nocturnal periodicity, in which they appear in the peripheral blood system (the outer blood vessels, such as those in the arms, legs, and skin) only at night, mostly between the hours of 10 P.M. and 2 A.M., and the remainder of the time they spend in the blood vessels of the lungs and other internal organs. This nighttime cycling into the peripheral blood is somehow related to the patient's sleeping habits, and although it is unknown exactly how or why the microfilariae do this, it is necessary for the survival of the worms. The microfilariae must develop through at least three different stages (called the first, second, and third larval stages) before they are ready to mature into adults; these stages take place not within humans, but within certain types of mosquitoes, which bite at night. Thus, the microfilariae appear in the peripheral blood just in time for the mosquitoes to bite an infected human and extract them so that they can continue their life cycle. It is important to note, therefore, that both humans and the proper type of mosquito are needed to keep a filariasis infection going in a particular area.

Female night-feeding mosquitoes of the genera *Culex*, *Aedes*, and *Anopheles* serve as intermediate hosts for *Wuchereria bancrofti*. The mosquitoes bite an infected person and ingest microfilariae from the peripheral blood. The microfilariae pass into the intestines of the mosquito, invade the intestinal wall, and within a day find their way to the thoracic muscles (the muscles in the middle part of the mosquito's body). There they develop from first-stage to third-stage larvae in about two weeks, and the new third-stage larvae move from the thoracic muscles to the head and mouth of the mosquito. Only the third-stage larvae are able to infect humans successfully, and the third stage can mature only inside humans. When the mosquito takes a blood meal, infective larvae make their way through the proboscis (the tubular sucking organ with which a mosquito bites a person) and enter the skin through the puncture wound. After they enter the skin, the larvae move by an unknown route to the lymphatic system, where they develop into adult worms. It takes about one year or longer for the larvae to grow into adults, mate, and produce more microfilariae.

A person contracts Bancroft's filariasis by being bitten by an infected mosquito. Various forms of the disease can occur, depending on the person's immune response and the number of times the person is bitten. The period of time from when a person is first infected with larvae to the time microfilariae appear in the blood can be between one and two years. Even after this time some persons, especially young people, show no symptoms at all, yet they may have numerous microfilariae in their blood. This period of being a carrier of microfilariae without showing any signs of disease may last several years, and such carriers act as reservoirs for infecting the mosquito population.

In those patients showing symptoms from the infection, there are two stages of the disease: acute and chronic. In acute disease, the most common symptoms are a recurrent fever and lymphangitis and/or lymphadenitis in the arms, legs, or genitals. These symptoms are caused by an inflammatory response to the adult worms trapped inside the lymphatic system. Lymphangitis, an inflammation of the lymph vessels, is characterized by a hard, cordlike swelling or a red superficial streak that is tender and painful. Lymphadenitis is characterized by swollen and painful lymph nodes. The attacks of fever and lymphangitis or lymphadenitis recur at irregular intervals and may last from three weeks up to three months. The attacks usually become less frequent as the disease becomes more chronic. In the absence of reinfection, there is usually a steady improvement in the victim, each relapse being milder. Thus, without specific therapy, this condition is self-limiting and presumably will not become chronic in those acquiring the infection during a brief visit to an area where the disease is endemic.

The most obvious symptoms caused as a result of *W. bancrofti* infection, such as elephantiasis, are noted in the chronic stage. Chronic disease occurs only after years of repeated infection with the worms. It is seen only in areas where the disease is endemic and only occurs in a small percentage of the infected population. The symptoms are the result of an accumulation of damage caused by inflammatory reactions to the adult worms. The inflammation causes tissue death and a buildup of scar tissue that eventually results in the blockage of the lymphatic vessels in which the worms live. One of the functions of lymphatic vessels is to carry excess fluid away from tissues and bring it back to the blood, where it enters the circulation again as the fluid portion of the blood. If the lymphatic vessels are blocked, the excess fluid stays in the tissues, and swelling occurs. When this swelling is extensive, grotesque enlargement of that part of the body occurs.

TREATMENT AND THERAPY

One way in which doctors can tell whether a person has Bancroft's filariasis is by taking a sample of peripheral blood between 10 P.M. and 2 A.M. and looking at the blood under a microscope to try to find microfilariae. Sometimes, the ability to find microfilariae is enhanced by filtering the blood to concentrate the possible microfilariae in a smaller volume of liquid. Many persons infected with *W. bancrofti* have no detectable microfilariae in their blood, so other methods are available. In the absence of microfilariae, a diagnosis can be made on the basis of a history of exposure, symptoms of the disease, positive antibody or skin tests, or the presence of worms in a sample of lymph tissue. It is important to note that occasionally a few other filarial worms and at least one bacteria can also cause elephantiasis; therefore, if symptoms of elephantiasis are observed, it is important to discover the correct cause so that the proper treatment can be given. Since chronic infection occurs after prolonged residence in areas where the disease occurs, patients with acute disease should be removed from those areas. They also should be reassured that elephantiasis is a rare complication that is limited to persons who have had constant exposure to infected mosquitoes for years.

The best way to avoid contracting filariasis when traveling to an affected area is to avoid being bitten by mosquitoes. Insect repellent, mosquito netting, and other methods are helpful in this regard. No drugs or vaccines are available to prevent infection once a person is bitten.

A problem in the treatment of all parasitic diseases is finding a drug that will kill the parasite without harming the human host. The drug diethylcarbamazine (DEC) is the drug of choice in treating Bancroft's filariasis. Its advantages are that it can be taken orally, patients have a relatively high tolerance to the drug, and it has relatively rapid, beneficial clinical effects. Generally, in the treatment of acute disease, excellent results are obtained when the proper dosage of the drug is given. There are only two relatively mild side effects of DEC. The first is nausea or vomiting. This symptom depends on the amount of the drug given; therefore, lower doses help alleviate this side effect. The second is fever and dizziness, the severity of which depends on the number of microfilariae a person has in his or her blood; the more microfilariae, the more severe the reac-

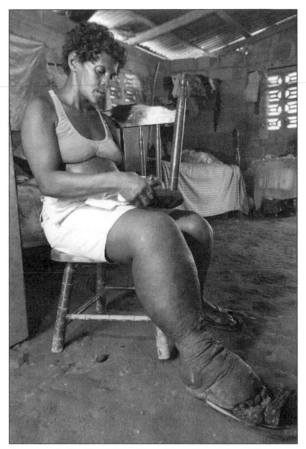

A woman in the Dominican Republic whose leg and foot have become crippled with elephantiasis, which affects many people in developing countries. (AP/Wide World Photos)

tion. It is important to warn patients ahead of time about the fever reaction and encourage them to continue taking their doses anyway. The fever reaction is a sign that the patient is being cured, but the cure will not completely work if the patient does not finish the whole regimen of drug doses. Other drugs have been used in the treatment of filariasis (suramin, metrifonate, levamisole) but are generally less effective or more toxic than DEC. Additional treatment measures include bed rest and supportive measures, such as using hot and cold compresses to reduce swelling. The administration of antibiotics for patients with secondary bacterial infections and painkillers as well as anti-inflammatory agents during the painful, acute stage is helpful. Sometimes, swollen limbs can be wrapped in pressure bandages to force the lymph from them. If the distortion is not too great, this method is successful. It should also be noted that, although drugs such as DEC might be effective in killing *W. bancrofti*, the chronic lesions resulting from the infection are mostly incurable. Signs of chronic filariasis, such as elephantiasis of the limbs or the scrotum, are usually unaffected or only incompletely cured by medication, and it sometimes becomes necessary to apply surgical or other symptomatic treatments to relieve the suffering of the patients. Chronic obstruction in less advanced stages is sometimes improved by surgery. The surgical removal of an elephantoid breast, vulva, or scrotum is sometimes necessary.

Theoretically, it should be possible first to control and eventually to eliminate Bancroft's filariasis. Conditions that are highly favorable for continued propagation of the infection include a pool of microfilariae carriers in the human population and the right species of mosquitoes breeding near human habitations. Thus, control can be effected by treating all microfilariae carriers in an affected area and eliminating the necessary mosquitoes. Microfilariae carriers can be effectively treated with DEC. The decision usually is between giving mass drug treatment to the entire population in an affected area or only treating those persons who are microfilariae positive. Usually, if the infection is at a high rate and very widespread in an area, it is best to treat the entire population, since it would be very time-consuming, difficult, and expensive to find all the microfilariae carriers. In other areas that are smaller or in which the pockets of infection are well defined, it is better to identify all the microfilariae-positive persons and treat only those persons until they are cured.

The second control measure is to eliminate the mosquito population. It is important to note that eliminating the mosquitoes alone will not control the disease, especially in tropical areas, since the breeding period and season in which the disease can be transmitted is so extensive. In some temperate areas, where Bancroft's filariasis used to be endemic, measures that removed the mosquitoes alone aided in the elimination of the disease from that area, since in temperate areas the breeding period and thus the season for transmission is so short. In tropical areas, both DEC therapy and mosquito control must be applied in order to control the disease.

The mosquito population can be controlled in four ways. First, general sanitation measures can be carried out in order to reduce the areas where the mosquitoes are breeding; for example, draining swamps. Second, insecticides can be used to kill the adult mosquitoes. Third, larvacides can be applied to sources of water where mosquitoes breed in order to kill the mosquito larvae. Finally, natural mosquito predators, such as certain species of fish, can be introduced into waters where mosquitoes breed to eat the mosquito larvae. Numerous problems stand in the way of eradication, such as poor sanitation, persons who do not cooperate with medical intervention, mosquitoes that become resistant to all known insecticides, increasing technology that yields increasing water supplies and therefore places for mosquitoes to breed, large populations, ignorance of the cause of the disease, and lack of medicine and a way of distributing that medicine.

PERSPECTIVE AND PROSPECTS

Dramatic symptoms of elephantiasis, especially the enormous swelling of legs or scrotum, were recorded in much of the ancient medical literature of India, Persia, and the Far East. The embryonic form of microfilariae was first discovered and described by a Frenchman in Paris in 1863. The organism was named for O. Wucherer, who also discovered microfilariae in 1866, and Joseph Bancroft, who discovered the adult worm in 1876. Two important facts about *W. bancrofti*—namely, its development in mosquitoes and the nocturnal periodicity of the microfilariae—were discovered by Patrick Manson between 1877 and 1879. This was the first example of a disease being transmitted by a mosquito, and its discovery earned for Manson the title of Father of Tropical Medicine. These and most of the other essential facts of the disease were discovered before the end of the nineteenth century. Progress in the epidemiology and control of filariasis came after World War II. In 1947, DEC was shown to kill filariae in animals, and this result was followed by the successful use of DEC in the treatment of humans. The first promising results in the control of Bancroft's filariasis by mass administration of DEC were reported in 1957 on a small island in the South Pacific. Through subsequent studies, it has become clear that effective control of the infection can be achieved if sufficient dosages of DEC are administered to infected populations.

Filariasis is a serious health hazard and public health problem in many tropical countries. Infection with *W. bancrofti* has been recorded in nearly all countries or territories in the tropical and subtropical zones of the world. The infection occurs primarily in coastal areas and islands that experience long periods of high humidity and heat. Infections have also been noted from some temperate zone districts, such as mainland Japan, central China, and some European countries. There is more Bancroft's filariasis now than there was a hundred years ago, principally because of increases in population in affected areas and in increased resistance of mosquitoes to insecticides. In 1947, it was estimated that 189 million people were infected with *W. bancrofti*. More recently, the World Health Organization estimated that 250 million people are infected and 400 million are at risk.

Bancroft's filariasis was introduced into and became endemic to Charleston, South Carolina, until 1920. It disappeared in the United States before World War II, presumably because of a reduction of mosquitoes resulting from improved sanitation. Servicemen in the Pacific in World War II were concerned about contracting elephantiasis; although several thousand showed signs of acute filariasis, only twenty had microfilariae in their blood, and no one developed elephantiasis. In the United States today, the infection is most frequently seen in immigrants, military veterans, and missionaries. It is important for physicians to be aware of this and other tropical diseases so that they can treat the occasional patient who is suffering from one of them, since most of these diseases are more successfully treated in the early stages of the disease.

—*Vicki J. Isola, Ph.D.*

See also Bites and stings; Edema; Inflammation; Insect-borne diseases; Lymphadenopathy and lymphoma; Lymphatic system; Parasitic diseases; Roundworms; Tropical medicine; Worms; Zoonoses.

FOR FURTHER INFORMATION:

Beaver, Paul C., and Rodney C. Jung. *Animal Agents and Vectors of Human Disease*. 5th ed. Philadelphia: Lea & Febiger, 1985. Discusses all major parasitic diseases. Chapter 12, "Filariae," which describes those diseases caused by filarial worms, contains helpful photographs and diagrams.

Biddle, Wayne. *A Field Guide to Germs*. 2d ed. New York: Anchor Books, 2002. This comprehensive book is easily accessible to the nonspecialist and includes a discussion of nearly every virus, bacterium, and fungus known to cause human and nonhuman animal disease. The history of the microbe and the treatment of diseases are included.

Frank, Steven A. *Immunology and Evolution of Infectious Disease*. Princeton, N.J.: Princeton University Press, 2002. Blends research from molecular biology, immunology, pathogen biology, and population dynamics to discuss how and why parasites vary to escape recognition by the immune system, vaccine design, and the control of epidemics.

Joklik, Wolfgang K., et al. *Zinsser Microbiology*. 20th ed. East Norwalk, Conn.: Appleton and Lange, 1992. The information presented in this textbook is thorough, logical, and supplemented by interesting diagrams, photographs, and charts. Contains a thorough description of Bancroft's filariasis.

Ransford, Oliver. *"Bid the Sickness Cease."* London: John Murray, 1983. Discusses the effect of disease on the development of Africa. Chapter 6, "The Father of Tropical Medicine," describes how Patrick Manson made the original discoveries of the cause of elephantiasis.

Roberts, Larry S., and John Janovy, Jr., eds. *Gerald D. Schmidt and Larry S. Roberts' Foundations of Parasitology*. 7th ed. Boston: McGraw-Hill Higher Education, 2005. Gives a good general description of all parasitic diseases and their causes, effects, and treatments. Deals specifically with diseases caused by filariae, including *Wuchereria bancrofti*.

Salyers, Abigail A., and Dixie D. Whitt. *Bacterial Pathogenesis: A Molecular Approach*. 2d ed. Washington, D.C.: ASM Press, 2002. Examines the molecular mechanism involved in bacterial-host interactions that can produce infectious disease. Introductory chapters discuss host-parasite relationships.

EMBOLISM

DISEASE/DISORDER

Anatomy or system affected: Blood vessels, brain, circulatory system, lungs, lymphatic system

SPECIALTIES AND RELATED FIELDS: Cardiology, internal medicine, neurology, vascular medicine

DEFINITION: A mass of undissolved matter traveling in the blood or lymphatic current.

CAUSES AND SYMPTOMS

An embolism is a mass of undissolved matter traveling in the vascular or lymphatic system. Although an embolism can be solid, liquid, or gaseous, the majority of emboli are solid. Likewise, emboli may consist of air bubbles, bits of tissue, globules of fat, tumor cells, or many other materials. The majority of emboli, however, are blood clots (thrombi) that originate in one portion of the body, then break loose and travel, eventually lodging in another part of the body. Where the traveling blood clot lodges will determine what kind of damage is done.

If the thrombus starts in the veins of the legs, it may break loose, travel up the veins of the leg and abdomen, pass through the right side of the heart, and lodge in the arteries in the lungs. This condition, called a pulmonary

INFORMATION ON EMBOLISM

CAUSES: Blood clot, air bubble, tissue, fat globules, tumor cells, or other material lodging in part of the body

SYMPTOMS: If in the lung, shortness of breath and chest pain; if in the heart, symptoms of heart attack; if in the brain, symptoms of stroke; if in the leg, pain, cold, numbness

DURATION: Acute

TREATMENTS: Depends on system affected; may include blood-thinners (heparin), thrombolytic drugs, bypass surgery

embolism, is often fatal. If the embolism is small, it may cause only shortness of breath and chest pain. If it is even smaller, the embolism may produce no symptoms at all.

If a blood clot forms in the chambers of the heart, breaks loose, and eventually lodges in an artery in the brain, then the patient will experience a stroke. If a clot breaks loose and lodges in an artery in the leg, then the patient will experience pain, coldness, or numbness in that leg. A blood clot that lodges in the coronary arteries, the arteries that feed the heart muscle, may cause a heart attack.

TREATMENT AND THERAPY

Treatment will vary depending on what system has been affected by the embolus. If the clot lodges in the lungs, then the patient will likely be placed on a blood-thinning drug such as heparin. In severe cases, thrombolytic drugs, which dissolve clots, may be used. If the clot lodges in a coronary artery, then open-heart surgery may be performed to bypass the occluded artery. If the clot lodges in the leg, a surgeon may remove the clot from the artery. This procedure is possible only when the clot is discovered early, when it has not yet formed a strong attachment to the vessel wall. Another approach to this problem may be to bypass the occluded artery using an artificial artery or a graft.

PERSPECTIVE AND PROSPECTS

The prevention and treatment of emboli are constantly improving. Venous thrombosis, the most common cause of pulmonary emboli, is becoming easier to diagnose thanks to major advances in ultrasound imaging. Also, magnetic resonance imaging (MRI) is being used to make the identification of emboli in the lungs more accurate and safer. Imaging procedures of the chambers of the heart, a common spot where emboli form, are improving as well, making prevention easier.

—*Steven R. Talbot, R.V.T.*

See also Arteriosclerosis; Blood and blood disorders; Cholesterol; Circulation; Heart; Heart attack; Lungs; Phlebitis; Pulmonary diseases; Pulmonary medicine; Pulmonary medicine, pediatric; Respiration; Strokes; Thrombolytic therapy and TPA; Thrombosis and thrombus; Varicose vein removal; Varicose veins; Vascular medicine; Vascular system.

FOR FURTHER INFORMATION:

Bick, Roger L. *Disorders of Thrombosis and Hemostasis: Clinical and Laboratory Practice.* 3d ed. Philadelphia: Lippincott Williams and Wilkins, 2002.

Kroll, Michael H. *Manual of Coagulation Disorders.* Malden, Mass.: Blackwell Science, 2001.

Reader's Digest, editors of. *ABC's of the Human Body: A Family Answer Book.* Pleasantville, N.Y.: Author, 1987.

Verstrate, Marc, Valentin Fuster, and Eric Topol, eds. *Cardiovascular Thrombosis: Thrombocardiology and Thromboneurology.* 2d ed. Philadelphia: Lippincott-Raven, 1998.

Virchow, Rudolf L. K. *Thrombosis and Emboli.* Translated by Axel C. Matzdorff and William R. Bell. Canton, Mass.: Science History, 1998.

EMBRYOLOGY

SPECIALTY

ANATOMY OR SYSTEM AFFECTED: All

SPECIALTIES AND RELATED FIELDS: Genetics, neonatology, obstetrics, perinatology

DEFINITION: The study of prenatal development from conception until the moment of birth.

KEY TERMS:

blastocyst: a small, hollow ball of cells which typifies one of the early embryonic stages in humans

cleavage: the process by which the fertilized egg undergoes a series of rapid cell divisions, which results in the formation of a blastocyst

congenital malformation: any anatomical defect present at birth

embryo: the developing human from conception until the end of the eighth week

fetus: the developing human from the end of the eighth week until the moment of birth

neural tube: the embryonic structure that gives rise to the central nervous system *teratogens:* substances that induce congenital malformations when embryonic tissues and organs are exposed to them

zygote: the fertilized egg; the first cell of a new organism

SCIENCE AND PROFESSION

The study of human embryology is the study of human prenatal development. The three stages of development are cleavage (the first week), embryonic development (the second through eighth weeks), and fetal development (the ninth through thirty-eighth weeks).

After an egg is fertilized by sperm in the uterine, or Fallopian, tube, the resulting zygote begins to divide rapidly. This period of rapid cell division is known as cleavage. By the third day, the zygote has divided into a solid ball containing twelve to sixteen cells. The small ball of cells resembles a mulberry and is called the morula, which is Latin for "mulberry." The morula moves from the uterine tube into the uterus.

The morula develops a central cavity as spaces begin to form between the inner cells. At this stage, the developing human is called a blastocyst. The ring of cells on the outer edge of the hollow ball is called the trophoblast and will form a placenta, while the cluster of cells within becomes the inner cell mass and will form the embryo. By the end of the first week, the surface of the inner cell mass has flattened to form an embryonic disc, and the blastocyst has attached to the lining of the uterus and begun to embed itself.

During the second week of development, the trophoblast makes connections with the uterus into which it has burrowed to form the placenta. Blood vessels from the embryo link it to the placenta through the umbilical cord, through which the embryo receives food and oxygen and releases wastes. Two sacs develop around the embryo: the fluid-filled amniotic sac that surrounds and cushions the embryo and the yolk sac that hangs beneath to provide nourishment. Finally, a large chorionic sac develops around the embryo and the two smaller sacs.

During the third week, the cells of the embryo are arranged in three layers. The outer layer of cells is called the ectoderm, the middle layer is the mesoderm, and the inner layer is the endoderm. The ectoderm gives rise to the epidermis (outer layer) of the skin and to the nervous system; the mesoderm gives rise to blood, bone, cartilage, and muscle; and the endoderm gives rise to body organ linings and glands.

Other significant events of the third week are the development of the primitive streak and notochord. The primitive streak is a thickened line of cells on the embryonic disk indicating the future embryonic axis. Development of the primitive streak stimulates the formation of a supporting rod of tissue beneath it called the notochord. The presence of the notochord triggers the ectoderm in the primitive streak above it to thicken, and the thickened area will give rise to the brain and spinal cord. Later, when vertebrae and muscles develop around the neural tissue, the notochord will disappear, leaving the center of the vertebral disk as its remnant.

The important event of the fourth week is the formation of the neural tube. After the thickened neural plate tissue has formed, an upward folding forms a groove, finally closing to form a neural tube. Closure begins at the head end and proceeds backward. The neural tube then sinks beneath surrounding ectodermal surface cells, which will become the skin covering the embryo.

Blocks of mesoderm cells line up along either side of

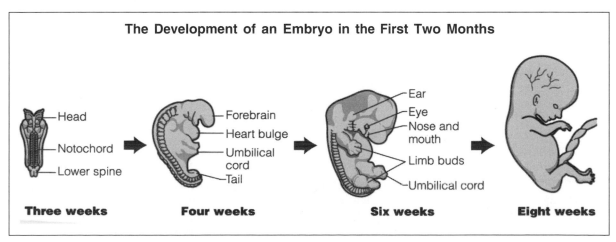

The Development of an Embryo in the First Two Months

Head
Notochord
Lower spine

Three weeks

Forebrain
Heart bulge
Umbilical cord
Tail

Four weeks

Ear
Eye
Nose and mouth
Limb buds
Umbilical cord

Six weeks

Eight weeks

the notochord and neural tube. These blocks are called somites, and eventually forty-two to forty-four pairs will form. They give rise to muscle, the cartilage of the head and trunk, and the inner layer of skin. At the same time, embryonic blood vessels develop on the yolk sac. Because the human embryo is provided little yolk, there is need for early development of a circulatory system to provide nutrition and gas exchange through the placenta.

The heart is formed and begins to beat in the fourth week, though it is not yet connected to many blood vessels. During the fourth through eighth weeks, all the organ systems develop, and the embryo is especially vulnerable to teratogens (environmental agents that interfere with normal development). A noticeable change in shape is seen during the fourth week because the rapidly increasing number of cells causes a folding under at the edges of the embryonic disk. The flattened disk takes on a cylindrical shape, and the folding process causes curvature of the embryo and it comes to lie on its side in a C-shaped position.

The beginnings of arms and legs are first seen in the fourth week and are called limb buds, appearing first as small bumps. The lower end of the embryo resembles a tail, and the swollen cranial part of the neural tube constricts to form three early sections of the brain. The eyes and ears begin to develop from the early brain tissue.

During the fifth through eighth weeks, the head enlarges as a result of rapid brain development. The head makes up almost half the embryo, and facial features begin to appear. Sexual differences exist but are difficult to detect. Nerves and muscles have developed enough to allow movement. By the end of the eighth week the limb buds have grown and differentiated into appendages with paddle-shaped hands and feet and short, webbed digits. The tail disappears, and the embryo begins to demonstrate human characteristics. By convention, the embryo is now called a fetus.

The fetal stage of development is the period between the ninth and thirty-eighth weeks, until birth. Organs formed during the embryonic stage grow and differentiate during the fetal stage. The body has the largest growth spurt between the ninth and twentieth weeks, but the greatest weight gain occurs during the last weeks of pregnancy.

In the third month, the difference between the sexes becomes apparent, urine begins to form and is excreted into the amniotic fluid, and the fetus can blink its eyelids. The fetus nearly doubles in length during the fourth month, and the head no longer appears to be so disproportionately large. Ossification of the skeleton begins, and by the end of the fourth month, ovaries are differentiated in the female fetus and already contain many cells destined to become eggs.

During the fifth month, fetal movements are felt by the mother, and the heartbeat can be heard with a stethoscope. Movements until this time usually go unnoticed. The average length of time that elapses between the first movement felt by the mother and delivery is twenty-one weeks.

During the sixth month, weight is gained by the fetus, but it is not until the seventh month that a baby usually can survive premature birth, when the body systems, particularly the lungs, are mature enough to function. During the eighth month, the eyes develop the ability to control the amount of light that enters them. Fat accumulates under the skin and fills in wrinkles. The skin becomes pink and smooth, and the arms and legs may become chubby. In the male fetus, the testes descend into the scrotal sac. Growth slows as birth approaches. The usual gestation length is 266 days, or thirty-eight weeks, after fertilization.

Diagnostic and Treatment Techniques

Knowledge of normal embryonic development is very important both in helping women provide optimal prenatal care for their children and in promoting scientific research for improved prenatal treatment, better understanding of malignant growths, and insight into the aging process.

Environmental stress to the embryo during the fourth through eighth weeks can cause abnormal development and result in congenital malformation, which may be defined as any anatomical defect present at birth. Environmental agents that cause malformations are known as teratogens. Malformations may develop from genetic or environmental factors, but most often they are caused by a combination of the two. Some of the common teratogens are viral infections, drug use, a poor diet, smoking, alcohol consumption, and irradiation.

The genetic makeup of some individuals makes them particularly sensitive to certain agents, while others are resistant. The abnormalities may be immediately apparent at birth or hidden within the body and discovered later. Embryos with severe structural abnormalities often do not survive, and such abnormalities represent an important cause of miscarriages. In fact, up to half of all conceptions spontaneously abort, with little or no notice by the prospective mother.

Genetic birth defects are passed on from one generation to another and result from a gene mutation at some time in the past. Mutations are caused by accidental rearrangement of deoxyribonucleic acid (DNA), the material of which genes are made, and range in severity from mild to life-threatening. They may cause such conditions as extra fingers and toes, cataracts, dwarfism, albinism, and cystic fibrosis. Gene mutations on a sex chromosome are described as sex-linked and are usually passed from mother to son; these include hemophilia, hydrocephalus (an excessive amount of cerebrospinal fluid), color blindness, and a form of baldness.

Abnormalities in the embryo may result because of unequal distribution of chromosomes in the formation of eggs or sperm. This imbalance can cause a variety of problems in development, such as Down syndrome and abnormal sexual development. The normal human cell contains twenty-three chromosomes, twenty-two pairs of which are nonsex chromosomes, or autosomes. The last pair consists of the two sex chromosomes. Females normally have two X chromosomes, and males have an X and a Y chromosome.

When females have only one X, a set of conditions known as Turner syndrome results. The embryo will develop as a normal female, though ovaries will not fully form and there may be congenital heart defects. Because the single X chromosome does not cause enough estrogen to be produced, sexual maturity will not occur. If a male embryo should receive only the Y chromosome, it cannot survive. Sometimes a male will receive two (or more) X chromosomes along with a Y chromosome (XXY), producing Klinefelter syndrome. The appearance of the child is normal, but at puberty the breasts may enlarge and the testes will not mature, causing sterility. Males receiving two Y chromosomes (XYY) develop normally, but they may be quite tall and find controlling their impulses to be difficult.

Viral infections in the mother during the embryonic stages can cause problems in organ formation by disturbing normal cell division, fetal vascularization, and the development of the immune system. The organs most vulnerable to infection will be those undergoing rapid cell division and growth at the time of infection. For example, the lens of the eye is forming during the sixth week of development, and infection at this time could cause the formation of cataracts.

While most microorganisms cannot pass through the placenta to reach the embryo or fetus, those that can are capable of causing major problems in the embryonic development. Rubella, the virus that causes German measles, often causes birth defects in children should infection occur shortly before or during the first three months of pregnancy. The developing ears, eyes, and heart are especially susceptible to damage during this time. When a rubella infection occurs during the first five weeks of pregnancy, interference with organ development is most pronounced. After the fifth week, the risks of infection are not as great, but central nervous system impairment may occur as late as the seventh month.

The most common source of fetal infection may be the cytomegalovirus (CMV), a form of herpes which causes abortion during the first three months of pregnancy. If infection occurs later, the liver and brain are especially vulnerable and impairment in vision, hearing, and mental ability may result. Evidence has also suggested that the immune system of the fetus is adversely affected.

Other viruses may affect fetal development as well. When herpes simplex infects the fetus several weeks before birth, blindness or mental retardation may result. *Toxoplasma gondii*, a parasite of animals often kept as pets, may adversely affect eye and brain development without the mother having known that she had the infection. Syphilis infection in the mother leads to death or serious fetal abnormalities unless it is treated before the sixteenth week of pregnancy; if it is untreated, the fetus may possess hearing impairment, hydrocephalus, facial abnormalities, and mental retardation. Women infected with acquired immunodeficiency syndrome (AIDS) may transmit the virus to their infants before or during birth.

Certain chemicals can cross the placenta and produce malformation of developing tissues and organs. During an embryo's first twenty-five days, damage to the primitive streak can cause malformation in bone, blood, and muscle. While bones and teeth are being formed, they may be adversely affected by antibiotics such as tetracycline.

At one time, thalidomide was widely used as an antinauseant in Great Britain and Germany and to some extent in the United States. Large numbers of congenital abnormalities began to appear in newborns, and the drug was withdrawn from the market after two years. Thalidomide caused failure of normal limb development and was especially damaging during the third to seventh weeks.

Exposure to other chemicals causes central nervous system disorders when the neural tube fails to close.

When the anterior end of the tube does not close, development of the brain and spinal cord will be absent or incomplete and anencephaly results. Babies can live no more than a few days with this condition because the higher control centers of the brain are undeveloped. If the posterior end of the tube fails to close, one or more vertebrae will not develop completely, exposing the spinal cord; this condition is called spina bifida. This condition varies in severity with the level of the defect and the amount of neural tissue that remains exposed, because exposed tissue degenerates.

It has been long believed that neural tube disorders accompanied maternal depletion of folic acid, one of the B vitamins, and research has substantiated that relationship. Anencephaly and spina bifida rarely occur in the infants of women taking folic acid supplements. One of the harmful effects of alcohol and anticonvulsants is their depletion of the body's natural folic acid. A decrease in the mother's folic acid levels in the first through third months of pregnancy can cause abortion or growth deformities.

Maternal smoking is strongly implicated in low infant birth weights and higher fetal and infant mortality rates. Cigarette smoke may cause cardiac abnormalities, cleft lip and palate, and a missing brain. Nicotine decreases blood flow to the uterus and interferes with normal development, allowing less oxygen to reach the embryo.

Alcohol use may be the number one cause of birth defects. Exposure of the fetus to alcohol in the blood results in fetal alcohol syndrome. Symptoms may include growth deficiencies, an abnormally small head, facial malformation, and damage to the heart and the nervous and reproductive systems. Behavioral disorders such as hyperactivity, attention deficit, and inability to relate to others may accompany fetal alcohol syndrome.

Radiation treatments given to pregnant women may cause cell death, chromosomal injury, and growth retardation in the developing embryo. The effect is proportional to the dosage of radiation. Malformations may be visible at birth, or a condition such as leukemia may develop later. Abnormalities caused by radiation include cleft palate, an abnormally small head, mental retardation, and spina bifida. Diagnostic X rays are not believed to emit enough radiation to cause abnormalities in embryonic development, but precautions should be taken.

Oxygen deficiency to the embryo or fetus occurs when mothers use cocaine. Maternal blood pressure fluctuates with the use of this drug, and the embryonic brain is deprived of oxygen, resulting in vision problems, lack of coordination, and mental retardation. Too little oxygen to the fetus may also cause death from lung collapse soon after birth.

Obvious physical malformations resulting from embryonic exposure to drugs have been recognized for a number of years, but recent investigators have found there are more subtle levels of effect that may show up later as behavioral problems. Physical abnormalities have been easily documented, but more attention is needed regarding the behavioral effects caused by teratogens.

PERSPECTIVE AND PROSPECTS

The first recorded observations of a developing embryo were performed on a chick by Hippocrates in the fifth century B.C.E. In the fourth century B.C.E., Aristotle wondered whether a preformed human unfolded in the embryo and enlarged with time, or whether a very simple embryonic structure gradually became more and more complex. This question was debated for nearly two thousand years until the early nineteenth century, when microscopic studies of chick embryos were carefully conducted and described.

Understanding human embryology is foundational for recognizing the relationships that exist between the body systems and congenital malformations in newborns. This field of study takes on new importance in the light of advances of modern technology, which have made prenatal diagnosis and treatment a reality.

The study of embryology is also making contributions toward finding the causes of malignant growth. Malignancy is a breakdown in the mechanisms for normal growth and differentiation first seen in the early embryo. Questions about uninhibited malignant growth may be answered by studying embryonic tissues and organs.

The study of old age is another area in which embryological research is valuable. Understanding the clock mechanisms of embryonic cells has led to greater understanding of the "winding down" of cells in old age. It is also important that researchers discover how environmental conditions modify rates of growth and affect the cell's clock. The degree to which the human life span can be expanded remains one of the most challenging questions in the area of aging.

In addition to the health benefits that may be derived from embryological research, this field is an important source of insight into some of the moral and ethical dilemmas facing humankind. Artificial insemination, contraception, and abortion regulations are some of the problems that will require close collaboration between ethicists and scientists, especially embryologists.

—*Katherine H. Houp, Ph.D.;*
updated by Alexander Sandra, M.D.

See also Abortion; Amniocentesis; Assisted reproductive technologies; Birth defects; Brain disorders; Cerebral palsy; Cesarean section; Chorionic villus sampling; Cloning; Conception; Down syndrome; Fetal alcohol syndrome; Fetal surgery; Gamete intrafallopian transfer (GIFT); Genetic counseling; Genetic diseases; Genetics and inheritance; Growth; Gynecology; In vitro fertilization; Miscarriage; Multiple births; Neonatology; Obstetrics; Perinatology; Placenta; Pregnancy and gestation; Premature birth; Reproductive system; Rh factor; Rubella; Sexual differentiation; Spina bifida; Stillbirth; Teratogens; Toxoplasmosis; Ultrasonography.

For Further Information:

Mader, Sylvia S. *Inquiry into Life.* 11th ed. New York: McGraw-Hill, 2004. An introductory-level college text designed to cover the entire range of biological topics. Gives a clear description of typical early developmental stages of all vertebrates and offers a section on human embryology and fetal development, adulthood, and aging.

Marieb, Elaine N. *Essentials of Human Anatomy and Physiology.* 8th ed. San Francisco: Pearson/Benjamin Cummings, 2006. This introductory anatomy and physiology textbook, easily accessible to those with little science background, is richly illustrated with diagrams and photographs, which help to illuminate body systems and processes.

Moore, Keith L., and T. V. N. Persaud. *The Developing Human.* 7th ed. Philadelphia: W. B. Saunders, 2003. An outstanding textbook on human embryonic development, with specific information about the causes of congenital malformations and common defects occurring in each of the body's systems. This widely used textbook gives a clear and careful description of normal human development during the entire prenatal period.

Riley, Edward P., and Charles V. Vorhees, eds. *Handbook of Behavioral Teratology.* New York: Plenum Press, 1986. An informative compilation of learning in the field of behavioral teratology. Covers historical context, general principles, and specific drugs and environmental agents that act as behavioral teratogens. Effects are listed for each agent that has been studied.

Tortora, Gerard J., and Bryan Derrickson. *Principles of Anatomy and Physiology.* 11th ed. Hoboken, N.J.: John Wiley & Sons, 2006. An intermediate-level college text widely used in fields of allied health. Chapters include overview of human prenatal development from fertilization through birth. Written in a very readable fashion; has excellent color diagrams and photographs on every page.

Tsiaras, Alexander, and Barry Werth. *From Conception to Birth: A Life Unfolds.* New York: Doubleday, 2002. Using state-of-the-art medical imaging technology, traces the development of a human life from conception through birth in spectacular, highly detailed photographs.

Emergency medicine
Specialty

Anatomy or system affected: All

Specialties and related fields: Cardiology, critical care, gastroenterology, geriatrics and gerontology, neurology, nursing, obstetrics, pediatrics, pharmacology, psychiatry, public health, pulmonary medicine, radiology, sports medicine, toxicology

Definition: The care of patients who are experiencing immediate health crises, a field defined by twenty-four-hour availability, the management of multiple patients simultaneously, and the need for broad-based skills and interventions.

Key terms:

diagnostic: relating to the determination of the nature of a disease

emergency medical services: the complete chain of human and physical resources that provides patient care in cases of sudden illness or injury

heuristics: methods used to aid and guide in the discovery of a disease process when incomplete knowledge exists

paramedic: a person trained and certified to provide prehospital emergency medical care

pathologic: pertaining to the study of disease and the development of abnormal conditions

pathophysiology: an alteration in function as seen in disease

patient assessment: the systematic gathering of information in order to determine the nature of a patient's illness

triage: the medical screening of patients to determine their relative priority for treatment

Science and Profession

The field of emergency medicine is defined as care to acutely ill and injured patients, both in the prehospital setting and in the emergency room. It is practiced as patient-demanded and continuously accessible care and is defined by the location of its practice rather than by an anatomical concern. Emergency medicine encompasses all medical specialties and physical systems. The commitment to rapid, prudent intervention under stressful and often chaotic conditions is of paramount importance to the critically ill patient. This branch of medicine is characterized by its complexity of problems, its twenty-four-hour availability to a variety of patients, and its effective and broad-based understanding of disease and injury. These features are used to orchestrate the response of multiple hands with the ultimate goal of referring the patient to ongoing care.

The hourglass is an appropriate symbol of the nature of this medical division. It not only portrays the importance of time and the need for quick intervention, but its shape—wide at either end and narrowing in the middle—also is an appropriate visualization of the pattern of emergency medical treatment. A large number of patients converge on a single area, the emergency room, where they are diagnosed, treated, and eventually released to other appropriate care, diverging on a wide range of follow-up options.

Unique to the field of emergency medicine is the importance of rapid definition and comprehension of the pathophysiology of the critically ill patient. Emergency care physicians must have a unique understanding of the practice of medicine, the nature of disease and injury, availing themselves of a host of clinical skills needed for the treatment of the variety of physical and psychological problems that require treatment. Emergency rooms are a melting pot of problems; most are medical, many are not. All of them reflect some person's perception of an emergency. Success in the emergency medical field often depends on the ability of personnel to use not only their medical knowledge but their knowledge of people as well.

Most often those seeking the assistance of emer-

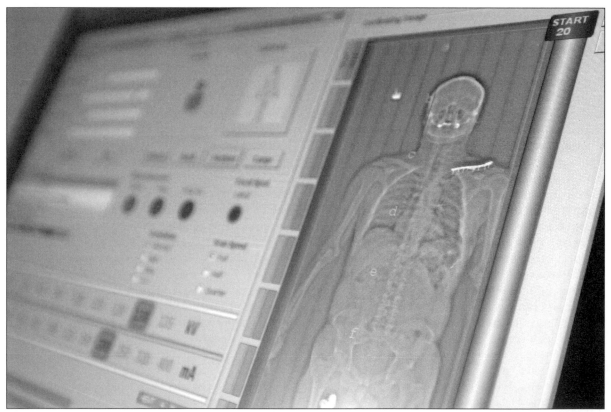

A monitor displays an image from Statscan, a low-dose, digital X-ray system that can provide a full-body scan in thirteen seconds without movement required from the patient. Such technology could prove lifesaving in emergency rooms. (AP/Wide World Photos)

gency medical providers are people suffering from pain of illness or trauma; however, any patient may seek treatment at the emergency room. Often loneliness, disability, or homelessness serves as the motivation to seek treatment. Regardless of what brought the patient, the emergency physician strives to recognize and deal with the patient's "emergency," remembering that not all patients are as ill as they might think and that not all are as well as they might appear. Physicians of this specialty sift through a multitude of information. It is necessary to know the patient's pertinent medical history and the history of the present illness or complaint before appropriate and effective treatment can be prescribed. Patients rarely follow a preconceived plan. Emergency medicine works best, therefore, when its practitioners follow heuristics—that is, incomplete guides that lead to greater knowledge, a holistic approach.

Emergency medicine is primarily a hospital-based specialty; however, it also involves extensive prehospital responsibilities. Many times, patients seeking emergency care are first the responsibility of police, fire, or ambulance personnel. In these situations, the role of emergency medicine must be viewed under the wider context of the emergency medical system. This system—beginning with the first aid administered by bystanders leading to initial treatment and transportation by trained certified emergency medical technicians, paramedics, or flight nurses and culminating with care at an emergency room or a highly equipped trauma center—forms a uniquely structured unit. The emergency medical system is designed to provide rapid quality intervention regardless of prehospital conditions. The emergency medical physician is best viewed as a central part of a team whose knowledge and understanding of the whole allow the best possible care to patients undergoing health crises.

Emergency physicians are charged with the responsibility of providing the highest standard of care in the hospital setting. They ensure that both staff members and equipment are maintained at their utmost level of quality. Trends, breakthroughs, and recent advances are monitored via journals and other medical publications. Training of personnel must keep pace with medical advancement. Developing an overall program depends as much on its planning as its dissemination. The emergency physician often plays the role of teacher, actively influencing the overall quality of the program through education and skills development. Thus, the exercise of emergency medicine is truly a team effort, with all members acting in accordance with their train-

ing and level of competence in order to minimize further injury or discomfort.

In practice, emergency medicine encompasses any person or structure involved in the immediate decision making and/or actions necessary to prevent death or further disability of a patient in the midst of a health crisis. It represents a chain of human and physical resources brought together for the purpose of providing total patient care. In this respect, everyone has a part to play in the delivery of emergency care. The bottom line of emergency medicine is the welfare of the patient. Thus, it is most appropriate to view the practice of emergency medicine in the context of the entire emergency medical system.

The components of the emergency medical system include recognition of the emergency, initiation of emergency medical response, treatment at the scene, transport by members of an emergency medical team to the appropriate facility, treatment in the emergency room or trauma center, and release of the patient. These components are only as strong as the weakest link.

DIAGNOSTIC AND TREATMENT TECHNIQUES

Recognition of an emergency is the first step in emergency care. Often this step is complicated by the patient's own denial and ignorance of basic symptoms. "Emergency" is in part defined by the patient's ability to identify, accept, and respond to a given situation. Regardless of the nature of the illness or injury, the sooner an emergency is defined, the sooner care can be provided. The typical heart attack victim, for example, waits an average of three hours after experiencing symptoms before seeking help. In such cases, treatment by bystanders who have been trained in first aid and cardiopulmonary resuscitation (CPR) has proven effective.

In the United States, the response of emergency medical personnel has been aided by the implementation of the 911 emergency system. While not all communities have this capability, its use is increasing. It has been documented that patients who receive treatment at an appropriate facility within sixty minutes of the onset of a life-threatening emergency are more likely to survive. This "golden hour" is precious time.

Operating under protocols developed and approved by the emergency medical director and emergency medical councils of a given locale, emergency medical technicians (EMTs) and paramedics are trained and authorized to deliver care to the patient in need at the scene. EMTs and paramedics are charged with the ini-

IN THE NEWS: EXEMPTION FROM INFORMED CONSENT REQUIREMENTS FOR EMERGENCY RESEARCH

Informed consent is a patient's competent, voluntary permission to undergo a proposed treatment plan or procedure. In order to obtain a patient's informed consent, the physician must provide the patient with sufficient information to assist the patient in making an informed decision. The information provided should include indications for the procedure, any risks, and any available alternatives. The patient should be given an opportunity to ask questions and to deny consent if, after a thorough explanation, the patient feels that that is the best option.

Federally mandated Institutional Review Boards (IRBs) must approve any research involving human subjects, including research in emergency departments. The IRBs aim to protect patients by ensuring that people who participate in research give adequate informed consent. In a medical emergency, however, it is unclear whether consent is sufficiently informed. So that critically ill and injured patients are not denied an opportunity to participate in beneficial research trials, the U.S. Food and Drug Administration (FDA) and the Department of Health and Human Services issued regulations that allow "emergency research" without informed consent. These regulations create an exception to the informed consent requirement when subjects are in a life-threatening situation, obtaining informed consent is not feasible, the research offers possible direct therapeutic benefit to the subjects, the investigation could not be carried out without the waiver, and additional protections of the rights and welfare of the subjects are provided. Because a waiver of informed consent undermines one of the most significant protections of human subjects, the guidelines attempt to compensate by providing additional precautions, including community consultation, public disclosure, and intensive oversight by an independent data and monitoring committee. The basis for these regulations is the premise that if the proposed research is not harmful, and particularly if it is potentially helpful, most "reasonable" patients would give their consent. Another instance in which consent may be waived involves minimal risk research, provided that the waiver will not adversely affect the rights and welfare of the subjects.

—Marcia J. Weiss, J.D.

tial assessment of the patient's condition, immediate stabilization prior to transport, delivery of care as far as their training allows, and the transport of the patient.

Unique to the field of emergency medicine is the special relationship of the paramedic with the doctor. Many people in need of emergency care are first treated outside the hospital. In these cases, emergency caregivers on the scene act as the eyes, ears, and hands of the physician. Through the EMT or paramedic, using telecommunications, an emergency doctor can speed the process of diagnosis. Signs and symptoms relayed through these trained professionals enable a doctor to make an accurate assessment of the patient's condition and to request a variety of treatments for a patient whom they cannot see or touch. Linked by telephone or radio, the medic and doctor can capitalize on the golden hour with the initiation of quality care.

Paramedics operate under the medical license of a medical command physician who has met all criteria set forth by the Department of Health and has been approved to provide medical directives to prehospital and interhospital providers. Protocols are the recognized practices that are within the training of the EMT and paramedic. They serve as standard procedures for prehospital treatment. While it is recognized that situations will arise which call for deviation from particular aspects of a given protocol, they are the standards under which the doctor and emergency personnel on the scene operate.

Treatment at the scene is followed by transport with advanced life support by members of the emergency medical system in 85 percent of all emergency cases. This requires much-needed equipment for the further treatment of patients. Deficiencies in the vehicle, equipment, or training of medical personnel can seriously endanger a patient. Thus, government agencies have been designated to grant permission for ambulance services and hospitals to engage in the practice of emergency medicine. This licensure process is designed to demand a level of competency for health care providers and ensure the public's protection.

Since only about 5 percent of all emergency department admissions constitute life-threatening situations, not all facilities stand at the same level of readiness for a given emergency. Transportation to the appropriate facility, therefore, requires a matching of patient's need to the hospital's capabilities. Hospitals are categorized according to their ability to render emergency intensive care, as well as to provide needed support services on a patient-demand basis. In general, they are viewed as emergency facilities, and trauma facilities, where trauma centers are designed to provide twenty-four-hour, comprehensive emergency intensive care, including operating rooms and intensive care nurses.

When the patient reaches the emergency facility, during the first five to fifteen minutes of care, many important decisions are made by the physician on duty. The process continues to overlap with needed diagnostic tests and consultations in an effort to provide quality care directed at the source of the illness or injury. The patient's immediate needs are cared for by emergency department staff until the patient is moved to a site of continued care or released to his or her own care.

Questions correctly phrased and sharply directed are effective tools for the rapid diagnosis needed in emergency medicine. The key to this field is the ability to triage, stabilize, prioritize, treat, and refer.

Triage is the system used for categorizing and sorting patients according to the severity of their problems. Emergency practitioners seek to ascertain the nature of the patient's problem and consider any life-threatening consequences of the present condition. This stage of triage allows for immediate care to the more seriously endangered person, relegating the more stable, less seriously ill or wounded patients to a waiting period. The emergency room, in other words, does not operate on a first come, first served basis.

Secondary to triage is stabilization. This term refers to any immediate treatment or intervening steps taken to alleviate conditions that would result in greater pain or defect and/or lead to irreversible or fatal consequences. Primary stabilization steps include ensuring an unobstructed airway and providing adequate ventilation and cardiovascular function.

Once patients have been stabilized, all illnesses must be looked at on the scale of their hierarchical importance. Life-threatening diseases or injuries are treated before more moderate or minor conditions. This system of prioritization can be illustrated from patient to patient: A heart attack victim, for example, is treated prior to the patient with an ankle sprain. It can also be applied for multiple conditions within the same patient. The heart attack victim with a sprained ankle receives treatment first for the life-threatening cardiovascular incident.

Treatment of the critically ill patient often poses a series of further questions. What is the primary disorder? Is there more than one active pathologic process present? How does the patient appear? Is the patient's presentation consistent with the initial diagnosis? Is a hospital stay warranted? What consultations are needed to diagnose and treat this patient?

The emergency physician's approach is to consider the most serious disease consistent with the patient's presentation and chief complaint. By rule of thumb, thinking the worst and hoping for the best is often the psychological stance of the emergency care provider. Only when more severe conditions have been ruled out are more minor processes considered. Often too, this broad view of patient assessment allows for multiple diagnosis. Through continued probing, alternate and additional conditions are often uncovered. It is not unlikely that the patient who seeks treatment for a head injury after a fall is diagnosed with a more serious condition which caused the fall. Focusing only on the immediate condition would endanger the patient. Success in this medical field therefore demands broad-based medical knowledge and diagnostic tools.

Emergency medicine is not practiced in a vacuum. Its very nature necessitates its interfacing with a variety of medical specialties. The emergency room is often only the first step in patient recovery. Initial diagnosis and stabilization must be coupled with plans for ongoing treatment and evaluation. Consultations and referrals play important roles in the overall care of a patient.

PERSPECTIVE AND PROSPECTS

Historians are unable to document specific systems for emergency patients before the 1790's. The need to provide care to the battlefield wounded is seen as the first implementation of emergency response. Early wartime treatment did not, however, include prehospital treatment. Clara Barton is credited with providing the first professional-level prehospital emergency care for the wounded as part of the American Red Cross. Ambulance services began in major cities of the United States at the beginning of the twentieth century, but it was not until 1960 that the National Academy of Sciences' National Research Council actually studied the problem of emergency care.

Emergency medicine as a specialty is relatively new. Not until 1975, when the House of Delegates of the American Medical Association defined the emergency physician, did the medical community even recognize this branch of medicine. In 1981, the American College of Emergency Physicians added further recognition through the development of the definition of emergency medicine. Since then, growth and changes have enabled this field to develop as a major specialty, evolving to accept greater responsibility in both education and practice.

The development of emergency medicine and the increasing number of health care providers in this field have been dramatic. In 1990, there were a total of 23,000 emergency physicians, 85,000 emergency nurses, and 521,734 emergency technicians. These health care providers delivered care to the nearly 87 million emergency department patients seen that year.

Emergency medicine developed at a time when both the general public and the medical community recognized the need for quality accessible care in the emergency situation. It has grown to include a gamut of services provided by a community. In addition to responding to the acutely ill or injured, emergency medicine has grown to accept responsibilities of education, administration, and advocacy.

Included in the role of today's emergency medical providers is the administration of the entire emergency medical system within a community. This system includes the development of public education programs such as CPR instruction, poison control education, and the introduction of the 911 system. Emergency management systems and coordinators are now part of every state and local government. Disaster planning for both natural and human-made accidents also comes under the heading of emergency medicine.

Research, too, plays an important role in emergency medicine. The desire to identify, understand, and disseminate scientific rationale for basic resuscitative interventions, as well as the need to improve preventive medical techniques, are often driving forces in scientific research.

Finally, emergency medicine plays a key role in many of society's problems. Homelessness, drug use and abuse, acquired immunodeficiency syndrome (AIDS), and rising health costs have all contributed to the increase in the number of patients seen in the emergency room. In response, those administering emergency medical care have tried to communicate such problems to the general public and legislative bodies, as well as educate them regarding preventive measures. Being on the front line of medicine brings a special obligation to improve laws and services to ensure public safety and well-being.

—*Mary Beth McGranaghan*

See also Abdominal disorders; Altitude sickness; Amputation; Aneurysms; Antibiotics; Appendectomy; Appendicitis; Asphyxiation; Avian influenza; Biological and chemical weapons; Bites and stings; Bleeding; Botulism; Burns and scalds; Cardiac arrest; Cardiology; Cardiology, pediatric; Cardiopulmonary resuscitation (CPR); Catheterization; Cesarean section; Choking; Coma; Concussion; Critical care; Critical care, pediatric; Drowning; Electrical shock; Electrocardiography (ECG or EKG); Electroencephalography (EEG); Emergency medicine, pediatric; Fracture and dislocation; Fracture repair; Frostbite; Grafts and grafting; Head and neck disorders; Heart attack; Heat exhaustion and heat stroke; Hospitals; Hyperbaric oxygen therapy; Hyperthermia and hypothermia; Intoxication; Laceration repair; Meningitis; Nursing; Obstetrics; Paramedics; Peritonitis; Pneumonia; Poisoning; Radiation sickness; Resuscitation; Reye's syndrome; Salmonella infection; Shock; Snakebites; Spinal cord disorders; Splenectomy; Sports medicine; Staphylococcal infections; Streptococcal infections; Strokes; Thrombolytic therapy and TPA; Tracheostomy; Transfusion; Unconsciousness; Veterinary medicine; Wounds.

FOR FURTHER INFORMATION:

Bledsoe, Bryan E., Robert S. Porter, and Bruce R. Shade. *Brady Paramedic Emergency Care*. 3d ed. Upper Saddle River, N.J.: Brady/Prentice Hall, 1997. A comprehensive guide to the practice of emergency medicine as it applies to and is practiced by the paramedic. A solid overview of the basics of prehospital care. This text focuses on advanced life support practices.

Caroline, Nancy L. *Emergency Care in the Streets*. 5th ed. Boston: Little, Brown, 1995. This text provides a sophisticated understanding of the fundamental concepts of advanced life support and the underlying physiology. A focused approach written by a physician who has spent many hours in the field as a prehospital care provider. Includes new chapters on AIDS and other communicable diseases.

Hamilton, Glenn C., et al. *Emergency Medicine: An Approach to Clinical Problem-Solving*. 2d ed. New York: W. B. Saunders, 2003. Addressed to students of medicine, this text provides a detailed, well-written script for the clinical setting. Facilitates the reader's understanding of the emergency scene. Actual medical cases are integrated into the chapters in order to reinforce concepts.

Limmer, Daniel, et al. *Emergency Care*. 9th ed. Upper Saddle River, N.J.: Brady/Prentice Hall Health, 2001. This simple text has been acclaimed for its comprehensive, accurate, and up-to-the-minute treatment of emergency care. Easy to read, this book provides the contemporary standards on CPR from the American Heart Association and a full treatment on many emergency medical protocols for prehospital treatment.

Marovchick, Vincent J., and Peter T. Pons, eds. *Emergency Medicine Secrets*. 4th ed. Philadelphia: Mosby Elsevier, 2006. Details all aspects of emergency medicine in a question-and-answer format. Topics include nontraumatic illness, hematology/oncology, infectious disease, environmental emergencies, neonatal and childhood disorders, toxicologic emergencies, emergency medicine administration and risk management, and disaster management.

Marx, John A., et al., eds. *Rosen's Emergency Medicine: Concepts and Clinical Practice*. 6th ed. Philadelphia: Mosby/Elsevier, 2006. A logical and straightforward presentation of current standards of emergency medicine. Intended to be a reference in busy emergency rooms. The writing is clear and to the point.

Tintinalli, Judith E., ed. *Emergency Medicine: A Comprehensive Study Guide*. 6th ed. New York: McGraw-Hill, 2004. This bible of emergency medicine provides a basic understanding of the field. Describes in detail key diagnostic techniques and treatments.

EMERGENCY MEDICINE, PEDIATRIC

SPECIALTY

ANATOMY OR SYSTEM AFFECTED: All

SPECIALTIES AND RELATED FIELDS: Critical care

DEFINITION: The decision making and actions necessary to prevent death or any further disability in children with life-threatening injuries, illnesses, and other health crises.

KEY TERMS:

abc's: the basics of survival—*a* is for airway obstruction/choking, *b* is for breathing/respiratory distress, and *c* is for circulatory collapse/shock

pediatric emergency specialists: emergency physicians who focus their practices on emergency care for children, including research and teaching pediatric emergency medicine

triage: the process of choosing who will receive medical treatment first because of dire illness or injury

SCIENCE AND PROFESSION

Physicians who specialize in pediatric emergency medicine have been trained to diagnose and treat patients in order to prevent death or any further disability for children in health crises. They are also skilled at health promotion and injury prevention efforts. For some young patients, emergency departments are increasingly the only source of routine medical care. Pediatric emergency physicians represent the front line of medicine.

Emergency medicine emphasizes the anticipation and recognition of a life-threatening process, rather than seeking a definitive diagnosis. The emergencies that these physicians treat are often the type parents hope never to see. The perceptions and complaints of the patients or the people who bring them to the emergency department or pediatric trauma center define the emergencies themselves. Most children treated in an emergency department will be seen in a general hospital whose staff is unlikely to include pediatric specialists. Each year, about one-third of the children who visit the emergency department are there because of an injury. Two-thirds of the visits are the result of illnesses such as debilitating asthma or life-threatening meningitis. Services are available twenty-four hours a day, seven days a week, 365 days a year in the hospital and in the field. They are provided by a network of health specialists, nurses, paramedics, emergency medical technicians, police officers, firefighters, and others dedicated to offering emergency medical services to children and adults.

Pediatric emergency specialists are needed because children are not little adults. The differences between children and adults are so great that they exist in virtually every organ system, body part, physiological process, and disease syndrome. For example, children's lungs are smaller and more fragile than those of adults, so that they require gentler thrusts during cardiopulmonary resuscitation (CPR). Children have faster heart and respiration rates than do adults, so that what may look like normal adult rates may be a sign of serious trouble in a child. Children require different and special equipment, different-sized instruments, different doses of different medicines, and different approaches to the psychological support and remedial care given to the ill or injured patient.

Physicians and other health care providers who lack pediatric emergency medical training and experience may find it difficult to recognize children who are critically ill and require the most urgent care. For example, infants may not develop a fever to signal infection. In children, respiratory arrest or shock signals the risk of cardiopulmonary arrest, rather than the arrhythmias that typically precede cardiac arrest in adults.

DIAGNOSTIC AND TREATMENT TECHNIQUES

A good medical outcome depends on the prompt identification and treatment of serious illness or injury in children. Emergency services personnel use a system called triage to decide whether patients are at risk for severe illness or imminent death, whether they have less urgent but still serious medical problems, or whether they have routine problems. Health care professionals use a system called the *abc*'s. Children who are choking (*a* for airway obstruction), in respiratory distress (*b* for breathing), or in shock (*c* for circulatory collapse) are treated immediately. The sickest patients always come first.

Doctors often make the most important decisions about a patient within the first five to fifteen minutes of care. The physician first determines whether the patient is in need of treatment and confirms or rules out the presence of catastrophic disease as quickly as possible. The doctor then stabilizes the patient's vital signs to reduce the risk of worsening symptoms or death. Next, the physician acts to relieve the most acute symptoms. The patient may then be hospitalized or discharged with directions about what to do next.

PERSPECTIVE AND PROSPECTS

Physicians have been treating pediatric emergencies for centuries. Only recently, however, has there been much recognition among the medical community or the public that pediatric emergency care requires unique training, equipment, and procedures.

Emergency medicine as a discipline in the United States dates to 1968, when the American College of Emergency Physicians was formed. During the 1970's, pediatricians and pediatric surgeons recognized that children's emergency care needs were not receiving adequate attention. The American Medical Association (AMA) and the American Board of Medical Specialties recognized emergency medicine as the twenty-third medical specialty in 1979. In the early 1980's, growing numbers of pediatric specialists and professional societies began to participate in the development of emergency medical systems. In 1993, a committee of the Institute of Medicine published a major study on the state of emergency care for children. The committee focused on standardizing the emergency care system so that the quality of emergency care would be consistent from state to state and community to community. It encouraged the creation of a nationwide 911 emergency response system and the establishment of minimum standards of care.

The tools, technologies, treatments, and problem-solving methods used by pediatric emergency physicians have been advancing rapidly. These specialists have gotten better at coping with the gamut of children's emergencies, including the medical and behavioral crises of newborns, infants, toddlers, young children, and adolescents. Emergency physicians have been and continue to be responsible for the development of new treatment techniques and the widespread availability of specialized pediatric equipment.

—*Fred Buchstein*

See also Allergies; Asthma; Biological and chemical weapons; Bites and stings; Bleeding; Burns and scalds; Cardiac arrest; Cardiology, pediatric; Cardiopulmonary resuscitation (CPR); Cardiovascular system; Choking; Critical care, pediatric; Dizziness and fainting; Drowning; Electrical shock; Fever; Food poisoning; Fracture and dislocation; Frostbite; Heat exhaustion and heat stroke; Meningitis; Physical examination; Pneumonia; Poisoning; Poisonous plants; Pulmonary medicine, pediatric; Rabies; Respiration; Respiratory distress syndrome; Seizures; Snakebites; Suicide.

FOR FURTHER INFORMATION:

Durch, Jane S., and Kathleen N. Lohr, eds. *Emergency Medical Services for Children.* Washington, D.C.: National Academy Press, 1993. This report of an Institute of Medicine study examines the nature and extent of acute illness and injury among children, reviews the origins and organization of emergency medical services (EMS) systems, describes the current state of effective care, and addresses data and standards needed for surveillance and evaluation of services and outcomes.

Hamilton, Glenn C., et al. *Emergency Medicine: An Approach to Clinical Problem-Solving.* 2d ed. New York: W. B. Saunders, 2003. A comprehensive textbook, in concise format, for residents and medical students.

Lynn, Stephan G., with Pamela Weintraub. *Medical Emergency! The St. Luke's-Roosevelt Hospital Center Book of Emergency Medicine.* New York: Hearst Books, 1996. This most helpful, informative, and well-arranged book tells how to be personally prepared for emergencies by having basic records and documents in a wallet or purse and others in known places for easy location. It clarifies emergency tests and treatments and explains how family members and friends can act as emergency patient advocates.

Soud, Treesa E., and Janice Steiner Rogers. *Manual of Pediatric Emergency Nursing.* St. Louis: Mosby, 1998. A portable handbook summarizing most of the conditions seen in a pediatric emergency department. Includes the essential points and priorities for diagnosis, management, and follow-up care, as well as indications for hospitalization.

Strange, Gary R., et al., eds. *Pediatric Emergency Medicine: A Comprehensive Study Guide.* 2d ed. New York: McGraw-Hill, 2002. A handbook for a range of emergency situations encountered in pediatric care.

EMOTIONS: BIOMEDICAL CAUSES AND EFFECTS

BIOLOGY

ANATOMY OR SYSTEM AFFECTED: Brain, endocrine system, gastrointestinal system, immune system, muscles, musculoskeletal system, nerves, nervous system, psychic-emotional system

SPECIALTIES AND RELATED FIELDS: Neurology, psychiatry, psychology

DEFINITION: Experiential events not characterized by any one sense and accompanied by complex physiological and mental changes.

KEY TERMS:

autonomic nervous system: the division of the nervous system that regulates involuntary action; comprises the sympathetic and parasympathetic systems

bipolar disorders: syndromes characterized by alternating periods of elevated and depressed mood; also discussed as manic-depressive disorder

Kluver-Bucy syndrome: a series of symptoms first observed in monkeys following temporal lobe removal, such as psychic blindness, abnormal oral tendencies, and changes in sexuality

loss-of-control syndrome: a pattern of behavior characterized by violent and emotional outbursts, occasionally associated with temporal lobe seizures

major depressive syndrome: a syndrome characterized by profound sadness and loss of pleasure in normal activities

sympathetic nervous system: the division of the autonomic nervous system concerned primarily with preparing the individual to expend energy

STRUCTURE AND FUNCTIONS

A central characteristic of being human is the ability to experience and express a wide range of emotions. Just what happens in the human brain and body to generate these feelings, however, is not completely clear. Over the years, it has been demonstrated that activity in the sympathetic nervous system is important in the expression and experience of emotional states, although the role of various regions of the brain in emotion has proved to be more elusive.

No consensus exists on how many different emotions humans are capable of experiencing, as so much depends on definitions and the type of evidence admitted. Most experts agree, however, that emotions have a significant impact on human behavior. The term "emotion" usually means some subjectively experienced effect. In addition, at least three other factors can be considered part of emotion: physiological arousal (increased heart rate, sweating palms), expressive changes of the muscles of the face and body (smiles, frowns), and behavior (striking with a fist, cringing). Debates persist about the degree to which there is a distinction between feelings and emotions; others argue about the degree to which cognition, or thinking, also affects emotion.

The best-studied physical responses characteristic of emotional states are those produced by the sympathetic nervous system, which controls many different internal organs of the body, as well as the salivary and sweat glands. Several of the responses produced by this system occur in emotional states. These responses are recorded in an attempt to study, measure, and evaluate emotion. The most commonly used responses include changes in heart rate, blood pressure, dilation of the pupils, and sweat gland activity. Physiological arousal in emotion also includes changes in the secretion of some hormones such as adrenaline, testosterone, and cortisol, measured from their presence in such body fluids as urine, saliva, and blood plasma.

The nervous system provides for rapid communication in the body, as it is concerned with events that occur on the order of milliseconds. Its structural and functional unit is the neuron, or nerve cell. Neurons have certain distinctive regions. The dendrites, or bushy protrusions, are the part specialized in receiving excitation, whether from an external stimulus or from another cell. The axon, or elongated part of the cell, takes care of distributing excitation away from the dendrite zone. Axons can be very long and form bundles that make up nerves.

The entire nervous system is a functional unit, and an impulse arising in any receptor can be transmitted to every effector in the body. Synapses are the functional junctions where connections between neurons form. In this region, one cell comes into contact, or near contact, with another cell, thus influencing it. Nerve impulses are propagated electrochemical reactions. The neural message must jump from the axon of one neuron to the dendrite of another for transmission to occur. The most common way of achieving this is through a chemical transmitter substance, also called a neurotransmitter. Chemical transmission at a synapse involves two steps. The first is the release of the specific chemical or neurotransmitter on the arrival of a nerve impulse. The chemical is released from its storage place in the tip of the axon into the narrow space between adjacent neurons. Once this has taken place, the specific transmitter substance is attached to a specific molecular site in the dendrite of the other neuron. This attachment produces a change in the properties of its cell membrane so that a new nerve impulse is set up, and the transmission continues.

The rapidly acting neurotransmitters include norepinephrine, epinephrine, dopamine, serotonin, acetylcholine, gamma aminobutyric acid (GABA), glycine, glutamate, and probably aspartate and adenosine triphosphate (ATP). The action of these neurotransmitters depends on the chemistry of the receptor to which they bind, and there are several types of receptor for each neurotransmitter. Receptors for neurotransmitters are important targets for toxins and drugs. For example, psychoactive drugs exert their effects at synapses, mostly by binding to specific receptors, but also by interfering with the degradation or removal of the transmitter from the synaptic cleft so that it lingers longer in the system.

From research on people with spinal cord injuries, it was found that while emotions may not be caused by feedback from sympathetic activity, this activity does play an important role in reinforcing emotional feelings, making them more intense and longer lasting.

Many different regions of the brain participate in emotions. The neocortex is responsible for dealing with symbolic manipulation, and bodily responses to emotion involve circuits located in lower brain regions such as the hypothalamus. Hormonal changes bring the endocrine system into play.

Dramatic changes in personality and emotional expression often occur following damage to various areas of the brain, such as weakening of emotional control with an injury to the frontal lobes. There is controversy, however, regarding where in the brain emotion is actually experienced. Research has pointed to certain parts of the brain below the cerebral cortex, such as the hypothalamus and the amygdala, as possible key participants. Two syndromes corroborate this finding. In loss-of-control syndrome, emotional outbursts are caused by abnormal electrical discharges in the region of the temporal lobe and amygdala. These spontaneous discharges are characteristic of epilepsy and are thought to result from congenital defects, high fever, brain infection, or trauma. Epilepsy can be controlled with drugs that inhibit the electrical discharges, since uncontrolled discharges result in epileptic seizures. Violent behavior and periods of intense emotion are common prior to an epileptic attack, although in some cases the sensations that take place before the seizure are interpreted by the individual as ecstasy of the highest order. Kluver-Bucy syndrome refers to a series of symptoms first observed in monkeys following temporal lobe removal: psychic blindness, abnormal oral tendencies, changes in sexuality, tameness (a significant lack of emotion), and hypermetamorphosis (a tendency to examine and react to virtually everything in the environment). Some or all of the symptoms described have been seen in human patients following strokes, brain injury, brain infections such as herpes, dementias, and other traumas, although the presence of all five in a single individual is very rare. Subsequent research has suggested that changes in emotionality and sexuality are probably caused by damage to the amygdala, while psychic blindness is more likely attributable to the removal of the neocortex of the temporal lobe.

Besides the temporal lobe and the amygdala, portions of the limbic system such as the septal area and the hypothalamus are involved in emotional responses. The pleasure centers of the brain are found in the limbic system (which includes the septal area, amygdala, cingulate cortex, and hippocampus), the hypothalamus, and the brain stem. Brain regions can be classified as positive, negative, or neutral with respect to whether animals will work to turn on or turn off electrical stimulation of these particular areas. Virtually all the cerebral neurocortex and cerebellum is neutral, much of the limbic system and hypothalamus is positive, and some regions of the brain stem and hippocampus are negative. In some cases, electrical stimulation of positive sites mimics the effects of a naturally rewarding event so well that animals prefer the electrical stimulation to the actual experience.

Some research has indicated possible differences between the brain hemispheres in the understanding and expression of emotion. Such data come from the examination of neurological patients having brain damage confined to either side of the brain. Those patients with damage to the left hemisphere are more likely to suffer catastrophic reaction, characterized by intense fear, depressions, and a generally negative outlook on life. The ones with damage on the right side show an attitude of indifference or even unusual cheerfulness. One possible interpretation is that the observed emotions are a result of dominance by the healthy hemisphere, suggesting that the right side is responsible for negative emotional states such as fear, anger, and depression and that the left side produces more positive emotional states. Another possible explanation can reverse this conclusion, simply by stating that the damaged hemisphere becomes dominant in these cases. Identifying emotions with one side of the brain or the other, however, ignores some important data. For example, some patients with frontal lobe damage in either hemisphere will display changes in personality and emotional reactions.

The relationship between behavioral and physiological response processes has long provided an important focus for both laboratory and clinical studies of emotion. For example, research concerned with shyness in children is aimed at investigating the role of sympathetic arousal in emotion. It has been shown that children who are inhibited and quiet when placed in an unfamiliar social situation show larger sympathetic responses than more relaxed, spontaneous children.

Emotions are also the focus of research in the detection of deception, especially as it relates to criminal investigations. A polygraph is a device used to measure involuntary body responses such as changes in respiration, heart rate, and blood pressure in relation to various kinds of questions. It can determine whether the individual is trying to be deceptive. The use of a polygraph is based on two main assumptions: first, that physiological responses during emotional arousal are involuntary, and second, that only individuals with guilty knowledge will display emotional arousal to certain questions asked by the tester. There are three types of questions: irrelevant questions, such as "What is your name?"; control questions, which deal with issues similar to those under consideration but not directly relevant; and relevant questions. The questions are asked in an unpredictable order, sometimes more than once. It is assumed that the person is being deceptive if the poly-

graph shows more arousal to relevant questions than to control ones. In a controlled laboratory setting, the polygraph is 80 to 90 percent effective in identifying guilty individuals and 90 to 95 percent effective in identifying innocent individuals. It is a process filled with interpretive problems that have to be solved.

Almost every drug found to be effective in altering affective states in humans has also been found to exert effects upon catecholamines (such as norepinephrine and epinephrine) in the brain. These effects would suggest that catecholamines are involved in the mediation of affective states and in the action of the drugs that affect them. Drugs that are associated with depressive phenomena in humans normally cause the loss of catecholamines, while drugs that elevate the mood (antidepressants) have the opposite effect by blocking the mechanisms that destroy the compounds.

DISORDERS AND DISEASES

Disorders of emotion may involve any of a variety of psychological disorders. The formal diagnostic class of mood disorders is one example. Mood disorders generally fall into one of two categories: those involving primarily depressed mood (such as major depression) and those involving both depressed and elevated mood (such as bipolar disorders).

Major depressive syndrome can often be treated without drugs. In many cases, however, drugs accelerate the recovery process. Three main families of antidepressant drugs are the tricyclics, the monoamine oxidase inhibitors (MAOIs), and the selective serotonin reuptake inhibitors (SSRIs). All these drugs help lift depression by increasing the availability of monoamine neurotransmitters at synapses in critical circuits in the brain. Monoamine neurotransmitters include norepinephrine, epinephrine, dopamine, and serotonin. Tricyclic compounds increase the time that the neurotransmitter is available in the synapse, and thus the duration of neurotransmitter action. MAOIs inhibit the action of the enzyme that normally degrades monoamines. SSRIs inhibit serotonin, thus making more of it available to brain cells.

Antidepressants, like any other drugs, can have bothersome side effects that may include constipation, urinary retention, blurred vision, and weight gain. More severe side effects include abnormalities in heart function and blood pressure. SSRIs have fewer and more easily tolerated side effects. As is evident from the list of symptoms, these drugs affect many systems in the body, raising again the question of where emotions reside and underscoring how profound their influence is on the body.

Bipolar mood disorder is much less common than major depressive syndrome. The main method of treatment is to administer lithium salts, although their mechanism of action is not known.

Anxiety disorders are another common emotional disorder. Included in this group is panic disorder. A panic attack includes shortness of breath, dizziness, acceleration of heart rate, and sweating. It can take place by anticipation of something or for no reason at all. Although attacks last only a few minutes, they are very disturbing. These symptoms involve activation of the sympathetic division of the nervous system.

Other anxiety disorders include conditions like phobias (chronic fears of certain situations), post-traumatic stress disorder, and obsessive-compulsive disorder. The benzodiazepines are drugs that are effective in the treatment of panic disorder. They include alprazolam (Xanax), chlordiazepoxide (Librium), and diazepam (Valium). These drugs enhance the inhibitory effect of GABA, a major inhibitory neurotransmitter, at synapses throughout the brain. Obsessive-compulsive disorder is characterized by stereotyped rituals or compulsions that develop in an attempt to deal with the anxiety produced by obsessions (such as the fear of germs). It has been successfully treated with some of the tricyclic drugs and also with SSRIs.

Perspective and Prospects

The word "passion" was frequently used by early philosophers to connote roughly what is now referred to as emotion: the phenomena of anger, fear, love, jealousy, and so on. In the fourth century B.C.E., Aristotle made a distinction between experiences that involve concurrent activity of both soul and body (such as appetites and passions) and those that involve activity of the soul alone (thinking). In the thirteenth century, Saint Thomas Aquinas was more explicit in affirming this belief in such a distinction, placing his argument within the context of Christian theology. In the seventeenth century, René Descartes directed his attention specifically to the passions. He reiterated that every passion experienced by the soul has its physical counterpart, and he emphasized the role of environmental stimulation in the generation of a passion and proposed a mechanism by which the environment created the passions. Descartes also established conceptual distinctions among passion (of the soul), bodily commotion (activity of the visceral organs), and action (motion of

the somatic musculature) and indicated close correspondence among the three.

About two centuries passed without significant development in theoretical ideas about emotion. Interest was renewed, however, as a result of the publication of Charles Darwin's *The Expression of Emotions in Man and Animals* (1872), in which he drew attention to emotional behavior as the biologically significant aspect of emotion and pointed out the causal role of stimulus events or situations in producing behavior.

The American philosopher and psychologist William James proposed the first explicit psychological theory of emotion in 1884. He claimed that emotions are the result, not the cause, of bodily arousal. According to James, bodily arousal is produced by the action of the sympathetic system. These reactions he believed to be reflexive responses to emotion-provoking situations. The emotion would then be produced by feedback from nerves bringing input from various internal organs (the heart and stomach) and blood vessels affected by the sympathetic system. This theory triggered the serious experimental study of emotion. Danish physiologist Carl Lange independently published a similar theory in 1885, and as a result, the theory is known as the James-Lange theory of emotion. Although it was frequently criticized, this theory dominated the field of emotion research for more than fifty years.

In 1915, Walter Cannon provided convincing experimental evidence of endocrine and autonomic participation in emotional response patterns. In 1927, he conducted a dramatic experiment by removing the sympathetic nervous system of a few cats. All the nerve connections between sympathetic neurons and internal organs and blood vessels were eliminated. According to the James-Lange theory, the cats should feel no emotions. They still displayed clear-cut emotional behaviors, however, and Cannon proposed that external stimuli caused emotion by simultaneously activating neural circuits in the neocortex and triggering responses in the sympathetic nervous system. Most modern theories are more closely aligned with Cannon's work than with the James-Lange hypothesis.

In 1962, Stanley Schachter and Jerome Singer followed up on Gregorio Maranon's 1924 experiment on the role of bodily responses in emotion. They proposed that people need to attribute their feelings to some emotional state and that the complete emotional experience is a joint product of cognition and feedback from sympathetic arousal. The role of sympathetic activity in emotion is still an active topic of research.

Various experiments have sought to discover the functions of certain regions of the brain, as they relate to emotional responses. In 1939, psychologist Heinrich Kluver and neurosurgeon Paul Bucy were interested in identifying the regions of the brain where drugs produce hallucinations. They speculated that the temporal lobe might be involved since brief hallucinations precede temporal lobe epileptic attacks. Both temporal lobes of monkeys were removed, and a constellation of dramatic behavioral changes was observed, proving their theory. In 1954, James Olds and Peter Milner published a report that rats would press a lever for the sole reward of passing electrical current into certain regions of their brains. This phenomenon is known as self-stimulation, and it led to the discovery of the pleasure centers of the brain. Fearlike responses have been elicited from electrical stimulation of three regions of a cat's brain: the tectum, the thalamus, and portions of the hippocampus. Such sites are called negatively reinforcing regions.

As additional information is accumulated, the complexity of the human brain becomes increasingly evident. Emotion is no exception. The biochemical aspects of emotional states have been studied extensively, and considerable information has been acquired, largely in terms of the biochemical changes that accompany and feed back into the central emotional state. Yet there are still many areas to be explored, including complete elucidation of the mechanism of action of some drugs and thus better treatment options for certain disorders.

—*Maria Pacheco, Ph.D.;*
updated by Nancy A. Piotrowski, Ph.D.

See also Addiction; Aging; Alcoholism; Antidepressants; Anxiety; Asperger's syndrome; Autism; Bipolar disorders; Bonding; Brain; Brain disorders; Death and dying; Depression; Developmental stages; Endocrinology; Endocrinology, pediatric; Epilepsy; Grief and guilt; Hormones; Hyperhidrosis; Hypochondriasis; Light therapy; Midlife crisis; Nervous system; Nightmares; Obsessive-compulsive disorder; Panic attacks; Paranoia; Phobias; Postpartum depression; Posttraumatic stress disorder; Psychiatric disorders; Psychiatry; Psychiatry, child and adolescent; Psychiatry, geriatric; Psychoanalysis; Psychosis; Psychosomatic disorders; Puberty and adolescence; Schizophrenia; Seasonal affective disorder; Separation anxiety; Sexual dysfunction; Shock therapy; Sibling rivalry; Stress; Thumb sucking; Toilet training.

FOR FURTHER INFORMATION:

Anders, S., et al., eds. *Understanding Emotions.* Boston: Elsevier Science, 2006. Provides overviews of different aspects of emotional perception and the underlying brain mechanisms. For researchers and advanced students.

Borod, Joan C. *The Neuropsychology of Emotion.* New York: Oxford University Press, 2000. Provides a discussion of the neural basis of emotional process, covering techniques, theory, emotional disorders, and treatments.

Breedlove, S. Marc, Mark R. Rosenzweig, and Neil V. Watson. *Biological Psychology: An Introduction to Behavioral, Cognitive, and Clinical Neuroscience.* 5th rev. ed. Sunderland, Mass.: Sinauer Associates, 2007. This new edition examines each major topic in psychobiology from the perspectives of the description, evolution, and development of behavior as well as biological mechanisms underlying it.

Cooper, J. R., F. E. Bloom, and R. H. Roth. *The Biochemical Basis of Neuropharmacology.* 8th ed. New York: Oxford University Press, 2002. A fine treatise on the drugs that affect the nervous system, such as psychotropic drugs that affect mood and behavior, sedatives, and other drugs that affect the autonomic nervous system.

Heilman, K. M., and Paul Satz, eds. *Neuropsychology of Human Emotion.* New York: Guilford Press, 1983. This book contains chapters by different authors on right-hemisphere involvement in emotion, the emotional changes associated with epilepsy, and other neurological and psychiatric diseases.

Henry, Helen L., and Anthony W. Norman, eds. *Encyclopedia of Hormones.* 3 vols. San Diego, Calif.: Academic Press, 2003. A comprehensive overview of the role of hormones, the major physiological systems in which they operate, and the biological consequences of an excess or deficiency of a particular hormone.

EMPHYSEMA

DISEASE/DISORDER

ANATOMY OR SYSTEM AFFECTED: Chest, lungs, respiratory system

SPECIALTIES AND RELATED FIELDS: Internal medicine, pulmonary medicine

DEFINITION: A disease of the lung characterized by enlargement of the small bronchioles or lung alveoli, the destruction of alveoli, decreased elastic recoil of these structures, and the trapping of air in the lungs, resulting in shortness of breath, reduced oxygen to the body, and a variety of serious and eventually fatal complications.

KEY TERMS:

alveoli: tiny, delicate, balloonlike air sacs composed of blood vessels that are supported by connecting tissue and enclosed in a very thin membrane; these sacs are found at the ends of the bronchioles

bronchioles: small branches of the bronchi, which are extensions of the trachea (the central duct that conducts air from the environment to the pulmonary system)

bullous emphysema: localized areas of emphysema within the lung substance

centrilobular (centriacinar) emphysema: a type of emphysema that destroys single alveoli, entering directly into the walls of terminal and respiratory bronchioles

diffusion: the passage of oxygen into the bloodstream from the alveoli and the return or exchange of carbon dioxide across the membrane between the blood vessels and the alveoli

panlobular (panacinar) emphysema: a type of emphysema that involves weakening and enlargement of the air sacs, which are clustered at the end of respiratory bronchioles

perfusion: the flow of blood through the lungs or other vessels in the body

ventilation: the transport of air from the mouth through the bronchial tree to the air sacs and back through the nose or mouth to the outside; ventilation includes both inspiration (breathing in) and expiration (breathing out)

CAUSES AND SYMPTOMS

Emphysema is a lung disease in which damage to these organs causes shortness of breath and can lead to heart or respiratory failure. A discussion of the structure and function of the normal lung can illuminate the nature and effects of this damage.

Gases, smoke, germs, allergens, and environmental pollutants pass from the nose and mouth into a large duct called the trachea. The trachea branches into smaller ducts, the bronchi and bronchioles (small branches of the bronchi), which lead to tiny air sacs called alveoli. The respiratory system is like a tree: The trachea is the trunk, the bronchi and bronchioles are similar to the branches, and the alveoli are similar to the leaves. The blood vessels of the alveoli carry red blood cells, which pick up oxygen and transport it to the rest of the body. The cellular waste product, carbon dioxide, is released to the alveoli from the bloodstream and then exhaled. The alveoli are supported by a framework of delicate elastic fibers and give the lung a very distensible quality and the ability to "snap back," or recoil.

The lungs and bronchial tubes are surrounded by the chest wall, composed of bone and muscle and functioning like a bellows. The lung is elastic and passively increases in size to fill the chest space during inspiration and decreases in size during expiration. As the lung (including the alveoli) enlarges, air from the environment flows in to fill this space. During exhalation, the muscles relax, the elasticity of the lung returns it to a normal size, and the air is pushed out. Air must pass through the bronchial tree to the alveoli before oxygen can get into the bloodstream and carbon dioxide can get out, because it is the alveoli that are in contact with blood vessels. The bronchial tree has two kinds of special lining cells. The first type can secrete mucus as a sticky protection against injury and irritation. The second type of cell is covered with fine, hairlike structures called cilia. These cells are supported by smooth muscle cells and elastic and collagen fibers. The cilia wave in the direction of the mouth and act as a defense system by physically removing germs and irritating substances. The cilia are covered with mucus, which helps to trap irritants and germs.

When alveoli are exposed to irritants such as cigarette smoke, they produce a defensive cell called an alveolar macrophage. These cells engulf irritants and bacteria and call for white blood cells, which aid in the defense against foreign bodies, to come into the lungs. The lung tissue also becomes a target for the enzymes or chemical substances produced by the alveolar macrophages and leukocytes (white blood cells). In a healthy body, natural defense systems inhibit the enzymes released by the alveolar macrophages and leukocytes, but it seems that this inhibiting function is impaired in smokers. In some cases, an individual may inherit a deficiency in an enzyme inhibitor. The enzymes vigorously attack the elastin and collagen of the lungs, the lung loses its elastic recoil, and air is trapped.

Emphysema, and a related disease, bronchitis, often work in concert. They are often lumped under the term "chronic obstructive pulmonary disease." Chronic bronchitis weakens and narrows the bronchi. Often, bronchial walls collapse, choking off the vital flow of air. Air is also trapped within the bronchial walls. Weakened by enzymes, the walls of the alveoli rupture

INFORMATION ON EMPHYSEMA

CAUSES: Long-term exposure to dry air, smoke, or other environmental toxins; infection; allergies
SYMPTOMS: Shortness of breath, labored breathing, discolored skin, wheezing, difficulty coughing and talking
DURATION: Chronic
TREATMENTS: Eliminating causes of irritation, cleaning out airways via nebulizers and intermittent positive pressure breathing machine, medications (theophylline, antibiotics, steroids)

and blood vessels die. Lung tissue is replaced with scar tissue, leaving areas of destroyed alveoli that appear as "holes" on an X ray. Small areas of destroyed alveoli are called blebs, and larger ones are called bullae.

As emphysema progresses, a patient has a set of large, overexpanded lungs with a weakened and partially plugged bronchial tree subject to airway collapse and air trapping with blebs and bullae. Breathing, especially exhalation, becomes a slow and difficult process. The patient often develops a "barrel chest" and is known, in medical circles, as a "blue bloater." The scientific world calls the mismatching of breathing to blood distribution a ventilation-to-perfusion imbalance; that is, when air arrives in the alveolus, there are no blood vessels there to transport the vital gaseous cargo to the cells (as a result of enzymatic damage). A person with chronic obstructive pulmonary disease has a bronchial tree with a narrow, defective trunk and sparse leaves.

The loss of elasticity of the lung and alveoli is a critical problem in the emphysemic patient. About one-half of the lungs' elastic recoil force comes from surface tension. The other half comes from the elastic nature of certain fibers throughout the lungs' structure. Emphysema weakens both of these forces because it destroys the elastic fibers and interferes with the surface tension. Fluid, a saline solution, bathes all the body's cells and surfaces. In the lung, this fluid contains surfactant, a substance that interferes with water's tendency to form a spherical drop with a pull into its center (and ultimate collapse). The tissue that gives shape to the lungs is composed of specialized fibers which contain a protein called elastin. These elastic fibers are also found in the alveolar walls and in the elastic connective tissue of the airways and air sacs. The amount of elastin in lung tissue determines its behavior. Healthy lungs maintain a proper balance between destruction of elastin and re-

newal. (Other parts of the body, such as bones, do this as well.) If too little elastin is destroyed, the lungs have difficulty expanding. If too much is destroyed, the lungs overexpand and cannot recoil properly.

The process of elastin destruction and renewal involves complex regulation. Specialized lung cells produce new elastin protein. Others produce elastase, an enzyme that destroys elastin. The liver plays a role in the production of a special enzyme known as alpha-1-antitrypsin, which controls the amount of elastase so that too much elastin is not digested. In emphysema, these regulatory systems fail: Too much elastin is destroyed because elastase is no longer controlled, apparently because alpha-1-antitrypsin production has been reduced to a trickle.

The loss of elastin (and thus elastic recoil) means that the lungs expand beyond the normal range during inspiration and cannot resume their resting size during expiration. Thus, alveoli overinflate and rupture. This further reduces elasticity because the loss of each alveolus further impairs the surface tension contribution to the lungs' ability to recoil. Thus, a state of hyperinflation is assumed in the emphysemic patient. This leads to stretched and narrowed alveolar capillaries, loss of elastic tissue, and dissolution of alveolar walls. The lungs increase in size, the thoracic (chest) cage assumes the inspiratory position, and the diaphragm becomes low and flat instead of convex. The patient becomes short of breath with any type of exertion. As the disease worsens, the patient's skin takes on a cyanotic color, as a result of poor oxygenation and perfusion. Wheezing is often present, and coughing is difficult and tiring. In the worst cases, even talking is enough exertion to produce a spasmodic cough. The hyperinflated chest causes inspiration to become a major effort, and the entire chest cage lifts up, resulting in considerable strain. The head moves with each inspiration while the chest remains relatively fixed.

Emphysema may be diagnosed by the early symptom of dyspnea (shortness of breath) on exertion. In advanced cases, the distended chest, depressed diaphragm, increased blood carbon dioxide content, and severe dyspnea clearly point to the disease.

TREATMENT AND THERAPY

The initial step in treating emphysema is to open the airways by eliminating the causes of irritation: smoke, dry air, infection, and allergies. The second treatment is to clean out the airways. There are several techniques and medicines for loosening airway mucus and expelling it. In most chronic obstructive lung diseases, including emphysema, the mucus becomes thick and purulent; coughing up mucus of this type is difficult. In addition, in emphysema the natural cleansing action of the cilia and lung elasticity are impaired. Thus, treatment is aimed at the patient consciously taking over the function of cleaning out the lungs. Coughing is nature's way of bringing up mucus (phlegm), and the emphysemic patient is urged to cough. Since the mucus is thick, one needs to do whatever is necessary to thin it out and to lubricate the airways so that the mucus slips up easily with coughing. The cough must come from deep within the chest in order to be "productive" (to raise mucus).

Moisture is helpful in loosening up thick mucus; hence, drinking large amounts of fluid is encouraged. Adding a humidifier or a vaporizer to a home is often helpful to the emphysemic patient. There are also machines known as nebulizers and intermittent positive pressure breathing (IPPB) machines that can help to add moisture to the airway of the patient with emphysema. Nebulizers are more effective in getting moisture beyond the throat and major airways than cold vaporizers. Nebulizers, which get their name from the Latin word for cloud or mist, create a mist that is a profusion of tiny droplets that keep themselves apart, even as they bump into one another. Nebulizers release only the smallest droplets—those which can penetrate far down into air passages, where thick mucus is likely to be. (Atomizers produce small droplets as well, but they also spray large droplets.) IPPBs have a special kind of valve that opens when one begins to breathe and allows the air to move into the lungs under mild pressure. As soon as the patient has come to the end of the inhalation, the valve closes and allows the patient to exhale freely.

When phlegm cannot be brought up by breathing mist, a technique called postural drainage is often combined with chest wall percussion or vibration. The idea is to move one's body to a position such that airways are perpendicular to the floor, or at least tilted down, so that gravity can help pull the mucus toward the larger airways, from which the phlegm can be coughed up. Percussion, or clapping the chest, is another way to loosen the mucus in the airways so that it can be coughed up.

A number of medications are useful in the treatment of emphysema. The bronchodilator drugs are xanthines, such as theophylline (Theo-Dur), that relieve bronchospasms, reduce wheezing and dyspnea, and improve respiratory muscle function. Theophylline is a drug that is similar chemically to caffeine. Whereas caffeine stimulates the skeletal muscles and the central nervous system, however, theophylline is potent as a cardiac stimulant and a smooth muscle relaxer. It has also been learned that theophylline stimulates mucociliary clearance of the airways, strengthens the diaphragm, and suppresses edema. Theophylline holds

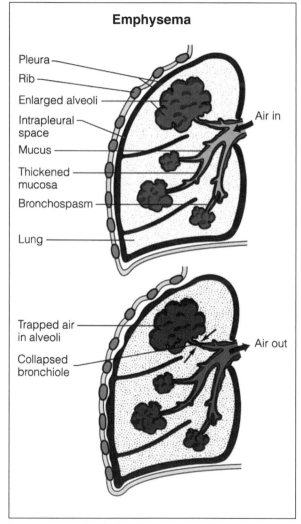

Emphysema

Pleura
Rib
Enlarged alveoli
Intrapleural space
Mucus
Thickened mucosa
Bronchospasm
Lung

Air in

Trapped air in alveoli
Collapsed bronchiole

Air out

In emphysema, the body releases enzymes in response to inhaling irritants in the air, such as cigarette smoke; these enzymes reduce the lungs' elasticity, compromising the bronchioles' ability to expand and contract normally. Air becomes trapped in the alveoli upon inhalation (top) and cannot escape upon exhalation (bottom). Over time, breathing becomes extremely difficult.

two benefits for the chronic obstructive pulmonary diseased patient: It helps get rid of mucus, and it strengthens the diaphragm, the main respiratory muscle. Common side effects are nausea, stomach pain, vomiting, insomnia, rapid heartbeat, loss of appetite, and restlessness. Another category of bronchodilator are the beta adrenergic stimulants such as metaproterenol (Alupent). Their side effects include nervousness, headache, nausea, and muscle cramps.

The antibiotics sometimes prescribed for emphysemic patients are used to combat bacterial infection. Common antibiotics include tetracycline, penicillin, cephalosporin, erythromycin, and sulfa drugs. Their side effects include a burning sensation in the stomach, vomiting, diarrhea, increased sensitivity to sunlight, rashes, itching, hives, fever, and weakness.

The steroid hormones, such as prednisone, decrease swelling, inflammation, and bronchospasms; they also relieve wheezing. Side effects include blurred vision, frequent urination, thirst, black stools, bone pain, mood changes, weight gain, swelling of the feet, muscle weakness, hoarseness, and a sore mouth.

Other drugs given for emphysema include digitalis, cardiac glycosides, diuretics, mast cell inhibitors, expectorants, and parasympatholytics. Digitalis and cardiac glycosides, such as digoxin, improve the strength of heart contractions and treat disturbances in heart rhythm. Side effects are loss of appetite, abdominal pain, nausea, slow uneven pulse, blurred vision, diarrhea, mood changes, and weakness. Diuretics, such as furosemide (Lasix), are often given to prevent excessive fluid retention. Such drugs cause loss of hearing, skin rashes, hives, bleeding, bruising, jaundice, an irregular or fast heartbeat, muscle cramps, light-headedness, dizziness, and weakness. Mast cell inhibitors are a unique category of drugs that inhibit the release of body chemicals that cause wheezing and bronchospasm; however, they also cause weakness, nosebleeds, and nasal congestion. Expectorants, such as Robitussin, are used to thin secretions and have no known side effects. The parasympatholytics are a type of bronchodilator drug that inhibits the nerves that cause bronchospasm. They are apparently free from the many side effects associated with other bronchodilator drugs.

The emphysemic patient should avoid both excessive heat and excessive cold. If body temperature rises above normal, the heart works faster, as do the lungs. Excessive cold stresses the body to maintain its normal temperature. Smog, air pollution, dusts, powders, and hairspray should be avoided. Finally, a healthy diet consisting of foods high in calcium, vitamins, complex carbohydrates, proteins, and fiber is advised for the patient with lung disease.

A healthy core diet is high in complex carbohydrates; is low in sugars, fats, and cholesterol; and has adequate protein for moderate stress. It should be high in fiber and contain approximately 1,000 milligrams of calcium, 15,000 milligrams of vitamin A, and 250 milligrams of vitamin C. Snack foods can include skim milk, fruit, popcorn, and fresh salads. The respiratory distress of the emphysemic patient uses vast amounts of energy, and the patient should eat several small meals a day so as not to distend the stomach and limit movement of the diaphragm. Liquids are important in keeping airways clear. Good nutrition is helpful in maintaining strength and improving the quality of life for the patient with lung disease.

PERSPECTIVE AND PROSPECTS

Chronic bronchitis and emphysema are responsible for at least fifty thousand deaths a year in the United States alone. An increase in air pollution and cigarette consumption are apparent causes for this rise. In males over forty, chronic obstructive pulmonary disease (COPD) is second to heart disease as a cause of disability. With more females and young people smoking, the incidence of lung disease is likely to increase. Aside from death, a disease such as emphysema can cause long years of disability, joblessness, loss of income, depression, hospitalization, and an inability to perform normal activities.

Smoking is, by far, the single most important risk factor for emphysema. In the United States especially, social acceptance of women smokers began after World War II and has increased the number of women being diagnosed with COPD. Socioeconomic status also influences smoking habits. In many countries in Europe, the mortality rate from lung disease for the lowest socioeconomic class has been six times higher than for the highest. In the United States, the COPD mortality rate among unskilled and semiskilled laborers is twice as high as among professionals. Families with lower incomes usually live in small, often overcrowded apartments; such overcrowding makes respiratory infections more frequent. Often, family members of the COPD patient also smoke, increasing the surrounding air pollution.

In the United States, COPD causes 3 percent of all deaths. In some cases, it causes another 100,000 Americans to be too weak to survive other, unrelated medical conditions. Therefore, an annual figure of 150,000 deaths from COPD-related diseases is more realistic. The expanding COPD population is a growing market for pharmaceutical firms. For example, greater amounts of bronchodilator medications will be needed; hence, pharmaceutical firms are eager to find longer-acting and more effective drugs for these patients to buy.

A number of economic pressures are likely to move COPD treatment from the hospital to the home. When effectively carried out by a well-trained health team, home care can lower medical costs. The COPD patient who finds a knowledgeable doctor and who begins a comprehensive rehabilitation program is the one who can look forward to a life that is more productive and more comfortable.

—Jane A. Slezak, Ph.D.

See also Asbestos exposure; Aspergillosis; Chronic obstructive pulmonary disease (COPD); Cyanosis; Environmental diseases; Lungs; Oxygen therapy; Pulmonary diseases; Pulmonary medicine; Pulmonary medicine, pediatric; Respiration; Wheezing.

FOR FURTHER INFORMATION:

American Lung Association. http://www.lungusa.org/. Includes in-depth information and recent research findings, a guide to local events and programs, and a section to share personal stories, among other features.

Bates, David V. *Respiratory Function in Disease*. 3d ed. Philadelphia: W. B. Saunders, 1989. Summarizes the effects of disease on pulmonary function. Also discussed are some of the more sophisticated pulmonary function tests. Exercise testing, obesity, and the effects of drugs are other topics reviewed in this work.

Decker, Caroline D. "Room to Breathe." *Saturday Evening Post* 266, no. 6 (November/December, 1994): 48-49. This article on emphysema discusses lung surgery. Illustrated with photographs.

Haas, François, and Sheila Sperber Haas. *The Chronic Bronchitis and Emphysema Handbook*. Rev. ed. New York: John Wiley & Sons, 2000. Helps patients with COPD learn to lead full and productive lives. Provides information pertinent to their disease and describes the treatments and medications available to them in order to improve their quality of life.

Hedrick, Hannah L., and Austin K. Kutscher, eds. *The Quiet Killer: Emphysema, Chronic Obstructive Pulmonary Disease*. Lanham, Md.: Scarecrow Press,

2002. Clinicians, researchers, and health educators combine their expertise in twenty-five chapters that discuss such topics as managing dyspnea, traveling with mechanical ventilation, encouraging patients to quit smoking, self-help groups, and hospice care.

Matthews, Dawn D. *Lung Disorders Sourcebook*. Detroit: Omnigraphics, 2002. A comprehensive overview of lung anatomy, physiology, and dysfunctions taken from government agencies, the American Academy of Family Physicians, the American Lung Association, and the Mayo Foundation. Discusses thirty-five lung disorders in depth.

National Emphysema Foundation. http://www.emphysemafoundation.org/. Site offers tips on exercises, inhaler uses, and other helpful items for those with emphysema.

West, John B. *Pulmonary Pathophysiology: The Essentials*. 6th ed. Baltimore: Lippincott Williams & Wilkins, 2003. Examines lungs afflicted with obstructive, restrictive, vascular, and environmental diseases.

Wolff, Ronald K. "Effects of Airborne Pollutants on Mucociliary Clearance." *Environmental Health Perspectives* 66 (April, 1986): 223-237. The role of mucociliary clearance as a lung defense mechanism is described in this article. The abnormal elimination of bronchial mucus is considered a possible factor in the pathogenesis of COPD. The role of certain pollutants, which pose a challenge to the mucociliary system, is detailed.

ENCEPHALITIS

DISEASE/DISORDER

ANATOMY OR SYSTEM AFFECTED: Brain, nerves, neck, nervous system, circulatory system, psychic-emotional system

SPECIALTIES AND RELATED FIELDS: Bacteriology, epidemiology, internal medicine, neurology, public health, virology

DEFINITION: A disease that involves inflammation of the brain.

KEY TERMS:

arbovirus: a virus transmitted by the bite of an arthropod, particularly a mosquito or a tick

central nervous system (CNS): in vertebrates, consisting of the brain and spinal cord

enterovirus: a virus that tends to multiply in the intestinal tract

CAUSES AND SYMPTOMS

In the United States, about twenty thousand cases of encephalitis are reported each year. The disease is sometimes classified according to the causative agent or the anatomic structures affected. Limbic encephalitis, for example, affects structures in the brain known as the limbic system. Exposure to lead often produces cerebral inflammation and edema (swelling) and is referred to as lead encephalitis. If the agent is bacterial, then the disease is referred to as bacterial encephalitis. In amebic encephalitis, patients with weakened immune systems become infected through certain protozoa (*Acanthamoeba*) found in water and moist soil.

The principal cause of encephalitis, however, is viral. In primary encephalitis, the virus directly invades the brain and spinal cord. Secondary encephalitis occurs as an aftereffect of such airborne diseases as measles and influenza (postinfectious) or of certain vaccinations (postvaccinal).

Though many viruses can produce encephalitis, only a limited number tend to recur. They fall into three major groups: enteroviruses; arboviruses, which include the four main agents common in the United States; and nonarthropod viruses. Nonarthropod viruses, transmitted without an insect vector, include the very common herpes simplex virus 1 (HSV-1).

Enteroviruses infect the gastrointestinal tract and are spread by a fecal-oral route. Hands come into contact with feces or bodily fluids in which the virus is present. If unwashed, the hands can transfer the virus to the mouth. Once ingested, the virus replicates in the intestines and then moves to the nervous system.

Arboviruses, which are responsible for epidemics, are spread by mosquitoes (such as in eastern equine encephalitis) and ticks (as in Powassan encephalitis, which occurs in the northeastern United States). For natural reasons related to their vectors (carriers), these infections, at least in northerly climes, peak in late summer. In 2002, West Nile virus caused the largest epidemic ever recorded, with nearly 4,200 cases and 300 deaths.

If a mosquito ingests a blood meal from an infected vertebrate, over a period of one to three weeks, the virus replicates in the mosquito's gut and then moves to its salivary glands. When the mosquito bites a human, the virus lurks in the person's visceral organs and then passes by means of the blood to the nervous system. A possible route to the central nervous system (CNS) is through the brain capillaries. Infection of neurons, and glial cells, which constitute the non-nervous tissue of the brain and spinal cord, follows, leading to cell dys-

---

INFORMATION ON ENCEPHALITIS

CAUSES: Viral infection, complications from another disease

SYMPTOMS: Headache, fever, stiff neck, loss of consciousness, seizures, sleep disturbances, blurred or double vision, vomiting, body aches

DURATION: Acute or chronic

TREATMENTS: Alleviation of symptoms

---

function and death. The body's own immune response, which includes infusing white blood cells into the cerebrospinal fluid, contributes to the brain edema and inflammation.

In diagnosis, physicians use blood and deoxyribonucleic acid (DNA) tests and analyze the cerebrospinal fluid for a too-high count of white blood cells and elevated protein levels and fluid pressure. Neuroimaging and electroencephalograms (EEGs), which record electrical activity in the brain, are used to eliminate other possibilities, such as clotting because of the rupture of a blood vessel (hematoma). Isolation of the virus itself, with some exceptions, is difficult. Biopsy of brain tissue for evidence of the virus has largely been replaced by less invasive procedures.

Symptoms may occur within a few hours or over the course of several days and initially are nonspecific, which complicates the diagnosis. Although they vary depending on the virus and the extent and length of infection, symptoms generally include fever, headache, muscle ache, stiff neck, respiratory symptoms, sensitivity to light, abdominal pain, vomiting, dizziness, an altered level of consciousness that may range from lethargy to coma, personality changes which may progress to behavior that appears psychotic, intellectual deficit, and a host of neurological deficiencies, such as tremors, loss of muscular coordination, partial paralysis, and ocular (eye) fixation.

TREATMENT AND THERAPY

For some types of encephalitis, such as Japanese encephalitis, effective vaccines exist. In bacterial cases, antibiotics are prescribed. In patients in whom the herpes simplex virus is implicated, the antiviral acyclovirin is useful. In general, however, treatment, often initially in an intensive care unit (ICU), is supportive and designed to control complications. For example, steroids are sometimes administered to reduce brain swelling and anticonvulsants, if seizures occur.

The disease runs its course in one to two weeks. Mortality rates depend on the type of virus and the age of the patient, the very young and elderly being more vulnerable. In eastern equine encephalitis, the mortality rate is about 33 percent; in western equine encephalitis, it is about 3 percent in older patients and as high as 30 percent in younger patients. Residual symptoms after recovery vary, again according to the agent and extent of infection. In eastern equine encephalitis, 80 percent of patients suffer neurologic aftereffects.

PERSPECTIVE AND PROSPECTS

Some historians of medicine believe that viral encephalitis appeared early in the Mediterranean area. The evidence is indirect, with the mention in the *Hippocratic corpus* (fifth century B.C.E. and later) of genital and labial lesions consistent with herpesvirus, a leading cause of the disease. It was not until the nineteenth and twentieth centuries that the numerous agents and vectors for encephalitis were successfully identified, such as the rabies virus (isolated by Louis Pasteur's dog experiments), the spirochete of syphilis, and more recently human immunodeficiency virus (HIV).

A firm connection between the great influenza pandemic of 1918 and the repeated global outbreaks of encephalitis lethargica in the 1920's was not established until 1982. In the 1990's, aspirin therapy in children's influenza was implicated in the sometimes fatal brain edema known as Reye's syndrome.

Research has focused on oral antiviral drug therapy. Interferon alpha-2b therapy and ribovarin, related to the vitamin B complex, have been tested on patients with West Nile virus, but their value has not been conclusively established. Emphasis therefore has remained on prevention: proper vaccinations and, for arboviruses, mosquito spraying campaigns, application of effective insect repellents, and limited outside exposure during the early evening hours.

—*David J. Ladouceur, Ph.D.*

See also Bites and stings; Brain; Brain damage; Brain disorders; Dementias; Hemiplegia; Insect-borne diseases; Lice, mites, and ticks; Nervous system; Neuroimaging; Neurology; Neurology, pediatric; Parasitic diseases; Sleeping sickness; Viral infections; West Nile virus.

FOR FURTHER INFORMATION:

American Medical Association. *American Medical Association Family Medical Guide.* 4th rev. ed. Hoboken, N.J.: John Wiley & Sons, 2004.

Goldman, Lee, and Dennis Ausiello, eds. *Cecil Textbook of Medicine.* 22d ed. Philadelphia: W. B. Saunders, 2004.

Kasper, Dennis L., et al., eds. *Harrison's Principles of Internal Medicine.* 16th ed. New York: McGraw-Hill, 2005.

Professional Guide to Diseases. 8th ed. Ambler, Pa.: Lippincott Williams & Wilkins, 2005.

ENDARTERECTOMY

PROCEDURE

ANATOMY OR SYSTEM AFFECTED: Blood vessels, circulatory system, neck

SPECIALTIES AND RELATED FIELDS: General surgery, vascular medicine

DEFINITION: A surgical procedure used to remove plaque from the lining of the carotid arteries in the neck.

INDICATIONS AND PROCEDURES

The internal carotid artery lies in the side of the neck, slightly in front of and beneath the sternocleidomastoid muscle. A skin incision is made anterior to this muscle. The branches of the carotid artery, adjacent blood vessels, and nerves are freed and inspected. A clamp is applied to the common carotid artery. Two additional clamps are applied to the external and internal carotid arteries to prevent bleeding and to prevent emboli from migrating to the brain during the procedure.

A lengthwise incision is made in the internal carotid artery from a point about 3.8 centimeters (1.5 inches) above the beginning of the vessel into the common carotid artery, about 2.5 centimeters (1 inch) below the beginning of the vessel. The edges of the artery are retracted, and the interior is exposed. The plaque can usually be scraped off the walls of the artery. The internal lining of the artery is carefully closed, and any tears are sutured. The carotid artery is then sewed together with fine suture material. If the underlying disease has been extensive or if the lining of the artery was damaged, a portion of the saphenous vein in the patient's leg is used to repair the arterial wall.

Restoring blood flow is crucial; it is important to avoid both leaks in the artery and the formation of emboli. The clamp on the external carotid artery is briefly released, and a small amount of blood is allowed to flow back into the repaired area to check for leaks under low pressure. This clamp is reapplied. The clamp on the common carotid artery is removed to check for leaks under high pressure. The clamp to the external carotid

Endarterectomy

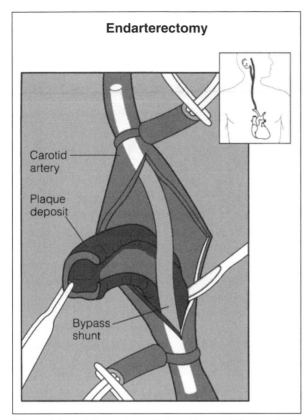

Carotid
artery

Plaque
deposit

Bypass
shunt

The excision of plaque deposits from the carotid artery in the neck is called endarterectomy; the inset shows the location of the carotid artery.

artery is removed next. Blood is allowed to flow, flushing any emboli from the operative site and away from the brain. If all is well, the clamp on the internal carotid artery is removed.

The structures that were pulled away from the carotid artery are released and briefly inspected to ensure that no damage has been done. The edges of the skin are then brought together and closed with sutures. The patient returns in about a week for a checkup and removal of the sutures.

USES AND COMPLICATIONS

Endarterectomy is used to restore adequate blood flow to the brain, thus preventing periods of ischemia that can result in loss of consciousness. Complications include emboli, which cause strokes by blocking important blood vessels.

Endarterectomy is successful in most patients and restores more normal circulation. It has decreased the incidence of strokes in younger patients.

—*L. Fleming Fallon, Jr., M.D., Ph.D., M.P.H.*

See also Angioplasty; Arteriosclerosis; Bypass surgery; Circulation; Embolism; Strokes; Vascular medicine; Vascular system.

FOR FURTHER INFORMATION:

Ancowitz, Arthur. *Strokes and Their Prevention: How to Avoid High Blood Pressure and Hardening of the Arteries.* New York: Van Nostrand Reinhold, 1975.

Browse, Norman L., A. O. Mansfield, and C. C. R. Bishop. *Carotid Endarterectomy: A Practical Guide.* Boston: Butterworth-Heinemann, 1997.

Loftus, Christopher M. *Carotid Endarterectomy: Principles and Technique.* 2d ed. New York: Informa Healthcare, 2007.

Loftus, Christopher M., and Timothy F. Kresowik. *Carotid Artery Surgery.* New York: Thieme, 2000.

Rutherford, Robert B., ed. *Vascular Surgery.* 6th ed. Philadelphia: W. B. Saunders, 2005.

ENDOCARDITIS

DISEASE/DISORDER

ANATOMY OR SYSTEM AFFECTED: Circulatory system, heart

SPECIALTIES AND RELATED FIELDS: Bacteriology, cardiology, internal medicine, vascular medicine

DEFINITION: Inflammatory lesions of the endocardium, the lining of the heart.

CAUSES AND SYMPTOMS

The lesions of endocarditis may be noninfective, as in rheumatic fever, or infective. The latter are characterized by direct invasion of the endocardium by microorganisms, most often bacteria. Bacterial endocarditis may occur on normal or previously damaged heart valves and also on artificial (prosthetic) heart valves. Rarely, endocarditis may occur on the wall (mural surface) of the heart or at the site of an abnormal hole between the pumping chambers of the heart, called a ventricular septal defect.

In areas of turbulent blood flow, platelet-fibrin deposition can occur, providing a nidus for subsequent bac-

---

INFORMATION ON ENDOCARDITIS

CAUSES: Bacterial infection
SYMPTOMS: Fever, malaise, fatigue, dyspnea, chest pain, heart murmurs
DURATION: Temporary
TREATMENTS: Antibiotics

terial colonization. Transient bacteremia may accompany infection elsewhere in the body or some medical and dental procedures, and these circulating bacteria can adhere to the endocardium, especially at platelet-fibrin deposition sites, and produce endocarditis. Intravenous drug abusers using unsterile equipment and drugs often inject bacteria along with the drugs, which can result in endocarditis. The lesions produced by these depositions plus bacteria are called vegetations. Clinical symptoms and signs usually begin about two weeks later.

Bacterial endocarditis usually involves either the mitral or the aortic heart valve. In intravenous drug abusers, the tricuspid heart valve is more commonly affected because it is the first valve to be reached by the endocardium-damaging drugs and contaminating bacteria. The pulmonic valve is only rarely the site of endocarditis. Occasionally, more than one heart valve is infected; this occurs most often in intravenous drug abusers or patients with multiple prosthetic heart valves.

Gram-positive cocci are the most common cause of bacterial endocarditis. Different species predominate in various conditions or situations: *Streptococcus viridans* in native valves, *Staphylococcus aureus* in the valves of intravenous drug abusers, and *Staphylococcus epidermidis* in prosthetic heart valves. Gram-negative bacilli are found in association with prosthetic heart valves or intravenous drug addiction.

The clinical manifestations of endocarditis are varied and often nonspecific. Early symptoms are similar to those encountered in most infections: fever, malaise, and fatigue. As the disease progresses, more cardiovascular and renal-related symptoms may appear: dyspnea, chest pain, and stroke. Fever and heart murmurs are found in most patients. Enlargement of the spleen, skin lesions, and evidence of emboli are commonly present.

The key to the diagnosis of bacterial endocarditis is to suspect the presence of the illness and obtain blood cultures. Febrile patients who have a heart murmur, cardiac failure, a prosthetic heart valve, history of intravenous drug abuse, preexisting valvular disease, stroke (especially in young adults), multiple pulmonary emboli, sudden arterial occlusion, unexplained prolonged fever, or multiple positive blood cultures are likely to have endocarditis. The hallmark of bacterial endocarditis is continuous bacteremia; thus, nearly all blood cultures will be positive. Other nonspecific blood tests, such as an erythrocyte sedimentation rate, or specific

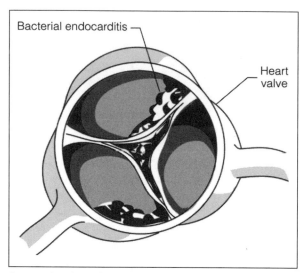

Bacterial endocarditis of a heart valve occurs when bacteria invade and cause inflammatory lesions; untreated, the condition is usually fatal.

blood tests, such as tests for teichoic acid antibodies, may be helpful in establishing a diagnosis.

TREATMENT AND THERAPY

Endocarditis may be prevented by administering prophylactic antibiotics to patients with preexisting heart abnormalities that predispose them to endocarditis when they are likely to have transient bacteremia. An example would be a patient with an artificial heart valve scheduled to have a dental cleaning.

Endocarditis is one of the few infections that is nearly always fatal if mistreated. Antibacterial therapy with agents capable of killing the offending bacteria, along with supportive medical care and cardiac surgery when indicated, cures most patients.

PERSPECTIVE AND PROSPECTS

The first demonstration of bacteria in vegetations associated with endocarditis was by Emmanuel Winge of Oslo, Norway, in 1869. Fifty years later, a fresh section was cut from the preserved heart valve described by Winge, and staining by modern methods revealed a chain of streptococci verifying his discovery. It was not until 1943, when Leo Loewe successfully treated seven cases of bacterial endocarditis with penicillin, that the era of modern therapy of this serious illness began.

Endocarditis accounts for approximately one case in every 1,000 hospital admissions in the United States. The incidence remained fairly constant between the 1960's and the 1990's, but the type of patient has changed: Heroin addicts, the elderly, and patients with prosthetic heart valves constitute an increasing percentage of endocarditis cases.

—*H. Bradford Hawley, M.D.*

See also Bacterial infections; Cardiac arrest; Cardiology; Cardiology, pediatric; Circulation; Echocardiography; Heart; Heart disease; Heart valve replacement; Mitral valve prolapse; Rheumatic fever; Vascular medicine; Vascular system.

For Further Information:

American Heart Association. http://www.american heart.org/. A group dedicated to reducing disability and death from cardiovascular diseases and stroke. Offers thorough information on a wide range of cardiovascular diseases, referrals to emergency cardiovascular care classes, and research statistics and articles.

Crawford, Michael, ed. *Current Diagnosis and Treatment in Cardiology.* 2d ed. New York: Lange Medical Books/McGraw-Hill, 2003. Discusses advances in cardiac diagnostics, treatments, and prognostic indicators and includes extensive information on prevention techniques.

Durack, David T., and Michael H. Crawford, eds. *Infective Endocarditis.* Philadelphia: W. B. Saunders, 2003. Covers all the features of endocarditis in the modern era.

Eagle, Kim A., and Ragavendra R. Baliga. *Practical Cardiology: Evaluation and Treatment of Common Cardiovascular Disorders.* Philadelphia: Lippincott Williams & Wilkins, 2003. Details advances in cardiac medicine.

Giessel, Barton E., Clint J. Koenig, Robert L. Blake, Jr. "Information from Your Family Doctor: Bacterial Endocarditis, a Heart at Risk." *American Family Physician* 61, no. 6 (March 15, 2000): 1705. This patient handout sheet contains information about bacterial endocarditis, an infection of the valves and inner lining of the heart. It includes information on prevention, complications, and treatment.

Magilligan, Donald J., Jr., and Edward L. Quinn, eds. *Endocarditis: Medical and Surgical Management.* New York: Marcel Dekker, 1986. Discusses the treatment of endocarditis and its complications.

Muirhead, Greg. "Targeting Therapy for Infective Endocarditis." *Patient Care* 33, no. 16 (October 15, 1999): 127-149. The diagnosis of infective endocarditis remains difficult, as does the treatment of this uncommon but potentially deadly disease. Dis-

cussed here are the better diagnostic criteria, developed in recent years, which allow for more effective therapy.

Endocrine disorders

Disease/disorder

Anatomy or system affected: Endocrine system, glands

Specialties and related fields: Endocrinology

Definition: Breakdowns in the normal functioning of the endocrine system, which controls the metabolic processes of the body.

Key terms:

cyclic AMP: a chemical that acts as a second messenger to bring about a response by the cell to the presence of some hormones at their receptors

endocrine: a secretion into the bloodstream rather than by way of a duct, such as hormones

feedback: the mechanism whereby a hormone inhibits its own production; often involves the inhibition of the hypothalamus and tropic hormones

hypothalamohypophysial: relating to the hypothalamus and the hypophysis (pituitary gland)

target cell or organ: a cell or organ possessing the specific hormone receptors needed to respond to a given hormone

tropic: hormones that feed a particular physiological state

tropin: hormones that cause a "turning toward" a particular physiological state

Process and Effects

Endocrine disorders include disturbances in the production of hormones that result from either insufficient or excessive activity and tissues unable to respond to hormones. In order to understand endocrine disorders, it is necessary to review briefly the location of the principal endocrine glands, the hormones secreted, and the normal functions of the hormones. The hormones are released into the bloodstream and are carried throughout the body, where they affect target cells or organs that have receptors for the given hormone.

The pituitary gland, or hypophysis, is sometimes called the master gland because of its widespread influences on many other endocrine glands and the body as a whole. It is located in the midline on the lower part of the brain just above the posterior part of the roof of the mouth. The pituitary has three lobes: the posterior lobe, the intermediate lobe, and the anterior lobe.

The posterior lobe does not synthesize hormones, but it does have nerve fibers coming into it from the hypothalamus of the brain. The ends of these axons release two hormones that are synthesized in the hypothalamus, oxytocin and antidiuretic hormone (ADH). Oxytocin causes the contraction of the smooth muscles of the uterus during childbirth and the contraction of tissues in the mammary glands to release milk during nursing. ADH causes the kidneys to reabsorb water and thereby reduce the volume of urine to normal levels when necessary.

The intermediate lobe of the pituitary secretes melanocyte-stimulating hormone (MSH), a hormone with an uncertain role in humans but known to cause the darkening of melanocytes in animals. Sometimes, the intermediate lobe is considered to be a part of the anterior lobe.

The anterior lobe of the pituitary is under the control of releasing hormones produced by the hypothalamus and carried to the anterior lobe by special blood vessels. In response to these releasing hormones, some stimulatory and some inhibitory, the anterior lobe produces thyroid-stimulating hormone (TSH), adrenocorticotropic hormone (ACTH), follicle-stimulating hormone (FSH), luteinizing hormone (LH), prolactin, and somatotropin or growth hormone (GH). TSH stimulates the thyroid to produce thyroxine, ACTH stimulates the adrenal cortex to produce some of its hormones, FSH stimulates the growth of the cells surrounding eggs in the ovary and causes the ovary to produce estrogen, LH induces ovulation (the release of an egg from the ovary) and stimulates the secretion of progesterone by the ovary, prolactin is essential for milk production and various metabolic functions, and GH is needed for normal growth.

The pineal gland, or epiphysis, is a neuroendocrine gland attached to the roof of the diencephalon in the brain. It produces melatonin, which is released into the bloodstream during the night and has important functions related to an individual's biological clock.

The thyroid gland is located below the larynx in the front of the throat. It produces the hormones thyroxine (T_3) and triiodothyronine (T_4), which are essential for maintaining a normal level of metabolism and heat production, as well as enabling normal development of the brain in young children. C cells in the thyroid produce calcitonin, which is involved in blood calcium regulation. This is also true for parathyroid hormone, a product of the nearby parathyroid glands. The thymus, located under the breast bone or sternum, produces the hormone thymosin that stimulates the immune system. Even the heart is an endocrine gland: It produces atrial natriuretic factor, which stimulates sodium excretion by the kidneys. The pancreas, located near the stomach and small intestine, produces digestive enzymes that pass to the duodenum, but also it produces insulin and glucagon in special cells called pancreatic islets. Insulin causes blood sugar (glucose) to be taken up from the blood into the tissues of the body, and glucagon causes stored starch (glycogen) to be broken down in the liver and thereby increases blood glucose levels.

The pair of adrenal glands, located on the kidneys, are made up of two components: first, a cortex that produces glucocorticoids, mineralocorticoids, and sex steroids or androgens; and second, a medulla, or inner part, that secretes adrenaline and noradrenaline. The gonads, testes or ovaries, are located in the pelvic region and produce several hormones, including the estrogen and progesterone that are essential for reproduction in females and the testosterone that is essential for reproduction in males. The kidneys and digestive tract also produce hormones that regulate red blood cell formation and the functioning of the digestive tract, respectively.

COMPLICATIONS AND DISORDERS

A wide variety of endocrine disorders can be treated successfully. In fact, the ability to restore normal endocrine function with replacement therapy has long been one of the techniques for showing the existence of hypothesized hormones.

The posterior pituitary releases both oxytocin and ADH. Chemicals similar to oxytocin are sometimes given to induce contractions in pregnant women so that birth will occur at a predetermined time. The other hormone released from the posterior pituitary, ADH, normally causes the reabsorption of water within the tubules of the kidney. A deficiency of ADH leads to di-

---

INFORMATION ON ENDOCRINE DISORDERS

CAUSES: Malfunction of endocrine system

SYMPTOMS: Wide ranging and dependent on region; may include precocious puberty, dwarfism, thyroid problems, diseases such as diabetes

DURATION: Chronic

TREATMENTS: Hormonal therapy, medications

abetes insipidus, a condition in which many liters of water a day are excreted by the urinary system; this necessitates that the patient drink huge quantities of water simply to stay alive. A synthetic form of ADH, desmopressin acetate, can be given in the form of a nasal spray that diffuses into the bloodstream and thus restores the reabsorption of water by the kidneys.

The anterior lobe of the pituitary produces six known hormones. The production of these hormones is stimulated and/or inhibited by special releasing hormones secreted by the hypothalamus and carried to the anterior lobe by the hypothalamo-hypophysial portal system of blood vessels. Thus, the source of some anterior pituitary disorders can reside in the hypothalamus. Tumors of anterior pituitary cells can result in the overproduction of a hormone, or if the tumor is destructive, the underproduction of a hormone. Radiation or surgery can be used to destroy tumors and thereby restore normal pituitary functioning.

Anterior pituitary hormones can be the basis of a variety of disorders. As with other hormones, there may be below-normal production of the hormone (hyposecretion) or overproduction of the hormone (hypersecretion). Because the pituitary hormones are often supportive of hormone secretion by the target organ or tissue, hyposecretion or hypersecretion of the tropic or supportive hormone leads to a similar change in the production of hormones by the target organ or tissue.

For example, hyperthyroidism, or Graves' disease, can be caused by excessive secretion of TSH by the pituitary, leading to hypersecretion of thyroxine, or by nodules within the thyroid that produce excessive thyroxine. In the diagnosis process, blood levels of both TSH and thyroxine are usually measured to determine the specific cause of the disorder. Similarly, hypothyroidism can be induced by deficits at several levels. The lack of iodine in the diet can prevent the production of thyroxine, which requires iodide as part of its molec-

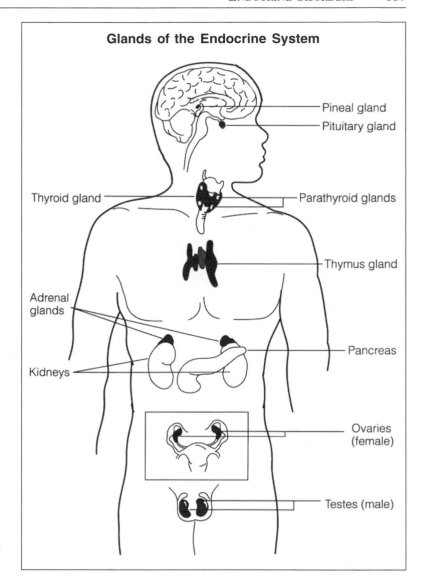

Glands of the Endocrine System

Pineal gland
Pituitary gland
Thyroid gland
Parathyroid glands
Thymus gland
Adrenal glands
Pancreas
Kidneys
Ovaries (female)
Testes (male)

ular composition. The production of thyroxine usually has a negative feedback effect on the hypothalamus and pituitary, reducing TSH production. The failure to produce thyroxine causes high blood levels of TSH and an abnormal growth of the thyroid that results in a greatly enlarged thyroid, called a goiter. The addition of iodine to salt has eliminated the incidence of goiter in developed countries. Even with an adequate supply of iodine in the diet, however, hypothyroidism can still develop from other sources. The usual treatment is to ingest a dose of thyroxine daily.

Other examples of anterior pituitary disorders include those involving changes in GH secretion. Undersecretion of GH can lead to short stature or even dwarfism, in which an individual has normal body proportions but is smaller than normal. Now it is possible to obtain human GH from bacteria genetically engineered to produce it. Replacement GH can be given during the normal growth years to enhance growth. A tumor sometimes develops in the pituitary cells that produce GH, and this can cause abnormally increased growth or gigantism. If the tumor develops during the adult years, only a few areas of abnormal growth can occur, such as in the facial bones and the bones of the hands and feet. This condition is called acromegaly. Abraham Lincoln is thought to have had abnormal levels of GH that caused gigantism in his youth and then acromegaly in his later years. Acromegaly can be treated by radiation or surgery of the anterior pituitary.

Pineal gland tumors have been associated with precocious puberty, in which children become sexually developed in early childhood. It is thought that melatonin normally inhibits sexual development during this period. The pineal gland is influenced by changes in the daily photo-period, so that the highest levels of melatonin appear in the blood during the night, especially during the long nights of winter. Seasonal affective disorder (SAD), a mental depression that occurs during the late fall and winter, has been linked to seasonally high melatonin levels. Daily exposure to bright lights to mimic summer has been used to treat SAD. The pineal gland and melatonin are also being studied with regard to jet lag and disorders associated with shift work. The pineal gland thus seems to be involved in the functioning of the body's biological clock.

The pancreatic islets, also called the islets of Langerhans, produce insulin and glucagon. Diabetes mellitus is caused by insufficient insulin production (type 1 or juvenile-onset diabetes) or by the lack of functional insulin receptors on body cells (type 2 or maturity-onset diabetes). Type 1 diabetes can be treated with insulin injections, an implanted insulin pump, or even a transplant of fetal pancreatic tissue. Type 2 diabetes is treated with diet and weight loss. Weight loss induces an increase in insulin receptors. In addition to the symptoms of high blood sugar levels in the diabetic, long-term damage to the kidneys, blood vessels to the retina, and blood vessels in the legs and feet are important concerns.

The adrenal cortex produces glucocorticoids, mineralocorticoids, and androgens, any of which can be the basis of hyposecretion or hypersecretion. Addison's disease is caused by hyposecretion, whereas Cushing's syndrome is caused by hypersecretion or more-than-sufficient replacement therapy. Similar to those of the thyroid, the adrenal cortex secretions have a negative feedback on the hypothalamus and the anterior pituitary. Addison's disease is characterized by low blood pressure and a poor physiological response to stress. The high levels of ACTH—high because of inadequate feedback of corticoids on the hypothalamus and anterior pituitary—cause a bronzing of the skin because ACTH is similar in its molecular composition to MSH. During an adrenal crisis, exogenous adrenal corticoids are essential to avoid death. Corticoids can be given to prevent inflammation, but their overuse can lead to adrenal cortex suppression by the negative feedback mechanism. The abuse of androgens by athletes wanting to build up their muscles can also result in adrenal suppression, sterility, and damage to the heart. Tumors of androgen-producing cells in women can cause beard growth, increased muscle development, and other changes associated with sex hormones.

Perspective and Prospects

The early history of endocrinology noted that boys who were castrated failed to undergo the changes associated with puberty. A. A. Berthold in 1849 described the effects of castration in cockerels. The birds failed to develop large combs and wattles and failed to show male behavior. He noted that these effects could be reversed if testes were transplanted back into the cockerels. W. M. Bayliss and E. H. Starling in 1902 first introduced the term "hormone" to refer to secretin. They found that secretin is produced by the small intestine in response to acid in the chyme and that secretin causes the pancreas to release digestive enzymes into the small intestine. Most important, F. G. Banting and G. H. Best in 1922 reported their extraction of insulin from the pancreas of dogs and their success in alleviating diabetes in dogs by means of injections of the insulin. Fredrick Sanger in 1953 established the amino acid sequence for insulin and later won a Nobel Prize for this achievement.

Another Nobel Prize was awarded to Earl W. Sutherland, Jr., in 1971 for his demonstration in 1962 of the role of cyclic AMP as a second messenger in the sequence involved in the stimulation of cells by many hormones. Andrew V. Schally and Roger C. L. Guillemin in 1977 received a Nobel Prize for their work in isolating and determining the structures of hypothalamic regulatory peptides.

More recent achievements in endocrinological research have centered on the identification of receptors that bind with the hormone when the hormone stimulates a cell and on the genetic engineering of bacteria to produce hormones such as human growth hormone. The use of fetal tissues in endocrinological research and therapy—the host usually does not reject fetal implants—continues to be an area for future research.

—John T. Burns, Ph.D.; updated by
Sharon W. Stark, R.N., A.P.R.N., D.N.Sc.

See also Addison's disease; Adrenalectomy; Amenorrhea; Corticosteroids; Cushing's syndrome; Diabetes mellitus; Dwarfism; Dysmenorrhea; Endocrinology; Endocrinology, pediatric; Endometriosis; Fructosemia; Gigantism; Glands; Goiter; Growth; Hashimoto's thyroiditis; Hormone replacement therapy (HRT); Hormones; Hyperhidrosis; Hyperparathyroidism and hypoparathyroidism; Hypoglycemia; Infertility, female; Infertility, male; Insulin resistance syndrome; Liver; Menopause; Menorrhagia; Metabolic disorders; Ovarian cysts; Pancreas; Pancreatitis; Parathyroidectomy; Pregnancy and gestation; Prostate gland; Prostate gland removal; Puberty and adolescence; Steroids; Testicular surgery; Thyroid disorders; Thyroid gland; Thyroidectomy.

FOR FURTHER INFORMATION:

Griffin, James E., and Sergio R. Ojeda, eds. *Textbook of Endocrine Physiology.* 5th ed. New York: Oxford University Press, 2004. A detailed account of normal and abnormal functioning of the endocrine system written by specialists. Intended for first year medical students.

Hadley, Mac E., and Jon E. Levine. *Endocrinology.* 6th ed. Upper Saddle River, N.J.: Pearson Prentice Hall, 2007. A college-level text covering the endocrine system, primarily in humans and mammals. Recommended for a technical but understandable coverage of the field.

Henry, Helen L., and Anthony W. Norman, eds. *Encyclopedia of Hormones.* 3 vols. San Diego, Calif.: Academic Press, 2003. A comprehensive overview of the role of hormones, the major physiological systems in which they operate, and the biological consequences of an excess or deficiency of a particular hormone.

Larsen, P. Reed, et al., eds. *Williams Textbook of Endocrinology.* 10th ed. Philadelphia: W. B. Saunders, 2003. Comprehensive information regarding endocrine diseases—their pathophysiology, diagnoses, treatment, and prognoses.

Martini, Frederic. *Fundamentals of Anatomy and Physiology.* 5th ed. Upper Saddle River, N.J.:

Prentice Hall, 2001. A good place to start for a solid overview of the anatomy and physiology of the endocrine system before considering the details of disease states.

Scanlon, Valerie, et al. *Essentials of Anatomy and Physiology.* 5th ed. Philadelphia: F. A. Davis, 2007. A text designed around three themes: the relationship between physiology and anatomy, the interrelations among the organ systems, and the relationship of each organ system to homeostasis.

Shaw, Michael, ed. *Everything You Need to Know About Diseases.* Springhouse, Pa.: Springhouse Press, 1996. This well-illustrated consumer reference, compiled by more than one hundred doctors and medical experts, describes five hundred illnesses and conditions, listing their causes, symptoms, diagnosis, treatment, and prevention. Of particular interest is chapter 12, "Hormone and Gland Disorders."

Wells, Ken R. "Endocrine System." In *Gale Encyclopedia of Nursing and Allied Health,* edited by Kristine Krapp. Detroit: Gale Group, 2002. A thorough examination of the endocrine system—its organs, role in health, and diseases and disorders.

ENDOCRINOLOGY

SPECIALTY

ANATOMY OR SYSTEM AFFECTED: Brain, endocrine system, glands, immune system, nervous system, pancreas, psychic-emotional system, reproductive system, uterus

SPECIALTIES AND RELATED FIELDS: Biochemistry, genetics, gynecology, immunology

DEFINITION: The science dealing with how the internal secretions from ductless glands in the body act both in normal physiology and in disease states.

KEY TERMS:

adrenal gland: an endocrine gland situated immediately above the upper pole of each kidney; it consists of an inner part or medulla, which produces epinephrine and norepinephrine, and an outer part or cortex, which produces steroid hormones

endocrine pancreas: specialized secretory tissue dispersed within the pancreas called islets of Langerhans, which are responsible for the secretion of glucagon and insulin

hypothalamus: the region of the brain called the diencephalon, forming the floor of the third ventricle, including neighboring associated nuclei

metabolism: the process of tissue change, which may be synthetic (anabolic) or degradative (catabolic)

parathyroid gland: one of four small endocrine glands situated underneath the thyroid gland, whose main product is parathyroid hormone, which is responsible for the regulation of serum calcium levels

pituitary gland: a small (0.5-gram), two-lobed endocrine gland that is attached by a stalk to the brain at the level of the hypothalamus

thyroid gland: a 20-gram endocrine gland that sits in front of the trachea and consists of two lateral lobes connected in the middle by an isthmus

SCIENCE AND PROFESSION

The rates of metabolic pathways in the body are controlled mainly by the endocrine system, in conjunction with the nervous system. These two systems are integrated in the neuroendocrine system, which controls the secretion of hormones by the endocrine glands. The study of endocrinology deals with the normal physiology and pathophysiology of endocrine glands. The endocrine glands that are typically the main focus of clinical endocrinologists are the hypothalamus, pituitary gland, thyroid, parathyroid, adrenal glands, endocrine pancreas, ovaries, and testes. The endocrine system regulates virtually all activities of the body, including growth and development, homeostasis, energy production, and reproduction.

The hypothalamus is a highly specialized endocrine organ that sits at the base of the brain and that functions as the master gland of the endocrine system. It is the main integrator for the endocrine and nervous systems. The hypothalamus produces a number of chemical mediators which have direct control over the pituitary gland. These chemicals are made in the cells of the hypothalamus and reach the pituitary gland, which sits just below it, by a special hypophyseoportal blood system. In adult humans, the pituitary is divided into two lobes: the anterior lobe (adenohypophysis) and the posterior lobe (neural lobe).

Vasopressin and oxytocin are the two main hormones that are made in the hypothalamus but stored in the posterior lobe of the pituitary for release when needed. Vasopressin (also known as antidiuretic hormone, or ADH) is a hormone that maintains a normal water concentration in the blood and is a regulator of circulating blood volume. Oxytocin is a hormone that is involved in lactation and obstetrical labor.

The hypothalamic-pituitary-thyroid axis is important in the control of basal metabolic rate. There are a number of releasing hormones secreted from the hypothalamus that control the release of anterior pituitary hormones, which then cause the release of hormone at the end organ. Most of these hormones have the chemical structures of peptides. Thyrotropin-releasing hormone (TRH) was the first hypothalamic releasing hormone that was synthesized and used clinically. TRH, secreted in nanogram quantities, is a cyclic tripeptide that causes release of thyrotropin-stimulating hormone (TSH) from the thyrotropic cells of the anterior pituitary gland. The release of TSH is in microgram quantities and leads to an increase in thyroid hormone release by the thyroid gland. The amount of thyroid hormone synthesized is on the order of milligrams. Therefore, the secretion of minute amounts of the TRH allows for the production of thyroid hormone that is a millionfold greater than the amount of TRH itself. This is an example of an amplifying cascade, a system by which the central nervous system can control all metabolic processes with the secretion of very small amounts of hypothalamic releasing hormones. This intricate system possesses controls to stop the production of too much hormone as well. Such negative feedback is an important concept in endocrinology.

In the case of the thyroid, an increased amount of thyroid hormone produced by the thyroid gland will cause the pituitary and hypothalamus to decrease the amounts that they produce of TSH and TRH, respectively. Many hormones are subject to the laws of negative feedback control. TRH also causes potent release of the anterior pituitary hormone called prolactin. Thyroid hormone is important in determining basal metabolism and is needed for proper development in the newborn child. The thyroid gland produces both thyroxine (T_4, also called tetraiodothyronine) and triiodothyronine (T_3), both of which it synthesizes from iodine and the amino acid tyrosine.

The hypothalamic-pituitary-adrenal axis is critical in the reaction to stress, both physical and emotional. Corticotropin-releasing hormone (CRH) is a polypeptide, consisting of forty-one amino acids, that causes the production of the proopiomelanocortin molecule by the corticotropic cells of the anterior pituitary. The proopiomelanocortin molecule is cleaved by proteolytic enzymes to yield adrenocorticotropic hormone (ACTH, also called corticotropin), melanocyte-stimulating hormone, and lipotropin. It is ACTH made by the anterior pituitary which then stimulates the adrenal cortex to produce steroid hormones. The main stress hormone produced by the adrenal cortex in response to ACTH is the glucocorticoid cortisol. ACTH also has some control over the production of the mineralocorticoid aldosterone and the androgens dehydroepiandrosterone and testosterone. These steroids are synthesized from cholesterol. The production of cortisol (also known as hydrocortisone) is subject to negative feedback by CRII and ACTH.

The hypothalamic-pituitary-gonadal axis is involved in the control of reproduction. Gonadotropin-releasing hormone (GnRH), also known as luteinizing hormone-releasing hormone (LHRH), is produced by the hypothalamus and stimulates the release of luteinizing hormone (LH) and follicle-stimulating hormone (FSH) from the gonadotrophic cells of the anterior pituitary. LH and FSH have different effects in men and women. In men, LH controls the production and secretion of testosterone by the Leydig's cells of the testes. The release of LH is regulated by negative feedback from testosterone. FSH along with testosterone acts on the Sertoli cells of the seminiferous tubule of the testis at the time of puberty to start sperm production. In women, LH controls ovulation by the ovary and also the development of the corpus luteum, which produces progesterone. Progesterone is a steroid hormone that is critically important for the maintenance of pregnancy. FSH in women stimulates the development and maturation of a primary follicle and oocyte. The ovarian follicle in the nonpregnant woman is the main site of production of estradiol. Estradiol is the principal estrogen made in the reproductive years by the ovary and is responsible for the development of female secondary sexual characteristics.

Growth hormone-releasing hormone (GHRH) is a polypeptide with forty-four amino acids that stimulates the release of growth hormone (GH) from the somatotrophic cells of the anterior pituitary. The regulation of GH secretion is under dual control. While GHRH positively releases GH, somatostatin (a polypeptide with fourteen amino acids, also released from the hypothalamus) inhibits the release of GH. Somatostatin has a wide variety of functions, including the suppression of insulin, glucagon, and gastrointestinal hormones. GH released from the pituitary circulates in the bloodstream and stimulates the production of somatomedins by the liver. Several somatomedins are produced, all of which have a profound effect on growth, with the most important one in humans being somatomedin C, also called insulin-like growth factor I (IGF I). Molecular biological techniques have shown that many cells outside the liver also produce IGF I; in these cells, IGF I acts in autocrine or paracrine ways to cause the growth of the cells or to affect neighboring cells.

Prolactin is a peptide hormone that is secreted by the lactotrophs of the anterior pituitary. It is involved in the differentiation of the mammary gland cells and initiates the production of milk proteins and other constituents. Prolactin may also have other functions, as a stress hormone or growth hormone. Prolactin is under tonic negative control. The inhibition of prolactin release is caused by dopamine, which is produced by the hypothalamus. Thus, while dopamine is normally considered to be a neurotransmitter, in the case of prolactin release it acts as an inhibitory hormone. Serotonin, also classically thought of as a neurotransmitter, may cause the stimulation of prolactin release from the anterior pituitary.

DIAGNOSTIC AND TREATMENT TECHNIQUES

One of the most common medical problems seen by specialists in the field of endocrinology is a patient with type I diabetes mellitus, sometimes also called juvenile-onset or insulin-dependent diabetes mellitus. "Insulin-dependent" is probably more appropriate, as not all patients with type I diabetes mellitus develop the disease in childhood. Type I diabetes is an autoimmune disease in which antibodies to different parts of the pancreatic beta cell, the cell that normally produces insulin, are produced. Some of these antibodies are cytotoxic; that is, they actually destroy the pancreatic beta cell. The most striking characteristic of patients with type I diabetes is that they produce very little insulin. The symptoms of type I diabetes include increased thirst, increased urination, blurring of vision, and weight loss. A doctor would confirm the diagnosis by running blood tests for glucose and insulin. The glucose level would be high, and the insulin level would be low. The treatment includes controlled diet, exercise, insulin therapy, and self-monitoring of blood glucose. With proper control of blood glucose, patients with type I diabetes can lead normal, productive lives.

Graves' disease is another autoimmune disease that is commonly seen by endocrinologists. Graves' disease is caused by the production of thyroid-stimulating immunoglobulin antibodies that bind to and activate TSH receptors. As a result, the thyroid gland produces too much thyroid hormone and the thyroid gland enlarges in size. The antibodies also commonly affect the eyes, causing a characteristic bulging. The clinical symptoms of hyperthyroidism include increased heart rate, anxiety, heat sensitivity, sleeplessness, diarrhea, and abdominal pain. Patients often lose considerable weight, despite having a great appetite and eating large amounts of food. Sometimes, the diagnosis is missed, leading to an extensive evaluation for a variety of other diseases. Often, a family history of thyroid disease or other endocrine disease can be found.

The usual method of screening for Graves' disease is with a simple blood test for thyroid function, which includes testing for T_4, T_3, and TSH. In patients with Graves' disease, both T_4 and T_3 will be elevated, and TSH will be very low. If the blood test reveals this pattern, the next usual step is to proceed to a radioactive iodine uptake and scan test, which involves giving a very small amount of radioactive iodine by mouth and having the patient return twenty-four hours later for a scan. The thyroid gland normally accumulates iodine and thus will accumulate the radioactive iodine as well. The radioactive iodine emits a gamma-ray energy that can be picked up by a solid-crystal scintillation counter placed over the thyroid gland. With this device, one can determine the percentage of iodine uptake and also obtain a picture of the thyroid gland. The normal radioactive iodine uptake is about 10 to 30 percent of the dose, depending somewhat on the amount of total body iodine, which is derived from the diet. Patients with Graves' disease will have high radioactive iodine uptakes.

Those who suffer from Graves' disease can be treated by three different means, depending on the circumstances. The first treatment that is often tried is antithyroid drugs, either propylthiouracil or methimazole. These drugs belong to the class of sulfonamides and inhibit the production of new thyroid hormone by blocking the attachment of iodine to the amino acid tyrosine. Another mode of therapy is the use of radioactive iodine. A dose of radioactive iodine (on the order of 5 to 10 millicuries) is used to destroy part of the thyroid gland. The gamma-ray energy emitted from the iodine molecule that has traveled to the thyroid gland is enough to kill some thyroid cells. An alternative way to destroy the thyroid gland is to remove it surgically (thyroidectomy). Endocrinologists rarely send patients for surgery, as the other therapies are often effective. The goal of all treatments is to bring the level of thyroid hormone into the normal range, as well as to shrink the thyroid gland. After treatment, the patient's level of thyroid hormone sometimes falls to levels that are below normal. The symptoms of hypothyroidism are the opposite of hyperthyroidism and include fatigue, weight gain, cold sensitivity, constipation, and dry skin. If this happens, the patient is treated with thyroid hormone replacement. The dose is adjusted for each individual to produce normal levels of T_4, T_3, and TSH.

A less common but important endocrine disorder is the existence of a pituitary tumor that secretes prolactin, called a prolactinoma. Prolactinomas are diagnosed earlier in women than in men, as women with the disorder often complain of a lack of menstrual periods and spontaneous milk production from the breasts, known as galactorrhea. These tumors, which can be quite small, are called microadenomas because they are less than 10 millimeters in size. They can affect men as well, causing decreased sex drive and impotence. Macroadenomas are tumors greater than 10 millimeters in size. When the tumors increase in size, they can cause symptoms such as headache and decreased vision. It is important to note that most microadenomas never progress to macroadenomas. Vision loss and/or decreased eye movement can be seen with a macroadenoma and are reason for immediate treatment.

Doctors screen patients for a prolactinoma by running a blood test for prolactin. There are other reasons for mild elevations in prolactin levels, including the use of certain psychiatric drugs such as phenothiazines or the antihypertensive drugs reserpine and methyldopa, primary hypothyroidism, cirrhosis, and chronic renal failure. If a pituitary tumor is suspected, then other biochemical tests of pituitary function are conducted to determine if the rest of the gland is functioning normally. At that time, imaging tests are often done to get a picture of the hypothalamic-pituitary area; this can be done with either computed tomography (CT) scanning or magnetic resonance imaging (MRI). Patients with macroadenomas will require treatment. In patients with little neurological involvement, medical therapy may be initiated. Bromocriptine, a semisynthetic ergot alkaloid which is an inhibitor of prolactin secretion, may be used. It has been shown that patients treated with this drug have reduction in tumor size. Patients can be maintained on the drug indefinitely because prolactin levels return to pretreatment levels when the drug is stopped. If there is severe neurologic involvement, with loss of vision and other eye problems, immediate surgery may be indicated. There is a very high incidence of tumor recurrence after surgery, requiring medical and/or radiation therapy.

PERSPECTIVE AND PROSPECTS

The field of endocrinology is a continuously evolving one. Advances in biomedical technology, including molecular biology and cell biology, have made it a demanding job for the clinician to keep up with all the breakthroughs in the field. The challenge for endocrinology will be to apply many of these new technologies to novel treatments for patients with endocrine diseases.

An example of the progression of the field of endocrinology can be seen in the history of pituitary diseases. The start of pituitary endocrinology is ascribed to Pierre Marie, the French neurologist who in 1886 first described pituitary enlargement in a patient with acromegaly (enlargement of the skull, jaw, hands, and feet) and linked the disease to a pituitary abnormality. During the first half of the twentieth century, many of the hypothalamic and pituitary hormones were isolated and characterized. The field of endocrinology was revolutionized by the development of the radioimmunoassay, which allows sensitive and specific measurements of hormones. The radioimmunoassay replaced bioassay techniques, which were laborious, time-consuming, and not always precise. This technique has allowed for rapid measurement of hormones and improved screening for endocrine diseases involving hormone deficiency or hormone excess.

The development of new hormone assays has been complemented by the development of noninvasive imaging techniques. Before the advent of CT scanning in the late 1970's, it was an ordeal to diagnose a pituitary tumor. Pneumoencephalography was often performed, which involved injecting air into the fluid-containing structures of the brain, with associated risk and discomfort to the patient. In the 1980's, with new generations of high-resolution CT scanners that were more sensitive than early scanners, smaller pituitary lesions could be detected and diagnosed. That decade also ushered in the use of MRI to diagnose disorders of the hypothalamic-pituitary unit. MRI has allowed doctors to evaluate the hypothalamus, pituitary, and nearby structures very precisely; it has become the method of choice for evaluating patients with pituitary disease. MRI can easily visualize the optic chiasm in the forebrain and the vascular structures surrounding the pituitary.

In patients who require surgery, advances have helped decrease mortality rates. Harvey Cushing pioneered the transsphenoidal technique in 1927 but abandoned it in favor of the transfrontal approach. This involves reaching the pituitary tumor by retracting the frontal lobes to visualize the pituitary gland sitting underneath. The modern era of transsphenoidal pituitary surgery was developed by Gérard Guiot and Jules Hardy in the late 1960's. Transsphenoidal surgery done with an operating microscope to visualize the pituitary contents allows for selective removal of the tumor, leaving the normal pituitary gland intact. The advantage of this approach from below, instead of from above, includes minimal movement of the brain and less blood loss. This technique requires a neurosurgeon with much skill and experience. There are also new drug treatments for patients with pituitary diseases, such as bromocriptine for use in patients with prolactinomas and octreotide (a somatostatin analogue) to lower growth hormone levels in patients with acromegaly.

—*RoseMarie Pasmantier, M.D.*

See also Addison's disease; Adrenalectomy; Chronobiology; Corticosteroids; Cushing's syndrome; Diabetes mellitus; Dwarfism; Endocrine disorders; Endocrinology, pediatric; Enzymes; Fructosemia; Gestational diabetes; Gigantism; Glands; Goiter; Growth; Gynecology; Hair loss and baldness; Hashimoto's thyroiditis; Hormone replacement therapy (HRT); Hormones; Hot flashes; Hyperhidrosis; Hyperparathyroidism and hypoparathyroidism; Hypoglycemia; Hysterectomy; Melatonin; Menopause; Menstruation; Metabolic disorders; Obesity; Obesity, childhood; Paget's disease; Pancreas; Pancreatitis; Parathyroidectomy; Pharmacology; Pharmacy; Prostate gland; Prostate gland removal; Puberty and adolescence; Sex change surgery; Sexual differentiation; Steroids; Thyroid disorders; Thyroid gland; Thyroidectomy; Weight loss and gain.

FOR FURTHER INFORMATION:

Bar, Robert S., ed. *Early Diagnosis and Treatment of Endocrine Disorders*. Totowa, N.J.: Humana Press, 2003. Reviews the early signs and symptoms of common endocrine diseases, surveys the clinical testing needed for a diagnosis, and presents recommendations for therapy.

Braverman, Lewis E., and Robert D. Utiger, eds. *Werner and Ingbar's The Thyroid: A Fundamental and Clinical Text*. 9th ed. Philadelphia: Lippincott Williams & Wilkins, 2005. An exhaustive textbook on all aspects of the thyroid, including history, anatomy, biology, pathology, basic and clinical research, and the thyroid in development and pregnancy.

Harmel, Anne Peters, and Ruchi Mathur. *Davidson's Diabetes Mellitus: Diagnosis and Treatment*. 5th ed. Philadelphia: W. B. Saunders, 2004. A very good, practical approach to the overall management of the endocrine patient with diabetes mellitus.

Imura, Hiroo, ed. *The Pituitary Gland*. 2d ed. New

York: Raven Press, 1994. Good discussion of the master gland, the hypothalamic-pituitary unit.

Larsen, P. Reed, et al., eds. *Williams Textbook of Endocrinology*. 10th ed. Philadelphia: W. B. Saunders, 2003. Text that covers the spectrum of information related to the endocrine system, including thyroid disorders, diabetes, endocrinology and aging, female reproduction and fertility control, sexual function and dysfunction, kidney stones, and endocrine hypertension.

Lebovitz, Harold E., ed. *Therapy for Diabetes Mellitus and Related Disorders*. 4th ed. Alexandria, Va.: American Diabetes Association, 2004. A comprehensive treatise on the treatment of various aspects of diabetes mellitus. The different chapters are written by experts in the field.

Speroff, Leon, and Marc A. Fritz. *Clinical Gynecologic Endocrinology and Infertility*. 7th ed. Philadelphia: Lippincott Williams & Wilkins, 2005. An excellent textbook which brings together all aspects of endocrinology in women from embryology to old age. Good discussion of the problems seen in infertile couples.

ENDOCRINOLOGY, PEDIATRIC

SPECIALTY

ANATOMY OR SYSTEM AFFECTED: Brain, endocrine system, glands, immune system, nervous system, pancreas, psychic-emotional system

SPECIALTIES AND RELATED FIELDS: Biochemistry, genetics, immunology, neonatology, pediatrics

DEFINITION: The study of the normal and abnormal function of the endocrine (ductless) glands in children and adolescents.

KEY TERMS:

hormone: a chemical molecule produced in either the hypothalamus or one of the endocrine glands that is secreted and travels (usually via the bloodstream) to a target organ or to specific receptor cells, causing a specific response

insulin: a hormone that is essential in regulating blood glucose, as well as in assimilating carbohydrates for growth and energy

pancreas: a large gland near the stomach which has both exocrine and endocrine functions and which produces insulin

pituitary gland: a very small gland at the base of the brain that is referred to as the master gland; with the hypothalamus, it regulates most of the endocrine systems

thyroid: a gland in the anterior neck which regulates the level of the body's metabolism and which is instrumental in normal physical and mental growth

SCIENCE AND PROFESSION

Pediatric endocrinology is a major subspecialty, limited to children and adolescents, which involves the study of normal as well as abnormal functions of the endocrine system, which comprises the glands of internal or ductless secretions. These practitioners, referred to as endocrinologists or pediatric endocrinologists, are doctors of medicine or osteopathy who have completed three years of pediatric residency training and an additional two to three years of fellowship training in endocrinology.

Endocrinology is one of the most interesting and challenging fields in pediatrics because it requires a blend of basic science and technology in the clinical setting. Some of the diagnoses are very difficult, yet they are almost always completely logical. Endocrinology is tightly related to other areas of pediatrics, such as adolescent medicine, genetics, growth, development, nutrition, and metabolism. These relationships make this field even more complex and intellectually stimulating.

Pediatric endocrinology and adult endocrinology are relatively young fields, probably beginning with the discovery in 1888 that "myxedema" (hypothyroidism) could be improved by feeding the patient thyroid extract. Both fields deal with the major endocrine glands and their disorders, such as diabetes mellitus or hypothyroidism, but there are several key differences, most related to growth (both physical and mental), potential, and genetics. Some major areas of specific emphasis in pediatric endocrinology include diabetes mellitus (which presents very differently in children), disorders of growth, disorders of sexual maturation and differentiation, genetic disorders, and adolescent medicine.

DIAGNOSTIC AND TREATMENT TECHNIQUES

In pediatric endocrinology, as in all medical fields, history taking and physical examination are the starting points and usually the most useful tools for diagnosis. Endocrinology is a specialty that is particularly aided by science. Blood and urine chemistries, hormone assays, chromosomal analyses, X rays, computed tomography (CT) scans, magnetic resonance imaging (MRI), and a host of other sophisticated tests have advanced diagnosis and treatment and have made this specialty one of the favorites for physicians who like science.

Virtually all the known hormones can be assayed accurately and quickly.

Since insulin was first available for injection in 1922, there have been amazing advances in treatment. Many of the treatments in endocrinology involve hormone therapy. In 1985, recombinant growth hormone was synthesized for the first time. This development has allowed endocrinologists to treat not only pituitary dwarfism but also other kinds of growth deficiencies, such as Turner syndrome.

Turner syndrome is a relatively common chromosomal abnormality affecting females and resulting in short stature and lack of sexual development. While these girls will never become fertile, the combination of growth hormone for stature and other hormonal therapy for the development of secondary sexual characteristics enables them to have a normal female body. Studies have shown that normal body image and the presence of menstruation is essential for the self-esteem of these patients.

Diabetes mellitus is the most common significant endocrine disorder in both adults and children. What was commonly referred to as juvenile diabetes years ago is now called diabetes mellitus, type I. Unlike type II, which usually presents insidiously in middle-aged and older adults, type I presents rapidly, and the patient will need daily injectable insulin treatments. Diabetes in children is complex to manage not only because of the insulin treatment but also because of the patients' growth, metabolism, fluctuating activity levels, and physiologic and psychological changes that occur, especially in adolescence.

Now small portable and quite accurate glucometers allow patients to measure blood glucose (sugar) at home, making diabetes management much simpler. Tighter control of blood glucose will decrease or delay the onset of long-term complications of the disease, such as blindness, heart disease, and kidney disease. In the United States, newborn screening, which is now performed in all fifty states, has virtually eliminated cretinism, which tragically resulted when congenital hypothyroidism was not diagnosed until later in childhood. These children were irreversibly mentally retarded.

Enhanced techniques in pediatric surgery and neurosurgery, greatly aided by scans, play a role in the treatment of some endocrine disorders. Very small tumors and masses can be identified and often removed successfully. Often, endocrinologists and oncologists work together in concert with the surgeon.

Although this subspecialty is one of the most scientific and laboratory-based in pediatrics, it is also a field where emotional support, counseling, and often mental health care are given. Children do not like being "different," and body image is very important in children and particularly in teenagers. Even when a child appears absolutely normal, the frustration of ongoing monitoring and treatment is resented and can result in rebellion, especially in children with diabetes. Often, a team approach is needed, which involves professionals, teachers, family, and peers.

PERSPECTIVE AND PROSPECTS

The future promises ever-advancing and dramatic tools for the diagnosis and treatment of endocrine disorders, as well as for their prevention. On the immediate horizon, an implantible glucose pump, which can serve as a substitute pancreas, can change the lives of diabetic patients dramatically. A method for rapidly analyzing blood glucose using the surface of the skin has been developed. In addition, genetic engineering may revolutionize the approaches to treating many of these diseases.

—C. Mervyn Rasmussen, M.D.

See also Addison's disease; Adrenalectomy; Chronobiology; Corticosteroids; Diabetes mellitus; Dwarfism; Endocrine disorders; Endocrinology; Enzymes; Fructosemia; Gigantism; Glands; Growth; Gynecology; Hormone replacement therapy (HRT); Hormones; Hyperparathyroidism and hypoparathyroidism; Hypoglycemia; Melatonin; Menstruation; Metabolic disorders; Obesity; Obesity, childhood; Pancreas; Pancreatitis; Parathyroidectomy; Pediatrics; Pharmacology; Pharmacy; Puberty and adolescence; Steroids; Thyroid disorders; Thyroid gland; Thyroidectomy; Weight loss and gain.

FOR FURTHER INFORMATION:

Bar, Robert S., ed. *Early Diagnosis and Treatment of Endocrine Disorders.* Totowa, N.J.: Humana Press, 2003. Reviews the early signs and symptoms of common endocrine diseases, surveys the clinical testing needed for a diagnosis, and presents recommendations for therapy.

Handwerger, Stuart, ed. *Molecular and Cellular Pediatric Endocrinology.* Totowa, N.J.: Humana Press, 1999. The chapters in this book reflect the genetic and molecular bases of many of the fundamental problems of differentiation and growth in a manner appropriate for a pediatrics textbook.

Larsen, P. Reed, et al., eds. *Williams Textbook of Endocrinology*. 10th ed. Philadelphia: W. B. Saunders, 2003. Text that covers the spectrum of information related to the endocrine system, including thyroid disorders, diabetes, endocrinology and aging, female reproduction and fertility control, sexual function and dysfunction, kidney stones, and endocrine hypertension.

Little, Marjorie. *Diabetes*. New York: Chelsea House, 1991. A clearly written overview directed toward a nonspecialized audience. Includes a fourteen-page chapter on type I (juvenile) diabetes.

Sperling, Mark A., ed. *Pediatric Endocrinology*. 2d ed. Philadelphia: W. B. Saunders, 2002. Discusses endocrine diseases in infancy and childhood. Includes a bibliography and an index.

Wales, Jeremy K. H., and Jan Maarten Wit. *Pediatric Endocrinology and Growth*. 2d ed. Philadelphia: W. B. Saunders, 2003. An illustrated text that outlines specific endocrine problems, from growth disorders to glucose homeostasis, early or late sexual development, abnormal genitalia, goiter, failure to thrive, and obesity.

ENDODONTIC DISEASE

DISEASE/DISORDER

ANATOMY OR SYSTEM AFFECTED: Mouth, teeth
SPECIALTIES AND RELATED FIELDS: Dentistry
DEFINITION: Disease of the dental pulp and sometimes also the soft tissues and bone around the tip of the root.

CAUSES AND SYMPTOMS

The most common cause of endodontic disease is infection of the dental pulp by the bacteria that cause tooth decay. The pulp is composed of connective tissue, nerves, blood vessels, and tooth regenerative cells. It fills the root canal, a narrow channel in the center of the tooth root, which is embedded in the jawbone. Teeth usually contain one to four root canals. Decay-causing bacteria reach the pulp after dissolving their way through the two, hard outer layers of the tooth—the enamel and dentin. Bacteria may also reach the pulp through a crack or fracture in a tooth and through tooth wear or abrasion. Many kinds of bacteria can infect the pulp.

Pulp infected by bacteria becomes inflamed and has no place to swell because it is surrounded by dentin, which is rigid. Pain may result. Eventually, the entire pulp may become infected and die. If not treated, the in-

---

INFORMATION ON ENDODONTIC DISEASE

CAUSES: Bacterial infection of dental pulp
SYMPTOMS: Gum inflammation and pain, which is severe if abscess forms
DURATION: Chronic if untreated
TREATMENTS: Root canal treatment

---

fection can spread to the soft tissue and bone surrounding the tip of the root and form an abscess, which often produces severe pain.

TREATMENT AND THERAPY

To treat damaged or dead pulp tissue and preserve the tooth, endodontic therapy, or root canal treatment, is required. Endodontists specialize in this procedure. One or two visits are usually required. A small hole is made in the top (crown) of the infected tooth, and all the pulp tissue is removed. Then an inert material, usually a piece of rubberlike gum called gutta percha, is inserted in place of the pulp and secured in place with a sealer or cement. A tooth that has had root canal treatment is commonly considered to be dead, but the fibers of the periodontal ligament that hold the tooth in the jawbone are still alive. Following this procedure, additional dental treatments are necessary to preserve the weakened tooth.

PERSPECTIVE AND PROSPECTS

Historically, the only remedy for endodontic disease was tooth extraction. Since the mid-twentieth century, endodontic research has yielded treatments that preserve infected teeth. Furthermore, there has been an increased appreciation of the role of dental hygiene in preventing tooth decay and the endodontic infections that can result from it. Research on the causes and prevention of endodontic disease, and treatments for it, is being conducted at dental schools and at the National Institute of Dental and Cranio-Facial Research.

—*Jane F. Hill, Ph.D.*

See also Cavities; Dental diseases; Dentistry; Gingivitis; Gum disease; Periodontal surgery; Periodontitis; Root canal treatment; Teeth; Tooth extraction; Toothache.

FOR FURTHER INFORMATION:

Beers, Mark H., et al., eds. *The Merck Manual of Medical Information, Second Home Edition*. Whitehouse Station, N.J.: Merck Research Laboratories, 2003.

Christensen, Gordon J. *A Consumer's Guide to Dentistry*. 2d ed. St. Louis: Mosby, 2001.

Kim, Syngcuk, ed. *Modern Endodontic Practice*. Philadelphia: Saunders, 2004.

Smith, Rebecca W. *The Columbia University School of Dental and Oral Surgery's Guide to Family Dental Care*. New York: W. W. Norton, 1997.

ENDOMETRIAL BIOPSY

PROCEDURE

ANATOMY OR SYSTEM AFFECTED: Genitals, reproductive system, uterus

SPECIALTIES AND RELATED FIELDS: Gynecology, histology, obstetrics, preventive medicine

DEFINITION: A procedure in which a tissue sample is taken from the lining of the uterus and examined.

KEY TERMS:

cervix: the entrance to the uterus

dilation and curettage (D&C): a prcedure in which the cervix is stretched and the lining of the uterus is scraped

endometrium: tissue lining the inside of the uterus

hysteroscopy: a procedure using a thin, lighted tube with a camera and tool to examine visually and remove part of the endometrium

uterus: the part of the reproductive tract that supports the development and nourishment of a developing fetus; also called the womb

vagina: the tube leading from the uterus to the outside of the body

INDICATIONS AND PROCEDURES

An endometrial biopsy is usually performed to identify the cause of abnormal uterine bleeding. Abnormal bleeding is that which is excessive in duration, frequency, or amount for the particular woman, and it includes bleeding at the wrong times (between menstrual periods) or after menopause. The biopsy may also be performed when there is no bleeding (or menstruation), or if a woman is having difficulty becoming pregnant.

Approximately 90 percent of women who have endometrial cancer have abnormal bleeding, so the biopsy is performed to rule out both cancer and hyperplasia, an excessive growth of tissue that could become cancerous. Women who are perimenopausal (prior to the actual end of menstrual cycles) may experience changes in their cycle that make it difficult to determine if there is abnormal bleeding or simply normal changes. Perimenopause usually lasts six to eight years, and then women become menopausal when menstrual cycles end. Women on hormone replacement therapy (HRT) are at greater risk of endometrial cancer, since they usually take the hormones estrogen and progesterone that their body is no longer producing at sufficient levels. Women who take estrogen but cannot take progesterone are at an even greater risk of endometrial cancer.

The biopsy may also be used as part of an infertility examination to determine if there are problems with the development of the endometrium. If the endometrium does not thicken in time to accept and support a fertilized egg, then the egg cannot implant properly, a condition called luteal phase defect (LPD). The biopsy can show whether the uterine lining is thickening and maturing by developing more blood vessels before menstruation, a definite sign that ovulation (the maturation and release of an egg by the ovary) has occurred and that the lining can support a pregnancy. Additionally, the biopsy may be performed to help evaluate the problem of repeated early miscarriages. Another use of the procedure is to obtain a sample for patients with suspected endometritis or polycystic ovary disease.

A gynecologist or obstetrician will perform the procedure in either the doctor's office or a local hospital. The procedure takes only about two minutes, and no anesthesia is needed, although a mild over-the-counter painkiller is recommended about one hour ahead of time to ease discomfort. Additionally, a local anesthetic may be injected into the cervix to decrease pain and discomfort.

After a pelvic examination, the doctor will insert a speculum into the vagina to hold the walls open. After the cervix is cleaned with antiseptic, a tiny hollow plastic tube is inserted into the vagina, through the cervix, and into the uterus. A plunger attached to the tube will suction out a sample of the inner layer of tissue in the uterine wall. The tube is turned clockwise or counterclockwise while being moved in and out of the uterine cavity in order to obtain specimens. The cells are then sent to a laboratory for testing and microscopic examination.

USES AND COMPLICATIONS

Mild cramping may occur during and after the procedure. Cramping, pressure, and discomfort may also occur when the instruments are inserted and the samples collected. A small amount of bleeding, or spotting, may occur afterward, although normal activities can be resumed immediately.

After the procedure, there are slight risks of infection or heavy bleeding. Heavy bleeding, severe pain or cramping, or a fever over 100 degrees Fahrenheit (about 38 degrees Celsius) requires immediate medical attention. Extremely rarely, the uterus may be injured or punctured by the tool, or the cervix torn, during the procedure. The procedure should not be performed if the patient is pregnant or suffers from acute pelvic inflammatory disease or acute cervical or vaginal infections.

Abnormal cells may indicate endometrial cancer, LPD, the presence of fibroids (a benign, or noncancerous, excessive growth of the smooth muscle wall of the uterus), or polyps (a usually benign growth of normal tissue attached to the lining of the uterus). Surgery and/or medication may be necessary to treat these conditions.

Patients with persistent symptoms may need additional tests and procedures. Because an endometrial biopsy often misses polyps and fibroids, alternative procedures such as dilation and curettage (D & C) or hysteroscopy may be used for further diagnostic purposes. Both D & C and hysteroscopy require a hospital visit and general or spinal anesthesia.

PERSPECTIVE AND PROSPECTS

The use of endometrial sampling to diagnose and treat problems has been practiced since at least 1843. The earliest tools were wide and required scraping the uterine lining. Later devices, such as the stainless-steel Novak, or Kevorkian, curet or Vabra aspirator, cause significant discomfort. The Novak curet requires a syringe to apply suction. The Vabra aspirator is a disposable device that uses an electric suction pump to obtain the sample.

By 2006, the most used tool for endometrial biopsies was the Pipelle curet, developed in France. The curet is narrower, more flexible, and easier to insert through the cervix, and it removes the sample by suction. This device is relatively inexpensive, causes little to no discomfort to the patient, and has been shown to obtain adequate specimens in 87 to 100 percent of patients.

—*Virginia L. Salmon*

See also Biopsy; Cancer; Cervical, ovarian, and uterine cancers; Cervical procedures; Genital disorders, female; Gynecology; Infertility, female; Oncology; Reproductive system; Women's health.

FOR FURTHER INFORMATION:

Berek, Jonathan S., ed. *Berek and Novak's Gynecology.* 14th ed. Philadelphia: Lippincott Williams & Wilkins, 2007.

Cherath, Lata. "Endometrial Biopsy." In *The Gale Encyclopedia of Medicine*, edited by Jacqueline L. Longe. 3d ed. Farmington Hill, Mich.: Thomson Gale, 2006.

Cunningham, F. Gary, et al., eds. *Williams Obstetrics.* 22d ed. New York: McGraw-Hill, 2005.

"Endometrial Biopsy: Finding the Cause of Uterine Bleeding." *Mayo Clinic Health Letter* 19, no. 8 (August, 2001): 6.

Minkin, Mary Jane, and Carol V. Wright. *The Yale Guide to Women's Reproductive Health: From Menarche to Menopause.* New Haven, Conn.: Yale University Press, 2003.

ENDOMETRIOSIS

DISEASE/DISORDER

ANATOMY OR SYSTEM AFFECTED: Reproductive system, uterus

SPECIALTIES AND RELATED FIELDS: Gynecology

DEFINITION: Growth of cells of the uterine lining at sites outside the uterus, causing severe pain and infertility.

KEY TERMS:

cervix: an oval-shaped organ that separates the uterus and the vagina

dysmenorrhea: painful menstruation

dyspareunia: painful sexual intercourse

endometrium: the tissue that lines the uterus, builds up, and sheds at the end of each menstrual cycle; when it grows outside the uterus, endometriosis occurs

Fallopian tubes: two tubes extending from the ovaries to the uterus; during ovulation, an egg travels down one of these tubes to the uterus

hysterectomy: surgery that removes part or all of the uterus

implant: an abnormal endometrial growth outside the uterus

laparoscopy: a surgical procedure in which a small incision made near the navel is used to view the uterus and other abdominal organs with a lighted tube called a laparoscope

laparotomy: a surgical procedure, often exploratory in nature, carried out through the abdominal wall; it may be used to correct endometriosis

laser: a concentrated, high-energy light beam often used to destroy abnormal tissue

oophorectomy (or *ovariectomy*): removal of the ovaries, which is often necessary in cases of severe endometriosis *prostaglandins:* fatlike hormones that control the contraction and relaxation of the uterus and other smooth muscle tissue

CAUSES AND SYMPTOMS

Endometriosis, the presence of endometrial tissue outside its normal location as the lining of the uterus, is a disabling disease in women that causes severe pain and in many cases infertility. The classic symptoms of endometriosis are very painful menstruation (dysmenorrhea), painful intercourse (dyspareunia), and infertility. Some other common endometriosis symptoms include nausea, vomiting, diarrhea, and fatigue.

It has been estimated that endometriosis affects between five million and twenty-five million American women. Often, it is incorrectly stereotyped as being a disease of upwardly mobile, professional women. According to many experts, the incidence of endometriosis worldwide and across most racial groups is probably very similar. They propose that the reported occurrence rate difference for some racial groups, such as a lower incidence in African Americans, has been a socioeconomic phenomenon attributable to the social class of women who seek medical treatment for the symptoms of endometriosis and to the highly stratified responses of many health care professionals who have dealt with the disease.

The symptoms of endometriosis arise from abnormalities in the effects of the menstrual cycle on the endometrial tissue lining the uterus. The endometrium normally thickens and becomes swollen with blood (engorged) during the cycle, a process controlled by female hormones called estrogens and progestins. This engorgement is designed to prepare the uterus for conception by optimizing conditions for implantation in the endometrium of a fertilized egg, which enters the uterus via one of the Fallopian tubes leading from the ovaries.

By the middle of the menstrual cycle, the endometrial lining is normally about ten times thicker than at its beginning. If the egg that is released into the uterus is not fertilized, pregnancy does not occur and decreases in production of the female sex hormones result in the breakdown of the endometrium. Endometrial tissue mixed with blood leaves the uterus as the menstrual flow and a new menstrual cycle begins. This series of uterine changes occurs repeatedly, as a monthly cycle, from puberty (which usually occurs between the ages of twelve and fourteen) to the menopause (which usually occurs between the ages of forty-five and fifty-five).

In women who develop endometriosis, some endometrial tissue begins to grow ectopically (in an abnormal position) at sites outside the uterus. The ectopic endometrial growths may be found attached to the ovaries, the Fallopian tubes, the urinary bladder, the rectum, other abdominal organs, and even the lungs. Regardless of body location, these implants behave as if they were still in the uterus, thickening and bleeding each month as the menstrual cycle proceeds. Like the endometrium at its normal uterine site, the ectopic tissue responds to the hormones that circulate through the body in the blood. Its inappropriate position in the body prevents this ectopic endometrial tissue from leaving the body as menstrual flow; as a result, some implants grow to be quite large.

In many cases, the endometrial growths that form between two organs become fibrous bands called adhesions. The fibrous nature of adhesions is attributable to the alternating swelling and breakdown of the ectopic tissue, which yields fibrous scar tissue. The alterations in size of living portions of the adhesions and other endometrial implants during the monthly menstrual cycle cause many afflicted women considerable pain. Because the body location of implants varies, the site of the pain may be almost anywhere, such as the back, chest, thighs, pelvis, rectum, or abdomen. For example, dyspareunia occurs when adhesions hold a uterus tightly to the abdominal wall, making its movement during intercourse painful. Many women report significant pain on a monthly basis with ovulation as well.

The presence of endometriosis is usually confirmed by laparoscopy, viewed as being the most reliable method for its diagnosis. Laparoscopy is carried out after a physician makes an initial diagnosis of probable endometriosis from a combined study including an examination of the patient's medical history and careful exploration of the patient's physical problems over a period of at least six months. During prelaparoscopy treatment, the patient is very often maintained on pain

---

INFORMATION ON ENDOMETRIOSIS

CAUSES: Unknown
SYMPTOMS: Painful menstrual periods, discomfort during sexual intercourse, localized pain, infertility
DURATION: Chronic
TREATMENTS: Chemotherapy, surgery

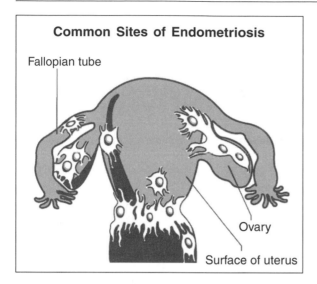

Common Sites of Endometriosis

Fallopian tube

Ovary

Surface of uterus

medication and other therapeutic drugs that will produce symptomatic relief.

For laparoscopy, the patient is anesthetized with a general anesthetic, a small incision is made near the navel, and a flexible lighted tube—a laparoscope—is inserted into this incision. The laparoscope, equipped with fiber optics, enables the examining physician to search the patient's abdominal organs for endometrial implants. Visibility of the abdominal organs in laparoscopic examination can be enhanced by pumping harmless carbon dioxide gas into the abdomen, causing it to distend. Women who undergo laparoscopy usually require a day of postoperative bed rest, followed by seven to ten days of curtailed physical activity. After a laparoscopic diagnosis of endometriosis is made, a variety of surgical and therapeutic drug treatments can be employed to manage the disease.

About 40 percent of all women who have endometriosis are infertile; contemporary wisdom evaluates this relationship as one of cause and effect, which should make this disease the second most common cause of fertility problems. The actual basis for this infertility is not always clear, but it is often the result of damage to the ovaries and Fallopian tubes, scar tissue produced by implants on these and other abdominal organs, and hormone imbalances.

Because the incidence of infertility accompanying endometriosis increases with the severity of the disease, all potentially afflicted women are encouraged to seek early diagnosis. Many experts advise all women with abnormal menstrual cycles, dysmenorrhea, severe menstrual bleeding, abnormal vaginal bleeding, and repeated dyspareunia to seek the advice of a physician

trained in identifying and dealing with endometriosis. Because the disease can begin to present symptoms at any age, teenagers are also encouraged to seek medical attention if they experience any of these symptoms.

John Sampson coined the term "endometriosis" in the 1920's. Sampson's theory for its causation, still widely accepted, is termed retrograde menstruation. Also called menstrual backup, this theory proposes that the backing up of some menstrual flow into the Fallopian tubes, and then into the abdominal cavity, forms the endometrial implants. Evidence supporting this theory, according to many physicians, is the fact that such backup is common. Others point out, however, that the backup is often found in women who do not have the disease. A surgical experiment was performed on female monkeys to test this theory. Their uteri were turned upside down so that the menstrual flow would spill into the abdominal cavity. Sixty percent of the animals developed endometriosis postoperatively—an inconclusive result.

Complicating the issue is the fact that implants are also found in tissues (such as in the lung) that cannot be reached by menstrual backup. It has been theorized that the presence of these implants results from the entry of endometrial cells into the lymphatic system, which returns body fluid to the blood and protects the body from many other diseases. This transplantation theory is supported by the occurrence of endometriosis in various portions of the lymphatic system and in tissues that could not otherwise become sites of endometriosis.

A third theory explaining the growth of implants is the iatrogenic, or nosocomial, transmission of endometrial tissue. These terms both indicate an accidental creation of the disease through the actions of physicians. Such implant formation is viewed as occurring most often after cesarean delivery of a baby when passage through the birth canal would otherwise be fatal to mother and/or child. Another proposed cause is episiotomy—widening of the birth canal by an incision between the anus and vagina—to ease births.

Any surgical procedure that allows the spread of endometrial tissue can be implicated, including surgical procedures carried out to correct existing endometriosis, because of the ease with which endometrial tissue implants itself anywhere in the body. Abnormal endometrial tissue growth, called adenomyosis, can also occur in the uterus and is viewed as a separate disease entity.

Other theories regarding the genesis of endometriosis include an immunologic theory, which proposes that women who develop endometriosis are lacking in antibodies that normally cause the destruction of endometrial tissue at sites where it does not belong, and a hormonal theory, which suggests the existence of large imbalances in hormones such as the prostaglandins that serve as the body's messengers in controlling biological processes. Several of these theories—retrograde menstruation, the transplantation theory, and iatrogenic transmission—all have support, but none has been proved unequivocally. Future evidence will identify whether one cause is dominant, whether they all interact to produce the disease, or whether endometriosis is actually a group of diseases that simply resemble one another in the eyes of contemporary medical science.

TREATMENT AND THERAPY

Laparoscopic examination most often identifies endometriosis as chocolate-colored lumps (chocolate cysts) ranging from the size of a pinhead to several inches across or as filmy coverings over parts of abdominal organs and ligaments. Once a diagnosis of the disease is confirmed by laparoscopy, endometriosis is treated by chemotherapy, surgery, or a combination of both methods. The only permanent contemporary cure for endometriosis, however, is the onset of the biological menopause at the end of a woman's childbearing years. As long as menstruation continues, implant development is likely to recur, regardless of its cause. Nevertheless, a temporary cure of endometriosis is better than no cure at all.

The chemotherapy that many physicians use to treat mild cases of endometriosis (and for prelaparoscopy periods) is analgesic painkillers, including aspirin, acetaminophen, and ibuprofen. The analgesics inhibit the body's production of prostaglandins, and the symptoms of the disease are merely covered up. Therefore, analgesics are of quite limited value except during a prelaparoscopy diagnostic period or with mild cases of endometriosis. In addition, the long-term administration of aspirin will often produce gastrointestinal bleeding, and excess use of acetaminophen can lead to severe liver damage. In some cases of very severe endometriosis pain, narcotic painkillers are given, such as codeine, Percodan (oxycodone and aspirin), or morphine. Narcotics are addicting and should be avoided unless absolutely necessary.

More effective for long-term management of the disease is hormone therapy. Such therapy is designed to prevent the monthly occurrence of menstruation—that is, to freeze the body in a sort of chemical menopause. The hormone types used, made by pharmaceutical companies, are chemical cousins of female hormones (estrogens and progestins), male hormones (androgens), and a brain hormone that controls ovulation

---

IN THE NEWS: LINK BETWEEN ENDOMETRIOSIS AND OTHER DISEASES

In the October, 2002, issue of *Human Reproduction*, the Endometriosis Association and the National Institutes of Health (NIH) announced the results of a study involving 3,680 women who were members of the Endometriosis Association and who had been diagnosed with endometriosis. The study suggested that women with endometriosis are significantly more likely than other women to contract a number of serious autoimmune diseases including lupus, Sjögren's syndrome, rheumatoid arthritis, and multiple sclerosis.

Although a study conducted in 1980 established a link between endometriosis and immune dysfunctions, the new study sought to identify specific diseases for which women with endometriosis are at higher risk. In addition to the connection between endometriosis and autoimmune diseases, researchers found that the women in the study were more than one hundred times more likely than women in the general population to suffer from chronic fatigue syndrome; twice as likely to suffer from fibromyalgia (recurrent pain in the muscles, tendons, and ligaments), and seven times as likely to suffer from hypothyroidism (which can also be an autoimmune disorder). Researchers also found that the women studied reported higher rates of allergies and asthma than women in the general population.

Researchers warn that the study may not be representative of all patients with endometriosis, both because members of the Endometriosis Association are most probably those patients suffering pain from their condition and because the survey was completed predominantly by white, educated women. Even so, this new information provides more light on an enigmatic disease and should help health care professionals treat patients.

—Cassandra Kircher, Ph.D.

(gonadotropin-releasing hormone, or GnRH). Appropriate hormone therapy is often useful for years, although each hormone class produces disadvantageous side effects in many patients.

The use of estrogens stops ovulation and menstruation, freeing many women with endometriosis from painful symptoms. Numerous estrogen preparations have been prescribed, including the birth control pills that contain them. Drawbacks of estrogen use can include weight gain, nausea, breast soreness, depression, blood-clotting abnormalities, and elevated risk of vaginal cancer. In addition, estrogen administration may cause endometrial implants to enlarge.

The use of progestins arose from the discovery that pregnancy—which is maintained by high levels of a natural progestin called progesterone—reversed the symptoms of many suffering from endometriosis. This realization led to the utilization of synthetic progestins to cause prolonged false pregnancy. The rationale is that all endometrial implants will die off and be reabsorbed during the prolonged absence of menstruation. The method works in most patients, and pain-free periods of up to five years are often observed. In some cases, however, side effects include nausea, depression, insomnia, and a very slow resumption of normal menstruation (such as lags of up to a year) when the therapy is stopped. In addition, progestins are ineffective in treating large implants; in fact, their use in such cases can lead to severe complications.

In the 1970's, studies showing the potential for heart attacks, high blood pressure, and strokes in patients receiving long-term female hormone therapy led to a search for more advantageous hormone medications. An alternative developed was the synthetic male hormone danazol (Danocrine), which is very effective. Danazol works by decreasing the amount of estrogen which is produced by the ovaries on a monthly basis to close to that which is present at menopause. The lack of estrogen prevents endometrial cells from growing, thereby eliminating most of the symptoms associated with endometriosis. One of its advantages over female hormones is the ability to shrink large implants and restore fertility to those patients whose problems arise from nonfunctional ovaries or Fallopian tubes. Danazol has become the drug of choice for treating millions of endometriosis sufferers. Problems associated with danazol use, however, can include weight gain, masculinization (decreased bust size, increased muscle mass, muscle cramping, facial hair growth, and deepened voice), fatigue, depression, and baldness. Those

women contemplating danazol use should be aware that it can also complicate pregnancy.

Because of the side effects of these hormones, other chemotherapy was sought. Another valuable drug that has become available is GnRH, which suppresses the function of the ovaries in a fashion equivalent to surgical oophorectomy (removal of the ovaries). This hormone produces none of the side effects of the sex hormones, such as weight gain, depression, or masculinization, but some evidence indicates that it may lead to osteoporosis.

Thus, despite the fact that hormone therapy may relieve or reduce pain for years, contemporary chemotherapy is flawed by many undesirable side effects. Perhaps more serious, however, is the high recurrence rate of endometriosis that is observed after the therapy is stopped. Consequently, it appears that the best treatment of endometriosis combines chemotherapy with surgery.

The extent of the surgery carried out to combat endometriosis is variable and depends on the observations made during laparoscopy. In cases of relatively mild endometriosis, conservative laparotomy surgery removes endometriosis implants, adhesions, and lesions. This type of procedure attempts to relieve endometriosis pain, to minimize the chances of postoperative recurrence of the disease, and to allow the patient to have children. Even in the most severe cases of this type, the uterus, an ovary, and its associated Fallopian tube are retained. Such surgery will often include removal of the appendix, whether diseased or not, because it is very likely to develop implants. The surgical techniques performed are the conventional excision of diseased tissue or the use of lasers to vaporize it. Many physicians prefer lasers because it is believed that they decrease the chances of recurrent endometriosis resulting from retained implant tissue or iatrogenic causes. In a new procedure, following the removal of endometrial tissue by surgical means, an intrauterine device containing Levonogestrel (a hormone which will decrease estrogen levels) is placed in order to prevent recurrence of endometriosis.

In more serious cases, hysterectomy is carried out. All visible implants, adhesions, and lesions are removed from the abdominal organs, as in conservative surgery. In addition, the uterus and cervix are taken out, but one or both ovaries are retained. This allows female hormone production to continue normally until the menopause. Uterine removal makes it impossible to have children, however, and may lead to profound psychological problems that require psychiatric help. Women planning to elect for hysterectomy to treat endometriosis should be aware of such potential difficulties. In many cases of conservative surgery or hysterectomy, danazol is used, both preoperatively and postoperatively, to minimize implant size.

The most extensive surgery carried out on the women afflicted with endometriosis is radical hysterectomy, also called definitive surgery, in which the ovaries and/or the vagina are also removed. The resultant symptoms are menopausal and may include vaginal bleeding atrophy (when the vagina is retained), increased risk of heart disease, and the development of osteoporosis. To counter the occurrence of these symptoms, replacement therapy with female hormones is suggested. Paradoxically, this hormone therapy can lead to the return of endometriosis by stimulating the growth of residual implant tissue.

Recently, more women have turned to complementary and alternative medicine in an attempt to relieve the symptoms of endometriosis. Acupuncture, homeopathy, and herbal therapy are currently being explored as means of treatment for endometriosis.

PERSPECTIVE AND PROSPECTS

Modern treatment of endometriosis is viewed by many physicians as beginning in the 1950's. A landmark development in this field was the accurate diagnosis of endometriosis via the laparoscope, which was invented in Europe and introduced into the United States in the 1960's. Medical science has progressed greatly since that time. Physicians and researchers have recognized the wide occurrence of the disease and accepted its symptoms as valid; realized that hysterectomy will not necessarily put an end to the disease; utilized chemotherapeutic tools, including hormones and painkillers, as treatments and as adjuncts to surgery; developed laser surgery and other techniques that decrease the occurrence of formerly ignored iatrogenic endometriosis; and understood that the disease can ravage teenagers as well and that these young women should be examined as early as possible.

Research into endometriosis is ongoing, and the efforts and information base of the proactive American Endometriosis Association, founded in 1980, have been very valuable. As a result, a potentially or presently afflicted woman is much more aware of the problems associated with the disease. In addition, she has a source for obtaining objective information on topics including state-of-the-art treatment, physician and hospi-

tal choice, and both physical and psychological outcomes of treatment.

Many potentially viable avenues for better endometriosis diagnosis and treatment have become the objects of intense investigation. These include the use of ultrasonography and radiology techniques for the predictive, nonsurgical examination of the course of growth or the chemotherapeutic destruction of implants; the design of new drugs to be utilized in the battle against endometriosis; endeavors aimed at the development of diagnostic tests for the disease that will stop it before symptoms develop; and the design of dietary treatments to soften its effects.

Regrettably, because of the insidious nature of endometriosis—which has the ability to strike almost anywhere in the body—some confusion about the disease still exists. New drugs, surgical techniques, and other aids are expected to be helpful in clarifying many of these issues. Particular value is being placed on the study of the immunologic aspects of endometriosis. Scientists hope to explain why the disease strikes some women and not others, to uncover its etiologic basis, and to solve the widespread problems of iatrogenic implant formation and other types of endometriosis recurrence.

—Sanford S. Singer, Ph.D.;
updated by Robin Kamienny Montvilo, Ph.D.
See also Amenorrhea; Cervical, ovarian, and uterine cancers; Childbirth complications; Dysmenorrhea; Endometrial biopsy; Genital disorders, female; Gynecology; Hysterectomy; Infertility, female; Menorrhagia; Menstruation; Pregnancy and gestation; Reproductive system; Women's health.

FOR FURTHER INFORMATION:

Berek, Jonathan S., ed. *Berek and Novak's Gynecology.* 14th ed. Philadelphia: Lippincott Williams & Wilkins, 2007. A standard text covering all aspects of gynecology with an emphasis on diagnosis and treatment. Topics include biology and physiology, family planning, sexuality, evaluation of pelvic infections, early pregnancy loss, benign breast disease, benign gynecologic conditions, malignant diseases of the reproductive tract, and breast cancer.

Endometriosis.org. http://www.endometriosis.org/. A Web site that offers FAQs about the disease, research articles, case histories, information about local support groups, diagnosis and treatment information, and a glossary.

Fernandez, I., C. Reid, and S. Dziurawiec. "Living with

Endometriosis: The Perspective of Male Partners." *Journal of Psychosomatic Research* 61, no. 4 (October, 2006): 433-438. This study explores the experience of the male partners of women with endometriosis.

Henderson, Lorraine, and Ros Wood. *Explaining Endometriosis*. 2d ed. St. Leonards, Australia: Allen and Unwin, 2001. Details possible causes, diagnosis, surgeries, and current treatment options for endometriosis.

Phillips, Robert H., and Glenda Motta. *Coping with Endometriosis: A Practical Guide to Understanding, Treating, and Living with Endometriosis*. New York: Putnam, 2000. Educates the reader on current research and addresses the psychological and emotional concerns brought on by a diagnosis.

Shaw, Michael, ed. *Everything You Need to Know About Diseases*. Springhouse, Pa.: Springhouse Press, 1996. This well-illustrated consumer reference, compiled by more than one hundred doctors and medical experts, describes five hundred illnesses and conditions, including their causes, symptoms, diagnosis, treatment, and prevention. Of particular interest is chapter 9, "Gynecologic Disorders."

Sherwood, Lauralee. *Human Physiology: From Cells to Systems*. 6th ed. Belmont, Calif.: Thomson/Brooks/Cole, 2007. This college text contains much useful biological information. Included are details about the menstrual cycle, hormones, the endometrium, and many helpful definitions. Clearly written, the book is a mine of information for interested readers.

2007 Physician's Desk Reference. Montvale, N.J.: Thomson PDR, 2006. This list of prescription drugs includes the drugs used against endometriosis, the companies that produce them, their useful dose ranges, their effects on metabolism and toxicology, and their contraindications.

Weinstein, Kate. *Living with Endometriosis*. Reading, Mass.: Addison-Wesley, 1991. The main divisions of this handy book are medical aspects, treatments and outcomes, emotional problems, and pain and psychiatric problems. Highlights include the complete description of the female reproductive system and menstruation, the glossary, and appendices on organizations, literature, and pain management centers.

Weschler, Toni. *Taking Charge of Your Fertility*. Rev. ed. New York: HarperCollins, 2001. Explores common health issues of women and their role in preventing pregnancy.

ENDOSCOPY

PROCEDURE

ANATOMY OR SYSTEM AFFECTED: Abdomen, anus, bladder, gastrointestinal system, intestines, joints, knees, lungs, stomach, urinary system

SPECIALTIES AND RELATED FIELDS: Gastroenterology, gynecology, obstetrics, orthopedics, proctology, pulmonary medicine, urology

DEFINITION: The use of a flexible tube to look into body structures in order to inspect and sometimes correct pathologies.

KEY TERMS:

biopsy: the collection and study of body tissue, often to determine whether it is cancerous

fiber optics: the transmission of light through thin, flexible tubes

pathology: a disease condition; also the study of diseases

INDICATIONS AND PROCEDURES

Early endoscopes were simply rigid hollow tubes with a light source. They were inserted into body orifices, such as the anus or the mouth, to allow the physician to look directly at structures and processes within. Modern instruments are more sophisticated. They use fiber optics in flexible cables to penetrate deep into body structures. For example, one form of colonoscope can be threaded though the entire lower intestine, allowing the physician to search for pathologies all the way from the anus to the cecum of the colon (large intestine).

There are eight basic types of endoscope: gastroscope, colonoscope, bronchoscope, cystoscope, laparoscope, colposcope, arthroscope, and amnioscope. Their primary uses are diagnostic; however, they can be fitted with special instruments to perform many different tasks, including taking bits of tissue for biopsy and carrying out surgical procedures.

USES AND COMPLICATIONS

The gastroscope and its variants are used to inspect structures of the gastrointestinal system. The name of one class of procedure gives an idea of how sophisticated the gastroscope has become: esophagogastroduodenoscopy. As the term implies, this technique can be used to investigate the esophagus (the tube leading to the stomach), the stomach itself, and the intestines all the way into the duodenum (the first link of the small intestine). Further, in a procedure called endoscopic retrograde cholangiopancreatography, the endoscope can be used to investigate processes in the gallbladder, the cystic duct, the common hepatic duct, and the common bile duct. By far the most common use of the gastroscope is in the diagnosis and management of esophageal and stomach problems. The gastroscope is used to confirm the suspicion of stomach ulcers and other gastroesophageal conditions and to monitor therapy.

The colonoscope and its variants are critical in the diagnosis of diseases in the lower intestine and in some aspects of therapy. The long, flexible fiber-optic tube can be threaded through the anus and rectum into the S-shaped sigmoid colon (flexible fiber-optic sigmoidoscopy). The tube can be made to rise up the descending colon, across the transverse colon, and down the as-

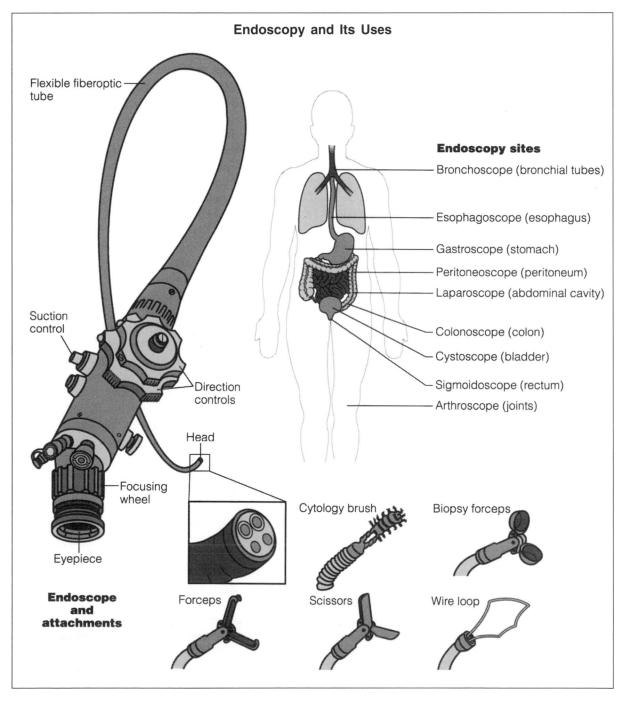

Endoscopy and Its Uses

Flexible fiberoptic tube

Endoscopy sites

Bronchoscope (bronchial tubes)

Esophagoscope (esophagus)

Gastroscope (stomach)
Peritoneoscope (peritoneum)
Laparoscope (abdominal cavity)

Colonoscope (colon)

Cystoscope (bladder)

Sigmoidoscope (rectum)

Arthroscope (joints)

Suction control

Direction controls

Head

Focusing wheel

Eyepiece

Endoscope and attachments

Forceps

Cytology brush

Biopsy forceps

Scissors

Wire loop

cending colon to the cecum. With the colonoscope, the physician can discover abnormalities such as polyps, diverticula, and blockages and the presence of cancer, Crohn's disease, ulcerative colitis, and many other diseases. The physician can also use the colonoscope to remove polyps; this is the major therapeutic use of colonoscopy.

Like most other forms of endoscopy, bronchoscopy is used for both diagnosis and treatment. The bronchoscope allows direct visualization of the trachea (the tube leading from the throat to the lungs) and the bronchi (the two main air ducts leading into the lungs). It will show certain forms of lung cancer, various infectious states, and other pathologies. The bronchoscope can also be used to remove foreign objects, excise local tumors, remove mucus plugs, and improve bronchial drainage.

The cystoscope is used for visual inspection of the urethra and bladder. The bladder stores urine; the urethra is the tube through which it is eliminated. Cystoscopy discovers many of the conditions that can afflict these organs: obstruction, infection, cancer, and other disorders.

The laparoscope is used to look into the abdominal cavity for evidence of a wide variety of conditions. It can inspect the liver, help evaluate liver disease, and take tissue samples for biopsy. Laparoscopy can confirm the diagnosis of ectopic pregnancy (a condition in which a fetus develops outside the womb, usually in one of the Fallopian tubes). It can confirm the presence or absence of abdominal cancers and diagnose disease conditions in the gallbladder, spleen, peritoneum (the membrane that surrounds the abdomen), and the diaphragm, as well as give some views of the small and large intestine. In an important, relatively new development, the laparoscope is being used to remove gallbladders (cholecystectomy). This procedure is far less traumatic than the old surgery, often permitting release of the patient a day or two after the operation rather than requiring weeks of recuperation.

The colposcope is used to inspect vaginal tissue and adjacent organs. Common reasons for colposcopy include abnormal bleeding and suspicion of tumors.

Arthroscopy, the investigation of joint structures by endoscopy, is now the most common invasive technique used on patients with arthritis or joint damage. In addition to viewing the area, the arthroscope can be fitted with various instruments to perform surgical procedures.

The term "amnioscope" comes from the amnion, the membrane that surrounds a fetus. This type of endoscope is used to enter the uterus and inspect the growing fetus in the search for any visible abnormalities.

Endoscopy is one of the most useful and most-used techniques for diagnosis because it permits the investigation of many internal body organs without surgery. It is extraordinarily safe in the hands of experienced practitioners and is relatively free of pain and discomfort. In addition, specialized endoscopes are assuming greater roles in therapy. Many procedures that once involved major surgery can now be conducted through the endoscope, saving the patient pain, trauma, and expense.

PERSPECTIVE AND PROSPECTS

Endoscopes have become highly sophisticated instruments with enormous range throughout the body and enormous potential. Colonoscopy, for example, promises to revolutionize the treatment of cancerous and precancerous polyps by helping physicians attain a clearer understanding of the polyp-to-cancer progression. The laparoscope has revolutionized gallbladder removal, as the arthroscope has revolutionized joint surgery. The gastroscope gives the physician new security and control in the management of gastrointestinal conditions, and the bronchoscope facilitates many lung procedures.

Similarly throughout the entire range of endoscopy, new opportunities are opening and leading to significant improvements in therapy, and these improvements will continue. Electronic and video techniques are being introduced into endoscopy, and this new technology promises to widen the applications and therapeutic range of endoscopy still further.

—*C. Richard Falcon*

See also Abdominal disorders; Arthritis; Arthroscopy; Biopsy; Cholecystectomy; Colon and rectal polyp removal; Colon cancer; Colonoscopy and sigmoidoscopy; Cystoscopy; Gallbladder diseases; Gastrointestinal disorders; Invasive tests; Laparoscopy; Pulmonary diseases; Stone removal; Stones.

FOR FURTHER INFORMATION:

Classen, Meinhard, G. N. J. Tytgat, and C. J. Lightdale, eds. *Gastroenterological Endoscopy*. New York: Thieme Medical, 2002. Text that examines such topics as the impact of endoscopy, its history of use, diagnostic procedures and techniques, therapeutic procedures, descriptions of diseases involving the upper and lower intestine, endoscopic features of infectious diseases of the GI tract, and pediatric endoscopy.

Emory, Theresa S., et al. *Atlas of Gastrointestinal Endoscopy and Endoscopic Biopsies*. Washington,

D.C.: Armed Forces Institute of Pathology, 2000. This resource is divided into four major sections that correspond to the major endoscopic divisions of the gastrointestinal tract. Each section begins with an overview of the endoscopic examination and the histology.

Litin, Scott C., ed. *Mayo Clinic Family Health Book*. 3d ed. New York: HarperResource, 2003. Perhaps the best general medical text for the layperson, this book covers the entire medical field. While the information is derived from a wide variety of highly technical sources, the articles are written to be easily understood by a general audience.

Scott-Conner, Carol E. H., ed. *The SAGES Manual: Fundamentals of Laparoscopy, Thoracoscopy, and GI Endoscopy*. 2d ed. New York: Springer, 2006. Explains the major laparoscopic and flexible endoscopic procedures.

ENEMAS

PROCEDURE

ANATOMY OR SYSTEM AFFECTED: Abdomen, anus, gastrointestinal system, intestines

SPECIALTIES AND RELATED FIELDS: Gastroenterology

DEFINITION: A procedure to assist the body in evacuating fecal material from the bowel.

INDICATIONS AND PROCEDURES

Enemas are used primarily for two purposes: cleansing and retention. Many solutions have been used to promote cleansing. The most commonly used is made up of mild soapsuds and tap water. Commercially prepared solutions containing premeasured mild soap and water are also available.

To receive an enema, the patient should lie on the left side of the body with the upper thigh drawn up to the abdomen. The solution should be slightly above body temperature. The source of the enema fluid should be 30 to 45 centimeters (12 to 18 inches) above the anus. All air should be removed from the tubing that connects the enema reservoir and the tip. The tip is warmed in the hands, lubricated with a commercial preparation or a bit of soapy water, and gently inserted into the anus with a combination of soft pressure and a twisting motion. The tip should not be inserted more than 10 centimeters (4 inches) into the rectum. The solution is allowed to flow slowly into the rectum to prevent cramping.

A towel may be held gently against the rectum to pre-

vent leakage. If cramping does occur, the flow should be interrupted by pinching the tubing. For an adult, approximately 1 liter (1 quart) of solution is probably sufficient; the patient should hold the solution for two to three minutes. The enema tube is tightly clamped and slowly withdrawn; a towel is again held against the anus to catch any leakage. A readily available bedpan or toilet stool is used while the patient evacuates the bowel. Depending on the need for the enema, the procedure may be repeated.

The procedure for administering a retention enema is similar except that the solution is instilled very slowly to promote retention. Lubricants or medicines are administered in this fashion. The patient holds the instilled solution as long as possible before evacuating the bowel.

USES AND COMPLICATIONS

Cleansing enemas are used to promote bowel evacuation by softening fecal material and stimulating the movement by bowel walls (peristalsis). Retention enemas are used to lubricate or soothe the mucosal lining of the rectum, to apply medication to the bowel wall or for absorption by the colon, and to soften feces.

There is no physiological need to have a bowel movement every day; normality is defined as from three to ten per week. Enemas should not be used routinely for cleansing because the bowel quickly becomes dependent on them. This problem is especially common among older individuals.

—L. Fleming Fallon, Jr., M.D., Ph.D., M.P.H.

See also Colon and rectal polyp removal; Colon and rectal surgery; Colon cancer; Colonoscopy and sigmoidoscopy; Gastroenterology; Gastrointestinal system; Hemorrhoid banding and removal; Hemorrhoids; Internal medicine; Intestines; Peristalsis; Proctology; Surgery, general.

FOR FURTHER INFORMATION:

Heuman, Douglas M., A. Scott Mills, and Hunter H. McGuire, Jr. *Gastroenterology*. Philadelphia: W. B. Saunders, 1997.

Icon Health. *Enemas: A Medical Dictionary, Bibliography, and Annotated Research Guide to Internet References*. San Diego, Calif.: Author, 2003.

Mitsuoka, Tomotari. *Intestinal Bacteria and Health*. Translated by Syoko Watanabe and W. C. T. Leung. Tokyo: Harcourt Brace Jovanovich, 1978.

Peikin, Steven R. *Gastrointestinal Health*. Rev. ed. New York: HarperCollins, 1999.

ENTEROCOLITIS
DISEASE/DISORDER

ALSO KNOWN AS: Acute infectious diarrhea

ANATOMY OR SYSTEM AFFECTED: Gastrointestinal system, intestines

SPECIALTIES AND RELATED FIELDS: Family medicine, gastroenterology, pediatrics

DEFINITION: Inflammation of the small and large intestines, which may be caused by a severe bacterial infection.

CAUSES AND SYMPTOMS

Enterocolitis is characterized by copious and sometimes bloody diarrhea, abdominal pain, vomiting, and dehydration. A high fever usually exists in young children. Cultures of the stool and blood can establish the exact organism involved.

Campylobacter enterocolitis, resulting from infection with *Campylobacter* bacteria, is the most common bacterial cause of diarrhea. It is endemic in developing countries, and epidemics are seen in Western countries in daycare centers. Salmonella enterocolitis is an infection in the lining of the small intestine caused by *Salmonella* bacteria acquired through the ingestion of contaminated food or water or exposure to reptiles. This type of enterocolitis can range from mild to severe and lasts from one to two weeks.

A different type of enterocolitis is necrotizing enterocolitis (NEC), the most common gastrointestinal medical emergency occurring in newborns. It is more prevalent in premature infants. NEC may begin with poor feeding, abdominal distention or tenderness, and decreased bowel sounds. If it becomes systemic, then symptoms can include apnea, lethargy, shock, and cardiovascular collapse. Outbreaks of NEC seem to follow an epidemic pattern, suggesting an infectious disease, but a specific causative organism has not been identified. Research suggests that several factors may be involved.

TREATMENT AND THERAPY

The treatment of bacterial enterocolitis involves intravenous fluids and antibiotics. In underdeveloped countries, where medical care is poor, enterocolitis is responsible for more than 60 percent of all deaths in children under age five.

Infants with NEC cannot take food by mouth and often must be fed through a central venous catheter. Those with severe disease may require surgical intervention such as intestinal resection. The mortality rate for NEC approaches 50 percent in infants weighing less than 1,500 grams.

—Connie Rizzo, M.D., Ph.D.;
updated by Tracy Irons-Georges

See also Antibiotics; Bacterial infections; Dehydration; Diarrhea and dysentery; Fever; Gastroenterology, pediatric; Gastrointestinal system; Intestinal disorders; Intestines; Nausea and vomiting; Salmonella infection.

FOR FURTHER INFORMATION:

Gilchrist, Brian F., ed. *Necrotizing Enterocolitis*. Georgetown, Tex.: Eurekah.com/Landes Bioscience, 2000.

Janowitz, Henry D. *Your Gut Feelings: A Complete Guide to Living Better with Intestinal Problems*. Rev. and updated ed. New York: Oxford University Press, 1994.

Stoll, Barbara J., and Robert M. Kliegman, eds. *Necrotizing Enterocolitis*. Philadelphia: W. B. Saunders, 1994.

Thompson, W. Grant. *Gut Reactions: Understanding Symptoms of the Digestive Tract*. New York: Plenum Press, 1989.

ENURESIS. *See* **BED-WETTING.**

ENVIRONMENTAL DISEASES
DISEASE/DISORDER

ANATOMY OR SYSTEM AFFECTED: All

SPECIALTIES AND RELATED FIELDS: All

DEFINITION: Sicknesses caused or exacerbated by human exposure to physical, chemical, biological, or social environmental conditions, the duration and in-

---

INFORMATION ON ENTEROCOLITIS

CAUSES: Bacterial infection; unknown for necrotizing enterocolitis

SYMPTOMS: For bacterial infection, copious and sometimes bloody diarrhea, abdominal pain, vomiting, dehydration, high fever in young children; for necrotizing enterocolitis, poor feeding, abdominal distention or tenderness, decreased bowel sounds, apnea, lethargy, shock, cardiovascular collapse

DURATION: Acute

TREATMENTS: For bacterial infection, intravenous fluids and antibiotics; for necrotizing enterocolitis, surgery (intestinal resection)

tensity of the exposure typically affecting the manifestation of symptoms and fatality-case ratios. Acute environmental diseases may result in rapid decline of health status and warrant emergency response, while chronic conditions often result from long-term exposures to low levels of environmental risk factors.

KEY TERMS:

acute: referring to exposure to hazardous environmental agents or conditions that occur once or over a short period of time (typically fourteen days or less); environmental disease symptoms that appear rapidly

chronic: referring to exposure to environmental risk factor or agent occurring over a long period of time, typically more than one year; symptoms of environmental diseases that take a long time to appear after first contact with the causative agent

dose-response: the relationship between the dose (a quantitative measurement of exposure usually expressed in terms of concentration and duration) and the quantitative expression of change to the status of human health and well-being resulting in disease

environmental epidemiology: the systematic study of the distribution and determinants of environmental diseases in a population

environmental infection: human exposure to infectious agents of diseases (including bacteria, fungi, parasites, and viruses) through contact with environmental media such as contaminated water, air, food, and soil

environmental radiation: human exposure to electromagnetic radiation at doses and durations that can produce adverse impacts on human health

environmental toxicity: human exposure to chemical or biochemical substances at doses that produce harmful modification to the body's physiological mechanisms, leading to diseases

exposure assessment: a systematic process of discovering the pathway through which humans are exposed to specific environmental agents and risk factors, and of ascertaining the quantity and duration of that exposure

CAUSES AND SYMPTOMS

The modern word "miasma" comes from the Greek *miasma* or *miainein*, meaning "pollution" or "to pollute." Before scientific theories of disease became entrenched in medical practice, miasma was used to connote bad environments to which human exposure led to various diseases. Even today, one of the most devastating human diseases, malaria, draws its name from references to "bad air." There is clearly a rich historical record of human recognition of the intimate connection between environmental quality and diseases. It is now known that serious human diseases are caused by numerous chemical, physical, and biological agents (risk factors) that occur naturally or as a result of human actions that modify the environment. In fact, the more that is learned about disease etiology, the more the complex interplay between environmental conditions and root causes of diseases within the body are recognized. Furthermore, some people are more sensitive to environmental risk factors because of their age, gender, occupation, culture, or genetic characteristics.

Environmental diseases are those illnesses for which cause and effect can be reasonably associated through epidemiological studies, preferably verified through laboratory experiments. Therefore, the recognition of environmental diseases draws upon two traditional postulates regarding causation in the study of human diseases, one ascribed to Robert Koch (1843-1910) and the other ascribed to Austin Bradford Hill (1897-1991). The more important set of guidelines for environmental diseases is generally known in epidemiology as Hill's criteria of causation, based on his landmark 1965 publication entitled "The Environment and Disease: Association or Causation?" Hill warned in the article that cause-effect decisions should not be based on a set of rules. Instead, he supported the view that cost-benefit analysis is essential for policy decisions on controlling environmental quality in order to avoid diseases. It is arguable that Hill's treatise initiated current trends characterized by the precautionary principle in environmental health science. Nevertheless, Hill's nine viewpoints for exploring the relationship between environment and disease are worth emphasizing. They are precedence, correlation, dose-response, consistency, plausibility, alternatives, empiricism, specificity, and coherence.

According to the precedence viewpoint, exposure must always precede the outcome in every case of the environmental disease. One of the most famous examples here is the classic epidemiological study of John Snow (1813-1858) on the spread of cholera and its association with exposure to contaminated water in the densely populated city of London.

According to the correlation viewpoint, a strong association or correlation should exist between the exposure and the incidence of the environmental disease. The clustering of diseases within neighborhoods or among workers at a specific occupation is frequently the beginning of investigations into environmental diseases. Clusters can provide strong evidence of correlations. Bernardino Ramazinni (1633-1714), considered by many to be one of the founders of the discipline of occupational and environmental health sciences, published his treatise *De Morbis Artificum* in 1700 following critical observations regarding the correlation between environmental exposures of and diseases in workers.

According to the dose-response viewpoint, the relationship between exposure and the severity of environmental disease should be characterized by a dose-response relationship, in which an increase in the intensity and/or duration of exposure produces a more severe disease outcome. "The dose makes the poison" is one of the central tenets of environmental toxicology. This phrase is attributed to Paracelsus (1493-1541). This tenet has proven difficult to interpret for formulating health policy in the case of environmental diseases because the variation in human genetics and physiology means that, in many situations, a single threshold of toxicity cannot be established as safe for every person. Exposure to ionizing radiation is an example of a situation in which it is difficult to establish dose-response relationships that are useful for setting uniformly applicable preventive health policy.

According to the consistency viewpoint, there should be consistent findings in different populations, across different studies, and at different times regarding the association between exposure and environmental disease. This means that the relationship should be reproducible. For example, exposure of people to mercury across civilizations, occupations, and age groups has been consistently associated with certain health effects that helped recognize the special hazards posed by this toxic metal. Mercury was used in various manufacturing processes for several centuries, and where precautions are not taken to prevent human exposure, disease invariably results.

Consistency should cut across not only generations but also occupations and different doses of exposure. For example, "mad hatter's" disease was associated with the use of mercury in the production of fur felt, in which mercurous nitrate was used to add texture to smooth fibers such as rabbit fur to facilitate matting (the process is called carroting because of the resulting orange color). More recently, the exposure of pregnant women to fish contaminated with methyl mercury from industrial sources in Japan produced developmental

diseases in fetuses. The societal repercussions of the so-called Minamata disease are still not completely settled after more than forty years. Mercury is now widely recognized as a cumulative toxicant with systemic effects and organ damage, with symptoms including trembling, dental problems, ataxia, depression, and anxiety.

According to the plausibility viewpoint, compelling evidence of "biological plausibility" should exist that a physiological pathway leads from exposure to a specific environmental risk factor to the development of a specific environmental disease. This does not exclude the possibility of multiple causes, some acquired through environmental exposures and others through genetic processes. For example, lead poisoning has been recognized since the 1950's as a pervasive and devastating environmental disease. The symptoms of lead poisoning vary, from specific organ effects such as kidney disease to systemic effects such as anemia and to cognitive effects such as intelligence quotient (IQ) deficiency. How a single environmental toxicant can produce such wide-ranging diseases was a puzzle until the molecular mechanisms underpinning lead poisoning and the pharmacokinetic distribution of lead in the human body was understood. Lead is temporarily stored in the blood, where it binds to a key enzyme, aminolevulinate dehydratase, which participates in the synthesis of heme. The by-products of that reaction produce anemia and organ effects, including kidney and brain diseases. Long-term storage of lead in the body occurs in bony tissue, where other effects are possible. These biological understandings have helped activists and scientists agitate for environmental policy to reduce lead exposure worldwide.

According to the alternatives viewpoint, alternative explanations for the development of diseases should be considered alongside the plausible environmental causes. These alternative explanations should be ruled out before conclusions are reached about causal relationship between environmental exposures and disease. For example, the typically low doses to which populations are exposed to pesticides, and the long time period between exposure and the typical chronic disease outcomes such as cancers and neurodegenerative disorders, makes it difficult to reconstruct the disease pathways and pinpoint causative agents. This is where it is important to consider all alternatives and to eliminate them before compelling arguments can be made about the effects of pesticide toxicity. Sometimes observing wildlife response to environmental risk factors help narrow down alternative explanations, as Rachel Carson taught in her timeless book *Silent Spring* (1965).

According to the empiricism viewpoint, the course of environmental disease should be alterable by appropriate intervention strategies verifiable through experimentation. In other words, the disease can be preventable or curable following manipulation of the environment and/or human physiology. For acute exposures, the emergency response is to eliminate the source of exposure. However, this is not always possible in cases where patients are unconscious or otherwise unable to articulate clearly the source of exposure, as is the case for many children. Nevertheless, standardized procedures exist for responding to environmental exposure beyond eliminating the source. For example, therapy based on chelation (from the Greek *chele*, meaning "claw") works for toxic metal exposure because the mode of action of the therapeutic agent, ethylene diamine tetra-acetic acid (EDTA), is well understood. It is possible to establish empirically the relative effectiveness of EDTA in dealing with various forms of toxic metal exposures. For example, under normal physiological conditions, EDTA binds metals in the following order: iron (ferric ion), mercury, copper, aluminum, nickel, lead, cobalt, zinc, iron (ferrous ion), cadmium, manganese, magnesium, and calcium. Based on this information, it is possible to design therapeutic processes that minimize adverse side effects.

According to the specificity viewpoint, when an environmental disease is associated with only one environmental agent, the relationship between exposure and environmental disease is said to be specific. This strengthens the argument for causality, but this situation is extremely rare. For example, the rarity of mesothelioma, a lung disease that afflicts people who have

---

IN THE NEWS: IRAQ WAR INCREASES DISEASE RISKS

Throughout the history of warfare, diseases have often caused more casualties among both soldiers and civilians than weaponry itself. The conflict in Iraq is no exception. A rare type of lung infection, acute eosinophilic pneumonia (AEP), is occurring at a higher rate among U.S. soldiers in Iraq than in any other segment of the population. The illness, characterized by fever, serious lung impairment, and eventually respiratory failure, has killed several soldiers since 2003. Of the individuals who contracted this pneumonia, all reported exposure to fine sand and dust particles, a common hazard in the desert environments of the Middle East. Administration of corticosteroids proved life-saving for most patients, but many who have recovered complain of residual lung problems.

Veterans of Operation Iraqi Freedom are not alone in fighting disabling illnesses. Brain cancer, amyotrophic lateral sclerosis (ALS), fibromyalgia, and multiple sclerosis are among the serious ailments plaguing the earlier Gulf War veterans from 1991. The demolition of weapons dumps in Iraq in March, 1991, released the deadly nerve agents sarin and cyclosarin. Many Gulf War veterans claim that this incident is to blame for the diseases from which they now suffer. A Department of Defense-sponsored study conducted by the Institute of Medicine of the National Academy of Sciences, published in *American Journal of Public Health* in August, 2005, focused on the nerve gas release event at Al Khamisiyah and subsequent increase in neurological illnesses in those exposed to the chemical contamination which followed.

Inflamed joints, heat and chemical sensitivities, severe headaches, hair loss, and recurrent skin rashes are just a few of the symptoms endured by affected troops who have returned from both Iraq conflicts. Nearly 200,000 Gulf War veterans are currently receiving disability payments from the Veterans Administration, and many of those payments are for battle-related illness rather than for injury.

—*Lenela Glass-Godwin, M.WS.*

---

been exposed to asbestos fibers, made it possible to use epidemiological evidence quickly to support policy in restricting the use of asbestos in commercial products and to protect employees from occupational exposures.

The recognition of new diseases often leads to speculation about causative agents or conditions. Occasionally, new ideas about causation challenge orthodox theories. According to the coherence viewpoint, it is important to conduct a rigorous assessment of coherence with existing information and scientific ideas before such causes are accepted in the case of environmental diseases. For example, the origin of neurodegenerative diseases currently associated with exposure to prion protein remains mysterious, and some environmental causes have been proposed, including exposure to toxic metal ions. Another example is the current concern with the introduction of nanoparticles into commercial products, with concomitant environmental dissemination. Although much has been learned from an understanding of the human health effects of respirable particulate matter, researchers should be sufficiently open-minded to the possibility that nanoparticles will behave differently in the environment and in the human body.

Hill's nine viewpoints were presented in the context of pitfalls associated with overreliance on statistical tests of "significance" as a justification to base health policy on epidemiological observations. Hill's viewpoints have been debated extensively, and it is worth noting the following caveats presented in the 2004 article "The Missed Lessons of Sir Austin Bradford Hill," by Carl V. Phillips and Karen J. Goodman: Statistical significance should not be mistaken for evidence of substantial association, association does not prove causation, precision should not be mistaken for validity, evidence that a causal relationship exists is not sufficient to suggest that action should be taken, and uncertainty about causation or association is not sufficient to suggest that action should not be taken.

The second set of guidelines regarding causality derives from what is generally known as Koch's postulates, but it is perhaps only useful for precautionary approaches to proactive assessment of potential health impacts of new agents about to be introduced into the environment. This approach complements the epidemiology-based inferences described by Hill, but further refinement is warranted to deal with complicated issues such as interactions between multiple environmental agents, which could have additive, neutral, or canceling effects. The question of dose is also difficult to subject to simple conclusions because of phenomena such as hormesis, in which small doses may show beneficial effects.

For environmental diseases, a modified version of Koch's postulates can be expressed as follows. First, exposure to an environmental agent must be demonstrable in all organisms suffering from the disease, but not in healthy organisms (assuming predisposition factors). Second, the identity, concentrations in different environmental and physiological compartments, and transformation pathways of the agent must be known as much as possible. Third, the agent should cause disease when introduced into healthy organisms. Fourth, biomarkers showing modification of the physiological target affected by the environmental agent must be observable in experimentally exposed organisms.

TREATMENT AND THERAPY

The symptoms of environmental diseases vary widely, and physiological, anatomical, and behavioral characteristics can succumb to the effects of environmental agents. In evaluating treatment and therapy, it is useful to consider two categories of symptoms. Acute symptoms are exhibited in response to human exposure to high doses of toxic agents within a short period of time. Essentially, the body is overwhelmed, and emergency therapy is necessary to avoid death or permanent disability. For toxic air contaminants, respiratory distress is a common symptom, and mortality can occur rapidly. Conversely, chronic symptoms of human exposures to low levels of environmental (particularly air) pollutants are difficult to diagnose, as in the case of cancers attributable to secondhand tobacco smoke or ambient exposure to respirable particulate matter. Similarly, exposure of the skin to rapidly absorbed toxins can produce rapid mortality, but the development of skin cancer due to ultraviolet (UV) light exposure may take decades to manifest. Ingestion of contaminated liquids or food may take minutes to provoke distress and vomiting, whereas it may take years for chronic symptoms to manifest in cases of carcinogenic water pollutants.

Treatment and therapy of environmental diseases requires accurate diagnosis of the causative agent. The first line of response is to limit exposure through flushing the body with clean air or liquids. Chelation therapy can be used to reduce the body burden of certain toxic metals. Curative measures follow the established procedures developed for specific organs. For example, chemotherapy, radiotherapy, and surgery are used to treat cancers regardless of the involvement of known environmental factors in their etiology. Skin diseases such as chloracne associated with exposure to chlorinated aromatic hydrocarbon pollutants, including polychlorinated biphenyls (PCBs), are managed to reduce the severity of lesions and enhance natural healing processes. Cognitive deficits associated with exposure to metals and other environmental pollutants are believed to be reversible as long further exposures are avoided. Finally, environmental diseases associated with infectious agents such as bacteria can be controlled through a combination of source disinfection and antibiotic therapy.

Perspective and Prospects

There has been a resurgence of interest in environmental diseases because of societal changes at regional and international levels. Industrialization demands the use of thousands of potentially hazardous chemicals that ultimately end up polluting human environments and remain an important source of causative agents for environmental diseases. Recent threats associated with global environmental change, bioterrorism, and chemical warfare have all contributed to the need for rapid detection of hazardous environmental agents and tougher laws to protect air, water, soil, and food resources. Prevention is still the crucial solution to reducing the human burden of environmental diseases worldwide.

On June 16, 2006, the World Health Organization (WHO) issued a landmark report estimating that environmental risk factors play a role in more than 80 percent of diseases regularly reported by WHO across fourteen regions globally. The environment has an impact on human health through exposures to physical, chemical, and biological risk factors and through changes in human behavior in response to environmental change at local and global levels. Globally, nearly 25 percent of all deaths and of the total disease burden (measured in disability-adjusted life years, or DALYs) can be attributed to environmental quality. The situation is more dire for children, with environmental risk factors accounting for more than 33 percent of the disease burden. These discoveries have important implications for national and international health policy, because many of the implicated environmental risk factors can be modified by established interventions. The lack of understanding on how to deploy these interventions globally has inspired the involvement of well-funded organizations and institutions in environmental health issues.

In the United States, the National Institute of Environmental Health Sciences (NIEHS), a subsidiary of the National Institutes of Health (NIH), is responsible for studying environmental diseases and guiding policy on how to protect vulnerable populations. A comprehensive five-year strategic plan developed by the NIEHS in 2006 outlined seven specific goals aimed at curtailing environmental exposures and reducing societal burden of environmental diseases.

The first goal is to expand the role of clinical research in environmental health sciences by emphasizing the use of environmental exposures to understand and better characterize complex diseases. This includes the development of research models for human diseases based on the coordinated knowledge of environmental sciences and human biology.

The second goal is to use environmental toxins to gaining more insight into the basic mechanisms in human biology. This goal involves tapping into the rapidly expanding knowledge of the biochemical mechanisms of disease progression and the influence of genetic factors in the path from environmental exposures to disease symptoms.

The third goal is to build an integrative multidisciplinary understanding of complex environmental systems and the various ways in which human diseases are manifested. The fourth goal is to improve the quality of community-based environmental health research. Much can be learned from studying populations that are exposed to high concentrations of environmental agents believed to cause human disease. The hope is to better understand disease clusters in communities and to link the understanding of regional prevalence of environmental diseases to global environmental health concerns.

The fifth goal is to improve the understanding and use of sensitive markers of exposure, susceptibility, and effects of environmental agents. There is also an urgent need to develop technologies for measuring exposures more accurately in order to link exposures more tightly to assessments of toxicity and other physiological impacts.

The sixth goal is to engage the broader biomedical community in research on environmental diseases and to support a pipeline for encouraging new researchers to enter the discipline of environmental health.

The seventh goal is to encourage pathways by which the results of research can inform policy quickly in order to protect vulnerable populations. This requires fostering cooperation with other agencies and organizations such as the U.S. Environmental Protection Agency (EPA), the Food and Drug Administration (FDA), the U.S. Department of Agriculture, and the Occupational Safety and Health Administration (OSHA). In addition, there must be straightforward communication paths between manufacturing industries where environmental agents of disease originate and the community of environmental health physicians, researchers, and regulatory agencies to ensure successful implementation of these laudable goals.

—*Oladele A. Ogunseitan, Ph.D., M.P.H.*

See also Allergies; Asbestos exposure; Aspergillosis; Asthma; Bronchitis; Cancer; Carcinogens; Carpal tunnel syndrome; Chronic obstructive pulmonary disease (COPD); *E. coli* infection; Emphysema; Environmental health; Epidemiology; Food poisoning; Gulf War syndrome; Lead poisoning; Lung cancer; Melanoma; Mercury poisoning; Multiple chemical sensitivity syndrome; Occupational health; Poisoning; Pulmonary diseases; Radiation sickness; Respiration; Skin cancer; Skin lesion removal; Teratogens; Toxicology; Tularemia.

For Further Information:

Carson, Rachel. *Silent Spring*. 40th anniversary ed. New York: Houghton Mifflin, 2002. A classic book that began the rewarding tradition of connecting ecosystems, environmental quality, and human health.

Hill, Austin Bradford. "The Environment and Disease: Association or Causation?" *Proceedings of the Royal Society of Medicine* 58 (1965): 295-300. A classic publication on causality in environmental epidemiology.

McMichael, Tony. *Human Frontiers, Environments, and Disease*. New York: Cambridge University Press, 2001. A general textbook on environmental quality and human diseases.

National Institute of Environmental Health Sciences (NIEHS). *New Frontier in Environmental Sciences and Human Health: The 2006-2011 NIEHS Strategic Plan*. http://www.niehs.nih.gov/external/plan2006. The comprehensive five-year strategic plan developed by the NIEHS.

Phillips, Carl V., and Karen J. Goodman. "The Missed Lessons of Sir Austin Bradford Hill." *Epidemiologic Perspectives & Innovations* 1, no. 3 (October 4, 2004). Presents the caveats on inferring causation based on epidemiological data. Also available online at http://www.epi-perspectives.com/content/1/1/3.

Solomon, Gina, Oladele A. Ogunseitan, and Jan Kirsch. *Pesticides and Human Health: A Resource for Health Care Professionals*. San Francisco: Physicians for Social Responsibility, Los Angeles and Californians for Pesticide Reform, 2000. A compendium on environmental diseases associated with pesticides in the human environment.

World Health Organization. *Preventing Disease Through Healthy Environments: Towards an Estimate of the Environmental Burden of Disease*. Edited by A. Pruss-Ustun and C. Corvalan. Geneva, Switzerland: Author, 2006. Provides a global outlook on environmental diseases.

Environmental health

Specialty

Anatomy or system affected: All

Specialties and related fields: Epidemiology, occupational health, preventive medicine, psychology, public health, toxicology

Definition: The control of all factors in the physical environment that exercise, or may exercise, a deleterious effect on human physical development, health, and survival and correcting and preventing those effects from adversely affecting future generations. The study of the influence of environment on health and disease.

Key terms:

community: a group of people living in the same locality

hygiene: the science of health and the prevention of disease

pollutant: a noxious substance that contaminates the environment

remediation: correcting an evil, fault, or error

sanitation: the application of measures designed to protect public health

Science and Profession

The environment is the sum of all external influences and conditions affecting the life and development of an organism. For humans, a healthy environment means that the surroundings in which humans live, work, and play meet some predetermined quality standard. The field of environmental health encompasses biological, chemical, physical, and psychosocial factors in the environment. This is the air that humans breathe, the water that they drink, the food that they consume, and the shelter that they inhabit. The definition also includes the identification of pollutants, waste materials, and other environmental factors that adversely affect life and health. The study of environmental health investigates how human health and disease are influenced by the environment. It encompasses the fields of environmental engineering and sanitation, public health engineering, and sanitary engineering. The majority of professionals working in the field of environmental health are trained as civil engineers, environmental engineers, geologists, toxicologists, or preventive medicine specialists. Many are also qualified in subspecialties such as hydrogeology, epidemiology, public sanitation, and occupational health.

Environmental health deals with the control of factors in the physical environment that cause (or may cause) a negative effect on the health and survival of communities. Consideration is given to the physical, economic, and social impact of the controlling measures. These measures include controlling, modifying, or adapting the physical, chemical, and biological factors of the environment in the interest of human health, comfort, and social well-being. Environmental health is concerned not only with simple survival and the prevention of disease and poisoning but also with the maintenance of an environment that is suited to efficient human performance and that preserves human comfort and enjoyment.

Diagnostic and Treatment Techniques

The field of environmental health covers an extremely broad area of human living space. For practical purposes, those involved in the profession of environmental health concern themselves with the impact of humans on the environment and the impact of the environment on humans, balancing their appraisals and allocations of available resources. The scope of environmental health research and community environmental health planning usually involves the following topics: water supplies, water pollution and wastewater treatment, solid waste disposal, pest control, soil pollution, food hygiene, air pollution, radiation control, noise control, transportation control, safe housing, land use planning, public recreation, abuse of controlled substances, resource conservation, postdisaster sanitation, accident prevention, medical facilities, and occupational health, particularly the control of physical, chemical, and biological hazards.

The implementation of effective environmental health strategies must take place within the context of comprehensive regional or area-wide community planning. Planning considerations for a community's environmental health are based on individual community aspirations and goals, priorities, local resources, and the availability of outside resources required to meet projected health standards. The planning and implementation of environmental health activities directly involve engineers, sanitarians, medical specialists, planners, architects, geologists, biologists, chemists, geophysicists, technicians, naturalists, and related personnel. The natural and physical scientists provide research necessary for communities to locate and use available resources responsibly, and they also identify potential and existing health hazards. The engineering specialties provide know-how to communities concerning the design, installation, and operation of equip-

ment. When a problem is identified or an emergency occurs, it is often the engineering professionals who direct remediation efforts. Medical specialists, with scientific backup, determine dangers to a community's physical health; if health problems arise, they concern themselves with treating and preventing disease and restoring health. The implementation of any environmental health strategy is clearly a team effort.

Perspective and Prospects

The concept of environmental health in modern society is considerably expanded from that of the past. Activities in the field of environmental health were once controlled only because they were known to be disease-related. The present concept of environmental health aims to provide a high quality of living.

The field of environmental health concerns itself with the control of physical factors affecting the health of humans and is different from the prevention and control of individual illness and the preservation of human health. Most environmental health problems are the direct result of human activities and interactions with natural and manufactured resources. Human manipulation of natural resources causes changes to the environment. These changes can be local or global, anticipated or unanticipated. At the present time, humans are living in a polluted environment, the result of centuries of lack of concern for and appreciation of the ecologic consequences of human activities. The cumulative effects of human actions on the environment have risen steeply and continuously, while human response to mounting problems of environmental quality has been sporadic and targeted toward high-profile or emergency problems. As a result, environmental programs have been developed to preserve wildlife, maintain clean groundwater supplies, manage resources, combat communicable disease, increase agricultural production, and ensure healthy and sanitary living conditions for human populations.

As a direct reflection of the public's concern about environmental degradation, environmental health has become a rapidly growing specialty in the fields of engineering, medicine, environmental science, geology, and resource management. As public awareness of the devastating effects of pollution and resource depletion grows, the demand for qualified environmental health professionals and administrators increases. Whether these sought-after professionals are asked to offer stopgap measures for environmental problems that have already progressed to dangerous, possibly unresolvable levels or whether they are employed to foster a new, more holistic approach to the natural world will depend on the environmental conscience of modern civilization.

—*Randall L. Milstein, Ph.D.; updated by Sharon W. Stark, R.N., A.P.R.N., D.N.Sc.*

See also Allergies; Asbestos exposure; Aspergillosis; Asthma; Bacteriology; Biological and chemical weapons; Carcinogens; Cholera; Chronic obstructive pulmonary disease (COPD); Environmental diseases; Environmental health; Epidemiology; Food poisoning; Frostbite; Gulf War syndrome; Heat exhaustion and heat stroke; Hyperthermia and hypothermia; Immune system; Immunization and vaccination; Immunology; Insect-borne diseases; Interstitial pulmonary fibrosis (IPF); Lead poisoning; Legionnaires' disease; Lice, mites, and ticks; Lung cancer; Lungs; Lyme disease; Malaria; Mercury poisoning; Microbiology; Nasopharyngeal disorders; Occupational health; Parasitic diseases; Plague; Poisoning; Poisonous plants; Preventive medicine; Pulmonary diseases; Pulmonary medicine; Pulmonary medicine, pediatric; Salmonella infection; Skin cancer; Snakebites; Stress; Stress reduction; Teratogens; Toxicology; Tropical medicine; Tularemia.

FOR FURTHER INFORMATION:

Environmental Defense. http://www.environmental defense.org/.

Friis, Robert H. *Essentials of Environmental Health.* Sudbury, Mass.: Jones and Bartlett, 2007.

Moeller, Dade W. *Environmental Health.* 3d ed. Cambridge, Mass.: Harvard University Press, 2005.

Morgan, Monroe T. *Environmental Health.* 3d ed. Belmont, Calif.: Thomson/Wadsworth, 2003.

National Institute for Environmental Health Sciences. *What Is Environmental Health?* http://www.niehs .nih.gov/oc/factsheets/pdf/e-health.pdf.

Philp, Richard B. *Ecosystems and Human Health: Toxicology and Environmental Hazards.* 2d ed. Boca Raton, Fla.: Lewis, 2001.

Raven, Peter H., and Linda R. Berg. *Environment.* 4th ed. Fort Worth, Tex.: Harcourt Brace College, 2004.

World Health Organization. *Public Health and Environment.* http://www.who.int/phe/en/.

Yassi, Annalee, et al. *Basic Environmental Health.* New York: Oxford University Press, 2001.

ENZYME THERAPY

TREATMENT

ALSO KNOWN AS: Enzyme replacement therapy

ANATOMY OR SYSTEM AFFECTED: All

SPECIALTIES AND RELATED FIELDS: Alternative medicine, biochemistry, genetics

DEFINITION: The use of enzymes as drugs to treat specific medical problems.

INDICATIONS AND PROCEDURES

Enzymes are large, complex protein molecules that catalyze chemical reactions in living organisms. The phrase "enzyme therapy" is sometimes used to refer to enzyme preparations given as dietary supplements, often as digestive aids. Such treatment is of questionable value because enzymes, like all proteins, are degraded in the stomach. Legitimate enzyme therapy is an innovative procedure based on emerging technology. Enzymes used to treat various medical conditions are delivered intravenously.

Enzyme therapy is used to dissolve clots in stroke and cardiac patients. Enzymes such as streptokinase, plasmin, and human tissue plasminogen activator (TPA) are able to dissolve clots when injected into the bloodstream.

Some types of adult leukemia can be treated by injection of the enzyme asparaginase, which destroys asparagine. Tumors in these patients require asparagine, and the asparaginase removes it from the blood, thus inhibiting the ability of these tumors to grow.

Enzyme therapy can also be used to treat certain inherited diseases. One of these is Fabry's disease. Patients with this disease are deficient in an enzyme called alpha-galactosidase A. Without this enzyme, harmful levels of a substance called ceremide trehexoside accumulate in the heart, brain, and kidneys. If left untreated, patients usually die in their forties or fifties after a lifetime of pain. On the other hand, patients injected with alpha-galactosidase A once every two weeks lead nearly normal lives.

Gaucher's disease is another severe inherited disease characterized by a deficiency in an enzyme that normally prevents the buildup of a chemical to injurious levels. It can be treated by injections of the enzyme glucocerebrosidase.

USES AND COMPLICATIONS

The use of enzymes to treat clotting problems and genetic diseases started in the early 1990's; thus, the long-term effects are unknown. Enzyme therapy does not cure genetic disease, so the therapy must be life-long.

Some people are encouraged to swallow enzyme preparations to aid digestion. For example, the enzyme papain is promoted as a digestive aid. Although papain is very effective at breaking down proteins in the laboratory or as a meat tenderizer in the kitchen, it does not function well in the stomach. Papain is most effective at a nearly neutral pH of 6.2, whereas the stomach is highly acidic with a pH of about 2.0. On the other hand, papain is active in the more neutral esophagus. Although normally little or no food is found in the esophagus, papain has the potential to damage the esophageal lining, especially in people with esophageal disorders.

—Lorraine Lica, Ph.D.

See also Blood and blood disorders; Digestion; Enzymes; Fatty acid oxidation disorder; Fructosemia; Galactosemia; Gaucher's disease; Genetic diseases; Glycogen storage diseases; Heart attack; Leukemia; Metabolism; Mucopolysaccharidosis (MPS); Niemann-Pick disease; Oncology; Pharmacology; Strokes; Tay-Sachs disease; Thrombolytic therapy and TPA; Thrombosis and thrombus; Tumors.

FOR FURTHER INFORMATION:

Cichoke, Anthony J. *The Complete Book of Enzyme Therapy.* Garden City Park, N.Y.: Avery, 1999.

Devlin, Thomas M., ed. *Textbook of Biochemistry: With Clinical Correlations.* 6th ed. Hoboken, N.J.: Wiley-Liss, 2006.

Rimoin, David L., et al., eds. *Emery and Rimoin's Principles and Practice of Medical Genetics.* 5th ed. New York: Churchill Livingstone, 2006.

Scriver, Charles R., et al., eds. *The Metabolic and Molecular Bases of Inherited Disease.* 8th ed. New York: McGraw-Hill, 2001.

ENZYMES

BIOLOGY

ANATOMY OR SYSTEM INVOLVED: Cells, immune system

SPECIALTIES AND RELATED FIELDS: Biochemistry, cytology, endocrinology, genetics, pharmacology

DEFINITION: Large molecules, produced by cells, that catalyze chemical reactions inside living organisms.

KEY TERMS:

active site: the part of an enzyme where the substrate is bound; this is the site where the reaction occurs

activity: a measure of the ability of an enzyme to catalyze its reaction

amino acid: the fundamental building blocks of proteins; there are twenty amino acids, each with a different chemistry

catalysis: increasing the speed of a chemical reaction

molecule: a collection of atoms bonded together; normally neutral because it has an equal number of protons and electrons

mutation: a substitution of one amino acid for another in the amino acid sequence of a protein

protein: large molecules made up of amino acids connected by peptide bonds; the sequence of amino acids in a protein determines its three-dimensional structure

substrates: reactants that enzymes convert into products; every enzyme is specific for one specific substrate

STRUCTURE AND FUNCTIONS

Enzymes are remarkable molecules because they increase rates of biochemical reactions. Each enzyme within a cell selectively speeds up, or catalyzes, one particular reaction or type of reaction. The vast majority of enzymes belong to the class of large molecules known as proteins. Proteins are built by combining amino acids. There are twenty amino acids, which can be divided into three classes: hydrophobic, charged, and polar. Hydrophobic amino acids behave chemically like oils, avoiding contact with water. Charged amino acids are ionic, containing one extra or one less electron than do neutral molecules. Polar amino acids are attracted to water and other polar amino acids. Each of these three classes of amino acids has a distinct chemistry. The specific order of the amino acid sequence defines the structure and function of every protein. Inside cells, enzymes catalyze reactions so that they occur millions of times faster than they would without the presence of these proteins. Each cell in the body produces many different enzymes. Different sets of enzymes are found in different tissues, reflecting the specialized function of each particular enzyme. Thousands of different enzymes are at work in the body; many have yet to be discovered.

Protein enzymes work by bringing the reactants in a chemical reaction together in the most favorable geometrical arrangement, so that bonds can be easily broken and reformed. This is possible because different enzymes have different three-dimensional shapes. It is the shape of the enzyme that determines its chemistry. Each enzyme combines with a specific substrate, or reactant, and catalyzes its characteristic reaction. When

The Function of Some Enzymes

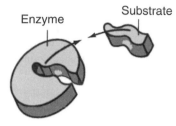

Enzyme   Substrate

An enzyme combines with a substrate that has molecules of a complementary shape.

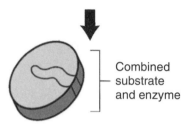

Combined substrate and enzyme

The interaction between the enzyme and substrate causes a chemical change in the substrate, splitting it in two.

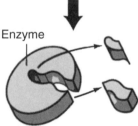

Enzyme

The enzyme is unchanged and can repeat the process with another substrate molecule.

the reaction is over, the substrate has been converted into products. The enzyme remains unchanged, ready to catalyze another reaction with the next substrate molecule it encounters.

Enzymes play a significant role in treating diseases. Because enzymes have specific functions, a particular enzyme that has the required function to treat the disorder can be administered. Modern methods of genetic engineering allow the production of desired enzymes. Scientists can use bacteria as factories to produce large amounts of enzyme from an organism by copying the gene from the organism of interest into bacterial cells. The bacteria are then grown in culture, producing the enzyme of interest as they grow. This procedure is a much safer method than the old procedure of isolating enzymes from animal tissues, because the enzymes produced are free of viruses and other contaminants present in animal tissues. Proteins produced by genetic engineering techniques are called recombinant proteins.

Sometimes enzymes can be used as drugs for the treatment of specific diseases. Streptokinase is an enzyme mixture that is useful in clearing blood clots that occur in the heart and the lower extremities. Another useful enzyme for dissolving blood clots that occur as a result of heart attacks is human tissue plasminogen activator (TPA). Recombinant TPA is produced by genetic engineering techniques, using bacteria cultures to produce large quantities of human TPA. The administration of TPA within an hour of the formation of a blood clot in a coronary artery dramatically increases survival rates of heart attack victims. Some types of adult leukemia are treated by intravenous administration of the asparaginase enzyme. Tumor cells require the molecule asparagine to grow, and they scavenge it from the bloodstream. Asparaginase drastically reduces the amount of asparagine in the blood, thus slowing the growth of the tumor. Because most enzymes do not last long in blood, huge amounts of enzymes are required for therapeutic effects. In classic hemophilia, the factor VIII enzyme is missing or is genetically mutated so that it has a very low activity. This enzyme is essential for inducing the formation of blood clots. In the past, it was a laborious task to collect a concentrated blood plasma sample containing factor VIII, which was administered to hemophiliacs to stop hemorrhages. This treatment carried the risk of infecting the patient with viruses that cause acquired immunodeficiency syndrome (AIDS), hepatitis, and other diseases. Purified recombinant factor VIII is now available. Because the recombinant human factor VIII is produced by bacteria, it cannot be infected with the viruses that cause hepatitis and AIDS.

A classic enzyme inhibitor used as a drug is penicillin. Penicillin was discovered in 1928 by Alexander Fleming, after he noticed that bacterial growth was prevented by a contaminating mold known as *Penicillium*. Ten years later, Howard Florey and Ernst Chain performed the key experiments that led to the isolation, characterization, and clinical use of this wonder drug antibiotic. In 1957, Joshua Lederberg showed that penicillin interferes with the synthesis of the cell walls of bacteria. In 1965, James Park and Jack Strominger independently discovered that penicillin blocks the last step in cell wall synthesis. The last step is the cross-linking of different strands of the wall and is catalyzed by the enzyme glycopeptide transpeptidase. The shape of penicillin resembles that of the normal substrate of glycopeptide transpeptidase, so that penicillin binds to the active site of the transpeptidase enzyme. Once bound to the active site, penicillin forms a permanent bond with one of the amino acid residues. This chemical reaction permanently inhibits the glycopeptide transpeptidase enzyme, thus preventing the transpeptidase from cross-linking the bacterial wall.

Several anticancer drugs work by blocking the synthesis of deoxythymidylate (dTMP), as an abundant supply of dTMP is required for rapid cell division to be sustained. Drugs that inhibit the enzymes thymidylate synthase and dihydrofolate reductase are very effective agents in cancer chemotherapy. Thymidylate synthase, which makes dTMP from deoxyuridylate, is irreversibly inhibited by the drug fluorouracil. This drug is converted into fluorodeoxyuridylate (F-dUMP), which chemically reacts with thymidylate synthase so that the enzyme can no longer function in its normal role of making dTMP from deoxyuridylate. The synthesis of dTMP can also be blocked by drugs that inhibit the enzyme dihydrofolate reductase. The normal substrate for dihydrofolate reductase is the molecule dihydrofolate. Drugs such as aminopterin and methotrexate bind to the active site of the reductase enzyme, inhibiting rapid cell growth. Methotrexate is very effective at inhibiting rapidly growing tumors such as acute leukemia and choriocarcinoma. Unfortunately methotrexate kills all rapidly dividing cells, including stem cells in bone marrow, epithelial cells of the intestinal tract, and hair follicles, which explains the many toxic side effects of this drug. Computer-aided drug design has been applied to the dihydrofolate reductase enzyme, with encouraging results.

The activity of an enzyme is a measure of how efficiently a particular enzyme catalyzes its reaction. A loss in activity corresponds to a decrease in catalytic efficiency, and an increase in activity corresponds to an increase in catalytic efficiency. Many drugs increase enzyme activity (enzyme induction), and many decrease enzyme activity (enzyme inhibition). Both enzyme induction and enzyme inhibition result from the interaction of the drug with the enzyme, altering the surface of the enzyme where the substrate normally is bound during catalysis. In enzyme induction, the surface is altered such that the substrate is bound tighter than usual, while in enzyme inhibition, the surface is altered so that the substrate cannot bind to the enzyme. The structures of many enzyme inhibitors are similar to the structures of substrates. Inhibitors bind at active sites of enzymes. Drugs that are enzyme inhibitors are very powerful medical tools, as they bind to the enzyme and are not easily removed.

Universities, government agencies, and pharmaceutical companies are continually seeking to develop drugs that specifically bind and inhibit enzymes responsible for disease. Much effort is spent trying to design drugs in a rational manner, using the most powerful tools of chemistry. Techniques such as X-ray crystallography, nuclear magnetic resonance (NMR) spectroscopy, and computational chemistry allow researchers to determine the shapes of enzymes, their substrates, and their inhibitors. These efforts allow the research team to design drugs that bind more specifically to the target enzyme, thus increasing the effectiveness and lowering the toxicity of the drug.

Disorders and Diseases

Defects in enzymes, known as mutations, can cause disease. A protein molecule is mutated when one or more of the original amino acids in the protein is replaced by a different amino acid. For example, if an enzyme consists of one hundred amino acids, and amino acid number 35 is changed from one kind of amino acid to a different kind, the protein is now a mutant. A mutated enzyme has a slightly altered shape compared to the original enzyme. If the change in shape causes the enzyme to perform its chemistry more slowly than the original enzyme, then the cell and tissue have an impaired function. In particular, if an amino acid is changed from one of the three classes (hydrophobic, charged, or polar) to a different class, then the mutation is more likely to cause a change in the structure and function of the enzyme. Not all mutations are harmful, but a single mutation in a key region of an enzyme can be fatal to a living organism.

Many diseases are diagnosed by measuring enzyme concentrations and activities in the body. Enzyme concentration refers to the amount of enzyme present, while enzyme activity refers to the ability of the enzyme to perform its chemistry. Enzyme concentrations and activities can be measured in blood or in tissue. Disease of tissues and organs can cause cellular damage, so that enzymes that are normally not present in significant quantities in blood are raised to very high levels as they flow from the damaged tissue into the blood plasma. Detection of particular enzymes in blood plasma indicates a diseased organ. The higher the concentration of enzyme in the blood, the more extensive the damage to that tissue or organ. The detection of these enzymes in the blood is a diagnostic tool, indicating a particular disorder. Genetic diseases caused by a mutation in an enzyme can be detected by laboratory tests that measure enzyme activity or enzyme shape.

Disease diagnosis is often made by measuring the concentration or activity of enzymes. Isozymes are enzymes that catalyze the same reaction but have slightly different structures. Most isozymes are enzymes consisting of two or more subunits, with different combinations of the subunits differentiating the isozymes. Isozymes of the enzymes lactate dehydrogenase, creatine kinase, and alkaline phosphatase are used for clinical applications. Monitoring of the isozyme concentrations and activities of lactate dehydrogenase and creatine kinase in the blood shows whether a patient has suffered a heart attack.

Creatine kinase consists of two subunits. The two possible subunits are M, which stands for muscle type, and B, which stands for brain type. There are three possible isozymes: MM, BB, and MB. The MM isozyme consists of two M subunits and is the only isozyme found in skeletal muscle, the BB isozyme consists of two B subunits and is the only isozyme found in the brain, and the MB isozyme consists of one M and one B subunit and is found only in the heart. Lactate dehydrogenase consists of four subunits, made from five combinations of two subunits. The two subunits are the heart subunit, designated by H, and the muscle subunit, designated by M. The HHHH and HHHM isozymes are found in the heart and in red blood cells, the HHMM isozyme is found in the brain and kidney, and the MMMM isozyme is found in the liver and skeletal muscle.

After a heart attack, the cellular breakup of heart tissue releases the MB isozyme of creatine kinase into the bloodstream within six to eighteen hours. Release of lactate dehydrogenase into the blood is slower than that of creatine kinase, occurring one to two days after the appearance of creatine kinase. In a healthy person, the activity of the HHHM isozyme of lactate dehydrogenase is higher than that of the HHHH isozyme. In heart attack victims, however, the activity of the HHHH isozyme becomes greater than that of the HHHM isozyme between twelve and twenty-four hours after the attack. Measurement of increased concentration of the MB isozyme a short while after a suspected heart attack, followed by the switch in lactate dehydrogenase activity between the HHHH and HHHM isozymes, indicates that a heart attack occurred. Secondary complications of a heart attack can also be followed with

isozyme measurements. For example, increased activity of the MMMM isozyme of lactate dehydrogenase is an indication of liver congestion.

Certain medical conditions can be screened by using immobilized enzymes as reagents in desktop clinical analyzers. For example, screening tests for cholesterol and triglycerides can be completed in a few minutes using 0.01 milliliter of blood plasma. The enzymes cholesterol oxidase and lipase are immobilized, or fixed in place, in a detection kit. If cholesterol is present, cholesterol oxidase breaks off hydrogen peroxide from the cholesterol. The enzyme peroxidase and a colorless dye are included in the detection kit, and peroxidase catalyzes the reaction of the colorless dye and hydrogen peroxide to form a colored dye that can be easily measured from the amount of light reflected from the solution. The enzyme lipase allows the accurate determination of triglycerides in blood.

A mutation in a protein that acts as a natural inhibitor of an enzyme can cause disease. For example, emphysema is a destructive lung disease in which the alveolar walls of the lungs are destroyed by an enzyme known as elastase. A person with emphysema breathes much harder to exchange the same volume of air because the alveoli, or air pockets, have become much less efficient. Normally, the elastase enzyme is prevented from destroying lung tissue by the protein antitrypsin. Antitrypsin is made in the liver and flows to the lungs, where it binds to the active site of elastase and prevents it from digesting lung tissue. Emphysema can occur when the negatively charged amino acid at position 53 of the amino acid sequence of antitrypsin is replaced with a positively charged amino acid. This mutation changes the chemical nature of antitrypsin such that the mutant antitrypsin is released from the liver at a much slower rate. The level of this mutant antitrypsin in the lungs is 15 percent of the normal level. The net result of this one amino acid mutation in the antitrypsin protein is that most of the elastase enzyme is free to destroy lung tissue. Cigarette smoking dramatically increases the incidence of emphysema in people who have the mutant antitrypsin. Cigarette smoke reacts with the hydrophobic amino acid at position 358 of antitrypsin, adding one oxygen atom at this position in the amino acid sequence. The addition of this one extra oxygen atom at this critical place in antitrypsin changes the chemical nature of the hydrophobic amino acid so that the antitrypsin no longer can bind to elastase. Because only 15 percent of the mutant antitrypsin gets from the liver to the lungs in the first place, cigarette smoking puts people with this particular mutation at grave risk for developing emphysema.

PERSPECTIVE AND PROSPECTS

Enzymatic reactions have been used by humankind since prehistoric times. It has been known for more than six thousand years that fermentation processes transform grapes into wine, but it was not until the nineteenth century that it was understood that the conversion of grape sugar to alcohol is a process catalyzed by enzymes found in yeast. In the 1700's, Antoine Lavoisier showed that a solution of sugar could be fermented if provided with the sediment of a previous fermentation and that the sugar was converted to alcohol and carbon dioxide in this process. At this time, it was thought that there was a vital force responsible for the workings of a living cell. This notion of a vital force slowed the development of the discipline of biochemistry considerably, as many good scientists struggled to understand the fermentation process. In 1828, Friedrich Wöhler synthesized urea in a test tube, providing strong evidence against the concept of a vital force. In 1833, Anselme Payen and Jean Persoz discovered the first enzyme, diastase (now known as amylase), which converted starch into sugar. The next year, Johann Eberle showed that the presence of a stomach is not required for gastric digestion to take place. In 1836, Theodor Schwann made the very important discovery that the active ingredient in digestion, which he called pepsin, could be extracted from the stomach wall.

The next year, Jöns Jakob Berzelius developed the idea of catalysis, making the point that both living and inorganic systems had catalysts. In the late 1850's, Louis Pasteur confirmed and extended the earlier experiments of Schwann. Despite his brilliant experimental abilities, however, Pasteur was handicapped in his research by his belief that fermentation could happen only within a living organism. In 1860, Marcelin Berthelot showed that a living being was not the ferment, but produced the ferment, in sharp contrast to Pasteur's vitalist ideas. Pasteur's response to this work was that Berthelot and he meant different things by the use of the word "ferment." Moritz Traube, a German wine merchant, realized that chemical processes and living bodies were mostly based on ferment actions, and he published these ideas in 1858 and again in 1878. In 1878, Friedrich Kühne proposed that to remove the discrepancy over the meaning of the word "ferment," the word "enzyme" should be used, as it means "in yeast." It was not until 1897 that Eduard Buchner showed that living cells are not essential for fermentation to occur, as he extracted from yeast a cell-free juice containing the entire fermentation system.

From 1894 to 1898, Emil Fischer used synthetic organic chemistry for the preparation of substrates of known structure and configuration. He showed that enzymes have a very high degree of specificity for their own particular substrate and developed the famous "lock-and-key" hypothesis. This theory, which has been only slightly modified, states that the shape of a substrate and the enzyme's active site must be complementary for catalysis to occur. Purification of enzymes remained a difficult problem, and it was not until 1926 that James Summer crystallized the first enzyme, jack bean urease. The sequence of protein enzymes could be determined experimentally after 1952, when Frederick Sanger developed his methods for amino acid sequencing. In 1965, David Phillips produced the first three-dimensional picture of an enzyme, determining the shape of lysozyme. The advent of genetic engineering techniques in the 1970's revolutionized the field of enzyme research and the use of enzymes in medical applications by enabling the production of copious amounts of recombinant proteins.

—*George C. Shields, Ph.D.*

See also Antibiotics; Bacteriology; Blood and blood disorders; Blood testing; Cholesterol; Digestion; Emphysema; Enzyme therapy; Fatty acid oxidation disorders; Food biochemistry; Fructosemia; Gaucher's disease; Genetic diseases; Genetic engineering; Genetics and inheritance; Glycogen storage diseases; Glycolysis; Hemophilia; Laboratory tests; Leukemia; Maple syrup urine disease (MSUD); Metabolic disorders; Metabolism; Mucopolysaccharidosis (MPS); Mutation; Niemann-Pick disease; Oncology; Pharmacology; Pulmonary medicine; Screening; Tay-Sachs disease; Thrombolytic therapy and TPA.

FOR FURTHER INFORMATION:

Campbell, Neil A., et al. *Biology: Concepts and Connections.* 5th ed. San Francisco: Pearson/Benjamin Cummings, 2006. This classic introductory textbook provides an excellent discussion of essential biological structures and mechanisms. Its extensive and detailed illustrations help to make even difficult concepts accessible to the nonspecialist. Of particular interest is the chapter on enzymes, titled "An Introduction to Metabolism."

Copeland, Robert A. *Enzymes: A Practical Introduction to Structure, Mechanism, and Data Analysis.* 2d ed. New York: Wiley, 2000. An introductory text that examines the structural complexities of proteins and enzymes and the mechanisms by which enzymes perform their catalytic functions.

Fruton, Joseph S. *Molecules and Life*. New York: Wiley-Interscience, 1972. Fruton, a Yale biochemist, has filled his book with historical essays on the interplay of chemistry and biology. The first part of the book, "From Ferments to Enzymes," is an interesting account of how science progressed from the known results of fermentation to the chemical knowledge that enzymes were the molecules responsible for this and all other biochemical processes.

Kornberg, Arthur. *For the Love of Enzymes: The Odyssey of a Biochemist*. Cambridge, Mass.: Harvard University Press, 1989. Both an autobiography of a great biochemist and a history of the study of enzymes. Arthur Kornberg won a Nobel Prize for the laboratory synthesis of deoxyribonucleic acid (DNA). An excellent scientific biography.

Liska, Ken. *Drugs and the Human Body, with Implications for Society*. 7th ed. Upper Saddle River, N.J.: Prentice Hall, 2004. An easy-to-read book about the effects of drugs on the human body. A good overview of how drugs interact with various molecules in the body, including many cases in which enzymes are drug targets.

Palmer, Trevor. *Understanding Enzymes*. 4th ed. New York: Prentice Hall, 1995. A standard text on enzymes and how they function. Includes a bibliography and an index.

Richard B. Silverman. *Organic Chemistry of Enzyme-Catalyzed Reactions*. Rev. ed. San Diego, Calif.: Academic Press, 2002. A text that examines the general mechanisms used by enzymes and stresses that enzymology is simply a biological application of physical organic chemistry.

Voet, Donald, and Judith G. Voet. *Biochemistry*. 3d ed. Hoboken, N.J.: John Wiley & Sons, 2004. A text that approaches biochemistry via organic chemistry reactions.

EPIDEMIOLOGY

SPECIALTY

ANATOMY OR SYSTEM AFFECTED: All

SPECIALTIES AND RELATED FIELDS: Public health

DEFINITION: The study of the distribution and determinants of diseases or health-related events in the human population. The main purpose of epidemiology is to prevent and control health problems.

KEY TERMS:

case-control study: an epidemiological study that starts with identification of a group of cases with the disease of interest and a control group of persons without the disease; the association between risk factors and the disease is examined by comparing the two groups with regard to how frequently the risk factors are present in each group

cohort study: an epidemiological study in which groups are identified by the status of exposure to risk factors of the disease of interest; the occurrences of the disease are observed during a follow-up and compared between different groups

cross-sectional study: an epidemiological study that describes disease distribution or frequency by person, place, and time in order to identify a population at risk

epidemiological triangle model: a model used to explain the interrelationship between agent, host, and environment, the three essential factors in the development of disease

population at risk: a group of people who have an increased risk for a particular disease

public health: the effort organized by society to protect, promote, and restore people health through programs that emphasize the prevention of diseases

risk factor: an aspect of behaviors, lifestyle, environmental exposure, or heredity that is known to be associated with a particular disease

SCIENCE AND PROFESSION

Although epidemiology is closely related to medicine, there are significant differences between the two fields. The main focus of medicine is to diagnose and to treat diseases in individuals, while the core purpose of epidemiology is to identify factors that cause health problems and to control diseases in populations. The health of a population is the responsibility of the field of public health, and epidemiology is a tool for public health. Epidemiology studies disease distribution in populations (for example, how often a disease occurs in different groups of people), examines determinants of diseases or risk factors that increase the risk for disease development, and evaluates strategies to prevent and control diseases in communities.

Diseases have certain patterns in populations. Some groups of people are at a higher risk for a particular disease. For example, smokers are at a higher risk for lung cancer. A key feature of epidemiology is the measurement of disease outcomes in relation to a population at risk. The concept of a population at risk can be explained by the traditional epidemiological triangle model. In this model, the three angles are agent, host, and environment. The interrelationship of these three factors is the basis of development of disease in the population.

In the triangle model, the agent is the cause of the disease and includes four main categories: biological, physical, chemical, and nutritive. Biological agents are often infectious. The common infectious agents that cause disease are bacteria, viruses, and parasites. Physical agents are related to mechanics, temperature, radiation, noise, and so forth. Chemical agents are often linked to poisons and air or water pollution. Nutritive agents are the macronutrients and micronutrients that the human body needs. Excess or deficiencies in these nutrients can cause health problems.

The second aspect in the triangle model is the host—the intrinsic factors which influence exposure, susceptibility, or response of an individual to an agent. Such intrinsic factors include age, gender, ethnic group, immunity, heredity, and personal behavior. For example, older age increases the risk for many diseases, such as heart disease and stroke. Certain ethnic groups also have increased risks for certain diseases, such as a high incidence of breast cancer in Jewish women.

The third component of the triangle model is the environment, which consists of the surroundings and conditions external to the individual that allow disease transmission or occurrence. The environment consists of physical, biologic, and socioeconomic components. Geology and climate are some examples of physical environment. Biologic environment may include population density, age distribution, and food sources. Socioeconomic environment may include degrees of industrialization and urbanization, use of technology, job security, cultural practices, and availability of health care.

The primary mission of epidemiology is to investigate the interrelationship among agent, host, and environment of a disease in a population and to disrupt the connection at some point in the triangle, so that the disease can be prevented. Some typical epidemiological activities include identification and surveillance of individuals and populations at risk for diseases, monitoring of diseases over time, identification of risk factors associated with diseases, recognition of disease transmission mode, and evaluation of the effectiveness of public health programs.

A specialist of epidemiology is an epidemiologist, who usually possesses a graduate degree in epidemiology with additional training in disease, public health, and biostatistics. The main responsibility of an epidemiologist is to investigate all elements contributing to the occurrence or absence of a disease in populations. Epidemiologists may work at all levels of communities, including academic or research institutions, federal governmental agencies, state health departments, or local health organizations or medical centers.

DIAGNOSTIC AND TREATMENT TECHNIQUES

The techniques or methods that epidemiologists use to investigate diseases in populations are epidemiological studies, which mainly consists of cross-sectional studies, case-control studies, and cohort studies.

Cross-sectional studies are also called descriptive epidemiology, because this method describes the distribution of diseases or health-related events and the exposure status of risk factors in terms of person, place, and time. Describing disease distribution by person allows discovery of disease frequency and the populations at greatest risk for the disease. Populations at a high risk can be identified by investigating such characteristics as age, gender, race, education, occupation, income, living arrangement, health status, smoking status, physical activity level, medication use, and access to health care. Disease frequencies can be observed specifically for any of these characteristics by different classifications. For example, hypertension occurrence can be observed by physical activity levels, such as low, medium, and high. Through comparisons of hypertension frequency among the three levels of physical activity, the group with the highest hypertension rate can be identified. Describing disease distribution by place can provide information associated with the geographic extent of the disease. This information includes county, state, country, birthplace, and workplace. Identifying place allows epidemiologists to examine where the causal agent of disease resides and how the disease is transmitted and spread. Describing distribution by time can reveal any seasonality of the disease and trends over time. Some diseases may be more common during a certain season; for example, influenza is more likely to be seen in winter and early spring. By tracking disease trends over time, changes in disease distribution, either emerging or declining, can be documented and corresponding measures can be taken to accompany these changes.

From a cross-sectional study, a group of people with an increased risk for a disease may be identified. Then, one would ask why this group of people has a higher risk for the disease. To answer this question, epidemiologists use case-control studies and cohort studies. Both of these methods are considered analytical studies, as they examine the relationship between a disease and its possible risk factors.

Case-control studies are one of the commonly used epidemiologic designs. A case-control study begins with the selection of a group of cases—the case group, individuals who have the disease or health-related outcome of interest. Then, through interviews or medical records, epidemiologists collect information about the previous exposure of cases (case group members) to possible risk factors. Because case-control studies obtain the information about risk factors in the past, they are also called retrospective studies. Certain demographic variables, such as age, gender, race, occupation, education, and residence, are collected as well and are used as the criteria to select the control group by matching the control subjects to the cases as closely as possible with respect to the demographic variables. No individuals of the control group exhibit the disease or health-related outcome under investigation. The information on previous exposure to risk factors is also collected from the controls.

Matching controls to cases allows the investigators to ignore the demographic variables and focus on risk factors in the analysis. Control subjects can match the cases individually or as a group. The ratio of cases to controls can be one to one or one to two or more. Increasing the number of controls can increase the power of the study to detect the differences between cases and controls; however, a large number of controls can increase the cost of the study as well.

The case and control groups are then compared for previous exposure to the risk factors of the disease using statistical analyses. The association and the strength of association between risk factors and the disease under investigation are evaluated. The results of a case control study may be a positive association, in which the risk factors increase the chance of seeing the disease; a negative association, in which the risk factors decrease the frequency of the disease; or no association, in which no relationship is found between the risk factors and the disease. For example, to study whether obesity is associated with type II diabetes, the researcher would select a group of diabetic cases and a group of controls who do not have diabetes but have similar demographic variables, such as age, gender, and occupation. Then, the history of weight would be assessed though interviews of both cases and controls. The information on weight history would then be compared between diabetic cases and nondiabetic controls. For this example, it is likely to see a positive association between obesity and diabetes, which means that obesity is more frequently seen in the diabetic cases.

Cohort studies are another type of analytical design of epidemiology. They are used to examine the causal relationship between a disease or health related outcome and its risk factors. The cohorts or study groups in a cohort study are identified by characteristics of risk factors exhibited by subjects prior to the appearance of the disease under investigation. Thus, one cohort may consist of subjects with risk factors for a disease, and another cohort may include subjects without such risk factors. In both cohorts, no subjects have the disease under investigation at the beginning of the study. Then, the research would follow both cohorts for a set period of time; therefore, cohort studies are also called prospective studies or longitudinal studies.

During the follow-up time, the difference in the occurrence of the disease under investigation will be recorded and compared between the two cohorts. The results of a cohort study may also be positive, negative, or no association, recognized through statistical analyses. A positive association means the incidence of the disease is increased in the cohort with the risk factors. A negative association indicates that the incidence of the disease is decreased in the cohort with the risk factors, which protect individuals from getting the disease—"good" risk factors. If no statistical differences are identified between the two cohorts, then the risk factors are not associated with the disease. A cohort study might study the relationship between cholesterol level and coronary artery disease. Individuals with a high cholesterol level would be included in one cohort, and individuals with a normal cholesterol level would be included in another cohort. Then, both cohorts would be followed up for a period of ten years. At the end of ten years, the incidence of coronary artery disease, which is diagnosed during those ten years, would be evaluated and compared between the two cohorts. For this study, it is very likely that the cohort with a high cholesterol level would have a higher incidence of coronary artery disease during the ten years of follow-up. A cohort study with only two cohorts is the simplest design. A study may use more than two cohorts, as long as each cohort has the unique risk factor characteristics.

There are advantages and disadvantages for both case-control studies and cohort studies. Cohort studies observe a disease from cause to effect and thus generate more accurate results; however, they are time-consuming and expensive. On the other hand, case-control studies are quick and inexpensive, but their results are less accurate since they are based on self-reported past experiences, which often encounter recall biases. In practice, epidemiologists often carry out a case-control study first. If a significant association is found from a case-control study, then a cohort study is used to confirm the association.

PERSPECTIVE AND PROSPECTS

Literally translated from Greek, "epidemiology" means "the study of people"—the population-level study of disease. The origins of epidemiology began with Dr. John Snow, a physician of London in the eighteenth century who investigated an epidemic of cholera. By observing and plotting the location of deaths related to the disease, Snow was able to legitimize his finding that cholera was spread through contaminated water and food.

In its early years, epidemiology was mainly used to study epidemics of infectious diseases, because infectious diseases were the major cause of death in populations at that time. Through improvements in nutrition and living standards, as well as advances in medicine, the major cause of death has been shifted from infectious diseases to noninfectious or chronic diseases, accompanied by a longer life expectancy in developed countries such as the United States. Epidemiology has now been applied to chronic diseases and other conditions as well, such as cancer, heart disease, diabetes, and injuries. The Framingham Heart Study is a famous epidemiological study of cardiovascular disease in the U.S. population. Epidemiologic methods have been approved as a powerful tool to study diseases or other conditions in populations and have been also applied to other fields, such as sociology.

In the future, the use of epidemiologic methods will continue to expand and allow an understanding of more human diseases and their causes. Because of improved medical technologies, epidemiology has been able to combine traditional observational methods with laboratory tests. New branches of epidemiology have been created, such as molecular epidemiology and genetic epidemiology. Research in these areas will yield knowledge about human diseases at a new level.

—*Kimberly Y. Z. Forrest, Ph.D.*

See also Acquired immunodeficiency syndrome (AIDS); Anthrax; Avian influenza; Bacterial infections; Bacteriology; Biological and chemical weapons; Biostatistics; Centers for Disease Control and Prevention (CDC); Childhood infectious diseases; Cholera; Creutzfeldt-Jakob disease (CJD); Disease; *E. coli* infection; Ebola virus; Elephantiasis; Environmental diseases; Environmental health; Epstein-Barr virus; Food poisoning; Forensic pathology; Hanta virus; Hepatitis; Human papillomavirus (HPV); Influenza; Insect-borne diseases; Kawasaki disease; Laboratory tests; Legionnaires' disease; Leprosy; Lice, mites, and ticks; Malaria; Marburg virus; Measles; Mercury poisoning; Microbiology; National Institutes of Health; Necrotizing fasciitis; Noroviruses; Occupational health; Parasitic diseases; Pathology; Plague; Poisoning; Poliomyelitis; Prion diseases; Pulmonary diseases; Rabies; Salmonella infection; Severe acute respiratory syndrome (SARS); Sexually transmitted diseases (STDs); Stress; Teratogens; Tropical medicine; Tularemia; Veterinary medicine; Viral infections; World Health Organization; Yellow fever; Zoonoses.

FOR FURTHER INFORMATION:

Day, Ian N. M., ed. *Molecular Genetic Epidemiology: A Laboratory Perspective*. New York: Springer, 2001. This book describes approaches to a series of methodologies in laboratories engaged in molecular and genetic epidemiological studies of population samples. It contains overviews of core topics and techniques that are widely available to researchers.

Fletcher, Robert H., and Suzanne W. Fletcher. *Clinical Epidemiology: The Essentials*. 4th ed. Baltimore: Lippincott Williams & Wilkins, 2005. Provides students and clinicians with the basic principles and concepts of clinical epidemiology, which helps develop a system observing and assessing outcomes in patients for the improvement of care for future patients.

Last, John M., et al., eds. *A Dictionary of Epidemiology*. 4th ed. New York: Oxford University Press, 2001. A standard English-language dictionary of epidemiology and many other related fields, including biostatistics, infectious disease control, health promotion, genetics, and medical ethics.

Lilienfeld, David E., and Paul D. Stolley. *Foundations of Epidemiology*. 3d ed. New York: Oxford University Press, 1994. A textbook commonly used by graduate students of epidemiology, with comprehensive information about concepts and methods of epidemiology. It provides numerous classical epidemiological study examples.

Newman, Stephen C. *Biostatistical Methods in Epidemiology*. New York: John Wiley & Sons, 2001. This book introduces the statistical methods used to analyze epidemiologic data. A reference book for students, health professionals, and epidemiologists.

EPIGLOTTITIS
DISEASE/DISORDER
ALSO KNOWN AS: Supraglottitis
ANATOMY OR SYSTEM AFFECTED: Respiratory system, throat
SPECIALTIES AND RELATED FIELDS: Bacteriology, emergency medicine, family medicine, internal medicine, pediatrics
DEFINITION: An acute, life-threatening inflammation of the epiglottis.

CAUSES AND SYMPTOMS
Epiglottitis is an acute, severe infection that commonly affects children between ages two and six. It is most commonly caused by the bacterium *Haemophilus influenzae*, but it can also be caused by other bacteria such as *Staphylococcus aureus* or *Streptococcus pneumoniae*, fungi such as *Candida albicans*, and viruses.

Epiglottitis presents classically with a fever and sore throat in a young child, who progresses rapidly within a few hours to an inability to eat and drooling, with signs of respiratory obstruction such as stridor. The epiglottis is a thin flap of cartilage at the back of the tongue that closes the respiratory tract while swallowing. When it is inflamed, considerable swelling and consequent respiratory obstruction result. Drooling occurs as the child is unable to swallow his or her own saliva. This is an emergency situation, as the respiratory distress can progress rapidly and become life-threatening within minutes.

It is strongly advised that the mouth and larynx not be examined using a tongue depressor, as this could precipitate a spasm of the epiglottis and exacerbate respiratory distress. Epiglottitis is diagnosed by a clinician through laryngoscopy, with efforts made to secure the airway first. Neck X rays reveal a characteristic "thumbprint" sign caused by an enlarged epiglottis. A blood culture may reveal the causative organism, and an elevated white blood cell count may be observed.

TREATMENT AND THERAPY
In most cases of epiglottitis, hospitalization is required, and the patient is usually admitted to the intensive care unit (ICU). The foremost concern is to secure and maintain an airway as soon as possible. Humidified oxygen, which has been moistened to help the patient breathe better, is administered. An emergency tracheostomy or needle cricothyrotomy may be needed to secure the airway. Antibiotics, intravenous fluids, and corticosteroids may also be administered to decrease the swelling. With proper and prompt treatment, the prognosis is very good.

PERSPECTIVE AND PROSPECTS
Epiglottitis, which was first described in 1848, is an acute inflammation of the epiglottis that should be distinguished from laryngotracheobronchitis or croup. Also, children ingesting hot liquids may present with similar symptoms. The disease must be managed efficiently and in a clinical setting only. Since the causative agent of the disease is infectious, family members must also be screened and treated for the disease. The aggressive immunization of children against *Haemophilus influenzae B* by the Hib vaccine has resulted in a significant decrease in the incidence of epiglottitis.

—*Venkat Raghavan Tirumala, M.D., M.H.A.*
See also Antibiotics; Bacterial infections; Childhood infectious diseases; Choking; Croup; Otorhinolaryngology; Pulmonary medicine, pediatric; Respiration; Sore throat; Tracheostomy.

INFORMATION ON EPIGLOTTITIS

CAUSES: Usually bacterial infection; sometimes fungal or viral infection
SYMPTOMS: Sore throat, fever, inability to eat, drooling, stridor
DURATION: Acute
TREATMENTS: Hospitalization, humidified oxygen, antibiotics, intravenous fluids, corticosteroids, emergency tracheostomy if needed

---

FOR FURTHER INFORMATION:
Kasper, Dennis L., et al., eds. *Harrison's Principles of Internal Medicine*. 16th ed. New York: McGraw-Hill, 2005.
Rakel, Robert E., ed. *Textbook of Family Practice*. 6th ed. Philadelphia: W. B. Saunders, 2002.
Tapley, Donald F., et al., eds. *The Columbia University College of Physicians and Surgeons Complete Home Medical Guide*. Rev. 3d ed. New York: Crown, 1995.

EPILEPSY

DISEASE/DISORDER

ANATOMY OR SYSTEM AFFECTED: Brain, head, nerves, nervous system

SPECIALTIES AND RELATED FIELDS: Neurology

DEFINITION: A serious neurologic disease characterized by seizures, which may involve convulsions and loss of consciousness.

KEY TERMS:

anticonvulsant: a therapeutic drug that prevents or diminishes convulsions

aura: a sensory symptom or group of such symptoms that precedes a grand mal seizure

clonic phase: the portion of an epileptic seizure that is characterized by convulsions

electroencephalogram (EEG): a graphic recording of the electrical activity of the brain, as recorded by an electroencephalograph

grand mal: a type of epileptic seizure characterized by severe convulsions, body stiffening, and loss of consciousness during which victims fall down; also called tonic-clonic seizure

idiopathic disease: a disease of unknown origin

petit mal: a mild type of epileptic seizure characterized by a very short lapse of consciousness, usually without convulsions; the epileptic does not fall down

psychomotor epilepsy: condition of impairment of consciousness with amnesia of the episode which may include movements of the arms and legs and hallucinations

seizure: a sudden convulsive attack of epilepsy that can involve loss of consciousness and falling down

seizure discharges: characteristic brain waves seen in the EEGs of epileptics; their strength and frequency depend upon whether a seizure is occurring and its type

status epilepticus: a rare, life-threatening condition in which many sequential seizures occur without recovery between them

tonic-clonic seizure: another term for a grand mal seizure

tonic phase: the portion of an epileptic seizure characterized by loss of consciousness and body stiffness

CAUSES AND SYMPTOMS

Epilepsy is characterized by seizures, commonly called fits, which may involve convulsions and the loss of consciousness. It was called the "falling disease" or "sacred disease" in antiquity and was mentioned in 2080 B.C.E. in the laws of the famous Babylonian king Hamurabi. Epilepsy is a serious neurologic disease that usually appears between the ages of two and fourteen. It does not affect intelligence, as shown by the fact that the range of intelligence quotients (IQs) for epileptics is quite similar to that of the general population. In addition, many suspected epileptics have achieved fame, such as Alexander the Great, Julius Caesar, Russian novelist Fyodor Dostoevski, and Dutch artist Vincent van Gogh.

In 400 B.C.E., Hippocrates of Cos proposed that epilepsy arose from physical problems in the brain. This origin of the disease is now known to be unequivocally true. Despite many centuries of exhaustive study and effort, however, only a small percentage (20 percent) of cases of epilepsy caused by brain injuries, brain tumors, and other diseases are curable. This type of epilepsy is called symptomatic epilepsy. In contrast, 80 percent of epileptics can be treated to control the occurrence of seizures but cannot be cured of the disease, which is therefore a lifelong affliction. In these cases, the basis of the epilepsy is not known, although the suspected cause is genetically programmed brain damage that still evades discovery. Most epilepsy is, therefore, an idiopathic disease (one of unknown origin), and such epileptics are thus said to suffer from idiopathic epilepsy.

A common denominator in idiopathic epilepsy, and also in symptomatic epilepsy, is that it is evidenced by unusual electrical discharges, brain waves, seen in the electroencephalograms (EEGs) of epileptics. These brain waves are called seizure discharges. They vary in both their strength and their frequency, depending on whether an epileptic is having a seizure and what type of seizure is occurring. Seizure discharges are almost always present and recognizable in the EEGs of epileptics, even during sleep.

There are four types of common epileptic seizures. Two of these are partial (local) seizures called focal motor and temporal lobe seizures, respectively. The

---

INFORMATION ON EPILEPSY

CAUSES: Brain injury, brain tumors, disease, possible genetic factors

SYMPTOMS: Seizures, loss of consciousness

DURATION: Typically chronic

TREATMENTS: Surgery to remove tumor or causative brain tissue abnormality, anticonvulsant drugs

others, grand mal and petit mal, are generalized and may involve the entire body. A focal motor seizure is characterized by rhythmic jerking of the facial muscles, an arm, or a leg. As with other epileptic seizures, it is caused by abnormal electrical discharges in the portion of the brain that controls normal movement in the body part that is affected. This abnormal electrical activity is always seen as seizure discharges in the EEG of the affected part of the brain.

In contrast, temporal lobe seizures (also known as psychomotor epilepsy), again characterized by seizure discharges in a distinct portion of the cerebrum of the brain, are characterized by sensory hallucinations and other types of consciousness alteration, a meaningless physical action, or even a babble of some incomprehensible language. Thus, for example, temporal lobe seizures may explain some cases of people "speaking in tongues" in religious experiences or in the days of the Delphic oracles of ancient Greece.

The term "grand mal" refers to the most severe type of epileptic seizure. Also called tonic-clonic seizures, grand mal attacks are characterized by very severe EEG seizure discharges throughout the entire brain. A grand mal seizure is usually preceded by sensory symptoms called an aura (probably related to temporal lobe seizures), which warn an epileptic of an impending attack. The aura is quickly followed by the grand mal seizure itself, which involves the loss of consciousness, localized or widespread jerking and convulsions, and severe body stiffness.

Epileptics suffering a grand mal seizure usually fall to the ground, may foam at the mouth, and often bite their tongues or the inside of their cheeks unless something is placed in the mouth before they lose consciousness. In a few cases, the victim will lose bladder or bowel control. In untreated epileptics, grand mal seizures can occur weekly. Most of these attacks last for only a minute or two, followed quickly by full recovery after a brief sense of disorientation and feelings of severe exhaustion. In some cases, however, grand mal seizures may last for up to five minutes and lead to temporary amnesia or to other mental deficits of a longer duration. In rare cases, the life-threatening condition of status epilepticus occurs, in which many sequential tonic-clonic seizures occur over several hours without recovery between them.

The fourth type of epileptic seizure is petit mal, which is often called generalized nonconvulsive seizure or, more simply, absence. A petit mal seizure consists of a brief period of loss of consciousness (ten to

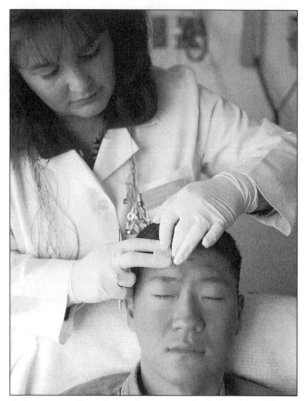

A doctor attaches electrodes to a patient's head in order to monitor his epilepsy. (PhotoDisc)

forty seconds) without the epileptic falling down. The epileptic usually appears to be daydreaming (absent) and shows no other symptoms. Often a victim of a petit mal seizure is not even aware that the event has occurred. In some cases, a petit mal seizure is accompanied by mild jerking of hands, head, or facial features and/or rapid blinking of the eyes. Petit mal attacks can be quite dangerous if they occur while an epileptic is driving a motor vehicle.

Diagnosing epilepsy usually requires a patient history, a careful physical examination, blood tests, and a neurologic examination. The patient history is most valuable when it includes eyewitness accounts of the symptoms, the frequency of occurrence, and the usual duration range of the seizures observed. In addition, documentation of any preceding severe trauma, infection, or episodes of addictive drug exposure provides useful information that will often differentiate between idiopathic and symptomatic epilepsy.

Evidence of trauma is quite important, as head injuries that caused unconsciousness are often the basis for later symptomatic epilepsy. Similarly, infectious diseases of the brain, including meningitis and encephalitis, can cause this type of epilepsy. Finally, excessive use of alcohol or other psychoactive drugs can also be a causative agent for symptomatic epilepsy.

Blood tests for serum glucose and calcium, electroencephalography, and computed tomography (CT) scanning are also useful diagnostic tools. The EEG will nearly always show seizure discharges in epileptics, and the location of the discharges in the brain may localize problem areas associated with the disease. CT scanning is most useful for identifying tumors and other serious brain damage that may cause symptomatic epilepsy. When all tests are negative except for abnormal EEGs, the epilepsy is considered idiopathic.

It is thought that the generation of epileptic symptoms occurs because of a malfunction in nerve impulse transport in some of the billions of nerve cells (neurons) that make up the brain and link it to the body organs that it innervates. This nerve impulse transport is an electrochemical process caused by the ability of the neurons to retain substances (including potassium) and to excrete substances (including sodium). This ability generates the weak electrical current that makes up a nerve impulse and that is registered by electroencephalography.

A nerve impulse leaves a given neuron via an outgoing extension (or axon), passes across a tiny synaptic gap that separates the axon from the next neuron in line, and enters an incoming extension (or dendrite) of that cell. The process is repeated until the impulse is transmitted to its site of action. The cell bodies of neurons make up the gray matter of the brain, and axons and dendrites (white matter) may be viewed as connecting wires.

Passage across synaptic gaps between neurons is mediated by chemicals called neurotransmitters, and it is now believed that epilepsy results when unknown materials cause abnormal electrical impulses by altering neurotransmitter production rates and/or the ability of sodium, potassium, and related substances to enter or leave neurons. The various nervous impulse abnormalities that cause epilepsy can be shown to occur in the portions of the gray matter of the cerebrum that control high-brain functions. For example, the frontal lobe—which controls speech, body movement, and eye movements—is associated with temporal lobe seizures.

TREATMENT AND THERAPY

Idiopathic epilepsy is viewed as the expression of a large group of different diseases, all of which present themselves clinically as seizures. This is extrapolated from the various types of symptomatic epilepsy observed, which have causes that include faulty biochemical processes (such as inappropriate calcium levels), brain tumors or severe brain injury, infectious diseases (such as encephalitis), and the chronic overuse of addictive drugs. As to why idiopathic epilepsy causes are not identifiable, the general biomedical wisdom states that present technology is too imprecise to detect its causes.

Symptomatic epilepsy is treated with medication and either by the extirpation of the tumor or other causative brain tissue abnormality that was engendered by trauma or disease or by the correction of the metabolic disorder involved. The more common, incurable idiopathic disease is usually treated entirely with medication that relieves symptoms. This treatment is essential because without it most epileptics cannot attend school successfully, maintain continued employment, or drive a motor vehicle safely.

A large number of anticonvulsant drugs are presently available for epilepsy management. It must, however, be made clear that no one therapeutic drug will control all types of seizures. In addition, some patients require several such drugs for effective therapy, and the natural history of a given case of epilepsy may often require periodic changes from drug to drug as the disease evolves. Furthermore, every therapeutic antiepilepsy drug has dangerous side effects that may occur when it is present in the body above certain levels or after it is used beyond some given time period. Therefore, each epileptic patient must be monitored at frequent intervals to ascertain that no dangerous physical symptoms are developing and that the drug levels in the body (monitored by the measurement of drug content in blood samples) are within a tolerable range.

More than twenty antiepilepsy drugs are widely used. Phenytoin (Dilantin) is very effective for grand mal seizures. Because of its slow metabolism, phenytoin can be administered relatively infrequently, but this slow metabolism also requires seven to ten days before its anticonvulsant effects occur. Side effects include cosmetically unpleasant hair overgrowth, swelling of the gums, and skin rash. These symptoms are particularly common in epileptic children. More serious are central nervous effects including ataxia (unsteadiness in walking), drowsiness, anemia, and marked thyroid deficiency. Most such symptoms are reversed by decreasing the drug doses or by discontinuing it. Phenytoin is often given together with other antiepilepsy drugs to produce optimum seizure prevention. In those cases, great care must be taken to prevent dangerous synergistic drug effects from occurring. High phenytoin doses also produce blood levels of the drug that are very close to toxic 25 micrograms per milliliter values.

Carbamazepine (Tegretol) is another frequently used antiepileptic drug. Chemically related to the drugs used as antidepressants, it is useful against both psychomotor epilepsy and grand mal seizures. Common carbamazepine side effects are ataxia, drowsiness, and double vision. A more dangerous, and fortunately less common, side effect is the inability of bone marrow to produce blood cells. Again, very serious and unexpected complications occur in mixed-drug therapy that includes carbamazepine, and at high doses toxic blood levels of the drug may be exceeded.

Phenobarbital, a sedative hypnotic also used as a tranquilizer by nonepileptics, is a standby for treating epilepsy. It too can have serious side effects, including a lowered attention span, hyperactivity, and learning difficulties. In addition, when given with phenytoin, phenobarbital will speed up the excretion of that drug, lowering its effective levels.

Four major lessons can be learned from these three drugs. First, individual antiepilepsy drugs have many different side effects. Second, there are concrete reasons that epileptics taking therapeutic drugs must be monitored carefully for physical symptoms. Third, at high antiepileptic drug doses, the blood levels attained may closely approximate and even exceed toxic values. Fourth, drug interactions in mixed-drug therapy can be counterproductive.

A new generation of antiepileptic medications that act by various mechanisms is now available. These drugs, which include gabapentin, lamotrigine, topiramate, tiagabine, levetiracetam, zonisamide, oxcarbazepine, and pregabalin, are often better tolerated, safer, and faster acting than the older generation of antiepileptics. However, the efficacy of both the newer and older drugs to prevent seizures remains highly dependent on the individual patient.

About 20 percent of idiopathic epileptics do not achieve adequate seizure control after prolonged and varied drug therapy. Another option for some—but not all—such people is brain surgery. This type of brain surgery is usually elected after two conditions are met. First, often-repeated EEGs must show that most or all of the portion of the brain in which the seizures develop is very localized. Second, these affected areas must be in a brain region that the patient can lose without significant mental loss (often in the prefrontal or temporal cerebral lobes). When such surgery is carried out, it is reported that 50 to 75 percent of the patients who are treated and given chronic, postoperative antiepilepsy drugs become able to achieve seizure control.

The most frequent antiepilepsy surgery is temporal lobectomy. The brain has two temporal lobes, one of which is dominant in the control of language, memory, and thought expression. A temporal lobectomy is carried out by removing the nondominant temporal lobe, when it is the site of epilepsy. About 6 percent of temporal lobectomies lead to a partial loss of temporal lobe functions, which may include impaired vision, movement, memory, and speech.

Another common type of antiepilepsy surgery is called corpus callosotomy. This procedure involves partially disconnecting the two cerebral hemispheres by severing some of the nerves in the corpus callosum that links them. This surgery is performed when an epileptic has frequent, uncontrollable grand mal attacks that cause many dangerous falls. The procedure usually results in reduced numbers of seizures and decreases in their severity.

Physicians now believe that many cases of epilepsy may be prevented by methods aimed at avoiding head injury (especially in children) and the use of techniques such as amniocentesis to identify potential epileptics and treat them before birth. Furthermore, the prophylactic administration of antiepilepsy drugs to nonepileptic people who are afflicted with encephalitis and other diseases known to produce epilepsy is viewed as wise.

Perspective and Prospects

A great number of advances have occurred in the treatment of epilepsy via therapeutic drugs and surgical techniques. With the exception of symptomatic epilepsy, drug therapy has been the method of choice because it is less drastic than surgery, is easier to manage, and rarely has the potential for irreversible damage to patients that can be caused by the removal of a portion of the brain. The main antiepileptic drugs are phenytoin, carbamazepine, and phenobarbital, but a tremendous variety of other chemical therapies has been investigated and utilized successfully.

Such treatments include the new generation of antiepileptic drugs, high doses of vitamins, injections of muscle relaxants, and changes in diet. The variety is unsurprising, considering the vast number of disease states that can cause seizures. For example, the rare genetic disease phenylketonuria (PKU) can cause epilepsy. Phenylketonuric epilepsy is often treated by use of a ketogenic diet rich in fats; the clear value of this treatment is unexplained. Readers are encouraged to investigate the many epilepsy treatments that have not been noted. Such an examination may be quite valuable because there are about a million epileptics in the United States alone, and some estimates indicate that four of every thousand humans are likely to develop some epileptic symptoms during their lifetime.

Modern surgical treatment of epilepsy reportedly began in 1828, with the efforts of Benjamin Dudley, who removed epilepsy-causing blood clots and skull fragments from five patients, who all survived despite primitive and nonsterile operating rooms. The next landmark in such surgery was the removal of a brain tumor by the German physician R. J. Godlee, in 1884, without the benefit of X rays or EEG techniques, which did not then exist.

By the 1950's EEGs were used to locate epileptic brain foci, and physicians such as the Canadians Wilder Penfield and Herbert Jasper pioneered their use to locate brain regions to remove for epilepsy remission without damaging vital functions. After considerable evolution over the course of forty years, antiepilepsy surgery by the 1990's had become widespread, commonplace, and relatively safe.

Nevertheless, because of the imperfections of all available methodologies, 5 to 8 percent of epileptics cannot achieve seizure control by any method or method combination, and even the "well-managed" epilepsy treatment regimen has its flaws. There is still much to be learned about curing epilepsy. Clinical and experimental perioperative studies are now possible during epilepsy surgery to examine the bioelectrical activity and molecular events of the affected neurons. It is hoped that the efforts of ongoing biomedical research, both in basic science and in clinical settings, will eliminate epilepsy through the development of new therapeutic drugs and sophisticated advances in surgery and other nondrug methods.

—Sanford S. Singer, Ph.D.;
updated by W. Michael Zawada, Ph.D.

See also Auras; Brain; Brain damage; Brain disorders; Brain tumors; Computed tomography (CT) scanning; Electroencephalography (EEG); Nervous system; Neuroimaging; Neurology; Neurology, pediatric; Neurosurgery; Phenylketonuria (PKU); Seizures; Unconsciousness.

FOR FURTHER INFORMATION:
Beers, Mark H., et al. *The Merck Manual of Diagnosis and Therapy*. 18th ed. Whitehouse Station, N.J.: Merck Research Laboratories, 2006. Contains a compendium of data on the characteristics, etiology, diagnosis, and treatment of adult epilepsy. Also discusses seizure disorders of children and newborns. Designed for physicians, the material is also useful to less specialized readers.
Bloom, Floyd E., M. Flint Beal, and David J. Kupfer, eds. *The Dana Guide to Brain Health*. New York: Simon & Schuster, 2003. An easy-to-understand health guide to the brain from neuroscience, neurology, and psychiatry perspectives. More than seventy psychiatric and neurological disorders, their diagnoses, and their treatments are covered.
Devinsky, Orrin. *Epilepsy: Patient and Family Guide*. 2d ed. Philadelphia: F. A. Davis, 2002. An excellent lay guide to the medical and social topics relevant to epilepsy. Topics include diagnosis and treatment, epilepsy in children and adults, legal and financial issues, and research resources.
Epilepsy Foundation. http://www.epilepsyfoundation.org/. A national organization dedicated to education, research, and advocacy. Web site offers information on careers and employment, parent support groups and children's programs, and online "Interest Groups," among many other features.
Freeman, John M., Eileen P. G. Vining, and Diana J. Pillas. *Seizures and Epilepsy in Childhood: A Guide*. 3d ed. Baltimore: Johns Hopkins University Press, 2002. Designed for parents, an overall guide to the symptoms, diagnosis, and treatment of children with epilepsy. Third edition includes new chapters on alternative therapies and medicines, routine health care, insurance issues, and research resources.
Gumnit, Robert J. *Living Well with Epilepsy*. 2d ed. New York: Demos Vermande, 1997. Designed to give people with epilepsy the outlook necessary to live successfully with the disease. Among the topics covered are causes and treatment, high-quality care, medical and surgical options, the problems of epileptic children, sexuality and pregnancy, the workplace, rights, and resources.
Hopkins, Anthony, and Richard Appleton. *Epilepsy: The Facts*. 2d ed. New York: Oxford University Press, 1996. The author wishes to eliminate misunderstanding about epilepsy and educate people about it. This is done nicely by clear coverage of topics including explanation of epilepsy, seizure types and

causes, epilepsy treatment methods, and information on living with the disease.

Nolte, John. *Human Brain: An Introduction to Its Functional Anatomy*. 5th ed. St. Louis: Mosby, 2001. Text covering major concepts and structure-function relationships in the human neurological system.

Weaver, Donald F. *Epilepsy and Seizures: Everything You Need to Know*. Toronto: Firefly Books, 2001. A lay guide covering research advances, history of the disease, different types, the mechanisms, diagnosis and treatment, and special situations, such as epilepsy in pregnant women, children, and the elderly.

EPISIOTOMY

PROCEDURE

ANATOMY OR SYSTEM AFFECTED: Anus, genitals, reproductive system

SPECIALTIES AND RELATED FIELDS: Gynecology, obstetrics

DEFINITION: A surgical cut made in the pelvic floor to enlarge the vagina for the facilitation of childbirth.

INDICATIONS AND PROCEDURES

An episiotomy is performed to enlarge the vaginal opening and ease the delivery of a baby during childbirth. While not a routine procedure, some circumstances which indicate the need for an episiotomy include macrosomia (large fetal size), rapid delivery, breech delivery, and presentation of the baby with face to the front of the birth canal, all of which prevent the perineum (the area between the vagina and the anus) from stretching rapidly enough to prevent tearing. Scarring from vaginal surgeries also limits the ability of the vagina to expand.

During the procedure, a local anesthetic is injected into the perineum. The obstetrician uses straight-bladed blunt scissors to snip the tissue between the vagina and anus, avoiding the anal sphincter muscle. After delivery, the incision is carefully stitched together, along with any minor tears in the birth canal.

USES AND COMPLICATIONS

The birth canal has very limited space to accommodate an infant, and situations such as feet-first or face-forward presentation can lead to compression of the umbilical cord and interruption of the oxygen supply to the baby, or even to potential crushing of the infant. An episiotomy can facilitate a rapid delivery in these circumstances, thereby preventing serious injury to the infant. Failure of the perineum to stretch sufficiently to accommodate the child can result in severe, irregular tears of the vagina and even of the anal sphincter muscles. Ragged tears are very difficult to repair surgically and are much more prone to infection. Tearing of the anal sphincter could lead to permanent incontinence. The easily repaired incisions of episiotomy eliminate these potential difficulties.

Healing of the incisions is rapid and straightforward, but the area may itch and be somewhat painful for a few weeks. Painkilling drugs may be prescribed, and ice packs can be used to alleviate pain. Women who do not desire episiotomies and have controlled, problem-free deliveries may try to stretch the perineum gradually by massaging it with warm oil during the delivery. While in the past, episiotomies were considered a routine part of delivery, they are now done less commonly, only as necessitated for conditions like those indicated above. Additionally, maternal satisfaction is increasing as episiotomies are being done more when they are necessary and to a lesser extent when they are avoidable.

—*Karen E. Kalumuck, Ph.D.;*
updated by Robin Kamienny Montvilo, Ph.D.

See also Childbirth; Childbirth complications; Incontinence; Obstetrics; Women's health.

FOR FURTHER INFORMATION:

Carlson, Karen J., Stephanie A. Eisenstat, and Terra Ziporyn. *The New Harvard Guide to Women's Health*. Cambridge, Mass.: Harvard University Press, 2004.

Cunningham, F. Gary, et al., eds. *Williams Obstetrics*. 22d ed. New York: McGraw-Hill, 2005.

Goldberg, Roger P. *Ever Since I Had My Baby: Understanding, Treating, and Preventing the Most Common Physical After-Effects of Pregnancy and Childbirth*. New York: Crown, 2003.

Gonik, Bernard, and Renee A. Bobrowski. *Medical Complications in Labor and Delivery*. Cambridge, Mass.: Blackwell Scientific, 1996.

Machisio, Sara, et al. "Care Pathways in Obstetrics: The Effectiveness in Reducing the Incidence of Episiotomy in Childbirth." *Journal of Nursing Management* 14, no. 7 (October, 2006): 538-543.

Reynolds, Karina, Christoph Lees, and Grainne McCarten. *Pregnancy and Birth: Your Questions Answered*. Rev. ed. New York: DK, 2002.

Sears, William, and Martha Sears. *The Birth Book*. Boston: Little, Brown, 1994.

Simkin, Penny, Janet Whalley, and Ann Keppler. *Pregnancy, Childbirth, and the Newborn: The Complete*

Guide. 3d ed. Minnetonka, Minn.: Meadowbrook Press, 2003.

Stoppard, Miriam. *Conception, Pregnancy, and Birth.* Rev. ed. New York: DK, 2000.

Warhus, Susan. *Countdown to Baby: Answers to the One Hundred Most Asked Questions About Pregnancy and Childbirth.* Omaha, Nebr.: Addicus Books, 2003.

EPSTEIN-BARR VIRUS

DISEASE/DISORDER

ALSO KNOWN AS: Human herpesvirus 4 (HHV-4)

ANATOMY OR SYSTEM AFFECTED: Blood, cells, glands, immune system, lymphatic system, mouth, muscles, nose, throat

SPECIALTIES AND RELATED FIELDS: Cytology, hematology, immunology, microbiology, oncology, pathology, pediatrics, virology

DEFINITION: An extensively occurring virus which infects almost all humans during their lifetime, often remaining latent in their systems but sometimes causing malignant tumors and various types of cancer.

KEY TERMS:

antibodies: protein molecules that detect antigens and destroy infected host cells

antigens: viral proteins that attract antibodies, which the immune system designs to attack them

B cells: also known as B lymphocytes; white blood cells that create antibodies

oncoviruses: viruses causing the growth of cancerous cells

replication: the viral insertion of genetic information into host cell nuclei to create additional similar viruses

T cells: also known as cytotoxic T lymphocytes; white blood cells that destroy cells hosting antigens or infected by pathogens which eluded antibodies

virion: a viral particle that contains genetic information inside a protective structure

CAUSES AND SYMPTOMS

Present only in humans, Epstein-Barr virus was the first documented oncovirus. The virus, resembling other human herpesviruses, consists of sphere-shaped, barbed virions approximately 120 to 220 nanometers in diameter. Each Epstein-Barr virus genome contains two strands of deoxyribonucleic acid (DNA). A protein shell protects the genome, and an envelope surrounds the protein shell. Various Epstein-Barr virus strains have evolved that can infect an individual at the same time.

The Epstein-Barr virus typically infects salivary gland cells or B cells. Usually, Epstein-Barr viral infections are transmitted through saliva. Seeking host cells in order to replicate, the Epstein-Barr virus proliferates, creating approximately one hundred types of antigens, including nuclear antigen EBNA 1, which the Epstein-Barr virus uses to put its DNA into new cells created during cell division.

T cells fight Epstein-Barr virus antigens by destroying infected host cells. T cells and antibodies stay in the immune system to continue protecting against infection, regulating latency, and developing immunity. EBNA1 is necessary for the Epstein-Barr virus genomes to endure being latent. T cells cannot detect the antigen EBNA1 and attack those host cells, which results in the Epstein-Barr virus often being invisible to immune protection. Latent infections are not apparent, usually remaining passive, but they can become active, potentially resulting in tumors and diseases.

The Epstein-Barr virus usually infects throat, blood, or immune system cells. Infectious mononucleosis, also known as glandular fever, is the most widely known Epstein-Barr viral infection. Physicians determine if people have been infected by Epstein-Barr virus by performing laboratory tests analyzing blood samples to detect if any of the antibodies to combat Epstein-Barr virus antigens are present and, if so, how many are present. Such antibodies might have existed for years and are not proof of an active infection.

People can contract the virus as children, adolescents, or adults, depending on their geographic location and socioeconomic factors. Some infants are born with the virus transmitted by their mothers. The Epstein-Barr virus usually infects people when they are chil-

---

INFORMATION ON EPSTEIN-BARR VIRUS

CAUSES: Viral infection spread primarily through saliva

SYMPTOMS: In children, usually none; in adolescents and adults, often mononucleosis; associated with a number of cancers and other diseases

DURATION: Acute and then chronic

TREATMENTS: None for viral infection; chemotherapy and radiation for resulting cancers

dren, without obvious signs. Often, these individuals never know that they are infected. Approximately half of the people who contract the Epstein-Barr virus as an adolescent or at an older age, however, develop infectious mononucleosis.

Activated Epstein-Barr virus can result in several serious diseases, and people with suppressed immune systems are vulnerable to developing such malignancies as cancerous tumors in smooth muscle tissue, stomach carcinomas, lymphomas, and sarcomas. Epstein-Barr virus often causes nasal and throat cancers known as nasopharyngeal carcinoma. In some individuals with acquired immunodeficiency syndrome (AIDS), Epstein-Barr virus replicates in tongue cells, resulting in oral hairy leukoplakia. Epstein-Barr virus has also been associated with leukemia.

Weak immune systems cause people to be vulnerable to Epstein-Barr virus infections, particularly after organ transplantation and the use of immunosuppressive drugs to lower the immune reaction and encourage acceptance of the new organ. In those cases, Epstein-Barr virus sometimes causes post-transplant lymphoproliferative disease to occur.

When it infects the nodes, Epstein-Barr virus might be a factor in people affected by Hodgkin's disease. Researchers have considered a possible role of Epstein-Barr virus in the development of multiple sclerosis and breast cancer. They have eliminated it as a factor in chronic fatigue syndrome.

TREATMENT AND THERAPY

Approximately 90 to 95 percent of humans globally at any time have been infected with Epstein-Barr virus, which remains latent and endures in their bodies until death. There is currently no way to eliminate the virus once infection has occurred. Treatment focuses instead on the diseases that Epstein-Barr virus causes.

Researchers have attempted to develop antiviral vaccines to stop the replication of Epstein-Barr virus. In the early twenty-first century, scientists at Queensland Institute of Medical Research developed a vaccine prototype to strengthen T cells combatting Epstein-Barr virus antigens.

PERSPECTIVE AND PROSPECTS

The Epstein-Barr virus was located as a result of researchers seeking viruses possibly associated with cancer in humans. In 1961, London researcher M. Anthony Epstein attended a lecture at which Denis P. Burkitt discussed his work with tumors, later called Burkitt's lymphoma, in African children's facial bones. Epstein, experienced with investigating viruses causing animal tumors, wanted to examine Burkitt's lymphoma tumor tissues to detect any viruses. The British Empire Cancer Campaign funded Epstein's travel to Uganda to acquire a consistent supply of tumor samples for his Middlesex Hospital Medical School laboratory. Epstein tried unsuccessfully to locate a virus for a couple of years.

The U.S. National Cancer Institute presented Epstein $45,000 for his investigations, and he hired doctoral student Yvonne M. Barr and colleague Bert G. Achong to expand his laboratory work attempting to culture viruses. The trio successfully grew a Burkitt's lymphoma cell line in culture. When cells from that sample were examined with an electron microscope, the London scientists saw viral particles with structural elements of herpesvirus. Scrutinizing the virions, the trio declared that they had isolated a previously unknown human herpesvirus. They published their results in a 1964 Lancet article. After Epstein-Barr virus was identified, additional investigators studied the virus to expand knowledge of its structure, replication, and the diseases associated with it, determining that it was an oncovirus.

Research into ways to fight Epstein-Barr virus is ongoing. Scientists at the European Molecular Biology Laboratory and Institut de Virologie Moléculaire et Structurale have focused on controlling a protein molecule known as ZEBRA which accompanies Epstein-Barr virus, helping activate it from the latent phase.

—Elizabeth D. Schafer, Ph.D.

See also Acquired immunodeficiency syndrome (AIDS); Burkitt's lymphoma; Cancer; Carcinoma; Carcinogens; Ewing's sarcoma; Herpes; Leukemia; Lymphadenopathy and lymphoma; Lymphatic system; Mononucleosis; Oncology; Sarcoma; Transplantation; Tumors; Viral infections.

FOR FURTHER INFORMATION:

Epstein, M. Anthony, and Bert G. Achong, eds. *The Epstein-Barr Virus*. New York: Springer-Verlag, 1979.

Robertson, Erle S., ed. *Epstein-Barr Virus*. Wymondham, Norfolk, England: Caister Academic Press, 2005.

Tselis, Alex C., and Hal B. Jenson, eds. *Epstein-Barr Virus*. New York: Taylor & Francis, 2006.

Umar, Constantine S., ed. *New Developments in Epstein-Barr Virus Research*. New York: Nova Science, 2006.

Wilson, Joanna B., and Gerhard H. W. May, eds. *Epstein-Barr Virus Protocols*. Totowa, N.J.: Humana Press, 2001.

Ergogenic aids

Biology

Also known as: Blood doping, steroids, caffeine, growth hormone, creatine

Anatomy or system affected: Blood, brain, cells, circulatory system, endocrine system, genitals, glands, heart, joints, kidneys, liver, musculoskeletal system

Specialties and related fields: Biochemistry, endocrinology, ethics, exercise physiology, family medicine, hematology, internal medicine, nephrology, orthopedics, pharmacology, psychology, sports medicine, toxicology

Definition: Substances used by athletes in an effort to gain an advantage. Most of these substances are illegal and unethical within competitive sports.

Introduction

In the history of sport, athletes have attempted to find a competitive advantage through advanced techniques in training, nutrition, and even in ergogenic aids, such as nutritional supplements and pharmacological aids. The use of these substances—such as anabolic-androgenic steroids (AAS), testosterone precursors (such as androstenedione), and nonsteroidal aids such as human growth hormone (GH) and creatine—have become increasingly popular in recent years, even without thorough scientific data supporting their efficacy and safety.

The population using such performance-enhancing drugs ranges from collegiate to professional athletes to adolescents and high school students. Recent meta-analyses estimate that 3 to 12 percent of adolescent boys have used an anabolic steroid at least once, and 28 percent of collegiate athletes admit to taking creatine. Other studies have suggested that the number may be closer to 41 percent.

Though such ergogenic aids are thought to improve strength, endurance, agility, and overall performance, most athletic improvement is anecdotal at best. Scientific evidence supporting these ideas is scarce and incomplete. Even with aids that may improve strength and/or performance, the safety of these substances has been seriously questioned, such as with the use of AAS, GH, and ephedra.

Types of Ergogenic Aids

Anabolic-androgenic steroids (AAS) as ergogenic aids in sports are chemical compounds that resemble the structure of testosterone, the naturally occurring male sex hormone that affects muscle growth and strength. "Anabolic" refers to the growth of cells, and "androgenic" refers to the stimulation of the growth of male sex organs and masculine sex characteristics. AAS bind to cells that are used for muscle repair and that can transform into muscle fibers.

AAS has been one of the most studied ergogenic aids, yet many of its mechanisms and adverse effects are still not well understood. Studies have shown that increased doses of testosterone can decrease total body adipose tissue in the body and can increase strength and fat-free mass. Adverse effects of AAS use include hypothalamic-pituitary dysfunction, gynecomastia, severe acne, infection as a result of sharing needles, aggressive and depressive behavior, and a possible association with premature death.

Androstenedione (andro) is a testosterone precursor produced by the adrenal glands and gonads. Its ergogenic effect occurs after it is converted to testosterone in the testes as well as in other tissues. It can also be converted to estrone and estradiol, which are steroid compounds that are primary female sex hormones (found in both men and women). The creation of testosterone is regulated by the amount of testosterone precursors in the body. Theoretically, an increase in androstenedione would increase the production of testosterone and thus can increase protein synthesis, lean body mass, and strength.

Older studies showed that andro supplementation results in increased serum testosterone levels. However, more recent studies have shown that andro supplementation fails to directly improve lean body mass, muscular strength, or serum testosterone levels. Possible side effects to andro use are suppressed testosterone production, liver dysfunction, cardiovascular disease, testicular atrophy, baldness, acne, and aggressive behavior.

Similar to androstenedione, dihydroepiandrosterone (DHEA) is a precursor of testosterone and is also formed in the adrenal glands and gonads. DHEA is the most abundant steroid hormone in circulation and is a precursor to androstenedione and other testosterone precursors (such as androstenediol). Studies of DHEA supplementation have not been shown to increase lean body mass, strength, or testosterone levels. Possible side effects are similar to andro and AAS use.

Human growth hormone (GH) is a metabolic hormone that is secreted into the blood by cells found in the anterior pituitary gland. After its secretion, GH stimulates the production of insulin-like growth factor (IGF)-1 in the liver. These hormones stimulate bone growth, protein synthesis, and the conversion of fat to energy. Athletes have been attracted to GH not only because of such theoretical benefits but also because of the limited techniques in detecting GH in the urine. GH levels vary in individuals of different, ages, sex, and activity and can vary throughout the day, so no reliable benchmark can be made to determine if illicit use has taken place.

Scientific studies have been unable to show that GH leads to increased muscle strength and exercise performance or changes in protein synthesis. Because of ethical limitations, it is difficult to study the effect of larger doses of GH on healthy individuals. Adverse effects of GH use include cosmetic damage, joint pain, muscle weakness, fluid retention, impaired glucose regulation (which may lead to diabetes mellitus), cardiomyopathy, hyperlipidemia, and possibly death.

Erythropoietin (EPO) is a hormone secreted by the kidneys that is a precursor to bone marrow. EPO increases the oxygen-carrying capacity of blood and, as a result, aids in endurance and aerobic respiration. The appeal of EPO among athletes is this endurance-enhancing effect. As a result, many abusers have been found to be skiers, cyclists, and other athletes who require high levels of endurance. Early use of EPO as an ergogenic aid, termed "blood doping," came in the form of autologous blood transfusions, in which athletes would harvest their own red blood cells and reintroduce them into their systems before events. Recently, the use of recombinant human erythropoietin (r-HuEPO) via injection has become more widespread.

Scientific studies have shown that EPO and r-HuEPO treatments do increase certain blood concentrations and can aid in endurance. EPO may also have serious and dangerous side effects, however, such as hypertension, seizures, thromboembolic events, and possibly death.

Creatine monohydrate is an amine synthesized in the kidneys, pancreas, and liver, and it can also be obtained through the diet from meat and fish. Approximately 90 to 95 percent of creatine in the body is found in skeletal muscle. Creatine, which is converted to creatine phosphate (PCr), is an important limiting factor in the resynthesis of adenosine triphosphate (ATP), which plays a significant role in energy reserves within the body. Theoretically, an increase of PCr in the body would in-

crease the regeneration of ATP, resulting in an increase in sustained maximal energy production for short-term exercise. This could lead to increased intensity and repetition frequency, and thus possible increases in skeletal muscle mass.

In 2002, A. M. Bohn and colleagues argued in an article in *Current Sports Medicine Reports* that there are "no studies demonstrating benefit with the relatively indiscriminant use of variable amounts of creatine by large numbers of athletes on a specific team." Nevertheless, creatine has been shown to enhance performance in small populations of athletes of various sports. Possible adverse effects of creatine include muscle cramping, dehydration, gastrointestinal distress, weight gain, increased risk of muscle tears, inhibited insulin and creatine production, renal damage, and possibly nephropathy.

Stimulants are drugs that increase nervous system activity. Examples of stimulants commonly used as ergogenic aids include the class of drugs called amphetamines, as well as specific chemical compounds such as caffeine and ephedrine. The use of caffeine has been shown to improve exercise time to exhaustion and may even significantly increase intestinal glucose absorption. It has been suggested that caffeine increases fat utilization for energy and delays the depletion of glycogen (the stored form of glucose). As a result, caffeine and other stimulants are popular ergogenic aids for extended aerobic activity.

Caffeine in small doses has been shown to increase performance. Possible adverse effects of caffeine may include anxiety, dependency, withdrawal, and possibly a diuretic effect (dehydration). Ephedrine may have similar adverse affects. Other stimulants, such as amphetamines or cocaine, have more serious and detrimental effects.

Perspective and Prospects

The use of ergogenic aids in the history of sport has progressively moved from primitive aids to more sophisticated performance enhancers. Crude natural concoctions and stimulants have paved the way for complex pharmacological agents (such as erythropoietin) and designer anabolic steroids (such as tetrahydrogestrinone). Athletes and trainers have utilized any and all means to gain a competitive edge, even if that results in damage to health and even a risk of death.

The biggest problem stemming from the use of such aids is the difficulty in detecting them. This is evident in recent media attention given to ergogenic aids and their popularity, as seen through the 1995 congressional hearings regarding steroid use in Major League Baseball as well as the recent discoveries of abuse by high-profile cyclists and track-and-field athletes. This media attention has also shown the difficulties among investigators, such as the International Olympic Committee (IOC) and United States Anti-Doping Agency, in detecting the use of new designer steroids and new ergogenic aids among elite athletes.

—*Julien M. Cobert and Jeffrey R. Bytomski, D.O.*

See also Blood and blood disorders; Blood testing; Caffeine; Ethics; Exercise physiology; Hormones; Hypertrophy; Metabolism; Muscles; Pharmacology; Sports medicine; Steroid use; Steroids.

FOR FURTHER INFORMATION:

Bhazin, S., et al. "The Effects of Supraphysiologic Doses of Testosterone on Muscle Size and Strength in Normal Men." *New England Journal of Medicine* 335 (1996): 1-7.

Bohn, Amy Miller, Stephanie Betts, and Thomas L. Schwenk. "Creatine and Other Nonsteroidal Strength-Enhancing Aids." *Current Sports Medicine Reports* 1, no. 4 (August, 2002): 239-245.

Foster, Zoë J., and Jeffrey A. Housner. "Anabolic-Andogenic Steroids and Testosterone Precursors: Ergogenic Aids and Sport." *Current Sports Medicine Reports* 3, no. 4 (August, 2004): 234-241.

Graham, T. E. "Caffeine and Exercise: Metabolism, Endurance, and Performance." *Sports Medicine* 31, no. 11 (November 1, 2001): 785-807.

Juhn, Mark S. "Ergogenic Aids in Aerobic Activity." *Current Sports Medicine Reports* 1, no. 4 (August, 2002): 233-238.

Powers, Michael E. "The Safety and Efficacy of Anabolic Steroid Precursors: What Is the Scientific Evidence?" *Journal of Athletic Training* 37, no. 3 (2002): 300-305.

Shekelle, Paul G., et al. "Efficacy and Safety of Ephedra and Ephedrine for Weight Loss and Athletic Performance: A Meta-analysis." *Journal of the American Medical Association* 289, no. 12 (March 26, 2003): 1537-1545.

Singbart, G. "Adverse Events of Erythropoietin in Long-Term and in Acute/Short-Term Treatment." *Clinical Investigation* 72 (1994): S36-S43.

Stacy, Jason J., Thomas R. Terrell, and Thomas D. Armsey. "Ergogenic Aids: Human Growth Hormone." *Current Sports Medicine Reports* 3, no. 4 (August, 2004): 229-233.

Yesalis, C. E., and M. S. Bahrke. "Doping Among Adolescent Athletes." *Baillieres Best Practice and Research in Clinical Endocrinology and Metabolism* 14, no. 1 (March, 2000): 25-35.

ESOPHAGEAL CANCER. *See* MOUTH AND THROAT CANCER.

ESTROGEN REPLACEMENT THERAPY. *See* HORMONE REPLACEMENT THERAPY (HRT).

ETHICS

ALSO KNOWN AS: Bioethics, medical ethics

DEFINITION: Ethics is a code of conduct based on established moral principles. Medical ethics is the study of the conduct of professionals in the field of medicine.

KEY TERMS:

autonomy: independence and self-reliance, especially referring to decision making

beneficence: doing good

informed consent: the dialogue between physician and patient prior to an invasive procedure

justice: the rationing of scarce resources according to a prearranged plan

nonmaleficence: avoiding evil

paternalism: acting in the manner of a father to his children

PRINCIPLES

Ethics deals with a code of conduct based on established moral principles. When applied to a particular professional field, abstract theories as well as concrete principles are considered. Often the consequences of a particular course of action dictate its rightness or wrongness. Bioethics is the study of ethics by professionals in the fields of medicine, law, philosophy, or theology. Some also refer to this area as applied ethics. The term "bioethics" is often used interchangeably with "medical ethics," but purists would define medical ethics as the study of conduct by professionals in the field of medicine. Codes of ethics promulgated by professional groups or associations define obligations governing members of a given profession.

Initial questions concerning medical ethics entail purpose, to whom a duty is owed (legal or moral) and how far that duty extends. Does it extend solely to patients, or does it extend to their families or to society as a whole? For example, public health obligations to society involve a duty to prevent disease, maintain the health of the populace, and oversee the delivery of health care.

In the 1972 article "Models for Ethical Practice in a Revolutionary Age," Robert M. Veatch proposed four models for ethical medicine. The first is the engineering model, in which the physician becomes an applied scientist interested in treating disease rather than caring for a patient. The Nazi physicians during World War II acting as so-called scientists and technicians are examples of the engineering model taken to its extreme. The second is the priestly model, in which the physician assumes a paternalistic role of moral dominance, treating the patient as a child. The main principle of this model is the traditional one of *primum non nocere*, or "first do no harm." It neglects principles of patient autonomy, dignity, and freedom. The third is the collegial model, in which physician and patient are colleagues cooperating in pursuing a common goal, such as preserving health, curing illness, or easing pain. This model requires mutual trust and confidence, demanding a continued dialogue between the parties. The fourth is the contractual model, in which the relationship between health care provider and patient is analogous to a legal contract, with rights and obligations on both sides. The contractual model can be modified to provide for shared decision making and cooperation between physician and patient and tailored to the particular physician-patient relationship involved, resulting in a collegial association.

Autonomy and informed consent. Since the Nuremberg trials, which presented horrible accounts of medical experimentation in Nazi concentration camps, the issue of consent has been one of primary importance. These basic concepts recognize an individual's uniqueness and inherent decision-making ability without coercion or undue influence from others. Respect for privacy and freedom are fundamental to human dignity. Even when people present difficult problems, such as being unconscious or in a coma, they must continue to be respected. Rational decision making by patients or their surrogates must be followed, and those with specialized knowledge or expertise are not authorized to impose their will on another person or limit that person's freedom.

Informed consent seeks to encourage open communication between patient and health care provider, to protect patients and research subjects from harm, and to encourage health care providers to act responsibly vis-à-vis patients and subjects, ultimately preserving autonomy and rational decision making. Especially applicable in invasive procedures, such as those involving surgery or treatments with serious risks, informed consent requires the presence of certain conditions, including a patient's competency or decision-making capacity, in order to understand the relative consequences of a proposed course of treatment and its effect on a patient's life and health. (Absent informed consent, an invasive procedure would constitute a legal cause of action in battery, or a harmful or offensive touching.) The health care provider must inform patients of alternative courses of action, if any, and the fact that patients have the option to refuse treatment, even if that alternative is contrary to the recommendation of the physician. The information conveyed to the patient must include the diagnosis, nature of the proposed treatment, known risks and consequences (excluding those that are too remote or improbable to bear significantly on the ultimate decision whether to proceed on a course of treatment, as well as those that are so well known that they are obvious to everyone), benefits from the proposed treatment, alternatives, prognosis without treatment, economic cost, and how the treatment plan will impact the patient's lifestyle. The patient should also be made aware that once given, an informed consent can be withdrawn. Hospital consent forms do not provide this type of information.

The information conveyed must be material and important to this patient, not a fictional reasonable and prudent person. A factor is material if it could change the decision of that patient. Inherent problems include speculation into the factors that would have a dramatic impact on the patient's life, requiring a dialogue between patient and health care provider. It is also important to recognize the role of the physician's time constraints as well as the patient's overall stress level while the information is being conveyed, including possible information overload. Not only must the information be conveyed adequately, but it must also be assimilated and understood. The ability of an individual to process information raises substantial issues about understanding. Comprehension is not always easily ascertainable. Sometimes a person's ability to make decisions is affected by problems of nonacceptance of information, even if it was comprehended. A patient may voluntarily waive informed consent, so that the patient asks not to be informed, thereby relieving the physician of the obligation to obtain informed consent and ultimately delegating decision-making authority to the physician.

Medical emergencies constitute exceptions to the informed consent requirement, provided that four conditions are met: The patient, whose wishes are unknown because no advance directive or living will exists, is incapable of giving consent because of the emergency; no surrogate is available; the medical condition poses a danger to the patient's life or seriously impairs the patient's health; and immediate treatment is required to avert the danger to life or health. This exception is justified on the grounds that consent can be assumed in cases in which a reasonable person would consent if informed. If the patient is not in imminent danger, or if consent can be obtained at a later time, the emergency exception does not apply. The second exception is the therapeutic privilege in which health care providers are justified in legitimately withholding information from a patient when they reasonably believe that disclosure will have an adverse effect on the patient's condition or health, as in the case of a depressed, emotionally drained, or unstable patient. Again, the decision is subjective, referring to this patient, decided on a case-by-case basis. The privilege does not apply if the health care provider withholds information based on the belief that the patient will refuse consent if told all the facts. In that instance, withholding information amounts to misrepresentation or deception.

Another ethical dilemma involving intentional deception or incomplete disclosure concerns the therapeutic use of placebos. One defense is that deception is moral when it is used for the patient's welfare.

Paternalism. From the Latin word *pater*, meaning "father," paternalism refers to controlling others as a father acts in his relationship with his children. In medical ethics, paternalism involves overriding one's own wishes in order to act to benefit or avert harm to the patient. Intervention by a health care provider to prevent competent patients from harming themselves is called strong paternalism. Strong paternalism is generally rejected by ethicists because of the view that health care providers do not know all the factors influencing the life of another person and therefore lack the competence to decide what is best for another person. Weak paternalism exists when the health care provider overrules the wishes of an incompetent or questionably competent patient. It is sometimes justified in nonemergencies without informed consent to relieve serious pain and suffering. Another example of weak paternalism is the temporary use of restraints, justified on the grounds that confused and disoriented patients are otherwise likely to injure themselves. When restraints are necessary, the surrogate is generally asked to give consent, recognizing that restraints, albeit temporary, constitute a limitation of one's liberty.

Beneficence and nonmaleficence. The principles of beneficence (doing good) and nonmaleficence (avoiding evil) are both expressed in the Hippocratic oath: "I will use treatment to help the sick according to my ability and judgment, but I will never use it to injure or wrong them." Each principle has a bearing on the other, and each is limited by the other. The obligations in beneficence are also limited by obligations to avoid evil. One may perform an act that risks evil if the following conditions are present (the principle of double effects): The action is good or morally indifferent; the agent intends a good effect; the evil effect is not the means to achieving good; and proportionality exists between good and evil. The principle of proportionality states that provided that an action does not go directly against the dignity of the individual, there must be a proportionate good to justify risking evil consequences. Items to be considered are the possible existence of an alternative means with less evil or no evil, the level of good intended and the level of evil risked, and the certitude or probability of good or evil. The latter is called the wedge principle, referring to the fact that putting the tip of a wedge into a crack in a log and striking the wedge will split the log and destroy it; by analogy, in defending a given position, even a small concession can destroy that position. The last element is the causal influence of the agent, recognizing that most effects result from many causes and that a particular agent is seldom the sole cause. For example, as noted by Thomas M. Garrett and colleagues in *Health Care Ethics: Principles and Problems* (2001), lung cancer can be triggered not only by smoking but also by conditions in the workplace, the environment, and heredity.

Obligations are imposed on the patient that demand the use of ordinary but not extraordinary means of preserving and restoring health. In other words, the patient should use means that produce more good than harm and evaluate the effects on the self, family, and society, including pain, cost, and health benefits to life, its meaning and quality. The health care provider's obligation demands that the benefits outweigh the burdens on the patient. An overarching obligation to society exists to provide health care information and leadership to ensure the equitable distribution of scarce medical resources accomplished in ways that allow the goals of health care to be achieved. Finally, the surrogate's obligation depends on whether the wishes of the once-competent patient are known or can be ascertained. If so, the surrogate should decide accordingly (the substituted judgment principle). Overruling the person's wishes would constitute a denial of the patient's autonomy. If the person has never been competent or has never expressed his or her wishes, the surrogate should act in the best interests of the patient alone, disregarding the interests of family, society, and the surrogate. Another approach requires the surrogate to choose what the patient would have chosen if and when competent after having considered all relevant information and the interests of others.

Certain conditions justify the decision to omit treatment, such as pointless or futile treatment, especially with regard to the dead or those who are dying, and situations in which the burdens of treatment outweigh the benefits. It should be noted that no bright line exists here because these cases are not decided easily. Ethicists as well as those in the medical professions debating these issues have not reached a clear-cut solution that applies in every case.

Justice. Also called distributive justice, justice establishes principles for the distribution of scarce resources in circumstances where demand outstrips supply and rationing must occur. Needs are to be considered in terms of overall needs and the dignity of members of society. Aside from the biological and physiological elements, the social context of health and disease may influence a given problem and its severity. Individual prejudices and presuppositions may enlarge the nature and scope of the disease, creating a demand for health care that makes it even more difficult to distribute scarce resources for all members of society. Principles of fair distribution in society often supersede and become paramount to the concerns of the individual. Questions about who shall receive what share of society's scarce resources generate controversies about a national health policy, unequal distributions of advantages to the disadvantaged, and the rationing of health care.

Similar problems recur with regard to access to and distribution of health insurance, medical equipment, and artificial organs. The lack of insurance as well as the problem of underinsurance constitutes a huge economic barrier to health care access in the United States. In *Principles of Biomedical Ethics* (2001), Tom L. Beauchamp and James F. Childress point out that the acquired immunodeficiency syndrome (AIDS) crisis

has presented dramatic instances of the problems of insurability and underwriting practices, in which insurers often appeal to actuarial fairness in defending their decisions while neglecting social justice. Proposals to alleviate the unfairness to those below the poverty line have been based on charity, compassion, and benevolence toward the sick rather than on claims of justice. The ongoing debate over the entitlement to a minimum of health care in the United States involves not only government entitlement programs but also complex social, political, economic, and cultural beliefs.

Decisions concerning the allocation of funds will dictate the type of health care that can be provided and for which problems. Numerous resources, supplies, and space in intensive care units (ICUs) have been allocated for specific patients or classes of patients. A life-threatening illness complicates this decision. In the United States, health care has often been allocated by one's ability to pay rather than by other criteria; rationing has at times been based on ranking a list of services or a patient's age.

Confidentiality and privacy. In the United States, the medical profession has always strived to maintain the confidentiality of physician-patient communications, as well as the privacy of a patient's medical records. While admirable, these values have not been absolute, and no uniformity exists among the fifty states regarding access to one's medical records. As technology improved, with computers and fax machines transmitting health care data to distant locations and medical records themselves existing in electronic form, no laws had been created to protect medical records adequately. In the late twentieth and early twenty-first centuries, the administrations of Bill Clinton and George W. Bush sought to enact legislation that would bridge the privacy gaps and create uniform standards, at the same time eliminating discrimination in employment and insurance coverage based on one's genetic predisposition. The Health Insurance Portability and Accountability Act (HIPAA) became law in 1997.

APPLICATION OF ETHICAL PRINCIPLES

Advances in medical technology have expanded the scope of what medicine can accomplish. As capabilities grow and become more sophisticated, medical ethics also seeks to resolve age-old dilemmas and to evaluate the use of new technologies. Certain ethical dilemmas have garnered sharp disagreement. Chief among these is the issue of death and dying, which brings into controversy two theories about the nature of health care. The "curing" approach is based on traditional medical ethical principles that date back to Hippocrates and include the principles of beneficence, nonmaleficence, and justice. The "caring" approach focuses on patient autonomy, proper bedside manners by health care providers, the preparation of advance directives, and the hospice movement.

The "curing" approach to medical ethics equates medicine with healing. The sanctity of life is important because it is a gift from God and must be sustained to the extent reasonably possible. All ordinary measures must be taken to preserve life. This tradition holds that only God can decide the time of death, and even in the face of suffering, the health care provider must not take measures to shorten life. Physicians are the primary decision makers and in the best position to recommend and advise the patient and to direct the treatment plan. The model is paternalistic.

In the "caring" approach, the health care provider's role is to minimize pain, to present alternatives and the relative consequences of various options, and ultimately to proceed according to the patient's determination. The "caring" approach is subjective, as each case is decided individually. The quality of life rather than the sanctity of life becomes the guiding principle.

Issues regarding futility of treatment arise, as well as the recognition that prolonging life does not always benefit patients. Physicians are not obligated to provide futile treatment, which may violate the physician's duty not to harm patients because such treatments are often burdensome and invasive, exacerbating the patient's pain and discomfort. Patients cannot ethically compel health care workers to provide treatment that violates the worker's own personal beliefs or the standards of the profession. Other issues in this area deal with physician-assisted suicide and whether to provide or withhold lifesaving treatments.

The transplantation of vital organs—notably the heart, liver, and kidney—raises difficult ethical questions. As organ transplantation has become routine at many medical centers, its success has opened a Pandora's box of ethical questions involving the allocation of scarce donor organs. One example is whether the sickest person on the waiting list for an organ should be the recipient, or whether it should go to someone more robust who may live longer. Another is whether live donors should be compensated for donating an organ, just as blood donors are compensated. Many countries outside the United States and the United Kingdom condone the sale of organs; the 1984 National Organ

Transplant Act makes selling organs illegal in the United States. Ethicists are debating animal-to-human organ transplants to alleviate the scarcity of human donor organs for transplantation.

Assisted reproduction in the form of in vitro fertilization (IVF), egg freezing, and sperm banking is largely an unregulated industry. Couples seeking help must make complex ethical decisions dealing with the preselection of embryos based on genetic traits through screening of a single cell. Other decisions deal with how many eggs should be fertilized and whether the remainder should be disposed of or frozen. The rights of the participants and the children created through assisted reproduction remain undefined. State laws vary widely regarding whether a child conceived by IVF or donor eggs or sperm has the right to know the identity of the biological parents.

The identification of human embryonic stem cells has been widely acknowledged as extremely valuable because it will assist scientists in understanding basic mechanisms of embryo development and gene regulation. It also holds the promise of allowing the development of techniques for manipulating, growing, and cloning stem cells to create designer cells and tissues. Stem cells are created in the first days of pregnancy. Scientists hope to direct stem cells to grow into replacement organs and tissues to treat a wide variety of diseases. Embryos are valued in research for their ability to produce stem cells, which can be harvested to grow a variety of tissues for use in transplantation to treat serious illnesses such as cancer, heart disease, and diabetes. In so doing, however, researchers must destroy days-old embryos, a procedure condemned by the Catholic Church, some antiabortion activists, and some women's rights organizations. Other research points to similar promise using stem cells harvested from adults, so that no embryos are destroyed.

PERSPECTIVE AND PROSPECTS

Medical ethics in Western culture has its roots in ancient Greek and Roman medicine, the Greek physician Hippocrates and the Roman physician Galen. In ancient Greece, as in most early societies, healing wounds and treating disease first appeared as folk practice and religious ritual. The earliest statement about ethics appears in a clinical and epidemiological book entitled *Epidemics I*, attributed to Hippocrates. It is in this work that the admonition "to help and not to harm" first appeared. The book itself deals with prognosis rather than treatment, which is the approach taken by Hippocrates.

Galen asserted that any worthwhile doctor must know philosophy, including the logical, the physical, and the ethical, and be skilled at reasoning about the problems presented to him, understanding the nature and function of the body within the physical world.

From the fourth to the fourteenth centuries, medicine became firmly established in the universities and in the public life of the emerging nations of Europe. During this time, the Roman Catholic Church had a strong influence on Western civilization. Medicine was deeply touched by the doctrine and discipline of the Church, and its theological influence shaped the ethics of medicine. The early Church endorsed the use of human medicine and encouraged care of the sick as a work of charity. One of the greatest physicians during this period was the Jewish Talmudic scholar Maimonides, whose writings sometimes dealt with ethical questions in medicine.

The duty to comfort the sick and dying was a moral imperative in Christianity and Judaism. As the bubonic plague swept across Europe over the following several centuries, Protestant leader Martin Luther urged doctors and ministers to fulfill the obligation of Christian charity by faithful service, but John Calvin argued that physicians and ministers could depart if the preservation of their lives was in the common interest.

The ethical debates surrounding the plague moved medical ethics ahead. As noted by Albert R. Jonsen in *A Short History of Medical Ethics* (2000), the question became, "Under what circumstances does a person who has medical skills have a special obligation to serve the community?" When syphilis emerged in epidemic proportions at the end of the fifteenth century, a similar question regarding service to the sick at the cost of danger to oneself resurfaced, and members of the medical profession struggled with the link between medical necessity and moral correctness. Not until the nineteenth century did a consensus appear, mandating that the physician should take personal risks to serve the needy without appraising the morality of a patient's behavior.

—*Marcia J. Weiss, M.A., J.D.*

See also Abortion; Aging: Extended care; Animal rights vs. research; Assisted reproductive technologies; Cloning; Contraception; Ergogenic aids; Euthanasia; Fetal tissue transplantation; Genetic engineering; Hippocratic oath; In vitro fertilization; Law and medicine; Malpractice; Medicare; Resuscitation; Screening; Stem cells; Suicide; Terminally ill: Extended care; Transplantation; Xenotransplantation.

For Further Information:
Beauchamp, Tom L., and James F. Childress. *Principles of Biomedical Ethics*. 5th ed. New York: Oxford University Press, 2001. Regarded as one of the basic texts of bioethics. An excellent source for a detailed discussion of fundamental principles.

Beauchamp, Tom L., and LeRoy Walters, eds. *Contemporary Issues in Bioethics*. 6th ed. Belmont, Calif.: Thomson/Wadsworth, 2003. A compilation of scholarly articles and major legal cases in bioethics.

Garrett, Thomas M., Harold W. Baillie, and Rosellen M. Garrett. *Health Care Ethics: Principles and Problems*. 4th ed. Upper Saddle River, N.J.: Prentice Hall, 2001. A basic and succinct text outlining the principles and problems of health care ethics.

Jonsen, Albert R. *A Short History of Medical Ethics*. New York: Oxford University Press, 2000. A concise and comprehensive chronicle of the history of ethics and medicine.

Pence, Gregory E. *Re-creating Medicine: Ethical Issues at the Frontiers of Medicine*. Lanham, Md.: Rowman & Littlefield, 2000. A subjective and skeptical (not balanced) discussion of the major bioethical issues at the beginning of the twenty-first century, such as organ donation, reproduction and its progeny, genetics, and other controversial subjects.

Torr, James D., ed. *Medical Ethics*. San Diego, Calif.: Greenhaven Press, 2000. Part of the Current Controversies series, this book presents reprints of articles illustrating both sides of controversial and contested issues in medical ethics.

Veatch, Robert M. "Models for Ethical Practice in a Revolutionary Age." *Hastings Center Report* 2, no. 3 (June, 1972): 5-7. A major figure in the bioethics movement, Veatch outlines four ethical medical models.

Euthanasia
Ethics

Definition: The intentional termination of a life, which may be active (resulting from specific actions causing death) or passive (resulting from the refusal or withdrawal of life-sustaining treatment), and voluntary (with the patient's consent) or involuntary (on behalf of infants or others who are incapable of making this decision, such as comatose patients).

Key terms:

active euthanasia: administration of a drug or some other means that directly causes death; the motivation is to relieve patient suffering

durable power of attorney: designation of a person who will have legal authority to make health care decisions if the patient becomes incapable of making decisions for himself or herself

living will: a legal document in which the patient states a preference regarding life-prolonging treatment in the event that he or she cannot choose

nonvoluntary euthanasia: a decision to terminate life made by another when the patient is incapable of making a decision for himself or herself

passive euthanasia: ending life by refusing or withdrawing life-sustaining medical treatment

voluntary euthanasia: a patient's consent to a decision which results in the shortening of his or her life

THE CONTROVERSY SURROUNDING EUTHANASIA

In the past, the role of the doctor was clear: The physician should minimize suffering and save lives whenever possible. In the present, it is possible for these two goals to be at odds. Saving lives in some situations seems to prolong the misery of the patient. In other cases, procedures or treatments may only marginally postpone the time of death. Advances in medical technology enable many to live who would have died just a few years ago, and massive amounts of money are spent each year on medical research with the goal of prolonging life. Experts in U.S. population trends indicate that by the year 2030, those over the age of sixty-five will comprise about 20 percent of the country's total population. These people will probably be healthy and alert well into their eighties; however, in the last years of their lives they will probably require significant medical care, putting financial stress on the health care system.

The complex issues surrounding death, suffering, and economics create demands for answers to difficult ethical questions. Does all life have value? Should one fight against death even when suffering is intense? Should suffering be lessened if the time of death is brought nearer? Should a patient be given the right to refuse medical treatment if the result is death? Should others be allowed to make this decision for the patient? Should other factors such as the financial or emotional burden on the family be part of the decision-making process? Once a decision has been made to terminate suffering by death, is there any ethical difference between discontinuing medical treatment and giving a lethal dosage of painkilling medication? Should laws be put into place that offer guidelines in these situations, or should each case be decided on an individual basis?

And who should decide? There is a wide range of opinion and much uncertainty involving euthanasia and what constitutes a "good" death.

Euthanasia comes from a Greek word that can be translated as "good death" and is defined in several ways, depending on the philosophical stance of the one giving the definition. Tom Beauchamp, in his book *Health and Human Values* (1983), defines euthanasia as

> putting to death or failing to prevent death in cases of terminal illness or injury; the motive is to relieve comatoseness, physical suffering, anxiety or a serious sense of burdensomeness to self and others. In euthanasia at least one other person causes or helps to cause the death of one who desires death or, in the case of an incompetent person, makes a substituted decision, either to cause death directly or to withdraw something that sustains life.

Most patients who express a wish to die more quickly are terminally ill; however, euthanasia is sometimes considered as a solution for nonterminal patients as well. An example of the latter would be seriously deformed or retarded infants whose futures are judged to have a poor "quality of life" and who would be a serious burden on their families and society.

When discussing the ethical implications of euthanasia, the types of cases have been divided into various classes. A distinction is made between voluntary and nonvoluntary euthanasia. In voluntary euthanasia, the patient consents to a specific course of medical action in which death is hastened. Nonvoluntary euthanasia would occur in cases in which the patient is not able to make decisions about his or her death because of an inability to communicate or a lack of mental facility. Each of these classes has advocates and antagonists. Some believe that voluntary euthanasia should always be allowed, but others would limit voluntary euthanasia to only those patients who have a terminal illness. Some, although agreeing in principle that voluntary euthanasia in terminal situations is ethically permissible, nevertheless oppose euthanasia of any type because of the possibility of abuses. With nonvoluntary euthanasia, the main ethical issues deal with when such an action should be performed and who should make the decision. If a person is in an irreversible coma, most agree that that person's physical life could be ended; however, arguments based on "quality of life" can easily become widened to include persons with physical or mental disabilities. Infants with severe deformities can sometimes be saved but not fully cured with medical technology, and some individuals would advocate nonvoluntary euthanasia in these cases because of the suffering of the infants' caregivers. Some believe that family members or those who stand to gain from the decision should not be allowed to make the decision. Others point out that the family is the most likely to know what the wishes of the patient would have been. Most believe that the medical care personnel, although knowledgeable, should not have the power to decide, and many are reluctant to institute rigid laws. The possibility of misappropriated self-interest from each of these parties magnifies the difficulty of arriving at well-defined criteria.

The second type of classification is between passive and active euthanasia. Passive euthanasia occurs when sustaining medical treatment is refused or withdrawn and death is allowed to take its course. Active euthanasia involves the administration of a drug or some other means that directly causes death. Once again, there are many opinions surrounding these two types. One position is that there is no difference between active and passive euthanasia because in each the end is premeditated death with the motive of prevention of suffering. In fact, some argue that active euthanasia is more compassionate than letting death occur naturally, which may involve suffering. In opposition, others believe that there is a fundamental difference between active and passive euthanasia. A person may have the right to die, but not the right to be killed. Passive euthanasia, they argue, is merely allowing a death which is inevitable to occur. Active euthanasia, if voluntary, is equated with suicide because a human being seizes control of death; if nonvoluntary, it is considered murder.

Passive euthanasia, although generally more publicly acceptable than active euthanasia, has become a topic of controversy as the types of medical treatment that can be withdrawn are debated. A distinction is sometimes made between ordinary and extraordinary means. Defining these terms is difficult, since what may be extraordinary for one patient is not for another, depending on other medical conditions that the patient may have. In addition, what is considered an extraordinary technique today may be judged ordinary in the future. Another way to assess whether passive euthanasia should be allowed in a particular situation is to weigh the benefits against the burdens for the patient. Although most agree that there are cases in which high-tech equipment such as respirators can be withdrawn, there is a question about whether administration of

food and water should ever be discontinued. Here the line between passive and active euthanasia is blurred.

RELIGIOUS AND LEGAL IMPLICATIONS

Decisions about death concern everyone because everyone will die. Eventually, each individual will be the patient who is making the decisions or for whom the decisions are being made. In the meantime, one may be called upon to make decisions for others. Even those not directly involved in the hard cases are affected, as taxpayers and subscribers to medical insurance, by the decisions made on the behalf of others. In a difficult moral issue such as this, individuals look to different institutions for guidelines. Two sources of guidance are the church and the law.

In 1971, the Roman Catholic Church issued a statement entitled *Ethical and Religious Directives for Catholic Health Facilities*. Included in this directive was the statement, "[I]t is not euthanasia to give a dying person sedatives and analgesics for alleviation of pain, when such a measure is judged necessary, even though they may deprive the patient of the use of reason or shorten his life." This thinking was reaffirmed by a 1980 statement from the Vatican which considers suffering and expense for the family legitimate reasons to withdraw medical treatment when death is imminent. Bishops from The Netherlands, in a letter to a government commission, state "[B]odily deterioration alone does not have to be unworthy of a man. History shows how many people, beaten, tortured and broken in body, sometimes even grew in personality in spite of it. Dying becomes unworthy of a man, if family and friends begin to look upon the dying person as a burden, withdraw themselves from him. . . ." When speaking of passive euthanasia, the bishops state, "We see no reason to call this euthanasia. Such a person after all dies of his own illness. His death is neither intended nor caused, only nothing is done anymore to postpone it." Christians from Protestant churches may reflect a wider spectrum of positions. Joseph Fletcher, an Episcopal priest, defines a person as one having the ability to think and reason. If a patient does not meet these criteria, according to Fletcher, his or her life may be ended out of compassion for the person he or she once was. The United Church of Christ illustrates this view in its policy statement: "When illness takes away those abilities we associate with full personhood . . . we may well feel that the mere continuance of the body by machine or drugs is a violation of their person. . . . We do not believe simply the continuance of mere physical existence is either morally defensible or socially desirable or is God's will."

These varied positions generally are derived from differing emphases on two truths concerning the nature of God and the role of suffering in the life of the believer. First is the belief that God is the giver of life and that human beings should not usurp God's authority in matters of life and death. Second, alleviation of suffering is of critical importance to God, since it is not loving one's neighbor to allow him or her to suffer. Those who give more weight to the first statement believe as well that God's will allows for suffering and that the suffering can be used for a good purpose in the life of the believer. Those who emphasize the second principle insist that a loving God would not prolong the suffering of people needlessly and that one should not desperately fight to prolong a life which God has willed to die.

C. Everett Koop, former surgeon general of the United States, differentiates between the positive role of a physician in providing a patient "all the life to which he or she is entitled" and the negative role of "prolonging the act of dying." Koop has opposed euthanasia in any form, cautioning against the possibility of sliding down a slippery slope toward making choices about death that reflect the caregivers' "quality of life" more than the patient's.

Dr. Jack Kevorkian, a Michigan physician, became the most well known advocate of assisted suicide in the United States. From 1990 to 1997, Kevorkian assisted at least sixty-six people in terminating their lives. According to Kevorkian's lawyer, many other assisted suicides have not been publicized. Kevorkian believes that physician-assisted suicide is a matter of individual choice and should be seen as a rational way to end tremendous pain and suffering. Most of the patients assisted by him spent many years suffering from extremely painful and debilitating diseases, such as multiple sclerosis, bone cancer, and brain cancer.

The American Medical Association (AMA) has criticized this view, calling it a violation of professional ethics. When faced with pain and suffering, the AMA asserts that it is a doctor's responsibility to provide adequate "comfort" care, not death. In the AMA's view, Kevorkian served as "a reckless instrument of death." Three trials in Michigan for assisting in suicide resulted in acquittals for Kevorkian before another trial delivered a guilty verdict on the charge of second-degree murder in March, 1999.

During the course of reevaluating the issues involved in terminating a life, the law has been in a state of flux. The decisions that are made by the courts act on the legal precedents of an individual's right to determine what is done to his or her own body and society's position against suicide. The balancing of these two premises has been handled legally by allowing refusal of treatment (passive euthanasia) but disallowing the use of poison or some other method that would cause death (active euthanasia). The latter is labeled suicide, and anyone who assists in such an act can be found guilty of assisting a suicide, or of murder. Following the Karen Ann Quinlan case in 1976, in which the family of a comatose woman secured permission to withdraw life-sustaining treatment, the courts routinely allowed family members to make decisions regarding life-sustaining treatment if the patient could not do so. The area of greatest legal controversy involves the withdrawal of food and water. Some courts have charged doctors with murder for the withdrawal of basic life support measures such as food and water. Others have ruled that invasive procedures to provide food and water (intravenously, for example) are similar to other medical procedures and may be discontinued if the benefit to the patient's quality of life is negligible.

In 1994, 51 percent of the voters in Oregon passed the world's first "death with dignity" law. It allowed physician-assisted suicide. Doctors could begin prescribing fatal overdoses of drugs to terminally ill patients. The vote was reaffirmed in 1997 by 60 percent of the state's voters, despite opposition from the Roman Catholic Church, the AMA, and various anti-abortion and right-to-life groups. The Ninth United States Circuit Court of Appeals in San Francisco then lifted a lower court order blocking implementation of the law. Since 1999, several states, including Hawaii, Vermont, New Hampshire, Maine, and North Carolina, have witnessed attempts to legalize physician-assisted suicide, but the cases have either been withdrawn or defeated by voters or in state legislature.

Doctors in Oregon became free to prescribe fatal doses of barbiturates to patients with less than six months to live. Physicians were required to file forms with the Oregon Health Division before prescribing the overdose. Then, there would be a fifteen-day waiting period between the request for suicide assistance and the approval of the prescription. Opponents of the Oregon law charged that it perverted the practice of medicine and forced many suffering people to "choose" an early death to save themselves from expensive medical care or pain that could be manageable if physicians were aware of new methods of pain control. The National Right to Life Committee indicated that it would continue to fight implementation of the law in federal courts.

Although the laws vary from state to state, most states allow residents to make their wishes known regarding terminal health care either by writing a living will or by choosing a durable power of attorney. A living will is a document in which one can state that some medical treatments should not be used in the event that one becomes incapacitated to the point where one cannot choose. Living wills allow the patient to decide in advance and protect health care providers from lawsuits. Which treatment options can be terminated and when this action can be put into effect may be limited in some states. Most states have a specific format that should be followed when drawing up a living will and require that the document be signed in the presence of two witnesses. Often, qualifying additions can be made by the individual that specify whether food and water may be withdrawn and whether the living will should go into effect only when death is imminent or also when a person has an incurable illness but death is not imminent. A copy of the living will should be given to the patient's physician and become a part of the patient's medical records. The preparation or execution of a living will cannot affect a person's life insurance coverage or the payment of benefits. Since the medical circumstances of one's life may change and a person's ethical stance may also change, a patient may change the living will at any time by signing a written statement.

A second way in which a person can control what kind of decisions will be made regarding his or her death is to choose a decision maker in advance. This person assumes a durable power of attorney and is legally allowed to act on the patient's behalf, making medical treatment decisions. One advantage of a durable power of attorney over a living will is that the patient can choose someone who shares similar ethical and religious values. Since it is difficult to foresee every medical situation that could arise, there is more security with a durable power of attorney in knowing that the person will have similar values and will therefore probably make the same judgments as the patient. Usually a primary agent and a secondary agent are designated in the event that the primary agent is unavailable. This is especially important if the primary agent is a spouse or a close relative who could, for example, be involved in an accident at the same time as the patient.

PERSPECTIVE AND PROSPECTS

Although large numbers of court decision, articles, and books suggest that the issues involved in euthanasia are recent products of medical technology, these questions are not new. Euthanasia was widely practiced in Western classical culture. The Greeks did not believe that all humans had the right to live, and in Athens, infants with disabilities were often killed. Although in general they did not condone suicide, Pythagoras, Plato, and Aristotle believed that a person could choose to die earlier in the face of an incurable disease and that others could help that person to die. Seneca, the Roman Stoic philosopher, was an avid proponent of euthanasia, stating:

> Against all the injuries of life, I have the refuge of death. If I can choose between a death of torture and one that is simple and easy, why should I not select the latter? As I choose the ship in which I sail and the house which I shall inhabit, so I will choose the death by which I leave life.

The famous Hippocratic oath for physicians acted in opposition to the prevailing cultural bias in favor of euthanasia. Contained in this oath is the statement, "I will never give a deadly drug to anybody if asked for it . . . or make a suggestion to this effect." Interestingly, the AMA has reaffirmed this position in a policy statement:

> the intentional termination of the life of one human being by another—"mercy killing"—is contrary to that for which the medical profession stands and is contrary to the policy of the American Medical Association.

Jewish and Christian theology has traditionally opposed any form of euthanasia or suicide, avowing that since God is the author of life and death, life is sacred. Therefore, a man rebels against God if he prematurely shortens his life, because he violates the Sixth Commandment, "Thou shalt not kill." Suffering was viewed not as an evil to be avoided at all costs but as a condition to be accepted. The Apostle Paul served as an example for early Christians. In 2 Corinthians, he prayed for physical healing, yet when it did not come, he accepted his weakness as a way to increase his dependence on God. This position was affirmed by Saint Augustine in his work *De Civitate Dei* (413-426; *The City of God*) when he condemned suicide as a "detestable and damnable wickedness" which was worse than murder because it left no room for repentance. These strong indictments from the Church against suicide and euthanasia were largely responsible for changing the Greco-Roman attitudes toward the value of human life. They were accepted as society's position until the advent of technologies that made it possible to extend life beyond what would have been the point of death a few years ago.

Although these issues have been debated among both physicians and philosophers for centuries, there is a heightened need for thoughtful discussion and resolution today. Clearly, the decisions surrounding the issue of euthanasia are very complicated. The choice is not simply between commitments to "sanctity of life" or "quality of life" viewpoints. No consensus has yet been reached across the spectrum of society, and instead a variety of alternatives are supported by groups of individuals. A clear understanding of all positions in the debate is the best preparation for making personal decisions at the time of death.

—Katherine B. Frederich, Ph.D.;
updated by Leslie V. Tischauser, Ph.D.

See also Aging: Extended care; Critical care; Critical care, pediatric; Death and dying; Ethics; Hippocratic oath; Law and medicine; Pain management; Psychiatry; Psychiatry, geriatric; Suicide; Terminally ill: Extended care.

FOR FURTHER INFORMATION:

Corr, Charles A., Clyde M. Nabe, and Donna M. Corr. *Death and Dying, Life and Living.* 5th ed. Belmont, Calif.: Wadsworth, 2005. This book provides perspective on common issues associated with death and dying for family members and others affected by life-threatening circumstances.

Dowbiggin, Ian Robert. *A Merciful End: The Euthanasia Movement in Modern America.* New York: Oxford University Press, 2003. Blends social history, medical knowledge, and political analysis to trace the evolution of euthanasia and its perception in the United States throughout the twentieth century.

Gorovitz, Samuel. *Drawing the Line: Life, Death, and Ethical Choices in an American Hospital.* Philadelphia: Temple University Press, 1993. This book reflects on the author's seven-week sabbatical-in-residence at Beth Israel Hospital. Gorovitz presents numerous insights drawn from conversations with patients and medical personnel.

Harron, Frank, John Burnside, and Tom Beauchamp. *Health and Human Values.* New Haven, Conn.: Yale University Press, 1983. Using a case-study approach, the authors consider the different types of euthanasia and report on policy statements from interested social groups.

Leone, Daniel A. *The Ethics of Euthanasia.* San Diego, Calif.: Greenhaven Press, 1998. This volume includes ten essays on the ethics and morality of euthanasia, potential abuse, distinctions between active and passive euthanasia, and whether euthanasia is consistent with Christian belief.

Magnusson, Roger, and Peter H. Ballis. *Angels of Death: Exploring the Euthanasia Underground.* New Haven, Conn.: Yale University Press, 2002. Explores the existence of a euthanasia underground in Australia and the United States using firsthand accounts of health professionals who have been involved in assisted death.

Rebman, Renée C. *Euthanasia and the Right to Die: Pro/Con Issues.* Berkeley Heights, N.J.: Enslow, 2002. Part of the "Hot Pro/Con Issues" series for young adults, offers a balanced perspective on a range of issues surrounding euthanasia.

Spring, Beth, and Ed Larson. *Euthanasia.* Portland, Oreg.: Multnomah Press, 1988. This book considers the spiritual, medical, and legal issues in terminal health care, citing numerous perspectives from the religious community. Contains two chapters detailing practical guidelines for writing living wills and durable powers of attorney.

Torr, James D. *Euthanasia: Opposing Viewpoints.* San Diego, Calif.: Greenhaven Press, 1999. Designed for students in grades nine through twelve, this volume brings together essays by authorities in diverse vocations. The four chapters explore whether euthanasia is ethical, if it should be legalized, if legalization would lead to involuntary killing, and under what circumstances, if any, doctors should assist in suicide.

Wennberg, Robert N. *Terminal Choices: Euthanasia, Suicide, and the Right to Die.* Grand Rapids, Mich.: Wm. B. Eerdmans, 1989. The author presents a helpful history of the euthanasia debate and also discusses possible moral distinctions between treatment refusal and treatment withdrawal.

EWING'S SARCOMA

DISEASE/DISORDER

ALSO KNOWN AS: Bone cancer

ANATOMY OR SYSTEM AFFECTED: Bones, musculoskeletal system

SPECIALTIES AND RELATED FIELDS: Oncology, orthopedics, pediatrics, radiology

DEFINITION: A rare bone cancer involving any part of the skeleton but found commonly in the long bones

(60 percent), the pelvis (18 percent), and the ribs (15 percent) of children and young adults.

CAUSES AND SYMPTOMS

The specific cause of Ewing's sarcoma is unknown, but it may be associated with recurrent trauma, metal implants, congenital anomalies, unrelated tumors, or exposure to ionizing radiation. Approximately 90 percent of patients are between five and twenty-five years of age; rarely are patients younger than five or older than forty.

The initial symptom is pain, discontinuous at first and then intense, in the long bones, vertebra, or pelvis. Swelling may follow. Neurological signs involving the nerve roots or spinal cord depression are characteristic of nearly one-half of patients with involvement of the axial skeleton. Weight loss may occur, with remittent fever and mild anemia.

The phases of Ewing's sarcoma are based on degree of metastasis: the local phase (a nonmetastatic tumor), the regional phase (lymph node involvement), and the distant phase (involvement of the lungs, bones, and sometimes the central nervous system).

TREATMENT AND THERAPY

Patients are of two types, those with localized tumors and those with metastasized tumors. Depending on where the tumor is located, the treatment of Ewing's sarcoma is complex in all stages of disease and requires a multidisciplinary perspective. It is best treated when diagnosed early. Obtaining a bone biopsy is recommended in nearly all cases.

Surgery may be used to remove a tumor, followed by chemotherapy administered to kill any remaining cancer cells. Radiation may be prescribed to kill cancer cells and shrink tumors.

INFORMATION ON EWING'S SARCOMA

CAUSES: Unknown; possibly related to recurrent trauma, metal implants, congenital anomalies, unrelated tumors, exposure to ionizing radiation

SYMPTOMS: Pain in long bones, vertebra, or pelvis; swelling; neurological disorders; weight loss; fever; mild anemia

DURATION: Long-term

TREATMENTS: Surgery, chemotherapy, radiation

PERSPECTIVE AND PROSPECTS

Ewing's sarcoma is one of the most malignant of all tumors. It may be localized or metastasize to the lungs and other bones. The primary tumor can be controlled by irradiation, but the prognosis is poor. Often, amputation is not justifiable. Recent developments in multiagent chemotherapy, however, are encouraging. Long-term survival of patients with Ewing's sarcoma is 50 to 70 percent or more with localized disease; the rate drops to less than 30 percent for metastatic disease.

—*John Alan Ross, Ph.D.*

See also Bone cancer; Bone disorders; Bones and the skeleton; Cancer; Orthopedics, pediatric.

FOR FURTHER INFORMATION:

Cady, Blake, ed. *Cancer Manual.* 7th ed. Boston: American Cancer Society, 1986.

Children's Cancer Web. http://www.cancerindex.org/ccw/.

Dollinger, Malin, et al. *Everyone's Guide to Cancer Therapy.* 4th rev. ed. Kansas City, Mo.: Andrews & McMeel, 2002.

Dorfman, Howard D., and Bogdan Czerniak. *Bone Tumors.* St. Louis: Mosby, 1998.

Eyre, Harmon J., Dianne Partie Lange, and Lois B. Morris. *Informed Decisions: The Complete Book of Cancer Diagnosis, Treatment, and Recovery.* 2d ed. Atlanta: American Cancer Society, 2002.

Grealy, Lucy. *Autobiography of a Face.* New York: Perennial, 2003.

Holleb, Arthur I., ed. *The American Cancer Society Cancer Book: Prevention, Detection, Diagnosis, Treatment, Rehabilitation, Cure.* Garden City, N.Y.: Doubleday, 1986.

Janes-Hodder, Honna, and Nancy Keene. *Childhood Cancer: A Parent's Guide to Solid Tumor Cancers.* 2d ed. Cambridge, Mass.: O'Reilly and Associates, 2002.

Morra, Marion, and Eve Potts. *Choices: Realistic Alternatives in Cancer Treatment.* Rev. ed. New York: Viking, 1997.

EXERCISE PHYSIOLOGY

SPECIALTY

ANATOMY OR SYSTEM AFFECTED: Circulatory system, heart, joints, knees, lungs, muscles, musculoskeletal system, respiratory system, tendons

SPECIALTIES AND RELATED FIELDS: Cardiology, family medicine, nutrition, physical therapy, preventive medicine, sports medicine

DEFINITION: The science that studies the effects on the body of various intensities and types of physical activity, including cellular metabolism, cardiovascular responses, respiratory responses, neural and hormonal adaptations, and muscular adaptations to exercise.

KEY TERMS:

adenosine triphosphate (ATP): a high-energy compound found in the cell which provides energy for all bodily functions

aerobic: metabolism involving the breakdown of energy substrates using oxygen

anaerobic: metabolism involving the breakdown of energy substrates without using oxygen

electrocardiogram (ECG): a graphic record of electrical currents of the heart

glycogen: the form that glucose takes when it is stored in the muscles and liver

heart rate: the number of times the heart contracts, or beats, per minute

maximal oxygen uptake: the maximum rate of oxygen consumption during exercise

metabolic equivalent (MET): a unit used to estimate the metabolic cost of physical activity; 1 MET is equal to 3.5 milliliters of oxygen consumed per kilogram of body weight per minute

SCIENCE AND PROFESSION

The primary focus of research in the field of exercise physiology is to gain a better understanding of the quantity and type of exercise needed for health maintenance and rehabilitation. A major goal of professionals in exercise physiology is to find ways to incorporate appropriate levels of physical activity into the lifestyles of all individuals.

Physiology is the science of physical and chemical factors and processes involved in the function of living organisms. The study of exercise physiology examines these factors and processes as they relate to physical exertion. The physical responses that occur are specific to the intensity, duration, and type of exercise performed.

Low or moderate exercise intensity relies on oxygen to release energy for work. This process is often referred to as aerobic exercise. In the muscles, carbohydrates and fats are broken down to produce adenosine triphosphate (ATP), the basic molecule used for energy. Aerobic exercise can be sustained for several minutes to several hours.

Higher-intensity exercise is predominantly fueled anaerobically (in the absence of oxygen) and can be sustained for up to two minutes only. Muscle glycogen is broken down without oxygen to produce ATP. Anaerobic metabolism is much less efficient at producing ATP than is aerobic metabolism.

During anaerobic metabolism, a by-product called lactic acid begins to accumulate in the blood as blood lactate. The point at which this accumulation begins is called the anaerobic threshold (AT), or the onset of blood lactate accumulation (OBLA). Blood lactate can cause muscle soreness and stiffness, but it also can be used as fuel during aerobic metabolism.

A third and less often used energy system is the creatine phosphate (ATP-CP) system. Utilizing the very limited supply of ATP that is stored in the muscles, phosphate molecules are exchanged between ATP and CP to provide energy. This system provides only enough fuel for a few seconds of maximum effort.

The type of muscle fiber recruited to perform a specific type of exercise is also dependent on exercise intensity. Skeletal muscle is composed of "slow-twitch" and two types of "fast-twitch" muscle fibers. Slow-twitch fibers are more suited to using oxygen than are fast-twitch fibers, and they are recruited primarily for aerobic exercise. One type of fast-twitch fiber also functions during aerobic activity. The second type of fast-twitch fiber serves to facilitate anaerobic, or high-intensity, exercise.

Exercise mode is also a factor in the physiological responses to exercise. Dynamic exercise (alternating muscular contraction and relaxation through a range of motion) using many large muscles requires more oxygen than does activity utilizing smaller and fewer muscles. The greater the oxygen requirement of the physical activity, the greater the cardiorespiratory benefits.

Many bodily adaptations occur over a training period of six to eight weeks, and other benefits are gradually manifested over several months. The positive adaptations include reduced resting and working heart rates. As the heart becomes stronger, there is a subsequent increase in stroke volume (the volume of blood the heart pumps with each beat), which allows the heart to beat less frequently while maintaining the same cardiac output (the volume of the blood pumped from the heart each minute). Another beneficial adaptation is increased metabolic efficiency. This is partially facilitated by an increase in the number of mitochondria (the organelles responsible for ATP production) in the muscle cells.

One of the most recognized representations of aerobic fitness is the maximum volume of oxygen (VO_{2max}) an individual can use during exercise. VO_{2max} is improved through habitual, relatively high-intensity aerobic activity. After three to six months of regular training, levels of high-density lipoproteins (HDLs) in the blood increase. HDL molecules remove cholesterol (a fatty substance) from the tissues to aid in protecting the heart from atherosclerosis.

Various internal and external factors influence the metabolic processes that take place during and after exercise. Internally, nutrition, degree of hydration, body composition, flexibility, sex, and age are some of the variables that play a role in the physiological responses. Other internal variables include medical conditions such as heart disease, diabetes, and hypertension (high blood pressure). Externally, environmental conditions such as temperature, humidity, and altitude alter how the exercising body functions.

Various modes of exercise testing and data collection are used to study the physiological responses of the body to exercise. Treadmills and cycle ergometers (instruments used to measure work and power output) are among the most common methods of evaluating maximum oxygen consumption. During these tests, special equipment and computers analyze expired air, heart rate is monitored with an electrocardiograph (ECG), and blood pressure is taken using a sphygmomanometer. Blood samples and muscle fiber samples can also be extracted to aid in identifying the fuel system and type of muscle fibers being used. Other data sometimes collected, such as skin temperatures and body core temperatures, can provide pertinent information.

Metabolic equivalent units, or METs, are often used to translate a person's capability into workloads on various pieces of exercise equipment or into everyday tasks. For every 3.5 milliliters of oxygen consumed per kilogram of body weight per minute, the subject is said to be performing at a workload of one MET. One MET is approximately equivalent to 1.5 kilocalories per minute, or the amount of energy expended per kilogram of body weight in one minute when a person is at rest.

Another factor greatly affecting the physical response to exercise is body composition. The three major structural components of the body are muscle, bone, and fat. Body composition can be evaluated using a

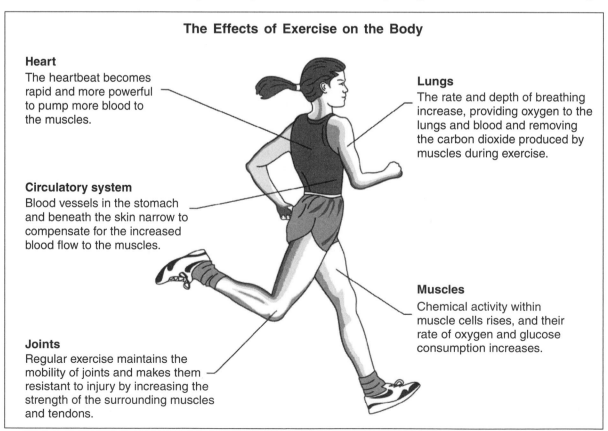

The Effects of Exercise on the Body

Heart
The heartbeat becomes rapid and more powerful to pump more blood to the muscles.

Lungs
The rate and depth of breathing increase, providing oxygen to the lungs and blood and removing the carbon dioxide produced by muscles during exercise.

Circulatory system
Blood vessels in the stomach and beneath the skin narrow to compensate for the increased blood flow to the muscles.

Muscles
Chemical activity within muscle cells rises, and their rate of oxygen and glucose consumption increases.

Joints
Regular exercise maintains the mobility of joints and makes them resistant to injury by increasing the strength of the surrounding muscles and tendons.

combination of anthropometric measurements. These measurements include body weight, standard height, measurements of circumferences at various locations using a tape measure, measurements of skeletal diameters using a sliding metric stick, and measurements of skinfold thicknesses using calipers.

Body fat can be estimated using several methods, the most accurate of which is based on a calculation of body density. This method is called hydrostatic weighing, which involves weighing the subject under water while taking into account the residual volume of air in the lungs. The principle underlying this measurement of body density is based on the fact that fat is less dense than water and will float, whereas bone and muscle, which are denser than water, will sink. One biochemical technique often used to determine levels of body fat is based on the relatively constant level of potassium 40 naturally existing in lean body mass. Another method utilizes ultrasound waves to measure the thickness of fat layers. X rays and computed tomography (CT) scanning can be used to provide images from which fat and bone can be measured. Bioelectrical impedance (BIA) is a method of estimating body composition based on the resistance imposed on a low voltage electrical current sent through the body. The most widely used and easily assessable method, however, involves measurement of skinfolds at various sites on the body using calipers. In all cases, mathematical formulas have been devised to interpret the collected data and provide the best estimate of an individual's body composition.

Other tests have been developed to determine muscular strength, muscular endurance, and flexibility. Muscular strength is often measured by performance of one maximal effort produced by a selected muscle group. Muscular endurance of a muscle or muscle group is often demonstrated by the length of time or number of repetitions a particular, submaximal workload or skill can be performed.

Two major types of flexibility have been identified. One type consists of the flexibility through the range of motion of a muscle group or joint. This is called static flexibility. It can be measured using a metric stick or a protractor-type instrument called a goniometer. Dynamic flexibility is the other major identified type of flexibility. It is the torque of or resistance to movement. Methods to measure dynamic flexibility have not been developed.

Overlapping the science of exercise physiology are the studies of biomechanics or kinesiology (sciences dealing with human movement) and nutrition. Only through an understanding of efficient body mechanics and proper nutrition can the physiological responses of the body to exercise be identified correctly.

DIAGNOSTIC AND TREATMENT TECHNIQUES

Exercise prescription is the primary focus in the application of exercise physiology. General health maintenance, cardiac rehabilitation, and competitive athletics are three major areas of exercise prescription.

Before making recommendations for an exercise program, an exercise physiologist must evaluate the physical limitations of the exerciser. In a normal, health maintenance setting—often called a "wellness" program—a health-related questionnaire can reveal relevant information. Such a questionnaire should include questions about family medical history and the subject's history of heart trouble or chest pain, bone or joint problems, and high blood pressure. The presence of any of these problems suggests the need for a physician's consent prior to exercising. After the individual has been deemed eligible to participate, an assessment of the level of physical fitness should be performed. Determining or estimating VO_{2max}, muscular strength, muscular endurance, flexibility, and body composition is usually included in this assessment. It is then possible to design a program best suited to the needs of the individual.

For the healthy adult participant, the American College of Sports Medicine (ACSM), a widely recognized authoritative body on exercise prescription, recommends three to five sessions of aerobic exercise weekly. Each session should include a five- to ten-minute warm-up period, twenty to sixty minutes of aerobic exercise at a predetermined exercise intensity, and a five- to ten-minute cool-down period.

In order to recommend an appropriate aerobic exercise intensity, the exercise physiologist must determine an individual's maximum heart rate. The best way to obtain this maximum heart rate is to administer a maximal exercise test. Such a test can be supervised by an exercise physiologist or an exercise test technician; it is advisable, especially for the older participant, that a cardiologist also be in attendance. An ECG is monitored for irregularities as the subject walks, runs, cycles, or performs some dynamic exercise to exhaustion or until the onset of irregular symptoms or discomfort.

Exercise prescription using heart rate as a measure can be achieved by various methods. A direct correlation exists between exercise intensity, in terms of oxygen consumption, and heart rate. From data collected

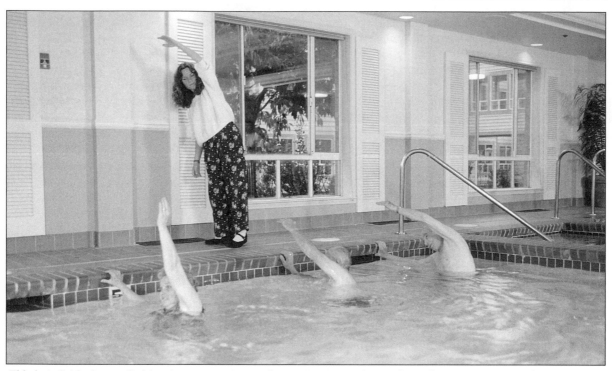

Elderly individuals may find low-impact exercise, such as swimming, to be a safer and easier way to stay fit. (PhotoDisc)

during a maximal exercise test, a target heart rate range of 40 percent to 85 percent of functional capacity can be calculated. Another method used to determine an appropriate heart rate range is based on the difference between an individual's resting heart rate and maximum heart rate, called the heart rate reserve (HRR). Values representing 60 percent and 80 percent of the heart rate reserve are calculated and added to the resting heart rate, yielding the individual's target heart rate range. A third method involves calculating 70 percent and 85 percent of the maximum heart rate. Although this method is less accurate than the other two methods, it is the simplest way to estimate a target heart rate range.

Intensity of exercise can also be prescribed using METs. This method relies on the predetermined metabolic equivalents required to perform activities at various intensities. Activity levels reflecting 40 percent to 85 percent of functional capacity can be calculated.

The rating of perceived exertion (RPE) is another method of prescribing exercise intensity. Verbal responses by the participant describing how an exercise feels at various intensities are assigned to a numerical scale, which is then correlated to heart rate. Through practice, the participant can correlate heart rate with the RPE, reducing the necessity of frequent pulse monitoring in the healthy individual.

Adequate physical fitness can be defined as the ability to perform daily tasks with enough reserve for emergency situations. All aspects of health-related fitness direct attention toward this goal. Aerobic exercise often provides some conditioning for muscular endurance, but muscular strength and flexibility need to be addressed separately.

The ACSM recommends resistance training using the "overload principle," which involves placing habitual stress on a system, causing it to adapt and respond. For this training, it is suggested that eight to twelve repetitions of eight to ten strengthening exercises of the major muscle groups be performed a minimum of two days per week.

Flexibility of connective tissue and muscle tissue is essential to maximize physical performance and to limit musculoskeletal injuries. At least one stretching exercise for each major muscle group should be executed three to four times per week while the muscles are warm. Three methods of stretching that have been designed to improve flexibility are ballistic stretching, static stretching, and proprioceptive neuromuscular facilitation (PNF). Ballistic stretching incorporates a bouncing motion and is generally prescribed only in sports that replicate this type of movement. During a static stretch, the muscles and connective tissue are passively stretched to their maximum lengths. PNF involves a contract-relax sequence of the muscle.

In addition to exercise prescription for cardiorespiratory fitness, muscular fitness, and flexibility, it is appropriate for the exercise physiologist to make recommendations concerning body composition. Exercise is an effective tool in fat loss. Dietary caloric restriction without exercise results in a greater loss of muscle mass along with fat loss than if exercise is part of a weight loss program.

For persons with special health concerns, such as diabetes mellitus or high blood pressure, the exercise physiologist works with the participant's physician. The physician is responsible for prescribing necessary medications and often decides which modes of exercise are contraindicated (those that should be avoided).

A second application, cardiac rehabilitation, takes exercise prescription a step further. Participation of the heart patient is more individualized than in wellness programs. The condition of the circulatory system, pulmonary system, and joints are only a few of the special concerns. Secondary conditions such as obesity, diabetes, and hypertension must also be considered. The responsibilities of cardiac rehabilitation specialists include monitoring blood sugar in diabetic patients and blood pressure in all patients, especially those with hypertension. Many drugs affect heart rate or blood pressure, and most of these participants are taking more than one type of medication. Patients with heart damage caused by a heart attack may display atypical heart rhythms, which can be seen on an ECG monitor. Furthermore, the stage of recovery of the postsurgical patient is a major factor in recommending the type, frequency, intensity, and duration of exercise.

Patient education is also important. Lifestyle is usually the main factor in the development of heart disease. Cardiac patients often have never participated in a regular exercise program. Frequently, they are smokers, are overweight, and have poor eating habits. Helping them to identify and correct destructive health-related behaviors is the focus of education for the heart patient.

A third application of the study of exercise physiology involves dealing with the competitive athlete. In this case, findings from the most recent research are constantly applied to yield the best athletic performance possible. A delicate balance of aerobic training, anaerobic training, strength training, endurance training, and flexibility exercises are combined with the optimum percentage of body fat, proper nutrition, and adequate sleep. The program that is designed must enhance the athletic qualities that are most beneficial to the sport in which the athlete participates.

The competitive athlete usually pushes beyond the boundaries of general exercise prescription in terms of intensity, duration, and frequency of exercise performance. As a result, the athlete risks suffering more injuries than the individual who exercises for health benefits. If the athlete sustains an injury, the exercise physiologist may work in conjunction with an athletic trainer or sports physician to return the athlete to competition as soon as possible.

PERSPECTIVE AND PROSPECTS

The modern study of exercise physiology developed out of an interest in physical fitness. In the United States, and possibly much of the world, that interest was primarily driven by a desire to prepare soldiers for war adequately.

In the United States, the concern for development and maintenance of physical fitness was well established by the end of the twentieth century. As early as 1819, Stanford and Harvard universities offered professional physical education programs. At least one textbook on the physiology of exercise was published by that time.

Much of the pioneer work in this field, however, was done in Europe. Nobel Prize-winning European research on muscular exercise, oxygen utilization as it relates to the upper limits of physical performance, and production of lactic acid during glucose metabolism dates back to the 1920's.

In the early 1950's, poor performance by children in the United States on a minimal muscular fitness test helped lead to the formation of what is now known as the President's Council on Physical Fitness and Sport. Concurrently, a significant number of deaths of middle-aged American males were found to be caused by poor health habits associated with coronary artery disease. A need for more research in the areas of health and physical activity was recognized by the mid-1960's. The subsequent research was facilitated by the existence of fifty-eight exercise physiology research laboratories in colleges and universities throughout the country. Organizations such as the American Physiological Society (APS), the American Alliance of Health, Physical Education, Recreation and Dance (AAHPERD), and the American College of Sports Medicine (ACSM) were established by the mid-1950's. In an effort to ensure that well-trained professionals were involved in cardiac rehabilitation programs, the ACSM developed a certification program in 1975. Certifications for fitness personnel were added later.

A better understanding of fundamental physiological mechanisms should stem from increasingly more sophisticated testing equipment, allowing practitioners to be more effective in measuring physical fitness and in prescribing exercise programs. Health maintenance has become a priority as the number of adults over the age of fifty continues to increase. Advances in medical techniques also increase the survival rate of victims of heart attacks, creating a need for more cardiac rehabilitation programs and practitioners. Health care professionals and the general population need to be made more aware of the benefits of exercise in the maintenance of good health and in the rehabilitation of individuals with medical problems.

—Kathleen O'Boyle;
updated by Bradley R. A. Wilson, Ph.D.

See also Biofeedback; Bones and the skeleton; Braces, orthopedic; Cardiac rehabilitation; Cardiology; Electrocardiography (ECG or EKG); Ergogenic aids; Glycolysis; Heart; Hyperbaric oxygen therapy; Kinesiology; Lungs; Metabolism; Muscle sprains, spasms, and disorders; Muscles; Nutrition; Orthopedics; Orthopedics, pediatric; Overtraining syndrome; Oxygen therapy; Physical rehabilitation; Physiology; Preventive medicine; Pulmonary medicine; Respiration; Sports medicine; Steroid abuse; Sweating; Tendinitis; Vascular system.

FOR FURTHER INFORMATION:

American College of Sports Medicine. *ACSM's Guidelines for Exercise Testing and Prescription.* 7th ed. Philadelphia: Lippincott Williams & Wilkins, 2006. This manual provides guidelines for professionals working in preventive exercise programs or in cardiac rehabilitation. The recommendations are based on the most up-to-date research available at the time of publication.

_____. *ACSM's Resource Manual for Guidelines for Exercise Testing and Prescription.* 5th ed. Baltimore: Lippincott Williams & Wilkins, 2005. Based on the objective of providing safe and effective exercise programs for all individuals, this publication provides an excellent overview of many of the topics of concern to the exercise physiologist. Specific recommendations regarding stress testing and exercise prescription are included in the text.

Brooks, George A., and Thomas D. Fahey. *Fundamen-*tals of Human Performance.* Mountain View, Calif.: Mayfield, 2000. This textbook was written for students of physical education, nursing, nutrition, and physical therapy who need a practical introduction to exercise physiology. The theoretical basis and practical application of physical activity are explained through a discussion of metabolic phenomena.

McArdle, William, Frank I. Katch, and Victor L. Katch. *Exercise Physiology: Energy, Nutrition, and Human Performance.* 6th ed. Philadelphia: Lippincott Williams & Wilkins, 2007. A wide-ranging text on exercise and the human body, covering topics such as nutrition, energy transfer, exercise training, systems of energy delivery and utilization, enhancement of energy capacity, the effect of environmental stress, and the effect of exercise on successful aging and disease prevention.

Powers, Scott K., and Edward T. Howley. *Exercise Physiology: Theory and Application to Fitness and Performance.* 6th ed. New York: McGraw-Hill, 2007. The upper-level undergraduate or beginning graduate student will find detailed information concerning exercise physiology in this useful textbook. Designed for students who are serious about the study of exercise science.

EXTENDED CARE FOR THE AGING. *See* **AGING: EXTENDED CARE.**

EXTENDED CARE FOR THE TERMINALLY ILL. *See* **TERMINALLY ILL: EXTENDED CARE.**

EXTREMITIES. *See* **FEET; FOOT DISORDERS; LOWER EXTREMITIES; UPPER EXTREMITIES.**

EYE INFECTIONS AND DISORDERS
DISEASE/DISORDER

ANATOMY OR SYSTEM AFFECTED: Blood vessels, brain, cells, eyes, glands, head, ligaments, muscles, nerves

SPECIALTIES AND RELATED FIELDS: Bacteriology, cytology, general surgery, geriatrics and gerontology, histology, neurology, nursing, nutrition, ophthalmology, optometry, pathology, pediatrics, radiology, virology

DEFINITION: Eye infections involve the invasion, multiplication, and colonization of microorganisms in the tissues of the eye. Eye disorders are derangement or abnormality of the functions of parts of the eye and the general impairment of function of the eye for precise and clear vision.

KEY TERMS:

allergy: abnormal reaction or increased sensitivity to a foreign substance

infection: invasion and multiplication of microorganisms in body tissues

inflammation: localized protective response provoked by injury or destruction of tissues

laser: an extremely intense small beam producing immense heat

ocular: pertaining to the eye

ophthalmologist: a physician who specializes in diagnosing and treating eye diseases and disorders

sign: a doctor's objective evidence of disease or dysfunction

symptom: any indication of disease perceived by the patient

CAUSES AND SYMPTOMS

Several varieties of eye problems exist worldwide. Among the most important are corneal infections, ocular herpes, trachoma, conjunctivitis, iritis, cataracts, glaucoma, macular degeneration, diabetic retinopathy, styes, ptosis, ectropion, entropion, either watery or dry eyes, astigmatism, myopia, hyperopia, presbyopia, amblyopia, and keratoconus.

Many organisms can infect the eye. In corneal infections, bacteria, fungi, or viruses invade the cornea and cause painful inflammation and corneal infections called keratitis. Visual clarity is reduced, and the cornea produces a discharge or becomes destroyed, resulting in corneal scarring and vision impairment.

Ocular herpes is a recurrent viral infection by the herpes simplex virus. Symptoms are a painful sore on the eyelid or eye surface and inflammation of the cornea. More severe infection destroys stromal cells and causes stromal keratitis, cornea scarring, and vision loss or blindness. It is the most common infectious cause of corneal blindness in the United States.

Trachoma is a chronic and contagious bacterial disease of the conjunctiva and cornea. The eye becomes inflamed, painful, and teary. Small gritty particles develop on the cornea. Conjunctivitis is the inflammation of the conjunctiva caused by virus or bacteria infection, chemical irritations, physical factors, and allergic reactions. Inflammation of the cornea accompanies viral forms. The eyes become very sensitive to light. The infectious form is highly contagious, especially acute

---

INFORMATION ON EYE INFECTIONS AND DISORDERS

CAUSES: Bacteria, viruses, or fungi in the eye; abnormal function of parts of the eye impairing vision

SYMPTOMS: Various; may include redness, itching, irritation, pain, swelling, sensitivity to light, blurred vision, vision loss, blindness

DURATION: Acute or chronic

TREATMENTS: Depends on cause; may include eyedrops or ointments, warm compresses, corrective lenses, surgery

---

contagious conjunctivitis (pinkeye). Signs are red, extremely itching, and irritating eyes with a gritty feeling; tearing; nasal discharge; sinus congestion; swollen eyelids (in severe cases); and eyelids that may stick together from dry mucus formed during the night.

Iritis is inflammation of the iris. The cause is still under investigation, but it is associated with rheumatoid arthritis, diabetes mellitus, syphilis, diseased teeth, tonsillitis, trauma, and infections. Symptoms are red eyes, contracted and irregularly shaped pupil, extreme sensitivity to light, tender eyeball, and blurred vision.

A cataract is a clouding of the lens that causes a progressive, slow, and painless loss of vision. Symptoms are reduced night vision, blurriness, poor depth perception, color distortion, problems with glare, and frequent eyeglass prescription changes. Cataracts are the world's leading cause of blindness. Causes are under investigation, but it could result from eye injury, prolonged exposure to drugs such as corticosteroids or to X rays, inflammatory and infectious eye diseases, complications of diseases such as diabetes, prolonged exposure to direct sunlight, poor nutrition, and smoking. Babies can be born with congenital cataracts.

Glaucoma is an optic nerve disease caused by fluid pressure that builds up abnormally within the eye because of very slow fluid production and draining. This can damage the optic nerve, retina, or other parts of the eye and result in vision loss. Early stages have no symptoms. Side (peripheral) vision is lost at an advanced point when irreversible damage makes vision restoration impossible. Blindness results if the condition is left untreated.

In macular degeneration, often called age-related macular degeneration (AMD or ARMD), the light-sensing cells of the macula, which is responsible for sharp and clear central vision, degenerates. The result is a slow, painless loss of central vision necessary for important activities such as driving and reading. Early signs are shadowy areas in the central vision, or fuzzy, blurry, or distorted vision. About 90 percent of cases are "dry" AMD, without bleeding, and 10 percent cases a more severe "wet" type, in which new blood vessels grow and leak blood and fluid under the macula, causing the most vision loss.

Diabetic retinopathy is damage to the blood vessels of the retina caused by uncontrolled diabetes. Early signs may not be exhibited, but blurred vision, pain in the eye, floaters, and gradual vision loss are the symptoms in advanced cases.

A number of disorders can affect the eyelids. A stye, or hordeolum, is a painful localized swelling produced by infection or inflammation in a sweat gland of the eyelids or the sebaceous glands that secrete oil to stop the eyelids from sticking together. Ptosis is drooping of the upper eyelid that obstructs the upper field of vision for one or both eyes. It produces blurred vision, refractive errors, astigmatism, strabismus (in which the eyes are not properly aligned), or amblyopia (lazy eye). Symptoms include aching eyebrows, difficulty in keeping the eyelids open, eyestrain, and eye fatigue, especially during reading.

With an ectropion, the lower eyelid and eyelashes turn outward and sag, usually because of aging. Scarring of the eyelid caused by thermal and chemical burns, skin cancers, trauma, or previous eyelid surgery can also cause the problem. Symptoms are eye irritation, excessive tearing, mucus discharge, and crusting of the eyelid. With an entropion, the lower eyelid and eyelashes roll inward toward the eye and rub against the cornea and conjunctiva. This condition is also primarily the result of aging. Symptoms are irritation of the cornea, excessive tearing, mucus discharge, crusting of the eyelid, a feeling of something in the eye, and

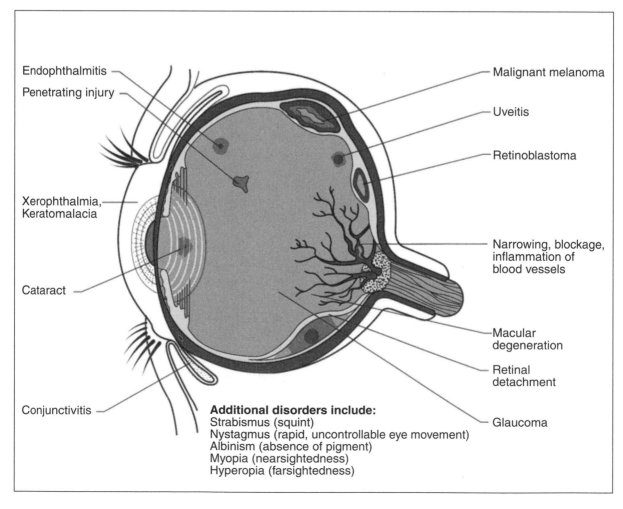

Endophthalmitis

Penetrating injury

Xerophthalmia, Keratomalacia

Cataract

Conjunctivitis

Malignant melanoma

Uveitis

Retinoblastoma

Narrowing, blockage, inflammation of blood vessels

Macular degeneration

Retinal detachment

Glaucoma

Additional disorders include:
Strabismus (squint)
Nystagmus (rapid, uncontrollable eye movement)
Albinism (absence of pigment)
Myopia (nearsightedness)
Hyperopia (farsightedness)

impaired vision. It can also be caused by allergic reactions, inflammatory diseases, and scarring of the inner surface of the eyelid caused by chemical and thermal burns.

Watery eyes are caused by the blockage of the lacrimal puncta (two small pores that drain tear secretions from lacrymal glands that bathe the conjunctival surfaces of the eye) or oversecretion of the lacrimal glands. Dry eyes result from inadequate tear production due to malfunction of the lacrymal (tear) glands, more common in women, especially after menopause. Symptoms are a scratchy or sandy feeling in the eye, pain and redness, excessive tearing following dry sensations, a stinging or burning feeling, discharge, heaviness of the eyelids, and blurred, changing, or decreased vision. Causes include dry air; the use of drugs such as tranquilizers, nasal decongestants, antidepressants, and antihistamines; connective tissue diseases such as rheumatoid arthritis; or the aging process.

Several refractive vision disorders are common. Astigmatism is blurred vision caused by a misshapen lens or cornea that makes light rays converge unevenly without focusing at any one point on the retina. In hyperopia (farsightedness), the eye can see distant objects normally but cannot focus at short distances because the eyeball is shorter than normal, causing the lens to focus images behind the retina. Presbyopia is farsightedness that develops with age. The lens gradually loses its ability to change shape and focus on nearby objects, creating difficulty in reading. In myopia (nearsightedness), the eye cannot focus properly on distant objects, although it can see well at short distances, because the eyeball is longer than normal. The lens cannot flatten enough to compensate and focuses distant objects in front, instead of on, the retina.

Amblyopia, commonly called lazy eye, is a neurologic disorder in which the brain favors vision in one eye. Misalignment of the eyes (strabismus) creates two different images for the brain. If the condition goes untreated, then the weaker eye ceases to function.

Keratoconus is the progressive thinning of the cornea, producing conical protrusion of the central part of the cornea. It results in astigmatism or myopia and swelling or scarring of cornea tissue that ultimately impairs sight. Its causes are heredity, eye injury, and systemic diseases.

TREATMENT AND THERAPY

The treatment of eye infections and disorders depends on their cause and severity. Minor corneal infections are treated with antibacterial eyedrops. Intensive antibiotic, antifungal, and steroid eyedrop treatments eliminate the infection and reduce inflammation in severe cases. With ocular herpes, prompt treatment with antiviral drugs stops the herpesvirus from multiplying and destroying epithelial cells. The resulting stromal keratitis, however, is more severe and therefore difficult to treat. The primary treatment for trachoma consists of three to four weeks of antibiotic therapy. Severe cases require surgical correction.

A conjunctivitis infection can clear without medical care, but sometimes treatment is necessary to avoid long-term effects of corneal inflammation and loss of vision. Treatment includes antibiotic eyedrops or ointments, antihistamine eyedrops or pills, decongestants, nonsteroidal anti-inflammatory drugs (NSAIDs), or mast-cell stabilizers. Artificial tears and warm compresses offer some relief. Tinted glasses reduce the discomfort of bright light.

With iritis, warm compresses can lessen the inflammation and pain. Certain steroid drugs produce quick reduction of the inflammation. A protective covering enables the eye to rest, and atropine drops could be used to dilate the pupils and prevent scarring or adhesions.

For cataracts, a stronger eyeglass prescription is recommended, but surgery that replaces the clouded lens with an artificial one is the only real cure. Drugs that keep the pupil dilated may help with vision.

Glaucoma detection is challenging because the disease is asymptomatic until it is advanced. Medical therapy is the first step for treatment. Glaucoma is difficult to cure, but some medications successfully lower pressure in the eye. If medication is ineffective, then laser surgery is applied to create openings and facilitate fluid draining in the eye.

One way to diagnose macular degeneration is by viewing a chart of black lines arranged in a graph pattern (Amsler grid). Early signs can be detected through retinal examination. No outright cure has been discovered, but some drug treatments may delay its progression or even improve vision.

Some cases of diabetic retinopathy can be treated with laser surgery that shrinks or seals leaking and abnormal vessels on the retina. Vision already lost cannot be restored. A vitrectomy is recommended for some advanced cases, in which the vitreous component of the eye is surgically removed and replaced with a clear solution.

In treating a stye, applying hot compresses for fifteen minutes every two hours may help localize the infection and promote drainage. Mild antiseptics may be applied to prevent spread of the infection. A small surgical incision may be necessary in some cases.

Surgery is the treatment for congenital ptosis. The procedure tightens the levator muscle to lift the upper eyelid to the required position, allowing a full field of vision. For ectropion and entropion, surgery, under local anesthesia, is used to repair the abnormal eyelid before the cornea becomes infected and scarred. This is followed by an overnight patch and application of antibiotics for a week.

For dry eyes, lubricating artificial tears in the form of eyedrops are the usual answer. Serious cases of watery eyes may be treated by surgically closing the lacrimal puncta (tear drain) temporarily or permanently. Sterile ointments prevent the eye from drying at night.

Astigmatism is corrected with asymmetrical lenses that compensate for the asymmetry in the eye. Surgery and laser treatments are used to reshape the cornea and change its focusing power. Myopia is corrected by concave-shaped glasses or contact lenses that diverge light rays from distant objects to focus on the retina. Hyperopia and presbyopia are corrected with convex-shaped eyeglasses or contact lenses that converge light rays from nearby objects slightly before entering the eye, in order to focus on the retina. For those with amblyopia, a patch over the preferred eye forces the brain to use the other eye, but the drug atropine, which temporarily blurs vision in the preferred eye, offers a better medical alternative to eye patches.

For keratoconus, vision is corrected with eyeglasses initially, followed by special contact lenses that reduce distortion if astigmatism worsens. Corneal transplantation becomes necessary when scarring becomes too severe. Preventive measures in strong sunlight are protective eyeglasses, sunglasses, and hats with brims.

PERSPECTIVE AND PROSPECTS

Ancient papyri indicate that physicians of Egypt were the first to establish clinical practices for the treatment of eye infections and disorders. Herbs and eye paints with bacteriocidal properties, such as malachite, were used to prevent infections. Medicated ointments were used by Arab and Greek physicians to treat trachoma. Leukoma (a white spot on the cornea) was treated with animal galls, especially the gall of tortoise. Antimony sulfite and copper solutions were used to treat eyelid disorders. Herbs have been used in Africa, Asia, and

Latin America to treat eye problems since ancient times.

In the twenty-first century, improved antibiotics and other chemicals are widely used to treat eye diseases. Technological advances in surgical procedures and laser techniques have provided additional options for treating vision disorders. Cataract surgery that once required several days of hospitalization is performed in less than thirty minutes on an outpatient basis. Multifocal lenses are designed to provide both near and distant vision that eliminates the use of reading glasses, advanced lens technology provide more foldable and flexible lens materials, and doctors use lasers to reduce secondary opacification in lenses. Immunotherapy is used to treat allergies that cause conjunctivitis.

Innovative research provides new knowledge and treatments for eye disorders. The Collaborative Longitudinal Evaluation of Keratoconus Study by the National Eye Institute (NEI) is investigating factors that influence the progression and severity of keratoconus. The NEI supported the clinical trials of the Herpetic Eye Disease Study that investigated treatments for severe ocular herpes, the most common infectious cause of corneal blindness in the United States.

Research that explored ayurvedic herbs of India has produced the isotine eyedrop, which effectively treats different eye disorders without surgery, including early stages of cataracts.

Functional MRI (fMRI) techniques allow researchers to create images of neurological activity in real time and to obtain insight into neurological eye diseases such as amblyopia. Scientists are conducting research to obtain implanted lens material that is able to form a new lens within the eye and that works efficiently with the original eye muscles. Investigations are in progress for glaucoma medications that reduce eye pressure and also protect the optic nerve. Research shows that antioxidants and nutrients such as zeaxanthin and lutein (found in green, leafy vegetables), zinc, and vitamins A, C, and E help to control AMD, and omega-3 fatty acids (abundant in coldwater fish) have a protective and healing effect against AMD.

The Food and Drug Administration (FDA) approved Lucentis in 2006 for treating the more severe "wet" AMD by monthly injections into the eye. Macugen (pegaptanib sodium), another AMD treatment medication that improves vision with six-week interval injections, was FDA-approved in 2004. In 2006, it was reported that a team of international research scientists discovered a protein called sVEGFR-1 that prevents blood vessels from forming in the cornea; it could become the basis of new treatments for cancer and macular degeneration.

Also in 2006, the *HealthDay News* reported that a visual aid invented by U.S. scientists comprising a tiny camera, a pocket-sized computer, and a transparent computer display mounted on a pair of glasses provides better vision and mobility for people with tunnel vision, who have lost their peripheral vision. Such innovations are welcome, since one in 200 Americans over age fifty-five has tunnel vision, which is caused by diseases such as retinitis pigmentosa and glaucoma.

Early detection of signs and symptoms is a primary key to the treatment of all eye infections and disorders. As preventive measures, people must avoid eyestrain, exercise their bodies, eat healthy foods, control their sugar levels and blood pressure, avoid smoking, protect the eyes from sunlight, and have regular medical checkups.

—*Samuel V. A. Kisseadoo, Ph.D.*

See also Albinos; Astigmatism; Blindness; Cataract surgery; Cataracts; Chlamydia; Color blindness; Conjunctivitis; Corneal transplantation; Diabetes mellitus; Dyslexia; Eye surgery; Eyes; Face lift and blepharoplasty; Glaucoma; Gonorrhea; Herpes; Jaundice; Keratitis; Laser use in surgery; Macular degeneration; Microscopy, slitlamp; Myopia; Ophthalmology; Optometry; Optometry, pediatric; Pigmentation; Ptosis; Refractive eye surgery; Sense organs; Sjögren's syndrome; Strabismus; Styes; Systems and organs; Trachoma; Transplantation; Vision disorders.

FOR FURTHER INFORMATION:

Boron, Walter F., and Emile L. Boulpaep. *Medical Physiology: A Cellular and Molecular Approach.* Rev. ed. Philadelphia: Elsevier Saunders, 2005. Up-to-date information on human functional and medical information, including that pertaining to the eye, for better understanding of structural and functional disorders.

Jenkins, Gail W., Christopher P. Kemnitz, and Gerard J. Tortora. *Anatomy and Physiology: From Science to Life.* Hoboken, N.J.: Wiley, 2007. Treats human body function, including the eye. With color photographs, illustrations, a DVD, an index, and a glossary.

McKinley, Michael, and Valerie O'Loughlin. *Human Anatomy.* 4th ed. New York: McGraw Hill, 2005. Provides updated anatomical information and describes the adaptive functions of the eye and other

human organs. With an appendix, a glossary, and an index.

Marieb, Elaine N., Jon Mallatt, and Patricia Brady Wilhelm. *Human Anatomy.* 4th ed. San Francisco: Pearson/Benjamin Cummings, 2005. Comprehensive treatment of parts and uses of the eye, with practice questions, color photographs, an appendix, a glossary, and an index.

Saladin, Kenneth S. *Human Anatomy.* 2d ed. New York: McGraw Hill, 2007. Updated treatment of eye anatomy and function. With color photographs, illustrations, an appendix, a glossary, and an index.

Tortora, Gerard J., and Bryan Derrickson. *Principles of Anatomy and Physiology.* 11th ed. Hoboken, N.J.: John Wiley & Sons, 2006. Excellent information on the structure and function of the eye and other organs. Includes color photographs, good illustrations, critical thinking exercises, an appendix, a glossary, and an index.

Van De Graaff, Kent M. *Human Anatomy.* 6th ed. New York: McGraw Hill, 2002. Excellent information on the eye and internal human structures. Includes an appendix listing useful Web sites, a glossary, and an index.

EYE SURGERY

PROCEDURE

ANATOMY OR SYSTEM AFFECTED: Eyes

SPECIALTIES AND RELATED FIELDS: General surgery, geriatrics, ophthalmology, optometry

DEFINITION: Surgical removals from or repairs to the eye.

KEY TERMS:

choroid: the vascular, intermediate coat furnishing nourishment to parts of the eyeball

cornea: the clear, transparent portion of the eye's outer coat, forming the covering of the aqueous chamber

iris: a colored circular membrane suspended behind the cornea and in front of the lens, regulating the amount of light entering the eye by changing the size of the pupil

lens: the transparent biconvex body of the eye

retina: the innermost coat of the eye, formed from sensitive nerve elements and connected with the optic nerve

sclera: the white part of the eye; with the cornea, it forms the eye's external protective coat

trabeculae: the portion of the eye in front of the canal of Schlemm and within the angle created by the iris and cornea

Indications and Procedures

Compared to surgery performed on internal organs and any number of outpatient procedures, eye surgery can fill patients with added fears, often concerned with great suffering and the possibility of permanent sight loss. Surgery to an internal organ is usually perceived as happening in a remote location in an unseen portion of the body, and most patients have little idea of the organ's function. Often, if an internal growth or organ is removed, the body continues to function quite well. Most patients have some knowledge of the eye, unlike most internal organs, and thus are more likely to develop anxiety about even common surgical procedures involving it. Patients know what eyes are and what they are used for and that they are extremely sensitive and painful to touch. A grain of sand or a hair touching the eye is painful, so the thought of contacting the eye with a needle or making an incision in it with a scalpel or laser can be almost unimaginable. Patients with ocular problems requiring surgery fear damage to the eye and know all too well the consequences of removal. In most instances, the general public has little to no knowledge or understanding of the function and mechanics of eye surgery. Common eye surgeries include, but are not limited to, cataract surgery, corneal transplantation, vision correction, pterygium removal, retinal detactment repair, and tear duct surgery.

A cataract is an opacity on the eye's lens. A cataract may be minimal in size and low in density, so that light transmission is not appreciably affected, or it may be large and opaque so that light cannot gain entry into the interior eye. When the cataract is pronounced, the interior of the patient's eye cannot be seen with clarity, and the patient cannot see out clearly. Over time, the lens takes on a yellowish hue and begins to lose transparency. As the lens thus becomes "cloudy," the patient needs brighter and brighter lights for visual clarity. If the lens becomes completely opaque, then the patient is functionally blind. A cataract is removed when it endangers the health of the eye or interferes with a patient's ability to function. Conditions such as contrast sensitivity, glare, pupillary constriction, and ambient light may significantly affect a patient's functionality.

The objective of cataract surgery is to remove the crystalline lens of the eye that has become cloudy. Modern surgical procedures involve removing the lens, either intact or in pieces after shattering it with high-frequency sound. The surgery is usually performed under an operating microscope because magnification is necessary. Many methods are used for cataract surgery, including an extracapsular procedure, an intracapsular procedure, and phacoemulsification. Most surgeons perform cataract surgery in freestanding surgical centers on an outpatient basis.

In extracapsular surgery, an incision is made at the superior limbus and a small opening is made into the anterior chamber. A viscoelastic substance is introduced and then a small, bent needle, or cystotome, is introduced. An incision is made into the anterior capsule in a circular, triangular, or D-shaped fashion. The wound is enlarged to a diameter of 10 to 11 millimeters, allowing removal of the cataractous nucleus.

The most common cataract surgical procedure is phacoemulsification, or small-incision cataract surgery. A stair-stepped incision of between 1.5 and 4.0 millimeters is made in the front of the eye. A cystotome is inserted to cut the anterior capsule of the lens. An emulsifier and aspirator is inserted to remove the collapsed lens. The missing lens is then replaced by an artificial substitute that is folded and inserted through the incision and rotated into place. The wound is sealed with a single suture or no suture at all. This procedure has become favored because it causes less tissue destruction, less wound reaction, and less astigmatism, and patients can resume normal activities immediately after surgery. Vision is then fine-tuned with glasses or contact lenses, if needed.

Another common eye surgery is corneal transplantation. The cornea is the clear portion in the front part of that eye. When injured, degenerated, or infected, the cornea can become cloudy and vision disrupted. Corneal surgery restores lost vision by replacing a portion of the cornea with a clear window taken from a donor eye. Usually, the donor cornea is taken from a recently deceased person. However, not everyone with corneal disease can be helped by corneal transplantation.

The cornea was one of the first structures of the body to be transplanted. Because the cornea is devoid of blood vessels, it is one of the few tissues in the human body that may be transplanted from one human to another with a high degree of success. The absence of blood vessels in the donor cornea reduces immune system reactions.

Two types of corneal transplants are performed: partial penetration, in which a half thickness of the cornea is transplanted, and penetrating transplantation, which involves the full thickness of the cornea. In partial penetration, the anterior of the eye is not entered; only the outer half or two-thirds of the cornea is transplanted. Union is made by several sutures around the periphery of the donor tissue. Depending on the extent of the disease, the donor tissue may be 6 to 10 millimeters in diameter. In a penetrating transplantation, surgery involves entering the anterior chamber of the eye, inserting the donor cornea, and establishing a tight fit with a continuous suture.

Glaucoma is an ocular disease affecting roughly 2 percent of the population over forty. The major characteristic of the condition is a sustained increase in intraocular pressure so great that the fibrous scleral coat cannot expand significantly and the eye cannot withstand the increasing pressures against surrounding soft tissue without damage to its structure and vision impairment. The results of this pressure increase include excavation of the optic disc, hardness of the eyeball, reduced vision, the appearance of colored halos around lights, visual field defects, and headaches. Surgical procedures are performed to relieve this pressure. Although many types of surgical procedures are performed to treat glaucoma, they are all basically fistulizing surgeries, attempting to create an opening between the anterior chamber and the subconjunctival space or between the surgically prepared layers of the sclera.

Glaucoma surgery involves a small incision made either directly through the cornea at the upper limbus or under a flap of conjunctival tissue. The iris is grasped with small forceps and pulled out of the eye, and a small portion of the trabecular meshwork is partially removed, allowing the aqueous fluid to filter out of the anterior chamber. The cornea is then sutured and the eye bandaged. The most popular procedure of this type is trabeculectomy. As a whole, glaucoma surgeries are performed less often today because of the success of nonsurgical treatments and management with drug therapies. A major consequence of some glaucoma surgery is the development of cataracts. For this reason, early surgery is advocated, especially if factors place patients at high risk.

A common early stage nonincisive procedure in treating glaucoma is laser trabeculoplasty. This procedure involves lasing the middle to anterior portion of the trabecular meshwork with eighty to one hundred equally spaced burns. The argon laser reopens blocked drainage channels and reduces fluid pressure in the eye. More than 90 percent of patients experience successful outcomes from this treatment. Surgery is performed only if patients continue to lose the visual field.

A pterygium is a fibrovascular membrane that extends from the medial aspect of the bulbar conjunctiva and invades the cornea. It is a progressive growth related to overexposure to ultraviolet (UV) light. In time, it can make its way to the central portion of the cornea and interfere with vision. Pterygia are most common in southern climates, where people have greater exposure to UV light. In northern regions, people who work outdoors, especially in open fields or on open water, are most prone to developing a pterygium growth.

The purpose of removing a pterygium is to excise the membrane before it can interfere with vision. The operation requires incision into the cornea as well as the conjunctiva, then removal of the pterygium tissue or its transplantation to another position to redirect its growth.

In a normal eye, the retina lies against the choroidal layer, from which it receives part of its blood supply and nourishment. The retina is loosely attached to the choroid, but when it becomes separated from the choroid, it flaps and hangs within the eye's vitreous fluid. Retinal detachment does not allow adequate nutrients to reach the retina and thus causes poor function, and it eventually leads to vision loss. Retinal detachment may be caused by injury, myopia, or previous eye surgeries. Often, a tear or hole permits fluid to collect under the retina, causing the detachment.

Retinal detachment surgery corrects the loose retina

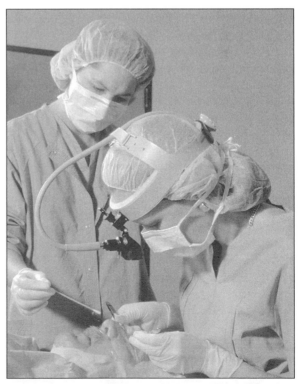

An eye surgeon performs an operation. (Digital Stock)

by bringing it back to the choroid or by pushing the choroid up to the retina. To bring the retina back into place, scleral punctures are made to drain fluids that lay between the retina and the choroid. When the retina returns to lie against the choroid, either electrocoagulation or cryotherapy with a cold probe against the sclera unites the retina to the choroid. Then the retina and choroid are brought together with a silicone buckling band to exert inward pressure. If the retina is not attached at this point, then air, special gases, or oil is injected into the vitreous fluid to push the retina back against the choroid.

Surgery involving corrective procedures to tear ducts is common, especially in older patients. A blockage in the nasolacrimal passage may result in a condition called epiphora, in which the tear ducts water constantly. Such a blockage of the tear canal may result from some form of obstruction. These obstructions are cleared by a surgical procedure called dacryocystorhinostomy. In this procedure, a large incision of 8 to 10 millimeters is made in the wall of the nose, and a union is created between the mucosal lining of the nose and the lacrimal sac. In this way, the lacrimal sac opens directly into the nose. The operation is usually successful in curing the tearing and infection problems arising from stagnation in the blocked tear duct.

Elective refractive eye surgery for the purpose of vision correction began in the Soviet Union in the 1970's and gained popularity in the United States in the 1990's with the use of lasers. It is performed for the relief of myopia, hypermyopia, and astigmatism, with the goal of eliminating the need for either eyeglasses or contact lenses. It is also used to correct refractive errors caused by cataract surgery and corneal transplantation.

Two of the most common refractive surgeries are radial keratotomy (RK) and photorefractive keratectomy (PRK), also known as excimer laser surgery. Myopic patients suffer from a cornea that is either too convex or has an axial length that is too long, causing light to converge at a focal point anterior to the retina. In refractive surgery, corneal reshaping is the important concept. The surgical goal is to flatten the center of the cornea so that light will focus more posteriorly.

RK reshapes the cornea by radial incisions made with a diamond knife. This process weakens the cornea, so normal intraocular pressure pushes the center of the cornea outward, flattening the central cornea. PRK uses a laser to remove the superficial layers of the central cornea, about 50 to 100 microns of tissue, to achieve a similar reshaping of the cornea.

USES AND COMPLICATIONS

The introduction of lasers to eye surgery has proved both beneficial and controversial, depending on its use. An excimer laser can remove any opacifications of the superficial layers of the cornea while retaining the health and clarity of deeper corneal layers. The laser can be used to remove injury-related and surgical corneal scars and to treat astigmatism that may follow implant cataract surgery. The excimer laser also enables surgeons to treat diseases such as fungal ulcers and to smoothe out pterygium irregularities.

Patients interested in pursuing elective refractive surgeries, however, should be aware of the inherent risks of the procedures and that some ophthalmologists are hesitant to use these procedures to correct nearsightedness. The leading cause of skepticism is a reluctance to operate on an essentially healthy eye, thus putting it at risk. These operative procedures have been developed to correct only refractive vision errors. Refractive surgery does not treat glaucoma, cataracts, or other disorders that affect or damage vision.

PERSPECTIVE AND PROSPECTS

As experience and long-term results from the use of laser energy as a surgical tool increase, other forms of therapy will be investigated. Noninvasive glaucoma procedures and laser disruptions of vitreous opacitites and retinal traction bands are already being performed. Ablation procedures to control late-stage glaucoma and techniques to emulsify and remove cataract lenses with lasers in a noninvasive procedure have undergone positive trials.

Today, lasers share space in many clinics and operating rooms along with traditional surgical techniques. Laser technology is providing new types of therapy and is treating more challenging forms of eye disease.

—*Randall L. Milstein, Ph.D.*

See also Blindness; Blurred vision; Cataract surgery; Cataracts; Corneal transplantation; Eye infections and disorders; Eyes; Glaucoma; Keratitis; Laser use in surgery; Myopia; Ophthalmology; Optometry; Refractive eye surgery; Sense organs; Surgery, general; Vision disorders.

FOR FURTHER INFORMATION:

Bartlett, Jimmy D., and Siret D. Jaanus, eds. *Clinical Ocular Pharmacology.* 4th ed. Boston: Butterworth-Heinemann, 2001. A well-illustrated and descriptive account of diseases of the eye, as well as surgical and pharmacological treatments. Though aimed at medical professionals, the book is a valuable reference for any interested reader.

Eden, John. *Physician's Guide to Cataracts, Glaucoma, and Other Eye Problems*. Yonkers, N.Y.: Consumer Reports Books, 1992. A book about eye problems and surgeries aimed at the general reader. The explanations and descriptions are easy to read and follow. The book contains no illustrations.

Johnson, Gordon J., et al., eds. *The Epidemiology of Eye Disease*. 2d ed. New York: Oxford University Press, 2003. A university-level text concerning eye disease. Very descriptive and richly illustrated with color images. The book is well referenced and provides researchers and interested readers with timely data sources.

Newell, F. W. *Ophthalmology: Principles and Concepts*. 8th ed. St. Louis: Mosby, 1996. A medical textbook of general ophthalmology. Written for the medical professional, it describes diagnostic and operational techniques for disorders of the eye.

Riordan-Eva, Paul, and John P. Whitcher. *Vaughan and Asbury's General Ophthalmology*. 16th ed. New York: Lange Medical Books/McGraw-Hill, 2004. An in-depth medical text on the general practice and science of ophthalmology. It is very technical and not for the general reader, though rich in information and illustrations.

Stein, Harold A., Raymond M. Stein, and Melvin I. Freeman. *The Ophthalmic Assistant: A Text for Allied and Associated Ophthalmic Personnel*. 8th ed. Philadelphia: Elsevier Mosby, 2006. A teaching text for ophthalmic surgical assistants. Very descriptive and well illustrated, with overviews of diseases, disorders, and infections, as well as most surgical procedures. Though written for students training in the field, the text is well referenced to the appendix and glossary.

EYES

ANATOMY

ANATOMY OR SYSTEM AFFECTED: Nervous system

SPECIALTIES AND RELATED FIELDS: Ophthalmology, optometry

DEFINITION: The body structures that receive and transform information about objects into neural impulses that can be translated by the brain into visual images.

KEY TERMS:

accommodation: adjustments of the crystalline lens that are necessary for clear vision at various distances

cornea: the transparent structure forming the anterior part of the fibrous tunic of the eye; light must pass through this structure to reach the retina

crystalline lens: the transparent focusing mechanism of the eye; it is a biconvex structure situated between the posterior chamber and the vitreous body of the eye

diopter: a unit of power of a lens equal to the reciprocal of the focal length of the lens in meters

iris: the circular pigmented membrane behind the cornea, perforated by the pupil; the most anterior portion of the vascular tunic of the eye

photoreceptor: a light-responsive nerve cell or receptor which is located in the retina of the eye

pupil: the opening at the center of the iris through which light passes

retina: the innermost of the three tunics of the eyeball, which is situated around the vitreous body and is continuous posteriorly with the optic nerve; it contains the photoreceptors

sclera: the tough outer coat or fibrous tunic of the eyeball, which covers the posterior five-sixths of its surface and is continuous anteriorly with the cornea

visual acuity: clarity or clearness in vision

STRUCTURE AND FUNCTIONS

The eye captures pictures from the environment and transforms them into neural impulses that are processed by the brain into visual images. The retina, with its light-sensitive cells, acts as a camera to "put the picture on film," while neural processing in the brain "develops the film" and forms a visual image that is meaningful and informative for the individual.

The human eye originates during development, that is, while the individual is being formed as an embryo in the uterus. Eye formation begins during the end of the third week of development when outgrowths of brain neural tissue, called the optic vesicles, form at the sides of the forebrain region. The optic vesicle induces overlying embryonic tissue to thicken in one region, forming a primitive lens structure called the lens placode. The lens placode, in turn, induces the optic vesicles to form a cuplike structure, the optic cup, while the brain's connection of the vesicles narrows into a slender stalk that forms the optic nerve. The inner part of the optic cup forms the neural or sensory retina, with its photoreceptors, while the outer part of the optic cup develops into the layers of tissues, or tunics, that make up the wall of the eyeball. The lens placode further condenses and solidifies by forming lens fibers that be-

The Anatomy of the Human Eye

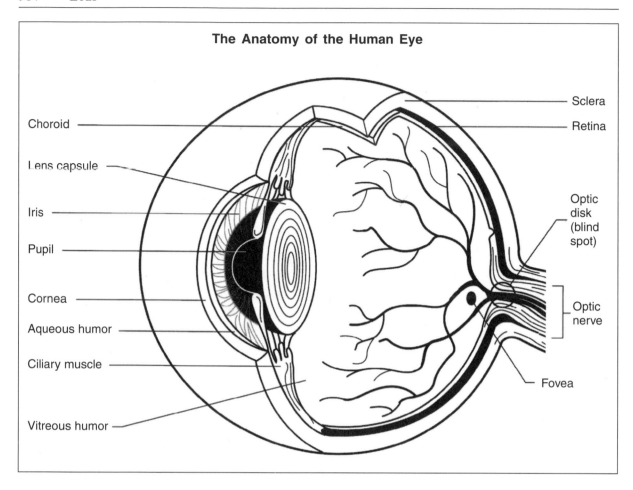

Choroid

Lens capsule

Iris

Pupil

Cornea

Aqueous humor

Ciliary muscle

Vitreous humor

Sclera

Retina

Optic disk (blind spot)

Optic nerve

Fovea

come transparent. The function of the lens will eventually be to focus light onto the retina. The major structures of the eye—the retina, lens, and eyeball coats—are initially formed by the fifth month of fetal development. During the remainder of the prenatal period, eye structures continue to enlarge, mature, and form increasingly complex neural networks with the visual processing regions of the brain.

At birth, an infant's eyes are about two-thirds the size of adult eyes. Until after their first month of life, most newborns lack complete retinal development, especially in the area that is responsible for visual acuity. As a result, infants cannot focus their eyes properly and typically have a vacant stare during their first weeks of life. Most of the subsequent eye growth occurs rapidly during the remainder of the first year of life. From the second year of life until puberty, the rate of eye growth progressively slows. After puberty, eye growth is negligible.

The adult human eye weighs approximately 7.5 grams and measures approximately 24.5 millimeters in its anterior-to-posterior diameter. All movement of the eyeball, or globe, is accomplished by six voluntary muscles attached anteriorly by ligaments to the outer coat of the globe and posteriorly to a tendinous ring located behind the globe. One voluntary muscle elevates the upper lid.

Three concentric tunics form the globe itself. The outermost fibrous tunic consists of two portions. In the small, anterior portion, the tunic fibrils are arranged in a regular pattern, forming the transparent cornea. Posteriorly, the tunic fibrils are irregularly spaced, forming the opaque, white sclera. The innermost tunic, or nervous tunic, consists of two parts: the pars optica, or retina, containing photoreceptor cells, and the pars ceca lining the iris and ciliary body. Tucked between the outer and inner tunics lies the vascular tunic, consisting of the pigmented iris, which gives the eye its distinctive color; the ciliary body, which forms the aqueous humor to provide nourishment for the anterior structures of the globe; and the highly vascular choroid, which provides nourishment for the retina and also acts as a cooling system by regulating blood flow to the chemically active retina. In the center of the circular, pigmented iris lies the pupil, which is a small opening into the posterior parts of the eyeball.

The cavity that contains the globe, circumscribed by the concentric tunics, is filled with a clear, jellylike substance called the vitreous body. This substance is anteriorly bounded in the vitreous cavity by the transparent crystalline lens that lies just posterior to the pupil. The crystalline lens is elastic in structure, allowing for variations in thickness that change the focusing power of the eye.

The eye can refract, or bend, light rays because of the curved surfaces of two transparent structures, the cornea and the crystalline lens, through which light rays must pass to reach the retina. Any curved surface, or lens, will refract light rays to a greater or lesser degree depending on the steepness or flatness of the surface curve. The steeper the curve, the greater the refracting power. If a curved surface refracts light rays to an intersection point one meter away from the refracting lens, this lens is defined as having 1 diopter of power. The human eye has approximately 59 diopters of power in its constituent parts, including the cornea and crystalline lens.

Light rays emitted from a distant point of light enter the eye in a basically parallel pattern and are bent to intersect perfectly at the retina, forming an image of the distant point of light. If the point of light is near the eye, the rays that are emitted are divergent in pattern. These divergent rays must also be refracted to meet at a point on the retina, but these rays require more bending—hence, a steeper curved surface is needed. By a process called accommodation, the human eye automatically adjusts the thickness of the crystalline lens, forming a steeper curve on its surface and thereby creating a perfect image on the retina. Variations from the normal in either the length of an eyeball or the curves of the cornea and crystalline lens will result in a refractive error or blurred image on the retina.

The major task of the eye is to focus environmental light rays on the photoreceptor cells, the rods and cones of the retina. These photoreceptors absorb the light energy, transforming it into electrical signals that are carried to the visual center of the brain. Cones are specialized for color or daylight vision and have greater visual discrimination or acuity than the rods, which are specialized for black-and-white or nighttime vision.

The fovea is a pin-sized depression in the center of the retina that contains only cone cells in high concentrations. This makes the fovea the point of the most distinct vision, or greatest visual acuity. When the eye focuses on an object, the object's image falls on the retina in the area of the fovea. Immediately surrounding the fovea is a larger area called the macula lutea that contains a relatively high concentration of cones. Macula lutea acuity, while not as great as in the fovea, is much greater than in the retina's periphery, which contains fewer cones. The concentration of cones is greatest in the fovea and declines toward the periphery of the retina. Conversely, the concentration of the rods is greater at the more peripheral areas of the retina than in the macula luteal area. The retina of each eye contains about 100 million rod cells and about 300 million cone cells.

The optic nerve carries impulses from the photoreceptors to the brain. This nerve exits the retina in a central location called the blind spot. No image can be detected in this area because it contains neither rods nor cones. Normally, an individual is not aware of the retinal blind spot because the brain's neural processing compensates for the missing information when some portion of a peripheral image falls across this part of the retina.

On a cellular level, rod and cone photoreceptors consist of three parts: an outer segment that detects the light stimulus, an inner segment that provides the metabolic energy for the cell, and a synaptic terminal that transmits the visual signal to the next nerve cell in the visual pathway leading to the brain. The outer segment is rod-shaped in the rods and cone-shaped in the cones (hence their names). This segment is made of a stack of flattened membranes containing photopigment molecules that undergo chemical changes when activated by light.

The rod photopigment, called rhodopsin, cannot discriminate between various colors of light. Thus rods provide vision only in shades of gray by detecting different intensities of light. Rhodopsin is a purple pigment (a combination of blue and red colors), and it transmits light in the blue and red regions of the visual spectrum while absorbing energy from the green region of the spectrum. The light that is absorbed best by a photopigment is called its absorption maximum. Thus at night, when rods are used for vision, a green car is seen far more easily than a red car, because red light is poorly absorbed by rhodopsin. Only absorbed light produces the photochemical reaction that results in vision.

When rhodopsin absorbs light, the photopigment

dissociates or separates into two parts: retinene, which is derived from vitamin A, and opsin, a protein. This separation of retinene from opsin, called the bleaching reaction, causes the production of nerve impulses in the photoreceptors. In the presence of bright light, practically all the rhodopsin undergoes the bleaching reaction and the person is in a light-adapted state. When a light-adapted person initially enters a darkened room, vision is poor since the light sensitivity of the rod photoreceptors is very low. After some time in the dark, however, a gradual increase in light sensitivity, called dark adaptation, occurs as increased amounts of retinene and opsin are recombined by the rods to form rhodopsin. The increased level of rhodopsin occurs after a few minutes in the dark and reaches a maximum sensitivity in about twenty minutes.

Each kind of cone—red, green, and blue—is distinguished by its unique photopigment, which responds to a particular wavelength or color of light. Combinations of cone colors provide the basis for color vision. While each type of cone is most sensitive to the particular wavelength of light indicated by its color—red, green, or blue—cones can respond to other colors with varying degrees. One's perception of color rests on the differential response of each cone type to a particular wavelength of light. The extent that each cone type is activated is coded and sent in separate parallel pathways to the brain. A color vision center in the brain combines and processes these parallel inputs to create the perception of color. Color is thus a concept in the mind of the viewer.

The intricacies of the human visual system require various methods to assess eye structure and function. Visual acuity is a measure of central cone function. Clinically, the most common method for testing visual acuity is by the use of a Snellen chart, consisting of a white background with black letters. All symbols on the chart create, or subtend, a visual angle at the approximate center of the eye. The smaller the symbol, the smaller the angle and the more difficult cone recognition becomes. At the standard distance of twenty feet, the smallest letters on the Snellen chart subtend an angle of five minutes of arc at the eye's center. The larger letters on the chart are calibrated such that each consecutively larger letter subtends a multiple unit of five minutes of arc. If the eye can detect the smallest letters on the chart, the patient is said to have normal (20/20) vision. The numerator of the clinical fraction designates the test distance of twenty feet. The denominator varies with the patient's visual function, identifying the

distance at which the smallest letter recognized by the patient subtends an angle of five minutes of arc. For example, if the smallest letter recognized is fifty minutes of arc in size, the fraction used to record this visual acuity is 20/200 because the letter with fifty minutes of arc is ten times as large as the smallest letters on the chart. Therefore, the distance needed for this letter to create five minutes of arc at the eye is ten times as far as the normal twenty feet. In this example, the patient is said to have a refractive error.

DISORDERS AND DISEASES

Commonly existing refractive errors are astigmatism, myopia, hyperopia, and presbyopia. Presbyopia is an anomaly that occurs with aging when the crystalline lens loses its ability to accommodate. Causes include thickening of the lens and changes in the attachment fibers that anchor the lens. Because of these alterations, the lens is not able to change its shape and the eye remains focused at a specific distance. To compensate for this problem, bifocal spectacles are normally prescribed, with the upper region of the lens focused for distant vision and the lower lens focused for near vision. Hyperopia, also called farsightedness, results when an eyeball is too short. Because light rays are not bent sufficiently by the lens system, the image is focused not on the retina but behind the retina. To compensate for this problem, spectacles with convex lenses are prescribed, which bring the focus point back on the retina. Conversely, myopia, or nearsightedness, results from an abnormally long eyeball. In this case, the lens system focuses in front of the retina. This abnormal vision can be corrected by spectacles with a concave lens. Astigmatism results from a refractive error of the lens system, usually caused by an irregular shape in the cornea or less frequently by an irregular shape in the lens. The consequence of this anomaly is that some light rays are focused in front of the retina and some behind the retina, creating a blurred image. To correct the focusing error, a special irregular spectacle must be made to correct the abnormal irregularity of the eye's lens system.

An examiner can assess the amount of refractive error based on a patient's verbal choice as to which of a given series of lenses sharpens the retinal image of the letters on the Snellen chart. Refractive error can also be determined when a patient is not capable of response. A retinoscope is often used to shine a light through the pupil onto the retina. An image of the light is reflected back out to the examiner who, in turn, can assess refractive error by the movement and shape of the image.

Visual field testing is a measure of the integrity of the neural pathways to the vision center in the brain. To test visual fields clinically, the patient focuses on a central target. While continuing to focus centrally, test targets are serially brought into the patient's peripheral vision, or visual field. The smaller and dimmer the test target, the more sensitive the test. The simplest visual field test technique is by confrontation. The patient and examiner sit facing each other one meter apart. If both patient and examiner cover their right eyes, the patient's left visual field is being tested. Since the patient's left visual field is congruent to the examiner's left visual field, the examiner can detect visual field defects when the patient is not responsive to a test target brought into view from the side. Lesions to some portion of the visual pathway to the brain will result in a scotoma, or blind area, in the corresponding visual field.

A biomicroscope, or slitlamp microscope, is commonly used to assess external eye structures, including the eyelids, lashes, conjunctiva, cornea, sclera, and one internal structure, the crystalline lens. The white part of the eye, or sclera, is covered with a thin, transparent covering called the conjunctiva. Infections and tumors often invade this external structure. Though the normally transparent crystalline lens is essentially free of infections and tumors, it can become cloudy or opaque and develop a cataract. Causes for cataract formation are multiple, the most common being the aging process; less frequently, trauma to the lens or a secondary symptom of systemic disease can result in cataracts. When the cataract is so dense that it obstructs vision, the crystalline lens is surgically removed and replaced with an artificial, plastic lens.

To view internal eye structures, the pupil is dilated to allow more light to be introduced into the interior and posterior regions of the eyeball. Two commonly used instruments are the handheld ophthalmoscope and the head-mounted indirect ophthalmoscope. Diseases of the retina include retinal tears, detachments, artery or vein occlusions, degenerations, and retinopathies secondary to systemic disease.

Glaucoma is an eye disease characterized by raised pressure inside the eye. Normal eye pressure is stabilized by the balance between the production and removal of the aqueous humor, the solution that bathes the internal, anterior structures of the eye. Abnormal pressures are often associated with defects in the visual, or optic, nerve and in the visual field. Approximately 300 people per 100,000 are affected by glaucoma. Clinically, intraocular pressure is assessed by numerous methods in a process called tonometry.

Abnormalities of the eye muscles constitute a significant portion of visual problems. Binocular vision and good depth perception are present when both eyes are aligned properly toward an object. A weakness in any of the six rotatory eye muscles will result in a tendency for that eye to deviate away from the object, resulting in an obvious or latent eye turn called strabismus. Associated signs are eye fatigue, abnormal head postures, and double vision. To alleviate objectionable double vision, a patient often suppresses the retinal image at the brain level, resulting in functional amblyopia (often called lazy eye), in which visual acuity is deficient.

Color blindness, a trait that occurs more frequently in men than in women, is caused by a hereditary lack of one or more types of cones. For example, if the green-sensitive cones are not functioning, the colors in the visual spectral range from green to red can stimulate only red-sensitive cones. This person can perceive only one color in this range, since the ratio of stimulation of the green-red cones is constant for the colors in this range. Thus this individual is considered to be green-red color-blind and will have difficulty distinguishing green from red.

Perspective and Prospects

Early physicians recognized the importance of good eyesight, but because of limited understanding they had minimal means to treat major eye disorders. During the Middle Ages, surgeons performed eye operations, including ones for cataracts in which the lens was pushed down and out of the way with a needle inserted into the eyeball. In the 1700's, this operation was improved when cataract lenses were extracted from the eye. In the early 1600's, Johannes Kepler described how light was focused by the lens of the eye on the retina, thus providing insight into why spectacles are valuable in cases of poor eyesight. In 1801, Thomas Young published a foundational text entitled *On the Mechanics of the Eye*. Hermann von Helmholtz in the 1800's invented the first ophthalmoscope, which allowed inspection of the interior structures of the eye. Young and Helmholtz also developed theories to explain the phenomenon of color vision. From the invention of the ophthalmoscope, the range of clinical observation was extended to the inside of the eyeball, allowing the diagnosis of eye disorders. The modern understanding of eyesight and vision is increasing with contributions from ongoing research.

Ophthalmology is the study of the structure, function, and diseases of the eye. An ophthalmologist is a physician who specializes in the diagnosis and treatment of eye disorders and diseases with surgery, drugs, and corrective lenses. An optometrist is a specialist with a doctorate in optometry who is trained to examine and test the eyes and treats defects in vision by prescribing corrective lenses. An optician is a technician who fits, adjusts, and dispenses corrective lenses that are based on the prescription of an ophthalmologist or optometrist.

Vision care personnel are vital to industry, public health, recreation, highway safety, education, and the community. Since 85 percent of learning is visual-based, good vision is extremely important in education, work, and play. Good vision enhances the production and morale of workers, and athletic performance is improved when vision problems are corrected. Vision care specialists work to promote the prevention of eye injuries and diseases while supporting practices that enhance good health and vision. Vision therapy may be used to correct many disorders of the eye such as amblyopia, reduced visual perception, reading disorders, poor eye coordination, and reduced visual acuity.

—*Elva B. Miller, O.D.,*
and Roman J. Miller, Ph.D.

See also Albinos; Astigmatism; Blindness; Cataract surgery; Cataracts; Chlamydia; Color blindness; Conjunctivitis; Corneal transplantation; Diabetes mellitus; Dyslexia; Eye infections and disorders; Eye surgery; Face lift and blepharoplasty; Glaucoma; Gonorrhea; Jaundice; Keratitis; Laser use in surgery; Macular degeneration; Microscopy, slitlamp; Myopia; Ophthalmology; Optometry; Optometry, pediatric; Pigmentation; Ptosis; Refractive eye surgery; Sense organs; Sjögren's syndrome; Strabismus; Styes; Systems and organs; Trachoma; Transplantation; Vision disorders.

For Further Information:

Buettner, Helmut, ed. *Mayo Clinic on Vision and Eye Health: Practical Answers on Glaucoma, Cataracts, Macular Degeneration, and Other Conditions.* Rochester, Minn.: Mayo Foundation for Medical Education and Research, 2002. A helpful handbook on all the medical, social, and emotional facets of vision impairment.

Guyton, Arthur C., and John E. Hall. *Human Physiology and Mechanisms of Disease.* 6th ed. Philadelphia: W. B. Saunders, 1997. Guyton is a nationally recognized authority on medical physiology, having written and edited numerous college-level and medical school textbooks on the subject. His writing style is understandable to the nonmedical specialist and student. This college-level text contains two chapters on the eye: The first deals with the optics of vision and the function of the retina; the second emphasizes the neurophysiology of vision.

Litin, Scott C., ed. *Mayo Clinic Family Health Book.* 3d ed. New York: HarperResource, 2003. Perhaps the best general medical text for the layperson, this book covers the entire medical field. While the information is derived from a wide variety of highly technical sources, the articles are written to be easily understood by a general audience.

National Foundation for Eye Research (NFER). http://www.nfer.org/. Site provides consumers and professionals with access to developing technology for treating impaired vision.

Prevent Blindness America. http://www.preventblindness.org/. Founded in 1908, this group is dedicated to fighting blindness and saving sight. Its efforts are focused on promoting a continuum of vision care, public and professional education, certified vision screening training, and community and patient service programs and research.

Riordan-Eva, Paul, and John P. Whitcher. *Vaughan and Asbury's General Ophthalmology.* 16th ed. New York: Lange Medical Books/McGraw-Hill, 2004. This well-illustrated textbook is an excellent reference for the serious student who desires more in-depth information on any aspect of the eye or its diseases.

Tortora, Gerard J., and Bryan Derrickson. *Principles of Anatomy and Physiology.* 11th ed. Hoboken, N.J.: John Wiley & Sons, 2006. An outstanding textbook of human anatomy and physiology, containing a well-written chapter on the special senses, emphasizing eyesight and vision.

FACE LIFT AND BLEPHAROPLASTY
PROCEDURES

ANATOMY OR SYSTEM AFFECTED: Eyes, skin
SPECIALTIES AND RELATED FIELDS: General surgery, plastic surgery
DEFINITION: Techniques used to remove unwanted wrinkles and other indicators of aging from the face.

INDICATIONS AND PROCEDURES

Aging may create serious problems among individuals for whom success in their occupations depends on appearance. Premature wrinkling of skin on the face and eyelids or premature looseness of these tissues can create an insurmountable psychological barrier. In these situations, cosmetic surgery such as face lift (rhytidectomy) and/or blepharoplasty (the removal of excess tissue around the eyelids) is indicated.

Surgical face lifting involves making an incision at the hairline and extending it downward in front of the ear toward the angle of the jaw; the length of the incision is dependent on the amount of skin sagging that is present. The skin is gently separated from the underlying fascia and is pulled back and tightened until the desired degree of wrinkle elimination is achieved. Excess skin at the posterior (back) margins is removed. The edges are carefully brought together and secured with fine sutures or adhesive closures. The patient returns to the plastic surgeon in seven to ten days for follow-up evaluation.

Blepharoplasty refers to the surgical alteration of the eyelids. The surgery is similar to that described for a total face lift. An incision is made along the lower margin of the eyebrow. Skin is separated from the fascia.

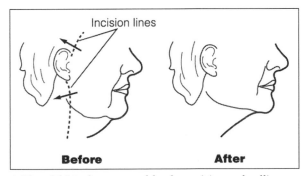

A "face lift" is the term used for the excision and pulling upward of sagging skin on the face. This cosmetic procedure can smooth wrinkles and provide a more attractive profile, but there are drawbacks: The patient's appearance may be changed too dramatically, and the procedure must be repeated periodically to maintain the desired results.

Sometimes, small amounts of fat are also removed. The skin of the upper eyelid is tightened. After excess tissue is removed, the free edges are attached with fine sutures. Cosmetic alteration of the lower eyelid can also be accomplished surgically. The incision is made along a natural crease in the skin just below the lower eyelid. The skin above the incision is separated from its underlying fascia. Some fat may be removed. Typically, excess skin is removed before the edges are reattached, again using very fine sutures. The patient returns to the plastic surgeon in approximately one week for removal of the sutures. Chemical peeling or dermabrasion are additional techniques that can be used to remove fine wrinkles and lines in skin.

USES AND COMPLICATIONS

A face lift is a form of cosmetic surgery and is usually undertaken for aesthetic reasons. Short-term problems include bruising and swelling. Possible long-term complications include infection, scarring, and insufficient removal of unwanted wrinkles. Proper techniques can reduce the first two problems. Realistic expectations can minimize disappointment.

Because of the eyelid's good blood circulation blepharoplasty performed under sterile conditions seldom results in serious infection. However, the procedure can result in a number of other complications: continued bleeding that requires reopening the eyelid wound and either the cauterization of the bleeding vessel or evacuation of a clot; the edges of the eyelid skin closure may separate, requiring either support tape or sutures; eyelid asymmetry, whereby the eyelids look fine individually but do not match as a pair; and finally, either insufficient or excessive skin removal.

PERSPECTIVE AND PROSPECTS

At birth, human skin contains relatively large amounts of a molecule called collagen. Collagen provides strength to the skin; this is technically called turgor. The function of collagen is similar to the fibers in fiberglass or steel reinforcement in concrete: strength. Living on Earth, people are constantly subjected to the effects of gravity and ultraviolet radiation, which over time cause slight damage to the collagen in skin. The turgor is slowly lost. Without sufficient collagen, the skin starts to sag under the influence of gravity. Excessive exposure to the sun accelerates this process. The use of tanning beds in salons can increase the amount of harmful ultraviolet radiation, which also accelerates the aging process. With sufficient time and

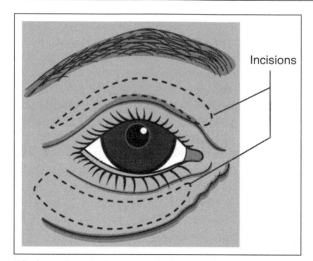

Incisions

Blepharoplasty is the removal of excess, baggy skin around the eyes.

exposure, the typical appearance of skin in old age is seen.

There is no way to stop the human body from aging; accepting this inevitable reality can reduce both stress and anxiety. Cosmetic surgical procedures such as blepharoplasty and face lifts are temporary and enable an individual to maintain only an approximation of youthfulness. Over time, the skin will continue to change, necessitating repeat procedures. Each time the procedure is repeated, the result is diminished in comparison to an earlier procedure. Cosmetic surgery can thus only retard the appearance of aging rather than re-create youth.

—*L. Fleming Fallon, Jr., M.D., Ph.D., M.P.H.*
See also Aging; Botox; Facial transplantation; Plastic surgery; Skin; Skin disorders.

FOR FURTHER INFORMATION:
Aston, Sherrell J., Robert W. Beasley, and Charles H. M. Thorne, eds. *Grabb and Smith's Plastic Surgery.* 5th ed. Philadelphia: Lippincott-Raven, 1997.

Bosniak, Stephen L., and Marian Cantisano Zilkha. *Cosmetic Blepharoplasty and Facial Rejuvenation.* 2d ed. Philadelphia: Lippincott-Raven, 1999.

Henry, Kimberly A. *The Face-Lift Sourcebook.* Los Angeles: Lowell House, 2000.

Lewis, Wendy. *The Beauty Battle: The Insider's Guide to Wrinkle Rescue and Cosmetic Perfection from Head to Toe.* Berkeley, Calif.: Laurel Glen Books, 2003.

Loftus, Jean. *The Smart Woman's Guide to Plastic Surgery.* New York: McGraw-Hill, 2000.

Marfuggi, Richard A. *Plastic Surgery: What You Need to Know Before, During, and After.* New York: Berkeley, 1998.

Narins, Rhoda, and Paul Jarrod Frank. *Turn Back the Clock Without Losing Time: Everything You Need to Know About Simple Cosmetic Procedures.* New York: Three Rivers Press, 2002.

Turkington, Carol, and Jeffrey S. Dover. *The Encyclopedia of Skin and Skin Disorders.* New York: Facts On File, 2002.

Wyer, E. Bingo. *The Unofficial Guide to Cosmetic Surgery.* New York: Wiley, 1998

FACIAL PALSY. *See* BELL'S PALSY.

FACIAL TRANSPLANTATION
PROCEDURE

ANATOMY OR SYSTEM AFFECTED: Blood vessels, bones, circulatory system, ears, eyes, head, immune system, mouth, muscles, neck, nerves, nervous system, nose, skin

SPECIALTIES AND RELATED FIELDS: Dermatology, ethics, physical therapy, plastic surgery, psychology

DEFINITION: A surgical procedure to transplant all or part of the face from a donor's corpse onto the severely disfigured face of a living person in order to provide a dramatic improvement in the appearance of the recipient.

KEY TERMS:

composite tissue allotransplantation (CTA): the grafting of several structures (such as skin, bones, muscles, and nerves) between two or more individuals

immunosuppressants: medications used to prevent the body from rejecting transplanted tissue and organs

transplant: to transfer organs or tissue from one part or individual to another

INDICATIONS AND PROCEDURES

Facial transplantation is a procedure that is reserved for people with extensive facial disfigurements who have exhausted all other options, including reconstructive surgery. Accidents such as burns, trauma, maulings, and gunshot wounds; diseases such as cancer and infection; and birth defects affect thousands of people each year, causing disfigurement to the face. For most people, surgery can correct all or most of the disfigurement. For the few people who experience a great loss of tissue, however, reconstructive surgery is very limited in returning normal function and appearance.

Facial transplantation is technically easier than other facial reconstruction surgeries, should involve fewer surgeries, and can improve appearance and mobility. In traditional facial reconstruction, tissue is surgically reattached or taken from another part of the person's own body. These reconstructions, however, do not transfer the subtle muscles needed for expression, which creates an expressionless, masklike appearance.

People with severe facial disfigurement may have limited facial movement, which can cause difficulty talking, eating, and even closing the eyes. People with facial disfigurement often have low self-esteem and experience social isolation, depression, anxiety, and poor quality of life. They may have difficulty making friends and finding employment.

The transplantation involves three separate surgeries. The first surgery, which takes ten to twelve hours, degloves the corpse of the donor. Degloving involves the removal of the face, whereby an incision is made across the hairline, down the temples, behind or around the ears, and around the jaw line. The face, including the eyebrows, eyelids, nose, mouth, and lips, is then detached, as is underlying fat and connective tissue. Surgeons must be careful not to damage the nerves controlling facial expression, eye movement, and facial sensation. If the donor's face is healthy enough for the transplant, then the surgeons begin the second surgery, in which they deglove the patient's face. This surgery takes longer, since the surgeons must clamp off the veins and arteries and take special care not to damage the nerves. Bone grafts would be performed if the patient needs bone replacement. The third surgery involves reattaching the face, including veins, arteries, and nerves, and could take twenty-four hours to complete.

Temporary tubing and drains are installed to remove fluid buildup. The patient would take immunosuppressants for life. After about two months, the patient's face would return to normal size. Depending on the nerve damage before the transplant and the success in nerve reattachment, the patient's facial movements may not be normal for several months to over a year.

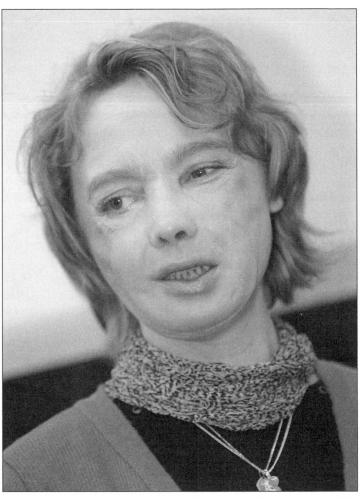

Isabelle Dinoire, the first person to undergo a partial face transplant. (AP/ Wide World Photos)

USES AND COMPLICATIONS

By the end of 2006, only two partial facial transplantations had been performed worldwide. No one yet knows of all the risks involved. In general, skin grafts are more susceptible to rejection than are most organ or other tissue transplants. In addition, skin transplants carry a life-threatening risk, and a rejected facial transplant would leave the patient in worse condition physically, emotionally, and psychologically.

Other risks include tissue damage that occurs because of cell death from the time of removal to reattachment, and a 10 percent loss of facial cells could result in lifelong sores. If the sensory nerves are not properly reconnected, then permanent numbness would occur. Long-term risks, including tissue mutation or psychological impact, are unknown. Short-term risks include infection, additional scarring, potential tissue rejection, and long-term healing. The side effects of immunosuppressants include infections, metabolic disorders such as diabetes, malignancies, and decreased kidney and lung function.

The new face would be a hybrid, a cross between the donor and recipient's faces. Most surgeons believe that, instead of completely removing any sign of disfigurement, a facial transplant would dramatically improve the appearance of the patient.

PERSPECTIVE AND PROSPECTS

With the introduction of immunosuppressive drugs in the 1980's, composite tissue allotransplantation (CTA) became possible. Prior to the introduction of these drugs, hand and face transplants had been considered almost impossible because of the tissue involved and the high risk of rejection.

In 1994, a surgeon successfully reattached the face of a nine-year-old in India whose face and scalp were ripped off by a threshing machine. Two other surgeries, one in Australia and one in the United States in 2002, also reattached entire faces. Facial transplantation was discussed as a serious therapeutic option in a 2002 meeting of the Plastic Surgical Research Council in Boston, Massachusetts, and, by early 2006, teams in the United States, France, and Great Britain had been working for years to develop surgical techniques, protocols for immunosuppression, psychological assessment, and informed consent for potential patients.

In France, on November 27, 2005, doctors transplanted a chin, lips, and nose onto Isabelle Dinoire, a woman who had been mauled by her dog while she was unconscious. In April, 2006, doctors in China grafted a nose, cheeks, and upper lip onto a man mauled by a bear years before.

The procedure is still very experimental, involves great risks, and raises numerous ethical questions. Patients are participating in research, not receiving traditional medical care. Additionally, most medical personnel agree that it will be years before anyone knows whether the partial transplants performed in France and China are successful. If these early attempts fail, with recipients dying or left more disfigured than before, then support for further attempts will decrease.

—*Virginia L. Salmon*

See also Bone grafting; Dermatology; Ethics; Grafts and grafting; Immune system; Plastic surgery; Skin; Transplantation.

FOR FURTHER INFORMATION:

Baylis, Françoise. "Changing Faces: Ethics, Identity, and Facial Transplantation." In *Cutting to the Core*, edited by David Benatar. New York: Rowman & Littlefield, 2006.

Concar, David. "The Boldest Cut." *New Scientist* 182 (May 29, 2004): 32-37.

"Crossing New Frontier: Paving the Way to Make Face Transplantation Reality." *Medical Ethics Advisor*, July 1, 2006.

McLaughlin, Sabrina. "Face to Face." *Current Science* 89, no. 2 (September 12, 2003): 8-9.

Wilson, Jim. "Trading Faces." *Popular Mechanics* 180, no. 11 (November, 2003): 76-79.

FACTITIOUS DISORDERS
DISEASE/DISORDER

ANATOMY OR SYSTEM AFFECTED: Psychic-emotional system, most bodily systems

SPECIALTIES AND RELATED FIELDS: Family medicine, internal medicine, psychiatry, psychology

DEFINITION: Psychophysiological disorders in which individuals intentionally produce their symptoms in order to play the role of patient.

CAUSES AND SYMPTOMS

Although factitious disorders cover a wide array of physical symptoms and are believed to be closely related to a subset of psychophysiological disorders (somatoform disorders), they are unique in all of medicine for two reasons. The first distinguishing factor is that whatever the physical disease for which treatment is sought and regardless of how serious, the patients who seek its treatment have deliberately and intentionally produced the condition. They may have done so in one of three ways, or in any combination of these three ways. First, patients fabricate, invent, lie about, and make up symptoms that they do not have; for example, they claim to have fever and night sweats or severe back pain that they actually do not have. Second, patients have the actual symptoms that they describe, but they intentionally caused them; for example, they might inject human saliva into their own skin to produce an abscess or ingest a known allergic food to cause the predictable reaction. Third, someone with a known condition such as pancreatitis has a pain episode but exaggerates its severity, or someone else with a history of migraines claims his or her headache to be yet another migraine when it is not. Factitious disorders may manifest as complaints about psychological problems, physical problems, or both.

The second element that makes these disorders unique (and at the same time both fascinating to study and frustrating to treat) is that the sole motivation for causing or claiming the symptoms is for these patients to become and remain patients, to assume the sick role wherein little can be expected from them. These patients are not malingerers, individuals who consciously use actual or feigned symptoms for some other gain (such as claiming a fever so one does not have to go to work or school, or insisting that one's post-traumatic stress is worse than it is to enhance the judgment in a lawsuit). In fact, it is the absence of any discernible external benefit that makes these disorders so intriguing.

Technically, psychiatrists and psychologists understand factitious disorders as having three subtypes. In the first, patients claim to have predominantly psychological symptoms such as memory loss, depression, contemplation of suicide, the hearing of voices, or false memory of childhood molestation. Characteristically, the symptoms worsen whenever the patients know themselves to be under observation. In the second, patients have predominantly physical symptoms that at least superficially suggest some general medical condition. In a more extreme form called Münchausen syndrome, individuals will have spent much of their lives getting admitted to medical facilities and, once there, remaining as long as possible. While common complaints include vomiting, dizziness, blacking out, generalized rashes, and bleeding, the symptoms can involve any organ and seem limited only to the individuals' medical knowledge and experience with the medical system. The third subtype combines both psychological and physical complaints in such a way that neither predominates.

Regardless of subtype, factitious disorders are difficult to diagnose. Usually, the diagnosis is considered when the course of treating either a medical or a mental illness becomes atypical and protracted. Often, the person with a factitious disorder will present in a way which seems odd to the experienced clinician. The person may have an unusually extensive history of traveling, much familiarity with medical procedures and terminology, a complex medical and surgical history, few visitors during the hospitalization, behavioral disruptions and disturbances while hospitalized, exacerbation of symptoms while under observation, and/or fluctuating illness with new symptoms and complications arising as the workup proceeds. When present, these traits along with others make suspicion of factitious disorders reasonable.

No one knows how many people suffer with factitious disorders, but the condition is generally regarded as uncommon. It is certainly rarely reported, but this in part may be attributable to the difficulties in determining the diagnosis. While brief episodes of the condition occur, most people who claim a factitious disorder have it chronically, and they usually move on to another physician or facility when they are confronted with the true nature of their illness. It is therefore likely that some individuals are reported more than once by different hospitals and providers.

There is little certainty about what causes factitious disorders. This is true in large measure because those who know the most about the subject—patients with the disorder—are notoriously unreliable in providing information about their psychological state and often seem only dimly aware of what they are doing to themselves. It may be that they are generally incapable of putting their feelings into words. They are unaware of having inner feelings and may not know, for example, that they are sad or angry. It is possible that they experience emotions more physically, behaviorally, and concretely than do most others.

Another view suggests that people learn to distinguish their primitive emotional states through the responsivity of their primary caretaker. A normal, healthy, average mother responds appropriately to her infant's differing affective states, thereby helping the infant, as he or she develops, to distinguish, define, and eventually name what he or she is feeling. When a primary caretaker is, for any of several reasons, incapable of responding in consistently appropriate ways, the infant's emotional awareness remains undifferentiated and the child experiences confusion and emotional chaos.

It is possible, too, that factitious disorder patients are motivated to assume what sociology defines as a sick role wherein people are required to acknowledge that they are ill and are required to relinquish adult responsibilities as they place themselves in the hands of designated caretakers.

TREATMENT AND THERAPY

In the United States, estimates suggest that factitious disorders may result in costs totaling well over $40 million per year. Understanding how to identify individuals with factitious disorders early in their treatment process is crucial to public health for three important reasons. First, early identification will help the individual obtain a more appropriate referral. Second, it will conserve valuable health care resources, so that clients who have pressing medical needs get the treatment that they deserve. Third, the earlier in the process these individuals can be identified, the sooner valuable health care dollars can be saved, lowering the cost of health care as a whole.

Internists, family practitioners, and surgeons are the specialists most likely to encounter patients with factitious disorder, although psychiatrists and psychologists are often consulted in the management of these patients. These patients pose a special challenge because, in a real sense, they do not wish to become well even as they present themselves for treatment. They are not ill in the usual sense, and their indirect communication and manipulation often make them frustrating to treat using standard goals and expectations.

Sometimes mental and medical specialists' joint, supportive confrontation of these patients results in a disappearance of the troubling and troublesome behavior. During these confrontations, the health professionals are acknowledging that such extreme behavior evidences extreme distress in these patients, and as such is its own reason for psychotherapeutic intervention. These patients are not psychologically minded, however; they also have trouble forming relationships that foster genuine self-disclosure, and they rarely accept the recommendation for psychotherapeutic treatment. Because they believe that their problems are physical, not psychological, they often become irate at the suggestion that their problems are not what they believe them to be. Taken from the patient's perspective, this anger makes some sense. For them, they have endured significant time in evaluation and often also a good bit of money, and if they are lacking insight into their condition, such a confrontation may leave them feeling helpless and misunderstood. As such, even in these circumstances, empathy remains an important element in successful intervention.

—Paul Moglia, Ph.D.;
updated by Nancy A. Piotrowski, Ph.D.

See also Hypochondriasis; Münchausen syndrome by proxy; Psychiatric disorders; Psychiatry; Psychiatry, child and adolescent; Psychiatry, geriatric; Psychoanalysis; Psychosomatic disorders.

FOR FURTHER INFORMATION:

American Psychiatric Association. *Diagnostic and Statistical Manual of Mental Disorders: DSM-IV-TR.* Rev. 4th ed. Washington, D.C.: Author, 2000. This reference book lists the clinical criteria for psychiatric disorders, including mood disorders.

Feldman, Marc D. *Playing Sick? Untangling the Web of Munchausen Syndrome, Munchausen by Proxy, Malingering, and Factitious Disorder.* New York: Brunner-Routledge, 2004. Fascinating case histories of people whose conditions lead them to fake illnesses, in themselves and others, sometimes to the point of death.

Phillips, Katherine A., ed. *Somatoform and Factitious Disorders.* Washington, D.C.: American Psychiatric Association, 2001. A comprehensive examination of such topics as epidemiology, etiology/pathology, and treatment modalities for somatoform and factitious disorders.

FAILURE TO THRIVE
DISEASE/DISORDER

ALSO KNOWN AS: Growth impairment, stunting, wasting

ANATOMY OR SYSTEM AFFECTED: Bones, brain, endocrine system, psychic-emotional system

SPECIALTIES AND RELATED FIELDS: Endocrinology, family medicine, gastroenterology, genetics, neonatology, pediatrics, psychiatry, psychology

DEFINITION: A disorder of early childhood growth that includes disturbances in psychosocial skills and development.

CAUSES AND SYMPTOMS

Failure to thrive may be organic or inorganic; in many children, the etiology is multifactorial. The onset of growth problems may be prenatal as a result of maternal substance abuse, most notably alcohol use, or of maternal infection, particularly with rubella, cytomegalovirus (CMV), or toxoplasmosis. Small size in infants secondary to prematurity resolves by two to three years of age unless there are complications.

Many children with failure to thrive are both stunted (linear growth-affected) and wasted (weight-affected). Assessing which of the two conditions predominates can be done using the body mass index (BMI), which is calculated by dividing weight in kilograms by height in meters squared. A low BMI is a sign of malnutrition. Children with environmental failure to thrive fall into this category.

A child who is small but has an appropriate BMI has short stature rather than failure to thrive. The two leading causes of short stature are familial short stature and constitutional delay.

**INFORMATION ON
FAILURE TO THRIVE**

CAUSES: Maternal substance abuse or infection during prenatal phase, familial short stature, constitutional delay
SYMPTOMS: Stunted growth, weight impairment
DURATION: Two to three years
TREATMENTS: Nurturing environment, nutritional intervention, family counseling

TREATMENT AND THERAPY

The main focus of the medical intervention with failure to thrive is to ensure a nurturing environment and adequate nutrition. Nutritional intervention can be achieved in many ways, such as by securing adequate access to food for the family and offering concentrated formulas, nutritional supplementation, and calorie-dense food, depending on the age of the child. Developmental intervention should also be provided if delay is detected. Likewise, family counseling, especially focusing on parenting skills, may be indicated.

PERSPECTIVE AND PROSPECTS

The term "failure to thrive" originated in 1933; it replaced the term "cease to thrive," which appeared in 1899. Initially, the condition was reported in institutionalized children, including those in orphanages. In the 1940's, it was recognized as a condition that could also affect children living at home with their biological or adoptive parents.

Although the list of conditions that can cause growth impairment in children is quite extensive, a systematic approach using history and both physical and psychosocial assessment will provide clues to the diagnosis. Intervention ensures an adequate outcome, with improved prospects for physical growth and brain development.

—*Carol D. Berkowitz, M.D.*

See also Bonding; Cognitive development; Cytomegalovirus (CMV); Developmental stages; Fetal alcohol syndrome; Growth; Malnutrition; Neonatology; Nutrition; Pediatrics; Rubella; Toxoplasmosis; Weight loss and gain.

FOR FURTHER INFORMATION:

Berk, Laura E. *Child Development.* 7th ed. Boston: Pearson/Allyn and Bacon, 2006.
Geissler, Catherine A., and Hilary J. Powers, eds. *Human Nutrition.* 11th ed. New York: Elsevier/Churchill Livingstone, 2005.
Kreutler, Patricia A., and Dorice M. Czajka-Narins. *Nutrition in Perspective.* 2d ed. Englewood Cliffs, N.J.: Prentice Hall, 1987.
Nathanson, Laura Walther. *The Portable Pediatrician: A Practicing Pediatrician's Guide to Your Child's Growth, Development, Health, and Behavior from Birth to Age Five.* 2d ed. New York: HarperCollins, 2002.
Shore, Rima. *Rethinking the Brain: New Insights into Early Development.* New York: Families and Work Institute, 1997.
Whitney, Ellie, and Sharon Rady Rolfes. *Understanding Nutrition.* 10th ed. Belmont, Calif.: Thomson/Wadsworth, 2005.
Winick, Myron, et al. *The Columbia Encyclopedia of Nutrition.* New York: G. P. Putnam's Sons, 1988.

FAINTING. *See* DIZZINESS AND FAINTING.

FAMILY MEDICINE
SPECIALTY

ALSO KNOWN AS: Family practice
ANATOMY OR SYSTEM AFFECTED: All
SPECIALTIES AND RELATED FIELDS: Geriatrics and gerontology, internal medicine, obstetrics, osteopathic medicine, pediatrics, preventive medicine, psychiatry, psychology
DEFINITION: The specialty concerned with the primary health maintenance and medical care of an undifferentiated patient population, in the context of family and community.

KEY TERMS:
ambulatory care: health care provided outside the hospital, usually in a clinic or office and sometimes in the patient's home
biopsychosocial model: a model that examines the effects of illness on all spheres in which the patient functions—the biological sphere, the psychological sphere, and the social sphere
general practice: a primary care field with care provided by physicians who usually have completed less than three years of residency training; the organization from which family medicine evolved
generalism: a medical and political movement concerned with primary care, often associated with the medical specialties of family medicine, general internal medicine, general pediatrics, and sometimes obstetrics and gynecology

health maintenance: the practice of anticipating, finding, preventing, and/or dealing with potential or established medical problems at the earliest possible stage to minimize adverse effects on the patient

internship: a synonym for the first year of residency training

patient advocacy: the representation of the patient's interest in medical diagnosis and treatment decisions, in which the physician acts as an information source and counselor for the patient

primary care: first-line or entry-level care; the health care that most people receive for most illnesses

residency training: medical training provided in a specialty after graduation from medical school; similar to an apprenticeship and designed to mimic real-life practice as closely as possible

specialist: any physician who practices in a specialty other than the generalist areas of family medicine, general internal medicine, general pediatrics, and obstetrics and gynecology

undifferentiated patient population: patients seen by family physicians regardless of age, sex, or type of problem

SCIENCE AND PROFESSION

From cradle to grave, family physicians have the ability to take care of patients from all age groups and manage a great variety of medical problems on a daily basis. As the primary care provider, they are central to a patient's care, either by providing it directly (85 percent of all medical problems) or by consulting specialists and following their management recommendations. They act as the patient's advocate even when healthy by providing preventive care services to find disease earlier in an attempt to eliminate it or slow its progression.

In the United States, there are 70,000 practicing family physicians, accounting for more than 200 million annual office visits. More than a third of all U.S. counties have access to only family physicians to provide medical care to their communities.

Family medicine is the direct descendant of general practice. For many years, most physicians were general practitioners. In the mid- to late twentieth century, however, the explosion of medical knowledge led to the specialization of medicine. For example, increased knowledge of the function and diseases of the heart seemed to demand creation of the specialty of cardiology. The model of the country doctor or jack-of-all-trades physician taking care of a wide range of medical problems seemed doomed to sink in the sea of sub-

specialization in medicine. The general practitioner, the venerable physician who hung out his or her shingle after medical school and one or more years of internship or residency training, appeared to be headed for extinction. Indeed, in their then-existent forms, the general practitioner and general practice would not have survived. Several forces came into play which did result in the passing of general practice but which also changed general practice into family medicine.

The primary force pushing for general practice to survive and improve was the desire of the general public to retain the family doctor. The services that these physicians rendered and the relationships developed between physician and patients were held in high esteem. Through such voices as the Citizen Commission on Graduate Medical Education appointed by the American Medical Association (AMA), the public requested the rescue of the family doctor.

Other major players in the movement to revive and reshape general practice included the AMA itself and the American Academy of General Practice. On February 8, 1969, approval was granted for the creation of family medicine as medicine's twentieth official specialty. The American Academy of General Practice became the American Academy of Family Physicians (AAFP), and a certifying board, the American Board of Family Practice (ABFP), was established. The name has since been changed to the American Board of Family Medicine (ABFM). After these steps were completed, three-year training programs (residencies) in family medicine were established in medical universities and larger community hospitals to provide the necessary training for family physicians.

Family physicians are trained to provide comprehensive ongoing medical care and health maintenance for their patients. Those people who choose to become family physicians tend to value relationships over technology and service over high financial rewards. Many family physicians find themselves providing service to underserved populations and in mission work both inside and outside the United States. Family physicians often become advocates, providing counseling and advice to patients who are trying to sort out medical treatment options. They generally enjoy close relationships with their patients, who often hold them in high esteem.

Following graduation from medical school, students interested in a career in family medicine begin a three-year residency in the specialty. During the residency, these physicians train in actual practice settings under the supervision of faculty physicians. Family medicine residency training consists of three years of rotations with other medical specialties, such as internal medicine, pediatrics, surgery, and psychiatry. The unifying thread in family medicine residency training is the continuity clinic. Throughout their training, the residents see their own patients several days a week under the supervision of family medicine faculty physicians. Every effort is made to make this training as close as possible to experiences in the real world. Family medicine residents will deliver their patients' babies, hospitalize their patients, and deal with the emotional issues of death and dying, chronic illness, and disability.

Family medicine residents receive intensive training in behavioral and psychosocial issues, as well as "bedside manner" training. Scientific research has shown that many patients who seek care from family physicians have problems that require the physician to be a good listener and a skilled counselor. Family medicine residency training emphasizes these skills. It also emphasizes the functioning (or malfunctioning) of the family as a system and the effect of major changes (such as the birth of a child or retirement) on the health and functioning of the family members.

The length of training (three years versus one year) and the emphasis on psychosocial and family systems training are two of the major differences in the training of a family physician and the training of a general practitioner. Moreover, family physicians spend up to 30 percent of their training time outside the hospital in a clinic. Family medicine was the first medical specialty to emphasize this type of training, and family physicians spend more time in ambulatory (clinic) training than virtually any other specialist.

Following the successful completion of a residency program, a family physician may take a competency examination devised and administered by the ABFM. Passing this examination allows the physician to assume the title of Diplomate of the American Board of Family Medicine and makes him or her eligible to join the American Academy of Family Physicians, the advocacy and educational organization of family medicine.

There are about 250 fellowships now available to graduating family medicine residents: faculty development (16 percent), geriatrics (14 percent), obstetrics (9 percent), preventive medicine (1 percent), research (19 percent), rural medicine (3 percent), sports medicine (28 percent), and others (24 percent) such as occupational medicine.

If family physicians wish to retain their diplomate status, they must take at least fifty hours per year of medical education. After a family physician fulfills all educational and other requirements of the ABFM, that physician must then retake the certifying examination every seven years or the certification will lapse. This periodic retesting is required by the ABFM to make sure that family physicians keep up their medical education and maintain their knowledge level and clinical skills. Family medicine was the first specialty to require periodic reexamination of its physicians. In fact, since family medicine has mandated reexaminations, many other medical specialty organizations now require periodic reexamination of their members or are considering such a move. Many former general practitioners who did not have a chance to do a three-year family medicine residency took the ABFM certifying examination and became diplomates based on their years of practice experience and successful completion of the certifying examination. This option was closed to general practitioners in 1988.

A new recertification program, called the Maintenance of Certification Program for Family Physicians (MC-FP), is being required by the ABFM starting with diplomates who recertified in 2003 and all diplomates phased in by 2010. To maintain certification, candidates must perform the following every seven years: submit an online application, maintain a valid medical license, verify completion of three hundred credits of accepted CME credits, and pass the cognitive exam.

Currently, the American Academy of Family Physicians requires new active physician members to be residency-trained in family medicine. Diplomate status reflects only an educational effort by the physician and does not directly affect medical licensure. Medical licensure is based on a different testing mechanism, and license requirements vary from state to state. There are more than fifty thousand family physicians providing health care in the United States, the District of Columbia, the Virgin Islands, Guam, and Puerto Rico. Family medicine residency programs are approximately four hundred in number and usually have about seven thousand residents in training.

DIAGNOSTIC AND TREATMENT TECHNIQUES
Service to patients is the primary concern of family medicine and all those who practice, teach, administer, or foster the specialty. Of all the family physicians in practice, more than 93 percent are involved in direct patient care. While family physicians by no means consti-

tute a majority of physicians, they are among the busiest when measured in terms of ambulatory patient visits. Family physicians see 30 percent of all ambulatory patients in the United States, which is more than the number of ambulatory visits to the next two specialty groups combined. Because of their training, family physicians can successfully care for more than 85 percent of all patient problems they encounter. Consultation with other specialty physicians is sought for the problems that are outside the scope of the family physician's knowledge or abilities. This level of consultation is not unique to family physicians, as other specialty physicians find it necessary to seek consultation for 10 to 15 percent of their patients as well.

Family physicians can be found in all areas of the United States and in virtually all types of practice situations, providing a wide range of medical services. Family physicians can successfully practice in metropolitan areas or rural communities of one thousand people (or less), and they can be found teaching or doing research in medical colleges. Because of their training and the fact that they see a truly undifferentiated patient population, family physicians deliver a wide range of medical services. Besides seeing many patients in their offices, family physicians care for patients in nursing homes, make house calls, and admit patients to the hospital. Within the hospital, many family physicians care for patients in intensive care and other special care units and assist in surgery when their patients have operations. A small number perform extensive surgical procedures in the hospital setting. A sizable minority of family physicians take care of pregnant women and deliver their children; some of these physicians also perform cesarean sections. Because family physicians see anyone that walks through the door, it is not unheard of for a family physician to deliver a child in the morning, see the siblings in the office in the afternoon, and make a house call to the grandparents in the evening. Over 80 percent of family physicians perform dermatologic procedures, musculoskeletal injections, and electrocardiograms (EKGs) in their own offices.

The thing that makes family physicians different from other physicians is their attention to the physician-patient relationship. The family physician has first contact with the patient and is in a position to bond with the patient. The family physician evaluates the patient's complete health needs and provides personal care in one or more areas of medicine. Such care is not limited to any particular type of problem, be it biological, behavioral, or social, and the patients seen are not screened according to age, sex, or illness. The family physician utilizes knowledge of the patient's functioning in the family and community and maintains continuity of care for the patient in a hospital, clinic, or nursing home or in the patient's own home. Thus, in family medicine, the patient-physician relationship is initiated, established, and nurtured for both sexes, for all ages, and across time for many types of problems.

Because of their training, family physicians are highly sought-after care providers. Small rural communities, insurance companies, and government agencies at all levels actively seek family physicians to care for patients in a wide variety of settings. In this respect, family medicine is the most versatile medical specialty. Family physicians are able to practice and live in communities that are too small to support any other types of physician.

In two reports released by Merritt Hawkins, a national recruiting company, requests for family physicians surged by 55 percent, more than all other specialties. According to data from the Massachussetts Medical Society, community hospitals reported family physicians constituted their "most critical shortage."

While the vast majority of family physicians find themselves providing care for patients, there is a minority of family physicians who serve in other, equally important roles. Roughly 3.5 percent of family physicians serve as administrators and educators. They can be found working in state, federal, and local governments; in the insurance industry; and in residency programs and medical schools. Family physicians in residency programs provide instruction and role modeling for family medicine residents in community-based and university-based residency programs. Family physicians in medical colleges design, implement, administer, and evaluate educational programs for medical students during the four years of medical school. The Society of Teachers of Family Medicine (STFM) is the organization that supports family physicians in their teaching role.

One problem facing the specialty of family medicine is the very small percentage who are dedicated to research: only 0.3 percent of all family physicians. There is a large need for research in family medicine to determine the natural course of illnesses, how best to treat them, and the effects of illness on the functioning of the family unit. The need for research in the ambulatory setting is especially acute because, while most medical research is done in the hospital setting, most medical care in the United States is provided in clinics and offices. This problem will not be easily solved because of the service focus of family medicine training and the small number of family physicians dedicated to research.

PERSPECTIVE AND PROSPECTS

Family medicine developed as a medical specialty because of the demands of the citizens of the United States; it is the only medical specialty with that claim. The ancestor of family medicine was general practice, and there is a direct link from the family physician to the general practitioner. Family medicine has grown and evolved into the specialty best suited to provide for the primary health care needs of most patients. Because of their broad scope of practice, cost-effective methods, and versatility, family physicians are found in virtually every type of medical and administrative setting. Family physicians provide a large portion of all ambulatory health care in the United States, and in some settings they are the sole providers of health care. General practice has been around as long as there have been physicians—Hippocrates was a general practitioner—but family medicine has a definite point of origin. It was created from general practice on February 8, 1969.

In January, 2000, a leadership team consisting of seven national family medicine organizations began the Future of Family Medicine (FFM) Project with its goal being "to develop a strategy to transform and renew the specialty of family medicine to meet the needs of patients in a changing health care environment." Six task forces were created as a result, with each one formed to address specific issues that aid in meeting the core needs of the people receiving care, the family physicians delivering that care, and shaping a quality health care delivery system. The FFM Leadership Committee has focused on improving the U.S. health care system by implementing the following strategies:

taking steps to ensure that every American has a personal medical home, has health care coverage for basic services and protection against extraordinary health care costs, promoting the use and reporting of quality measures to improve performance and service, advancing research that supports the clinical decision making of family physicians, developing reimbursement models to sustain family medicine and primary care offices, and asserting family medicine's leadership to help transform the U.S. health care system.

The present role of the family physician is and will continue to be to seek to improve the health of the people of the United States at all levels. Major problems exist for family medicine, including attrition as older family physicians retire or die, lack of medical student interest in family medicine as a career choice, and the lack of a solid cadre of researchers to advance medical knowledge in family medicine. The major strengths supporting family medicine are its service ethic, attention to the physician-patient relationship, and cost-effectiveness.

After their near demise as a recognizable group in the mid-twentieth century, family physicians have a number of reasons to expect that they will have expanded opportunities to provide for the health care needs of their patients in the future. As the United States, for example, examines its system of health care, which is the most costly and the least effective of any health care system in the developed world, many medical and political leaders look to generalism, and particularly family medicine, to provide answers. Research has shown that, for many medical problems, family physicians can provide outcomes very similar to those provided by specialists. When one couples that fact with the versatility and cost-effectiveness of generalist physicians, it can be argued that to save health care dollars the nation must reverse the 30 percent to 70 percent ratio of generalist to specialist physicians. A ratio of 50 percent to 50 percent generalist to specialist physicians has been proposed at many levels in medicine and government.

As the population ages due to improved mortality statistics and the addition of baby boomers to the geriatric age group, a further shortage of general practitioners such as family physicians is inevitable. This situation will force the United States to deal with its health care issues in order to provide its citizens with cost-effective and adequate coverage. The shortage of family physicians specifically in rural areas has led to 22 million Americans living in federally designated rural health professions shortage areas (HPSAs), defined as less than 1 primary care physician per 3,500 people. A growing challenge exists for those physicians living in rural areas as a lack of training and preparation for practice in their medical education and residency training has led to a steady decline in their choosing to practice there.

—Paul M. Paulman, M.D.;
updated by Kenneth Dill, M.D.

See also African American health; Allergies; American Indian health; Anemia; Asian American health; Athlete's foot; Bacterial infections; Bronchitis; Bruises; Chickenpox; Childhood infectious diseases; Cholesterol; Common cold; Constipation; Coughing; Cytomegalovirus (CMV); Death and dying; Diarrhea and dysentery; Digestion; Dizziness and fainting; Domestic violence; Ear infections and disorders; Exercise physiology; Eye infections and disorders; Fatigue; Fever; Fungal infections; Geriatrics and gerontology; Grief and guilt; Halitosis; Headaches; Healing; Heartburn; Hypercholesterolemia; Hyperlipidemia; Hypertension; Hypoglycemia; Indigestion; Infection; Inflammation; Influenza; Laryngitis; Measles; Men's health; Mercury poisoning; Mononucleosis; Mumps; Muscle sprains, spasms, and disorders; Nutrition; Obesity; Obesity, childhood; Osteopathic medicine; Over-the-counter medications; Pain; Pediatrics; Pharmacology; Pharmacy; Physical examination; Pneumonia; Poisonous plants; Preventive medicine; Psychology; Puberty and adolescence; Rashes; Rheumatic fever; Rubella; Scabies; Scarlet fever; Sciatica; Shingles; Shock; Sinusitis; Sleep disorders; Sore throat; Strep throat; Stress; Telemedicine; Tetanus; Tonsillitis; Toxicology; Ulcers; Viral infections; Vitamins and minerals; Wheezing; Whooping cough; Women's health; Wounds.

FOR FURTHER INFORMATION:

American Academy of Family Physicians. http://www.aafp.org/. A Web site with a wealth of information regarding the field of family medicine and the organization as well as links to the journals *Family Practice Management* and *The Journal of Family Practice.*

American Academy of Family Physicians' Membership Directory, 1973- . Available from the American Academy of Family Physicians, this annual publication provides a state-by-state, city-by-city listing of family physicians by name.

American Board of Family Medicine. http://www.theabfm.org/. A Web site about the requirements of the ABFM for family physicians.

Behrman, Richard E., Robert M. Kliegman, and Hal B. Jenson, eds. *Nelson Textbook of Pediatrics*. 17th ed. Philadelphia: Saunders, 2004. Text covering all medical and surgical disorders in children with authoritative information on genetics, endocrinology, etiology, epidemiology, pathology, pathophysiology, clinical manifestations, diagnosis, prevention, treatment, and prognosis.

Rakel, Robert E., ed. *Essential Family Medicine: Fundamentals and Case Studies*. 3d ed. Philadelphia: Saunders Elsevier, 2006. This book outlines the core content essentials for family medicine training.

Scherger, Joseph E., et al. "Responses to Questions by Medical Students About Family Practice." *The Journal of Family Practice* 26, no. 2 (1988): 169-176. Although aimed at medical students, this popular medical article provides good background information about the scope and socioeconomic aspects of family medicine.

Sloane, Philip D., et al., eds. *Essentials of Family Medicine*. 4th ed. Philadelphia: Lippincott Williams & Wilkins, 2002. A basic introductory reference text to family medicine with three sections: "Principles of Family Medicine," "Preventive Care," and "Common Problems."

FATIGUE

DISEASE/DISORDER

ANATOMY OR SYSTEM AFFECTED: All

SPECIALTIES AND RELATED FIELDS: Family medicine, geriatrics and gerontology, internal medicine, psychiatry

DEFINITION: A general symptom of tiredness, malaise, depression, and sometimes anxiety associated with many diseases and disorders; in some cases, no specific cause can be found.

KEY TERMS:

physical deconditioning: a condition that results when a person who has previously been exercising (has become conditioned) stops exercising

psychogenic fatigue: fatigue caused by mental factors, such as anxiety, and not attributable to any physical cause

sleep apnea: cessation of breathing during sleep, which may result from either an inhibition of the respiratory center (central apnea) or an obstruction to the flow of air (obstructive apnea)

sleep disorders: conditions resulting in sleep interruption, interfering with the restorative functions of sleep

syndrome: a collection of complaints (symptoms) and signs (abnormal findings on clinical examination) which do not match any specific disease

CAUSES AND SYMPTOMS

Almost all people suffer from fatigue at some point in their lives. It is a nonspecific complaint including tiredness, lack of energy, listlessness, or malaise. Patients often confuse fatigue with weakness, breathlessness, or dizziness, which indicate the existence of other physical disorders. Rest or a change in the daily routine ordinarily alleviates fatigue in healthy individuals. Though normally short in duration, fatigue occasionally lasts for weeks, months, or even years in some individuals. In such cases, it limits the amount of physical and mental activity in which the person can participate.

Long-term fatigue can have serious consequences. Often, patients begin to withdraw from their normal activities. They may withdraw from society in general and may gradually become more apathetic and depressed. As a result of this progression, a patient's physical and mental capabilities may begin to deteriorate. Fatigue may be aggravated further by a reduced appetite and inadequate nutritional intake. Ultimately, these symptoms lead to malnutrition and multiple vitamin deficiencies, which intensify the fatigue state and trigger a vicious circle.

This fatigue cycle ends with a person who lacks interest and energy. Such patients may lose interest in daily events and social contacts. In later stages of fatigue, they may neglect themselves and lose track of their goals in life. The will to live and fight decreases, making them prime targets for accidents and repeated infections. They may also become potential candidates for suicide.

Physical and/or mental overactivity commonly cause recent-onset fatigue. Management of such fatigue is simple: Adequate physical and/or mental relaxation typically relieve it. Fortunately, many persistent fatigue states can be easily diagnosed and successfully treated. In some cases, however, fatigue does not respond to simple measures.

Fatigue can stem from depression. Depressed individuals often reflect boredom and a lack of interest, and frequently express uncertainty and/or anxiety about the future. These people usually appear "down." They may walk slowly with their head down, slump their shoulders, and sigh frequently. They often take unusually long to respond to questions or requests. They also show little motivation. Depressed individuals typically relate feelings of dejection, sadness, worthlessness, or helplessness. Often, they complain of feeling tired when they wake up in the morning, and no amount of sleep or rest improves their condition. In fact, they feel weary all day and frequently complain of feeling weak. They often have poor appetites and sometimes lose weight. Once these patients are questioned by a physician, however, it may become apparent that their state of fatigue actually fluctuates. At times they feel exhausted, while at other times (sometimes only minutes later) they feel refreshed and full of energy.

INFORMATION ON FATIGUE

CAUSES: Disease, depression, sleep disorders, physical and/or mental overactivity, excessive intake of stimulants, medications
SYMPTOMS: Tiredness, malaise, depression, anxiety, withdrawal
DURATION: Typically short-term but can be chronic
TREATMENTS: Rest and relaxation, medications, counseling

Other manifestations of depression include sleep disorders (particularly early morning waking), reduced appetite, altered bowel habits, and difficulty concentrating. Depressed individuals sometimes fail to recognize their condition. They may channel their depression into physical complaints such as abdominal pain, headaches, joint pain, or vaguely defined aches and pains. In older people, depression sometimes manifests itself as impaired memory.

Anxiety, another major cause of fatigue, interferes with the patient's ability to achieve adequate mental and physical rest. Anxious individuals often appear scared, worried, or fearful. They frequently report multiple physical complaints, including neck muscle tension, headaches, palpitations, difficulty in breathing, chest tightness, intestinal cramping, and trouble falling asleep. In some cases, both depression and anxiety may be present simultaneously.

Medications also constitute a major cause of fatigue. All drugs—prescription, over-the-counter, or recreational—can cause fatigue. Sleeping medications, antidepressants, antianxiety medications, muscle relaxants, allergy medications, cold medications, and certain blood pressure medications can lead to problems with fatigue.

An excessive intake of stimulants, paradoxically, sometimes leads to easy fatigability. Stimulants can interfere with proper sleeping habits and relaxation. Common culprits include caffeine and medications (such as some diet pills and nasal decongestants) that can be purchased without a prescription. So-called recreational drugs can also contribute to chronic fatigue. Depending on their tendencies, they function to cause fatigue in much the same way as the prescription and over-the-counter drugs already discussed. Cocaine and amphetamines, for example, act as stimulants. Narcotics such as heroin and barbiturates (downers) possess strong sedative qualities. Alcohol consumption in an attempt to escape loneliness, depression, or boredom may further exacerbate a sense of fatigue. Alcohol produces fatigue in two ways. It has sedative qualities, and it also intensifies the sedative effects of other medications, if taken with them.

Other drugs that may induce fatigue include diuretics and those that lower blood pressure. These medications increase the excretions of many substances through the kidneys. If inappropriately given or regulated, these drugs may alter the blood concentration of other medications taken concurrently.

Painkillers can lead to fatigue in a different way. In some individuals, they irritate the lining of the stomach and cause it to bleed. Such bleeding usually occurs in small amounts and goes unnoticed by the patient. This slight blood loss can gradually lead to anemia and fatigue.

Medications are particularly likely to cause fatigue in elderly individuals. With many drugs, their elimination from the body through metabolism or excretion may decrease with age. This often leads to higher drug concentrations in the blood than intended, resulting in a state of constant sedation and lethargy. Also, elderly individuals' brains may be more sensitive to sedation than those of younger individuals. Finally, the elderly tend to take more medication for more illnesses than younger adults. The additive side effects of multiple medicines can add to fatigue problems.

Sleep deprivation or frequent sleep interruptions lead to fatigue. A change in environment can induce sleep disorders, especially if accompanied by unfamiliar noises, excessive lighting, uncomfortable temperatures, or an excessive degree of humidity or dryness. Total sleep time may be adequate under such conditions, but quality of sleep is usually poor. Nightmares can also interrupt sleep, and if numerous and recurring, they also cause fatigue.

Some sleep interruptions are not so readily apparent. In sleep apnea, a specific and increasingly diagnosed sleep disorder, the patient temporarily stops breathing while sleeping. This results in reduced oxygen levels and increased carbon dioxide levels in the blood. When a critical level is reached, the patient awakens briefly, takes a few deep breaths, and then falls asleep again. Many episodes of sleep apnea may occur during the night, making the sleep interrupted and less refreshing than it should be. The next day, the patient often feels tired and fatigued but may not recognize the source of the problem. Obstructive sleep apnea normally develops in grossly overweight patients or in those with large tonsils or adenoids. Patients with obstructive sleep apnea usually snore while sleeping, and typically they are unaware of their snoring and/or sleep disturbance.

A number of diseases can lead to easy fatigability. In most illnesses, rest relieves fatigue and individuals awake refreshed after a nap or a good night's sleep. Unfortunately, they also tire quickly. Unlike psychogenic fatigue or fatigue induced by drugs, disease-related fatigue is not usually the patient's main symptom. Other symptoms and signs frequently reveal the underlying diagnosis. Individuals who suffer from severe malnutrition, anemia, endocrine system malfunction, chronic infections, tuberculosis, Lyme disease, bacterial endocarditis (a bacterial infection of the valves of the heart), chronic sinusitis, mononucleosis, hepatitis, parasitic infections, and fungal infections may all experience chronic fatigue.

In early stages of acquired immunodeficiency syndrome (AIDS), fatigue may be the only symptom. Persons at high risk for contracting the human immunodeficiency virus (HIV)—those with multiple sexual partners, homosexual men, those with a history of blood transfusion, or intravenous drug users—who complain of persistent fatigue should be tested for HIV infection.

Abnormalities of mineral or electrolyte concentrations—potassium, sodium, chloride, and calcium are the most important of these—may also cause fatigue. Such abnormalities may result from medications (diuretics are frequently responsible), diarrhea, vomiting, dietary fads, and endocrine or bone disorders.

Some less common medical causes of chronic fatigue include dysfunction of specific organs such as kidney failure or liver failure. Allergies can also produce chronic fatigue. Cancer can cause fatigue, but other symptoms usually surface and lead to a diagnosis before the patient begins to notice chronic weariness.

TREATMENT AND THERAPY

When an individual's fatigue persists in spite of adequate rest, medical help becomes necessary in order to determine the cause. Common diseases known to be associated with fatigue should be considered. Initially, the physician makes detailed inquiries about the severity of the fatigue and how long ago it started. Other important questions include whether it is progressive, whether there are any factors that make it worse or relieve it, or whether it is worse during specific times of the day. An examination of the patient's psychological state may also be necessary.

The physician should ask about the presence of any symptoms that occur along with the general sense of fatigue. For example, breathlessness may indicate a cardiovascular or respiratory disease. Abdominal pain might arouse the suspicion of a gastrointestinal disease. Weakness may point to a neuromuscular collagen disease. Excessive thirst and increased urine output may suggest diabetes mellitus, and weight loss may accompany metabolic or endocrinal abnormalities, chronic infections, or cancer.

Whether they have been prescribed by a physician or purchased over-the-counter, the medications taken regularly by a patient should be reviewed. The doctor should also inquire about alcohol and tobacco use and dietary fads. A thorough physical examination may be required. During an examination, the doctor sometimes uncovers physical signs of fatigue-inducing diseases. Blood tests and other laboratory investigations may also be needed, especially because a physical examination does not always reveal the cause.

Often, however, despite an extensive workup, no specific cause for the persistent fatigue appears. At this stage, the diagnosis of chronic fatigue syndrome should be considered. In order to fit this diagnosis, patients must have several of the symptoms associated with this syndrome. They must have complained of fatigue for at least six months, and the fatigue should be of such an extent that it interferes with normal daily activities. Since many of the symptoms associated with chronic fatigue syndrome overlap with other disorders, these other fatigue-inducing conditions must be considered and ruled out.

In order to fit the diagnosis of chronic fatigue syndrome, patients must have at least six of the classic symptoms. These include a mild fever and/or sore throat, painful lymph nodes in the neck or axilla, unexplained generalized weakness, and muscle pain or discomfort. Patients may describe marked fatigue lasting for more than twenty-four hours that is induced by levels of exercise that would have been easily tolerated before the onset of fatigue. They may suffer from generalized headaches of a type, severity, or pattern that is different from headaches experienced before the onset of chronic fatigue. Patients may also have joint pain without swelling or redness and/or neuropsychologic complaints such as a bad memory and excessive irritability. Confusion, difficulty in thinking, inability to concentrate, depression, and sleep disturbances are also on the list of associated symptoms.

No one knows the exact cause of chronic fatigue syndrome. Researchers continue to study the disease and come up with hypotheses, though none have proven entirely satisfactory. One theory argues that since patients with chronic fatigue syndrome appear to have a reduced aerobic work capacity, defects in the muscles may cause the condition. This, however, constitutes only one of many theories concerning the syndrome and its origin.

Many patients with chronic fatigue syndrome relate that they suffered from an infectious illness immediately preceding the onset of fatigue. This pattern causes some scientists to suspect a viral origin. Typically, the illness that precedes the patient's problems with fatigue is not severe, and resembles other upper respiratory tract infections experienced previously. The implicated viruses include the Epstein-Barr virus, Coxsackie B virus, herpes simplex virus, cytomegalovirus, human herpesvirus 6, and the measles virus. It should be mentioned, however, that some patients with long-term fatigue do not have a history of a triggering infectious disease before the onset of fatigue.

Patients with chronic fatigue syndrome sometimes have a number of immune system abnormalities. Laboratory evidence exists of immune dysfunction in many patients with this syndrome, and there have been reports of improvement when immunoglobulin (antibody) therapy was given. The significance of immunological abnormalities in chronic fatigue syndrome, however, remains uncertain. Most of these abnormalities do not occur in all patients with this syndrome. Furthermore, the degree of immunologic abnormality does not always correspond with the severity of the symptoms.

Some researchers believe that the acute infectious disease that often precedes the onset of chronic fatigue syndrome forces the patient to become physically inactive. This inactivity leads to physical deconditioning, and the progression ends in chronic fatigue syndrome. Experiments in which patients with chronic fatigue syndrome were given exercise testing, however, do not support this theory completely. In the case of physical deconditioning, the heart rates of patients with chronic fatigue syndrome should have risen more rapidly with exercise than those without the syndrome. The exact opposite was found. The data were not determined consistent with the suggestion that physical deconditioning causes chronic fatigue syndrome.

A high prevalence of unrecognized psychiatric disorders exists in patients with chronic fatigue, especially depression. Depression affects about half of chronic fatigue syndrome patients and precedes other symptoms in about half of them as well. Yet a critical question remains unanswered concerning chronic fatigue syndrome: Are patients with this syndrome fatigued because they have a primary mood disorder, or has the mood disorder developed as a secondary component of the chronic fatigue syndrome?

No completely satisfactory treatment exists for chronic fatigue syndrome, since the cause remains a mystery. A group of researchers using intravenous immunoglobulin therapy met with varying degrees of success, but other investigators could not reproduce these results. Other therapeutic trials used high doses of medications such as acyclovir, liver extract, folic acid, and cyanocobalamine. A mixture of evening primrose oil and fish oil was also administered with some degree of success. Claims have also been made that patients administered magnesium sulfate improved to a larger extent than those receiving a placebo. Other therapeutic options include cognitive behavioral therapy, programs of gradually increasing physical activity, analgesics, nonsteroidal anti-inflammatory drugs (NSAIDs), and antidepressants. Finally, a number of self-help groups exist for chronic fatigue sufferers.

The prognosis and natural history of chronic fatigue syndrome are still poorly defined. Chronic fatigue syndrome does not kill patients, but it does significantly decrease the quality of life for sufferers. For the physician, management of this syndrome remains challenging. In addition to correcting any physical abnormalities present, the physician should attempt to find an activity that interests the patient and encourage him or her to become involved in it.

Perspective and Prospects

Fatigue is generally considered a normal bodily response, protecting the individual from excessive physical and/or mental activity. After all, the normal levels of performance for individuals who do not rest usually decline. In the case of overactivity, fatigue should be viewed as a positive warning sign. Using relaxation and rest (mental and/or physical), the individual can often alleviate weariness and optimize performance.

In some cases, however, fatigue does not derive from physical or mental overactivity, nor does it respond adequately to relaxation and rest. In these instances, it interferes with an individual's ability to cope with everyday life and enjoy usual activities. The patient begins referring to fatigue as the reason for not participating in normal physical, mental, and social activities.

Unfortunately, physicians, health care professionals, society, and even the patients themselves dismiss fatigue as a trivial complaint. As a result, sufferers seek medical help only after the condition becomes advanced. This dangerous, negative attitude can delay the correct diagnosis of the underlying pathology and threaten the patient's chances for a quick recovery.

The diagnosis and management of chronic fatigue syndrome prove challenging for both physician and patient. It is important to note that chronic fatigue syndrome often stems from nonmedical causes. While the possibility of a serious medical illness should be addressed, illness-related fatigue usually occurs along with other, more prominent symptoms. The causes of chronic fatigue syndrome are numerous and can take time to define. Patients need to answer all questions related to their complaints as thoroughly and accurately as possible, so that their physicians can reach accurate diagnoses using the minimum number of tests. Extensive testing for rare medical causes of fatigue can become extraordinarily expensive and uncomfortable, so doctors select the tests that they are ordering cautiously. They must balance the benefit, the cost, and the risk of each test to the patient. Such decisions should be based on their own experience and on the available data.

Open communication between the patient and doctor is of paramount importance. It ensures a correct diagnosis, followed by the most effective treatment. Follow-up visits and reassurance may be the best therapy in many cases. Professional counselors can offer assistance with fatigue-inducing psychological disorders. Examination of sleep and relaxation habits can reveal potential problems, and steps can be taken to ensure adequate rest.

Persistent fatigue should not be regarded lightly, and serious attempts should be made to determine its underlying causes. In this respect, it may be appropriate to recall one of Hippocrates' aphorisms, "Unprovoked fatigue means disease."

—*Ronald C. Hamdy, M.D., Mark R. Doman, M.D., and Katherine Hoffman Doman*

See also Aging; Anemia; Anxiety; Apnea; Chronic fatigue syndrome; Depression; Dizziness and fainting; Epstein-Barr virus; Fibromyalgia; Malnutrition; Multiple chemical sensitivity syndrome; Narcolepsy; Overtraining syndrome; Sleep; Sleep disorders; Sleeping sickness; Stress; Stress reduction.

For Further Information:

Archer, James, Jr. *Managing Anxiety and Stress.* 2d ed. New York: Routledge, 1991. Anxiety is a common cause of persistent fatigue. This text examines the nature of anxiety. Contains several methods to combat anxiety and stress, ranging from management skills, personal relations, nutrition, and exercise to meditation and relaxation techniques.

DePaulo, J. Raymond, Jr., and Leslie Ann Horvitz. *Understanding Depression: What We Know and What You Can Do About It.* New York: Wiley, 2003. A leading expert on depression examines the disease's nature, causes, effects, and treatments.

Feiden, Karyn. *Hope and Help for Chronic Fatigue Syndrome: The Official Guide of the CFS-CFIDS Network.* New York: Prentice Hall, 1990. A complete review of chronic fatigue syndrome, presenting the many aspects of this disease. The history of this syndrome, symptomatology, theories of causation, and experimental therapies are addressed.

Goroll, Allan H., and Albert G. Mulley, eds. *Primary Care Medicine.* 5th ed. Philadelphia: Lippincott Williams & Wilkins, 2006. The essential text for the medical office practice of adult medicine. It is problem-oriented and easily read even by individuals without medical training. The section on the causes of fatigue is one of the best available.

Patarca-Montero, Roberto. *Chronic Fatigue Syndrome and the Body's Immune Defense System.* New York: Haworth Medical Press, 2002. Patarca-Montero, a leading immunologist, examines the connections between the disease and immunology, reviews how therapeutic tools such as herbal medicine, vaccines, and cell therapy are being used in CFS research, and discusses the connection between CFS and fibromyalgia, Gulf War syndrome, sick building syndrome, and multiple chemical sensitivity.

Talley, Joseph. *Family Practitioner's Guide to Treating Depressive Illness.* Chicago: Precept Press, 1987. Depression is probably the most common cause of persistent fatigue. This well-written text examines the multiple facets of depression. It also reviews the various therapies available, different philosophies of depressive treatments, and the use of psychotherapy.

Wilson, James L. *Adrenal Fatigue: The Twenty-first Century Stress Syndrome.* Petaluma, Calif.: Smart, 2001. The author, a clinician for more than two decades, helps readers assess their condition and symptoms and determine causes, and suggests treatment of the condition through lifestyle and dietary modification.

Zgourides, George D., and Christie Zgourides. *Stop Feeling Tired! Ten Mind-Body Steps to Fight Fatigue and Feel Your Best.* Oakland, Calif.: New Harbinger, 2003. A self-help book that stresses holistic tools for eliminating tension and improving quality of life. Explores relaxation methods adapted from both Western and Eastern disciplines, such as cognitive-behavioral strategies, simple meditation, visualization, and energy-balancing techniques.

Fatty acid oxidation disorders

Disease/disorder

Anatomy or system affected: Heart, liver, muscles

Specialties and related fields: Biochemistry, biotechnology, nutrition, pediatrics, perinatology

Definition: Inherited metabolic defects that prevent the breakdown of fatty acids in the liver, muscles, and heart.

Causes and Symptoms

Fatty acid oxidation disorders are inherited defects in the enzymes that break down fatty acids to generate metabolic energy. Defects in at least eleven of the twenty enzymes involved with this process have been identified and can be diagnosed by enzymatic analysis of a tissue biopsy. Some generate unique profiles of metabolites in the blood or urine that can be used for diagnosis. These disorders are inherited as autosomal recessive traits, and, in many cases, the causative deoxyribonucleic acid (DNA) mutations have been determined. Fatty acid oxidation disorders can affect the liver, which breaks down fatty acids for its own needs and, by converting them to ketone bodies, for energy

---

Information on
Fatty Acid Oxidation Disorders

Causes: Genetic enzyme deficiency

Symptoms: Only under fasting conditions (overnight or when exacerbated by infection or fever), vomiting, coma, and sometimes death; some disorders largely asymptomatic

Duration: Chronic with acute episodes

Treatments: Minimizing of fasting (snacking before sleep), intravenous glucose for acute episodes

generation in other body tissues; they can also affect muscles and the heart, which use fatty acids as a source of energy.

Symptoms appear only under fasting conditions, either overnight or when exacerbated by infection or fever. Under these conditions, as glycogen stores are depleted, the body depends increasingly on fatty acids for energy. If fatty acids cannot be broken down completely, an energy deficit and the accumulation of deleterious intermediates lead to vomiting, coma, and, in severe cases, death. The levels of blood glucose are low because the energy needed for its synthesis is lacking. The first episode may occur in the first two years of life; such an episode can be fatal and may be mistakenly attributed to sudden infant death syndrome (SIDS). Some fatty acid oxidation disorders, however, are largely asymptomatic.

Treatment and Therapy

The general treatment for fatty acid oxidation disorders is to minimize fasting, as by snacking before sleep, and, in acute episodes, to administer intravenous glucose. This treatment restores depleted blood glucose and reduces the demand for fatty acid oxidation. Some defects also benefit from a low intake of dietary fat. Fasting or low carbohydrate diets, for weight loss or other reasons, are contraindicated for individuals with these disorders.

One of these diseases is attributable to the defective cellular uptake of carnitine, which is needed to transport fatty acids into mitochondria, where they are oxidized; this type can be treated with supplemental carnitine. In acute episodes with some other disorders, treatment with carnitine has proven beneficial in increasing the urinary excretion of deleterious intermediates.

Perspective and Prospects

The first observation of a defect in fatty acid oxidation was made in 1972. Although not reported until 1982, one such disorder, medium-chain acyl-coenzyme A dehydrogenase (MCAD) deficiency, is among the most common inborn errors of metabolism, with a frequency of 1 in 9,000 live births. Each disorder of fatty acid oxidation is a candidate for enzyme replacement therapy or gene replacement therapy, although these remain experimental treatments.

—*James L. Robinson, Ph.D.*

See also Enzyme therapy; Enzymes; Food biochemistry; Glycogen storage diseases; Metabolic disorders; Metabolism.

For Further Information:
Devlin, Thomas M., ed. *Textbook of Biochemistry: With Clinical Correlations*. 6th ed. Hoboken, N.J.: Wiley-Liss, 2006.
Hay, William W., Jr., et al., eds. *Current Diagnosis and Treatment in Pediatrics*. 18th ed. New York: McGraw-Hill, 2006.
Roe, C. R., and J. Ding. "Mitochondrial Fatty Acid Oxidation Disorders." In *The Metabolic and Molecular Bases of Inherited Disease*, edited by Charles R. Scriver et al. 8th ed. New York: McGraw-Hill, 2001.

Feet

Anatomy

Anatomy or system involved: Bones, musculoskeletal system

Specialties and related fields: Orthopedics, podiatry

Definition: The lowest extremities, composed of a complex system of muscles and bones, that act as levers to propel the body and that must support the weight of the body in standing, walking, or running.

Key terms:

distal: referring to a particular body part that is farther from the point of attachment or farther from the trunk than another part

extension: movement that increases the angle between the bones, causing them to move farther apart; straightening or extension of the ankle occurs when the toes point away from the shin

flexion: a bending movement that decreases the angle of the joint and brings two bones closer together; flexion of the ankle pulls the foot closer to the shin

hallucis: a term referring to the big toe; the flexor hallucis longus is a muscle which flexes the big toe

inferior: situated below another part; the ankle bones are inferior to the bones of the lower leg

lateral: toward the side with respect to the body's imaginary midline; away from the midline of the body, a limb, or any understood point of reference

medial: closer to an imaginary midline dividing the body into equal right and left halves than another part

plantar: having to do with the sole of the foot (for example, a plantar wart)

podiatry: the branch of medicine that deals with the study, examination, diagnosis, treatment, and prevention of diseases and malfunctions of the foot

proximal: referring to a particular body part that is closer to a point of attachment than another part *superior:* above another part or closer to the head; the ankle bones are superior to the bones of the feet

STRUCTURE AND FUNCTIONS

The anatomy of the foot is very similar to that of the hand; however, the foot is adapted to perform very different functions. The human hand has the ability to perform fine movements such as grasping and writing, while the foot is involved mainly in support and movement. Therefore, the bones and muscles of the foot tend to be heavier and function without the same dexterity as the hand.

The twenty-six bones of the foot include the tarsals, metatarsals, and phalanges. The proximal portion of the foot next to the ankle is composed of seven tarsal bones: the calcaneus, talus, navicular, cuboid, medial cuneiform, intermediate cuneiform, and lateral cuneiform. The bones are rather irregular in shape and form gliding joints; these joints allow only a limited movement when compared to other joints in the body. The calcaneus forms the large heel bone, which serves as a major attachment for the muscles that are located in the back of the lower leg. Just above the calcaneus is another large foot bone called the talus. The talus rests between the tibia and the fibula, the two lower leg bones. Interestingly, the talus is the single bone that receives the entire weight of the body when an individual is standing; it must then transmit this weight to the rest of the foot below. The cuboid and the three cuneiform bones meet the proximal end of the long foot bones, the metatarsals.

The five separate metatarsal bones are relatively long and thin when compared to the tarsal bones. Anatomists distinguish between the five metatarsals by number. If one begins numbering from the medial (or inside) part of the foot, that metatarsal is number one and the lateral (or outside) metatarsal is number five. The distal portion of each metatarsal articulates (meets) with the toe bones, or phalanges.

Humans have toes that are very similar to their fingers. In fact, the numbers and names of the toe and finger bones, phalanges, are identical. The major differences lie in the fact that the finger phalanges are longer than the phalanges that make up toes. Hinge joints are located between each phalanx and allow for flexion and extension movements only. Human toes (or fingers) are made up of fourteen different phalanges. Each toe (or finger) has three phalanges except for the big toe (or thumb), which has only two. The toes are named in a similar way as the metatarsals; that is, the big toe is number one and the little toe is number five. The three phalanges that make up each toe (except for the big toe) are named according to location. The phalanx meeting the metatarsal is referred to as the proximal phalanx. The bone at the tip of the toe is the distal phalanx, and the one in between is the middle phalanx. Since the big toe only has two phalanges, they are called proximal and distal phalanges.

Although it seems that there is only a single arch in each foot, podiatrists and anatomists identify three arches: the medial and lateral longitudinal arches and the transverse, or metatarsal, arch. The medial longitudinal arch, as the name implies, is located on the medial surface of the foot and follows the long axis from the calcaneus to the big toe. Likewise, the lateral longitudinal arch is on the lateral surface and runs from the heel to the little toe. The transverse, or metatarsal, arch crosses the width of the foot near the proximal end of the metatarsals. The bones are only one factor that maintains arches in the feet and prevents them from flattening under the weight of the body. Ligaments (which connect bones), muscles, and tendons (which attach muscles to bones) are primarily responsible for the support of the arches. The arches function to distribute body weight between the calcaneus and the distal end of the metatarsals (the balls of the feet). They also are flexible enough to absorb some of the shock to the feet from walking, running, and jumping.

While the feet seem to be composed of only bones, tendons, and ligaments, the movements of the toes and feet require an extensive system of muscles. Most of the larger muscles that act on the foot and toes are actually located in the lower leg. Anatomists divide these muscles into separate compartments: anterior, posterior, and lateral.

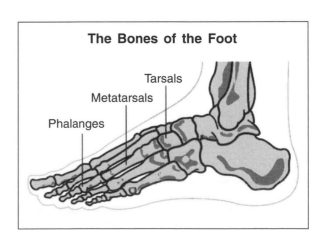

The Bones of the Foot

Tarsals

Metatarsals

Phalanges

The muscles of the anterior compartment move the foot upward (dorsiflex) and extend the toes. These muscles include the tibialis anterior, extensor digitorum longus, extensor hallucis longus, and peroneus tertius. The tibialis anterior is attached to the top of the first metatarsal and pulls the medial part of the foot upward and slightly lateral. All the toes except the big toe are pulled up (extended) by the extensor digitorum longus. The extensor hallucis longus moves only the big toe upward, while the peroneus tertius is attached to the fifth metatarsal and moves the foot upward.

The muscles of the lateral compartment act to move the foot in a lateral or outward direction. The peroneus longus and peroneus brevis are attached to the first and fifth metatarsal, respectively. Using these attachments, the muscles can pull the foot laterally.

The muscles of the posterior compartment are the largest group and act to flex the foot and toes. All these muscles share a common tendon, the calcaneus (or Achilles) tendon. As the name suggests, this large tendon attaches to the calcaneus bone. The larger, more superficial muscles include the gastrocnemius, soleus, and plantaris; these powerful muscles are commonly called the calf muscles. Also in the posterior compartment are four smaller muscles located beneath the calf muscles: the popliteus (located directly behind the knee joint), flexor hallucis longus, flexor digitorum longus, and tibialis posterior. The popliteus rotates the lower leg medially. The flexor hallucis longus flexes the big toe. The remaining toes are flexed by the flexor digitorum longus, while the tibialis posterior acts opposite the tibialis anterior to flex the foot.

Within the foot itself are some muscles known as the intrinsic foot muscles. All but one of these muscles are located on the bottom surface of the foot. This one muscle extends all the toes except the little toe. The remaining intrinsic muscles are on the plantar (bottom) surface and serve to flex the toes.

The major vessels that provide blood to the foot include branches from the anterior tibial artery. This relatively large artery is located along the anterior surface of the lower leg and branches into the dorsalis pedis artery, which serves the ankle and upper part of the foot. Physicians often check for a pulse in this foot artery to provide information about circulation to the foot and circulation in general, as this is the point farthest from the heart. The bottom parts of the feet are supplied with blood by branches of the peroneal artery. At the ankle, this artery branches into plantar arteries, which supply the structures on the sole of the foot. The human toes re-

ceive most of their blood from branches of the plantar arteries called the digital arteries.

DISORDERS AND DISEASES

Even though the anatomy of the foot is resistant to the tremendous amount of force that the body places on it, it can be injured. Force injuries to the foot commonly result in fractures or breaks of the metatarsals and phalanges. Occasionally, the calcaneus may fracture from a fall on a hard surface. More commonly, patients complain of painful heel syndrome.

Because the shock-absorbing pads of tissue on the heel become thinner with age, repeated pressure on the heel can cause pain. Prolonged standing, walking, or running can add to the pressure, as can being overweight. One cause of pain is plantar fasciitis, an inflammation of the tough band of connective tissue on the sole. The inflammation occurs when the muscles located on the back of the lower leg that are attached to the connective tissue at the calcaneus pull under stress. This may even be associated with small fractures. X rays may show small spurs of bone near the site of stress; however, these spurs are not believed to be the cause of pain.

Deformities of the foot at birth are fairly common and include clubfoot, flat foot, and clawfoot. The cause of these anomalies is abnormal development. The foot of the fetus normally goes through stages where it is turned outward and inward but gradually assumes a normal position by about the seventh month of gestation. In the case of clubfoot, arrested development in the stage when the foot is turned inward causes the muscles, bones, and joints to develop in this abnormal anatomical position. At the time of birth, the deformity is readily observable and the foot immobile. Treatment includes splints, casting, and surgery. If treatment is begun at birth, the foot may look relatively normal after approximately one year.

Almost everyone is born with feet that are flat because the arches do not begin to develop until the ligaments and muscles function normally. In most people, the arches are fully formed by the age of six. In some individuals, however, the ligaments and muscles remain weak and the feet do not develop a normal arch. Flat feet can also develop in adult life, at which time they are called "fallen arches." Body weight moves along a precise path during walking or running, beginning with the heel touching the ground. Then, as the foot steps, the arch receives the forces pushing down on the foot. Because the bones, muscles, and ligaments form an arch in the foot, the arch can deform slightly and absorb some of the downward force. With further movement, the weight passes to the ball of the foot (the distal metatarsals). A fallen arch has lost this flexibility and shock-absorbing capability. The arch "falls" because of improper weight distribution along the foot, causing the arch to stretch excessively and to weaken with time. Without proper arch support, the foot begins to twist inward, or medially, causing the body weight to be transmitted to the inside of the foot rather than in a straight line toward the toes. This problem often occurs in runners who have improperly fitted shoes or a poor running style (although anyone can suffer from fallen longitudinal arches, regardless of the individual's level of physical activity). As a runner increases distance and speed without correcting his or her shoes or running form, the force applied to the feet increases. Fallen arches appear to occur particularly in runners or joggers who exercise on hard surfaces without proper technique or arch support.

A number of disorders can affect the skin of the foot. Corns are small areas of thickened skin on a toe that are usually caused by tight-fitting shoes. People with high arches are affected most because the arch increases the pressure applied to the toes during walking. If the corn becomes painful, the easiest treatment is for the person to wear better-fitting shoes. If the pain persists, a clinician can pare down the growth with a scalpel.

Plantar warts appear on the skin of the sole and are caused by a papillomavirus. Because of pressure from the weight of the body, the plantar wart is often flattened and forced into the skin of the sole. The wart may disappear without treatment. If it persists, surgery or chemical therapy can be used to relieve the discomfort.

Athlete's foot is a common fungal infection which causes the foot to become itchy, sore, and cracked. It is usually treated with antifungal agents such as miconazole. Preventive measures including keeping the feet dry and disinfecting areas where the fungus may live, such as shower stalls.

Another common deformity is a bunion, which is a bursa (fluid-filled pad) overlying the joint at the base of the big toe. Normal structure of the first metatarsal, first phalange, and their joint is necessary to withstand the force applied to them in everyday activities. A bunion is caused by an abnormal outward projection of the joint and an inward projection of the big toe. Treatment involves correcting the position of the big toe and keeping it in a normal position. Sometimes surgery is neces-

sary if the tissues become too swollen. In fact, some severe cases of bunions have required complete reconstruction of the toe. Unless treated, a bunion will get progressively worse.

Gout is a metabolic disorder, mainly found in men, which causes uric acid crystals to form in joints. Even though any joint can be affected, the big toe joint is likely the major site for gout because it is under chronic stress from walking. The joint is usually red, swollen, and very tender and painful. The first attack usually involves only one joint and lasts a few days. Some patients never experience another attack, but most have a second episode between six months and two years after the first. After the second attack, more joints may become involved. Treatment includes anti-inflammatory drugs and colchicine. These drugs help reduce the pain by decreasing the amount of inflammation around the joint. Physicians may also prescribe allopurinol to reduce the amount of uric acid that the body produces. Drugs are also available that increase the kidneys' ability to excrete uric acid; examples of these agents are probenecid and sulfinpyrazone.

PERSPECTIVE AND PROSPECTS

Even though the feet constitute a relatively small area of the body, ailments of the feet afflict more than half the world's population. For a long time, disorders of the foot were not taken as seriously as those found in other parts of the body. It is now known, however, that poor foot health can have serious effects. For example, in children a painful foot condition not properly diagnosed and treated can result in lost school days and decreased participation in other activities. More important, an uncorrected congenital abnormality, if neglected, could have irreversible consequences. For the elderly, foot problems hinder or prevent normal activities such as taking care of personal needs, exercising, and socializing. Anything that affects the feet affects that individual's overall health and well-being.

Because of the potentially devastating problems of improper foot care, a branch of medicine developed that specifically addresses problems of the feet. Physicians known as podiatrists practice a specialized branch of medicine called podiatry. It is the job of the podiatrist to assess the cause of the foot problem and the patient's general medical condition in determining the need for and the course of treatment. This assessment often calls for contact with the patient's primary care physician for access to the patient's medical records, as many diseases affect the whole body but present signs and symptoms in the feet. The podiatrist or other physician, such as an orthopedist, will evaluate a disorder through physical exams, laboratory tests, and anatomical tests to examine the internal structures; the latter may include X rays, computed tomography (CT) scans, or magnetic resonance imaging (MRI). The physician will then diagnose and begin treating the disorder using surgery, medical therapy, or physical therapy.

As more individuals become physically active throughout their lives, clinicians who practice sports medicine are paying closer attention to problems of the foot. Many people seek to improve their health by walking, jogging, and bicycling. All these activities have proven to be excellent for maintaining cardiovascular health, but all place additional stress on the foot. Physicians who counsel patients on physical fitness programs attempt to identify individuals who may be injury-prone. Failure to recognize an anatomical anomaly of the feet could lead to an injury or series of injuries that restrict certain activities or even cause permanent damage. Occasionally, individuals are too enthusiastic about their exercise program and experience overuse injuries involving the feet. Such injuries may cause a sudden cessation of the physical activity and may have a significant demoralizing effect on individuals who finally decide to take steps to improve their health and well-being.

People commonly neglect their feet and underemphasize the importance of the normal functional anatomy of the foot. Individuals who experience a foot injury, however, begin to appreciate the absolute importance of this rather complex but often overlooked structure.

—*Matthew Berria, Ph.D.*

See also Anatomy; Athlete's foot; Bones and the skeleton; Bunions; Cysts; Flat feet; Foot disorders; Frostbite; Ganglion removal; Gout; Hammertoe correction; Hammertoes; Heel spur removal; Lower extremities; Nail removal; Nails; Orthopedic surgery; Orthopedics; Orthopedics, pediatric; Podiatry; Sports medicine; Tendon repair; Warts.

FOR FURTHER INFORMATION:

Currey, John D. *Bones: Structures and Mechanics.* Princeton, N.J.: Princeton University Press, 2002. Very accessible overview of a range of information related to whole bones, bone tissue, and dentin and enamel. Topics include stiffness, strength, viscoelasticity, fatigue, fracture mechanics properties, buckling, impact fracture, and properties of cancellous bone.

Hales, Dianne. *An Invitation to Health.* 12th ed. New York: Brooks Cole, 2006. This text should be read by anyone who wishes an overview of health topics. Chapter 7 deals with exercise and contains a section on the importance of wearing the correct shoes for a given activity.

Lippert, Frederick G., and Sigvard T. Hansen. *Foot and Ankle Disorders: Tricks of the Trade.* New York: Thieme, 2003. Details common foot disorders and their causes and treatment.

Mader, Sylvia S. *Human Biology.* 9th ed. Dubuque, Iowa: McGraw-Hill, 2006. Provides an excellent overview of lower limb anatomy and physiology. It also addresses common medical terminology relating to foot movement.

Marieb, Elaine N., and Katja Hoehn. *Human Anatomy and Physiology.* 7th ed. San Francisco: Pearson Benjamin Cummings, 2007. This text discusses the functional significance of various anatomical structures, including the foot. Readers will enjoy the excellent pictures and diagrams of the foot and associated body parts.

Shier, David N., Jackie L. Butler, and Ricki Lewis. *Hole's Essentials of Human Anatomy and Physiology.* 9th ed. New York: McGraw-Hill, 2004. The authors do an excellent job of describing the rather complex anatomy of the foot and lower leg. Several views of the internal and external anatomy of the foot are given.

Van De Graaff, Kent M., and Stuart I. Fox. *Concepts of Human Anatomy and Physiology.* 5th ed. Dubuque, Iowa: Wm. C. Brown, 2000. Van De Graaff has taught human anatomy for years, and anyone would appreciate the approach that he has taken in presenting human structures. Chapters 7, 9, and 10 cover the anatomy of the foot and some problems that can occur if the anatomy is abnormal. Chapter 10 includes the surface anatomy of the lower leg and foot.

FETAL ALCOHOL SYNDROME
DISEASE/DISORDER

ALSO KNOWN AS: Fetal alcohol spectrum disorder (FASD), alcohol-related neurodevelopmental disorder (ARND), alcohol-related birth defects (ARBD), fetal alcohol effects (FAE)

ANATOMY OR SYSTEM AFFECTED: Brain, ears, eyes, hands, head, heart, mouth

SPECIALTIES AND RELATED FIELDS: All

DEFINITION: Prenatal alcohol exposure of the fetus, resulting in specific facial and central nervous system abnormalities, impairment of physical growth (especially linear growth), and other associated anomalies.

CAUSES AND SYMPTOMS

Fetal alcohol syndrome was first described in 1973 after recognition of a specific pattern of craniofacial, limb, and cardiac defects in unrelated infants born to alcoholic mothers.

Alcohol is a potent teratogen. Ethanol toxicity was initially suspected and has since been proven as the etiology of this syndrome. Fetal alcohol syndrome is not genetically inherited but rather is an acquired syndrome.

Alcohol induces abnormalities in neurogenesis and synaptogenesis and is the leading cause of preventable mental retardation and developmental disabilities in the United States. These processes result in central nervous system structural anomalies and microcephaly (small head size). Attention-deficit, hyperactivity, behavioral and learning difficulties; planning difficulties; memory problems; receptive language skill deficits; and math and verbal processing difficulties are common with fetal alcohol syndrome. Alcohol also has lifelong negative effects on fine motor coordination and balance. Prenatal and postnatal growth is below the 10th percentile for age and ethnicity.

Additionally, prenatal alcohol exposure results in numerous cardiovascular problems and facial and limb anomalies. Distinguishing features include short palpebral (eyelid) fissures, a thin vermilion (upper edge of the lip), and a long, smooth philtrum (vertical groove in the upper lip). Underdeveloped ears, clinodactyly (curvature of the little fingers), camptodactyly (bent fingers that cannot straighten), "hockey stick" palmar creases, and cardiac defects are common.

TREATMENT AND THERAPY

Primary prevention is the optimal treatment. Programs to educate health care providers and the general public regarding the adverse effects of alcohol usage during pregnancy may be effective in reducing the incidence of fetal alcohol syndrome. For individuals with this disorder, lifelong therapy directed toward educational planning, including improving cognitive, motor, behavioral, and psychosocial skills, is warranted. In addition, medical care is required for various associated anomalies such as cardiac defects.

INFORMATION ON FETAL ALCOHOL SYNDROME

CAUSES: Alcohol consumption by mother during pregnancy

SYMPTOMS: Growth retardation, certain facial anomalies, central nervous system impairment, clumsiness, behavioral problems, brief attention span, poor judgment, impaired memory, diminished capacity to learn from experience

DURATION: Chronic

TREATMENTS: None; preventive measures during pregnancy

PERSPECTIVE AND PROSPECTS

Alcohol exposure—as a fetus, adolescent, or adult—leads to an increased probability of further alcohol ingestion at other developmental stages. An interruption of this cycle is imperative in order to reduce the incidence of fetal alcohol syndrome. Prevention of alcohol-affected pregnancies depends on developing and implementing evidence-based tools for fetal alcohol syndrome prevention, diagnosis, and treatment. There is no safe dose of alcohol during pregnancy, and current recommendations note that no alcohol should be ingested at conception and throughout gestation.

—*Wanda Bradshaw, R.N.C., M.S.N., N.N.P./P.N.P.*

See also Addiction; Alcoholism; Birth defects; Brain disorders; Childbirth; Childbirth complications; Embryology; Learning disabilities; Mental retardation; Neonatology; Obstetrics; Perinatology; Pregnancy and gestation.

FOR FURTHER INFORMATION:

Calhoun, Faye, et al. "National Institute on Alcohol Abuse and Alcoholism and the Study of Fetal Alcohol Spectrum Disorders: The International Consortium." *Annali dell'Istituto superiore di sanità* 42, no. 1 (2006): 4-7.

Chudley, Albert, et al. "Fetal Alcohol Spectrum Disorder: Canadian Guidelines for Diagnosis." *Canadian Medical Association Journal* 172, suppl. 5 (2005): S1-21.

Gerberding, Julie Louise, Jose Cordero, and R. Louise Floyd. *Fetal Alcohol Syndrome: Guidelines for Referral and Diagnosis.* Atlanta: CDC National Task Force on Fetal Alcohol Syndrome and Fetal Alcohol Effect, 2004.

Hoyme, H. Eugene, et al. "A Practical Clinical Approach to Diagnosis of Fetal Alcohol Spectrum Disorders: Clarification of the 1996 Institute of Medicine Criteria." *Pediatrics* 115, no. 1 (2005): 39-47.

National Organization on Fetal Alcohol Syndrome. http://www.nofas.org/.

Wattendorf, Daniel, and Maximilian Muenke. "Fetal Alcohol Spectrum Disorders." *American Family Physician* 72 (2005): 279-282, 285.

FETAL SURGERY

PROCEDURE

ANATOMY OR SYSTEM AFFECTED: Bladder, blood, brain, liver, lungs, respiratory system, urinary system

SPECIALTIES AND RELATED FIELDS: Cardiology, ethics, genetics, neonatology, obstetrics, pediatrics, urology

DEFINITION: Surgical intervention in utero, before birth, if the fetus has a life-threatening condition or congenital abnormality that can be alleviated.

KEY TERMS:

amniocentesis: the drawing of amniotic fluid through the abdominal wall of a pregnant woman in the fifteenth or sixteenth week of pregnancy to test for fetal abnormalities, particularly Down syndrome

diaphragmatic hernia: a protrusion of the stomach into the diaphragm

hiatal hernia: a protrusion of the stomach into the opening normally occupied in the diaphragm by the esophagus

hydronephrosis: swelling (distension) of the kidney

hypotonic: the presence of a low osmotic pressure

in utero: the Latin term for "inside or within the womb"

neonatologist: a physician who specializes in treating newborn infants

osmotic pressure: the pressure between two solutions separated by a membrane

teratoma: a tumor composed of tissue not normally found at that site

thorax: the bone and cartilage cage attached to the sternum; generally referred to as the rib cage

uropathy: any disease of the urinary tract

INDICATIONS AND PROCEDURES

As early as the 1960's, some unborn infants suffering from progressive anemia caused by antibodies that drew away their strength were saved by receiving blood transfusions in utero. These early procedures marked the beginnings of invasive medical intervention in dealing with fetal problems.

Not until the technical advances of the 1970's and beyond, however, was it possible to observe human fetuses in the uterus. With the development of ultrasound imaging, it became possible to examine in considerable detail the size, growth, and contour of fetuses. The use of ultrasound enabled physicians to assess with considerable accuracy the age of fetuses, their probable date of birth, and a number of congenital abnormalities, such as spina bifida.

Laparoscopes with diameters of less than 0.1 inch make it possible to examine the fetal stomach. The use of lasers and tiny instruments guided by computers has allowed methods of fetal surgery that were inconceivable at mid-twentieth century. These instruments greatly reduce blood loss in all types of surgery, including fetal surgery, and greatly improve the prognosis in such procedures. They are used to repair ruptured membranes in fetuses, to install shunts to relieve blockages, and, with the laser excision of placental vessels, to equalize osmotic pressure in twin-twin transfusion syndrome.

It has become possible for obstetricians to observe all significant fetal organs. Whereas physicians earlier could barely hear the beat of the fetal heart, they now can monitor all four of its chambers in the unborn to detect defects early, and, in some cases, to repair them surgically. Ultrasound enables physicians to observe fetal movement within the uterus and to monitor fetal breathing and swallowing.

Because physicians can now gather specific information about the fetus and its health, abnormalities and life-threatening physical problems can be detected several months prior to delivery. Whereas neonatologists have regularly encountered such problems as intestinal and urinary tract obstructions, heart defects, protrusions of the wall of the stomach into the thorax (diaphragmatic hernia) or into the esophageal region (hiatal hernia), swelling of the kidney (hydronephrosis), tumors (sacrococcygeal teratomas), hydrocephalus (water on the brain), and defects of the chromosomes shortly after the birth of a child, it is now possible to detect and, in some cases, to treat these defects surgically in utero.

In cases where fetal surgery appears to offer the most reasonable solution to a difficult problem, the mother may be sent to one of the few centers in the United States where this highly specialized and controversial form of surgery is performed regularly. With the development of sophisticated computer-operated instrumentation, surgeons geographically distant from their patients can perform highly specialized surgery on them. Eventually, such surgery will likely be performed without uprooting mothers.

The current success rate of fetal surgery is not encouraging, although some remarkable outcomes have occurred through its use. Fetal surgical procedures often result in miscarriages and sometimes in the death of both the mother and the fetus.

Two conditions that frequently require fetal surgery are obstructions in the urinary tract that, if untreated until birth, may lead to kidney failure, and hydrocephalus, in which cerebral swelling makes it difficult or impossible for brain cerebrospinal fluid to circulate. Both conditions, which occur in 1 of every 5,000 to 10,000 births, require immediate attention to prevent long-term problems or death. Stents can overcome blockages. Instruments have been developed to drain fluid from the brain in instances of hydrocephalus.

When surgery is performed to allow fetal lungs to develop normally, the fetus, attached to the mother through the umbilical cord, exists in the most protective environment it is ever likely to know. If corrections are made in the uterus, then the fetal lungs are in the safest possible environment for becoming stronger before they are forced to function on their own.

In cases of obstructive urinopathy (obstruction of the urinary tract), surgery may help injured kidneys to recover and develop. Hypotonic urine found in fetal samples indicates that normal kidney function might be restored and suggests that surgery may permit the affected kidneys to gain strength within the uterus. On the other hand, the presence of isotonic urine in fetal samples indicates kidneys that are too badly compromised to regain normal function. Treatments currently available offer no solution to this problem.

One of the more routine procedures connected with pregnancy is amniocentesis, testing for chromosomal abnormalities through the analysis of amniotic fluid drawn through the abdominal wall of the mother and of blood drawn from the umbilical cord. This procedure is not without risks to mothers and fetuses. It is commonly used, however, because the benefits derived from it are generally thought to outweigh the risks.

Nevertheless, amniocentesis remains a controversial procedure, and major ethical questions surround its use. If the test reveals a chro-

mosomal abnormality, the parents are left with the decision of whether to seek a therapeutic abortion to terminate the pregnancy, which in many jurisdictions would be considered a realistic option. With many such abnormalities, however, the fetus might be delivered alive and, although significantly handicapped, have a life expectancy of many years.

Fetal surgery is indicated when physicians are convinced that a fetus will not survive long enough to be delivered or when it appears certain that the newborn will be unable to survive long after its birth. For example, if it appears through ultrasound that a fetus suffers from a severe kind of congenital diaphragmatic hernia in which the liver is in the chest, then it is obvious that the development of the lungs will be seriously compromised without surgical intervention. Fetal surgery becomes a stopgap measure in such cases to lessen the severity of the problem so that the fetus can grow to term and be delivered, after which corrective surgery outside the uterus can be undertaken. This procedure involves substantial risk, however, because the liver can be destroyed in the process of trying to restore it to its normal position below the diaphragm.

Sometimes ultrasound reveals noncancerous sacro-

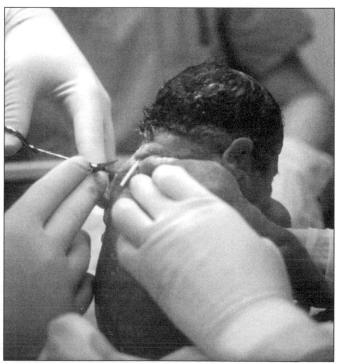

Shortly after birth, doctors examine the shunt that was inserted into a baby two months earlier in an effort to correct his hydrocephalus. (AP/ Wide World Photos)

coccygeal tumors. Such tumors, if untreated, can become large enough in a fetus to put a strain on the heart sufficient to cause heart failure. This severely compromises the survival of the fetus. Guided by ultrasound imagery, surgeons can cut off the blood supply to such tumors and starve them before they do irreparable damage to the fetus. When this procedure is used, the destroyed tumor can be removed surgically after birth.

Another growing use of fetal surgery is in cases where spina bifida, usually identified through ultrasound around the sixteenth week of pregnancy, is present. This congenital defect involves a malformation in the vertebral arch, in which the neural tube connected to the brain and the spine is exposed. When this condition is diagnosed and treated early in the development of the fetus, considerable spinal cord function can be preserved. This makes postnatal treatment more effective than it would be were the condition not discovered until after delivery.

There are essentially two major forms of fetal surgery. The more drastic of these involves performing a cesarean section, after which the fetus is carefully removed from the uterus and treated. It is then returned to the uterus, which is closed with sutures. The umbilical cord is not cut, so that the fetus is still receiving oxygen and need not breathe on its own before its lungs have developed sufficiently. This procedure is indicated when some congenital defect, possibly a teratoma (tumor), blocks the airway. Clearing the fetal airway enables the baby to breathe independently upon delivery. The other form of fetal surgery is done without removing the fetus from the uterus and is made possible by the use of laparoscopes and other specialized instruments. This is the preferred method if a choice is offered.

Uses and Complications

As fetal surgery becomes more significant and more common in the treatment and elimination of many threatening prenatal conditions, numerous complications, both ethical and physical, necessarily arise. Any surgery involves risk, and in fetal surgery a dual risk exists: risk to the fetus and risk to the mother. Therefore, physicians who perform fetal surgery have simultaneously as patients both prospective mothers and fetuses. Because fetuses cannot speak for themselves or make their own decisions, fetal surgeons often find themselves in an ethical quagmire. Most physicians hestitate to recommend fetal surgery except in such extreme cases that fetal death or severe disability without such surgery seems inevitable.

Sometimes wrenching decisions must be made about whether to save the life of the mother or the life of the fetus. Questions also arise about whether to allow a fetus to come to term if it is obvious that it will suffer from birth defects that will either severely limit the length of its life or adversely compromise its quality of life, which in some cases may involve a normal life span. Many notable people who suffered from severe birth defects have made significant contributions to society and have led productive and rewarding lives.

One of the more significant uses of fetal surgery is in the treatment of twin-twin transfusion syndrome. In the United States, this syndrome occurs in about one thousand pregnancies each year. Twin-twin transfusion syndrome results in a pair of twins being of unequal size in the fetal state because of abnormal circulation of amniotic fluid between them within the placenta that they share. The larger of the two is surrounded by considerably more amniotic fluid than the smaller one. This disproportion can result in the death of one or both of the fetuses. Attempts can be made to equalize the amniotic fluid by inserting a hollow needle through the mother's abdomen and drawing out excess fluid, a procedure that can threaten the viability of one or both of the fetuses.

Another more sophisticated treatment of twin-twin transfusion syndrome involves inserting a fetoscope into the uterus and using heat from a laser to seal off the blood vessels between the fetuses. This treatment is directed toward separating the circulation between the twins, which accounts for the condition. Regardless of which treatment is employed, the mortality rate is currently quite high in such cases, and premature delivery is a virtual certainty in them. Without intervention, however, these fetuses inevitably die in the uterus.

One of the greatest complications of fetal surgery is premature delivery. Fetuses were once thought to be viable only in the seventh month and beyond. Now the means are available to make survival outside the uterus possible earlier than that, although extraordinary care, attention, and equipment are required for extended periods following the delivery of a baby short of seven months and hospitalization in the neonatal intensive care unit (NICU) may continue for many months following such a birth.

When fetal surgery is performed, the mother is routinely medicated with drugs that will both reduce her pain and substantially decrease the possibility of miscarriage or premature delivery. As the field grows and becomes increasingly sophisticated, many of the current problems that it poses will surely be overcome.

PERSPECTIVE AND PROSPECTS

The development of highly specialized instruments, including fiber-optic telescopes and instruments specially designed to enter the uterus through minute incisions, has made possible the field of fetal surgery. Obstetrical surgeons can now correct life-threatening defects and malformations through the smallest, least invasive of openings while the fetus remains within the protection of the mother's body. This procedure, referred to as fetoscopic surgery, is the method preferred whenever it is possible because it reduces substantially the danger of bringing about premature labor at a time when the fetus cannot breathe on its own.

Because fetal surgery is in its infancy, relatively few surgeons specialize in it and the full range of its uses and promises has yet to be explored. The two major centers in the United States that have pioneered development in this field are the Children's Hospital in Philadelphia and the University of California Hospital in San Francisco.

Considerable research in fetal surgery is being conducted at both of these institutions and in laboratories and hospitals throughout the country. It is a matter of time before improved technology will exist to eradicate some of the major barriers to more extensive fetal surgery. Surgery of all kinds is becoming less invasive, which reduces considerably the shock that it delivers to patients' bodies, including blood loss and recovery time. Noninvasive fetal surgery is particularly important to ensure the physical welfare of both the fetus and the mother.

—*R. Baird Shuman, Ph.D.;*
updated by Alexander Sandra, M.D.
See also Abortion; Amniocentesis; Birth defects; Brain disorders; Cesarean section; Chorionic villus sampling; Down syndrome; Embryology; Ethics; Genetic diseases; Genetics and inheritance; Hernia; Hernia repair; Hydrocephalus; Laparoscopy; Miscarriage; Multiple births; Neonatology; Obstetrics; Perinatology; Pregnancy and gestation; Premature birth; Spina bifida; Stillbirth; Teratogens; Ultrasonography; Umbilical cord.

FOR FURTHER INFORMATION:

Barron, S. L., and D. F. Roberts, eds. *Issues in Fetal Medicine: Proceedings of the Twenty-ninth Annual Symposium of the Galton Institute, London, 1992.* New York: St. Martin's Press, 1995. Chapter 7, "Fetal Surgery," by Don K. Nakauyama, and chapter 8, "Fetal Therapy," by Martin J. Whittle, deal directly with matters relating to fetal surgery, clearly outlining the medical problems that it is generally directed toward treating. In chapter 1, "The Galton Lecture for 1992: The Changing Status of the Fetus," Barron also touches briefly on intravenous transfusion and limited exchange transfusion in utero.

Harrison, Michael, et al. *The Unborn Patient: The Art and Science of Fetal Therapy.* 3d ed. Philadelphia: W. B. Saunders, 2001. Deals with correcting hydrocephalus through fetal surgery that results in the reduction of fluid in the brain.

O'Neill, J. A., Jr. "The Fetus as a Patient." *Annals of Surgery* 213 (1991): 277-278. This brief editorial raises cogent ethical concerns surrounding fetal surgery.

Wise, Barbara, et al., eds. *Nursing Care of the General Pediatric Surgical Patient.* Gaithersburg, Md.: Aspen, 2000. Of particular relevance is chapter 9, "Fetal Surgery," by Lori J. Howell, Susan K. Von Nessen, and Kelli M. Burns, which explores the varieties of surgeries generally performed on fetuses.

FETAL TISSUE TRANSPLANTATION
PROCEDURE

ANATOMY OR SYSTEM AFFECTED: Blood, brain, eyes, immune system, nervous system, pancreas, spine

SPECIALTIES AND RELATED FIELDS: Embryology, ethics, immunology, neurology

DEFINITION: The experimental and controversial use of tissue from aborted human fetuses to replace damaged tissue in patients with diseases in which the patient's own tissue has been destroyed (such as Parkinson's disease or diabetes mellitus).

KEY TERMS:

allograft: a transplanted tissue or organ from a genetically different member of the same species as the recipient

autograft: tissue transplanted from one site to another in the same patient

cannula: a narrow tube used in surgery to drain fluid or to deliver cell suspensions for a transplant

fetal: in humans, a term normally referring to the developmental period following eight weeks of gestation; in fetal tissue transplantation, refers to tissue from earlier developmental stages as well

in utero: a Latin term meaning "in the womb"

isograft: a transplanted tissue or organ from a genetically identical individual (identical twin)

Parkinson's disease: a disease in which the dopamine-secreting cells of the midbrain degenerate, resulting in reduced levels of the neurotransmitter dopamine, tremors, uncontrolled and slow movement, and rigidity

stereotaxic computed tomography (CT): a method of imaging using a series of X rays that are compiled by a computer to give a three-dimensional image of internal structures

xenograft: a transplanted tissue or organ obtained from a member of a species different from that of the recipient

INDICATIONS AND PROCEDURES

Advances in technology sometimes catapult a society into ethical arenas that are not yet circumscribed by laws and clear moral boundaries. Fetal tissue transplantation is one of these advances. It is a technology that carries the hope of curing a diverse array of severe, often tragic, ailments but one that raises many difficult questions. Tissues from aborted fetuses have been shown in experimental trials to be an excellent source of replacement tissue for patients whose diseases have destroyed their own vital tissues. Parkinson's, Huntington's, and Alzheimer's diseases (in which regions of the brain deteriorate) or juvenile-onset diabetes mellitus (in which insulin-secreting cells of the pancreas degenerate) theoretically could be cured with suitable tissue replacement.

The two sources of tissue used in transplantations, donations from adult cadavers and from aborted fetuses, differ significantly in their suitability. Tissues from cadavers have the severe disadvantage of being immunologically rejected when grafted into anyone who is not an identical twin. The body's surveillance system that protects against infection is designed to attack and destroy any cells that carry molecular markers identifying them as foreign. Patients receiving tissue transplants from other individuals, therefore, will tolerate the tissue graft only if their immune systems are first suppressed with a battery of potent drugs, leaving the patient dangerously unarmed against infection.

Other disadvantages of cadaveric tissues are cell death due to extended postmortem interval (time between individual's death and collection of the tissue) and poor integration into the recipient organ. Porcine xenografts into patients with Parkinson's disease have also been attempted, but they were unsuccessful because of the rejection of the majority of transplanted cells despite aggressive immunosuppression. Taken to-

gether, allografts, a transplanted tissue or organ from a genetically different member of the same species, are generally much better tolerated than are xenografts, a transplanted tissue or organ obtained from a member of a species different from that of the recipient. In contrast, isografts, which utilize tissue from a genetically identical twin, are not rejected. Of note is that transplant rejection decreases with the recipient's age, possibly due to immunosenescence and the increased effectiveness of immunosuppressive drugs.

Fetal tissues, however, do not induce a full-scale immune response when transplanted. This is particularly true when cells are transplanted into an organ such as the brain, which is considered an immunologically privileged site along with other locations in the body, such as the anterior chamber of the eye, testis, renal tubule, and uterus. At these sites, the immune response to antigens is reduced and/or not destructive to the transplanted tissue. Nevertheless, transplanted fetal tissues do attract lymphocytes (a type of white blood cell of the immune system) and other immune cells, but the role of this process in graft survival and function is not well understood.

Other properties add to the suitability of fetal tissue for transplantation. Because it is not yet fully differentiated, fetal tissue is said to be very plastic in its abilities to adapt to new locations. Moreover, once placed in a patient, it secretes factors that promote its own growth and those of the new blood vessels at the site. Tissue from an adult source does not have these properties and consequently is slow-growing and poorly vascularized. Though growth factors can be added along with the graft, adult tissue is less responsive to these hormones than is fetal tissue.

It is the source of fetal tissue that has fired such debate over its use for transplantation. Though there has been general acceptance of using tissue from spontaneous abortions or from ectopic pregnancies which, because of their location outside of the womb, endanger the life of the mother and must be terminated, these sources are not well suited to transplantation. Spontaneous abortions rarely produce viable tissue, since in most cases the fetus has died two to three weeks before it is expelled. In addition, there are usually major genetic defects in the aborted fetus. In ectopic pregnancies as well, more than 50 percent of the fetuses are genetically abnormal, and most resolve themselves in spontaneous abortion outside a clinic setting. These types of abortions are almost always accompanied by a sense of tragic loss felt by the parents. Many researchers find it unacceptable to request permission from these parents to transplant tissue from the lost fetus.

The alternative source of fetal tissue is elected abortions. One-and-a-half million of these abortions occur in the United States every year. The debate over the ethical correctness of elected abortions has left a cloud of confusion over the issue of using this tissue for transplantation.

When an elective abortion is performed in a clinic, the tissue is removed by suction through a narrow tube. Normally, the tissue would be thrown away. If it is to be used for transplantation, written permission must be obtained from the woman after the abortion is completed. No discussion of transplantation is to take place prior to the abortion, and no alteration in the abortion procedure, except to keep the tissue sterile during collection, is to be made. The donor may not be paid for the tissue, and both the donor and the recipient of the tissue must remain anonymous to each other.

Once collected, the tissue is searched through to locate suitable tissue for transplantation. Although the size of the transplanted tissue varies depending on the type of cell replacement, often only a small block of tissue is used, about eight cubic millimeters (the size of a thin slice of pencil eraser). The tissue is screened for infectious diseases such as hepatitis B and human immunodeficiency virus (HIV). Tissue that is collected is washed a number of times in a sterile solution to ensure that there is no bacterial contamination, and then it is maintained in a sterile, buffered salt solution until it is used. In order to increase the amount of usable tissue, the tissue may be grown in culture on a nutritive medium under carefully controlled conditions of humidity (95 percent), temperature (37 degrees Celsius), and gas (5 percent carbon dioxide in air) to stimulate normal growing conditions. Preservation of the tissue for long-term storage has been made possible by the highly refined technique of freezing the tissue in liquid nitrogen (cryostorage). Fetal tissue has been kept for as long as ten months in this manner before being used successfully in transplantation. Although the technique should provide methods of maintaining tissue indefinitely, not all types of cells contained in such tissues survive cryopreservation well. For example, despite many attempts to optimize storage conditions, fetal neurons are severely harmed by freezing.

The actual transplantation of the tissue is usually relatively quick and in some cases relatively noninvasive. Often the tissue is injected into the patient as a suspension of individual cells. This permits the use of a small-bore tube called a cannula to deliver the cells to the target organ, thereby avoiding large surgical incisions. Because of modern stereotaxic imaging equipment such as computed tomography (CT) scanning and ultrasound, the physician is able to determine with extreme precision exactly where the cells are to be delivered and can visualize the position of the transplant cannula as the cells are injected. In this way, an entire region of an organ can be seeded with fetal cells. Often the patient is under only a local anesthetic. This aspect of the surgery is especially important when fetal cells are being inserted into the brain, since the physicians can then monitor the patient's ability to speak and move, to ensure that no major damage to the brain is occurring. Usually, antibiotics are given on the day of the transplantation procedure and for two additional days to avoid infection. Although the procedure is relatively safe and recovery is quick—patients often go home in less than three days—transplantation into the central nervous system (CNS) carries risk of hemorrhage (bleeding) and blood clot formation that can damage neurons in the affected area.

Fetal tissue transplantation is still considered an experimental procedure, and further trials are needed to fine-tune the techniques. For example, the precise age of fetal tissue that would be most effective in various cases is uncertain, though it is generally agreed that tissue from a first-trimester fetus is optimal, and six to eight weeks of gestation is most suitable for grafts into brains of Parkinson's sufferers. Often it is not known which patients would respond best to the therapy, but in case of neurotransplantation in Parkinson's disease patients, those with good response to levodopa (L-dopa), a precursor of dopamine, benefit the most. Researchers are also uncertain about whether immunosuppressive drugs should be administered. In animal trials using mice, rats, and monkeys, fetal tissue allografts, but not xenografts, have been well tolerated in the absence of immunosuppression. In humans as well, fetal tissue appears to be readily accepted, with no signs of rejection, and in one study, patients did better without immunosuppression. Some surgeons, however, unwilling to risk tissue rejection, routinely give the transplant patient immunosuppressive drugs, such as cyclosporine and prednisone.

USES AND COMPLICATIONS

The major focus for fetal tissue transplantation has been the treatment of patients with Parkinson's disease, and results have been encouraging. The disease is caused by a deterioration of dopamine-producing regions of the midbrain, the substantia nigra, so named because of the presence of pigmented neurons, which secrete dopamine, in the putamen and caudate nucleus of the basal ganglia. There these neurons send their processes (projecting parts). There is an accompanying loss of motor control causing slowness of movement (bradykinesia), tremors, rigidity, and finally paralysis. Death is most typically a result of accompanying illnesses, such as infections, or caused by the loss of balance and falls. The key drug used to treat the disorder, L-dopa, produces side effects that cause unrelenting and uncontrolled movement of the limbs (dyskinesias) and hallucinations, and the drug loses its effectiveness over time. Advanced patients, who are no longer taking the medication, often remain in a "frozen" state.

A number of patients who have received fetal tissue transplants have shown remarkable improvement and diminished requirements for drug treatment. The first case in the United States to be treated was a man with a twenty-year history of parkinsonian symptoms. He had frequent freezing spells, could not walk without a cane, and suffered from chronic constipation. He also was unable to whistle, a beloved hobby of his. He was operated on by Dr. Curt R. Freed and his associates in 1988. Following the operation, initial improvement was slow, but within a year, he was walking without a cane, his speed of movement had considerably improved, and his constipation had resolved itself. He also had regained his ability to whistle. Even after four years, improvements continued. Such results have occurred with many parkinsonian patients receiving fetal tissue transplants.

Beneficial effects of transplants have also been obtained in patients with induced Parkinson-like symptoms. In 1982, some intravenous drug users developed Parkinson-like symptoms after using a homemade preparation of "synthetic heroin" that was contaminated with 1-methyl-4-phenyl-1,2,5,6-tetrahydropyridine (MPTP). MPTP destroys dopamine-secreting cells of the substantia nigra. Two of these patients received fetal tissue transplants in Sweden. Within a year after their operation, they were able to walk with a normal gait, resume chores, and be virtually free of their previously uncontrollable movements.

Because no patient with Parkinson's disease or with Parkinson-like symptoms has yet been cured by a fetal tissue transplant, some have considered the results of such experiments to be disappointing. The expectation of complete cures from a technique that is still in its early experimental phase, however, is overly optimistic. Many patients themselves are encouraged, and many have resumed driving and the other tasks of normal daily life. Altogether, more than two hundred patients with Parkinson's disease have received fetal tissue transplants worldwide. It is important to note that fetal tissue transplants are not stem cell transplants, or grafts of tissue produced from stem cells. Coincidentally, fetal tissue usually contains some stem cells, but the transplant effects are thought to be mostly mediated by the mature or maturing cells in the donor tissue (dopamine neurons or pancreatic beta cells, for example).

That transplanted fetal brain tissue can replace damaged brain tissue to any extent has opened the doors of hope for many diseases. For example, Huntington's disease, a genetic disorder that destroys a different set of neurons but in the same region as that affected by parkinsonism, brings a slow death to those carrying the dominant trait. Its severe dementia and uncontrollable jerking and writhing that steadily progress have had no treatment and no cure. In animal studies in which fetal brain tissue was transplanted into rats with symptoms mimicking Huntington's disease, results have been encouraging enough to warrant human trials, and one human trial, reported by a surgeon in Mexico, has shown limited success. Another such study is ongoing in France. Researchers are hopeful, though less optimistic, that Alzheimer's disease, a form of dementia that is characterized by neuronal death within the brain, also may be treatable with fetal tissue transplants. Because the destruction is so widespread, however, it is difficult to determine where the transplants should be placed.

Type I insulin-dependent diabetes, often called juvenile-onset diabetes, also has been treated with fetal tissue transplants. More than a million people in the United States suffer from this disease caused by the destruction of pancreatic beta cells, the insulin-secreting cells that regulate sugar metabolism. Though the disease can be controlled with regular insulin shots, the long-term effects of diabetes can lead to blindness, premature aging, and renal and circulatory problems. After animal tests showed a complete reversal of the disease when fetal pancreatic tissue was transplanted into diabetic rats, human trials were initiated with great expectations. Though complete success has not been achieved, the sixteen diabetic patients who were given fetal pancreatic tissue transplants by Dr. Kevin Lafferty between 1987 and 1992 all showed significant drops in the amount of insulin needed to manage their disease. The transplanted tissue continued to pump out insulin.

An unusual variation of such procedures has been to transplant fetal tissue into fetuses diagnosed with severe metabolic diseases. It is more effective to treat the condition while the fetus is still in the womb than to wait until after birth, when damage from the disease may already be extensive. Fetuses with Hurler's syndrome and similar "storage" diseases have been treated in this way. Hurler's syndrome is a lethal condition in which tissues become clogged with stored mucopolysaccharides, long-chain sugars that the body is unable to break down because it lacks the appropriate enzyme. One of the fetuses to receive this treatment was the child of a couple who had lost two children to the disease. With the transplanted tissue, the child lived and by one year of age was producing therapeutic levels of the enzyme. It has been estimated that there are at least 155 other genetic disorders that could be similarly treated by fetal tissue transplants in utero.

The list of ailments that fetal tissue transplants may alleviate includes some of the major concerns of modern medicine. In addition to those already mentioned are macular degeneration, sickle cell disease, thalassemias, metabolic disorders, immune deficiencies, myelin disorders, and spinal cord injuries. In interpreting the value of these applications, however, it is important to separate the politics of abortion from the medical issue of fetal tissue transplantation.

PERSPECTIVE AND PROSPECTS

Though controversy surrounds the use of fetal tissue for transplantation, such controversy has not included all facets of fetal tissue research. Indeed, fetal cells were used in the 1950's to develop the Salk polio vaccine and later the vaccine against rubella (German measles). With the scourge of acquired immunodeficiency syndrome (AIDS), in the 1990's fetal cells were first used to help design treatments against the AIDS virus. Even the early attempts at fetal tissue transplantation occurred quietly. Reports date as far back as 1928, when Italian surgeons attempted unsuccessfully to cure a patient with diabetes using fetal pancreatic tissue, a procedure repeated, again unsuccessfully, in the United States in 1939. In 1959, American physicians tried to cure leukemia with fetal tissue transplants, but again without success.

The first real indicator that such techniques might work came in 1968, when fetal liver cells were used to treat a patient with DiGeorge syndrome. The success of

this procedure resulted in its becoming the accepted treatment for this usually fatal genetic disorder, which results from a deletion of a part of chromosome 22. Because many of the DiGeorge patients are athymic (fail to develop a thymus), they lack T cells, making them immunodeficient. Because the fetal liver supports hematopoiesis (the production of blood cells, including immune cells) during development, fetal liver cells have some value in the treatment of immunodeficiency. However, fetal thymus transplantation can promote more complete immune system reconstitution and is now used as a treatment in athymic patients.

Because suitable fetal tissues are often very difficult to obtain, recently the focus on donor cells for transplantation has shifted toward stem cell-derived cells. Stem cells can be relatively easily expanded in numbers in culture and have the potential to generate a large supply of different cell types for transplantation, thereby averting some of the issues that have decelerated the field of fetal transplantation. Donor cells differentiated from one's own stem cells could be used in an autograft and thereby circumvent both immunological and ethical issues. Studies to explore the potential of such technologies are ongoing. Thus the next chapter in the fetal tissue transplantation story may involve the fast-evolving fields of stem cell research and regenerative medicine.

It was not until 1987 that ethical issues over fetal tissue transplants truly surfaced in the United States. Debate was precipitated when the director of the National Institutes of Health (NIH) submitted a request to the Department of Health and Human Services to transplant fetal tissue into patients with Parkinson's disease. Rather than receiving approval, the request was tabled, pending a thorough study of the issue by an NIH panel on fetal tissue transplantation. The panel made a detailed report on the ethical, legal, and scientific implications of fetal tissue transplantation, concluding that it was acceptable public policy. Despite the report, however, the Secretary of Health and Human Services instituted a ban against the use of government funds for transplanting fetal tissue derived from elective abortions. While in effect, the ban influenced private funding as well. Physicians who performed fetal tissue transplants, unable to obtain grant money, were forced to charge their patients—a bill that could reach as high as forty thousand dollars per transplant. President Bill Clinton's lifting of the ban in 1993, on his third day in office, paved the way for research advances, including isolating and propagating human stem cells. However, the opposition of Clinton's successor, George W. Bush, to the use of fetal tissue and stem cells for scientific purposes led to several legislative battles and cast some doubts on the future of this field.

The debates over fetal tissue transplantation are far from over. Though a strict set of guidelines are in place concerning the procurement of fetal tissue, ensuring that the needs never influence decisions concerning abortion, other issues have not been addressed. Some ask whether a fetal tissue bank should be established and, if so, whether it should be government-funded to avoid commercialization. As technology continues to create increasingly complicated ethical issues, society's responsibility increases, as does its need to be scientifically informed.

—Mary S. Tyler, Ph.D.;
updated by W. Michael Zawada, Ph.D.

See also Abortion; Alzheimer's disease; Brain; Brain disorders; Diabetes mellitus; Ethics; Genetic diseases; Genetic engineering; Neurology; Pancreas; Parkinson's disease; Stem cells; Transplantation.

FOR FURTHER INFORMATION:

Beardsley, Tim. "Aborting Research." *Scientific American* 267, no. 2 (August, 1992): 17-18. An excellent encapsulation of the debate over fetal tissue transplantation and the instances in which it has been used.

Beauchamp, Tom, and James F. Childress. *Principles of Biomedical Ethics*. 5th ed. New York: Oxford University Press, 2001. A classic text that introduces the field of ethics, its theories, and their application to biomedical issues and presents ten cases covering a wide range of issues in biomedical ethics, some of which have led to landmark decisions.

Begley, Sharon. "From Human Embryos, Hope for 'Spare Parts.'" *Newsweek*, November 16, 1998, 73. Researchers have teased out clumps of cells from human embryos and induced them to burst into a veritable cellular symphony, forming most of the 210 kinds of cells that constitute the human body. These colonies could revolutionize transplantation medicine.

Brundin, Patrik, and C. Warren Olanow, eds. *Restorative Therapies in Parkinson's Disease*. New York: Springer, 2006. Covers in depth the ethical, clinical, and scientific issues surrounding neural grafting in Parkinson's disease and prospects for the future use of stem cell-derived grafts. The book is appropriate for clinicians, scientists, and anyone interest in restorative therapies for the brain.

Clinical Trials. http://www.clinicaltrials.gov/ct/. A Web site of the National Institutes of Health (NIH) and the National Library of Medicine that provides information on current and completed federally and privately supported clinical trials in human volunteers. The purposes of the research, as well as details on how to participate, are included.

"Fetal Cell Study Shows Promise for Parkinson's." *Los Angeles Times*, April 22, 1999, p. 29. The first federally funded trial to study the effectiveness of fetal cell transplants for Parkinson's disease has proved that it works for some patients, mainly those under the age of sixty.

Freed, Curt R., Robert Breeze, and Neil Rosenberg. "Transplantation of Human Fetal Dopamine Cells for Parkinson's Disease." *Archives of Neurology* 47, no. 5 (May 1, 1990): 505-512. A historically important paper describing the techniques used by Freed, an American doctor who has been a pioneer in the technique of fetal tissue transplantation. Though written for a medical audience, most of the paper is readily understandable to a lay audience.

Freed, Curt R., and Simon LeVay. *Healing the Brain: A Doctor's Controversial Quest for a Cell Therapy to Cure Parkinson's Disease*. New York: Times Books/Henry Holt, 2002. A thrilling story about the development of a new cell transplantation therapy for Parkinson's disease and the controversies surrounding it. A must read for anyone interested in cell replacement therapies.

Holland, Suzanne, Karen Lebacqz, and Laurie Zoloth, eds. *The Human Embryonic Stem Cell Debate: Science, Ethics, and Public Policy*. Cambridge, Mass.: MIT Press, 2001. Tackles difficult questions such as the nature of human life, the limits of intervention into human cells and tissues, who should approve controversial research, and what constitutes human dignity, respect, and justice.

Lindvall, Olle, Patrik Brundin, and Håkan Widner. "Grafts of Fetal Dopamine Neurons Survive and Improve Motor Function in Parkinson's Disease." *Science* 247 (February 2, 1990): 574-577. A landmark reference describing the technique of a group of physicians led by Lindvall of Sweden. This and the paper by Freed's group encompass the extent of variation in the technique, and the degrees of success.

Marshak, Daniel R., Richard L. Gardner, and David Gottlieb, eds. *Stem Cell Biology*. Cold Springs Harbor, N.Y.: Cold Springs Harbor Press, 2002. An excellent, multidisciplinary examination of recent advances in the field and their impact on medicine and science.

Singer, Peter, et al., eds. *Embryo Experimentation*. New York: Cambridge University Press, 1993. This text provides an excellent discussion of the moral questions raised by the use of fetal tissue for transplantation.

U.S. Congress. Senate. Committee on Labor and Human Resources. *Finding Medical Cures: The Promise of Fetal Tissue Transplantation Research*. 102d Congress, 1st session, 1992. Senate Report 1902. A surprisingly readable and gripping set of testimonies from physicians, interest groups, and citizens concerning the debate over the use of fetal tissue for transplantations.

Wade, Nicholas. "Primordial Cells Fuel Debate on Ethics." *The New York Times*, November 10, 1998, p. 1. Two groups of scientists, one led by James A. Thomson of the University of Wisconsin at Madison and the other led by John D. Gearhart of The Johns Hopkins University in Baltimore, have reported success in the attempt to grow primordial human cells outside the body.

FEVER

DISEASE/DISORDER

ANATOMY OR SYSTEM AFFECTED: All

SPECIALTIES AND RELATED FIELDS: Family medicine, internal medicine, pediatrics, virology

DEFINITION: A symptom associated with a variety of diseases and disorders, characterized by body temperature above normal (98.6 degrees Fahrenheit, or 37 degrees centigrade or Celsius); considered very serious at 104 degrees Fahrenheit (40 degrees Celsius) and higher.

KEY TERMS:

antipyretic drugs: drugs that are employed to reduce fevers, such as sodium salicylate, indomethacin, and acetaminophen

ectotherms: organisms that rely on external temperature conditions in order to maintain their internal temperature

endotherms: organisms that control the internal temperature of their bodies by the conversion of calories to heat

febrile response: an upward adjustment of the thermoregulatory set point

metabolic rate: a measurement of the Calories (kilocalories) that are converted into heat energy in order to maintain body temperature and/or for physical exertion

pyrogens: protein substances that appear at the outset of the process that leads to a fever reaction

thermoregulatory set point: the ultimate neural control that maintains the human internal body temperature at 37 degrees Celsius and can either raise or lower it

CAUSES AND SYMPTOMS

Although the symptoms that often accompany a fever are familiar to everyone—shivering, sweating, thirst, hot skin, and a flushed face—what causes fever and its function during illness are not fully clear even among medical specialists. Considerable literature exists on the differences between warm-blooded organisms (endotherms) and cold-blooded organisms (ectotherms) in what is called the normal state, when no symptoms of disease are present. Cold-blooded organisms depend on temperature conditions in their external environment to maintain various levels of temperature within their bodies. These fluctuations correspond to the various levels of activity that they need to sustain at given moments. Thus, reptiles, for example, may "recharge" themselves internally by moving into the warmth of the sun. Warm-blooded organisms, on the other hand, including all mammals, utilize energy released from the digestion of food to maintain a constant level of heat within their bodies. This level—a "normal" temperature—is approximately 37 degrees Celsius (98.6 degrees Fahrenheit) in humans. An internal body temperature which rises above this level is called a febrile temperature, or a fever.

If the temperature in the surrounding environment is low, warm-blooded organisms must raise their metabolic rate (a measurement, in Calories, of converted energy) accordingly to maintain a normal internal body temperature. In humans, this rate of energy expenditure is about 1,800 Calories per day. If insufficient food is taken in to supply the necessary potential energy for this metabolic conversion into heat, the body will draw on its storage resource—fat—to fulfill this vital need. The potentially fatal condition called hypothermia, in which the body is too fatigued to maintain metabolic functions or has exhausted all of its stores of Calories, occurs when the internal temperature falls below normal. Although cold-blooded animals must also protect themselves against the danger that their body heat may fall too low to sustain life functions, they can support adjustments in their own internal temperature down to about 20 degrees Celsius. At the same time, metabolic expenditures, as measured in Calories, are very low in cold-blooded animals; for example, alligators must expend only 60 Calories per day to create the same amount of heat as 1,800 Calories per day in warm-blooded humans.

The question of internal temperature in warm-blooded animals is closely tied to management efficiency in the body. This function becomes critical when one considers abnormally high internal temperature, or fever. Generally speaking, all essential biochemical functions in the human body can be carried out at optimal levels of efficiency at the set point of 37 degrees Celsius. In the simplest of terms, any increase or decrease in temperature creates either more or less kinetic energy and has the potential to affect the chemistry of all body functions.

Endotherms are able to tolerate a certain range of involuntary change in their internal body temperature (brought about by disease or illness), but there is an upper limit of 45 degrees Celsius, which constitutes a high fever. If the self-regulating higher set point associated with fever goes beyond this point, destructive biochemical phenomena will occur in the body—in particular, a breaking down of protein molecules. If these phenomena are not checked, they can bring about death.

Modern scientific approaches to the internal body processes that lead to fever, like a medical discussion of the effects that occur once fever is operating in the body, are much more complicated. They revolve around the concept of a change in the set point monitored in the brain. When this change in the brain's normal (37 degree) thermostatic signal is called for, a process called phagocytosis begins, leading to a higher internal body heat level throughout the organism.

Phagocytosis, the ingestion of a solid substance (especially foreign material such as invading bacteria), involves the appearance in the host's system of large numbers of leukocyte cells. When these cells ingest the bacteria, small quantities of protein called leukocytic

pyrogens are produced. According to most modern theories, these protein pyrogens trigger the biochemical reactions in the brain that alter the body's temperature set point. After this point, changes that occur throughout the system and raise the body's internal temperature depend on a component of the bacterial cell wall called endotoxin. By the end of the 1960's, researchers had drawn attention to at least twenty effects that activated endotoxins may have on the host organism. Key effects include enhancement of the production of new white blood cells (leukocytosis), enhancement of various forms of immunological resistance, reduction of serum iron levels, and lowering of blood pressure.

Most, if not all, of these effects brought about by endotoxins are accompanied by higher levels of heat throughout the body, the definition of fever. Closer biochemical examination of the source of the added heat yielded the suggestion, made by P. B. Beeson in 1948, that the host's endotoxin-affected cells begin to produce a distinct form of protein, now called endogenous pyrogens. Pyrogens are thought to induce the first stage of fever by interacting with cells in tissues very close to the brain, specifically in the brain stem itself. Laboratory experiments in the first half of the twentieth century allowed researchers to produce almost immediate fever reactions when they injected pyrogen protein material into rabbits. Studies of the induced febrile state in laboratory animals, and therefore presumably also in humans, linked fever to immunological (virus-resistant and bacteria-resistant) reactions, not necessarily in the initially affected tissues around the brain but in various places throughout the organism.

Although scientific research has produced many hypotheses concerning the origins of fever in the body, experts admit that the process is not well understood. Matthew J. Kluger, in *Fever: Its Biology, Evolution, and Function* (1979), claims that "the precise mechanism behind endogenous pyrogens' effect on the thermoregulatory set-point is unknown."

TREATMENT AND THERAPY

The febrile response has been noted in five of the seven extant classes of vertebrates on earth (Agnatha, such as lampreys, and Chondrichthyes, such as sharks, are excluded). Scientists have determined that its function as a reaction to bacterial infection can be traced back as far as 400 million years in primitive bony fishes. The question of whether the natural phenomenon of fever actually aids in combating disease in the body, however, has not been fully resolved.

In ancient and medieval times, it was believed that fever served to "cook" and separate out one of the four essential body "humors"—blood, phlegm, yellow bile, and black bile—that had become excessively dominant. Throughout the centuries, such beliefs even caused some physicians to try to induce higher internal body temperatures as a means of treating disease. Use of modern antipyretic drugs to reduce fever remained unthinkable until the nineteenth century.

It was the German physician Carl von Liebermeister who, by the end of the nineteenth century, set some of the guidelines that are still generally observed in deciding whether antipyretic drugs should or should not be used to reduce a naturally occurring fever during illness. Liebermeister insisted that the phenomenon of fe-

ver was not one of body temperature gone "out of control" but rather a sign that the organism was regulating its own temperature. He also demonstrated that part of the process leading to increased internal temperature could be seen in reactions that actually reduce heat loss at the body's surface, notably decreases in skin blood flow and evaporative cooling through perspiration. Liebermeister determined that one of the positive effects of higher temperatures inside the body was to impede the growth of harmful microorganisms. At the same time, however, other side effects of fever during illness were deemed to be negative, such as loss of appetite and, in some cases, actual degeneration of key internal organs. Liebermeister's generation of physicians, therefore, tended to rely on antipyretic drugs

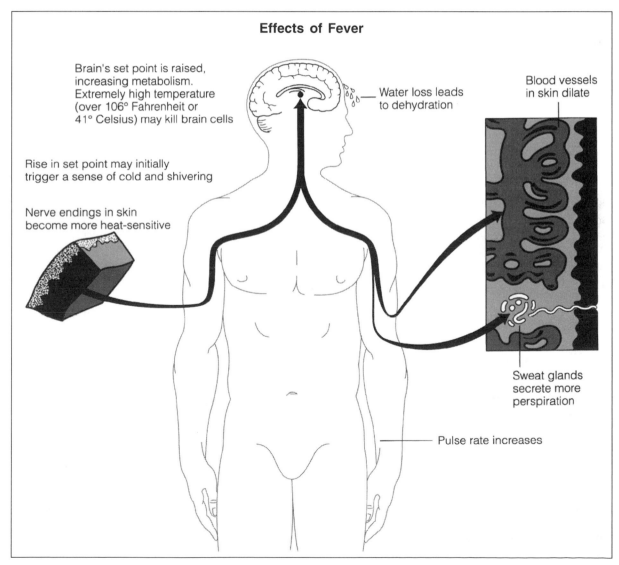

Effects of Fever

Brain's set point is raised, increasing metabolism. Extremely high temperature (over 106° Fahrenheit or 41° Celsius) may kill brain cells

Water loss leads to dehydration

Blood vessels in skin dilate

Rise in set point may initially trigger a sense of cold and shivering

Nerve endings in skin become more heat-sensitive

Sweat glands secrete more perspiration

Pulse rate increases

only when high fevers persisted for long periods of time. Moderate fevers or even high fevers, if they did not continue too long, were deemed to contribute to the overall process of natural body resistance to disease.

In fact, a limited school of physicians followed the teaching of 1927 Nobel laureate Julius Wagner-Jauregg, who claimed that "fever therapy" methods should be adopted for the treatment of certain diseases. Wagner-Jauregg himself had pioneered this theory by inoculating victims of neurosyphilis with fever-producing malaria. Part of his argument in favor of this experimental therapy was that malaria, with its accompanying fever, was a treatable disease (through the use of quinine) and could be controlled at regular intervals during its "service" as a fighter against a disease that still had no known cure. Later use of fever therapy for treatment of other sexually transmitted diseases, specifically gonorrhea, proved to be moderately successful. When typhoid vaccine was used to induce fevers in some patients, however, side effects such as hypotension (low blood pressure) or cardiovascular shock introduced what some considered to be dangerous risk factors. Nevertheless, certain fields of medicine, especially those involved with eye diseases and related eye ailments, have proved that fever-inducing agents (specifically those contained in typhoid and typhoid-paratyphoid vaccines) also induce beneficial secretion of the anti-inflammatory hormone cortisol.

By the second half of the twentieth century, the medical use of antipyretic drugs, containing such components as salicylates and indomethacin, had become widespread. This phenomenon was not caused by any compelling reversal of earlier general assumptions that moderate levels of fever, being a natural body reaction, were not necessarily harmful to patients suffering from a wide variety of diseases. Rather, physicians may have opted to use such drugs as much for their pain-relieving qualities as for their fever-reducing characteristics. Although patients receiving such drug treatment notice a diminishing of severe pains or general aching, the cause of the disease has not been combated merely by the removal of such symptoms as fever and pain.

Modern medical science has tended to support further study of particular circumstances in which induced fevers can actually produce disease-combating reactions. A newly emerging field by the late 1970's, for example, involved studying the benefits of higher temperatures in newborn infants fighting viral infections. Although specific circumstances and the nature of disease prevent a generalized conclusion in terms of the

use of induced fevers as a form of treatment, researchers have shown that an elevated body temperature serves to increase the speed at which white blood cells, the body's natural enemies against disease, move to infected areas.

Perspective and Prospects

Although doctors have been aware of the symptoms of fever since the beginnings of medical history, centuries passed before its importance as an indicator of disease was accepted. A certain degree of sophistication in the study of fevers became possible largely as a result of the development of the common thermometer, in a rudimentary form in the seventeenth century and then with greater technical accuracy in the eighteenth century. Systematic use of the thermometer in the eighteenth century enabled doctors to observe such phenomena as morning remission and evening peaking of fever intensity. Studies involving the recording of temperature in healthy individuals also yielded important discoveries. One such discovery was made in 1774, when use of the thermometer showed that, even in a room heated to the boiling point of water (100 degrees Celsius), healthy subjects maintained an internal body heat that was very close to the normal 37-degree level.

Medical reports as late as the end of the eighteenth century, however, indicate that even internationally recognized pioneers of science were still not close to understanding the causes of fever. The English doctor John Hunter, for example, declared himself opposed to the prevailing view that rising body heat came from the circulation of warmer blood throughout the body. Hunter suspected that the warmth was produced by an entirely different agent that was independent of the circulatory system. He never learned what that agent might be, however, and failed in defense of his theory that the source of added body heat was in the stomach. Even the famous French chemist Antoine-Laurent Lavoisier erred when he tried to explain fever in terms of some form of chemical "combustion" involving hydrogen and carbon. Lavoisier identified the lungs as the possible location for this spontaneous production of internal body heat.

Although these theories were identified as erroneous, the late eighteenth and early nineteenth centuries left one legacy that would develop into the twentieth century and is still practiced by physicians: systematic thermometry. In essence, thermometry involves the tracing of the upward or downward direction of fever during illness in order to judge the course of the disease and the effects brought about by different stages of treatment. In many diseases, for example, clinical records of the full course of previous cases can be studied by doctors responsible for treating an individual patient. With thermometry, the doctor is able to determine how far the body's struggle against a certain disease has progressed. If thermometry shows a marked departure from what clinical records have charted as the normal course of disease under certain forms of treatment, then the physician may look for signs of another disease.

—Byron D. Cannon, Ph.D.

See also Avian influenza; Bacterial infections; Common cold; Heat exhaustion and heat stroke; Hyperthermia and hypothermia; Influenza; Kawasaki disease; Reye's syndrome; Rheumatic fever; Scarlet fever; Sweating; Typhoid fever; Typhus; Viral infections; Yellow fever; *other specific diseases.*

FOR FURTHER INFORMATION:

Kemper, Kathi J. *The Holistic Pediatrician: A Pediatrician's Comprehensive Guide to Safe and Effective Therapies for the Twenty-five Most Common Ailments of Infants, Children, and Adolescents.* New York: HarperCollins, 2002. Integrates mainstream and alternative medicine to aid parents in dealing with the most common childhood health problems such as fever, diaper rash, ear infections, and allergies.

Kluger, Matthew J. *Fever: Its Biology, Evolution, and Function.* Princeton, N.J.: Princeton University Press, 1979. An accessible book-length study of the phenomenon of fever. Although some parts of the discussion are more technical in nature, the general level is comprehensible.

Kluger, Matthew J., Tamas Bartfai, and Charles A. Dinarello, eds. *Molecular Mechanisms of Fever.* New York: New York Academy of Sciences, 1998. The authors place major emphasis on recent advances using molecular tools such as cytokine knockout mice, cloned cytokines, descriptions of molecular pathways for signal transduction, and heat shock proteins.

Litin, Scott C., ed. *Mayo Clinic Family Health Book.* 3d ed. New York: HarperResource, 2003. Perhaps the best general medical text for the layperson, this book covers the entire medical field. While the information is derived from a wide variety of highly technical sources, the articles are written to be easily understood by a general audience.

Mackowiak, Philip A., ed. *Fever: Basic Mechanisms and Management.* 2d ed. Philadelphia: Lippincott-Raven, 1997. This text explains the physiology behind fever and addresses ways to treat it. Includes a bibliography and an index.

Nathanson, Laura Walther. *The Portable Pediatrician: A Practicing Pediatrician's Guide to Your Child's Growth, Development, Health, and Behavior from Birth to Age Five.* 2d ed. New York: HarperCollins, 2002. An engaging, easy-to-read guide for parents to assess their child's development, medical symptoms, and behavioral problems.

FIBROCYSTIC BREAST DISEASE. *See* BREAST DISORDERS.

FIBROMYALGIA
DISEASE/DISORDER
ANATOMY OR SYSTEM AFFECTED: Brain, head, muscles, musculoskeletal system, nerves, nervous system, psychic-emotional system

SPECIALTIES AND RELATED FIELDS: Rheumatology

DEFINITION: A connective, soft tissue disease involving chronic, spontaneous, and widespread musculoskeletal pain, as well as recurrent fatigue and sleep disturbance.

KEY TERMS:
connective tissue: the supporting framework of the body, particularly tendons and ligaments

fibrositis: an earlier, less common term for fibromyalgia

flare-up: an episode of heightened pain and debilitation in fibromyalgia; sometimes flare-ups do not have an immediate, precipitating cause that is identifiable, while other times they are associated with humidity, cold, physical exertion, or psychological stress

functional somatic syndromes: a continuum or spectrum of disorders (such as chronic fatigue syndrome, Epstein-Barr virus, and primary headaches) characterized by complex interactions between symptoms and patients' personal stress

tender points: specific, precise, and localized areas of moderately to severely intense pain

CAUSES AND SYMPTOMS
The cause of fibromyalgia is unknown. Some researchers believe that an injury or trauma to the central nervous system causes the disorder. Other researchers believe that changes in muscle and connective tissue metabolism produce decreased blood flow, beginning a

pathological cycle of weakness, fatigue, and decreased strength that eventually results in the full-blown syndrome. Still others believe that an as-yet-undiscovered virus or infectious agent attacks people who are naturally susceptible to the infection, who then develop the syndrome.

The most salient feature of fibromyalgia syndrome is pain. Described by sufferers as "having no boundaries," the pain is characteristically variable. The same sufferer experiences pain ranging from deep muscle aching to throbbing, stabbing, or shooting pains to a burning sensation that has been called "acid running through blood vessels." The pain frequently causes joint and muscle stiffness. Pain and stiffness may be worse in the morning and may be more intense in the joints and muscle groups that are used more often. Patients may have tender points, as in the knee, hips, spine, shoulders, and neck. There are typically eighteen potential tender points, and at least eleven must be painful for a diagnosis of fibromyalgia to be made.

Sufferers also experience fatigue and weakness, ranging from mild to debilitating. Patients liken the fatigue to having their arms and legs tied to concrete, and many feel that they are living in a kind of mental fog, unable to focus or concentrate. Between 40 and 70 percent of patients also have some variation of irritable bowel syndrome (IBS): frequent abdominal cramping, nausea, and chronic constipation or diarrhea. About half of all sufferers also experience concurrent migraine or tension headaches. The condition is often mental as well as physical, as sufferers may also suffer from major depressive disorder and anxiety.

Less common, but readily found, are a constellation of symptoms that, in order of prevalence, include jaw, face, and head pain, which is easily misdiagnosed as temporomandibular joint syndrome (TMJ); hypersensitivities to odors, bright lights, and even fibromyalgia medications; painful menstruation; memory problems; and muscle twitching. Weather (particularly exposure to cold), normal hormonal fluctuation, stress, anxiety, depression, and physical exertion can aggravate fibromyalgia and produce flare-ups.

TREATMENT AND THERAPY

Because the cause of fibromyalgia is unknown, only its symptoms can be addressed. The treatment plan must be individualized and flexible and is considered long-term management. Rigid, stereotyped approaches can be worse than no management at all.

Because difficulty sleeping and pain can be both contributors to and outcomes of fibromyalgia, traditional treatment approaches focus on improving quality of sleep and reducing pain. Physicians commonly prescribe medications that increase the neurotransmitters serotonin and norepinephrine, which modulate sleep, pain, and the immune system. Amitriptyline (Elavil), paroxetine (Paxil), doxepin (Sinequan), cyclobenzaprine (Flexeril), clonazepam (Klonopin), and similar medications may be prescribed in low doses; they benefit one-third to one-half of patients. Alone or in combination, these medicines improve sleep staging, elevate mood, and relax overtense, stiff, and spasm-prone muscle groups.

More comprehensive are approaches that use medications as part of a well-rounded treatment plan. Physical therapy, massage therapy, acupuncture, and behavioral health are other treatment options. Physical therapy and aerobic exercises such as swimming and walking reduce muscle tenderness and pain while improving muscle conditioning and fitness. Because of fibromyalgia sufferers' sensitivity to cold and frequent stiffness, applied heat and therapeutic massage can render short-term relief. Though acupuncture is less well studied, anecdotal accounts claim its effectiveness, making it a sought-after therapy. Psychological counseling, or psychotherapy, can be effective for patients who are overwrought, overstressed, often wrongly blamed for having fibromyalgia, and in need of lifestyle adjustments.

PERSPECTIVE AND PROSPECTS

Until the 1990's, fibromyalgia syndrome—or fibrositis, as it was then more often called—

INFORMATION ON FIBROMYALGIA

CAUSES: Unknown; possibly injury or trauma to central nervous system, changes in muscle and connective tissue metabolism, or infectious agent

SYMPTOMS: Severe muscle pain; joint and muscle stiffness; tender points in knee, hips, spine, shoulders, and neck; fatigue; weakness; sometimes concurrent irritable bowel syndrome (IBS) and migraine or tension headaches

DURATION: Chronic with acute episodes

TREATMENTS: Alleviation of symptoms through medications, physical therapy, massage therapy, acupuncture, behavioral therapy

was not widely accepted by primary care specialists as a legitimate condition. Difficult to diagnose, it was often mistaken as chronic fatigue syndrome (itself a condition not widely recognized in primary care medicine), a sort of chronic pain syndrome, or some condition that was completely psychosomatic (that is, all in the patient's head). Fibromyalgia syndrome was often thought of as a "garbage can diagnosis": a little bit of everything, but not a real syndrome that could be treated. Sufferers had difficulty finding sympathetic medical help and were often at odds with family, friends, and coworkers who misattributed the causes of this connective, soft tissue disease whose existence could not be proven.

Advances in rheumatological research and the American College of Rheumatology's establishment of diagnostic criteria for fibromyalgia have made it a legitimate medical condition for which treatment can be sought. Previously, fibromyalgia patients often suffered from this painful, fatiguing condition and felt blamed for causing it—or worse, "making it up." Even today, the Fibromyalgia Network, a grassroots informational clearinghouse, underscores research that proves fibromyalgia syndrome is real.

Despite differing theories about the cause of fibromyalgia, ongoing research has produced some results that all investigators consider reliable. This syndrome seems to involve a relationship among the nervous system, the endocrine system, and sleep. When sleep electroencephalograms (EEGs) for patients known to have fibromyalgia are compared with those for nonpatient subjects, disturbances in the non-rapid eye movement (non-REM) stages become evident. There are five well-known and easily recognized stages of sleep: four non-REM stages and then a REM stage. Most people effortlessly progress through non-REM and REM stages. When they reach stage 4, a non-REM stage, they have reached sleep at its deepest. This is the stage during which tissue repair, antibody production, and possibly neurotransmitter regulation occur. Fibromyalgia EEGs show that these patients revert to stage 2 after stage 3, without having reached stage 4. Specialists refer to this sleep disorder as the alpha-EEG anomaly.

This EEG finding corresponds directly with fibromyalgia patients' anecdotal reports that they frequently do not feel rested or refreshed after a night's sleep. This result also contributes to an understanding of why sufferers are fatigued so often. The disturbance of non-REM sleep helps to produce the symptoms of insufficient sleep: tiredness, reduced mental acuity, irri-

tability, and autoimmune susceptibilities. The various stages of sleep also have corresponding hormonal activity, with different hormones and different levels released during each. Stages 3 and 4 are when growth hormones, including insulin growth factor (IGF), are primarily released. Fibromyalgia patients have low IGF levels.

A few other characteristic findings in these patients are not related to sleep. First, the neurotransmitter cerebrospinal fluid P (CSF P), also called substance P, is found in fibromyalgia patients at three times the normal level. Significantly, CSF P is associated with enhanced pain perception. Second, sufferers have low cortisol levels, suggesting that the hypopituitary-adrenal axis is adversely altered. Among much else, this axis mediates the fight-or-flight response and relaxation. Third, using an office procedure called tilt table testing, fibromyalgia symptoms can be provoked, accompanied by a rapid lowering of blood pressure in fibromyalgia patients but not in nonpatients. These findings all provide evidence that problems in the autonomic and endocrine systems cause fibromyalgia. What would set these problems into motion in the first place, however, is unknown, although many sufferers have experienced significant physical and/or psychological trauma before any syndrome-specific symptoms began.

—Paul Moglia, Ph.D.

See also Anxiety; Chronic fatigue syndrome; Depression; Fatigue; Headaches; Irritable bowel syndrome (IBS); Migraine headaches; Muscle sprains, spasms, and disorders; Muscles; Pain; Pain management; Sleep; Sleep disorders; Stress; Stress reduction.

For Further Information:

Fibromyalgia Network. http://www.fmnetnews.com/.

Goldenberg, Don L. *Fibromyalgia: A Leading Expert's Guide to Understanding and Getting Relief from the Pain That Won't Go Away*. Berkeley, Calif.: Berkeley Publishing Group, 2002.

Pellegrino, Mark. *Inside Fibromyalgia*. Columbus, Ohio: Anadem, 2001.

Wallace, Daniel J., and Daniel J. Clauw, eds. *Fibromyalgia and Other Central Pain Syndromes*. Philadelphia: Lippincott Williams & Wilkins, 2005.

Wallace, Daniel J., and Janice Brook Wallace. *All About Fibromyalgia: A Guide for Patients and Their Families*. 2d ed. New York: Oxford University Press, 2007.

FIFTH DISEASE
DISEASE/DISORDER

ALSO KNOWN AS: Erythema infectiosum

ANATOMY OR SYSTEM AFFECTED: Nose, skin, throat

SPECIALTIES AND RELATED FIELDS: Family medicine, pediatrics

DEFINITION: An infectious disease of children characterized by an erythematous (reddish) rash and low-grade fever.

CAUSES AND SYMPTOMS

Fifth disease is caused by infection with the human parvovirus (HPV) B19. The disease is more prevalent during late winter or early spring. Fifth disease is most commonly observed in young children, with the peak attack rate between five and fourteen years of age. Adults may become infected, but they rarely show evidence of disease.

The virus is spread from person to person through nasal secretions or sneezing. Following an incubation period of several days, a rash develops on the face, which has the appearance of slapped cheeks. The bright red color fades as the rash spreads over the rest of the body. An erythematous, pimply eruption may also appear on the trunk or extremities. A mild fever, sore throat, and nasal stuffiness may also be apparent. The rash generally lasts from ten days to two weeks. Often, it will fade only to reappear a short time later. Sunlight may aggravate the skin during this period, also causing a reappearance of the rash.

The diagnosis of fifth disease is primarily clinical, based on the symptoms. Laboratory tests for the virus are generally not performed.

TREATMENT AND THERAPY

No antibiotic therapy is available for fifth disease. Since the disease is rarely serious, treatment is mainly symptomatic. Bed rest and the administration of liquids, as commonly used in treating mild illness in children, are generally sufficient. Isolation is unnecessary since transmission is unlikely following appearance of the rash.

PERSPECTIVE AND PROSPECTS

Fifth disease was first described during the late nineteenth century as the fifth in the series of erythematous illnesses often encountered by children; the others are measles, mumps, chickenpox, and rubella. HPV B19 was isolated in 1975 and shown to be the etiological agent of the disease in the mid-1980's.

The disease is common and generally benign. HPV B19 has been implicated, however, in certain forms of hemolytic anemias and arthritis in adults, and research continues on the virus.

—*Richard Adler, Ph.D.*

See also Childhood infectious diseases; Fever; Rashes; Sneezing; Sore throat; Viral infections.

FOR FURTHER INFORMATION:

Behrman, Richard E., Robert M. Kliegman, and Hal B. Jenson, eds. *Nelson Textbook of Pediatrics*. 17th ed. Philadelphia: Saunders, 2004.

Burg, Fredric D., et al., eds. *Treatment of Infants, Children, and Adolescents*. Philadelphia: W. B. Saunders, 1990.

Kemper, Kathi J. *The Holistic Pediatrician: A Pediatrician's Comprehensive Guide to Safe and Effective Therapies for the Twenty-five Most Common Ailments of Infants, Children, and Adolescents*. New York: HarperCollins, 2002.

Kumar, Vinay, Abul K. Abbas, and Nelson Fausto, eds. *Robbins and Cotran Pathologic Basis of Disease*. 7th ed. Philadelphia: Elsevier Saunders, 2005.

Sompayrac, Lauren. *How Pathogenic Viruses Work*. Boston: Jones and Bartlett, 2002.

FINGERNAIL REMOVAL. *See* NAIL REMOVAL.

FISTULA REPAIR
PROCEDURE

ANATOMY OR SYSTEM AFFECTED: Abdomen, anus, bladder, blood, gallbladder, gastrointestinal system, intestines, reproductive system, urinary system, uterus

SPECIALTIES AND RELATED FIELDS: Gastroenterology, general surgery, pediatrics, proctology

DEFINITION: The removal of any abnormal passage associated with body sites or tissues.

INFORMATION ON FIFTH DISEASE

CAUSES: Viral infection

SYMPTOMS: "Slapped cheek" rash, fever, sore throat, achiness, malaise

DURATION: Ten to fourteen days

TREATMENTS: Alleviation of symptoms through bed rest, administration of liquids

KEY TERMS:

anorectal: associated with the anal portion of the large intestine

arteriovenous: associated with arteries and/or veins

Crohn's disease: a chronic inflammation of the bowel, often as a result of an autoimmune disease

crypt: a pit or depression in the body

fistulectomy: the surgical elimination of a fistula

INDICATIONS AND PROCEDURES

A fistula represents any abnormal opening or passage between internal organs or between an internal organ and the surface of the body. Fistulas can occur nearly anywhere in the body, but they are most commonly associated with the anorectal portion of the anatomy. Some fistulas may result from congenital defects, while others may be created surgically in association with specific procedures. For example, an arteriovenous fistula may be created to allow the insertion of a cannula (tube) for hemodialysis.

Anorectal fistulas usually begin as an abscess within the anal region or internal crypt that then spreads to adjacent tissue or to the surface of the body. Pain, itching, or tenderness in the region is often the first sign of a problem. The discomfort may be aggravated by bowel movements. Since infection is common, the opening may become purulent (pus-producing).

Treatment of anorectal fistulas usually requires surgery. A crypt hook may be used if the site of the original crypt must be located, an observation which is often unnecessary. The crypt may also be observed through an anoscope, or as part of a proctoscopic examination. Often, digital examination of the anal canal may detect a nodule, representing the abscess itself.

Any abscess must first be drained and treated. If the fistula is small, it may heal itself. The surgical procedure, commonly referred to as a fistulectomy, is a relatively simple operation carried out under general anesthesia. The fistula must be reduced or removed. Surgical repair begins at the primary opening, and generally the entire tract is opened, both to allow for proper drainage of infectious material and to promote healing. If the surgery is carried out properly, the incision should heal relatively quickly.

Difficult labor in women may create a variety of fistulas. A vesicovaginal fistula, created between the urinary bladder and the vagina, may be indicated by the presence of urine in the vaginal tract. As with any opening to the surface of the body, infection may develop. Likewise, a rectovaginal fistula, between the rectum

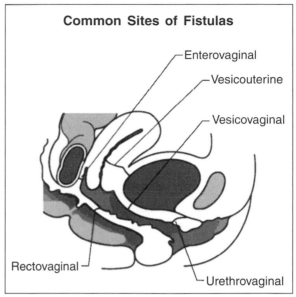

Common Sites of Fistulas

Enterovaginal

Vesicouterine

Vesicovaginal

Rectovaginal

Urethrovaginal

Fistulas are abnormal passages between organs or an organ and the outside of the body. They are more common in the rectal and genital regions of women, such as between the intestines and vagina (enterovaginal), the bladder and uterus (vesicouterine), the bladder and vagina (vesicovaginal), the urethra and vagina (urethrovaginal), and the rectum and vagina (rectovaginal).

and vagina, was formerly a possible serious complication of difficult childbirth. As with any fistulas, such openings have to be opened, drained, and sutured for healing.

Fistula formation may also be internal, as in biliary fistulas between the gallbladder and intestine. Such connections can occur as a consequence of gallstones, ulcers, or tumor formation. Often, the major symptom may be an intestinal blockage resulting from the stone or tumor itself. Bile may leak from the gallbladder into the peritoneum or body cavities, resulting in infection. Therapy for such fistula formation first requires an analysis of the channel itself. If the fistula is external, contrast material may be injected into the site to analyze the tract. If the fistula is internal, the extent of the tract may require cholangiography, the injection of a radiopaque material to outline the bile duct. General surgery is required for the proper correction of any underlying problem.

USES AND COMPLICATIONS

Surgical repair of a fistula has a number of functions, in addition to the elimination of the fistula itself. The goal of repair is to support the healing process, while at the same time attempting to maintain the normal function (and appearance, when applicable) of the tissue.

The anal fistula represents one of the more common types. Frequently, it begins as an abscess or break in the anal or rectal wall. Not infrequently, the underlying cause may be inflammation of the colon as a result of ulcerative colitis or Crohn's disease, an autoimmune disease which can cause ulceration of the intestinal wall. The fistula itself may become chronically infected, resulting in pain and discomfort. Cancer development in the area of the fistula, while uncommon, has been known to occur.

The major complication of anorectal surgery to repair the fistula is delayed healing. If not completely drained or covered, the area may continue to become infected. If the fistula is deep, damage to muscles during surgical repair may result in incontinence. Assuming that the fistula does not recur and postoperative care is properly provided, however, the prognosis is generally excellent.

Surgical procedures can also be used in the intentional formation of a fistula. For example, a site must be prepared for insertion of a cannula to carry out hemodialysis, the removal of waste from the blood under conditions of renal insufficiency. Generally, such a fistula between an artery and a vein is prepared one to two months prior to insertion of the cannula. The fistula is created either by grafting a section of bovine carotid artery into the site or by using a graft prepared from synthetic material. Proper circulation through the fistula must be monitored to ensure that infection does not develop.

PERSPECTIVE AND PROSPECTS

The development and widespread use of antibiotics in the mid-twentieth century provided a means for the effective treatment of the major complication associated with fistula development: infection. Fistulas may result in abscess formation or may be secondary to problems elsewhere, as with Crohn's disease. Better treatment of those infections associated with fistula formation, such as tuberculosis, has reduced their incidence. Likewise, proper prenatal care has largely controlled fistula development secondary to difficult labor in women.

—*Richard Adler, Ph.D.*

See also Abscess drainage; Abscesses; Childbirth complications; Colon and rectal surgery; Crohn's disease; Gastroenterology; Gastroenterology, pediatric; Gastrointestinal disorders; Gastrointestinal system; Grafts and grafting; Gynecology; Infection; Proctol-

ogy; Reproductive system; Stone removal; Stones; Tumor removal; Tumors; Ulcer surgery; Ulcers; Urinary system; Urology; Urology, pediatric.

FOR FURTHER INFORMATION:

American Medical Association. *American Medical Association Family Medical Guide*. 4th rev. ed. Hoboken, N.J.: John Wiley & Sons, 2004. An excellent reference for the beginner. The scientific accuracy of the text is not compromised by its accessibility.

Doherty, Gerard M., and Lawrence W. Way, eds. *Current Surgical Diagnosis and Treatment*. 12th ed. New York: Lange Medical Books/McGraw-Hill, 2006. A reference work on general surgery for physicians, this tome is nevertheless comprehensible to laypersons familiar with medical terminology. Presents succinct overviews of the stoma procedures and their potential complications and contains finely detailed illustrations.

Peikin, Steven R. *Gastrointestinal Health*. Rev. ed. New York: HarperCollins, 1999. Examines a range of gastrointestinal ailments in depth, including diarrhea and colitis, and offers tips for managing them via diet, stress management, and drugs.

Saibil, Fred. *Crohn's Disease and Ulcerative Colitis: Everything You Need to Know*. Rev. ed. Toronto: Firefly Books, 2003. A leading expert on IBD, Saibil covers topics such as signs and symptoms, how the gastrointestinal system works normally and how IBD affects it, procedures and instruments used to diagnose IBD, effects of diet, children and IBD, and effects on sexual activity and child-bearing.

Tierney, Lawrence M., Stephen J. McPhee, and Maxine A. Papadakis, eds. *Current Medical Diagnosis and Treatment 2007*. New York: McGraw-Hill Medical, 2006. This text, updated yearly, is the point of reference for physicians and other health care practitioners. It incorporates each year's biomedical research discoveries that have immediate, relevant, and applicable use for the patient.

FLAT FEET

DISEASE/DISORDER

ALSO KNOWN AS: Pes planus, talipes planus

ANATOMY OR SYSTEM AFFECTED: Feet, ligaments, muscles, musculoskeletal system

SPECIALTIES AND RELATED FIELDS: Orthopedics, podiatry

DEFINITION: A congenital or acquired flatness of the longitudinal arch of the foot.

INFORMATION ON FLAT FEET

CAUSES: Congenital weakness of muscles in arches, changes in shape of foot bones, short Achilles tendon, injury
SYMPTOMS: Delays in learning how to walk, pain, clumsiness in walking
DURATION: Typically short-term
TREATMENTS: Depends on severity; ranges from orthopedic shoes with arch supports, foot exercises, and rest to casts or surgery

CAUSES AND SYMPTOMS

Congenital flat feet are considered to be hereditary. Acquired flat feet can be caused by stretching of the arch ligaments and a weakness of the muscles found in the arches; this produces flexible flat feet. Rigid flat feet are caused by changes in the shape of the foot bones or a short Achilles tendon. Other causes of flat feet include injury and a lack of muscle tone or weak foot muscles that cannot sustain the body's weight.

All infants appear to be flat-footed because of a pad of fat under each instep. Arch formation in the feet takes place once they begin walking. Flat feet are often detected by parents when an infant experiences delays in learning how to walk.

Flat feet usually are painless and do not contribute to changes in posture or the ability to walk. Adolescents and adults are occasionally prone to fallen arches, or temporary foot strain caused by an activity that overstretches the ligaments in the arch; this condition is accompanied by pain. Rigid flat feet caused by a short Achilles tendon and spastic flat feet caused by a deformity of the heel result in pain and clumsiness in walking.

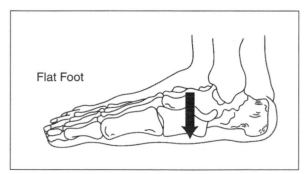

Flat Foot

Flat feet, or abnormally flat arches, can arise from muscle weakness, improper walking, or developmental defects.

TREATMENT AND THERAPY

Flexible, pain-free flat feet require no treatment. Special orthopedic shoes with arch supports do not change the shape of the feet over time, while foot exercises and prescribed changes in gait are hard to enforce in children.

In cases of fallen arches accompanied by fatigue or pain, however, rest, foot exercises, and the use of arch supports are recommended. If the Achilles tendon is too short or tight, it can be stretched by placing the foot in a cast. Severe cases of flat feet require surgery that removes excess bone or reconstructs the soft tissue of the foot.

—*Rose Secrest*

See also Arthritis; Bone disorders; Bones and the skeleton; Foot disorders; Lower extremities; Orthopedics; Orthopedics, pediatric; Podiatry.

FOR FURTHER INFORMATION:

Copeland, D. P. M. Glenn, and Stan Solomon. *The Foot Doctor: Lifetime Relief for Your Aching Feet.* Emmaus, Pa.: Rodale Press, 1986.

Currey, John D. *Bones: Structures and Mechanics.* Princeton, N.J.: Princeton University Press, 2002.

Lippert, Frederick G., and Sigvard T. Hansen. *Foot and Ankle Disorders: Tricks of the Trade.* New York: Thieme, 2003.

Lorimer, Donald L., et al., eds. *Neale's Disorders of the Foot.* 7th ed. New York: Elsevier Churchill Livingstone, 2006.

Van De Graaff, Kent M. *Human Anatomy.* 6th ed. New York: McGraw Hill, 2002.

FLUIDS AND ELECTROLYTES
BIOLOGY

ANATOMY OR SYSTEM AFFECTED: Blood, cells, respiratory system
SPECIALTIES AND RELATED FIELDS: Biochemistry, cytology, hematology, histology, pharmacology, pulmonary medicine, serology, urology
DEFINITION: Body fluids are intracellular or extracellular solutions of water and other substances, the concentrations of which must be regulated to achieve proper physiological functioning; electrolytes are chemicals that become electrically charged particles when they dissolve in water.

KEY TERMS:

adenosine triphosphate: a chemical that, when it reacts to lose a phosphate group, gives off free energy that is available for bodily processes

edema: the abnormal accumulation of fluid in tissues or cavities of the body

electrolyte: a chemical that, when it dissolves in water, dissociates to form positive and negative ions so that the resulting solution is an electrical conductor

homeostasis: the tendency of the body to maintain a beneficial balance among its parts

physiology: the study of the processes and mechanisms by which living organisms function

resorption: the process in which bones dissolve and return their components to the body fluids

semipermeable membrane: a barrier that allows some materials to pass but blocks others

solute: a material that has gone into solution and in so doing has changed its phase

STRUCTURE AND FUNCTIONS

Humans live in a wide variety of environmental conditions. Some days are hot and wet, others are cold and dry, and most are somewhere between. At the same time, as foods and liquid are taken in, the body is exposed to a variety of chemical substances over a wide range of concentrations. Amid these widely changing circumstances, the internal environment, to which the body's cells are exposed, remains essentially unchanged. This regulation of the internal environment, which is called homeostasis, is necessary for the correct functioning of the body. Essentially, all the organs and tissues of the body play roles in the homeostatic processes, and the main control mechanism operates through the movement of body fluids.

There are several different body fluids, but they are all solutions of solutes in water. The identity of the solutes and their concentrations differentiates one body fluid from another. Among the solutes, two categories exist. Some solutes dissociate into electrically charged particles when they dissolve and are thus called electrolytes. Others remain as neutral particles dissolved in the water and are nonelectrolytes. Both types of solutes play important roles in the correct physiological functioning of the body, but it is the electrolytes that draw the most attention. This is the case because the fluids and the electrolytes are interdependent and because imbalances of these factors are associated with a vast array of illnesses.

Although subject to some variation with age, gender, and physical condition, the body is composed of about 60 percent water by weight. For purposes of classification, this water is considered to be present in compartments. It is important to recognize that this terminology is conceptual only and does not refer to the existence of any real, separate, water-containing compartments in the body. Approximately 25 cubic decimeters of water are contained within the body's cells; this is the intracellular fluid. Most of the remaining fluid, about 12 cubic decimeters, is termed extracellular and exists in the regions exterior to cells. The extracellular fluid is further subdivided into the categories of interstitial fluid, which surrounds the cells; intravascular fluid, which is located within the blood vessels; and transcellular fluid, which includes the fluid found in the spinal column, the region of the lungs, the area surrounding the heart, the sinuses, and the eyes, along with sweat and digestive secretions. These subcategories are listed in order of the amount of fluid present. Of all these types, only the intravascular fluid is directly affected when a person drinks or eliminates fluid. Alterations in the other regions occur in response to that change, however, and there is a continual dynamic exchange of fluid among all compartments. The balance of conditions created by this exchange determines the state of health of the individual.

The solutes that are electrolytes generate positively charged ions called cations and negatively charged ions called anions. The amount of positive charge present in a solution is always equal to the amount of negative charge. The major cations present are hydrogen, sodium, potassium, calcium, and magnesium. The most important anions are chloride, hydrogen carbonate, hydrogen phosphate, sulfate, and those derived from organic acids such as acetic acid. Several other ions of both types are present at very low levels. The nonelectrolytes present include urea, creatinine, bilirubin, and glucose. All these solutes are involved with particular biological changes in the body, so their presence at the correct concentration is vital.

The fluid and its solutes move within the body by means of several transport mechanisms, some of which move solutes through the fluid and some of which move either water or the solutes from one side of a cell membrane to the other. The mechanisms available are diffusion, active transport, filtration, and osmosis. Diffusion is the movement of particles through a solution from a region in which the concentration of the particles is high to a region in which it is lower. The energy that drives this motion is thermal energy, and the transport rate is increased by increasing the temperature, which increases the concentration difference from point to point and is faster for smaller particles. Cell walls are a barrier to this type of transport unless the solute particles are small enough to pass through pores in the wall or are soluble in the cell wall itself. Active transport provides another means of moving solutes across cell walls. The energy for such movement is provided by a series of chemical reactions involving adenosine triphosphate. The movement of sodium out of and potassium into cells, as well as the transport of amino acids into cells, occurs in this manner. Filtration is a means by which both water and some solutes are transported through a porous membrane. The solutes transported are those that are small enough to pass through the pores in the membrane. The driving force for filtration is provided by a difference in pressure on the two sides of the membrane, and the motion occurs from the high-pressure side to the low-pressure side. The pressure in this case results from gravity and from the pumping action of the heart. Osmosis is a process by which water is moved across a semipermeable membrane as the result of the influence of a different type of pressure. When two solutions of different concentrations of solute particles are separated by a semipermeable membrane, an osmotic pressure develops that acts as the driving force to move water from the side of the membrane where the concentration of solute particles is lower to the side where the solute particle concentration is higher.

A solute's concentration in the body fluid has a great effect on the transport of materials and thus on the body's health. Concentrations in body fluids are expressed in several ways. Electrolyte concentration is often expressed in terms of milliequivalents of solute per cubic decimeter of solution. This is a measure of the amount of change, positive or negative, provided by that solute. A solution with twice the number of milliequivalents per cubic decimeter will have twice the concentration of change. This also measures the solute's combining power, because one milliequivalent of cations will chemically combine with one milliequivalent of anions. Osmolality, osmolarity, and tonicity refer to a solution's ability to provide an osmotic pressure. Osmolality and osmolarity are proportional to the number of particles of solute present in the solution. When solutions of different osmolalities or osmolarities are separated by a semipermeable membrane, there will be a flow of solvent across the membrane. Isotonic solutions have equal osmotic effects. Tonicity is a way of comparing the osmotic potential of solutions by referring to one as being hypotonic, isotonic, or hypertonic to the other.

Disorders and Diseases

There are two ways to approach thinking about the health role of body fluids and electrolytes. One is to consider one particular fluid component, such as sodium, that is out of balance and proceed to trace possible causes of the imbalance and appropriate treatment modes. It must be noted, however, that there are many possible illnesses that could cause any particular imbalance. The second approach is to consider a representative number of specific diseases and to look at their effect on the fluid and electrolyte balance and how such effects may be treated.

The first of these two approaches is adopted here because it highlights the fluids and electrolytes themselves rather than the diseases. Two imbalances will be considered as examples of the types of effects seen. First to be considered is the volume of fluid itself. Second, the balance of calcium will be given attention because of the connection of calcium deficiency with the bone brittleness that often occurs during aging.

Volume imbalance that is larger than the system's normal regulatory ability to control may occur in either the intracellular or extracellular fluid or both and may be in the direction of too little fluid (dehydration) or too much (overhydration). Both of these effects may result from a number of underlying illnesses, but each is, by itself, life-threatening and requires direct treatment. Often, this treatment precedes the diagnosis of the root cause.

The body apparently senses fluid volume imbalance with receptors near the heart, and several coping responses are triggered. Dehydration can be the result of vomiting, diarrhea, excessive perspiration, or blood loss. In such cases, the body's responses are in the direction of maintaining the flow of blood to vital organs. Vessels at the extremities are constricted, and those in the regions of the vital organs are dilated. Kidney function is greatly slowed, the reabsorption of sodium is increased, and the production of urine is markedly decreased, ensuring water retention. Centers in the hypothalamus respond and cause the individual to become thirsty. Thus, the body acts to protect its most important functions while at the same time stimulating actions from the individual that will bring additional fluid volume into the system. The manner in which the individual responds to being thirsty will determine other bodily changes. If plain water is used to quench the thirst, the extracellular fluid becomes less concentrated in electrolytes than is the intracellular fluid, causing an osmotic pressure imbalance that the body regulates by transporting more water into the cells, producing overhydration there and aggravating the original dehydration in the extracellular fluid. Notice that this means that drinking large amounts of water can, strange though it may seem, cause dehydration. If saltwater is ingested, the reverse occurs, with a resulting dehydration of the cells that in turn triggers extreme thirst but few cardiovascular problems. Proper volume replacement thus requires that the water brought into the system be of the same electrolyte concentration as the cellular fluids—that is, that they be isotonic. In that case, the osmotic pressure remains balanced and the fluid volumes in both of the major compartments can be built up.

Overhydration is a less common occurrence that is usually associated with cardiovascular disease, severe malnutrition and kidney disease, or surgical stress. When the heart is not able to act as an effective pump, a back pressure builds in the circulatory system that causes fluid to be filtered through the walls of the vessels and that results in the accumulation of fluid in the interstitial regions around the heart and lungs. A decrease in proteins in the bloodstream, resulting from either malnutrition or kidney malfunction, lowers the osmotic pressure in the blood and causes water retention in the interstitial spaces. Accumulation of excess fluid in the interstitial spaces is called edema. This same end condition also arises when the kidney excessively filters fluid from the bloodstream into the interstitial spaces. The treatment of overhydration takes the form of fluid intake restriction, restriction of dietary sodium, and the use of diuretic therapy to stimulate urine production.

Calcium, much of which comes from milk and milk products, is the fifth most abundant ion in the body and is involved with the formation of the mineral component of teeth and bones, the contraction of muscles, proper blood clotting, and the maintenance of cell wall permeability. Calcium is added to extracellular fluid as a result of the intestinal absorption of dietary calcium and bone resorption. It is lost from the extracellular fluid via secretion into the intestinal tract, urinary excretion, and deposition in bone. The maintenance of a proper calcium level mainly depends on processes occurring in the intestinal tract. Only a very small part of the body's total calcium is in fluids. Both hypocalcemia and hypercalcemia, the shortage and the overabundance of calcium in the fluids, may occur. Unlike the case of water shortage or excess, however, there are few direct visual consequences of a calcium imbalance;

one must rely on laboratory testing of the fluid and on indirect physical assessment.

Hypocalcemia in the blood is associated with reduced intake, increased loss, or altered regulation, as in hypoparathyroidism. Bone, a living material, continually absorbs and desorbs calcium. The parathyroid gland secretes a hormone that regulates bone resorption and thus can raise the calcium level in the extracellular fluid at the expense of decreasing the amount of bone. Obviously, this cannot be a long-term mechanism to provide calcium. The same hormone also regulates the absorption of calcium from the intestines and the kidneys. Vitamin D is an essential, although indirect, factor in permitting the absorption of calcium from the intestine. A deficiency of this vitamin is a major cause of hypocalcemia. When the calcium level in the extracellular fluid falls below normal, the nervous system becomes increasingly excited. If the level continues to fall, the nerve fibers begin to discharge spontaneously, passing impulses to the peripheral skeletal muscles, where they cause a contractive spasm. Often, this is first seen in a contracting of the fingers. Generalized muscular spasming can be lethal if the calcium imbalance is not corrected quickly. Immediate calcium deficiency is treated with the administration of either oral or intravenous calcium compounds, with vitamin D therapy, and with the inclusion of foods of high calcium content in the diet. In the longer term, treatment of the underlying illness is necessary.

The opposite imbalance, hypercalcemia, can occur as a result of an excessive intake of calcium supplements and vitamin D, in conjunction with a high-calcium diet. Calcium excess is also associated with some tumors and with kidney or glandular diseases. It has also been found to be caused by prolonged immobility, in which case the bones resorb because of the lack of bone stress. This latter effect has been of major concern in the space program. Too high a level of calcium in the intercellular fluid causes a depression of the nervous system and a slowing of reflexes. Lack of appetite and constipation are also common results. At very high levels, calcium salts may precipitate in the blood system, an effect that can be rapidly lethal. Again, in the long term, the underlying cause of the imbalance must be corrected, but treatments do exist for more immediate alleviation. As long as the kidneys are functioning correctly, intravenous treatment with saline serves as a means of flushing out excess calcium. Calcium also can be bound to phosphate that is delivered intravenously, but there is a risk of causing soft tissue precipitation of the calcium phosphate compound. Dietary control is used, at times in concert with steroid therapy, to counter high calcium levels. If resorption is the cause of the excess, there are therapies, both chemical and physical, that are effective in increasing bone deposition.

PERSPECTIVE AND PROSPECTS

From the earliest times, those concerned with the treatment of illnesses have had their attention drawn to the fluids present in or exuded by the human body. The color, smell, and texture of fluids being given off by a sick or injured person provided clues to the nature of the illness or injury. Bleeding was commonly practiced as a means of venting the illness so that health could be restored. Lancing of ulcerative conditions was also practiced by early healers. These early attempts at understanding and of treatment have been greatly refined, and the search for better understanding and improved treatment modes continues.

This concern with fluids and electrolytes is easy to understand. The fluids and their components constitute both the external and the internal environment for all the body's tissues and cells. Any abnormality in the cells or tissues is reflected in a variation from normal conditions in the fluids. All major illnesses and many minor ones have associated with them a fluid and electrolyte disorder. Fluids are more readily accessible for study than are tissues from deep within the body; hence, a considerable effort has been directed at measuring fluid constituents and interpreting the findings. The testing of fluids has evolved from highly labor intensive measurements of a few components to highly automated testing procedures applied to dozens of components. The reliability and precision of the measurements continue to increase, and the scope of measurements continues to expand.

Not all that is to be known about fluids and electrolytes, however, depends on laboratory testing. Some knowledge can be collected from close observation of the patient. Although the resulting measurements are not precise, they are nevertheless important because they are much more immediately available. Physical symptoms that carry information about fluids and electrolytes include the following: sudden weight gain or loss; changes in abdominal girth; changes in either the intake or output of fluids; body temperature; depth of respiration; heart rate; blood pressure; skin moisture, color, and temperature; the skin's ability to relax to normal after being pinched; the swelling of tissue; the con-

dition of the tongue; the appearance of visible veins; reflexive responses; apparent mental state; and thirst. Each of these observations, and more, is readily available to one who is monitoring the health of an individual.

As is the case with most testing and data-gathering situations, interpreting the test and observation results is the critical step. Any one measure, by itself, points to a vast array of possible illnesses. Only by considering the whole and recognizing the existence of patterns in the information can a health professional narrow the possibilities. It is this recognition of patterns that develops with education and experience, and it is this step that relies on judgment that makes medicine an art as well as a science.

—*Kenneth H. Brown, Ph.D.*

See also Acid-base chemistry; Blood and blood disorders; Cells; Circulation; Cytology; Dehydration; Edema; Fever; Hyperhidrosis; Hypertension; Hypotension; Lipids; Physiology; Sweating; Vascular system; Weight loss and gain.

FOR FURTHER INFORMATION:

Campbell, Neil A., et al. *Biology: Concepts and Connections.* 5th ed. San Francisco: Pearson/Benjamin Cummings, 2006. This classic introductory textbook provides an excellent discussion of essential biological structures and mechanisms.

Chambers, Jeanette K., Marilyn J. Rantz, and Meridean Maas, eds. *Common Fluid and Electrolyte Disorders, Nursing Diagnoses: Implementation.* Philadelphia: W. B. Saunders, 1987. The first part of this two-part book contains twelve short chapters, each targeted to an aspect of the subject. The book is designed for nurses, and the material is presented on a very practical level.

Guyton, Arthur C., and John E. Hall. *Human Physiology and Mechanisms of Disease.* 6th ed. Philadelphia: W. B. Saunders, 1997. This college-level physiology text contains several chapters relevant to the appreciation of the importance of body fluids and electrolytes. Although written at an advanced level, the writing is well done, and the major points are clearly presented. The text allows the subject to be placed in context of the whole of human physiology.

Horne, Mima M., Ursula Easterday Heitz, and Pamela L. Swearingen. *Fluid, Electrolyte, and Acid-Base Balance: A Case Study Approach.* St. Louis: Mosby Year Book, 1991. This book, written for nursing students but readable by those with minimum science background, provides an excellent summary of the subject and places the material in the context of human health. Its particular strength is in relating fluids and electrolytes to specific illnesses and in discussing treatment modes.

Kee, Joyce LeFever, Betty J. Paulanka, and Larry D. Purnell. *Fluids and Electrolytes with Clinical Applications: A Programmed Approach.* 7th ed. Clifton Park, N.Y.: Delmar, 2004. This is a well-presented self-instruction text that begins with the basics and then refines the topic. The thrust is the connection of the assessment of fluid and electrolyte imbalance with an understanding of illness and treatment.

Lee, Carla A. Bouska, C. Ann Barrett, and Donna D. Ignatavicius. *Fluids and Electrolytes: A Practical Approach.* 4th ed. Philadelphia: F. A. Davis, 1996. The authors have aimed for a pragmatic and simplified treatment of the subject matter that is related directly to the clinical situation. Following sections that summarize the principles, the book uses a case study approach to connect principles and practice.

Speakman, Elizabeth, and Norma Jean Weldy. *Body Fluids and Electrolytes.* 8th ed. New York: Elsevier, 2002. A classic text that details clinical conditions such as pH imbalance, electrolyte imbalance, and fluid overload or underload.

FLUORIDE TREATMENTS
PROCEDURE

ANATOMY OR SYSTEM AFFECTED: Gums, mouth, teeth

SPECIALTIES AND RELATED FIELDS: Bacteriology, biochemistry, dentistry, microbiology

DEFINITION: Treatment of the teeth with a fluoride-releasing substance to help the enamel resist tooth decay.

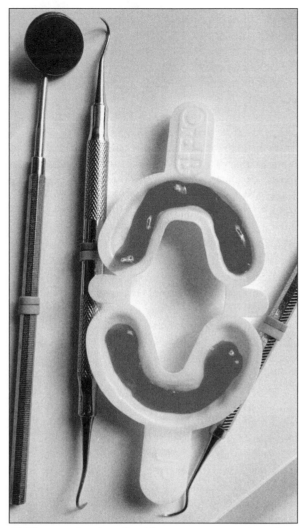

Children may be given fluoride treatments as a gel in a foam mouthpiece in order to protect against the formation of cavities. (AP/Wide World Photos)

INDICATIONS AND PROCEDURES

Tooth decay involves the solubility of food during eating. Consumed carbohydrates are oxidized to organic acids, such as lactic acid, by the action of specific bacteria that adhere to the teeth. These acids dissolve tooth enamel, which mainly consists of a mineral called hydroxyapatite and is considered to be the hardest substance in the body. The protection of the enamel, and thus the inner part of the tooth, from decomposition can be achieved through fluoride treatments.

Fluoride treatment involves the ingestion of fluoride ions in drinking water, toothpaste, and other sources to change the nature and composition of hydroxyapatite by producing a new compound called fluorapatite. Because it is less basic than hydroxyapatite, fluorapatite forms a more resistant enamel. Because of its effectiveness in preventing cavities, fluoride is added in the form of sodium fluoride or sodium hexafluorosilicate to the public water supply of many municipalities in the United States in concentrations of about 1 milligram per milliliter, or 1 part per million.

USES AND COMPLICATIONS

As a result of this so-called fluoridation process, a drastic reduction in dental decay has been observed. In addition, more than 80 percent of all toothpastes and gels now sold in the United States contain fluoride, in the form of stannous fluoride, sodium monofluoro-phosphate, and/or sodium fluoride in concentrations of about 0.1 percent fluoride by weight.

The recommended annual or semiannual dental cleaning by a dentist or oral hygienist removes accumulated plaque and may include further application with a fluoride substance. Generally, only children and teenagers receive such a fluoride treatment, although some adults may also have it.

It must be noted that fluoride ions are toxic in large quantities. As a result, when the fluoride concentration in water is about 2 to 3 parts per million, discoloration (mottling) or damage of the teeth may occur.

—*Soraya Ghayourmanesh, Ph.D.*

See also Cavities; Dental diseases; Dentistry; Dentistry, pediatric; Teeth; Wisdom teeth.

FOR FURTHER INFORMATION:

Ash, Major M., Jr., and Stanley J. Nelson. *Wheeler's Dental Anatomy, Physiology, and Occlusion.* 8th ed. St. Louis: Saunders, 2003.

Foster, Malcolm S. *Protecting Our Children's Teeth: A Guide to Quality Dental Care from Infancy Through Age Twelve.* Cambridge, Mass.: Perseus, 1992.

Smith, Rebecca W. *The Columbia University School of Dental and Oral Surgery's Guide to Family Dental Care.* New York: W. W. Norton, 1997.

Woodall, Irene R., ed. *Comprehensive Dental Hygiene Care.* 4th ed. St. Louis: C. V. Mosby, 1993.

FLUOROSCOPY. *See* IMAGING AND RADIOLOGY.

FOOD AND DRUG ADMINISTRATION (FDA)

ORGANIZATION

ALSO KNOWN AS: Bureau of Chemistry (1906-1927); Food, Drug, and Insecticide Administration (1927-1931)

DEFINITION: An agency in the United States Department of Health and Human Services whose responsibilities include protecting citizens against harmful or falsely labeled foods, food additives, drugs, cosmetics, or medical devices.

KEY TERMS:

Generally Recognized as Safe (GRAS) list: food ingredients or chemicals designated by the FDA as harmless to human beings when used as intended

generic drugs: copycat versions of brand-name originals that are no longer protected by patents

orphan drug: a drug developed for a very rare disease (legally, drugs for two hundred thousand or fewer potential users)

thalidomide: a sedative and sleep-inducing drug that was found to produce phocomelia (a birth defect in which hands or feet are attached to the body by short, flipperlike stumps) in developing fetuses and newborns

STRUCTURE AND FUNCTION

The mission of the Food and Drug Administration (FDA) is to protect the nation's health. Consequently, the U.S. Congress empowered this agency to prevent the sale of harmful products. The FDA's specific duty is to enforce the numerous federal laws that have been passed to ensure that foods and drugs are pure and safe and that all such products are correctly labeled. With the multiplication of its responsibilities over time came a concomitant growth in the FDA's administrative, technical, and service staffs both in Washington, D.C., and in ten regions around the country. Officials in each region are responsible for enforcing the relevant laws in their jurisdictions, and they are helped in this by inspectors and scientists.

The activities of FDA personnel include research, inspection, and legal action. In FDA laboratories scientists verify manufacturers' claims of the safety and effectiveness of food additives, drugs, and cosmetics before they are put onto the market. In addition to studying the long-term effects of various products, FDA workers also study how foods are processed, preserved, packaged, and stored. Using their field staffs, FDA officials send their inspectors to monitor manufacturing facilities and assist industrial employees in setting up procedures to prevent violations of the law. The FDA also has the duty of enforcing laws against illegal sales of prescription drugs, and FDA employees periodically examine imports of foods, drugs, cosmetics, and therapeutic devices to make sure that they comply with federal laws.

Even though the FDA has the responsibility of protecting consumers from various lawbreakers, its enforcement of relevant laws is limited by the courts. In fact, the agency must have the cooperation of attorneys and judges to prosecute persons or firms, impose fines, or seize products. FDA inspectors collect evidence of violations, and administrators review this evidence before deciding which cases will be presented to the federal courts for action. As a federal agency, the FDA is restricted to products involved in interstate commerce.

IN THE NEWS:
CREATION OF DRUG SAFETY OVERSIGHT BOARD

On February 15, 2005, the FDA announced the creation of a Drug Safety Oversight Board that would be independent of the existing Office of Drug Safety. The board would be responsible for overseeing drug safety policies and resolving disputes involving drug risks.

The board was the result of several scientific controversies regarding the safety of drugs that the FDA had approved for public sale. Recall of the popular and widely advertised painkiller Vioxx by Merck, amid revelations that continued use increased the risk of heart attack or stroke, as well as disclosure that frequently prescribed antidepressants increased suicidal desires among children, shook the agency. In each case, the FDA was accused of being slow to act, of ignoring warnings from its own Office of Drug Safety, and of being reluctant to inform the public about problems with drugs already on the market.

The board has fifteen voting members appointed by the FDA commissioner; thirteen are senior scientific managers at the FDA and the other are two staff physicians at the National Institutes of Health and the Department of Veterans Affairs. In its first year, the board held five private meetings and issued safety alerts on forty-four drugs, of which three were suspended and two withdrawn.

Criticism of the board's composition and methods of operation came quickly and continued. Lawmakers and consumer groups argued that since all members came from within the FDA, the board lacked true independence, which was not possible as long as the same agency approved drugs and evaluated their postmarket safety. The FDA defended holding closed meetings on the grounds that the board considered proprietary information of drug companies, but lawmakers complained that the lack of transparency meant they did not know what the board actually did. The original FDA announcement said that medical experts and patient and consumer groups would act as consultants to the board, but no consultations were held during the first year. Although the FDA promised to set up a Web site where actions of the board would be posted, it did not do so.

—*Milton Berman, Ph.D.*

nate in pharmaceutical or chemical companies, government laboratories, medical schools, or universities. An inventor or discoverer of a new drug can be granted a patent for the drug itself or for how it is made or used. Patents give the developer exclusive rights to a drug for seventeen years. After a patent has expired, other companies may sell a generic version of the drug, usually at a much lower price. The FDA's approval of a generic drug is based on laboratory studies to guarantee that the copy has the safety and effectiveness of the original. Since the generic drug manufacturer who is first to market a new generic drug reaps huge financial rewards, great pressures exist on the FDA to facilitate this process.

In 1988 generic drugs became the focus of a congressional subcommittee. It discovered that three generic drug companies were receiving accelerated approval of their applications in exchange for payoffs to FDA employees. When this generic drug scandal was over, federal courts had convicted ten companies and forty-two people of corruption. This scandal also revealed a potentially corrupting collusion between FDA workers and pharmaceutical companies, since FDA employees often leave their government jobs for highly paid positions at the companies they had formerly regulated.

CONTROVERSIES AND ETHICAL DEBATES

As the federal agency charged with protecting the health of Americans, the FDA is often entangled in controversial and ethical issues. For example, it is responsible for the regulation of investigational new drugs (INDs)—drugs approved for testing but not for sale. For a drug to become an IND, it must first be given to animals, since a correlation often exists between a drug's adverse effect on animals and its similar effect on humans. The FDA's procedure for testing INDs in-

Because of physicians' professional concerns with nutrition, prescription and nonprescription drugs, and medical technologies, they have a vested interest in the FDA and its activities. According to several studies, physicians are protective of their independence and the integrity of the doctor-patient relationship, and many doctors are wary of governmental involvement in how they practice medicine. On the other hand, critics have pointed out the dangers of the close relationship that has developed between doctors and drug companies.

The FDA supervises the development and marketing of all drugs sold in the United States. New drugs origi-

cludes three phases: In Phase I, small groups of healthy volunteers are given the IND to help researchers study its effectiveness, dosage, and metabolism; in Phase II, one to two hundred patients with the drug-targeted disease are monitored for the drug's safety, efficacy, and side effects; in Phase III, even larger numbers of patients take the drug to refine optimum dosages and, with the use of placebos, to make sure that the IND's effects are not due to chance or the developer's optimism.

In the 1970's, the FDA's handling of INDs came under attack. The General Accounting Office (GAO) studied ten of the more than six thousand drugs then classified as INDs, concluding that in eight cases the FDA failed to halt human tests after receiving indications that the new drugs were unsafe. Furthermore the GAO found that drug companies delayed reporting adverse drug effects to the FDA. Others pointed out that the FDA tested INDs singly, whereas some drugs have the potential of causing great harm when they interact with other drugs (the so-called synergistic effect). Some criticized the FDA for approving too many drugs too quickly, thereby increasing risks, while others blamed the FDA for increasing risks by approving too few drugs too slowly. Defenders of the FDA responded by saying that it is impossible to eliminate all risks from the use of medicines.

A specific example of what some see as the FDA's excessive regulation of foods and drugs is the controversy over dietary supplements. Initially the FDA tried to restrict the public's right to choose these supplements. Some scientists thought that the FDA's vitamin regulations were reasonable, but public discontent forced Congress to pass a law guaranteeing consumers freedom to choose nutritional supplements. In the 1970's, this debate centered on laetrile (also known as vitamin B_{17}), a substance found naturally in apricot pits. Many countries permitted the sale of laetrile as a supplement, but the FDA banned it, pointing out that it causes the release of cyanide in the body. Advocates believed that laetrile relieved the symptoms and slowed the growth of cancers, and some states legalized laetrile, challenging the FDA ban. However, in 1979, the Supreme Court ruled unanimously that the FDA had the power to ban the interstate sale and distribution of laetrile. This and such controversies as disputes over artificial hearts, cigarettes as "drug-delivery devices," and various acquired immunodeficiency syndrome (AIDS) drugs helped define the FDA's role in American society, just as similar controversies have throughout the history of the agency.

PERSPECTIVE AND PROSPECTS

Most scholars trace the history of the FDA to the Pure Food and Drug Act of 1906. This law, like many that would follow it, originated from public outrage over tragedies caused by impure foods and drugs. More than a century ago, food producers commonly added water to milk and adulterated coffee with charcoal. They colored foods and drinks with harmful dyes, and they used such injurious preservatives as formaldehyde, sodium benzoate, and borax. Consumers had to choose drugs based on false or misleading labels. This intolerable situation inspired the crusade of Harvey Wiley, who, because of his attacks on adulterated or pernicious foods and drugs, became known as the "Father of the Pure Food and Drug Law." In his position as chief of the Bureau of Chemistry of the Department of Agriculture, Wiley gathered a group of idealistic young chemists, nicknamed the "Poison Squad," to study the physiological effects of various chemical additives in foods. Their studies aroused public concern over food additives, but "Wiley's Law" would never have become a reality were it not for Upton Sinclair, whose novel *The Jungle* (1906) dramatized unsanitary practices in the meatpacking industry, and for President Theodore Roosevelt, who, disgusted by scandals in the drug trade, prodded members of Congress to pass the law. The Food and Drug Act of 1906 prohibited the "manufacture, sale, or transportation of adulterated or misbranded or poisonous or deleterious foods, drugs, medicines, and liquors." The Bureau of Chemistry administered the new law, and Wiley and his successors developed an organization that won many victories for pure foods and drugs in the courts.

In 1928, Congress authorized the creation of the Food, Drug, and Insecticide Administration as the executor of the Pure Food and Drug Act. The Agricultural Appropriation Act of 1931 changed the agency's name to the Food and Drug Administration. When Franklin D. Roosevelt became president in 1933, he and his team of "New Dealers" tried to get through Congress a number of fiscal and social reforms, including an expansion of the FDA's mission, since companies were continuing to make dangerous medicines. Little was accomplished until 1937, when the Massengill Company shipped its Elixir Sulfanilamide to pharmacists. This drug, which was intended to cure infections, eventually caused the deaths of 107 people. Within months of this tragedy, Congress finally passed the Federal Food, Drug, and Cosmetic Act of 1938. This law required drug manufacturers to provide scientific proof, through tests on animals and humans, that all their new drugs were safe before they were put on the market.

To isolate the FDA from advocacy groups, it became part of the Federal Security Agency in 1940. World War II expanded the FDA's workload, especially with the discovery of new "wonder drugs" that had to be tested. After the war, the number, variety, and power of new drugs increased dramatically. With the FDA's emphasis on prescription drugs, new industries emerged and, because of high profits, these companies grew in size and influence. The profitability of the postwar food and drug industries brought both abuses and legislative remedies.

During the 1950's and 1960's the 1938 act was periodically amended, including the Humphrey-Durham Drug Prescription Act (1951), the Food Additives Amendment (1958), the Color Additives Amendment (1961), and the Kefauver-Harris Drug Amendment (1962). After the FDA became part of the Department of Health, Education, and Welfare in 1953, it used these new laws to concentrate control of powerful new drugs in the hands of FDA officials and doctors. Some of these new laws gave the FDA responsibility for determining the safety of food ingredients, even those on the Generally Recognized as Safe (GRAS) list that had previously been used with no apparent ill effects. For example, sodium cyclamate, an additive used as an artificial sweetener, had originally been classified as GRAS but was later banned as being possibly carcinogenic. The Delaney Clause (1958) prohibited the use of substances in food if they caused cancer in laboratory animals. This law led to a controversial ban of another artificial sweetener, saccharin, a weak carcinogen (the Delaney Clause was replaced, in 1996, by a less stringent standard).

In the late 1950's, the thalidomide tragedy in Europe, during which thousands of deformed infants were born, helped to enhance public support for legislation strengthening the Food, Drug, and Cosmetic Act. Widespread use of thalidomide in America was prevented by Dr. Frances Kelsey, an FDA examiner, who used the pretext of insufficient information to turn down a company's repeated applications to market this drug in the United States. Congress responded to the thalidomide tragedy by passing the Kefauver-Harris Amendment in 1962. This law changed the ways in which drugs were created, tested, developed, prescribed, and sold. The burden was now on the companies sponsoring a new drug to show that it was safe and effective. The FDA also issued new regulations that

made the drug review process extremely stringent; some said too stringent, because FDA officials, fearful of another thalidomide-like tragedy, delayed new drug approval by asking for study after study.

During the 1970's, 1980's, and 1990's, the Food, Drug, and Cosmetic Act of 1938 was constantly revised and amended. For example, an amendment in 1976 strengthened the FDA's authority to regulate medical devices, and in 1980 serious illnesses in babies caused Congress to pass an Infant Formula Act requiring strict controls over the nutritional content and safety of commercial baby foods. In 1982 seven deaths from cyanide poisoning later traced to Tylenol capsules caused the FDA to issue regulations requiring tamper-resistant packaging. The Orphan Drug Act of 1983 offered economic inducement to encourage pharmaceutical companies to develop drugs for rare diseases affecting small populations. However, the multiplication of regulations did not prevent the generic drug scandals of the late 1980's. In fact, for many critics, the FDA had become an inefficient agency, under constant attack from congressional subcommittees, newspaper reporters, public interest groups, and industry executives.

In the 1990's, the FDA struggled to retrieve its credibility and authority by becoming once again the guardian of the nation's health. In 1992, the Prescription Drug User Fee Act required $100,000 for each new drug application, rising to $233,000 per application in five years. In return, the FDA hired six hundred new examiners to cut the review time for important new drugs. The FDA also improved standards of risk assessment for food additives, drugs, and medical devices, and it increased inspections of food and drug factories. By the end of the twentieth century, the FDA was an agency trying to keep up with the revolutionary advances in the chemical, biological, and medical sciences.

The beginning of the twenty-first century introduced an interesting era for the FDA. Because of a slowdown in the creation of innovative drugs and medical devices, the FDA rolled out new guidelines to help pharmaceutical companies better prove how a drug works in efforts to streamline the process of approval and get new treatments to the consumer market faster. Noting that drug companies went from sending a high of sixty never-before-seen drugs in 1995 for FDA approval down to just seventeen in 2002, the agency decided to make their requirements for approval more clear so that companies could do better research faster and be more willing to take chances on truly novel treatments instead of safer "copycat" medications. Some of these requirements included helping companies avoid incomplete applications, developing special guidelines for brand-new technology so that companies can design the right studies from the beginning, and providing more training of FDA reviewers.

The terrorist attacks on the World Trade Center and the Pentagon in 2001 also introduced a change in the FDA's approval process. In order to help in the development of bioterrorism antidotes, the agency announced that it would approve certain drugs based only on animal studies if human drug testing would be impossible. The new approach to the evaluation process includes only those drugs that would treat or prevent the potentially lethal or disabling toxicity of chemical, biological, or nuclear substances.

—Robert J. Paradowski, Ph.D.

See also Animal rights vs. research; Antibiotics; Anti-inflammatory drugs; Clinical trials; Creutzfeldt-Jakob disease (CJD); Food biochemistry; Food poisoning; Iatrogenic disorders; Over-the-counter medications; Pharmacology; Pharmacy; Screening.

FOR FURTHER INFORMATION:

Hickmann, Meredith A. ed. *The Food and Drug Administration (FDA)*. Hauppauge, N.Y.: Nova Science, 2003. Explains how the FDA is responsible for ensuring the safety of foods, drugs, medical devices, cosmetics, and other products.

Hilts, Philip J. *Protecting America's Health: The FDA, Business, and One Hundred Years of Regulation*. New York: Alfred Knopf, 2003. Provides a thorough history of the FDA and its battles with self-serving political and industrial interests.

Jackson, Charles O. *Food and Drug Legislation in the New Deal*. Princeton, N.J.: Princeton University Press, 1970. A political and historical analysis of the complex struggle leading to the Food, Drug, and Cosmetic Act of 1938.

Liska, Ken. *Drugs and the Human Body with Implications for Society*. Englewood Cliffs, N.J.: Prentice Hall, 2003. Examines the use of drugs in the North American culture by discussing such topics as what constitutes a drug and where drugs come from, drug metabolism, the different classifications of drugs, and federal laws that can be applied generally to many drug categories, including over-the-counter and prescription drugs.

O'Reilly, James T. *Food and Drug Administration*. 2d ed. St. Paul, Minn.: Thomson/West, 2005. This au-thoritative guide explains the practice of law within the FDA.

Parrish, Richard. *Defining Drugs: How Government Became the Arbiter of Pharmaceutical Fact*. Somerset, N.J.: Transaction, 2003. Traces the development of drug regulation in the United States, explains the social construction of this system, and argues for a "therapeutic reformation."

Pisano, Douglas. *Essentials of Pharmacy Law*. Boca Raton, Fla.: CRC Press, 2003. A clear, user-friendly text that compiles and comments on selected federal laws and regulations pertaining to the general practice of pharmacy in the United States.

Young, James Harvey. *Pure Food: Securing the Federal Food and Drugs Act of 1906*. Princeton, N.J.: Princeton University Press, 1989. A historical study of how pure-food advocates, chemists, and politicians helped make the Pure Food and Drug Law into a reality.

FOOD BIOCHEMISTRY

BIOLOGY

ANATOMY OR SYSTEM AFFECTED: Cells, gastrointestinal system, pancreas, stomach

SPECIALTIES AND RELATED FIELDS: Biochemistry, cytology, gastroenterology, nutrition, pharmacology

DEFINITION: The breakdown of food by cells, a process in which nutrients are converted to energy and other components needed by the body.

KEY TERMS:

amino acids: the organic compounds that make up proteins; twenty are necessary for growth, nine of which must be obtained in the diet

Calorie: the basic unit of energy; the amount of heat needed to change the temperature of one liter of water from 14.5 degrees Celsius to 15.5 degrees Celsius

carbohydrates: a group of organic compounds that includes the sugars and the starches; one of three classes of nutrients and a basic source of energy

fats: a group of organic compounds, also called lipids, that store energy; one of three classes of nutrients

glycolysis: a metabolic pathway that converts the sugar glucose to pyruvate for energy without the use of oxygen

metabolism: the totality of a cell's biochemical processes; the process by which food molecules release their stored energy

minerals: inorganic compounds that are essential for human life; seventeen are required in the diet

proteins: organic compounds that are composed of amino acids and function as enzymes, speeding up metabolic reactions; one of three classes of nutrients

vitamins: organic compounds, essential for life but required in very minute quantities, that participate in biochemical reactions and help to release energy from the three classes of nutrients

STRUCTURE AND FUNCTIONS

Food biochemistry is concerned with the breakdown of food in the cell as a source of energy. Each cell is a factory that converts the nutrients of the food one eats to energy and other structural components of the body. The amount of energy that these nutrients supply is expressed in Calories (kilocalories). The number of Calories consumed will determine the energy balance of the individual and whether one loses or gains weight. The nutrients come in a variety of forms, but they can be divided into three major categories: carbohydrates, lipids (fats), and proteins. These nutrients are broken down by the cell metabolically to produce energy for cellular processes. Other components are used by the cell and the entire body for structure and transport. Each of these nutrients is essential to a well-balanced diet and good health. Two other components of a successful diet are vitamins and minerals.

Carbohydrates are molecules composed of carbon, hydrogen, and oxygen. They range from the simple sugars all the way to the complex carbohydrates. The simplest carbohydrates are the monosaccharides (one-sugar molecules), primarily glucose and fructose. The simple monosaccharides are usually joined to form disaccharides (two-sugar molecules), such as sucrose (glucose and fructose, or cane sugar), lactose (glucose and galactose, or milk sugar), and maltose (two glucoses, which is found in grains). The complex carbohydrates are the polysaccharides (multiple sugar molecules), which are composed of many monosaccharides, usually glucose. There are two main types: starch, which is found in plants such as potatoes, and glycogen, in which form humans store carbohydrate energy for the short term (up to twelve hours) in the liver.

The next major group of molecules is the lipids, which are made up of the solid fats and liquid oils. These molecules are primarily composed of carbon and hydrogen. They form three major groups: the triglycerides, phospholipids, and sterols. The triglycerides are composed of three fatty acids attached to a glycerol (a three-carbon molecule); this is the group that makes up the fats and oils. Fats, which are primarily of animal or-igin, are triglycerides that are solid at room temperature; such triglycerides are saturated, which means that there are no double bonds between their carbon molecules. Oils are liquid at room temperature, primarily of plant origin, and either monounsaturated or polyunsaturated (there are one or more double bonds between the carbon molecules in the chain). This group provides long-term energy in humans and is stored as adipose (fat) tissue. Each gram of fat stores approximately 9 Calories of energy per gram, which is about twice that of carbohydrates and proteins (4 Calories per gram). The adipose tissue also provides important insulation in maintaining body temperature. Phospholipids are similar to triglycerides in structure, but they have two fatty acids and a phosphate attached to the glycerol molecule. Phospholipids are the building blocks of the cell membranes that form the barrier between the inside and the outside of the cell. Sterols are considered lipids, but they have a completely different structure. This group includes cholesterol, vitamin D, estrogen, and testosterone. The sterols function in the structure of the cell membrane (as cholesterol does) or as hormones (as do testosterone and estrogen).

The last major group of molecules is that of the proteins, which are composed of carbon, hydrogen, oxygen, and nitrogen. Proteins are long chains of amino acids; each protein is composed of varying amounts of the twenty different amino acids. Proteins are used in the body as enzymes, substances that catalyze (generally, speed up) the biochemical reactions that take place in cells. They also function as transport molecules (such as hemoglobin, which transports oxygen) and provide structure (as does keratin, the protein in hair and nails). The human body can synthesize eleven of the twenty amino acids; the other nine are considered essential amino acids because they cannot be synthesized and are required in the diet.

Two other groups of essential compounds are necessary in the diet for the body's metabolism: vitamins and minerals. The vitamins are organic compounds (made up of carbon) that are required in only milligram or microgram quantities per day. The vitamins are classified into two groups: the water-soluble vitamins (the B vitamins and vitamin C) and the fat-soluble vitamins (vitamins A, D, E, and K). Vitamins are vital components of enzymes.

The minerals are inorganic nutrients that can be divided into two classes, depending on the amounts needed by the body. The major minerals are required in amounts greater than 100 milligrams per day; these minerals are calcium, phosphorus, magnesium, sodium, chloride, sulfur, and potassium. The trace elements, those needed in amounts of only a few milligrams per day, are iron, zinc, iodine, fluoride, copper, selenium, chromium, manganese, and molybdenum. Although they are required in small quantities, the minerals play an important role in the human body. Calcium is involved in bone and teeth formation and muscle contractions. Iron is found in hemoglobin and aids in the transportation of oxygen throughout the body. Potassium helps nerves send electrical impulses. Sodium and chloride maintain water balance in tissues and vascular fluid.

An adequate diet is one that supplies the body and cells with sources of energy and building blocks. The first priority of the diet is to supply the bulk nutrients—carbohydrates, fats, and proteins. An average young adult requires between 2,100 and 2,900 Calories per day, taking into account the amount of energy required for rest and work. Carbohydrates, fats, and proteins are taken in during a meal and digested—that is, broken into smaller components. Starch is broken down to glucose, and sucrose is broken down to fructose and glucose and absorbed by the bloodstream. Fats are broken down to triglycerides, and proteins are divided into their separate amino acids, to be absorbed by the bloodstream and transported throughout the body. Each cell then takes up essential nutrients for energy and to use as building parts of the cell.

Once the nutrients enter the cell, they are broken down into energy through a series of metabolic reactions. The first step in the metabolic process is called glycolysis. Glucose is broken down through a series of reactions to produce adenosine triphosphate (ATP), a molecule used to fuel other biochemical pathways in the cell. Glycolysis gives off a small amount of energy and does not require oxygen. This process can provide the energy for a short sprint; lactic acid buildup in the muscles will lead to fatigue, however, if there is insufficient oxygen.

Long-term energy requires oxygen. Aerobic respiration can metabolize not only the sugars produced by glycolysis but triglycerides and amino acids as well. The molecules enter what is called the Krebs cycle, an aerobic pathway that provides eighteen times more energy than glycolysis. The waste products of this pathway are carbon dioxide and water, which are exhaled.

DISORDERS AND DISEASES

Diet plays a major role in the metabolism of the cells. One major problem in diet is the overconsumption of

Calories, which can lead to weight gain and eventual obesity. Obesity is defined as being 20 percent over one's ideal weight for one's body size. A number of problems are associated with obesity, such as high blood pressure, high levels of cholesterol, increased risk of cancer, heart disease, and early death.

At the other end of the scale is malnutrition. Carbohydrates are the preferred energy source in the form of either blood glucose or glycogen, which is found in the liver and muscles. This source gives a person approximately four to twelve hours of energy. Long-term storage of energy occurs as fat, which constitutes anywhere from 15 percent to 25 percent of body composition. During times of starvation, when the carbohydrate reserve is almost zero, fat will be mobilized for energy. Fat will also be used to make glucose for the blood because the brain requires glucose as its energy source. In extreme starvation, the body will begin to degrade the protein in muscles down to its constituent amino acids in order to produce energy.

Malnutrition can also occur if essential vitamins and minerals are excluded from the diet. Vitamin deficiencies affect the metabolism of the cell since these compounds are often required to aid the enzymes in producing energy. A number of medical problems are associated with vitamin deficiencies. A deficiency in thiamine will result in the metabolic disorder called beriberi. A loss of the thiamine found in wheat and rice can occur in the refinement process, making it more difficult to obtain enough of this vitamin from the diet. Alcoholics have an increased thiamine requirement, to help in the metabolism of alcohol, and usually have a low level of food consumption; thus, they are at risk for developing beriberi. Lack of vitamin A results in night blindness, and lack of vitamin D results in rickets, in which the bones are weakened as a result of poor calcium uptake.

One interesting feature about diet and the metabolic pathways concerns how different molecules are treated. Some people mistakenly believe that it is better to eat fruit sugar than other sugars. Fruit sugar, the simple sugar fructose, is chemically related to glucose. Because glucose and fructose are converted to each other during glycolysis, it does not matter which sugar is eaten. Far more important to proper nutrition is what accompanies the sugar. Table sugar provides only calories, while a piece of fruit contains both fruit sugar and vitamins, minerals, and fiber for a more complete diet.

Many errors in metabolism occur because genes do

not carry the proper information. The result may be an enzyme that, although critical to a biochemical pathway, does not function properly or is missing altogether. One disorder of carbohydrate metabolism is called galactosemia. Mother's milk contains lactose, which is normally broken down into galactose and glucose. With galactosemia, the cells take in the galactose but are unable to convert it to glucose because of the lack of an enzyme. Thus, galactose levels build up in the blood, liver, and other organs, impairing their function. This condition can lead to death in an infant, but the effects of galactosemia are usually detected and the diet modified by use of a milk substitute.

Amino acid metabolism can also be defective, leading to the accumulation of toxic by-products. One of the best-known examples involves the amino acid phenylalanine. About one in ten thousand infants is born with a defective pathway, a disorder called phenylketonuria (PKU). If PKU is not discovered in time, by-products can accumulate, causing poor brain development and severe mental retardation. PKU must be diagnosed early in life, and a special, controlled diet must be given to the infant. Because phenylalanine is an essential amino acid, limited amounts are included in the diet for proper growth, but large amounts need to be excluded. The artificial sweetener aspartame (NutraSweet) poses a problem for those with PKU. Aspartame is composed of two amino acids, phenylalanine and aspartic acid. When aspartame is broken down during digestion, phenylalanine enters the bloodstream. Individuals with PKU should not ingest aspartame; there is a warning to that effect on products containing this chemical.

Other errors of metabolism are noted later in life. One example is lactose intolerance, in which lactose is cleaved by the enzyme lactase into glucose and galactose. The enzyme lactase, found in the digestive tract, is very active in suckling infants, but only Northern Europeans and members of some African tribes retain lactase activity into adulthood. Other groups, such as Asian, Arab, Jewish, Indian, and Mediterranean peoples, show little lactase activity as adults. These people cannot digest the lactose in milk products, which then cannot be absorbed in the intestinal tract. A buildup of lactose can lead to diarrhea and colic. Usually in those parts of the world milk is not used by adults as food. In the United States, one can purchase milk that contains lactose which has been partially broken down into galactose and glucose. One can also purchase the lactase enzyme itself and add it to milk.

Another error of metabolism results in diabetes mellitus, which means "excessive excretion of sweet urine." A telltale sign of this condition is sugar, specifically glucose, in the urine. In normal people, blood glucose levels remain relatively stable. After a meal, when the blood glucose levels rise, the pancreas starts to secrete the hormone insulin. Insulin causes the cells to take in the extra blood glucose and convert it to glycogen or fat, thus storing the extra energy. In diabetics, there is little or no insulin production or release, or the target cells may have faulty receptors. As a result, the blood glucose level remains high. The excess glucose is then excreted in the urine, leading to the symptom of excess thirst. The body is forced to rely much more heavily on fats as an energy source, leading to high levels of circulating fats and cholesterol in the blood. These substances can be deposited in the blood vessels, causing high blood pressure and heart disease. Excess fats, in levels that exceed the body's ability to metabolize and burn them, may produce acetone, which gives the breath of diabetics a sweet odor. A buildup of acetone can lead to ketoacidosis, a pathologic condition in which the blood pH drops from 7.4 to 6.8. Complications arising from diabetes also include blindness, kidney disease, and nerve damage. Furthermore, resulting peripheral vascular disease, in which the body's extremities do not get enough blood, leads to tissue death and gangrene.

PERSPECTIVE AND PROSPECTS

The study of food biochemistry has evolved over the years from a strictly biochemical approach to one in which diet and nutrition play a major role. An understanding of diet and nutrition required vital information about the metabolic processes occurring in the cell, supplied by the field of biochemistry.

This information started to become available in 1898 when Eduard Buchner discovered that the fermentation of glucose to alcohol and carbon dioxide could occur in a cell-free extract. The early 1900's led to the complete discovery of the glycolytic pathway and the enzymes that were involved in the process. In the 1930's, other pathways of metabolism were elucidated.

In conjunction with Buchner's discovery, British physician Archibald Garrod in 1909 hypothesized that genes control a person's appearance through enzymes that catalyze certain metabolic processes in the cell. Garrod thought that some inherited diseases resulted from a patient's inability to make a particular enzyme, and he called them "inborn errors of metabolism." One example he gave was a condition called alkaptonuria, in which the urine turns black upon exposure to the air.

Some of the earliest nutritional studies date back to the time of Aristotle, who knew that raw liver contained an ingredient that could cure night blindness. Christiaan Eijkman studied beriberi in the Dutch East Indies and traced the problem to diet. Sir Frederick Hopkins was an English biochemist who conducted pioneering work on vitamins and the essentiality of amino acids in the early 1900's. Hopkins realized that the type of protein is important in the diet as well as the quantity. Hopkins hypothesized that some trace substance in addition to proteins, fats, and carbohydrates may be required in the diet for growth; this substance was later identified as the vitamin. Hopkins was the first biochemist to explore diet and metabolic function.

Working with this broad base, scientists have made tremendous advances in the study of diet and nutrition based on the biochemistry of the cell. In 1943, the first recommended daily (or dietary) allowances (RDAs) were published. They provide standards for diet and good nutrition and are revised every five years as new information becomes available. The RDAs suggest the amounts of protein, fats, carbohydrates, vitamins, and minerals required for adequate nutrient uptake. The major uses of the RDAs are for schools and other institutions in planning menus, obtaining food supplies, and preparing food labels.

Since the 1970's, research has consistently associated nutritional factors with six of the ten leading causes of death in the United States: high blood pressure, heart disease, cancer, cardiovascular disease, chronic liver disease, and non-insulin-dependent diabetes mellitus. This research has led to improvements in the American diet.

—Lonnie J. Guralnick, Ph.D.

See also Antioxidants; Appetite loss; Caffeine; Cholesterol; Cytology; Diabetes mellitus; Digestion; Enzymes; Fatty acid oxidation disorders; Glycogen storage diseases; Glycolysis; Lactose intolerance; Malnutrition; Metabolism; Nutrition; Phenylketonuria (PKU); Phytochemicals; Supplements; Vitamins and minerals.

FOR FURTHER INFORMATION:

Bonci, Leslie. *American Dietetic Association Guide to Better Digestion*. New York: Wiley, 2003. A user-friendly guide to help analyze one's eating habits, map out a dietary plan to manage and reduce the uncomfortable symptoms of digestive disorders, and find practical recommendations for implementing lifestyle changes.

Campbell, Neil A., et al. *Biology: Concepts and Connections*. 5th ed. San Francisco: Pearson/Benjamin Cummings, 2006. An introductory college textbook geared for the biology major but easily understood by the high school student. One chapter covers the process of digestion and nutritional requirements. References at the end of the chapter are provided for further reading. Contains useful tables and diagrams.

Clark, Nancy. *Nancy Clark's Sports Nutrition Guidebook*. 3d ed. Champaign, Ill.: Human Kinetics, 2003. An easy-to-read book that covers the subject of nutrition for the sports-minded reader. Dispels a number of nutritional myths. Explores many applications of food biochemistry, and offers recipes and references in the appendix.

Duyff, Roberta Larson. *American Dietetic Association Complete Food and Nutrition Guide*. 3d ed. Hoboken, N.J.: John Wiley & Sons, 2006. Experts from the American Dietetic Association detail advances in nutrition research and provide authoritative answers to questions regarding food and nutrition.

Margen, Sheldon. *Wellness Foods A to Z: An Indispensable Guide for Health-Conscious Food Lovers*. New York: Rebus, 2002. In encyclopedic format, offers a nutritional and market profile of the health benefits of myriad foods; a guide to food groups, vitamins and minerals, and herbs and spices; how to read food labels; and a cooking glossary.

Nasset, Edmund S. *Nutrition Handbook*. 3d ed. New York: Harper & Row, 1982. A small, easy-to-read book that describes the three classes of nutrients. Covers digestion and absorption, and discusses how the body utilizes nutrients and vitamins. A valuable glossary is provided at the end of the book.

Nelson, David L., and Michael M. Cox. *Lehninger Principles of Biochemistry*. 4th ed. New York: W. H. Freeman, 2005. A well-written elementary biochemistry college textbook. Easy to read even for the beginner who has little understanding of biochemistry.

Nieman, David C., Diane E. Butterworth, and Catherine N. Nieman. *Nutrition*. Rev. ed. Dubuque, Iowa: Wm. C. Brown, 1992. A good textbook that links food biochemistry to health and nutrition. Covers the basics on carbohydrates, lipids, and proteins. Easy to read. Tables and diagrams are included.

FOOD POISONING

DISEASE/DISORDER

ANATOMY OR SYSTEM AFFECTED: Gastrointestinal system, intestines, stomach

SPECIALTIES AND RELATED FIELDS: Environmental health, epidemiology, gastroenterology, public health, toxicology

DEFINITION: Food-borne illness caused by bacteria, viruses, or parasites consumed in food and resulting in acute gastrointestinal disturbance that may include diarrhea, nausea, vomiting, and abdominal discomfort.

KEY TERMS:

contamination: infection of a food item by a pathogen

food-borne infection: disease caused by eating foods contaminated by infectious microorganisms, with onset occurring within twenty-four hours (for example, salmonellosis)

food-borne intoxication: disease caused by eating foods containing microorganisms that produce toxins, with onset occurring within six hours (for example, botulism)

microorganism: an organism which is too small to be seen with the naked eye

parasite: an organism which lives on another organism (the host) and causes harm to the host while it benefits

pathogen: a disease-causing organism

thermal death point: the lowest temperature that can destroy a food-borne organism

CAUSES AND SYMPTOMS

Often a person feeling the symptoms of nausea, vomiting, diarrhea, and abdominal discomfort assumes that he or she has contracted influenza. The presence of a true influenza virus, however, is uncommon. More likely, these symptoms are caused by eating food that contains undesirable bacteria, viruses, or parasites. This is called food-borne illness, or food poisoning. Most food-borne pathogens are colorless, odorless, and tasteless. Fortunately, there are recommendations based on scientific principles to help prevent food-borne illness.

Food poisoning is a worldwide problem. In developing countries, diarrhea is a factor in child malnutrition and is estimated to cause 3.5 million deaths per year. Despite advances in modern technology, food-borne illness is a major problem in developed countries as well. In the United States, an estimated 24 million cases of food-borne diarrheal disease occur each year, which

means that about one of ten people experience a food-associated illness in a given year.

Certain foods, particularly foods with a high protein and moisture content, provide an ideal environment for the multiplication of pathogens. The foods with high risk in the United States are raw shellfish (especially mollusks), underdone poultry, raw eggs, rare meats, raw milk, and cooked food that another person handled before it was packaged and chilled. In addition to those foods listed, some developing countries could add raw vegetables, raw fruits that cannot be peeled, foods from sidewalk vendors, and tap water or water from unknown sources. Most of the documented cases of food-borne illness are caused by only a few bacteria, viruses, and parasites.

Bacteria known as *Salmonella* are ingested by humans in contaminated foods such as beef, poultry, and eggs; they may also be transmitted by kitchen utensils and the hands of people who have handled infected food or utensils. Once the bacteria are inside the body, the incubation time is from eight to twenty-four hours. Since the bacteria multiply inside the body and attack the gastrointestinal tract, this disease is known as a true food infection. The main symptoms are diarrhea, abdominal cramps, and vomiting. The bacteria are killed by cooking foods to the well-done stage.

The major food-borne intoxication in the United States is caused by eating food contaminated with the toxin of *Staphylococcus* bacteria. Because the toxin or poison has already been produced in the food item that is ingested, the onset of symptoms is usually very rapid (between one-half hour and six hours). Improperly stored or cooked foods (particularly meats, tuna, and potato salad) are the main carriers of these bacteria. Since this toxin cannot be killed by reheating the food items to a high temperature, it is important that foods are properly stored.

Botulism is a rare food poisoning caused by the toxin of *Clostridium botulinum*. It is anaerobic, meaning that it multiplies in environments without oxygen, and is mainly found in improperly home-canned food items. Originally one of the sources of the disease was from eating sausages (the Latin word for which is *botulus*)—hence, the name "botulism." A very small amount of toxin, the size of a grain of salt, could kill hundreds of people within an hour. Danger signs include double vision and difficulty swallowing and breathing.

Though everyone is at risk for food-borne illness, certain groups of people develop more severe symptoms and are at a greater risk for serious illness and death. Higher-risk groups include pregnant women, very young children, the elderly, and immunocompromised individuals, such as patients with acquired immunodeficiency syndrome (AIDS) and cancer.

Bacteria known as *Listeria* were first documented in 1981 as being transmitted by food. Most people are at low risk of becoming ill after ingesting these bacteria; however, pregnant women are at high risk. *Listeria* infection is rare in the United States, but it does cause serious illness. It is associated with consumption of raw (unpasteurized) milk, nonreheated hot dogs, undercooked chicken, various soft cheeses (Mexican style, feta, Brie, Camembert, and blue-veined cheese), and food purchased from delicatessen counters. *Listeria* cause a short-term illness in pregnant women; however, this bacteria can cause stillbirths and spontaneous abortions. A parasite called *Toxoplasma gondii* is also of particular risk for pregnant women. For this reason, raw or very rare meat should not be eaten. (In addition, since cats may shed these parasites in their feces, it is recommended that pregnant women avoid cleaning cat litter boxes.)

As the protective antibodies from the mother are lost, infants become more susceptible to food poisoning. Botulism generally occurs by ingesting the toxin or poison; however, in infant botulism it is the spores that germinate and produce the toxin within the intestinal tract of the infant. Since honey and corn syrup have been found to contain spores, it is recommended that they not be fed to infants under one year of age, especially those under six months.

Determining whether a disease is caused by a food-borne organism is highly skilled work. The Centers for Disease Control and Prevention (CDC) in Atlanta, Georgia, investigate diseases and their causes. It has been estimated that the true incidence of food-borne illness in the United States is ten to one hundred times greater than that reported to the CDC. The CDC report some of the more interesting cases and outbreaks in narrative form in the *Morbidity and Mortality Weekly Report*.

TREATMENT AND THERAPY

In cases of severe food poisoning marked by vomiting, diarrhea, or collapse—especially in cases of botulism and ingestion of poisonous plant material such as suspicious mushrooms—emergency medical attention should be sought immediately, and, if possible, specimens of the suspected food should be submitted for analysis. Identifying the source of the food is especially important if that source is a public venue such as a restaurant, because stemming a widespread outbreak of food poisoning may thereby be possible. In less severe cases of food poisoning, the victim should rest, eat nothing, but drink fluids that contain some salt and sugar; the person should begin to recover after several hours or one or two days and should see a doctor if not well after two or three days.

The best "treatment" for food poisoning is prevention. While there is ample information regarding the prevention of food poisoning, many outbreaks still occur as a result of carelessness in the kitchen. Good food safety is basically good common sense, yet it can make sense only when one has acquired some knowledge of how food-borne pathogens spread and how to apply food safety steps to prevent food-borne illness. Based on the research literature, as well as on the suggestions made by the World Health Organization (WHO) and other groups, the recommendations are to cook foods well, to prevent cross-contamination, and to keep hot foods hot and cold foods cold.

Cooking foods well means cooking them to a high enough temperature in the slowest-to-heat part and for a long enough time to destroy pathogens that have already gained access to foods. Cooking foods well is only a concern when they have become previously contaminated from other sources or are naturally contaminated. There are a number of possible sources of contamination of food products.

Coastal water may contaminate seafood. Filter-feeding marine animals (such as clams, scallops, oysters, cockles, and mussels) and some fish (such as anchovies, sardines, and herring) live by pumping in seawater and sifting out organisms that they need for food. Therefore, they have the ability to concentrate suspended material by many orders of magnitude. Shellfish grown in contaminated coastal waters are the most frequent carriers of a virus called hepatitis A.

INFORMATION ON FOOD POISONING

CAUSES: Bacteria, viruses, or parasites consumed in food
SYMPTOMS: Diarrhea, nausea, vomiting, fever, abdominal discomfort
DURATION: One to three days
TREATMENTS: Rest, avoidance of food, extra fluid intake

Contaminated eggs can be another vehicle of food-borne illness. Contamination of eggs can occur from external as well as internal sources. If moist conditions are present and there is a crack in the shell, the fecal material of hens carrying the microorganism can penetrate the shell and membrane of the egg and can multiply. In the early 1990's, *Salmonella enteritidis* began to appear in the intact egg, particularly in the northeastern part of the United States. It is hypothesized that contamination occurs in the oviduct of the hen before the egg is laid. Food vehicles in which *Salmonella enteritidis* has been reported include sandwiches dipped in eggs and cooked, hollandaise sauce, eggs Benedict, commercial frozen pasta with raw egg and cheese stuffing, Caesar salad dressing, and blended food in which cross-contamination had occurred. Foods such as cookie or cake dough or homemade ice cream made with raw eggs are other possible vehicles of food-borne illness.

Milk, especially raw milk, can be contaminated. Sources of milk contaminants could be an unhealthy cow (such as from mastitis, a major infection of the mammary gland of the dairy cow) or unclean methods of milking, such as not cleaning the teats well before attaching them to the milker or unclean utensils (milking tanks). If milk is not cooled fast enough, contaminants can multiply.

Modern mechanized milking procedures have reduced but not eliminated food-borne pathogens. Postpasteurization contamination may occur, especially if bulk tanks or equipment have not been properly cleaned and sanitized. In 1985 in Chicago, one of the largest salmonellosis outbreaks occurred, with the causal food being pasteurized milk. More than sixteen thousand people were infected, and ten died. A small connecting piece in the milk tank which allowed milk and microorganisms to collect was determined to be the source of the contamination. Bulk tanks should be properly maintained and piping should be inspected regularly for opportunities for raw milk to contaminate the pasteurized product.

Recommendations for cooking temperatures are based not only on the temperature required to kill food-borne pathogens but also on aesthetics and palatability. Generally, a margin of safety is built into the cooking temperature because of the possibility of nonuniform heating. Based on generally accepted temperature requirements, cooking red meat until 71 degrees Celsius (160 degrees Fahrenheit) will reach the thermal death point. Hamburger should be well cooked so that it is medium-brown inside. If pressed, it should feel firm and the juices that run out should be clear. Cooking poultry to the well-done stage is done for palatability. Tenderness is indicated when there is a flexible hip joint, and juices should run clear and not pink when the meat is pierced with a fork. Fish should be cooked until it loses its translucent appearance and flakes when pierced with a fork. Eggs should be thoroughly cooked until the yolk is thickened and the white is firm, not runny. Cooked or chilled foods that are served hot (that is, leftovers) should be reheated so that they come to a rolling boil.

Cross-contamination occurs when microorganisms are transmitted from humans, cutting boards, and utensils to food. Contamination between foods, especially from raw meat and poultry to fresh vegetables or other ready-to-eat foods, is a major problem.

One of the best ways to prevent cross-contamination is simply washing one's hands with soap and water. Twenty seconds is the minimum time span that should be spent washing one's hands. In order to prevent the spread of disease, it is also recommended that the hands be dried with a paper towel, which is then thrown away. Thoroughly washed hands can still be a source of bacteria, however, so one should use tongs and spoons when cooking to prevent contamination.

It is especially important to wash one's hands after certain activities, such as blowing the nose or sneezing, using the lavatory, diapering a baby, smoking, petting animals or pets, and before cooking or handling food.

Other sources of cross-contamination include utensils and cutting surfaces. If people use the same knife and cutting board to cut up raw chicken for a stir-fry and peaches for a fruit salad, they are putting themselves at great risk for food-borne illness. The bacteria on the cutting board and the knife could cross-contaminate the peaches. While the chicken will be cooked until it is well done, the peaches in the salad will not be. In this situation, one could cut the fruit first and then the chicken, and then wash and sanitize the knife and cutting board.

Cleaning and sanitizing is actually a two-step process. Cleaning involves using soap and water and a scrubber or dishcloth to remove the major debris from the surface. The second step, sanitizing, involves using a diluted chloride solution to kill bacteria and viruses.

Wooden cutting boards are the worst offenders in terms of causing cross-contamination. Since bacteria and viruses are small, they can adhere to and grow in the grooves of a wooden cutting board and spread to other foods when the cutting board is used again. Use of a plastic or acrylic cutting board prevents this problem.

The danger zone in which bacteria can multiply is a range of 4.4 degrees Celsius (40 degrees Fahrenheit) to 60 degrees Celsius (140 degrees Fahrenheit). Room temperature is generally right in the middle of this danger zone. The danger zone is critical because, even though they cannot be seen, bacteria are increasing in number. They can double and even quadruple in fifteen to thirty minutes. Consequently, perishable foods such as meats, poultry, fish, milk, cooked rice, leftover pizza, hard-cooked eggs, leftover refried beans, and potato salad should not be left in the danger zone for more than two hours. Keeping hot foods hot means keeping them at a temperature higher than 60 degrees Celsius. Keeping cold foods cold means keeping them at a temperature lower than 4.4 degrees Celsius.

Other rules are helpful for preventing contamination. When shopping, the grocery store should be the last stop so that foods are not stored in a hot car. When meal time is over, leftovers should be placed in the refrigerator or freezer as soon as possible. When packing for a picnic, food items should be kept in an ice chest to keep them cold or brought slightly frozen. Much serious illness and death could be prevented if such food safety rules were followed.

PERSPECTIVE AND PROSPECTS

When the lifestyle of people changed from a hunting-and-gathering society to a more agrarian one, the need to preserve food from spoilage was necessary for survival. As early as 3000 B.C.E., salt was used as a meat preservative and the production of cheese had begun in the Near East. The production of wine and the preservation of fish by smoking also were introduced at that time. Even though throughout history people had tried many methods to preserve foods and keep them from spoiling, the relationship between illness and pathogens or toxins in food was not recognized and documented until 1857. It was then that the French chemist Louis Pasteur demonstrated that the microorganisms in raw milk caused spoilage.

Stories from the American Civil War (1860-1865) demonstrate the problems of institutional feeding of many people for long periods of time. Gastrointestinal diseases were rampant during that time period. During the first year of the war, of the people who had diarrhea and dysentery, the morbidity rate was 640 per 1,000 and increased to 995 per 1,000 in 1862. More men died of disease and illness than were killed in battle.

Food can be contaminated by disease-causing organisms at any step of the food-handling chain, from the farm to the table. An important role of government and industry is to ensure a safe food supply. In the United States, setting and monitoring of food safety standards are the responsibility of the Food and Drug Administration (FDA) under the auspices of the U.S. Department of Health and Human Services and the Food Safety and Inspection Service (FSIS) under the auspices of the U.S. Department of Agriculture (USDA). The FDA is responsible for the wholesomeness of all food sold in interstate commerce, except meat and poultry, while the USDA is responsible for the inspection of meat and poultry sold in interstate commerce and internationally. Some major food safety laws and policies that have guided the provision of safe food are the Federal Food and Drugs Act in 1906; the Federal Meat Inspection Act in 1906-1907; the Food, Drug, and Cosmetic Act in 1938; and the Poultry Products Inspection Act in 1957. The food supply in the United States has been credited as being among the safest in the world.

Historically, the diseases of tuberculosis, scarlet fever, strep throat, typhoid fever, and diphtheria have been associated with raw or unpasteurized milk. The reporting of food-borne illness was initiated in the 1920's by the U.S. Public Health Service (USPHS) when annual summaries of outbreaks of milk-borne disease were recorded and reported. Later, reports of waterborne and food-borne diseases were added.

The public attitude about what is hazardous in the food supply and that of the FDA have often differed. The public generally believes that the safety of additives and chemical contaminants in food is of a higher priority than that of the microbiological and nutritional hazards—the exact opposite of the FDA's priorities. (For example, in the mid-1980's, the story about Alar, a chemical used to slow the ripening of apples, represented a very emotional topic. There was particular concern about the risks that this chemical might pose to children who ate large amounts of apple products.) As more reliable information is available about both areas of concern, the situation regarding priorities is likely to change.

—Martha M. Henze, M.S., R.D.;
updated by Maria Pacheco, Ph.D.

See also Bacterial infections; Biological and chemical weapons; Botulism; Diarrhea and dysentery; *E. coli* infection; Enterocolitis; Gangrene; Gastroenterology; Gastroenterology, pediatric; Gastrointestinal disorders; Gastrointestinal system; Indigestion; Intestinal disorders; Intestines; Lead poisoning; Mercury poisoning; Nausea and vomiting; Noroviruses; Parasitic diseases; Poisoning; Rotavirus; Salmonella infection; Shigellosis; Trichinosis; Tularemia; Ulcers; Viral infections.

FOR FURTHER INFORMATION:

Cliver, Dean O., and Hans P. Riemann, eds. *Foodborne Diseases.* 2d ed. San Diego, Calif.: Academic Press, 2002. An exceptional college textbook providing chapters written by experts in the field. This important work provides not only background information but also in-depth reference information on the most common food-borne pathogens.

Food and Drug Administration Center for Food Safety and Applied Nutrition. http://vm.cfsan.fda.gov/list.html. Site provides information on food safety, nutrition, and wholesomeness, as well as the regulation of cosmetics safety.

Gaman, P. M., and K. B. Sherrington. *The Science of Food: An Introduction to Food Science, Nutrition, and Microbiology.* 4th ed. Boston: Butterworth-Heinemann, An easy-to-read book dealing with food composition and microbiology. Includes good bibliographical references and an index.

Hobbs, Betty C., and Diane Roberts. *Food Poisoning and Food Hygiene.* 6th ed. San Diego, Calif.: Singular, 1993. A nontechnical handbook of the causes of food poisoning and other food-borne diseases for those in the fields of food microbiology and food hygiene. Emphasis is given to the main aspects of hygiene necessary for the production, preparation, sale, and service of safe and palatable food.

Jay, James M., Martin J. Loessner, and David A. Golden. *Modern Food Microbiology.* 7th ed. New York: Springer, 2005. This excellent textbook summarizes the current state of knowledge of the biology and epidemiology of the microorganisms that cause food-borne illness.

Leon, Warren, and Caroline Smith DeWaal. *Is Our Food Safe? A Consumer's Guide to Protecting Your Health and the Environment.* New York: Crown, 2002. Focuses on three themes—food safety and food-borne illnesses, environmental aspects of food choices, and sound diet and nutrition—and answers common questions about the safety of meat, dairy products, fish, fruits, and other foods that make up American diets.

Longrée, Karla, and Gertrude Armbruster. *Quantity Food Sanitation.* 5th ed. New York: John Wiley & Sons, 1996. An excellent reference guide on food safety for quantity cooking in institutions such as hospitals and restaurants.

Marriot, Norman G., and Robert B. Gravani. *Principles of Food Sanitation.* 5th ed. New York: Springer, 2006. A reference work that provides students and food industry personnel with the information necessary to ensure hygienic practices in food production and specific directions for applying these fundamentals to attain hygienic conditions in various food processing and food preparation facilities.

Nestle, Marion. *Safe Food: Bacteria, Biotechnology, and Bioterrorism.* Berkeley: University of California Press, 2003. Argues that ensuring safe food involves politics, its connections with industry, government, and consumers, and issues of values, economics, and political power.

Ray, Bibek. *Fundamental Food Microbiology.* 3d ed. Boca Raton, Fla.: CRC Press, 2004. A comprehensive text on the basic principles of food microbiology. Includes bibliographical references and an index.

U.S. Department of Agriculture/Food and Drug Administration Foodborne Illness Education Information Center. http://www.nal.usda.gov/foodborne/index.html. Site provides information on foodborne illnesses.

Wilson, Michael, Brian Henderson, and Rod McNab. *Bacterial Virulence Mechanisms.* New York: Cambridge University Press, 2002. Basing their discussion on research advances in microbiology, molecular biology, and cell biology, the authors describe the interactions that exist between bacteria and human cells both in health and during infection.

FOOT DISORDERS

DISEASE/DISORDER

ANATOMY OR SYSTEM AFFECTED: Bones, feet, muscles, musculoskeletal system

SPECIALTIES AND RELATED FIELDS: Orthopedics, podiatry

DEFINITION: Disorders involving the muscles, bones, nerves, or skin of the feet.

Because of the constant and heavy use of feet by humans as bipeds, they are prone to many problems. In spite of what is commonly believed, most cases of foot bone and joint abnormalities are developmental in origin instead of being caused by poorly fitting footwear.

INFORMATION ON FOOT DISORDERS

CAUSES: Congenital and developmental factors, improper footwear, muscle weakness, incorrect weight-bearing, short Achilles tendon, nerve disorders, dermatologic disorders
SYMPTOMS: Pain, swelling, limping, numbness, tingling
DURATION: Short-term or chronic
TREATMENTS: Medication, ointments, surgery, orthopedic footwear

Developmental, muscle, and bone disorders of the feet. Clubfoot, also called talipes, is one of the developmental, or congenital, disorders affecting the feet. It occurs in approximately 1 of every 1,000 live human births and is characterized by deformities such as the foot turning down and under, such that a child will walk on the top of his or her foot. Over time, tendon and ligament contraction reinforces the deformity; thus, either casting or surgery is needed for realignment.

Flat foot, or pes planus, is an abnormally flat arch in the foot, accompanied by a characteristic gait, both of which can occur in varying degrees. Muscle weakness, incorrect weight-bearing, a short Achilles tendon, and developmental defects may all contribute to this deformity. Flat foot may or may not produce a pathologic condition such as arthritis.

A bunion is the relocation of bone from the first metatarsal to the inner portion of the joint connecting it to the big toe. This prominence at the base of the big toe makes the soft tissue in the area subject to pressure from shoes, causing swelling and pain in the protective sac above the metatarsophalangeal joint in a condition called bursitis. Cortisone injections may relieve symptoms, but surgery is required in extreme cases to realign the first metatarsal. Flat foot usually accompanies bunions and is a factor in their development.

Muscular imbalances inherent in the foot are the reason for the curvature of the individual bones of the toes. Abnormally curved bones produce hammertoe, or claw toe, which usually requires little treatment other than a padding of the shoes to avoid corn or callus development. Excessive muscle tension at the heel can produce bony growths called heel spurs or calcaneal exostoses. Inflammation may develop in a neighboring joint's bursa, causing a throbbing pain.

Apophysitis of the calcaneus or heel bone can occur in childhood while the heel is still in the process of fusing from two bones. Injury can result because the connecting, softer cartilage between the two bones has not yet been replaced with bone. This affliction usually disappears as a child grows.

Nerve and skin disorders of the feet. Factors including footwear, the structures of the foot itself, and harmful external forces acting on the foot may all contribute to the irritation and/or damage to the nerves of the foot. Morton's neuroma is the thickening of the nerve located between the metatarsals of the third and fourth toes, followed by the formation of a small benign tumor. Painful burning, numbness, or tingling sensations may be alleviated by wearing more comfortable footwear or by the surgical removal of the tumor. Tarsal tunnel syndrome occurs when a nerve traveling along the bottom of the foot through a channel called the tar-

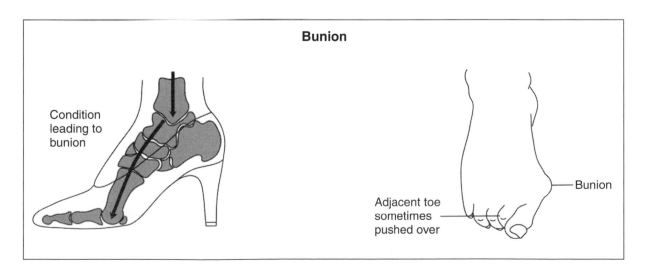

Bunion

Condition leading to bunion

Adjacent toe sometimes pushed over

Bunion

sal canal becomes compressed and damaged. Cortisone injections into this canal can relieve pressure on the nerve, and surgery can be used to treat severe cases.

The skin of the foot is subject to much pressure and rubbing; thus, it responds by producing changes, termed dermatologic disorders, which themselves cause pain. A corn, or heloma, is a small, sharply defined, raised area of thickened skin containing much of the fibrous protein called keratin. Calluses are also composed of keratin but are flatter and do not possess the defined borders of corns. Both types of thickened keratinized skin are usually attributed to incorrect positioning of the underlying bone.

Warts, or verrucae, are actually skin tumors caused by the human papillomavirus. They occur most commonly on the sole of the foot, where they are named plantar warts. Warts can be transmitted from person to person, and the lymphatic communication between warts within an individual explains their ability to spread. Warts on the foot are invariably benign, however, and should not be treated with X-ray or radium therapy lest the surrounding areas undergo change themselves and eventually produce tumors.

Dermatitis venenata is often caused by chemicals used in the binding or dyeing of shoes. Angiokeratoma is a lesion on the bottom of the foot commonly mistaken for a wart. Fibroma is the name of the benign growth that may spread under the toenails as a result of insect bites in the vicinity or manifestations of other skin diseases.

Ingrown toenails, or onychocryptoses, occur when the free end of the toenail penetrates the surrounding soft tissue. Reasons for this painful disorder are commonly badly fitted footwear, nail disease, and foot or nail structural abnormalities.

Systemic diseases affecting the feet. Rheumatoid arthritis is a condition involving connective tissue, unknown in origin, in which the synovial membrane of joints proliferates while invading and even destroying cartilage and bone. Women acquire this disease three times more often than do men. Steroid hormones are sometimes applied to aid in the treatment of rheumatoid arthritis, but gold salt injection is the only therapy resulting in a permanent cure. The chances of a cure are greater when this disease occurs in children. The condition is then known as juvenile rheumatoid arthritis, or Still's disease.

Several normally fatal diseases may accompany rheumatoid arthritis. Systemic lupus erythematosus can be masked by the arthritic condition until inflam-

mation spreads to small arteries of the body's organs. Polyarteritis nodosa also involves arteries throughout the body, and its true diagnosis may be prevented by the misleading arthritic condition. Scleroderma involves the thickening of the skin on the face, hands, and feet; depigmentation; loss of hair; and lesions. Sarcoidosis manifests itself in the hands and feet and causes microscopic lesions in the bone that eventually become visible by X-ray examination. Schönlein-Henoch syndrome is an allergic reaction that can resemble the synovitis of rheumatic fever.

Rheumatic fever affects fibrous tissues in a widespread fashion involving the joints and later the heart. It is related to streptococcal infections and occurs as a migrating arthritis producing no lasting joint damage in the feet, but it can cause permanent damage to the cardiac valve. Osteoarthritis causes the degeneration of cartilage and the overgrowth of bone surfaces. The effects of this condition are limited to the joints, unlike rheumatoid arthritis, which can spread to nearby cartilage and bone. Staphylococci, streptococci, and coliform bacteria are the infective agents involved in pyogenic arthritis. In this condition, the organism is carried by the blood to the joint interior. Ulcers of the feet may be caused by a variety of conditions, including diabetes mellitus, syphilis, anemia, and leprosy.

If there is sustained pain in the foot or ankle with no known cause such as injury, a continuously low leukocyte count, and negative laboratory tests for the presence of bacteria, then a viral infection is likely present. An elevated leukocyte count is often indicative of a bacterial infection.

—*Ryan C. Horst and Roman J. Miller, Ph.D.*

See also Athlete's foot; Birth defects; Bones and the skeleton; Bunions; Feet; Flat feet; Fracture and dislocation; Frostbite; Fungal infections; Ganglion removal; Gout; Hammertoe correction; Hammertoes; Heel spur removal; Lower extremities; Nail removal; Nails; Orthopedic surgery; Orthopedics; Orthopedics, pediatric; Osteonecrosis; Podiatry; Tendon repair; Warts.

For Further Information:

American Podiatric Medical Association. http://www .apma.org/.

Copeland, D. P. M. Glenn, and Stan Solomon. *The Foot Doctor: Lifetime Relief for Your Aching Feet.* Emmaus, Pa.: Rodale Press, 1986.

Lippert, Frederick G., and Sigvard T. Hansen. *Foot and Ankle Disorders: Tricks of the Trade.* New York: Thieme, 2003.

Lorimer, Donald L., et al., eds. *Neale's Disorders of the Foot.* 7th ed. New York: Elsevier Churchill Livingstone, 2006.

Van De Graaff, Kent M. *Human Anatomy.* 6th ed. New York: McGraw Hill, 2002.

FORENSIC PATHOLOGY

SPECIALTY

ANATOMY OR SYSTEM AFFECTED: All

SPECIALTIES AND RELATED FIELDS: Dentistry, epidemiology, hematology, histology, pathology, psychology, public health, pulmonary medicine, serology, toxicology

DEFINITION: A science that brings medical knowledge to bear in order to resolve legal issues, usually through the performance of an autopsy.

KEY TERMS:

anthropology: the study of human remains, especially skeletal ones

autopsy: the examination of a body to determine the cause and circumstances of death

forensic: having to do or in connection with the operation of the law, usually criminal law

histology: the microscopic study of plant and animal tissue

odontology: the study of teeth

pathology: the study of disease and the deviations from normalcy that it causes

psychiatry: the medical discipline concerned with mental, emotional, and behavioral disorders

serology: the study of body fluids

toxicology: the study of poisons and their effects

trace evidence: minute, often microscopic, signs or indications of an event or a presence

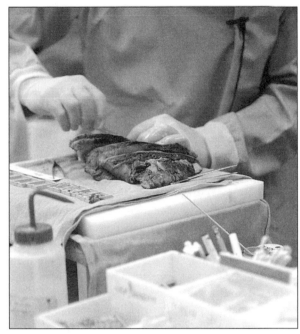

A pathologist studies a tissue sample. (PhotoDisc)

SCIENCE AND PROFESSION

Forensic medicine probably is best known to most people because of the work of forensic pathologists, principally for the autopsies that they perform as coroners and medical examiners. Other experts, however, also are key participants in the field. They include anthropologists, histologists, odontologists, psychiatrists, serologists, toxicologists, police officers, and specialists in trace evidence. Except for the forensic psychiatrist, who is called on to determine the sanity of an accused individual and thus that person's fitness to stand trial, the above-listed specialists generally do not become involved in the work of forensic medicine until a death has occurred that obviously is other than from natural causes.

In the United States, a forensic pathologist is a medical doctor who typically will spend three to four years preparing in that field after being graduated from medical school and two or so years beyond that before being certified by the American Society of Clinical Pathologists. Other forensic specialties generally require a four-year college degree as well as specialized training after that.

Forensic medicine is not a crowded field. Indeed, there is a shortage of trained and qualified people because most such jobs are in the public sector, where salaries are good but not as high as similar skills and knowledge will command in the private sector. Those who choose careers in forensic medicine, however, find the fascinating and exciting work, intellectual challenge, and personal satisfaction that private-sector jobs seldom offer.

DUTIES AND INVESTIGATIVE TECHNIQUES

As a general rule, the coroner, supported to a greater or lesser extent by one or more of the specialists listed above, will become involved in a death when a person dies of criminal or other violent means, by suicide, suddenly when in apparent good health, or in any suspicious or unusual manner. In such a case, the coroner typically is charged by law with determining the cause, mode, and manner of death, with each of those terms having a specific meaning. The physical cause of death is a purely medical determination. Legal considerations, on the other hand, are broader and more inclusive.

Both medical and legal aspects, however, are so interrelated that they cannot be separated. For example, to determine the physical cause of death, it would be sufficient to show a penetrating wound to the heart. To determine the mode of death, however, it would be necessary to establish whether the wound was caused by a bullet or a sharp instrument. An autopsy would reveal the mode of death. The next question is legal: What was the manner of death? In other words, how was the wound inflicted? Was it self-inflicted? If it was, was it intentional (suicide) or accidental? If it was inflicted by another person, was it an accident or was it homicide? Investigation of the scene where the injury was sustained, examination of the evidence found there, and statements of witnesses would furnish information as to the circumstances of the incident.

The actual autopsy involves the dissection and examination of a dead body—surgery performed postmortem. It begins with what is called a gross examination—that is, a visual examination with the naked eye, first externally and then internally. For the internal examination, a Y-shaped incision is made beginning at each shoulder, running down to and meeting just below the sternum or breastbone and continuing as a single cut down to the lower portion of the abdomen just above the genital area. Rib cutters are used to expose the thoracic area. The internal organs are removed and examined. Fluids are drawn for laboratory tests, and tissue samples are taken for microscopic examination. Access to the brain is gained by using a small powersaw to remove the top part of the skull. The third portion of the autopsy involves the toxicological examination of body fluids, including blood, urine, and the vitreous humor of the eye. After examination, the body is restored, and the incisions are carefully sewn.

PERSPECTIVE AND PROSPECTS

Probably the first well-known person to be the subject of a postmortem examination was Julius Caesar. A physician named Antisius determined that of the twenty-three wounds that Caesar sustained, the one that perforated the thorax was the cause of death. The Justinian Code of the sixth century required the opinion of a physician in certain circumstances and often is credited as the first recognition of the correlation of law and medicine in effecting legal justice. By the sixteenth century in England, investigations were being made by a representative of the king, who had the title of Custos

Placitorum Coronae (guardian of the decrees of the crown), from which comes the word "coroner." It is believed that William Penn appointed the first coroner in the American colonies. In the nineteenth century, forensic medicine became established as a distinct specialty and has continued to mature into the advanced and sophisticated field that it is today.

The capabilities of and advances in forensic medicine traditionally are tied to those of science in general and applicable medical specialties. They set the pace for the development of forensic medicine. The future should prove no different. The advances in overall knowledge of deoxyribonucleic acid (DNA), the development of scanning electron microscopy, improvements in spectrographic analysis, and advances in computer graphics capabilities, for example, occurred outside the field of forensic medicine and subsequently were adopted by it.

—John M. Shaw;
updated by Karen E. Kalumuck, Ph.D.

See also Anatomy; Autopsy; Death and dying; DNA and RNA; Histology; Laboratory tests; Law and medicine; Pathology; Suicide; Toxicology.

FOR FURTHER INFORMATION:

Browning, Michael, and William R. Maples. *Dead Men Do Tell Tales: The Strange and Fascinating Cases of a Forensic Anthropologist.* New York: Main Street Books, 1995. From a skeleton, a skull, a mere fragment of burnt thighbone, Dr. Maples can deduce the age, gender, and ethnicity of a murder victim, the manner in which the person was dispatched, and, ultimately, the identity of the killer.

Camenson, Blythe. *Opportunities in Forensic Science Careers.* New York: McGraw-Hill, 2001. Provides those seeking a career in forensics with information on training and education requirements and salary statistics, and lists professional and Internet resources.

Evans, Colin. *The Casebook of Forensic Detection: How Science Solved One Hundred of the World's Most Baffling Crimes.* New York: John Wiley & Sons, 1996. This book describes the development of forensics from the nineteenth century to the present. Cases are classified by fifteen forensic types and then arranged chronologically.

Genge, N. E. *The Forensic Casebook: The Science of Crime Scene Investigation.* New York: Random House, 2002. Uses true crime stories and draws on interviews with police personnel and forensic scientists—including animal examiners, botanists, zoologists, firearms specialists, and autoposists—to provide an encyclopedic view of the underworkings of criminal investigation.

James, Stuart H., and Jon J. Nordby. *Forensic Science: An Introduction to Scientific and Investigative Techniques.* Boca Raton, Fla.: CRC Press, 2002. An introductory text that covers a range of topics, including trace evidence, forensic toxicology, DNA analysis, crime scene investigation, fingerprints, traumatic death, forensic anthropology, bloodstain patterns, and criminal profiling, among many others.

Joyce, Christopher, and Eric Stover. *Witnesses from the Grave: The Stories Bones Tell.* Boston: Little, Brown, 1991. Journalists Joyce and Stover explore the history and investigative methods of forensic anthropology, focusing on one of its foremost practitioners, Clyde Snow, who has participated in civil, criminal, and human rights investigations, and who was called upon in 1985 to identify the skeletal remains of Nazi doctor Josef Mengele.

Klawans, Harold L. *Trials of an Expert Witness: Tales of Clinical Neurology and the Law.* Boston: Little, Brown, 1998. This book is written by a physician who has learned the ropes of the court system and who entertains the reader with forensic medical tales. Although Dr. Klawans is a frequent medical expert witness for both sides of the versus, he does not hesitate to use the term "hired gun" for impartial medical experts and minces no words in describing the shortcomings of the tort system.

Miller, Hugh. *What the Corpse Revealed: Murder and the Science of Forensic Detection.* New York: St. Martin's Press, 1999. This resource examines a number of cases in which forensic medicine played a role in criminal investigations. Each chapter is devoted to a different case. Includes an index.

Ubelaker, Douglas H., and Henry Scammel. *Bones: A Forensic Detective's Casebook.* New York: M. Evans, 2000. Among the dozens of true stories in this volume are accounts of homicide, cannibalism, ritual sacrifice, and other horrific crimes, solved and unsolved, from Ubelaker's own personal casebooks and those of the Smithsonian.

FRACTURE AND DISLOCATION
DISEASE/DISORDER

ANATOMY OR SYSTEM AFFECTED: Arms, bones, hands, hips, joints, knees, legs, musculoskeletal system

SPECIALTIES AND RELATED FIELDS: Emergency medicine, orthopedics

DEFINITION: A fracture is a break in a bone, which may be partial or complete; a dislocation is the forceful separation of bones in a joint.

KEY TERMS:

anesthesia: a state characterized by loss of sensation, caused by or resulting from the pharmacological depression of normal nerve function

callus: a hard, bonelike substance made by osteocytes which is found in and around the ends of a fractured bone; it temporarily maintains bony alignment and is resorbed after complete healing or union of a fracture occurs

ecchymosis: a purplish patch on the skin caused by bleeding; the spots are easily visible to the naked eye

embolus: an obstruction or occlusion of a vessel (most commonly, an artery or vein) caused by a transported blood clot, vegetation, mass of bacteria, or other foreign material

epiphysis: the part of a long bone from which growth or elongation occurs

instability: excessive mobility of two or more bones caused by damage to ligaments, the joint capsule, or fracture of one or more bones

ischemia: a local anemia or area of diminished or insufficient blood supply due to mechanical obstruction, commonly narrowing of an artery

osteoblast: a bone-forming cell

osteocyte: a bone cell

paralysis: the loss of power of voluntary movement or other function of a muscle as a result of disease or injury to its nerve supply

petechiae: minute spots caused by hemorrhage or bleeding into the skin; the spots are the size of pinheads

prone: the position of the body when face downward, on one's stomach and abdomen

pulse: the rhythmical dilation of an artery, produced by the increased volume of blood forced into the vessel by the contraction of the heart

transection: a partial or complete severance of the spinal cord

CAUSES AND SYMPTOMS

A fracture is a linear deformation or discontinuity of a bone produced by the application of a force that exceeds the modulus of elasticity (ability to bend) of a bone. Normal bones require excessive force to fracture. Bones may be weakened by disease or other pathology such as a tumor or tumor-related disease that reduces their ability to withstand an impact. Bones respond to stresses made upon them and can thus be strengthened

---

INFORMATION ON FRACTURE AND DISLOCATION

CAUSES: Usually injury, sometimes disease or infection
SYMPTOMS: Varies widely; typically pain, swelling, deformity, bruising
DURATION: Acute
TREATMENTS: Reduction (return of fractured bone to normal position), immobilization, surgery, orthopedic appliances

---

through physical conditioning and made more resistant to fracture. This is a normal part of training in many athletic activities.

Fractures are classified according to the type of break or, more correctly, by the plane or surface that is fractured. A break that is at a right angle to the axis of the bone is called transverse. A fracture that is similar but at an angle, rather than perpendicular to the main axis of the bone, is called oblique. If a twisting force is applied, the break may be spiral, or twisted. A comminuted fracture is a break that results in two or more fragments of bone. If the pieces of bone remain in their original positions, the fracture is undisplaced. In a displaced fracture, the portions of bone are not properly aligned.

If bones do not penetrate the skin, the fracture is called closed, or simple. When bones protrude through the skin, the result is an open, or compound, fracture. Other types of fractures are associated with pathologic or disease processes. A stress fracture results from repeated stress or trauma to the same site of a bone. None of the individual stresses is sufficient to cause a break. If these stresses cause a callus to form, the bone will be strengthened and actual separation of fragments will not occur. A pathologic fracture occurs at the site of a tumor, infection, or other bone disease. A compression fracture results when bone is crushed; the force applied is greater than the ability of the bone to withstand it. A greenstick fracture is an incomplete separation of bone.

The diagnosis of a fracture is based on several criteria: instability, pain, swelling, deformity, and ecchymosis. The most reliable diagnostic criterion is instability. Pain is not universally present at a fracture site. Swelling may be delayed and occur at some time after a fracture is sustained. Deformity is obvious with open fractures but may not be apparent with other, undisplaced breaks.

Ecchymosis is a purplish patch caused by bleeding into skin; it will not be present if blood vessels are not broken. A definitive diagnosis is made with two plane film X rays taken at the site of a fracture and at right angles to each other. If the fracture site is visually examined and palpated shortly after the injury occurs, an accurate tentative diagnosis may be made; this should be confirmed with X rays as soon as is convenient. Occasionally, an X ray will not show undisplaced or chip fractures. If a patient experiences symptoms of pain, swelling, or ecchymosis but has a negative X ray for fracture, the site should be immobilized and X-rayed again in two to three weeks.

Fractures occur most commonly in extremities: arms or legs. Such fractures must be evaluated to determine if injuries have occurred to other tissues such as nerves or blood vessels. The presence of bruising or ecchymosis indicates blood vessel damage. The existence of peripheral pulses indicates that arteries are not injured. Venous flow is more difficult to evaluate. For a relatively short period of time, however, venous bleeding may be of lesser importance and therefore tolerated.

Neurologic functioning may be assessed by the ability of the patient to contract muscles or sense skin touches or pinpricks. Temporary immobilization may be necessary before nerve status can be evaluated accurately.

An open fracture creates a direct pathway between the skin surface and underlying tissues. If the site becomes contaminated by bacteria, an opportunity for osteomyelitis (infection of the bone) is created. Inadequate treatment by the initial surgeon may result in skin loss, delayed union, loss of joint mobility, osteomyelitis, and even amputation.

Skin damage may or may not be related to a fracture. When skin integrity is broken over or near a fracture site, bone involvement must be assumed. The problem is infection of the fracture site; appropriate antibiotics are normally administered. If skin damage is extensive, final surgical reduction of the underlying fracture may have to be delayed until the skin is healed.

Delayed union refers to the inability of a fractured bone to heal. This is a potentially serious problem, as normal stability is not possible as long as a fracture exists. Joints may not function normally in the presence of a fracture. If a fracture heals improperly, bones may be misaligned and cause pain with movement, leading to limitations of motion. If the bones are affected by osteomyelitis, the infection may spread to the joint capsule and reduce the normal range of motion for the bones or the joint. Amputation may become necessary if infection becomes extensive in the area of a fracture. An infection which becomes firmly established in bones or spreads widely into adjacent muscle tissue may lead to cellulitis or gangrene and may compromise a portion of an extremity. Amputation may be performed if the pathologic process cannot be treated with antibiotics.

Adequate blood supply to tissues is critical for survival. In an extremity, the maximum time limit for complete ischemia (lack of blood flow) is six to eight hours; after that time, the likelihood of later amputation increases. Pain, pallor, pulselessness, and paralysis are indicators of impaired circulation associated with a fracture. When two of these signs are present, the possibility of vascular damage must be thoroughly explored.

Dislocations occur at joints and are caused by an applied force that is greater than the strength of the ligaments and muscles that keep a joint intact. The result is a stretching deformity or injury to a joint and abnormal movement of a bone out of the joint. Accidental trauma, commonly the result of an athletic injury or automobile accident, is the most common cause of a dis-

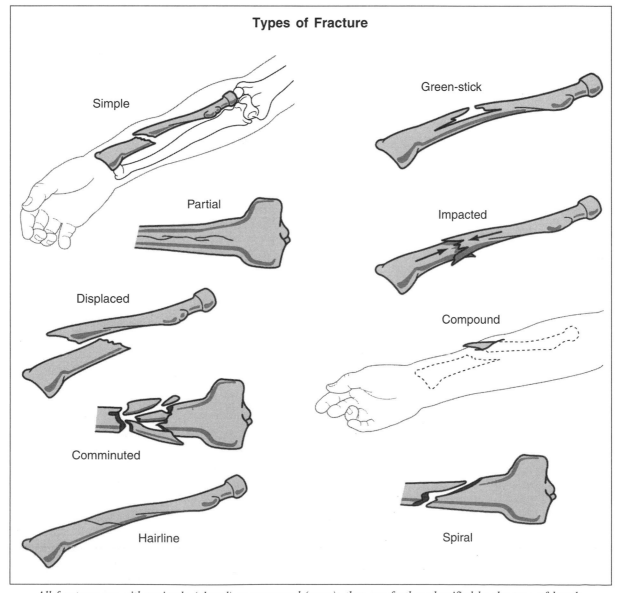

Types of Fracture

Simple

Green-stick

Partial

Impacted

Displaced

Compound

Comminuted

Hairline

Spiral

All fractures are either simple (closed) or compound (open); they are further classified by the type of break.

location. Joints that are frequently dislocated include the shoulder and digits (fingers and toes). Dislocations of the ankle and hip are infrequent but serious; they require immediate management. Dislocations may accompany fractures, but the two injuries need not occur together.

When dislocations are reduced, the bones of the joint are returned to normal position. Reduction is accomplished by relaxing adjacent muscles and applying traction or a pulling force to the bone until it returns to its normal position in the joint. For most dislocations of the shoulder, the victim lies in a prone position and the dislocated arm hangs down freely. Gradual traction is applied until reduction occurs. This can be accomplished by bandaging a pail to the arm and slowly filling it with water. Alternatively, a heavy book can be held by the victim and the muscles of the arm allowed to relax until the dislocation is reduced. Such treatments are usually reserved for situations in which medical assistance is unavailable. Digits are reduced in a similar manner, by gentle pulling of the end of the finger or toe. Ankle and hip dislocations are potentially more serious because these joints are more complex and have extensive blood supplies. Reduction of dislocated ankles and hips should be undertaken by qualified medical personnel in an expedited manner.

After reduction, all dislocations should be evaluated by competent medical personnel. With dislocated digits, later damage is relatively unlikely but can occur because of ligament damage sustained in the initial injury. Dislocations of the shoulder may be accompanied by a fracture of the clavicle or collar bone and may involve nerve damage in the shoulder joint. Dislocations of the ankle and hip may lead to avascular necrosis (damage to the bone as a result of inadequate blood supply) if not evaluated and reduced promptly.

TREATMENT AND THERAPY

Fractures are usually treated by reduction and immobilization. Reduction, which refers to the process of returning the fractured bones to normal position, may be either closed or open. Closed reduction is accomplished without surgery by manipulating the broken bone through overlying skin and muscles. Open reduction requires surgical intervention in which the broken pieces are exposed and returned to normal position. Orthopedic appliances may be used to hold the bones in correct position. The most common of these appliances are pins and screws, but metal plates and wires may also be employed. Orthopedic appliances are usually

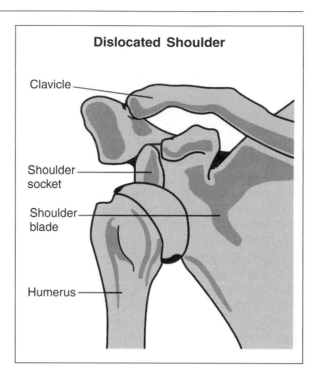

Dislocated Shoulder

Clavicle

Shoulder socket

Shoulder blade

Humerus

made of stainless steel. These may be left in the body indefinitely or may be surgically removed after healing is complete. Local anesthesia is usually used with closed reductions; open reductions are performed in an operating room, under sterile conditions using general anesthesia.

Immobilization is generally accomplished by the use of a cast. Casts are often made of plaster, but they may be constructed of inflatable plastic. It is important to hold bones in a rigid, fixed position for a sufficient length of time for the broken ends to unite and heal. The cast must be loose enough, however, to allow blood to circulate. Padding is usually put in place before plaster is applied to form a cast. Whenever possible, the newly immobilized body part is elevated to reduce the chance of swelling in the cast, which would compromise the blood supply to the fracture site and body portion beyond the cast. Casts should be checked periodically to ensure that they do not impair circulation.

The broken bone and accompanying body part must be placed in an anatomically neutral position. This is done to minimize postfracture disability and improve the prospect for rehabilitation. The length of time that a fractured bone is immobilized is highly variable and dependent on a number of factors.

Traction may also be used to immobilize a fracture. Traction is the external application of force to overcome muscular resistance and hold bones in a desired position. Commonly, holes are drilled through bones and pins are inserted; the ends of these pins extend through the surface of the skin. Part of the body is fixed in position through the use of a strap or weights, and wires are attached to the pins in the body part to be stretched. Weights or tension is applied to the wires until the broken bone parts move into the desired position. Traction is maintained until healing has occurred.

Individual ends of a single fractured bone are sometimes held in position by external pins and screws. Holes are drilled through the bone, and pins are inserted. The pins on opposite sides of the fracture site are then attached to each other with threaded rods and locked in position by nuts. This process allows a fractured bone to be immobilized without using a cast.

Different bones require different amounts of time to heal. Further, age is a factor in fracture healing. Fractures in young children heal more quickly than do broken bones in adults. Older adults typically require even more time for healing. The availability of calcium and other nutrients also affects the speed with which a fracture heals.

Delayed union of fractures is a term applied to fractures that either do not heal or take longer than normal to heal; there is no precise time frame associated with delayed union. Nonunion refers to fractures in which healing is not observed and cannot be expected even with prolonged immobilization. X-ray analysis of a nonunion will show that the bone ends have hardened (sclerosed), that the ends of the marrow canal have become plugged, and that a gap persists between the ends of a fractured bone. Nonunion may be caused by inadequate blood supply to the fracture site, which leads to the formation of cartilage instead of new bone between the broken pieces of bone. Nonunion may also be caused by injury to the soft tissues that surround a fracture site. This damage impairs the formation of a callus and the reestablishment of an adequate blood supply to the fracture site; it is frequently seen in young children. Inadequate immobilization may also allow soft tissue to enter the fracture site by slipping between the bone fragments, and may lead to nonunion. Respect for tissue and minimizing damage in the vicinity of a fracture, especially with open reduction, will minimize problems of nonunion. Subjecting the nonuniting fracture site to a low-level electromagnetic field will usually stimulate osteoblastic activity and lead to healing.

The epiphyseal plate is the portion of bone where growth occurs. Bony epiphyses are active in children until they attain their adult height, at which time the epiphyses become inactive and close. Once an epiphysis ceases to function, further growth does not occur. In children, a fracture involving the epiphyseal plate is potentially dangerous because bone growth may be interrupted or halted. This situation can lead to inequalities in the length of extremities or impaired range of movement in joints. Accurate reduction of injuries involving an epiphyseal plate is necessary to minimize subsequent deformity. A key factor is blood supply to the injured area: If adequate blood supply is maintained, epiphyseal plate damage is minimized.

Fractures of the spinal vertebrae are potentially very dangerous because they can cause injury to the nerves and tracts of the spinal cord. Fractures of the vertebrae are commonly sustained in automobile accidents, athletic injuries, falls from heights, and other situations involving rapid deceleration. When vertebrae are fractured, the spinal cord can be compromised. Spinal cord injury can be direct and cut all or a portion of the spinal nerves at the site of the fracture. The extent of the damage is dependent on the level of the injury. An accident that completely severs the spinal cord will lead to a complete loss of function for all structures below the level of injury. Since spinal nerves are arranged segmentally, cord damage at a lower level involves compromise of fewer structures. As the level of injury becomes higher in the spinal cord, more vital structures are involved. Transection of the spinal cord in the neck usually leads to complete paralysis of the entire body; it can cause death if high enough to cut the nerves controlling the lungs. Individuals in whom vertebral fractures and thus spinal cord injuries are suspected must have the spinal column immobilized before they are moved. Reduction of spinal cord fractures must be undertaken by a highly skilled person.

When bones having large marrow cavities such as the femur (thigh bone) are fractured, fat globules may escape from the marrow and enter the bloodstream. Such a fat globule is then called an embolus (plural is emboli). Fat emboli are potentially dangerous in that they can become lodged in the capillaries of the lungs. This causes pain and can lead to impaired oxygenation of blood, a condition called hypoxemia. About 10 to 20 percent of individuals sustaining a fractured femur also have central nervous system depression and skin petechiae (minute spots caused by hemorrhage or bleeding into the skin) in addition to hypoxemia in the two to three days after the injury. This triad of signs is called fat embolism syndrome. It is treated medically with oxygen, steroids, and anticoagulant drugs.

Perspective and Prospects

Fractures rarely threaten a patient's life directly, and injuries to the brain, heart, circulatory system, and abdominal cavity must receive priority of treatment. It is imperative, however, not to move a patient in whom a fracture is suspected without first immobilizing the potential fracture site. This is especially true with suspected fractures of the spine. Instability may not be apparent when a patient is lying down but can become catastrophic if the person is moved without proper preparation and immobilization.

Crush injuries of the spinal cord are relatively common among victims of osteoporosis. Osteoporosis is a pathological syndrome defined by a decrease in the density of a bone below the level required for mechanical support and is frequently associated with a deficiency of calcium, problems related to calcium in the body, or a rate of bone cell breakdown that is greater than the rate of bone cell remodeling. Crush fractures occur when the bones become so weak that the weight of the upper portion of the body is greater than the ability of the vertebrae to support it. These crush injuries may occur slowly over time and cause no serious injury to the underlying spinal cord. The resulting deformity of the spine, however, impairs movement. There is no treatment for osteoporotic crush fractures of the vertebrae.

Occupational exposures may lead to fractures and dislocations. Professional athletes are clearly at increased risk for skeletal injuries. These individuals are also usually well conditioned, however, and so can withstand increased impacts and blows to the body. Many are also trained in methods that minimize the force of impact; they know how to fall properly.

The vast proportion of workers are not conditioned and are given minimal training to avoid situations that lead to fractures. Accident analysis reveals that carelessness is the most common predisposing factor. Workers operating without safety equipment such as belaying lines or belts may become overconfident. In such a situation, slips or falls can occur, and fractures result. Unsafe equipment can lead to hazardous situations and cause fractures or dislocations. Machinery that is not properly maintained can fail; parts may become detached, hit nearby workers, and cause fractures.

Recreational activities also result in fractures. Individuals who once were well conditioned may engage in sports without proper equipment and sustain fractures or dislocations. Contact sports such as hockey, football, and basketball are primary examples of such activities. Riding bicycles and motorized recreational vehicles without proper safety equipment can lead to serious skeletal injuries. Activities such as rock climbing are inherently dangerous. With proper training and use of safety equipment, accidents can be reduced or their severity minimized. The keys to avoiding fractures and dislocations when participating in recreational activities are receiving proper instruction and training, employing adequate safety equipment, and using common sense by avoiding difficult or hazardous situations that are beyond one's physical abilities or skill level.

—*L. Fleming Fallon, Jr., M.D., Ph.D., M.P.H.*

See also Bone disorders; Bone grafting; Bones and the skeleton; Fracture repair; Head and neck disorders; Hip fracture repair; Orthopedic surgery; Orthopedics; Orthopedics, pediatric; Osteonecrosis; Osteoporosis; Physical rehabilitation; Spinal cord disorders; Spine, vertebrae, and disks; Wounds.

For Further Information:

Brunicardi, F. Charles, et al., eds. *Schwartz's Principles of Surgery*. 8th ed. New York: McGraw-Hill, 2005. A standard textbook of surgery containing sections on fractures and dislocations. Its intended audience is practicing surgeons, and thus the language is sometimes technical. Nevertheless, the serious reader can obtain much useful detail from this work.

Currey, John D. *Bones: Structures and Mechanics*. Princeton, N.J.: Princeton University Press, 2002. Very accessible overview of a range of information related to whole bones, bone tissue, and dentin and enamel. Topics include stiffness, strength, viscoelasticity, fatigue, fracture mechanics properties, buckling, impact fracture, and properties of cancellous bone.

Doherty, Gerard M., and Lawrence W. Way, eds. *Current Surgical Diagnosis and Treatment*. 12th ed. New York: Lange Medical Books/McGraw-Hill, 2006. The diagnosis and treatment of fractures and dislocations is discussed in a brief and concise format emphasizing treatment modalities. The different section authors are recognized experts in their fields. The material is accessible to the general reader, but the sections are brief.

Marieb, Elaine N., and Katja Hoehn. *Human Anatomy and Physiology*. 7th ed. San Francisco: Pearson Benjamin Cummings, 2007. Nonscientists at the advanced high school level or above will be able to understand this fine textbook. The chapters titled "Bones and Bone Tissue," "The Skeleton," and "Joints" are very well illustrated.

Townsend, Courtney M., Jr., et al., eds. *Sabiston Textbook of Surgery*. 17th ed. Philadelphia: Elsevier Saunders, 2005. A standard textbook of surgery which contains an extensive discussion of different types of fractures and dislocations and how they are treated. Intended for practicing professionals but can be generally understood by the layperson.

Wilmore, Douglas W., et al., eds. *Scientific American Surgery 2006*. New York: Scientific American, 2007. Annual book sponsored by the American College of Surgeons. Sections discuss fractures and dislocations. The reputation of Scientific American for style and clarity is evident. Written for professionals, but a good source for the general reader.

FRACTURE REPAIR

PROCEDURE

ANATOMY OR SYSTEM AFFECTED: Arms, bones, hips, legs, musculoskeletal system, teeth

SPECIALTIES AND RELATED FIELDS: Dentistry, orthopedics

DEFINITION: The placement and fixation of broken portions of bones in their correct positions until they have grown together.

INDICATIONS AND PROCEDURES

A fracture is a break in a bone, either partial or complete, resulting from an applied force that is greater than the bone's internal strength. The most common causes of fractures are accidents or trauma.

Fractures are usually treated by reduction and immobilization. Reduction, which may be either closed or open, refers to the process of returning the fractured bones to normal position. Closed reduction is accomplished without surgery by manipulating the broken bone through overlying skin and muscles. Open reduction requires surgical intervention. The broken pieces are exposed and returned to their normal positions. Orthopedic appliances may be used to hold the bones in the proper position (internal fixation); the most common appliances are stainless steel pins and screws, but metal plates and wires may also be employed. These devices can be left in the body indefinitely or may be surgically removed after healing is complete. Local anesthesia is usually used with closed reductions; open reductions are performed in an operating room under sterile conditions, using general anesthesia.

After reduction, the broken bone and accompanying body part must be placed in an anatomically neutral position. Immobilization is generally accomplished by the use of a cast. Casts are usually made of plaster, but they may be constructed of inflatable plastic.

Individual ends of a single fractured bone are sometimes held in position by external pins and screws (external fixation). Holes are drilled through the bone, and pins are inserted as described above. The pins on opposite sides of the fracture site are then attached to each other with threaded rods and locked in position by nuts. This process allows a fractured bone to be immobilized without using a cast.

Traction, the external application of force to overcome muscular resistance and hold bones in a desired position, may also be used to immobilize a fracture. Commonly, holes are drilled through bones and pins are inserted; the ends of these pins extend through the surface of the skin. Part of the body is fixed in position through the use of a strap or weights. Wires are attached to the pins in the body part to be stretched. Force through weights or tension is applied to the wires until the broken bone parts are in the desired position. Traction is maintained until complete healing has occurred.

USES AND COMPLICATIONS

All broken bones must be held in position until healing takes place. The complications associated with repairing fractures include infection, which is rare, and loss of function. The potential for loss of function is minimized by placing the limb into an anatomically neutral position prior to the application of a cast.

The techniques of fracture repair have not changed radically in decades. New methods, however, are being tried. For example, electromagnetic fields are used with fractures that do not heal spontaneously. Such a field induces the growth of osteoblasts, which are bone-forming cells.

—*L. Fleming Fallon, Jr., M.D., Ph.D., M.P.H.*

See also Bone grafting; Bones and the skeleton; Dentistry; Emergency medicine; Fracture and dislocation; Hip fracture repair; Jaw wiring; Orthopedic surgery; Orthopedics; Orthopedics, pediatric; Osteoporosis; Teeth.

FOR FURTHER INFORMATION:

Browner, Bruce D., et al. *Skeletal Trauma: Basic Science, Management, and Reconstruction*. 3d ed. Philadelphia: W. B. Saunders, 2003.

Eiff, M. Patrice, Robert L. Hatch, and Walter L.

Types of Fracture Repair

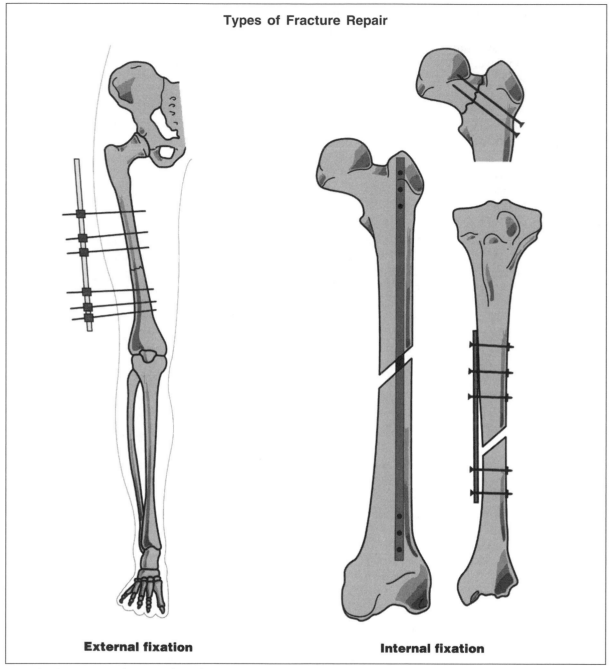

External fixation   **Internal fixation**

Severe leg fractures can be immobilized through external fixation or internal fixation. External fixation involves the use of long pins that are inserted through the bone and held in place with a steel rod on the outside of the body. Internal fixation involves the use of screws, pins, and plates that are attached directly to the bones and often left there permanently.

Calmbach. *Fracture Management for Primary Care.* 2d ed. Philadelphia: Saunders, 2003.

Gregg, Paul J., Jack Stevens, and Peter H. Worlock. *Fractures and Dislocations: Principles of Management.* Cambridge, Mass.: Blackwell Science, 1996.

Gustilo, Ramon B., Richard F. Kyle, and David C. Templeman, eds. *Fractures and Dislocations.* St. Louis: C. V. Mosby, 1993.

Hodgson, Stephen F. *Mayo Clinic on Osteoporosis: Keeping Bones Healthy and Strong and Reducing the Risk of Fractures.* New York: Kensington, 2003.

Magee, David J. *Orthopedic Physical Assessment.* 4th rev. ed. Philadelphia: Elsevier Saunders, 2006.

Ruiz, Ernest, and James J. Cicero, eds. *Emergency Management of Skeletal Injuries.* St. Louis: C. V. Mosby, 1995.

Salter, Robert Bruce. *Textbook of Disorders and Injuries of the Musculoskeletal System.* 3d ed. Baltimore: Williams & Wilkins, 1999.

FRAGILE X SYNDROME

DISEASE/DISORDER

ALSO KNOWN AS: Martin-Bell syndrome

ANATOMY OR SYSTEM AFFECTED: Brain, ears, feet, genitals, hands, joints

SPECIALTIES AND RELATED FIELDS: Genetics

DEFINITION: A genetic disorder of variable expression, with mental retardation being the most common feature.

CAUSES AND SYMPTOMS

Fragile X syndrome is caused by a change in a gene located on the long arm of the X chromosome. It is a sex-linked inherited disease, transmitted from parent to child, with boys being affected much more often and more severely than girls. The prevalence of the disorder is estimated to be 1 in 1,200 males and 1 in 2,500 females.

While symptoms and their severity vary widely, common physical features of fragile X syndrome include a long, thin face, a prominent jaw and ears, a broad nose, a high palate, large testicles (macroorchidism) in males, and large hands with loose finger joints. Physical features are more subtle in females.

INFORMATION ON FRAGILE X SYNDROME

CAUSES: Genetic

SYMPTOMS: Thin face, prominent jaw and ears, broad nose, large testicles in males, large hands with loose finger joints, mental impairment ranging from severe retardation to learning disabilities, unusual speech patterns, problems with attention span and hyperactivity, motor delays, occasional autistic-type behaviors

DURATION: Chronic

TREATMENTS: None; alleviation of symptoms

Nonphysical features include mental impairment ranging from severe retardation to learning disabilities, with the majority of affected males demonstrating a mental impairment ranging from low-normal intelligence to severe retardation. More recent research has found that the intelligence quotients (IQs) of males with fragile X syndrome appear to decline throughout childhood. Associated behavioral symptoms include unusual speech patterns, problems with attention span, hyperactivity, motor delays, and occasional autistic-type behaviors, such as poor eye contact, hand-biting, or hand-flapping.

TREATMENT AND THERAPY

While there is no cure for fragile X syndrome, a number of possible interventions can address various symptoms. Medications can be administered to assist with attention span and hyperactivity, as well as with aggressive behavior. Schools can provide children with assistance in speech, physical therapy, and vocational planning. Early childhood special education services for children prior to school age can provide necessary early intervention that may prove most helpful if indeed the rate of learning for children with fragile X syndrome slows with age. Genetic counseling is advised for families who carry the gene.

PERSPECTIVE AND PROSPECTS

In 1969, the discovery was made of a break or fragile site on the long arm of the X chromosome. It was not until the 1980's, however, that consistent diagnoses of fragile X syndrome were made. In 1991, the responsible gene was sequenced and named the FMR-1 (fragile X mental retardation 1) gene. Cytogenetic and deoxyribonucleic acid (DNA) testing are now available to identify affected persons.

—*Robin Hasslen, Ph.D.*

See also Autism; Genetic diseases; Genetics and inheritance; Learning disabilities; Mental retardation; Motor skill development; Speech disorders.

FOR FURTHER INFORMATION:

FRAXA Research Foundation. http://www.fraxa.org/.

Hagerman, Randi Jensen, and Paul J. Henssen. *Fragile X Syndrome: Diagnosis, Treatment, and Research.* 3d ed. Baltimore: Johns Hopkins University Press, 2002.

Maxson, Linda, and Charles Daugherty. *Genetics: A Human Perspective.* Dubuque, Iowa: Wm. C. Brown, 1992.

Moore, Keith L., and T. V. N. Persaud. *The Developing Human.* 7th ed. Philadelphia: W. B. Saunders, 2003.

Parker, James N., and Philip M. Parker, eds. *The 2002 Official Parent's Sourcebook on Fragile X Syndrome.* San Diego, Calif.: Icon Health, 2002.

Sherwood, Lauralee. *Human Physiology: From Cells to Systems.* 6th ed. Belmont, Calif.: Thomson/Brooks/Cole, 2007.

Webb, Jayne Dixon, ed. *Children with Fragile X Syndrome: A Parents' Guide.* Bethesda, Md.: Woodbine House, 2000.

FROSTBITE

DISEASE/DISORDER

ANATOMY OR SYSTEM AFFECTED: Hands, feet, skin and adjacent tissues

SPECIALTIES AND RELATED FIELDS: Emergency medicine, environmental health

DEFINITION: Frostbite is localized freezing of tissue, usually of extremities exposed to low temperatures, that results in ice crystals forming within cells, thereby killing them.

KEY TERMS:

anticoagulant: a drug that reduces the clotting of the blood

basal metabolic rate: the rate at which the body burns calories and produces heat energy while the body is at rest or not active

gangrene: the death of part of the body (such as an arm or leg) caused by the death of the cells in that structure

hypothermia: the process by which the body core temperature falls below that needed for the body to function normally

hypoxia: a lack of an adequate amount of oxygen to the tissues; results in a reduction of mental and physical capabilities

maceration: the process of breaking down tissue to a soft mass, either by soaking it or through infection or gangrene

necrosis: the death of body tissue cells

sludging: an increase in red blood cell structures, known as platelets, which slows down the blood flow through vessels and promotes clotting of the blood

sympathectomy: the surgical process of removing or destroying nerves that may be afflicted by frostbite or other injury

vascoconstriction: a decrease in the diameter of vessels transporting blood throughout the body, reducing blood flow and oxygen transport

windchill: the effect of wind blowing across exposed flesh; increased heat is lost from the skin's surface, as if the air were much colder than the actual temperature indicates

CAUSES AND SYMPTOMS

The effect of cold on the human body is to reduce the circulation of blood to surface areas, such as the feet, hands, and face. This reduction restricts the amount of heat lost by the body and helps to prevent the development of hypothermia. Blood constriction may become so severe in severely chilled areas of the body, however, that circulation almost totally ceases. People with poorer circulation, such as the elderly and the exhausted, are not as resistant to low temperatures as are fit or younger people.

If the skin's temperature falls below −0.53 degree Celsius, the tissue actually freezes and frostbite occurs. Rapid freezing causes ice crystals to form within a cell. These crystals rupture the cell wall and destroy structures within the cell, effectively killing it. If freezing is slow, ice crystals form between the cells; they grow by extracting water from the cells. The tissue may be injured physically by the ice crystals or by dehydration and the resulting disruption of osmotic and chemical balance within the cells; however, tissue death following frostbite is more likely to be attributable to interruption of the blood supply to the tissue than to the direct action of freezing. Cold also damages the capillaries in the affected areas, causing blood plasma to leak through their walls, thus adding to tissue injury and further impairing circulation by allowing the blood to sludge (to clot because of an increase in red blood cells) inside the vessels. All sensation of cold or pain is lost as circulation becomes seriously impaired. Unless the tissue is warmed quickly, the skin and superficial tissues actually begin to freeze. With continual chilling, the frozen area enlarges and extends to deeper areas. This condition is known as frostbite.

Frostbite was common among soldiers during Napoleon's campaign in Russia in the early 1800's, during World War II in Northern Europe, in the Korean War, and in fighting between Indian and Chinese troops in the Himalayas. Air crews, especially waist-gunners in the U.S. Air Force in World War II, were particularly prone to frostbite. In 1943, frostbite injuries among these bomber crews were greater than all other casualties combined.

Polar travelers before the 1920's suffered severely from frostbite. Mountain climbers are at risk from frostbite at higher elevations. Lower oxygen availability increases the danger of frostbite because the body cannot take in sufficient oxygen in this thinner air. The resulting condition, called hypoxia, reduces mental abilities, and precautions normally taken against the cold may be either inadequate or neglected altogether. High winds, often experienced in the mountains, speed heat loss from exposed skin surfaces. This windchill can be deadly to mountaineers and often produces hypothermia. Poor appetite at high elevations reduces the energy available for the production of body heat. The insulating layer of subcutaneous fat also decreases with longer periods of time spent at higher elevations; this in turn decreases the insulation of the surface areas of the body against freezing. Inadequate food intake while mountain climbing increases the danger of frostbite, as the body does not have enough calories to keep its temperature constant. The occurrence of hypothermia also increases the risk of frostbite as heat is drawn away from extremities to protect the body's core temperature. At higher elevations, most humans function at only about 60 percent of the physiological efficiency that they have at sea level. Women have more resistance to cold and may be less likely to experience frostbite than are men.

Frostbite at high altitudes seems to be more common for the same temperature than at lower altitudes. More red blood cells are found in the blood of persons working at higher elevations, thickening the blood and reducing circulation to the extremities. This reduced circulation lowers the temperature of these extremities. The basal metabolic rate and cardiac output of the body also decrease as one goes higher; both of these actions reduce the body's ability to keep its feet, hands, and face warm.

Blood vessels move heat from the central body core to the skin; it radiates into the air from exposed surfaces. This heat loss is greatest in the hands, feet, and head, where the vessels are close to the skin's surface. Respiration loses body heat when cold air is inhaled into the lungs and body heat warms it; this heat is lost when the air is exhaled. Evaporation, moisture leaving the skin's surface, also draws heat from the body. In low temperatures, spilling gasoline on exposed skin will create frostbite because the evaporation of the fuel draws heat away from the body quickly. Convection carries body heat away by wind currents. This windchill factor, calculated for Fahrenheit temperatures by subtracting two times the wind speed from the air temperature, determines the amount of heat energy lost

INFORMATION ON FROSTBITE

CAUSES: Exposure to freezing temperatures, causing impaired circulation to nearly cease
SYMPTOMS: Tingling and pain in afflicted tissues, slightly flushed skin before freezing begins followed by white or blotchy blue color, skin that is firm and insensitive to the touch
DURATION: Acute
TREATMENTS: Manual or medical rewarming, antibiotics, hyperbaric oxygen, occasionally surgery

from the body's surface. Conduction transfers heat from one substance to another; for example, contact between the body and snow or metal will cause the skin to lose heat. Although many people work and live in subzero temperatures, frostbite is uncommon. Nevertheless, an accident that prevents one from moving, loss of the ability to shiver in order to generate heat, or inactivity may increase the chance of developing frostbite. Frostbite can occur in any cold environment. Warning symptoms of frostbite initially include tingling and pain in the afflicted tissues. The skin may be slightly flushed before freezing. It then turns white or a blotchy blue in color and is firm and insensitive to the touch. Tissue that is painful and then becomes numb and insensitive is frozen.

TREATMENT AND THERAPY

Slight cases of frostbite, often termed frostnip or superficial frostbite, can be treated outdoors or in the field with little or no medical help. Such cases are usually reversible, with no permanent damage, as only skin and subcutaneous tissues are involved. The frozen part, although white and frozen on the surface, is soft and pliable when pressed gently before thawing. The area is often a cheek or the tip of the nose or the fingers. The frozen area, usually small, can be warmed manually. A hand is placed over the frostnipped area if it is a cheek or nose, and frozen fingers can be placed under the armpit or on a partner's bare stomach for warming. Tissue that has had only a minor amount of frostnip soon returns to normal color. A tingling sensation is felt when frostnipped tissue is thawed. After thawing, areas that have had more serious superficial frostbite become numb, mottled, or blue or purple in color and then will sting, burn, or swell for a period of time. Blisters, small ones called blebs, may occur within twenty-four to forty-eight hours. Blistering is more common where the skin is loose. Blister fluid is absorbed slowly; the skin may harden, become black (from gangrene), and be insensitive to touch. Throbbing or aching may persist for weeks. Gangrene occurring after frostnip is essentially superficial and extends only a few millimeters deep into the tissue. In two or three months, this type of frostbite will be mostly healed. With immediate treatment, frostnipped tissue will not progress to the much more serious injury of deep frostbite.

Tissues vary in their resistance to frostbite. Skin freezes at −0.53 Celsius, while muscles, blood vessels, and nerves are also highly subject to freezing. Connective tissue, tendons, and bones are relatively resistant to freezing, which explains why the blackened extremities of a frostbitten hand or foot can be moved: The tendons under the gangrenous skin remain intact and functional.

Deep frostbite includes not only skin and subcutaneous tissue but also deeper structures, including muscle, bone, and tendons. The affected area becomes cold, mottled, and blue or gray in color and may remain swollen for months. With deep frostbite, the tissues become quite hard to the touch. One to three days after thawing, the affected area becomes quite painful. Blisters, initially small blebs and then large, coalescing ones, may take weeks to develop. The patient should not be allowed to become alarmed about his or her condition; even mild cases of frostbite have a frightening appearance during blistering. Initially, the frozen part may be painless, but shooting and throbbing pains may occur for several months after thawing. Permanent loss of tissue is almost inevitable with deep frostbite. The affected extremity has a severely shriveled look. A limb may return to almost normal over some months, however, and amputation should never be carried out until a considerable period, probably at least six to nine months, has elapsed.

In cases of frostbite, surgical intervention must be minimal. Blackened frostbitten tissue will gradually separate itself from healthy, unfrozen tissue without interference; no efforts should be taken to hasten separation. Most cases of deep frostbite seem to heal in six to twelve months, and the gangrenous tissue, if it has not become infected with bacteria, is essentially superficial. Many unnecessary amputations have been carried

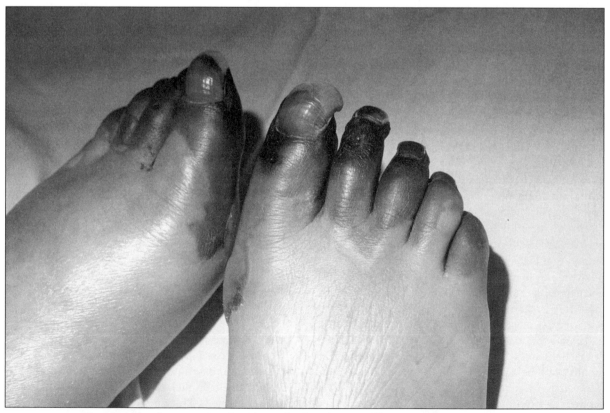

Frostbite that has progressed to tissue death (necrosis). (Custom Medical Stock Photo)

out because of impatience at the slow recovery rate of tissue that has suffered deep frostbite; amputation is only necessary when infection has set in and it cannot be controlled with antibiotics.

If possible, deep frostbite should be treated under hospital care, not in the field or outdoors. The deep frozen tissue should remain frozen until hospital care is available. If frozen tissues are thawed, the patient will most likely be unable to move as the pain will be severe with any movement. Walking on feet that have been thawed after being frozen will cause permanent damage; however, walking on a frozen foot for twelve to eighteen hours or even longer produces less damage than inadequate warming. As frozen tissue thaws, cells exude fluid. If this tissue is refrozen, ice crystals form and cause more extensive, irreparable damage.

Rapid rewarming is the recommended treatment for deep frostbite and is a proven method of reducing tissue loss. Rubbing the frostbitten area with the hand or snow—akin to rubbing the area with broken glass— should never be done. This treatment does not melt the intracellular ice crystals, nor does it increase circulation to the frozen area. It breaks the skin and allows infection to enter into the system. Vasodilator agents do not improve tissue survival. Local antibiotics in aerosol form can be used, but it is unwise to rely on this method alone for combating infection. Sympathectomy, the removal or destruction of affected nerves, does not improve cell survival. The use of the drug dextran early to prevent sludging has limited use and may have dangerous side effects. The use of hyperbaric oxygen or supplementary oxygen may increase the tissue tension of oxygen and save some cells partially damaged by cold injury.

Rewarming should be carried out in a water bath with water temperatures ranging from 37.7 to 42.2 degrees Celsius (100 to 108 degrees Fahrenheit). Higher temperatures will further damage already injured tissues. Rewarming in a large bathtub warms the frozen extremity more rapidly, resulting in less tissue loss in many cases, particularly where frostbite has been deep and extensive. A large container also permits more accurate control of the water temperature. If a bathtub is not available, a bucket, large wastebasket, dishpan, or other similar container can be used. During rewarming, hot water usually must be added to the bath occasionally to keep the temperature correct; in such cases the injured extremity should be removed from the bath and not returned to it until the water has been thoroughly mixed and its temperature measured. An open flame

must not come into contact with the area to which heat is applied, since sensation is lost as a result of the frostbite and the tissue could be seriously burned.

For rewarming, the extremity should be stripped of all clothing, and any constricting bands, straps, or other objects that might stop circulation should be removed. The injured area should be suspended in the center of the water and not permitted to rest against the side or bottom. Warming should continue for thirty to forty minutes. The frostbitten tissues may become quite painful during this process, so it may be necessary to give painkillers to the patient in order to reduce discomfort during or after thawing of the frostbitten area. Aspirin (as well as codeine, morphine, or meperidine, if needed) may be given for pain. Aspirin or an anticoagulant increases blood circulation by reducing red blood cell platelet formation and thus reducing sludging. Phenoxybenzamine reduces vasoconstriction.

Following rewarming, the patient must be kept warm and the injured tissue elevated and protected from any kind of trauma. One should avoid rupturing blisters that have formed. Blankets or bedclothes should be supported by a framework to avoid pressure or rubbing of the injured area.

Subsequent care is directed primarily toward preventing infection. Cleanliness of the frostbitten area is extremely important. It should be soaked daily in a water bath at body temperature to which a germicidal soap has been added. If contamination of the water supply is a possibility, the bath water should be boiled and cooled before use. Dead tissue should not be cut or pulled away; the water baths remove such tissue more efficiently.

The afflicted area should be immobilized and kept sterile. Even contact with sheets can be damaging to a frostbitten limb. Sterile, dry cotton may be placed between the fingers or toes to avoid maceration. If infection appears present, as indicated by the area between the frostbitten tissue and healthy tissue becoming inflamed and feeling tender or throbbing, antibiotics such as ampicillin or cloxicillin should be given every six hours. Wet, antiseptic dressings should be applied if gangrene occurs in the damaged tissue. A tetanus toxoid booster shot, or human antitoxin if the patient has not been previously immunized against tetanus, should be given. Complete rest and a diet high in protein will help healing. Moderate movement of the afflicted area should be encouraged but should be limited to that done by a physical therapist, without assistance by the patient. Considerable reassurance and emotional support may be required by the patient, as the appearance of the frostbitten area can be alarming.

Amputation in response to infected, spreading gangrene may be needed eventually, but it should be delayed until the natural separation of dead from living tissue and bone has taken place. Radionucleotide scanning helps save frostbitten limbs. These scans accurately demonstrate blood flow in frostbitten extremities, thus predicting what tissue will survive.

PERSPECTIVE AND PROSPECTS

Frostbite is an injury that can affect anyone who works or plays under cold conditions. Increased knowledge about what causes this injury, better equipment, and techniques that minimize its effect, however, have reduced its occurrence. Advances in medical knowledge regarding how the injury occurs within the afflicted tissues have produced treatment protocols that reduce the extent of permanent injury from frostbite.

Prevention is the most effective treatment for frostbite, which can occur only when the body lacks enough heat to keep the extremities above freezing. The overall body heat deficit results from inadequate clothing or equipment, reduced food consumption, exhaustion, injury or inactivity causing a lack of body movement, or some combination of these factors. Those playing or working in a cold environment should know the conditions under which frostbite may develop. For frostnip to occur, the windchill index must exceed 1,400 and the air temperature must be below the freezing point of exposed skin (−0.53 degree Celsius). An ambient temperature of −10 to −15 degrees Celsius is usually necessary for deep frostbite to develop.

Adequate clothing—especially boots that allow circulation to occur freely, mittens (not gloves) that cover the hands, and a head covering that protects the face, ears, and neck—must be worn. Boots should be well broken in and large enough to fit comfortably with several pairs of socks. The laces at the top of the boots should not be tight. Gaiters or overboots should be worn if deep or wet snow is anticipated. Windproof or insulated pants protect the legs from cold and help keep the feet warm. Dry socks and mitten liners should be carried. Moisture greatly reduces the insulative value of clothing, so it is necessary to stay dry; if clothing becomes wet or damp, one should change into dry items. Plastic bags, worn over bare feet, provide a vapor barrier liner that is effective in helping keep one's feet dry and warm under cold conditions. Adequate ventilation avoids dampness from excessive perspiration. Dress-

ing in layers—having several light shirts, jackets, or a windbreaker—is better than wearing only one heavy jacket.

Heat production, resulting from exercise or the protective mechanism of shivering, is just as important as clothing in maintaining body temperature. Injuries that cause the victim to go into shock or lie immobilized, even though adequate clothing may be worn, predispose the victim to frostbite.

Eating high-energy foods and taking in 6,000 or more kilocalories (Calories) a day may be necessary to keep body temperatures constant under very cold or physically demanding conditions. Adequate rest, including eight or more hours of sleep, helps to reduce fatigue, which in turn increases the body's ability to produce heat. Alcohol and tobacco should be strictly avoided. Alcohol dilates the blood vessels and, although this action temporarily warms the skin, results in increased loss of total body heat. Smoking constricts the blood vessels in the skin and so reduces heat flow to surface areas; this may be sufficient to initiate frostbite in exposed tissue. A person who has sustained frostbite in the past is usually more susceptible to more cold injury. Problems with arthritis may develop in extremities that have been frostbitten.

—*David L. Chesemore, Ph.D.*

See also Amputation; Cyanosis; Gangrene; Hyperbaric oxygen therapy; Hyperthermia and hypothermia; Skin; Skin disorders.

FOR FURTHER INFORMATION:

Calvert, John H., Jr. "Frostbite." *Flying Safety* 54, no. 10 (October, 1998): 24-25. Frostbite can be a painful and disfiguring injury, caused by the freezing of the moisture in one's body tissues. Steps for taking care of frostbite injuries are presented.

Phillips, David. "How Frostbite Performs Its Misery." *Canadian Geographic* 115, no. 1 (January/February, 1995): 20-21. This article explains the progression of frostbite and discusses its causes. Illustrated with photographs.

Tilton, Buck. *Backcountry First Aid and Extended Care.* 5th ed. Guilford, Conn.: Falcon, 2007. A small, portable guide to the myriad emergencies and medical problems encountered in the wilderness.

_____. "The Chill That Bites." *Backpacker* 28, no. 7 (September, 2000): 27. Tilton offers important information about windchill, frostbite, and appropriate attire for braving the cold.

Tredget, Edward E., ed. *Thermal Injuries.* Philadelphia: W. B. Saunders, 2000. Examines wounds such as burns and frostbite and their surgical treatments.

Wilkerson, James A., ed. *Medicine for Mountaineering and Other Wilderness Activities.* 5th ed. Seattle: The Mountaineers Books, 2001. This book is a first-aid manual that goes beyond traditional treatment protocols. It was written for those who need information to care for serious injuries when organized medical help is not available.

FRUCTOSEMIA
DISEASE/DISORDER

ANATOMY OR SYSTEM AFFECTED: Gastrointestinal system, intestines, kidneys, liver

SPECIALTIES AND RELATED FIELDS: Biochemistry, genetics, nutrition, pediatrics

DEFINITION: An inborn error of metabolism in which eating foods containing fructose or sucrose will result in high blood fructose levels.

CAUSES AND SYMPTOMS

Fructosemia may also be called hereditary fructose intolerance; it literally means "fructose in the blood." Fructosemia occurs as a result of a hereditary lack of an enzyme called fructose-1-phosphate aldolase B. This autosomal recessive disease is rare, although some researchers suspect that more people have the disorder than are diagnosed. These individuals may naturally avoid fructose after becoming ill following the consumption of fructose-containing foods. The infant, child, or adult with undiagnosed fructosemia will be normal unless foods containing fructose, sucrose, or sorbitol are eaten. If foods containing these carbohydrates are eaten, then fructose levels will increase in the patient's blood and urine and the person will become ill. Symptoms include vomiting and low blood glucose and may progress to failure to thrive and/or coma. The severity of the disease appears to be variable, being rather mild in some individuals and causing death in others. In severe cases, the liver, kidneys, and intestines may be affected, although this damage usually reverses with the elimination of dietary fructose.

TREATMENT AND THERAPY

Treatment for this disorder is entirely dietary. Foods containing fructose, sucrose, or sorbitol must be eliminated from the diet. Fructose is often thought of as "fruit sugar," but far more foods than fruits and juices must be eliminated. Honey contains fructose. Because

---

INFORMATION ON FRUCTOSEMIA

CAUSES: Genetic enzyme deficiency

SYMPTOMS: Variable; may include vomiting, low blood glucose, failure to thrive, and coma if foods containing fructose, sucrose, or sorbitol are eaten

DURATION: Chronic

TREATMENTS: Avoidance of foods containing fructose, sucrose, or sorbitol

---

half of sucrose becomes fructose when sucrose is metabolized, all foods containing sucrose (sugar) must be eliminated as well. This includes all sugar, whether from cane, beets, or sorghum. Sucrose is also part of maple syrup. Sorbitol metabolism also produces fructose, and so this sugar substitute must be avoided as well. Some infant formulas and baby foods may contain fructose, and many sweetened fruit beverages do. Reading food labels and being familiar with the ingredients of restaurant food is imperative for those with fructosemia.

PERSPECTIVE AND PROSPECTS

Cases of fructosemia were first described in the mid-1950's. Soon after, the biochemical pathway defect was discovered. Today, genetic counseling may be of benefit to those who have fructosemia and want to have children, although strict avoidance of the three carbohydrates fructose, sucrose, and sorbitol will prevent symptoms.

—*Karen Chapman-Novakofski, R.D., L.D., Ph.D.*

See also Endocrine disorders; Endocrinology; Endocrinology, pediatric; Enzyme therapy; Enzymes; Galactosemia; Genetic diseases; Lactose intolerance; Metabolic disorders; Metabolism; Nutrition.

FOR FURTHER INFORMATION:

Ali, M., et al. "Hereditary Fructose Intolerance." *Journal of Medical Genetics* 35, no. 5 (May, 1998): 353-365.

Cox, T. M. "Aldolase B and Fructose Intolerance." *FASEB Journal* 8, no. 1 (January, 1994): 62-71.

Steinmann, Beat, René Santer, and Georges van den Berghe. "Disorders of Fructose Metabolism." In *Inborn Metabolic Diseases: Diagnosis and Treatment,* edited by John Fernandes et al. 4th rev. ed. New York: Springer, 2006.

FUNGAL INFECTIONS

DISEASE/DISORDER

ANATOMY OR SYSTEM AFFECTED: Immune system, nails, respiratory system, skin

SPECIALTIES AND RELATED FIELDS: Dermatology, family medicine, immunology, internal medicine, microbiology, pulmonary medicine

DEFINITION: Infections caused by fungi—simple, plantlike organisms—that range from minor skin diseases to serious, disseminated diseases of the lungs and other organs; patients whose immune systems are impaired are at greater risk of serious fungal infections.

KEY TERMS:

asexual reproduction: the production of new individuals without the mating of two parents of unlike genotype, such as by budding

mycelium: a collection of threadlike fungal strands (hyphae) making up the thallus, or nonreproductive portion, of a fungus

mycosis: a disease of humans, plants, or animals caused by a fungus; the prefix myco- means "fungus," hence mycology (the study of fungi)

pleomorphic fungus: a fungus whose morphology changes markedly from one phase of its life cycle to another, or according to changes in environmental conditions

tinea: a medical term for fungal skin diseases, such as ringworm and athlete's foot, caused by a variety of fungi

yeast: a unicellular fungus which reproduces by budding off smaller cells from the parent cell; yeasts belong to several different groups of fungi, and some fungi are capable of growing either as a yeast or as a filamentous fungus

TYPES OF FUNGUS

The term "fungus" is a general one for plantlike organisms that do not produce their own food through photosynthesis but live as heterotrophs, absorbing complex carbon compounds from other living or dead organisms. Fungi were formerly classified in the plant kingdom (together with bacteria, all algae, mosses, and green plants); more recently, biologists have realized that there are fundamental differences in cell structure and organization separating the lower plants into a number of groups which merit recognition as kingdoms. Fungi differ from bacteria and actinomycetes in being eukaryotic, that is, in having an organized nucleus with chromosomes within the cell. One division of fungi, which is believed to be distantly related to certain aquatic algae, has spores that swim by means of flagella. These water molds include pathogens of fish and aquatic insect larvae and a few economically important plant pathogens, but none have yet been recorded as causing a defined, nonopportunistic human disease. The other division of fungi lacks flagellated spores at any stage in its life cycle. It encompasses most familiar fungi, including molds, mushrooms, yeasts, wood-rotting fungi, leaf spots, and all fungi reliably reported to cause disease in humans.

Fungi that lack flagellated stages in their life cycles are further divided into three classes and one form-class according to the manner in which the spores are produced. The first of these, the Zygomycetes (for example *Rhizopus*, the black bread mold), produce thick-walled, solitary sexual spores as a result of hyphal fusion; they are a diverse assemblage including many parasites of insects. Species in the genus *Mucor* cause a rare, fulminating, rapidly fatal systemic disease called mucormycosis, generally in acidotic diabetic patients. The Basidiomycetes, characterized by the production of sexual spores externally on a club-shaped structure called a basidium, include mushrooms, plant rusts (such as stem rust of wheat), and most wood-rotting fungi. There is one important basidiomycetous human pathogen (*Filobasidiella neoformans*) and a few confirmed opportunists. The Ascomycetes, including most yeasts and lichens, many plant pathogens (such as Dutch elm disease and chestnut blight), and a great diversity of saprophytes growing on wood and herbaceous material, produce sexual spores in a saclike structure called an ascus. One ascomycete, *Piedraia nigra*, regularly produces its characteristic fruiting bod-

---

INFORMATION ON FUNGAL INFECTIONS

CAUSES: Invasion of body tissues or organs by fungi

SYMPTOMS: Varies; can include vascular constriction leading to gangrene of limbs, hallucinations, discolored patches on skin, localized inflammation, thrush, chronic localized tumors, pulmonary infection, miscarriage

DURATION: Acute or chronic with recurring episodes

TREATMENTS: Antifungal agents, antibiotics, chemotherapy

ies on its human host; others do so in culture. In addition, there is a form-class Deuteromycetes consisting of fungi that produce only asexual spores. Most are suspected of being stages in the life cycle of Ascomycetes, but some are Basidiomycetes or are of uncertain affinity. Human pathogens, at least as they occur on the host or in typical laboratory culture, are mostly Deuteromycetes.

Medical mycology would occupy only a single chapter in a book on the relationship of fungi to human affairs. Relatively few fungi have become adapted to living as parasites of human (or even mammalian) hosts, and of these, the most common ones cause superficial and cutaneous mycoses with annoying but scarcely life-threatening effects. Serious fungal diseases are mercifully rare among people with normally functioning immune systems.

The majority of fungi are directly dependent on green plants, as parasites, as symbionts living in a mutually beneficial association with a plant, or as saprophytes on dead plant material. One large, successful group of Ascomycetes lives in symbiotic association with algae, forming lichens. Fungi play a critical ecological role in maintaining stable plant communities. As plant pathogens, they cause serious economic loss, leading in extreme cases to famine. The ability of saprophytic fungi to transform chemically the substrate on which they are growing has been exploited by the brewing industry since antiquity and has been expanded to other industrial processes. Penicillin, other antibiotics, and some vitamins are extracted from fungi, which produce a vast array of complex organic compounds whose potential is only beginning to be explored and which constitutes a fertile field for those interested in genetic engineering.

This same chemical diversity and complexity also enable fungi to produce mycotoxins—chemicals that have an adverse effect on humans and animals. Saprophytic fungi growing on improperly stored food are a troublesome source of toxic compounds, some of which are carcinogenic. The old adage that "a little mold won't hurt you" is true in the sense that common molds do not cause acute illness when ingested, but it is poor advice in terms of long-term health.

A mycotoxicity problem of considerable medical and veterinary interest is posed by Ascomycetes of the order Clavicipitales, which are widespread on grasses. Some species of grasses routinely harbor systemic, asymptomatic infections by these fungi, which produce compounds toxic to animals that graze on them. From the point of view of the grass, the relationship is symbiotic, since it discourages grazing; from the point of view of range management, the relationship is deleterious to stock. *Claviceps purpurea*, a pathogen of rye, causes a condition known as ergotism in humans, with symptoms including miscarriage, vascular constriction leading to gangrene of the limbs, and hallucinations. Outbreaks of hallucinatory ergotism are thought by some authors to be responsible for some of the more spectacular perceptions of witchcraft in premodern times. Better control of plant disease and a decreased reliance on rye as a staple grain have virtually eliminated ergotism as a human disease in the twentieth century.

Fungi exhibit a bewildering variety of forms and life cycles; nevertheless, certain generalizations can be made. A fungus starts life as a spore, which may be a single cell or a cluster of cells and is usually microscopic. Under proper conditions, the spore germinates, producing a filament of fungal cells oriented end to end, called a hypha. Hyphae grow into the substrate, secreting enzymes that dissolve structures to provide food for the growing fungus and to provide holes through which the fungus can grow. In an asexually reproducing fungus, some of the hyphae become differentiated, producing specialized cells (spores) which differ from the parent hypha in size and pigmentation and are adapted for dispersal, but which are genetically identical to the parent. In a sexually reproducing fungus, two hyphae (or a hypha and a spore from different individuals) fuse, their nuclei fuse, and meiosis takes place before spores are formed. Spores are often produced in a specialized fruiting body, such as a mushroom.

Fungus spores are ubiquitous. Common saprophytic fungi produce airborne spores in enormous quantities; thus it is difficult to avoid contact with them in all but the most hypersterile environments. In culture, fungi (including pathogenic species) produce large numbers of dry spores that can be transmitted in the air from host to host, making working with fungi in a medical laboratory potentially hazardous.

FUNGAL DISEASES AND TREATMENTS
Human fungal diseases are generally placed in four broad categories according to the tissues they attack, and they are further subdivided according to specific pathologies and the organisms involved. The categories of disease are superficial mycoses, cutaneous mycoses, subcutaneous mycoses, and systemic mycoses.

Superficial mycoses affect hair and the outermost layer of the epidermis and do not evoke a cellular response. They include tinea versicolor and tinea nigra, deutermycete infections that cause discolored patches on skin, and black piedra, caused by an ascomycete growing on hair shafts. They can be treated with a topical fungicide, such as nystatin, or, in the case of piedra, by shaving off the affected hair.

Cutaneous mycoses involve living cells of the skin or mucous membrane and evoke a cellular response, generally localized inflammation. Dermatomycoses (dermatophytes), which affect skin and hair, include tinea capitis (ringworm of the scalp), tinea pedis (athlete's foot), and favus, a scaly infection of the scalp. Domestic animals serve as a reservoir for some cutaneous mycoses. The organisms responsible are generally fungi imperfecti in the genera Microsporon and Trichophyton. Cutaneous mycoses can be successfully treated with topical nystatin or oral griseofulvin.

Candida albicans, a ubiquitous pleomorphic fungus with both a yeast and a mycelial form, causes a variety of cutaneous mycoses as well as systemic infections collectively named candidiasis. Thrush is a *Candida* yeast infection of the mouth which is most common in infants, especially in infants born to mothers with vaginal candidiasis. Vaginal yeast infections periodically affect 18 to 20 percent of the adult female population and more than 30 percent of pregnant women. *Candida* also causes paronychia, a nailbed infection. Small populations of *Candida* are normally present in the alimentary tract and genital tract of healthy individuals; candidiasis of the mucous membranes tends to develop in response to antibiotic treatment, which disturbs the normal bacterial flora of the body, or in response to metabolic changes or decreasing immune function.

None of the organisms causing cutaneous mycoses elicits a lasting immune response, so recurring infections by these agents is the rule rather than the exception. Even in temperate climates, under modern standards of hygiene, cutaneous mycoses are extremely common.

Subcutaneous mycoses, affecting skin and muscle tissue, are predominantly tropical in distribution and not particularly common. Chromomycosis and maduromycosis are caused by soil fungi that enter the skin through wounds, causing chronic localized tumors, usually on the feet. Sporotrichosis enters through wounds and spreads through the lymphatic system, causing skin ulcers associated with lymph nodes. Amphotericin B, a highly toxic systemic antifungal agent, has been used to treat all three conditions; potassium iodide is used to treat sporotrichosis, and localized chromomycosis and maduromycosis lesions can be surgically removed.

Systemic mycoses, the most serious of fungal infections, have the ability to become generally disseminated in the body. The main nonopportunistic systemic mycoses known in North America are histoplasmosis, caused by *Histoplasma capsulatum*; coccidiomycosis, caused by *Coccidiodes immitis*; blastomycosis, caused by *Ajellomyces* (or *Blastomyces*) *dermatidis*; and cryptococcosis, caused by *Cryptococcus* (or *Filobasidiella*) *neoformans*. Similar infections, caused by related species, occur in other parts of the world.

Coccidiomycosis, also called San Joaquin Valley fever or valley fever, will serve as an example of the etiology of systemic mycoses. The causative organism lives in arid soils in the American southwest; its spores are wind-disseminated. When inhaled, the fungus grows in the lungs, producing a mild respiratory infection which is self-limiting in perhaps 95 percent of the cases. The mild form of the disease is common in rural areas. In a minority of cases, a chronic lung disease whose symptoms resemble tuberculosis develops. There is also a disseminated form of the disease producing meningitis; chronic cutaneous disease, with the production of ulcers and granulomas; and attack of the bones, internal organs, and lymphatic system. A chronic pulmonary infection may become systemic in response to factors that undermine the body's immune system. Factors involved in individual susceptibility among individuals with intact immune systems are poorly understood.

Histoplasmosis (also known as summer fever, cave fever, or Mississippi Valley fever) is even more common; 90 percent of people tested in the southern Mississippi Valley show a positive reaction to this fungus, indicating prior, self-limiting lung infection. The fungus is associated with bird and bat droppings, and severe cases sometimes occur when previously unexposed individuals are exposed to high levels of innoculum in caves where bats roost. A related organism, *Histoplasma duboisii*, occurs in central Africa. Blastomycosis causes chronic pulmonary disease, chronic cutaneous disease, and systemic disease, all of which were usually fatal until the advent of chemotherapy with amphotericin B. The natural habitat of the fungus is unclear. *Cryptococcus neoformans* occurs in pigeon droppings and is worldwide in distribution. The subclinical pulmonary form of the disease is probably common; invasive disease occurs in patients with collagen diseases, such as lupus, and in patients with weakened immune systems. It is the leading cause of invasive fungal disease in patients with acquired immunodeficiency syndrome (AIDS).

Systemic fungal diseases are notoriously difficult to treat. Chemotherapy of systemic, organismally caused diseases depends on finding a chemical compound which will selectively kill or inhibit the invading organism without damaging the host. Therefore, the more closely the parasite species is related biologically to the host species, the more difficult it is to find a compound which will act in such a selective manner. Fungi are, from a biological standpoint, more like humans than they are like bacteria, and antibacterial antibiotics are ineffective against them. If a fungus has invaded the skin or the digestive tract, it can be attacked with toxic substances that are not readily absorbed into the bloodstream, but this approach is not appropriate for a systemic infection. Amphotericin, intraconazole, and fluconazole, the drugs of choice for systemic fungal infections, are highly toxic to humans. Thus, dosage is critical, close clinical supervision is necessary, and long-term therapy may not be feasible.

Perspective and Prospects

Medical mycology textbooks written before 1980 tended to focus on two categories of fungal infection: the common, ubiquitous, and comparatively benign superficial and cutaneous mycoses, frequently seen in clinical practice in the industrialized world, and the subcutaneous and deep mycoses, treated as a rare and/ or predominantly tropical problem. Opportunistic systemic infections, if mentioned at all, were regarded as a rare curiosity.

The rising population of patients with compromised immune systems, including cancer patients undergoing chemotherapy, people being treated with steroids for various conditions, transplant patients, and people with AIDS, has dramatically changed this clinical picture. Between 1980 and 1986, more than a hundred fungi, a few previously unknown and the majority common inhabitants of crop plants, rotting vegetable debris, and soil, were identified as causing human disease. The number continues to increase steadily. Compared to organisms routinely isolated from soil and plants, these opportunistic fungi do not seem to have any special characteristics other than the ability to grow at human body temperature; however, the possibility that an opportunistic pathogen might mutate into a form capable of attacking healthy humans is worrisome.

Systemic opportunistic human infections have been attributed to *Alternaria alternata* and *Fusarium oxysporum*, common plant pathogens that cause diseases of tomatoes and strawberries, respectively. Several species of *Aspergillus*, saprophytic molds (many of them thermophilic), have long been implicated in human disease. Colonizing aspergillosis, involving localized growth in the lungs of people exposed to high levels of aspergillus spores (notably agricultural workers working with silage), is not particularly rare among people with normal immune systems, but the more severe invasive form of the disease, in which massive lung lesions form, and disseminated aspergillosis, in which other organs are attacked, almost always involve immunocompromised patients. *Ramichloridium schulzeri*, described originally from wheat roots, causes "golden tongue" in leukemia patients; fortunately this infection responds to amphotericin B. *Scelidosporium inflatum*, first isolated from a serious bone infection in an immunocompromised patient in 1984, is being isolated with increasing frequency in cases of disseminated mycosis; it resists standard drug treatment.

Oral colonization by strains of *Candida* is often the first sign of AIDS-related complex or full-blown AIDS in an individual harboring the human immunodeficiency virus (HIV). Drug therapy with fluconazole is effective against oral candidiasis, but relapse rates of up to 50 percent within a month of the cessation of drug therapy are reported. Reported rates of disseminated candidiasis in AIDS patients range from 1 to 10 percent. Invasive procedures such as intravenous catheters represent a significant risk of introducing *Candida* and other common fungi into the bloodstream of patients.

Pneumocystis carinii, the organism causing a form of pneumonia which is the single most important cause of death in patients with AIDS, was originally classified as a sporozoan—that is, as a parasitic protozoan—but detailed investigations of the life cycle, metabolism, and genetic material of *Pneumocystis* have convinced some biologists that it is actually an ascomycete, although an anomalous one that lacks a cell wall. Unfortunately, it does not respond to therapy with the antifungal drugs currently in use.

In general, antifungal drug therapy for mycoses in AIDS patients is not very successful. In the absence of significant patient immunity, it is difficult to eradicate a disseminated infection from the body entirely, making a resurgence likely once drug therapy is discontinued. Reinfection is also likely if the organism is a common component of the patient's environment.

Given the increasing number of lethal systemic fungal infections seen in clinical practice, there is substantial impetus for a search for more effective, less toxic antifungal drugs. A number of compounds, produced by bacteria and chemically dissimilar to both antibacterial antibiotics and the most widely used antifungal compounds, have been identified and are being tested. It is also possible that the plant kingdom, which has been under assault by fungi for all its long geologic history, may prove a source for medically useful antifungal compounds.

—*Martha Sherwood-Pike, Ph.D.*

See also Acquired immunodeficiency syndrome (AIDS); Aspergillosis; Athlete's foot; Candidiasis; Diaper rash; Food poisoning; Immune system; Immunodeficiency disorders; Immunology; Immunopathology; Microbiology; Mold and mildew; Nail removal; Nails; Pneumonia; Poisonous plants; Ringworm; Skin; Skin disorders.

FOR FURTHER INFORMATION:

Alcamo, I. Edward. *Microbes and Society: An Introduction to Microbiology.* Sudbury, Mass.: Jones and Bartlett, 2002. A nonscientific text for the liberal arts student that explores the importance of microbes to human life and their role in food production and agriculture, in biotechnology and industry, in ecology and the environment, and in disease and bioterrorism.

Biddle, Wayne. *A Field Guide to Germs.* 2d ed. New York: Anchor Books, 2002. This comprehensive book is easily accessible to the nonspecialist and includes a discussion of nearly every virus, bacterium, and fungus known to cause human and nonhuman animal disease. The history of the microbe and the treatment of diseases are included.

Carlile, Michael J., Sarah Watkinson, and Graham W. Gooday. *Fungi.* 2d ed. San Diego, Calif.: Academic Press, 2001. Text that takes a microbiological perspective and introduces the importance of fungi in the natural world and in practical applications. The diversity of fungi as organisms and their roles in relation to people, animals, and plants are clearly described.

Crissey, John Thorne, Heidi Lang, and Lawrence Charles Parish. *Manual of Medical Mycology.* Cambridge, Mass.: Blackwell Scientific, 1995. This handbook discusses the diagnosis and treatment of fungal infections. Includes a bibliography and an index.

Kumar, Vinay, Abul K. Abbas, and Nelson Fausto, eds. *Robbins and Cotran Pathologic Basis of Disease.* 7th ed. Philadelphia: Elsevier Saunders, 2005. A leading medical textbook that covers the major topics of general and systemic pathology.

Mandell, Gerald L., John E. Bennett, and Raphael Dolin, eds. *Mandell, Douglas, and Bennett's Principles and Practice of Infectious Diseases.* 6th ed. New York: Elsevier/Churchill Livingstone, 2005. An outstanding textbook on infectious diseases, with chapters on the various diseases caused by *Candida*, illnesses and conditions associated with this fungus, and antifungal agents.

Murray, Patrick R., Ken S. Rosenthal, and Michael A. Pfaller. *Medical Microbiology.* 5th ed. Philadelphia: Elsevier/Mosby, 2005. Focuses on microbes that cause disease in humans. Each chapter consistently presents the etiology, epidemiology, host defenses, identification, diagnosis, prevention, and control of each disease.

Rippon, John Willard. *Medical Mycology: The Pathogenic Fungi and Pathogenic Actinomycetes.* 3d ed. Philadelphia: W. B. Saunders, 1988. A standard medical mycology textbook for students of medicine and microbiology, with detailed descriptions of common mycoses and the organisms that cause them, as an aid to clinical diagnosis.

Shaw, Michael, ed. *Everything You Need to Know About Diseases.* Springhouse, Pa.: Springhouse Press, 1996. This well-illustrated consumer reference, compiled by more than one hundred doctors and medical experts, describes five hundred illnesses and conditions, their causes, symptoms, diagnosis, treatment, and prevention. Of particular interest is chapter 19, "Infection."

Weedon, David. *Skin Pathology.* 2d ed. New York: Harcourt, 2002. Text with extensive photographs, covering tissue reaction patterns; the epidermis, dermis and subcutis; the skin in systemic and miscellaneous diseases; infections and infestations; and tumors, among other topics.

GALACTOSEMIA

DISEASE/DISORDER

ANATOMY OR SYSTEM AFFECTED: Eyes, liver

SPECIALTIES AND RELATED FIELDS: Biochemistry, genetics, nutrition, pediatrics

DEFINITION: An inherited disorder of carbohydrate metabolism in which an infant is unable to utilize galactose from food.

CAUSES AND SYMPTOMS

In classic I galactosemia, a congenital deficiency of the enzyme galactose-1-phosphate uridyl transferase (GALT) causes galactose to accumulate instead of being converted to glucose for energy production. As galactose accumulates in the child's tissues and organs, it will have a toxic effect and cause various signs and symptoms. Galactosemia means "galactose in the blood." Galactose is a sugar that may be found alone in foods but is usually associated with lactose, a milk sugar.

A gene mutation on the short arm of chromosome 9 has been identified in babies with galactosemia. About 1 in 40,000 newborns is affected with this autosomal recessive disorder. Both parents serve as carriers; they are not themselves affected, but there is a one in four chance that one of their children will be born with galactosemia. Prenatal diagnosis is possible in cultured fibroblasts from amniotic fluid. Mandatory screening programs in many states test all newborns for galactosemia during the first week of life.

Galactosemia is an example of a multiple-allele system. In addition to the normal allele (G) and the recessive allele (g), a third allele, known as G^D, has been found. The D allele is named after Duarte, California, where it was discovered. The existence of three alleles produces six possible genotypic combinations in the deoxyribonucleic acid (DNA). These enzymatic activities may range from 0 to 100 percent. Consequently, it is very important to monitor each patient with biochemical studies.

Homozygous recessive infants (gg) are unaffected at birth but develop symptoms a few days later, including jaundice, vomiting, an enlarged liver from extensive fatty deposits, cataracts, and failure to thrive. Mental retardation and death may also occur if dietary treatment has not been started.

TREATMENT AND THERAPY

Galactosemia is treated by removing foods that contain galactose from the diet. Since milk and milk products are the most common source of galactose, infants with galactosemia should not be given these foods. Serious problems can be prevented through this early exclusion of galactose.

While it is not possible for a child with galactosemia to have an entirely galactose-free diet, all persons with galactosemia should limit galactose intake from foods to a very low level. The galactose-1-phosphate levels determine the degree of dietary restriction for each individual. Advice from a dietician is needed.

—Phillip A. Farber, Ph.D.

See also Endocrine system; Endocrinology; Endocrinology, pediatric; Enzyme therapy; Enzymes; Fructosemia; Gaucher's disease; Genetic diseases; Glycogen storage diseases; Lactose intolerance; Mental retardation; Metabolic disorders; Metabolism; Nutrition.

FOR FURTHER INFORMATION:

Cummings, Michael R. *Human Heredity: Principles and Issues.* 7th ed. Belmont, Calif.: Thomson/Brooks/Cole, 2006.

Icon Health. *Galactosemia: A Medical Dictionary, Bibliography, and Annotated Research Guide to Internet References.* San Diego, Calif.: Author, 2004.

Kasper, Dennis L., et al., eds. *Harrison's Principles of Internal Medicine.* 16th ed. New York: McGraw-Hill, 2005.

Rudolph, Colin D., et al., eds. *Rudolph's Pediatrics.* 21st ed. New York: McGraw-Hill, 2003.

INFORMATION ON GALACTOSEMIA

CAUSES: Genetic enzyme deficiency

SYMPTOMS: Varies; may include jaundice, vomiting, liver enlargement, cataracts, failure to thrive, and mental retardation if foods containing galactose (milk sugar) are eaten

DURATION: Chronic

TREATMENTS: Avoidance of foods containing galactose

GALLBLADDER CANCER

DISEASE/DISORDER

ALSO KNOWN AS: Biliary cancer, biliary tract cancer

ANATOMY OR SYSTEM AFFECTED: Gallbladder, gastrointestinal system

SPECIALTIES AND RELATED FIELDS: Gastroenterology, general surgery, oncology, radiology

DEFINITION: A rare type of cancer affecting the gallbladder (a muscular, membranous sac containing bile) and its surrounding organs.

KEY TERMS:

adenocarcinoma: a malignant tumor originating in glandular epithelium

bile: a yellowish-green, viscous fluid secreted by the liver and passed into the duodenum to aid in the breakdown and absorption of fats

cholecystectomy: surgical removal of the gallbladder

gallstones: crystalline accumulations of bile salts within the gallbladder

jaundice: yellowing of the skin, eyes, and other tissues that occurs when bile salts are deposited in these areas of the body

resectable: able to be surgically removed and/or repaired

CAUSES AND SYMPTOMS

The gallbladder is an accessory organ of digestion which stores bile, a yellowish-green, thick fluid produced by the liver. Bile aids in the breakdown and absorption of fats, and it also helps to eliminate waste metabolic products, excess cholesterol, and drugs. Food intake, especially the ingestion of fatty foods, stimulates the release of a hormone, cholecystokinin (CCK), from the small intestine. CCK then stimulates the gallbladder to contract and send bile through the common bile duct and into the duodenum, where fat emulsification and absorption continues.

A rare disease, gallbladder cancer usually occurs in patients who have gallstones. Gallstones form within the gallbladder when bile salts crystallize into hard, rocklike accumulations. These stones may then block the common bile duct, resulting in intense gastrointestinal pain when the gallbladder contracts and tries to squeeze bile into this duct during the process of digestion.

Besides the presence of gallstones, gallbladder cancer has also been associated with high alcohol intake, smoking, obesity, high levels of estrogen, and inflammatory bowel disease (IBD). Patients who have taken certain medications, such as oral contraceptives and methyldopa, may have a higher incidence of this type of cancer. Recent research also indicates that exposure to carcinogens such as asbestos, dioxin, polychlorinated biphenyls (PCBs), and azotoluene may cause gallbladder cancer. The presence in the body of *Salmonella typhi*, a bacterium, may cause chronic gallbladder infections that can lead to cancer.

INFORMATION ON GALLBLADDER CANCER

CAUSES: Possibly gallstones, high alcohol intake, smoking, obesity, high levels of estrogen, inflammatory bowel disease (IBD), carcinogens

SYMPTOMS: Jaundice, extreme itching, nausea, weight loss, abdominal pain

DURATION: Depends on stage, from five or more years to between two and four months; often fatal

TREATMENTS: Surgery

Patients with gallbladder cancer often suffer from jaundice, extreme itching, nausea, unexplained weight loss, and pain in the upper right abdomen or more generalized abdominal pain. Diagnosis of this cancer may sometimes be made with simple tests, such as a complete blood count, liver function test, or chest X ray. More bloodwork may be ordered by a physician to search for a specific tumor marker, CA 19-9, which detects the adenocarcinomas of gallbladder cancer. Usually, however, more extensive testing with ultrasound, computed tomography (CT) scans, and magnetic resonance imaging (MRI) is required. Ultrasonography is useful for detecting gallstones and a "porcelain" (highly calcified) gallbladder. CT scans may show invasion of the cancer into the liver, while MRI can also reveal extension into other tissues. A very specific test for biliary tract cancers called endoscopic retrograde cholangiopancreatography (ERCP) is used to check for blockages in the bile ducts. If a tumor is found to be blocking ducts, then a fine tube may be inserted into the area in an attempt to clear the blockage.

Gallbladder cancer affects about 8,600 adults in the United States each year, with deaths from this ailment occurring in more than 3,000 of these cases. Most patients are female and Native American or Mexican American. Native Americans are five times more likely than the general population to develop gallstones and gallbladder cancer. Women are twice as likely to develop the disease than are men because estrogen, the female sex hormone, causes more cholesterol to be excreted into the bile. High rates of this cancer also occur in Mexico, South America, and Israel. This cancer is usually diagnosed in patients who are in their mid-sixties.

TREATMENT AND THERAPY

Surgical removal of the gallbladder, known as cholecystectomy, is the only cure for gallbladder cancer. Unfortunately, only about 25 percent of patients are able to have successful surgery. Because the symptoms of gallbladder cancer mimic those of many other diseases, a majority of patients come to their doctors with a well-advanced stage of cancer. Of the patients diagnosed with this condition, 40 percent to 60 percent have cancer that has already spread to surrounding tissues. For these patients, surgical removal of the gallbladder is essential, and removal of parts of the liver, small intestine, colon, and nearby lymph nodes may also be required. Approximately 30 percent of patients who are diagnosed already have metastatic disease.

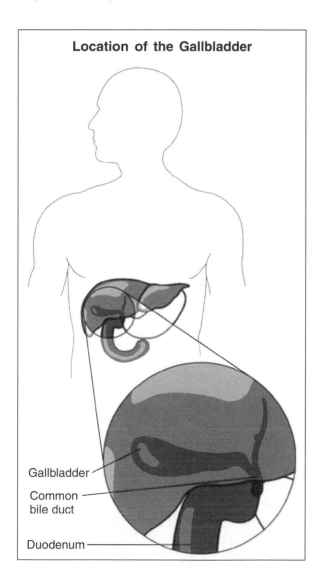

Location of the Gallbladder

Gallbladder

Common
bile duct

Duodenum

As with other cancers, gallbladder cancer is "staged" (the degree of progression of the disease is categorized) according to the tumor, node, metastases (TNM) system of the American Joint Committee on Cancer (AJCC). Stage I and II cancers are localized within the gallbladder and surgically resectable. Stage III cancers have spread to surrounding tissues and are not generally cured by surgery. Stage IV cancers have metastasized.

Radiation therapy is often used as a follow-up to surgery and may help to kill remaining cancer cells. Chemotherapy may also be used after surgery, but oncologists report that it does not work very well for this type of cancer.

PERSPECTIVE AND PROSPECTS

Gallbladder cancer was first diagnosed in 1777. More than two hundred years later, the prognosis for patients with this disease is still generally poor, depending upon the stage of the disease when the patient is first diagnosed. Of patients with stage I and II cancers, 70 percent to 85 percent survive five years or longer. For those with stage III cancer, the five-year survival rate drops to 12 percent, and for those with stage IV, only 1 to 2 percent survive. In the advanced stages of gallbladder cancer, the survival period is usually very short, about two to four months. Hospice referral is considered essential for these patients.

—*Lenela Glass-Godwin, M.WS.*

See also Abdomen; Abdominal disorders; American Indian health; Cancer; Chemotherapy; Cholecystectomy; Cholecystitis; Gallbladder diseases; Gastroenterology; Gastrointestinal diseases; Internal medicine; Jaundice; Radiation therapy; Stone removal; Stones.

FOR FURTHER INFORMATION:

Clavien, Pierre-Alain, and John Baillie, eds. *Diseases of the Gallbladder and Bile Ducts: Diagnosis and Treatment.* 2d ed. Malden, Mass.: Blackwell, 2006.

Gunderson, L. L., and C.G. Willett. "Pancreas and Hepatobiliary Tract." In *Principles and Practice of Radiation Oncology,* edited by C. A. Perez and L. W. Brady. 3d ed. Philadelphia: Lippincott-Raven, 1997.

Laczano-Ponce, E. C., et al. "Epidemiology and Molecular Pathology of Gallbladder Cancer." *CA: A Cancer Journal for Clinicians* 51 (2001): 349-364.

Toner, C. B., et al. "Surgical Treatment of Gallbladder Cancer." *Journal of Gastrointestinal Surgery* 8, no. 1 (January, 2004): 83-89.

GALLBLADDER DISEASES
DISEASE/DISORDER

ANATOMY OR SYSTEM AFFECTED: Abdomen, gallbladder, gastrointestinal system

SPECIALTIES AND RELATED FIELDS: Gastroenterology, internal medicine

DEFINITION: A family of disorders affecting the gallbladder and causing abdominal pain or occasionally symptomless.

KEY TERMS:

bile: a complex solution formed by liver cells which is composed mainly of bile salts, fats, and cholesterol, which aids in fat digestion; it is secreted by the liver into a system of ducts connecting the liver, gallbladder, and intestinal tract

biliary colic: a distinct pain syndrome characterized by severe intermittent waves of right-sided, upper abdominal pain, often brought on by the ingestion of fatty foods; pain occurs when a gallstone obstructs the outflow of bile and usually resolves when the gallstone moves away from the outflow area

cholecystectomy: the surgical procedure that results in the removal of the gallbladder in its entirety; the two main techniques are the traditional open method and the laparoscopically aided method

cholecystitis: the disease that occurs when the gallbladder becomes inflamed or infected, which produces severe right-sided, upper abdominal pain, fever, and other signs of infection; a frequent indication for removal of the gallbladder

cholelithiasis: the presence of gallstones in the gallbladder

gallbladder: a muscular, walled sac located on the under surface of the liver which stores and concentrates bile; under stimulus from the intestine in response to a meal, the gallbladder contracts and expels bile into the digestive tract to aid in fat digestion

gallstones: particles that form in the gallbladder when the solubility of the components of bile is somehow altered, also resulting in the precipitation of cholesterol; the gallstones, which can grow very large, are made up mostly of cholesterol but can be pigmented or contain other substances

laparoscopic cholecystectomy: a procedure in which the gallbladder is removed with the help of a telescopic eyepiece which is attached to a tube inserted into the patient's body; the surgery is done using four small incisions and allows the patient to recover much faster than the traditional method of open surgery

CAUSES AND SYMPTOMS

Gallbladder diseases affect a large number of patients and are among the most common causes of abdominal pain. Most gallbladder problems stem from the presence of gallstones, which may be present in as many as one of every ten adults. In the past, anyone with gallstones was advised to have the gallbladder taken out, but this is no longer the case. It is now known that many people with gallstones never experience difficulty because of them.

A very common gallbladder disease is biliary colic. This is usually manifested by severe right-sided, upper abdominal pain that is fairly repetitive in nature. The pain may literally take the patient's breath away, but an episode usually lasts less than thirty minutes. The patient may also complain of right-sided shoulder or back pain, often caused by irritation of the diaphragmatic nerves, which are located just above the liver on the right side. Many people may confuse the pain of biliary colic with indigestion, because in some patients it may be experienced in the middle of the upper abdomen. This pain is almost always brought on by eating, since the gallbladder contracts in response to food in the intestinal tract. The meal triggering such an episode often is described as rich and fatty, and many patients soon learn what types of food to avoid. Biliary colic does not occur unless gallstones are present, because they tend to obstruct the outflow of bile from the gallbladder. The treatment for biliary colic usually consists of dietary manipulation, that is, the avoidance of fatty foods or other foods known to trigger the pain. Surgery is performed if the patient so desires, and removing the gallbladder should cure the problem.

When a diagnosis of gallstones is suspected, the physician will take down the patient's medical history and perform a physical examination. In most cases, however, such actions will yield no physical findings that are indicative of gallstone disease. Thus the diagnosis

---

INFORMATION ON GALLBLADDER DISEASES

CAUSES: Presence of gallstones

SYMPTOMS: Varies; often includes severe and repetitive right-sided, upper abdominal pain; inflammation and infection; chills or fever

DURATION: Acute

TREATMENTS: Surgery, dietary management

is usually confirmed by an imaging study of the gall-bladder, in which the gallstones are either directly or indirectly visualized. The most commonly used imaging modality is the ultrasound test, which can be easily and rapidly performed with very reliable results. While the gallstones cannot actually be seen, they have a density which reflects, rather than transmits, sound waves. As a result, they create specific echoes and shadows that can be interpreted by the radiologists as gallstones. No patient should be treated for gallstone disease without such imaging to confirm the presence of gallstones.

A potentially serious type of gallbladder disease caused by gallstones is acute cholecystitis. In this condition, the outflow of bile is obstructed, usually by a gallstone that is stuck in the outflow tract, and severe inflammation and infection may develop. A patient with acute cholecystitis often complains of pain that does not go away promptly, may have chills or fever, and is usually found to have a very tender abdomen on the upper right side. The treatment of this condition is not controversial, and most physicians would probably recommend removing the gallbladder surgically. The only question remaining is whether the gallbladder should be removed immediately or electively, at a later date, if the patient recovers from acute cholecystitis with conservative management, including the use of antibiotics and the avoidance of eating until the inflammation subsides.

Inflammation and infection can also occur, although rarely, in gallbladders that do not produce gallstones. This happens in very select circumstances and is called acute acalculous cholecystitis. It usually afflicts very ill patients who have been in an intensive care unit for a long time, patients who have needed a heart-lung machine as a result of open heart surgery, or patients who are unable to eat for an extended period of time because of other problems. These patients are often fed only intravenously, which can lead to severe gallbladder problems. The exact mechanisms are not entirely known, but alterations in blood flow and an impaired ability to fight infection may play a role. Whatever the cause, the treatment often remains the same: removal of the gallbladder that does not respond to conservative therapy.

Gallstones can also move out of the gallbladder and cause serious problems. The main outflow tract of bile from the gallbladder and liver is the common bile duct, and this is a place gallstones frequently lodge. The end of this duct is surrounded by a small muscle called the sphincter of Oddi, which may not allow the passage of gallstones. If they become stuck there, they can com-

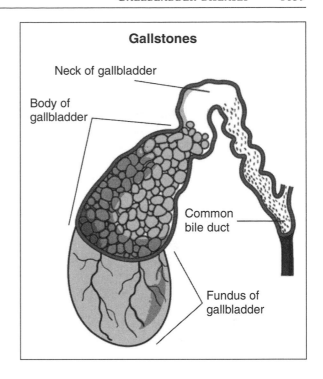

Gallstones

Neck of gallbladder

Body of gallbladder

Common bile duct

Fundus of gallbladder

pletely obstruct the biliary system, and the patient will appear jaundiced. Removal of the gallstones will cure the problem. The presence of gallstones in the common bile duct is also associated with the development of pancreatitis, an inflammation of the pancreas that can be severe and life-threatening. Removal of the gallbladder at an appropriate time will prevent future bouts of pancreatitis.

The gallbladder can also be a source of cancer. Although cancer of the gallbladder is not common, it is estimated that one of every one hundred gallbladders removed will contain cancer. Therefore, all specimens removed must be examined by a qualified pathologist and all reports must be reviewed in their entirety by the surgeon. If the disease is limited to a minor thickness of the gallbladder, no further therapy is needed, but if the tumor is larger, further surgery—including removal of part of the liver—may be necessary. Gallbladder cancer grows silently in many patients, and it is often not detected until late in its course.

TREATMENT AND THERAPY

Because there is no simple way to prevent gallbladder problems, surgery plays a large role in their management. Removing the gallbladder, a relatively routine operation, results in a complete cure, with acceptably low complication rates and few long-term problems.

While several exciting new ways of treating gallbladder and gallstone problems have been developed, the classic and standard method of therapy for gallbladder disease has been open cholecystectomy. This procedure entails making an incision across the upper right side of the abdomen a few inches below and parallel to the bottom of the rib cage. The muscles of the abdominal wall are cut, and the abdominal cavity is opened. The gallbladder, which is usually located right under this incision, is then removed and the incision closed in layers. This method of gallbladder removal has acceptable complication rates and is relatively safe and extremely effective. It allows the surgeon to inspect the entire abdomen and rule out other problems. One must consider, however, that this procedure constitutes major surgery. Most patients need to be in the hospital for a minimum of three to five days, and there is a considerable amount of pain with this incision. These problems have prompted surgeons to find a less invasive way of removing the gallbladder, thereby achieving better pain control and reducing the length of the hospital stay and the time lost from work and other activities.

A laparoscope is an optical instrument, composed of a tube connected to a telescopic eyepiece, that allows the surgeon to perform a procedure inside the patient's body. Although it has been employed in surgeries for many years, mainly in gynecological procedures, it was adapted only recently for removal of the gallbladder, as well as in other types of surgeries. Since then, laparoscopic cholecystectomy has become a procedure that all surgeons must know in order to stay current with the profession. The laparoscope and other surgical instruments are inserted directly into the abdomen through several small incisions, and the gallbladder is removed without a large incision having been made. The patients are often discharged the same day of the surgery, and they return to work much faster than with the open technique.

Despite its advantages, there are some pitfalls with laparoscopic cholecystectomy, and it cannot be used for all patients. There is an increased incidence of certain injuries to other organs and bile ducts at the time of the operation because less of the area can be seen than with an open operation. In addition, patients who have had previous upper abdominal surgery are not candidates for this procedure, and for those with acute cholecystitis, severe inflammation may make this technique unsafe. For most patients, however, laparoscopic cholecystectomy can be performed easily and safely with minimal complications and excellent results. It is be-

coming the standard of care and will continue to change the way gallbladder surgery is performed. The laparoscope is also being used to perform appendectomies, ulcer surgeries, cancer surveillance, and all types of intra-abdominal surgery.

Radiologists and internists may play an important role in the management of gallbladder disease. In certain circumstances, the techniques performed by these specialists may be indicated for extremely ill patients who might not be able to tolerate an operation, or for whom the anesthesia might be too hazardous. Invasive radiologists can actually place a tube into the gallbladder with help from their imaging equipment and remove infection or troublesome gallstones from the gallbladder. This procedure can alleviate symptoms in some patients, who may not even require any additional intervention. These practices are not common, however, and they are usually reserved for the very ill patient who might not survive an open operation or is at extremely high risk to develop a certain complication.

Gallstones can migrate out of the gallbladder and cause problems if they lodge in and obstruct the common bile duct. This places the patient at high risk for developing jaundice and infection in the biliary system. The standard method for dealing with this problem continues to be open surgery. In this procedure, the gallbladder is removed through an incision and the common bile duct is also opened. The gallstones are removed through a variety of techniques, and the duct is then closed. A tube is placed in the duct to keep it open, because otherwise it could scar and become narrowed. Many of these patients must be hospitalized for a number of days, making this surgery an expensive one.

Internists who specialize in the diseases of the abdomen have become proficient at performing endoscopic techniques. These techniques came about after the development of fiber optics, which allow one to see through a tube, even if it is bent at a variety of angles. An endoscope, composed of surgical instruments, a light source, and fiber-optic cables, can be used to examine the lining of the stomach and intestines, allowing the diagnosis of many conditions.

Endoscopy is performed by inserting the endoscope through the mouth and into the patient's stomach and the first part of the intestines. From this location, the area where the common bile duct opens into the intestines can be seen, and this is often where gallstones become lodged. The gallstones can be removed with instruments attached to the scope, thus solving the patient's problem. Unfortunately, this technique does not remove the gallbladder, the source of the gallstones, and the patient is at some risk for a recurrence. This risk can be minimized by enlarging the opening where the duct enters the intestinal tract. This technique, too, is advantageous for patients who are elderly or ill and cannot withstand the trauma of surgery and anesthesia.

There are other options besides surgery or dietary changes for the treatment of patients with gallstones. Medicines are available that can dissolve the gallstones by changing the chemical nature and solubility of bile. Such drugs, however, are not ideal: They work only for certain types of gallstones, are expensive, and may produce side effects. In addition, there may be a recurrence of the gallstones when a patient stops taking these medicines. Such a result indicates that the bile-concentrating action of the gallbladder combines with a given patient's bile composition to create a gallstone-forming environment. Thus, gallstones will continue to form unless the gallbladder is removed or the bile is again altered when the taking of such medicines is resumed. Patients can also have the gallstones broken up into very small pieces, as is often done with kidney stones, by high-frequency sound waves aimed at the gallstones. This procedure, however, known as lithotripsy, has drawbacks: It works in only a small percentage of patients (those with a limited number of small gallstones), and the results have not been uniformly consistent or satisfactory.

PERSPECTIVE AND PROSPECTS

Diseases of the gallbladder and biliary system are common in modern industrialized societies. The exact etiologies are not entirely clear, but they may involve dietary mechanisms or other customs of the Western lifestyle. There is also evidence that genetic factors are important, as gallbladder disease often runs in families. Traditionally, the treatment of non-life-threatening gallbladder disease has been conservative, with dietary discretion being the most important factor. When that failed, or if the condition was more serious, the gallbladder was removed. Open cholecystectomy was long considered the best method for dealing with these problems. This operation has been recently challenged by endoscopic and laparoscopic techniques, which have become widely available and enjoyed great success. These new treatment options will become more important as increasing medical costs promote the refinement of less invasive and better techniques. Nevertheless, open cholecystectomy is sometimes the only option for a patient, and less invasive techniques can have limitations as well as complications.

Basic scientific research is also important in this field. Investigations into the mechanisms of gallstone formation are critical to the understanding of gallbladder diseases, as gallstones are the cause of many of these problems. As with many other diseases, prevention might be the key to eliminating many gallbladder diseases, making biliary colic, cholecystitis, and common bile duct diseases rare.

—*Mark Wengrovitz, M.D.*

See also Abdomen; Abdominal disorders; Cholecystectomy; Cholecystitis; Gallbladder cancer; Gastroenterology; Gastroenterology, pediatric; Gastrointestinal disorders; Internal medicine; Jaundice; Kidney stones; Laparoscopy; Liver; Liver cancer; Liver disorders; Liver transplantation; Obesity; Pain; Pancreatitis; Stone removal; Stones; Ultrasonography.

FOR FURTHER INFORMATION:

Blumgart, L. H., and Y. Fong, eds. *Surgery of the Liver and Biliary Tract*. 3d ed. 2 vols. New York: W. B. Saunders, 2000. This authoritative text offers a comprehensive, detailed description of the subject.

Cameron, John L., ed. *Current Surgical Therapy*. 8th ed. Philadelphia: Elsevier Mosby, 2004. An excellent textbook that covers all surgical problems, including those related to gallbladder and gallstone removal.

Krames Communications. *The Gallbladder Surgery Book*. San Bruno, Calif.: Author, 1991. This helpful book provides the general reader with an understanding of the symptoms of gallbladder diseases, their most common causes, and treatment options.

_____. *Laparoscopic Gallbladder Surgery*. San Bruno, Calif.: Author, 1991. This work offers information regarding laparoscopic cholecystectomy to patients who are facing gallbladder surgery.

Zinner, Michael J., et al., eds. *Maingot's Abdominal Operations*. 10th ed. Stamford, Conn.: Appleton & Lange, 1997. This textbook has long been considered the classic work on all surgical disciplines. Contains an excellent section on gallbladder diseases.

GALLBLADDER REMOVAL. *See* CHOLECYSTECTOMY.

GALLSTONES. *See* GALLBLADDER DISEASES; STONE REMOVAL; STONES.

GAMETE INTRAFALLOPIAN TRANSFER (GIFT)

PROCEDURE

ALSO KNOWN AS: Gamete intrafallopian tube transfer

ANATOMY OR SYSTEM AFFECTED: Reproductive system

SPECIALTIES AND RELATED FIELDS: Embryology, endocrinology, obstetrics

DEFINITION: A treatment for infertility in which sperm and eggs are introduced surgically into a Fallopian tube, where fertilization (and subsequent implantation in the uterus) are expected to occur naturally.

KEY TERMS:

assisted reproductive technology: any treatment or procedure involving the manipulation of sperm or eggs outside the body in order to achieve pregnancy

Fallopian tube: one of the pair of open-ended ducts branching from the top of the uterus, which collects eggs released from the ovary and in which fertilization usually occurs

fertilization: the union of egg and sperm

gamete: any reproductive cell, either egg or sperm

in vitro fertilization (IVF): the fertilization of eggs outside the body with subsequent implantation of embryos in the uterus

laparoscope: a thin, needlelike medical instrument containing a fiber-optic light source that is inserted through the skin and used both to visualize internal organs and to perform certain surgical procedures

ovulation: the release of a mature egg from an ovary

uterus: the female organ in which the embryo/fetus develops

zygote: a fertilized egg before cell division occurs; after the first division, it is called an embryo

INDICATIONS AND PROCEDURES

Couples who have sexual intercourse for a year without contraception and do not achieve pregnancy are defined as infertile. So too are couples who conceive but, because of repeated miscarriages, have not had a child. There are many possible causes of infertility. In the female, they include abnormal or irregular ovulation, blocked or constricted Fallopian tubes, and growths, scarring, or abnormalities of the uterus. In the male, infertility may result from failure to ejaculate, low sperm count, abnormalities in sperm cells, or a blocked sperm tube. In many cases, no cause of infertility can be determined.

In order to have a child, some infertile couples turn to clinics offering assisted reproductive technology (ART) services. The most common form of ART is in vitro fertilization (IVF). Gamete intrafallopian transfer (GIFT) is similar to IVF, but it does not involve fertilization outside the body. Gametes (sperm and egg) are collected and then surgically introduced into a Fallopian tube, where fertilization and subsequent implantation in the uterus are expected to occur naturally. GIFT is the least frequently done of all ARTs. In 2000, it accounted for less than 1 percent of the ART procedures performed in the United States.

Women who have at least one Fallopian tube open are considered candidates for any of the ARTs, if sufficient numbers of healthy sperm can be collected from the male. (Women with blocked Fallopian tubes are candidates for IVF.) GIFT may be the ART of choice for young women who have never undergone laparoscopy and for men with weak or few sperm. GIFT is sometimes employed in cases of unexplained infertility.

To perform the procedure, egg maturation in the ovaries is stimulated with fertility drugs. With ultrasound guiding the probe, the physician retrieves eggs using a laparoscope. Sperm are collected several hours before the procedure. A laparoscope is also used to inject eggs and sperm into a Fallopian tube. The patient may be awake or under general anesthesia for GIFT, which is typically done as a same-day, outpatient procedure. The American Society for Reproductive Medicine recommends that GIFT be performed only in a facility capable of performing IVF, in case GIFT fails or excess eggs are recovered.

USES AND COMPLICATIONS

All ART procedures involve risks, including general surgical risks, pregnancy complications, multiple fetuses, low birth weight, and possibly certain birth defects. The rate of ectopic pregnancy (implantation outside the uterus) is also slightly higher. Multiple fetuses, which are present in nearly one-third of ART pregnancies, are associated with increased risk of prematurity, low birth weight, and neonatal death in the infant and of cesarean section and hemorrhage in the mother. Although ARTs are emotionally taxing, physically demanding, and expensive, thousands of infertile couples seek them annually. In 2000, more than 35,000 babies were born in the United States as a result of ART.

The possible side effects of the hormonal drugs used to induce ovulation include hot flashes, changes in vision, ovarian cysts (sacs of fluid forming in the ovary), ovarian enlargement, and leakage of fluid into the abdominal cavity, which can trigger kidney failure, strokes, and heart attacks if not treated. IVF entails a slightly increased risk of chromosomal birth defects; whether GIFT carries a similar risk is unknown. Some studies conclude that ART increases a woman's risk of ovarian cancer, but other studies dispute that claim. ARTs do not appear to increase the overall risk of birth defects, although specific defects, such as vision problems, have been uncovered in some studies. While some experts claim that the risk of miscarriage increases, others refute that assertion.

Some couples want GIFT because they consider it more "natural" than IVF. However, GIFT is a riskier procedure than IVF, because laparoscopic surgery is required. Also, because fertilization is not confirmed before the injection of gametes, there is no way of knowing whether it occurred unless pregnancy is achieved. Nevertheless, GIFT carries a success rate approximately equal to that of other ARTs—roughly one in every four attempts. The mother's age is an important factor: the younger the mother, the better the chance of success.

Perspective and Prospects

Before the 1970's, infertility treatment was limited mostly to the surgical repair of blocked Fallopian tubes and the insertion of sperm into the uterus (artificial insemination). In the early 1960's, Min Chang, a scientist at the Worcester Foundation in Shrewsbury, Massachusetts, performed the first IVF. He used sperm and eggs from black rabbits to grow embryos in vitro (meaning literally "in glass," or in a laboratory dish). He then placed the embryos in the uterus of a white rabbit. A litter of black pups was born.

In 1969, English physician Robert G. Edwards successfully fertilized human eggs in vitro. Cell division was achieved a year later. He next collaborated with English physician Patrick Steptoe, who specialized in laparoscopic surgery. Together, they developed reliable techniques for retrieving eggs and maintaining embryos. The result was Louise Brown, the first "test tube baby." She was born in England in 1978. In 1981, the breakthrough was replicated in the United States. During the following twenty years, more than one million IVF babies were born.

After that, the field of reproductive endocrinology flourished, as did the development of ART techniques. Dr. Ricardo H. Asch of the University of Texas at San Antonio performed the first successful GIFT in 1984. Another, similar development was zygote intrafallopian transfer (ZIFT), first successfully performed in 1986. ZIFT involves mixing sperm and eggs together outside the body, then confirming fertilization before the zygote is surgically placed in a Fallopian tube. Another ART, intracytoplasmic sperm injection (ICSI), was introduced in 1992. It involves injecting a single sperm directly into an egg. It is often used in conjunction with IVF to fertilize eggs before embryo transplantation.

Research and development activities continue to improve ART methods and techniques. Certain conditions within the Fallopian tube that interfere with ART can now be treated, and better culture media have been developed for growing and maintaining embryos. The selection of smaller numbers of higher-quality embryos may cut the rate of multiple pregnancies, and improved methods for identifying those couples most likely to benefit from ART are being perfected. New blastocyst culture methods allow laboratories to grow embryos through the sixth day of development, when they contain one hundred fifty to two hundred cells. Researchers hope that implanting smaller numbers of more mature embryos will reduce the number of multiple births and diminish the risks that they entail.

ARTs raise ethical and social issues. Some churches and religious leaders oppose ARTs, because they are "unnatural" or because some of the embryos produced in vitro are subsequently destroyed. Other controversies include pregnancies achieved in women past their natural reproductive age and legal issues surrounding the ownership of reproductive cells and frozen embryos.

—*Faith Hickman Brynie, Ph.D.*

See also Assisted reproductive technologies; Conception; Embryology; Ethics; Genetic engineering; Gynecology; In vitro fertilization; Infertility, female; Infertility, male; Multiple births; Obstetrics; Pregnancy and gestation; Reproductive system; Women's health.

For Further Information:

Meniru, Godwin I. *Cambridge Guide to Infertility Management and Assisted Reproduction.* New York: Cambridge University Press, 2001.

Peoples, Debby, and Harriette Rovner Ferguson. *Experiencing Infertility: An Essential Resource.* New York: W. W. Norton, 2000.

U.S. Department of Health and Human Services. *2002 Assisted Reproductive Technology Success Rates: National Summary and Fertility Clinic Reports*. Atlanta: Author, 2004.

GANGLION REMOVAL

PROCEDURE

ANATOMY OR SYSTEM AFFECTED: Feet, hands, tendons

SPECIALTIES AND RELATED FIELDS: Dermatology, family medicine, general surgery

DEFINITION: The removal of fluid-filled sacs which usually develop on the tendons of the wrists, fingers, or feet.

INDICATIONS AND PROCEDURES

Sacs containing synovial fluid surround tendons to reduce the friction on adjacent tissues during movement. These sacs can form cysts, known as ganglions, that range in size from a pea to a golf ball. Smaller ganglions are more common and often spontaneously disappear. A ganglion is not harmful unless it causes pain or the patient desires its removal for cosmetic reasons. Ganglion formation typically occurs around the tendons of the wrist.

In order to remove a ganglion, the physician will disinfect the skin overlying the cyst and insert a needle attached to a syringe in order to aspirate the fluid from the ganglion. Unfortunately, this procedure usually reduces the ganglion's size only temporarily. Some physicians will make an incision into the skin and remove the whole ganglion. This procedure requires thorough disinfection of the skin using alcohol and/or povidone-iodine and may require a local anesthetic such as lidocaine to be injected under the skin. Surgical instruments are used to dissect the cyst wall from the tendon and surrounding tissues. The total removal of the ganglion usually prevents recurrence.

USES AND COMPLICATIONS

As with any invasive procedure, the physician performing the surgical removal of a ganglion must be cautious so as to prevent infections or damage to surrounding healthy tissues.

The larger the ganglion, the greater are the potential complications. A longer incision must be made, which allows a large site for potential bacterial invasion and infection. The larger ganglion also requires more extensive dissection from surrounding tissues, which increases the possibility of injury to these structures. Although it is rare, tendons, ligaments, and nerves can be permanently damaged in ganglion removal. For example, if the ganglion was located in the wrist and the underlying tendons and nerves were severely damaged, the result may be a limited use or loss of use of the hand.

—*Matthew Berria, Ph.D.,*
and Douglas Reinhart, M.D.

See also Abscess removal; Abscesses; Cyst removal; Cysts; Nervous system; Neurology; Tendon disorders; Tendon repair.

FOR FURTHER INFORMATION:

Icon Health. *Ganglions: A Medical Dictionary, Bibliography, and Annotated Research Guide to Internet References*. San Diego, Calif.: Author, 2004.

Kikuchi, Kenji, and Masahiro Saito. "Ganglion-Cell Tumor of the Filum Terminale: Immunohistochemical Characterization." *Tohoku Journal of Experimental Medicine* 188, no. 3 (July, 1999): 245-256.

Lenfant, C., R. Paoletti, and A. Albertini, eds. *Growth Factors of the Vascular and Nervous Systems: Functional Characterization and Biotechnology*. New York: S. Karger, 1992.

McLendon, Roger E., et al. *Pathology of Tumors of the Central Nervous System: A Guide to Histological Diagnosis*. New York: Oxford University Press, 2000.

GANGLIONS. *See* CYSTS; GANGLION REMOVAL.

GANGRENE

DISEASE/DISORDER

ALSO KNOWN AS: Gas gangrene

ANATOMY OR SYSTEM AFFECTED: Heart, muscles, skin

SPECIALTIES AND RELATED FIELDS: Bacteriology, dermatology, emergency medicine

DEFINITION: Gas gangrene is an infectious disease usually caused by *Clostridium perfringens*, a spore-producing bacterium that is usually found in soil and the gastrointestinal tract of humans and other animals.

KEY TERMS:

aerobic: living or growing only in the presence of air

anaerobic: living without air

exotoxin: a poisonous substance that is secreted by a microorganism and released into the surrounding environment

myo-: a prefix that refers to muscle

necrosis: death of a cell or tissue as a result of injury or trauma

organism: a form of life that contains mutually independent components

sepsis: local or generalized invasion of the body by an organism or its toxins, which can cause death

spontaneous: growing naturally without cultivation

spore: a walled-off cell that can reproduce directly or indirectly

---

INFORMATION ON GANGRENE

CAUSES: Trauma, bacterial infection
SYMPTOMS: Pain, fever, blisters, sweating, rapid heart rate
DURATION: Acute
TREATMENTS: Antibiotics, surgery, amputation

CAUSES AND SYMPTOMS

Gas gangrene involves tissue necrosis (death) and severe bacterial infection. (Dry gangrene refers to necrosis caused by blood flow interruption without bacterial infection.) Gas gangrene is generally the result of trauma (injury) or surgery. However, it can occur spontaneously. The disease is known for its quick progression, muscle and tissue death, gas production, and ultimately sepsis. Not every wound that is infected with Clostridia bacteria will progress to gas gangrene. Gas gangrene occurs only if there is sufficient tissue death. The dead tissue provides an excellent environment for the organism to grow and flourish. The organism grows well in anaerobic conditions. Clostridia is the cause of 80 to 90 percent of gangrene cases.

With gas gangrene that is the result of surgery or trauma, bacteria enter the body through an opening in the skin. When the involved tissue becomes compromised because of a lack of blood, infection occurs and the process of tissue necrosis begins. Spontaneous gas gangrene occurs when the organism spreads from the gastrointestinal tract (stomach and intestines) in people with colon cancer. When there is a small tear in the gastrointestinal tract, the organism enters the bloodstream and spreads to the muscles. Spontaneous gas gangrene is caused by *Clostridium septicum. C. septicum* is different from *C. perfringens* because it can survive and grow in conditions that are aerobic. In both types of gas gangrene, the real cause of the associated problems are the exotoxins that are released. These exotoxins destroy cells, resulting in tissue death that can also affect the heart muscle.

Gas gangrene can occur within twenty-four hours of exposure. It also can take up to six hours or more after exposure for symptoms to occur. The pain associated with gas gangrene is greater than the initial symptoms. Gas gangrene involves very subtle signs in the early phases of the disease. Because gas gangrene affects the deep muscle tissues, the skin over the affected area may appear normal in the early phases of the disease. Over time, the skin of the affected area will change from normal to pale, and eventually gray to purplish-red. Once the disease advances, the skin can be "crackly" and tense, experience drainage, form blisters, and then turn black. There is also a low-grade fever (99 to 100 degrees Fahrenheit), a fast heart rate, changes in mentation, and significant sweating.

In order to diagnose gas gangrene properly, several laboratory tests must be completed. These tests are aimed at addressing all the possible areas that gas gangrene can affect. The first study is a Gram stain culture of the affected tissue. This test helps to identify the causative organism and determine how it will respond to antibiotics. A complete blood count will help health care providers determine if there is anemia. Anemia occurs when the exotoxins have been released into the bloodstream. Additional tests that may be taken are liver function tests, electrolytes, blood gases, renal tests, coagulation studies, myoglobin, and blood cultures. Plain X rays can show where gas has formed in the affected area. A tissue biopsy will provide the most information in terms of reaching a diagnosis.

TREATMENT AND THERAPY

Gas gangrene is an infectious disease emergency, and the patient should be evaluated immediately. Laboratory tests should be performed, along with careful monitoring of the ABCs of airway, breathing, and circulation. The airway (mouth and neck areas) should be monitored to ensure that the patient is able to breathe without obstruction. Oxygen should be administered to make sure that the body is receiving enough air to sustain life. Lastly, circulation is maintained via intravenous (IV) fluids. An IV will also make it easier for other medications to be administered.

Clostridia are sensitive (easily killed) by the antibiotic penicillin. Patients who are suspected of having gas gangrene should have their tetanus status reviewed. If it is unclear when their last tetanus immunization was given, then it should be given immediately. Individuals who have never had a tetanus immunization should also receive tetanus immunoglobulin. Admittance to the hospital for pain management, wound care, and IV antibiotics helps ensure that the disease does not progress and become fatal.

In order to prevent the disease, early wound care is mandatory. The use of antibiotics to prevent infection is also important in the care of a patient who has sustained trauma. Once the diagnosis of gas gangrene has been made, aggressive management that includes cutting away the dead tissue, managing the basic life support parameters, antibiotics, and surgery if needed, will improve the prognosis. Therefore, the mainstay of treatment is early identification and aggressive treatment.

—*Rosslynn S. Byous, D.P.A., PA-C*

See also Amputation; Bacterial infections; Embolism; Food poisoning; Frostbite; Hernia; Hernia repair; Hyperbaric oxygen therapy; Infection; Poisoning; Thrombosis and thrombus; Wounds.

FOR FURTHER INFORMATION:

Folstad, Steven G. "Soft Tissue Infections." In *Emergency Medicine: A Comprehensive Study Guide*, edited by Judith E. Tintinalli. 6th ed. New York: McGraw Hill, 2004. A chapter in an excellent medical textbook that provides a vast amount of information regarding this topic.

Urschel, John D. "Necrotizing Soft Tissue Infections." *Postgraduate Medical Journal* 75 (November, 1999): 645-649. Discusses the various types of diseases that can destroy the skin and its underlying structures.

Wong, Jason K., et al. *Gas Gangrene*. http://www .emedicine.com/emerg/topic211.htm. This online article provides all the basic medical information regarding gas gangrene: what symptoms will be manifested, what an examination will entail, and how to best take care of the disease once it has been identified.

GASTRECTOMY

PROCEDURE

ANATOMY OR SYSTEM AFFECTED: Abdomen, gastrointestinal system, stomach

SPECIALTIES AND RELATED FIELDS: Gastroenterology, general surgery, oncology

DEFINITION: The surgical removal of all or part of the stomach.

KEY TERMS:

anesthesia: the use of drugs to inhibit pain and alter consciousness

duodenum: the first part of the small intestine, located just after the stomach and before the jejunum

hemostasis: the control of bleeding

incision: a cut made with a scalpel

jejunum: a region of the small intestine located after the duodenum

suture: a thread used to unite parts of the body

INDICATIONS AND PROCEDURES

The stomach is an important organ in the gastrointestinal system. It receives the food that has been swallowed from the esophagus and immediately begins to process it. The stomach produces and secretes gastric juices, which include hydrochloric acid and an enzyme called pepsin for digestion. As the stomach collects it, food is churned and mixed with the gastric fluid before it is passed to the first region of the small intestine, the duodenum. Occasionally, the stomach becomes cancerous or has an ulcer that will not heal and thus must be surgically removed.

Complete removal of the stomach, a total gastrectomy, is a relatively rare operation usually performed to treat stomach cancer. Partial gastrectomy, however, in which only the diseased portion of the stomach is removed surgically, is fairly common. A partial gastrectomy is often performed to treat a peptic ulcer that fails to heal after medical treatment. Peptic ulcers, which include gastric and more commonly duodenal ulcers, may not respond to drug therapy and can place the patient at risk for bleeding into the gastrointestinal tract or even complete perforation of the stomach or duodenal wall. Therefore, the indications for gastrectomy include perforation, obstruction, massive bleeding, and severe abdominal pain.

Gastrectomy requires hospitalization, general anesthesia, and postoperative care. An anesthesiologist will administer a general anesthetic, rendering the patient unconscious and insensible to pain during the operation. A nasogastric tube is passed into the stomach via the nose and nasal cavity so that any stomach contents can be removed using suction before an incision is made into the stomach.

During total gastrectomy, the whole stomach is removed and the esophagus is attached to the jejunum. The two most common types of partial gastrectomy surgeries are the Billroth I and Billroth II. A surgeon performing a Billroth I will remove the diseased part of the stomach and attach the remaining healthy stomach to the duodenum. The Billroth I is also known as gastroduodenostomy. This operation preserves most of the

The Three Major Kinds of Gastrectomy

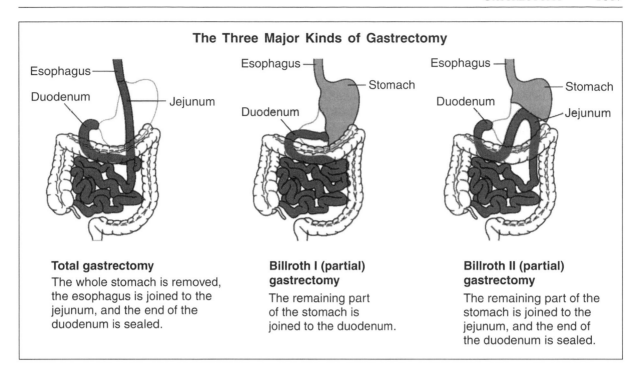

Total gastrectomy
The whole stomach is removed, the esophagus is joined to the jejunum, and the end of the duodenum is sealed.

Billroth I (partial) gastrectomy
The remaining part of the stomach is joined to the duodenum.

Billroth II (partial) gastrectomy
The remaining part of the stomach is joined to the jejunum, and the end of the duodenum is sealed.

digestive functions. Billroth II gastrectomy requires the surgeon to perform a gastrojejunostomy in which the remaining stomach is joined with the jejunum and bypasses the duodenum. Thus the opening of the duodenum must be closed to prevent the digestive contents from escaping into the abdominal cavity.

During the recovery period, the nasogastric tube is left in place to help drain the secretions from the gastrointestinal system until the body is recovered enough to eliminate these secretions normally. Once the normal movement of the digestive tract (peristalsis) is detected, the patient is given very small amounts of fluid. If the intestines can process the ingested fluids, then the nasogastric tube is removed and the amount of fluid ingested is gradually increased. Typically, if there is no pain or nausea and vomiting, the patient can be started on a diet containing small amounts of solid food.

USES AND COMPLICATIONS

The risk of complications is relatively high in a total gastrectomy and lessens if smaller portions of the stomach are removed. The overall rate of complications is approximately 10 percent.

Since the stomach has such an important role in the process of digestion, it is not surprising that complications and adverse effects occur postsurgically. Some of the most common symptoms noted after gastrectomy include a feeling of discomfort and fullness after in-

gesting a relatively small meal. This feeling is attributable to the fact that the stomach volume has been reduced in a partial gastrectomy or eliminated in a total gastrectomy. New ulcers may also form and necessitate further drug treatment. Gastritis (inflammation of the stomach lining) may also occur after surgery, as well as a condition called dumping syndrome. Patients with dumping syndrome feel weak, nauseated, and lightheaded after a meal because the food moves too rapidly out of the stomach. Most of these side effects can be treated with medications and dietary changes.

Long-term complications include malabsorption problems. Occasionally after gastrectomy, the digestive system cannot compensate adequately for the loss of the stomach, leading to poor digestion and absorption of nutrients. The most common malabsorptive disorder following gastrectomy is the inability to absorb vitamin B_{12}. The stomach produces a substance called intrinsic factor which is required for the absorption of this essential vitamin. Without intrinsic factor and the ability to absorb vitamin B_{12}, the patient must receive monthly injections of the vitamin for the rest of his or her life.

PERSPECTIVE AND PROSPECTS

Early detection of stomach cancers and ulcers may help reduce the need for gastrectomies. Endoscopic examinations in which the physician can observe the lining of

inflame the membrane. Aside from causing a burning sensation, the juices can erode through the membrane, creating ulcers. If the membrane is eaten through entirely, a hole opens into the body cavity around the gut, spilling food, blood, and digestive juices. Emergency surgery is then needed. Although conventional wisdom has long attributed ulcers to emotional stress or bad habits, such as too much alcohol, recent research has determined that virtually all people with stomach or duodenum ulcers have a bacterium known as *Helicobacter pylori* in their gut. Most scientists now believe that *H. pylori* may be necessary for ulcers to form, although there is still some question about whether high levels of acid or long-term use of aspirin can produce ulcers independently of the bacteria. *H. pylori* may also play a role in the development of gastroenterological cancers. Patients with symptoms of ulcers or with cancers of the gastrointestinal tract should be tested for this bacteria and treated with antibiotics. Ulcers can also occur in the stomach and duodenum as a result of motility disorders, excess acid, or drugs, especially alcohol and aspirin, that irritate the membrane. Regardless of cause, symptoms of ulcers are exacerbated by motility disorders, excess acid, or drugs, especially alcohol and aspirin, that irritate the membrane.

Colitis and Crohn's disease are serious inflammations of the gut lining, especially in the colon; except for some forms of colitis that are caused by bacteria, the mechanism behind such inflammation remains unknown, but the disorders frequently require surgery to remove damaged and inflamed areas.

Similarly, tears in the gut lining, strictures, passages blocked by chunks of food, exposed veins (varices), infected sacs in the colon (diverticula), and communicable diseases such as dysentery and hepatitis produce potentially deadly symptoms.

DIAGNOSTIC AND TREATMENT TECHNIQUES

An extensive battery of tests, procedures, and medications enable gastroenterologists to cure or palliate many GI diseases. In addition to the traditional physician's tools of the physical examination and the patient's medical history, high-tech instruments let gastroenterologists see inside parts of the gut, produce images of it, remove tissue and stones, stop bleeding, and destroy tumors. Medicines kill bacteria, help regulate motility, speed the healing of damaged tissue, and control diarrhea and constipation. Yet the GI tract is a very intricate system, and at times the gastroenterologist's most effective remedy is sympathy and advice

about changing behavior or diet so that patients learn to live with their diseases.

Before treatment can begin, the disease must be identified. An interview with the patient and a medical examination constitute the first step in narrowing the range of possible causes of distressing symptoms. Symptoms described by the patient or discovered by the physician are clues to the underlying causes and suggest the kinds of tests that will most likely isolate the actions of a specific disease. Blood tests can reveal abnormal levels of white cells or chemicals and the presence of infection. Samples of digestive juices likewise can show chemical imbalances, infections, and bleeding, as can stool samples. Biopsies of the gut membrane, liver, and tumors allow pathologists to inspect tissue damage and look for viruses or bacteria. For example, a patient with yellowish skin (jaundice) and a tender liver who complains of nausea and chills may lead a physician to suspect hepatitis. The physician will then order a blood serum test, looking for specific proteins typical of hepatitis infection, and a liver biopsy to learn the type of hepatitis.

Some diseases, especially those destroying or inflaming tissue or involving motility problems, require imaging to identify, as do blockages and strictures. To obtain pictures of the gut, physicians use ultrasonography, X rays, magnetic resonance imaging (MRI), and computed tomography (CT) scans. Ultrasonographs transmit sound waves through the body and judge the density of tissues by the intensity and pattern of reflection; they are particularly useful for spotting gallstones. X rays, MRIs, and CT scans pass radiation through the body and record it on film or by sensors that feed data to a computer to construct an image. Plain X rays show the pattern of air and gas distribution in the digestive tract and can detect obstructions; X rays may also be taken after barium, a radioopaque element, has been swallowed or inserted in the colon so that it coats the GI tract's walls and makes them easier to see. Such imaging helps the physician to locate strictures, perforations, cancers, diverticula, blockages, and distended areas.

Few tests are more revealing, however, than a direct look inside the GI tract. Until the 1960's, this could not be done without exploratory surgery. At that time, the endoscope became widely available. Developed by British, American, and Japanese scientists, the endoscope is a long, flexible, maneuverable tube filled with fiber optic strands and a central channel for inserting various instruments. A light source at its tip illuminates the area ahead of the scope; the fiber optics collect the reflected light and pass it directly to the eye of the examining physician at the scope's opposite end, to a television monitor, or to a camera. There are many types of endoscopes, of which three are most common: The meter-long upper gastrointestinal panendoscope (or gastroscope), inserted through the mouth, can be used for seeing well into the duodenum; the 60-centimeter flexible sigmoidoscope is used in the rectum and sigmoid colon; and the lower panendoscope (or colonoscope)—180, 140, 100, or 70 centimeters long—inserted through the anus, can be worked through the entire colon and as much as 30 centimeters into the ileum. Most of the small intestine cannot be seen by endoscopy.

With endoscopy, gastroenterologists can spot and examine a diseased or damaged area of the gut and perform a biopsy so that tissue can be examined under a microscope. Yet endoscopes can do even more than that. They can push a wad of food obstructing the esophagus into the stomach, stretch open a stricture, or clear a clogged duct with wires inserted through the scope's channel; small balloons can be inflated inside the gut to widen constricted passages. Similarly, endoscopes with wire attachments can open a passage between the surface skin and the stomach, allowing food to be put directly in the stomach for patients incapable of swallowing, a procedure called percutaneous endoscopic gastrostomy (PEG). With looped and electrified wires, they can remove polyps, cut away tissue, and cauterize bleeding vessels and ulcers. One such procedure, endoscopic retrograde-cholangiopancreatography (ERCP), can image the biliary and pancreatic ducts and allow removal of gallstones without surgery. Drugs may also be injected through the endoscope to control bleeding from varicose veins (sclerotherapy), and fiber optics permit the use of lasers to vaporize cancerous tissue. Endoscopic treatments exist for chronic heartburn, including EndoCinch, a procedure that strengthens the lower esophageal sphincter (LES) by putting in stitches that pleat the tissue, and the Stretta procedure, which increases the thickness of the LES using radiofrequency energy. Endoscopy can also be used to treat GERD.

Gastroenterologists use drugs to sedate patients during procedures and to treat dysfunctions and diseases. Other medications available are too numerous and their administration too complex to describe in detail, but basically they ease pain, check diarrhea and vomiting, decrease acid production to permit ulcers to heal,

soften the stool of constipated patients, control motility problems (such as spasms), regulate secretions, speed coagulation at bleeding sites, or kill harmful bacteria and parasites. GI pain, especially from irritable bowel syndrome, is notoriously difficult to treat because of the diversity of contributing causes, including emotional problems. Researchers turn out a steady supply of new drugs each year, but improvements are slow, and new drugs require extensive clinical trials to determine proper dosage and detect harmful side effects. Sometimes, a placebo—that is, a pill with no active ingredient, a "sugar pill"—is enough to make a patient feel better. The interaction between a patient's gut, nervous system, and personality is intricate and sometimes highly idiosyncratic.

Gastroenterologists do not simply react to disease and trauma with treatments; they also try to prevent trouble from starting in the first place. A large part of their job involves educating patients. They discuss diets that can reduce GI pain and warn against the abuse of drugs, especially alcohol and tobacco, that are known to contribute to heartburn and ulcers. They routinely screen patients over the age of fifty for cancer, sometimes by endoscopic examination, especially if there is a family history of cancer.

PERSPECTIVE AND PROSPECTS

Jan Baptista van Helmont, a seventeenth century medical chemist, was the first to describe the diseases and digestive juices of the GI tract scientifically. Gastroenterology can be said to have started with his studies (he also coined the word "gas"). Yet no one directly observed the operations of digestion until 1833, when U.S. Army surgeon William Beaumont cared for a French Canadian with a bullet wound to the stomach. The wound remained open, and Beaumont could watch the action of gastric juices and the stomach's mixing and grinding action. Throughout the nineteenth century, there were advances in the understanding and treatment of the GI tract, including the introduction of enemas and gastric lavage (washing out), X rays, and an early form of endoscopy.

As it did for most branches of medicine, twentieth century technology greatly expanded the role of gastroenterology in diagnosing, preventing, and treating disease. Imaging and endoscopy especially have revolutionized the field. In 1932, Rudolph Schindler developed a flexible gastroscope, and in 1943, Lester Dragstedt performed the first vagotomy (surgically cutting the vagus nerve) to reduce stomach acid secretions. Advances were also made to heal peptic ulcers with a special diet. The second half of the twentieth century saw an escalating number of refinements and innovations in procedures but was most remarkable for the development of drugs.

This progress has meant that far fewer surgical procedures are needed for common GI diseases. Because of new medicines, ulcer disease rarely requires surgery. Gallstones in the common bile duct that once necessitated surgical removal now may be taken out during an ERCP; a stent (perforated tube) can be inserted into a blocked bile duct under a gastroenterologist's guidance to keep bile flowing from the liver. Screenings for colon cancer and the removal of polyps, which can become cancerous, often identify cancerous or precancerous areas early and permit surgeons to remove tumors before the cancer spreads, sometimes making surgery unnecessary. Patients who once might have died because of a blocked or strictured esophagus can now be relieved and quickly released from the hospital. The overall trend has been shorter hospital stays and lower medical costs for common ailments. The sophistication of equipment and the training needed to treat difficult problems, however, have correspondingly inflated costs, as has the tendency to medicate painful ailments that sufferers once had to steel themselves to endure, such as irritable bowel syndrome.

Despite the expansion of gastroenterology's procedures and knowledge, it is far from an independent field. Gastroenterologists typically act as consultants, caring for patients only after they have been screened by family practitioners, emergency room doctors, and internists. Moreover, gastroenterologists rely on pathologists to decipher the information in biopsied tissue samples, radiologists to interpret imaging, neurologists to trace nervous system problems, and surgeons to repair perforated gut walls and remove diseased organs or transplant new ones. Finally, specially trained nurses and technicians must help them with many procedures and ensure that patients follow prescribed dietary and drug regimens.

—*Roger Smith, Ph.D.;*
updated by Caroline M. Small

See also Abdomen; Abdominal disorders; Acid reflux disease; Appendectomy; Appendicitis; Appetite loss; Bariatric surgery; Bulimia; Bypass surgery; Celiac sprue; Cholecystectomy; Cholecystitis; Cholera; Colic; Colitis; Colon and rectal polyp removal; Colon and rectal surgery; Colon cancer; Colonoscopy and sigmoidoscopy; Constipation; Crohn's disease; Diarrhea and dysentery; Digestion; Diverticulitis and diverticulosis; *E. coli* infection; Emergency medicine; Endoscopy; Enemas; Enzymes; Fistula repair; Food biochemistry; Food poisoning; Gallbladder cancer; Gallbladder diseases; Gastrectomy; Gastroenterology, pediatric; Gastrointestinal disorders; Gastrointestinal system; Gastrostomy; Glands; Heartburn; Hemorrhoid banding and removal; Hemorrhoids; Hernia; Hernia repair; Hirschsprung's disease; Ileostomy and colostomy; Indigestion; Internal medicine; Intestinal disorders; Intestines; Irritable bowel syndrome (IBS); Lactose intolerance; Liver; Liver cancer; Liver disorders; Liver transplantation; Malabsorption; Malnutrition; Metabolism; Nausea and vomiting; Noroviruses; Nutrition; Obstruction; Pancreas; Pancreatitis; Peristalsis; Pinworms; Poisonous plants; Proctology; Pyloric stenosis; Rotavirus; Roundworms; Salmonella infection; Shigellosis; Soiling; Stomach, intestinal, and pancreatic cancers; Stone removal; Stones; Tapeworms; Taste; Toilet training; Trichinosis; Ulcer surgery; Ulcers; Vagotomy; Weight loss and gain; Worms.

FOR FURTHER INFORMATION:

Brandt, Lawrence J., ed. *The Clinical Practice of Gastroenterology.* 2 vols. Philadelphia: Current Medicine, 1999. Details virtually all of the adult and pediatric gastroenterologic problems encountered in practice. Features a full section on liver disease and synthesizes new advances in molecular immunology and imaging techniques.

Heuman, Douglas M., A. Scott Mills, and Hunter H. McGuire, Jr. *Gastroenterology.* Philadelphia: W. B. Saunders, 1997. This volume in the Saunders text and review series discusses digestive system diseases, the physiology of the digestive system, and the methods employed in the field of gastroenterology. Includes a bibliography and an index.

Janowitz, Henry D. *Indigestion: Living Better with Upper Intestinal Problems from Heartburn to Ulcers and Gallstones.* New York: Oxford University Press, 1994. Janowitz discusses common ailments of the upper GI tract with special attention to degenerative diseases afflicting people as they age. His style is clear and straightforward, aimed at general readers who want to prevent illness or to manage an existing one. Accompanied by charts and illustrations.

Massoni, Margaret. "Nurses' GI Handbook." *Nursing 20* (November, 1990): 65-80. Intended as a primer on GI problems for nurses, this article contains many illustrations of the gut, surgical techniques, and physical examination methods; lists of symptoms and the disorders they suggest; and tables of biochemical tests.

Peikin, Steven. *Gastrointestinal Health*. Rev. ed. New York: HarperCollins, 1999. Concerned almost completely with the effect of nutrition on GI maladies, the author offers a self-help guide for the afflicted. After explaining the GI tract's workings and describing common symptoms, Peikin specifies diets that he argues will relieve symptoms.

Steiner-Grossman, Penny, Peter A. Banks, and Daniel H. Present, eds. *The New People, Not Patients: A Source Book for Living with Inflammatory Bowel Disease*. Rev. ed. Dubuque, Iowa: Kendall/Hunt, 1997. This book is for those suffering from ulcerative colitis or Crohn's disease. Easy-to-understand, detailed discussions of the diseases are accompanied by illustrations and photographs.

GASTROENTEROLOGY, PEDIATRIC
SPECIALTY

ANATOMY OR SYSTEM AFFECTED: Abdomen, gallbladder, gastrointestinal system, intestines, liver, pancreas, stomach, throat

SPECIALTIES AND RELATED FIELDS: Internal medicine, neonatology, nutrition, pediatrics

DEFINITION: The diagnosis and treatment of diseases and disorders of the digestive tract in infants and children.

KEY TERMS:

biopsy: a small sample of tissue, such as from the lining of the gastrointestinal tract, which is removed for laboratory study to aid in diagnosis

endoscopy: the use of a small-diameter, flexible tube of optical fibers with an external light source to examine visually the interior of the body, such as the gastrointestinal tract

SCIENCE AND PROFESSION

The pediatric gastroenterologist is a pediatrician who has received extra training in the diagnosis and treatment of gastrointestinal diseases and disorders. The full course of training requires a medical degree followed by three years of pediatric residency, plus an additional three years of solely studying children's gastrointestinal diseases. The six years of postdoctoral training are almost always conducted at a large teaching hospital.

The gastrointestinal tract extends from the mouth to the anus. It is responsible for the ingestion, digestion, and absorption of food and for the elimination of unusable waste from the diet. Its principal parts are the esophagus, the stomach, the small intestine and colon, and the liver, gallbladder, and pancreas.

Children suffer the same wide range of gastrointestinal problems that afflict adults. Each age group, however, has its own special problems. For example, children very rarely have stomach or colon cancer, both relatively common in adults. On the other hand, diarrhea is a very common cause of infant death worldwide but is seldom life-threatening for adults.

Childhood gastrointestinal disease varies widely in its severity, from simple constipation needing only a change in diet to liver disease so severe that the child must undergo a liver transplant in order to survive. Common problems that a pediatric gastroenterologist might treat include gastroenteritis, constipation, chronic diarrhea, gastroesophageal reflux (especially in infants), and infections such as bacterial dysentery or viral hepatitis. Less common disorders are peptic ulcers, inflammatory bowel diseases (IBDs) such as ulcerative colitis and Crohn's disease, and malabsorption disorders involving the ability of the intestines to absorb nutrients from digested food.

The liver, gallbladder, and pancreas are abdominal organs that connect directly with the gastrointestinal tract. They are important in the digestion and absorption of food and in the metabolism of the basic sugars, fats, and proteins that are absorbed by the intestines. The diagnosis and treatment of disorders of these organs are part of gastroenterology.

Anatomical defects of the gastrointestinal tract can occur, such as intestinal malformations, obstructions, imperforate anus, and congenital fistulas between the trachea and esophagus. They are generally treated both by the gastroenterologist and by a general or pediatric surgeon, who performs any necessary surgery.

Since the gastrointestinal tract is critical in the digestion and absorption of food, a pediatric gastroenterologist must know much about nutrition. The physician will often prescribe the proper diet for a particular ailment. Occasionally, this program includes parenteral nutrition, in which a patient is fed intravenously with a complex solution of nutrients.

Most of the gastroenterologist's time is spent in the clinic, examining patients and prescribing medications, or performing procedures such as endoscopy of the stomach or colon. A minority of this specialist's patients require hospitalization, few of whom will be seriously or terminally ill.

A child's intestinal disease, especially if serious, can be very stressful for the patient's parents. The pediatric gastroenterologist must be able to communicate clearly with parents and to support them emotionally during the child's illness.

Diagnostic and Treatment Techniques

Much of the pediatric gastroenterologist's work involves obtaining a thorough, detailed history of the ailment from the child and parent. Often, skillful questioning will lead to the proper diagnosis and suggest the best treatment. A careful physical examination of the entire child, not simply the abdomen, is also important.

The pediatric gastroenterologist conducts a wide variety of laboratory tests in evaluating the nature and severity of the illness, such as complete blood counts and liver enzyme measurements. Bowel movement specimens often provide important data, such as the presence of blood or infectious bacteria in the intestines.

The pediatric gastroenterologist performs several diagnostic and therapeutic procedures. Flexible endoscopy is the use of a thin, bendable tube of optic fibers to view the interior of the esophagus, stomach, or colon. The physician can obtain biopsies, small samples of gastric or intestinal tissue, through the endoscope and can remove benign intestinal growths called polyps. The gastroenterologist may place a pH probe, a small electrode on a wire, in the esophagus to test acidity levels for periods as long as twenty-four hours. This probe is used to monitor acid reflux from the stomach into the esophagus. This disease, called gastroesophageal reflux, can lead to weight loss, recurrent pneumonia, or a scarred esophagus if left untreated.

Liver transplantation may be necessary when a child suffers irreversible liver failure as a result of severe hepatitis, congenital abnormalities such as biliary atresia (failure of the bile ducts to form properly), or some disorders of the body's metabolism. The pediatric gastroenterologist is an important member of the transplant team.

Perspective and Prospects

Subspecialties of pediatrics began to be recognized in the middle of the twentieth century. The first organization for pediatricians interested in gastroenterology was formed in the early 1970's.

In adult gastroenterology, diagnostic tools such as endoscopy and therapies such as antirejection medications for transplantation procedures improved rapidly in the last quarter of the twentieth century. Taking advantage of this new knowledge, pediatric gastroenterologists were also able to diagnose accurately more disorders in their own patients and to treat them effectively.

—*Thomas C. Jefferson, M.D.*

See also Abdomen; Abdominal disorders; Appendectomy; Appendicitis; Appetite loss; Bulimia; Bypass surgery; Celiac sprue; Cholera; Colic; Colitis; Colon and rectal surgery; Constipation; Crohn's disease; Diarrhea and dysentery; Digestion; *E. coli* infection; Emergency medicine; Endoscopy; Enemas; Enzymes; Fistula repair; Food biochemistry; Food poisoning; Gastroenterology; Gastrointestinal disorders; Gastrointestinal system; Glands; Heartburn; Hernia; Hernia repair; Hirschsprung's disease; Ileostomy and colostomy; Indigestion; Internal medicine; Intestinal disorders; Intestines; Lactose intolerance; Liver; Liver disorders; Malabsorption; Malnutrition; Metabolism; Nausea and vomiting; Noroviruses; Nutrition; Obstruction; Pancreas; Pancreatitis; Pediatrics; Peristalsis; Pinworms; Poisonous plants; Proctology; Pyloric stenosis; Rotavirus; Roundworms; Salmonella infection; Shigellosis; Soiling; Tapeworms; Taste; Toilet training; Trichinosis; Weight loss and gain; Worms.

For Further Information:

Cunningham, Carin L., and Gerard A. Banez. *Pediatric Gastrointestinal Disorders: Biopsychosocial Assessment and Treatment*. New York: Springer, 2006. Discusses the prevalence and etiology of pediatric gastrointestinal disorders. Covers psychological and behavioral symptoms, treatment strategies, and case studies.

Kirschner, Barbara S., and Dennis D. Black. "The Gastrointestinal Tract." In *Nelson Essentials of Pediatrics*, edited by Richard E. Behrman and Robert M. Kliegman. 4th ed. Philadelphia: W. B. Saunders, 2002. A chapter in a great text for medical students rotating through pediatrics. It has thorough explanations of diseases and treatments.

Walker, W. Allan, et al., eds. *Pediatric Gastrointestinal Disease: Pathophysiology, Diagnosis, Management*. 4th ed. Lewiston, N.Y.: BC Decker, 2004. This reference textbook deals extensively with the pathophysiologic basis of gastrointestinal disease in children of all ages. An approach to dealing with the families of children with gastrointestinal diseases augments the in-depth approach to disease manifestations and management. A careful approach to diagnosis follows.

GASTROINTESTINAL DISORDERS

DISEASE/DISORDER

ANATOMY OR SYSTEM AFFECTED: Abdomen, gastrointestinal system, intestines, stomach

SPECIALTIES AND RELATED FIELDS: Gastroenterology, internal medicine, microbiology

DEFINITION: The many problems that can affect the gastrointestinal tract, such as infections, injuries, dysfunctions, tumors, congenital defects, and genetic abnormalities.

KEY TERMS:

gastroenterologist: a medical specialist in diseases of the gut

endoscope: any of several flexible fiber-optic scopes used to examine the inside of the gut; it is equipped with tools to cauterize wounds or remove tissue or gallstones

intestines: the section of the gut between the anus and the stomach, consisting of the rectum, colon, and small bowel (subdivided into the ileus, jejunum, and duodenum)

motility: the spontaneous movements of the gut during swallowing, digestion, and elimination

mucosa: the tissue lining the interior of the gastrointestinal tract, through which nutrients pass into the bloodstream

stool: the waste products excreted from the body upon defecation; feces

tumor: a mass of abnormal cells that can be cancerous

CAUSES AND SYMPTOMS

What and how people eat, their digestion, and their toilet habits affect their health more than any other voluntary daily activity. Breathing, circulation, the brain's control of most bodily functions—these normally take place without conscious thought. The intake of nourishment and elimination of wastes, by contrast, afford a great variety of choices. Accordingly, poor or self-destructive eating and toilet habits lie behind many gastrointestinal (GI) disorders. Yet not all disorders result from an individual's habits. Many arise because of a person's cultural or physical environment, some are hereditary or congenital, and a fair amount have no known cause. All told, more than one hundred disorders may originate in the GI tract and its organs, including infections, cancer, dysfunctions, obstructions, autoimmune diseases, malabsorption of nutrients, and reactions to toxins taken in during eating, drinking, or breathing. Furthermore, diseases in other organs, systemic infections such as lupus, immune suppression such as that caused by acquired immunodeficiency syndrome (AIDS), reactions to altered body conditions as during pregnancy, and psychiatric problems can all reverberate to the gut.

The symptoms of GI disorders range from mildly annoying to life-threatening, although seldom does any single symptom except massive bleeding lead quickly to death. Indigestion, bloating, and gas send more people to gastroenterologists than any other set of symptoms, and they often reflect nothing more than overeating. Pain anywhere along the gut, aversion to food (anorexia), and nausea are general symptoms common to many disorders, although pain in the chest is likely to come from the esophagus while pain in the abdomen points to a stomach or intestinal problem. Red blood in the stool indicates bleeding in the intestines, black (digested) blood suggests bleeding in the upper small bowel or stomach, and vomited blood indicates injury to the stomach or esophagus—all dangerous signs indeed. Chronic diarrhea, fatty stool, constipation, difficulty in swallowing, hiccuping, vomiting, and cramps point to disturbances in the GI tract's orderly, wavelike contractions or absorption of nutrients and fluid. Pruritus (intense itching) can come from something as transient as a mild drug reaction or as serious as cancer. Dysentery (bloody diarrhea) usually comes from severe inflammation or lesions caused by viruses, bacteria, or other parasites. Malnourishment is a sign of badly disordered digestion, and ascites (fluid accumulation in body cavities) can result from serious disease in the liver or pancreas. Likewise, jaundice, the yellowing of the skin or eyes because of excess bile, signals problems in the liver, pancreas, or their ducts.

INFORMATION ON GASTROINTESTINAL DISORDERS

CAUSES: Congenital and hereditary factors, infection, cancer, obstructions, autoimmune diseases, malabsorption of nutrients, reactions to toxins

SYMPTOMS: Varies; can include abdominal discomfort and pain, constipation, diarrhea, fever, nausea, weight loss, fatigue, indigestion, bloating, aversion to food, difficulty swallowing

DURATION: Ranges from acute to chronic

TREATMENTS: Drug therapy, surgery, dietary regulation, lifestyle changes

The large number and complexity of GI disorders do not allow a quick, comprehensive summary. Fortunately, many are uncommon, and the most frequent problems can be described through a tour of the GI tract. The GI tract is basically a tube that moves food from one end to the other, extracting energy and biochemical building blocks for the body along the way. So a disorder that interrupts the flow in one section of the intestines can have secondary effects on other parts of the gut. Disorders seldom affect one area alone.

The esophagus. The GI tract's first section, the esophagus, is simply a passageway from the mouth to the stomach. Although it rarely gets infected, the esophagus is the site of several common problems, usually relatively minor, if painful. Muscle dysfunctions, including slow, weak, or spasmodic muscular movement, can impair motility and make swallowing difficult, as can strictures, which usually occur at the sphincter to the stomach. The mucosal lining of the esophagus is not as hardy as in other parts of the gut. When acid backflushes from the stomach into the esophagus, it inflames tissue there and can cause burning and even bleeding, a condition popularly known as heartburn and technically called gastroesophageal reflux disease (GERD). Retching and vomiting, usually resulting from alcohol abuse or associated with a hiatal hernia, can tear the mucosa. Smokers and drinkers run the risk of esophageal cancer, which can spread down into the gut early in its development and then becomes deadly; however, it accounts for only about 1 percent of cancers. Most of these conditions can be cured or controlled if diagnosed early enough.

The stomach. In order to store food and prepare it for digestion lower in the gut, the stomach churns it into a homogenous mass and releases it in small portions into the small bowel; meanwhile, the stomach also secretes acid to kill bacteria. Bacteria that are acid-resistant, however, can multiply there. One type, *Helicobacter pylori*, is thought to be involved in the development of ulcers and perhaps cancer. Overuse of aspirins and other nonsteroidal anti-inflammatory drugs (NSAIDs) can also cause stomach ulcers. A variety of substances, including alcohol, can prompt inflammation and even hemorrhaging. Stomach cancer has been shown to strike those who have a diet high in salted, smoked, or pickled foods; the most common cancer in the world, although not in the United States, it has a low survival rate. When stomach muscle function fails, food accumulates until the stomach overstretches and rebounds, causing vomiting. Some foods can coalesce into an in-digestible lump, and hair and food fibers can roll into a ball, called a bezoar; such masses can interfere with digestion.

The small intestine. The five to six meters of looped gut between the stomach and colon is called the small intestine. It secretes fluids, hormones, and enzymes into food passing through, breaking it down chemically and absorbing nutrients. Although cancers seldom develop in the small intestine itself, they frequently do so in the organs connected to it, the liver and pancreas. The major problem in the small bowel is the multitude of diseases causing diarrhea, dysentery, or ulceration: They include bacterial, viral, and parasitic disease; motility disorders; and the chronic, progressive inflammatory illness called Crohn's disease, which also ulcerates the bowel wall. Although most diarrhea is temporary, if it persists diarrhea severely weakens patients through dehydration and malnourishment. For this reason, diarrheal diseases caused by toxins in water or food are the leading cause of childhood death worldwide. Furthermore, the small bowel can become paralyzed, twisted, or kinked, thereby obstructing the passage of food. Sometimes its contents rush through too fast, a condition called dumping syndrome. All these disorders reduce digestion, and if they are chronic, then malnutrition, vitamin deficiency, and weight loss ensue.

The large intestine. The small intestine empties into the large intestine, or colon, the last meter of the GI tract; here the water content of digestive waste matter (about a liter a day) is reabsorbed, and the waste becomes increasingly solid along the way to the rectum, forming feces. Unlike the small bowel, which is nearly sterile under normal conditions, the colon hosts a large population of bacteria that ferments the indigestible fiber in waste matter, and some of the by-products are absorbed through the colon's mucosa. Bacteria or parasites gaining access from the outside world can cause diarrhea by interfering with this absorption (a condition called malabsorption) or by irritating the mucosa and speeding up muscle action. For unknown reasons, the colon can also become chronically inflamed, resulting in cramps and bloody diarrhea, an illness known as ulcerative colitis; Crohn's disease also can affect the colon. Probably because it is so often exposed to a variety of toxins, the colon is particularly susceptible to cancer in people over fifty years old: Colorectal cancer accounted for the second highest number of cancer deaths in 1993, with an equal proportion of men and women. As people age, the muscles controlling the colon deteriorate, sometimes forming small pouches in the bowel wall, called diverticula, that can become infected (diverticulitis). In addition, small knobs called polyps can grow, and they may become cancerous. One of the most common lower GI disorders is constipation, which may derive from a poor diet, motility malfunction, or both.

The rectum. The last segment of the colon, the rectum collects and holds feces for defecation through the anus. The rectum is susceptible to many of the diseases affecting the colon, including cancer and chronic inflammation. The powerful anal sphincter muscle, which controls defecation, can be the site of brief but intensely painful spasms called proctalgia fugax, which strikes for unknown reasons. The tissue lining the anal canal contains a dense network of blood vessels; straining to eliminate stool because of constipation or diarrhea or simply sitting too long on a toilet can distend these blood vessels, creating hemorrhoids, which may burn, itch, bleed, and become remarkably annoying. If infected, hemorrhoids or anal fissures may develop painful abscesses (sacs of pus). Extreme straining can cause the rectum to turn inside out through the anus, or prolapse.

The liver. The GI tract's organs figure prominently in many disorders. The liver is a large spongy organ that filters the blood, removing toxins and dumping them with bile into the duodenum. A number of viruses can invade the liver and inflame it, a malady called hepatitis. Acute forms of the disease have flulike symptoms and are self-limited. Some viruses, however, as well as alcohol or drug abuse and worms, cause extensive cirrhosis (the formation of abnormal, scarlike tissue) and chronic hepatitis. Although only recently common in the United States, viral hepatitis has long affected a large percentage of people in Southeast Asia; because hepatitis can trigger the mutation of normal cells, liver cancer is among the most common cancers worldwide. Hepatitis patients often have jaundice, as do those who, as a result of drug reactions, cancer, or stones, have blocked bile flow. Because of congenital or inherited errors of metabolism, excess fat, iron, and copper can build up in the liver, causing upper abdominal pain, skin discolorations, weakness, and behavioral changes; complications can include cirrhosis, diabetes mellitus, and heart disease.

The gallbladder. A small sac that concentrates and stores bile from the liver, the gallbladder is connected to the liver and duodenum by ducts. The concentrate often coalesces into stones, which seldom cause prob-

lems if they stay in one place. If they block the opening to the gallbladder or lodge in a duct, however, they can cause pain, fever, and jaundice. Although rare, tumors may also grow in the gallbladder or ducts, perhaps as a result of gallstone obstruction.

The pancreas. Lying just behind the stomach, the pancreas produces enzymes to break down fats and proteins for absorption and insulin to metabolize sugar; a duct joins it to the duodenum. The pancreas can become inflamed, either because of toxins (largely alcohol) or blockage of its duct, usually by gallstones. Either cause precipitates a painful condition, pancreatitis, that may last a few days, with full recovery, or turn into a life-threatening disease. If the source of inflammation is not eliminated, then chronic pancreatitis may develop and with it the gradual loss of the pancreas' ability to make enzymes and insulin. Severe abdominal pain, malnutrition, diarrhea, and diabetes may develop. Pancreatic cancer, once rare in the United States, ranked fifth among cancers causing death during 1993. Scientists are unsure of the causes; pancreatitis, gallstones, diabetes, and alcohol have been implicated, but only smoking is well attested to increase the risk of contracting pancreatic cancer, which is very lethal and difficult to treat. Only about 1 percent of patients live more than a year after diagnosis.

Functional diseases. Finally, some disorders appear to upset several parts of the GI tract at the same time, often with no identifiable cause but with chronic or recurrent symptoms. Gastroenterologists call them functional diseases, and they afflict as much as 30 percent of the population in Western countries. People with irritable bowel syndrome (IBS) complain of abdominal pain, urgency in defecation, and bloating from intestinal gas; they often feel that they cannot empty their rectums completely, even after straining. Functional dyspepsia manifests itself as upper abdominal pain, bloating, early feelings of fullness during a meal, and nausea. Also included in this group are various motility disorders in the esophagus and stomach, whose typical symptom is vomiting, and pseudo-obstruction, a condition in which the small bowel acts as if it is blocked but no lesion can be found. Many gastroenterologists believe that emotional disturbance plays a part in some of these diseases.

TREATMENT AND THERAPY

The majority of GI disorders are transient and pose no short-term or long-term threat to life. The body's natural defenses can combat most bacterial and viral infections in the gut without help. Even potentially dangerous noninfectious conditions, such as pancreatitis, resolve on their own if the irritating agent is eliminated. Many disorders require a gastroenterologist's help, however, and even despite help can make people semi-invalids. Regulation of diet and the use of drugs to combat infections or relieve pain are important treatments. If these fail, as is likely to happen in such serious conditions as chronic inflammatory disease and cancer, cures or palliation is yet possible because of gastroenterological technology, particularly endoscopy, and surgical techniques developed in the twentieth century.

While it is not true that GI disorders would necessarily disappear with improved diet, since genetic disorders would remain, gastroenterologists stress that proper nourishment is the first line of defense against trouble. For example, incidence of stomach cancer plummets in countries where people eat fresh foods and use refrigeration rather than salting and smoking to preserve food. Regions where fiber makes up a high percentage of the diet, such as Africa, have a far lower incidence of inflammatory bowel disease. Last, and certainly not least, groups that do not drink alcohol or smoke (such as Mormons) have far lower incidences of cancer and inflammatory disease throughout the GI tract.

—Roger Smith, Ph.D.

See also Abdomen; Abdominal disorders; Acid reflux disease; Appendectomy; Appendicitis; Appetite loss; Bacterial infections; Bariatric surgery; Botulism; Bypass surgery; Candidiasis; Celiac sprue; Cholecystitis; Cholera; Cirrhosis; Colic; Colitis; Colon and rectal polyp removal; Colon and rectal surgery; Colon cancer; Colon therapy; Colonoscopy and sigmoidoscopy; Constipation; Crohn's disease; Diabetes mellitus; Diarrhea and dysentery; Digestion; Diverticulitis and diverticulosis; Enemas; Enterocolitis; Fistula repair; Food poisoning; Gallbladder cancer; Gallbladder diseases; Gastrectomy; Gastroenterology; Gastroenterology, pediatric; Gastrointestinal system; Gastrostomy; Heartburn; Hemorrhoid banding and removal; Hemorrhoids; Hernia; Hernia repair; Hirschsprung's disease; Ileostomy and colostomy; Incontinence; Indigestion; Internal medicine; Intestinal disorders; Intestines; Irritable bowel syndrome (IBS); Jaundice; Kwashiorkor; Lactose intolerance; Liver; Liver cancer; Liver disorders; Malabsorption; Malnutrition; Metabolism;

Nausea and vomiting; Nonalcoholic steatohepatitis (NASH); Noroviruses; Nutrition; Obstruction; Pancreas; Pancreatitis; Peristalsis; Peritonitis; Pinworms; Poisoning; Poisonous plants; Proctology; Protozoan diseases; Pyloric stenosis; Rotavirus; Roundworms; Salmonella infection; Shigellosis; Soiling; Stomach, intestinal, and pancreatic cancers; Tapeworms; Toilet training; Trichinosis; Tumor removal; Tumors; Typhoid fever; Typhus; Ulcer surgery; Ulcers; Vagotomy; Weight loss and gain; Worms.

FOR FURTHER INFORMATION:

Feldman, Mark, Lawrence S. Friedman, and Lawrence J. Brandt, eds. *Sleisenger and Fordtran's Gastrointestinal and Liver Disease: Pathophysiology, Diagnosis, Management.* 8th ed. 2 vols. Philadelphia: W. B. Saunders, 2006. A comprehensive textbook of gastrointestinal diseases and physiology. Contains excellent chapters on all disorders mentioned in the text, as well as some beautiful endoscopic photographs.

Heuman, Douglas M., A. Scott Mills, and Hunter H. McGuire, Jr. *Gastroenterology.* Philadephia: W. B. Saunders, 1997. A review of digestive system diseases and methods of treating them. Includes a bibliography and an index.

Janowitz, Henry D. *Indigestion: Living Better with Upper Intestinal Problems from Heartburn to Ulcers and Gallstones.* New York: Oxford University Press, 1994. Clear explanations of common ailments, especially those related to aging, to help people prevent or manage GI disorders. With charts and illustrations.

Sachar, David B., Jerome D. Waye, and Blair S. Lewis, eds. *Pocket Guide to Gastroenterology.* Rev. ed. Baltimore: Williams & Wilkins, 1991. In detailed outlines intended for physicians, this handbook contains a wealth of information from which general readers can profit despite the extensive use of medical terminology.

Thompson, W. Grant. *The Angry Gut: Coping with Colitis and Crohn's Disease.* New York: Plenum Press, 1993. In addition to highlighting the significant similarities and differences of these two syndromes and stressing the importance of a correct diagnosis, Thompson broaches more sensitive topics that seem to be ignored by the medical profession.

GASTROINTESTINAL SYSTEM

ANATOMY

ANATOMY OR SYSTEM AFFECTED: Abdomen, gallbladder, intestines, liver, pancreas, stomach, teeth, throat

SPECIALTIES AND RELATED FIELDS: Dentistry, gastroenterology, internal medicine, nutrition, oncology, otorhinolaryngology

DEFINITION: A compartmentalized tube that is equipped to reduce food, both mechanically and chemically, to a state in which it is absorbed and used by the body; this system includes the mouth, esophagus, stomach, small intestine, and colon (large intestine), as well as the salivary glands, pancreas, liver, and gallbladder.

KEY TERMS:

absorption: the movement of digested food from the small intestine into blood vessels and from blood into body cells

bolus: food that has been mixed with saliva and formed into a ball; the bolus passes from the mouth to the stomach through a process called swallowing or deglutition

chyme: the semiliquid state of food as it is found in the stomach and first part of the small intestine

digestion: the mechanical and chemical breakdown of food into physical and molecular units that can be absorbed and used by cells

enzymes: substances that aid in the chemical digestion of food; enzymes are produced and secreted by glands found in digestive organs

peristalsis: a muscular contraction that helps to move food through the digestive tube

sphincter: a circular muscle that controls the opening and closing of an orifice

villus: a fingerlike projection in the small intestine that provides a site for the absorption of digested food into the circulatory and lymph systems

STRUCTURE AND FUNCTIONS

The gastrointestinal system or alimentary canal exists as a tube that runs through the body from mouth to anus. The wall of the tube is composed of four layers of tissue. The outermost layer, the serosa, is part of a large tissue called the peritoneum, which covers internal organs and lines body cavities. Extensions of the peritoneum called mesenteries anchor the organs of digestion to the body wall. Fatty, apronlike structures that hang in front of the abdominal organs are also modifications of the peritoneum. They are called the lesser and the greater omentum. The muscular layer, composed of circular and longitudinal muscles, makes up the bulk of the wall of the tube. The contractions of this layer aid in moving materials through the tube. Nerves, blood vessels, and lymph vessels are found in the third layer, the submucosa. The innermost or mucous layer has glands for secretion and modifications for absorption.

The tube is compartmentalized, and each section is equipped to accomplish some part of the digestive process. The mechanical phase of digestion involves the physical reduction of food to a semiliquid state; this is accomplished by tearing, chewing, and churning the food. Chemical digestion utilizes enzymes to reduce food to simple molecules that can be absorbed and used by the body to provide energy and to build and repair tissue.

The mouth (also called the buccal or oral cavity) marks the beginning of the gastrointestinal system and the digestive process. The mouth is divided into two areas. The vestibule is the space between the lips, cheeks, gums, and teeth. Lips, or labia, are the fleshy folds that surround the opening to the mouth. The skin covers the outside, while the inside is lined with mucous membrane. The colored part of the lips, called the vermilion, is a juncture of these two tissues. Because the tissue at this point is unclouded, underlying blood vessels can be seen. A membrane called the labial frenulum attaches each lip to the gum, or gingivalum.

The oral cavity occupies the space posterior to the teeth and anterior to the fauces or opening to the throat. It is bounded on the sides by cheeks and on the roof by an anterior bony structure called the hard palate and a posterior muscular area, the soft palate. The uvula, a cone-shaped extension of the soft palate, can be seen hanging down in front of the fauces. The floor of the oral cavity is formed by the tongue and associated muscles. Taste buds are found on the surface of the tongue. The bottom of the tongue is anchored posteriorly to the hyoid bone. Anteriorly, the membranous frenulum lingua anchors the tongue to the floor of the mouth. The tongue's movement is controlled by extrinsic muscles that form the floor of the mouth and by intrinsic muscles that are part of the tongue itself. The movements of the tongue assist in speaking, swallowing, and forming food into a bolus.

Teeth, found in gum sockets, are the principal means of mechanical digestion in the mouth. Human teeth appear in two sets. The deciduous or milk teeth are the first to appear. There are usually ten in each jaw, and they are replaced by the second, permanent set during childhood. The permanent set consists of sixteen teeth in each jaw. The four incisors and two canines have sharp chiseled edges, which permit biting and tearing of food. The four premolars and six molars have flat surfaces that are used in grinding the food. Frequently, the third pair of molars or wisdom teeth do not erupt until later in adolescence. The crown of a tooth appears above the gum line while the roots are embedded in the gum socket. The small area between the crown and the root is called the neck. The crown is covered with enamel and the root with cementum. Dentin is beneath the covering in both areas and forms the bulk of the tooth. The central cavity of the tooth is filled with a soft membrane called pulp. Blood vessels and nerves are embedded in the pulp.

At the rear of the mouth, the fauces or opening leads to the pharynx. The pharynx is a common passageway for the movement of air from nasal cavity to trachea and food from mouth to esophagus. The esophagus is a tube approximately 25 centimeters long. Most of the esophagus is located within the thoracic cavity, although the lower end of the tube pierces the diaphragm and connects with the stomach in the abdominal cavity. Both ends of the esophagus are controlled by a circular muscle called a sphincter. The movement of food through the esophagus is assisted by gravity and the contrac-

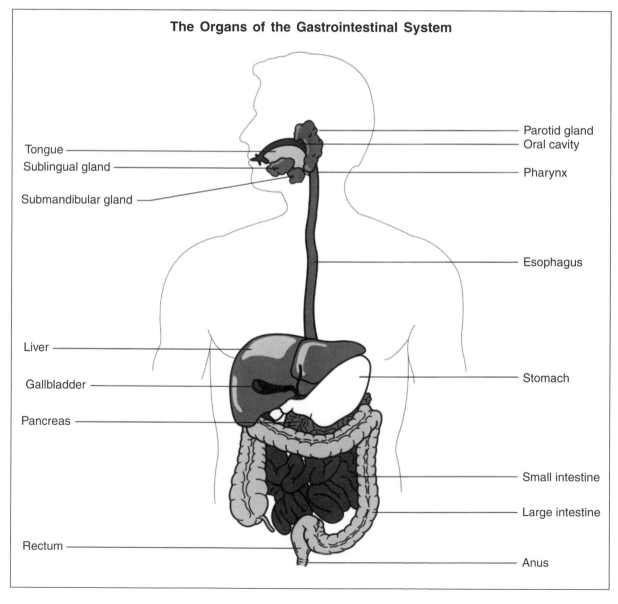

The Organs of the Gastrointestinal System

Tongue

Sublingual gland

Submandibular gland

Liver

Gallbladder

Pancreas

Rectum

Parotid gland
Oral cavity

Pharynx

Esophagus

Stomach

Small intestine

Large intestine

Anus

tions of the muscularis layer. No digestion is accomplished in either the pharynx or the esophagus.

The stomach, a J-shaped organ, is divided into four areas: the cardia, fundus, body, and pyloris. The cardia lies just below the sphincter at the juncture of esophagus and stomach, while the fundus is a pouch that pushes upward and to the left of the cardia. The large central area is the body, and the lower end of the stomach is the pyloris. Here another sphincter, the pyloric valve, controls the opening between stomach and intestine. The mucosa of the stomach is arranged in folds called rugae. The rugae permit distension of the organ as it fills. Gastric and mucus glands are present in the mucosa. The gastric glands produce and secrete enzymes that are specific for protein digestion, as well as hydrochloric acid, which creates the proper acid environment for enzyme action. The muscularis of the stomach wall has three layers of muscle with a circular, longitudinal, and oblique arrangement. The muscle arrangement facilitates the churning action that reduces the food to a semiliquid called chyme. The pyloric valve relaxes under neuronal and hormonal influence, and the chyme is moved into the small intestine.

The site for the completion of digestion and the absorption of digested material is the small intestine. This tube, with a 2.5-centimeter diameter and a length of 6.4 meters, is coiled into the mid and lower abdomen. The first 25 centimeters of the small intestine constitute the duodenum. This is followed by the jejunum, which is 2.5 meters long. The ileum, at 3.6 meters, terminates at the ileocecal valve, which connects the small to the large intestine. The interior of the small intestine is characterized by the presence of fingerlike projections of the mucosa called villi that contain blood and lymph capillaries and circular folds of submucosa (the plicae circularis), both of which provide absorption surface for the digested food. Mucosal glands produce enzymes that contribute to the digestion of carbohydrates, lipids, and proteins. Enzymes from the pancreas and bile from the liver enter the small intestine at the duodenum and aid the chemical digestion.

The final compartment in the gastrointestinal system is the large intestine, sometimes called the bowel or colon. This tube, with a diameter of 6.5 centimeters and a length of 1.5 meters, is divided into the cecum; the ascending, transverse, and descending colon; the rectum; and the anal canal. The cecum is a blind pouch located just below the ileocecal valve. The fingerlike appendix is attached to the cecum. The ascending colon extends from the cecum up the right side of the abdomen to the

underside of the liver, where it turns and runs across the body. The colon descends along the left side of the abdomen. The last few centimeters of colon form an S-shaped curve that gives the section its name, sigmoid colon. Three bands of longitudinal muscle called taeniae coli run the length of the colon. Contraction of these bands causes pouches or haustra to form in the colon, giving the tube a puckered appearance. The sigmoid colon leads into the rectum, a 20-centimeter segment that terminates in a short anal canal. The anus is the opening from the anal canal to the exterior of the body.

DISORDERS AND DISEASES

Because the primary function performed in the gastrointestinal system is the physical and chemical preparation of food for cellular absorption and use, any malfunction of the process has implications for the overall metabolism of the body. Structural changes or abnormalities in the anatomy of the system interfere with the proper mechanical and chemical preparation of the food.

Teeth are the principal agents of mechanical digestion or mastication in the mouth. Dental caries or tooth decay involves a demineralization of the enamel through bacterial action. Disrupted enamel provides an entrance for bacteria to underlying tissues, resulting in infection and inflammation of the tissues. The resulting pain and discomfort interfere with the biting, chewing, and grinding of food. Three pairs of salivary glands secrete the water-based, enzyme-containing fluid called saliva. These glands can be the target of the virus that causes mumps. (Although the pain and swelling that are typical of this disease can prevent swallowing, the more important effect of the virus in males is the possible inflammation of the testes and subsequent sterility.)

The gastroesophageal sphincter at the lower end of the esophagus controls the movement of materials from the stomach into the esophagus. Relaxation of this sphincter allows a backflow of food (gastroesophageal reflux) to occur. The acidity of the stomach contents damages the esophageal lining, and a burning sensation is experienced. Substances such as citric fruits, chocolate, tomatoes, alcohol, and nicotine as well as body positions that increase abdominal pressure, such as bending or lying on the side, induce heartburn or indigestion. A hiatal hernia occurs when a defect of the diaphragm allows the lower portion of the esophagus and the upper portion of the stomach to enter the chest cavity; it causes heartburn and difficulty in swallowing.

Pathologies and abnormalities of the stomach and intestines are studied in the medical science called gastroenterology. The stomach is the site of both mechanical and chemical digestion. Although small amounts of digested food begin to pass into the small intestine within minutes following a meal, the chyme usually remains in the stomach for three to five hours. Relaxation of the gastroesophageal sphincter will result in reflux; and stimulation by nerves from the medulla of the brain can cause the forceful emptying of stomach contents through the mouth. This is called vomiting and may be brought about by irritation, overdistension, certain foods, or drugs. Excessive vomiting results in dehydration, which in turn upsets electrolyte and fluid balance.

Chemical digestion in the stomach requires an acidic environment. This is provided by gastric glands, which secrete hydrochloric acid. The tissue lining the stomach protects it from this acidity and prevents self-digestion. Oversecretion of the gastric juices or a breakdown of the stomach lining can cause lesions or peptic ulcers to form in the mucosal lining. Gastritis, the inflammation of the stomach mucosa brought on by the ingestion of irritants such as alcohol and aspirin or an overactive nervous stimulation of the gastric glands, may be the underlying cause of ulcer formation. Ulcers can form in the lower esophagus, stomach, and duodenum because these are the organs that come in contact with gastric juice. The terms "gastric ulcer" and "duodenal ulcer" refer to peptic ulcers located in the stomach and the first portion of the small intestine, respectively.

Gastroenteritis could involve the stomach, the small intestine, or the large intestine. It is a disorder marked by nausea, vomiting, abdominal discomfort, and diarrhea. The condition has various causes and is known by several names. Bacteria are a common cause of the condition known as food poisoning. Amoebas, parasites, and viruses can bring about the symptoms associated with intestinal influenza or travelers' diarrhea. Allergic reactions to food or drugs may cause gastroenteritis.

Although diverticulitis may be found anywhere along the gastrointestinal tract, it is most commonly found in the sigmoid colon. This disorder results from the formation of pouches or diverticula in the wall of the tract. Undigested food and bacteria collect in the diverticula and react to form a hard mass. The mass interferes with the blood supply to the area and ultimately irritates and inflames surrounding tissue. Abscess, obstruction, and hemorrhage may develop. A diet lacking in fiber appears to be the major contributor to this disorder.

Colitis, or inflammation of the bowel, is accompanied by abdominal cramps, diarrhea, and constipation. It may be brought about by psychological stress, as in irritable bowel syndrome, or may be a manifestation of such disorders as chronic ulcerative colitis and Crohn's disease.

A change in the rate of motility through the colon or large intestine results in one of two disorders: diarrhea or constipation. As food passes through the colon, water is reabsorbed by the body. If the food moves too quickly through the colon, then much of the water will remain in the feces and diarrhea results. Severe diarrhea affects electrolyte balance. Viral, bacterial, and parasitic organisms may initiate the rapid motility of substances through the colon. Another condition, called constipation, develops from sluggish motility. When the food remains for too long a time in the bowel, too much water is reabsorbed by the body. The feces then become dry and hard, and defecation is difficult. Lack of fiber in the diet and lack of exercise are the leading causes of constipation.

Hemorrhoids are varicose veins that develop in the rectum or anal canal. Varicose veins are the result of weakened venous valves. Factors such as pressure, lack of muscle tone as a result of aging, straining at defecation, pregnancy, and obesity are among the common contributors. Hemorrhoids become irritated and bleed when hard stools are passed.

Disorders in the accessory organs contribute to the malfunctioning of the gastrointestinal system. Gallstones, cirrhosis of the liver, pancreatitis, and pancreatic cancer are among the major diseases affecting the digestive process. These disorders generally involve the obstruction of tubes or the destruction of glands, so that enzymes do not reach the intended site of digestion.

PERSPECTIVE AND PROSPECTS

The proper functioning of the gastrointestinal system is dependent on the anatomical structure and health of the organs. The organs provide the site for the mechanical and chemical digestion of food, the absorption of food and water, and the elimination of waste material. Two factors play a primary role in causing anatomical abnormalities in digestion: aging and eating disorders.

The aging process gradually changes anatomical structure. In order for food to be chewed properly, teeth must be in good health. Dental caries, periodontal disease, and missing teeth prevent the proper mastication of food. Because of these problems, older people tend to avoid foods that require chewing. This may lead to an unbalanced diet. Another age-related change in the mouth is the atrophy of the salivary glands and other secretory glands, which interferes with chemical digestion and swallowing. A loss of muscle tone in the organ walls impedes mechanical digestion and slows down the movement of food through the system. Often, the elimination of waste material becomes difficult and constipation results.

Eating disorders such as anorexia nervosa and bulimia contribute to digestive malfunctioning. These disorders are most often associated with but are not limited to young women. Anorexia is self-imposed starvation, while bulimia is characterized by a binge-purge cycle that incorporates vomiting and/or abuse of laxatives. Both conditions induce nutrient deficiencies and upset water and electrolyte balances. The vomiting of the acid contents of the stomach damages esophageal, pharyngeal, and mouth tissue. It also destroys tooth enamel. In addition to the harm done to the gastrointestinal system, eating disorders affect several other systems, such as the reproductive system.

The field of medical science that studies and diagnoses digestive system disorders is gastroenterology. Gastroenterologists use several investigative techniques. Blood tests and stool examination are used to detect internal bleeding and deficiency disorders. For a time, X rays were the only nonsurgical means of obtaining information on the structure of internal organs. The advent of nuclear medicine in the 1950's led to the use of radioisotopes in body scanning procedures. Instruments capable of a more detailed and direct visualization were developed, such as fiber optics and the fluoroscope. Fiber optics involves the use of long, threadlike fibers of glass or plastic that transmit light into the organ and reflect the image back to the viewer; this method allows the physician to detect ulcers, lesions, neoplasms, and structural abnormalities. The fluoroscope uses X rays to permit continuous observation of motion within the organs.

The 1970's saw the development of more sophisticated scanning and imaging techniques. Computed tomography (CT) scanning uses X-ray techniques to scan very thin slices of tissue and presents a defined, unobstructed view. Magnetic resonance imaging (MRI) can provide detailed information even to the molecular level; energies from powerful magnetic fields are translated into a visual representation of the structure being studied. Another technique, ultrasonography, passes sound waves through a body area, intercepts the echoes

that are produced, and translates them into electrical impulses, which are recorded and interpreted by the physician.

—Rosemary Scheirer, Ed.D.

See also Abdomen; Acid reflux disease; Bariatric surgery; Constipation; Diarrhea and dysentery; Digestion; Endoscopy; Enzymes; Food biochemistry; Gastroenterology; Gastroenterology, pediatric; Gastrointestinal disorders; Glands; Hemorrhoids; Hernia; Host-defense mechanisms; Indigestion; Internal medicine; Intestinal disorders; Intestines; Laparoscopy; Lipids; Liver; Malnutrition; Metabolism; Muscles; Nausea and vomiting; Nutrition; Obstruction; Peristalsis; Proctology; Sense organs; Systems and organs; Taste; Teeth.

FOR FURTHER INFORMATION:

Abrahams, Peter H., Sandy C. Marks, Jr., and Ralph Hutchings. *McMinn's Color Atlas of Human Anatomy.* 5th ed. New York: Mosby, 2003. Although this atlas is intended for an advanced student of human anatomy, the average reader can profit from the marvelous diagrams and pictures. The pictures are especially helpful in visualizing the organs as they actually appear in the human body.

Moog, Florence. "The Lining of the Small Intestine." *Scientific American* 245 (November, 1981): 154-176. This article incorporates a historical perspective in the detailed explanation of absorption as it occurs in the small intestine. The article requires some scientific literacy but is not beyond the comprehension of a reader with a high school science background.

Tortora, Gerard J., and Bryan Derrickson. *Principles of Anatomy and Physiology.* 11th ed. Hoboken, N.J.: John Wiley & Sons, 2006. This highly readable text gives a clear and accurate description of the anatomy and physiology of the gastrointestinal system. The illustrations and diagrams are excellent. The authors include descriptions of major disorders and clinical applications.

GASTROSTOMY

PROCEDURE

ANATOMY OR SYSTEM AFFECTED: Abdomen, gastrointestinal system, stomach

SPECIALTIES AND RELATED FIELDS: Gastroenterology, oncology

DEFINITION: The creation of a hole through the wall of the abdomen into the stomach in order to feed a patient who is unable to swallow.

INDICATIONS AND PROCEDURES

Gastrostomies are carried out during situations in which a patient is unable to swallow food. This condition may result from cancer or strictures of the esophagus; when an esophageal fistula is present, causing the diversion of swallowed food; or when a patient is unconscious. In some cases, the patient is a child who has swallowed a caustic substance, causing damage to the esophagus. Under such circumstances in which a gastrostomy is warranted, an artificial opening is prepared through the abdominal wall into the stomach, and a tube is inserted through the opening.

The gastrostomy tube, which is usually made of plastic or nylon, may be permanently inserted or removed after each feeding. The development of the Barnes-Redo prosthesis has alleviated some of the problems associated with permanent gastrostomies. The device, which is permanently installed, has a cap placed over the opening between feedings. When it is time to eat, the cap is removed, and a catheter is placed through the tube into the stomach, allowing food or liquids to be fed to the patient. When the meal is finished, the catheter is removed and the cap replaced on the gastrostomy tube.

Food for gastrostomy patients cannot be solid. It is recommended that any food first be thoroughly cooked and then blended into a mushy consistency. Patients should smell and taste the food prior to feeding, both to minimize difficulty in adjustment to the situation and to stimulate gastric secretions, which will aid in digestion.

USES AND COMPLICATIONS

Care must be taken with gastrostomy patients to minimize the chance of infection. Any tubes that will be inserted into the stomach must be sterilized prior to use. In addition, the skin around the gastrostomy tube must be protected from gastric juices such as stomach acid, which could cause irritation. The major adjustment for these patients, however, is often psychological—particularly for those with permanent gastrostomies, since meals are often times for social gatherings.

—*Richard Adler, Ph.D.*

See also Cancer; Catheterization; Critical care; Critical care, pediatric; Gastroenterology; Gastroenterology, pediatric; Gastrointestinal disorders; Gastrointestinal system; Nutrition; Stomach, intestinal, and pancreatic cancers.

FOR FURTHER INFORMATION:

Barrett, Catherine, ed. *Gastrostomy Care: A Guide to Practice*. San Francisco: Ausmed, 2004.

Breckman, Brigid, ed. *Stoma Care and Rehabilitation*. New York: Elsevier Churchill Livingstone, 2005.

Broadwell, Debra C., and Bettie S. Jackson, eds. *Principles of Ostomy Care*. St. Louis: Mosby, 1982.

Gauderer, Michael W. L., and Thomas A. Stellato. *Gastrostomies: Evolution, Techniques, Indications, and Complications*. Chicago: Year Book Medical, 1986.

Ponsky, Jeffrey L., ed. *Techniques of Percutaneous Gastrostomy*. New York: Igaku-Shoin, 1988.

GATES FOUNDATION

ORGANIZATION

DEFINITION: A private charitable foundation, founded in 2000 and headquartered in Seattle, which aids in global health.

ESTABLISHMENT AND PURPOSE

In January, 2000, Microsoft founder and chief executive officer (CEO) Bill Gates and his wife Melinda established what has become the world's most lavishly funded charitable foundation. The Gateses earmarked five billion dollars for the foundation in June, 1999, following this with a contribution of $106 million in 2000. By June, 2006, with additional funding from the Gateses, the foundation's endowment reached $29.2 billion.

The endowment was enhanced substantially on June 25, 2006, when Warren Buffett pledged to the Gates Foundation ten million shares of Berkshire Hathaway class B stock, worth $30.7 billion on June 23, 2006, the most substantial charitable donation in American history. This contribution, spread over several years, gives the Gates Foundation the largest endowment of any existing foundation. Even before Buffett's gift, its assets exceeded the gross national product (GNP) of more than one hundred nations.

The Gates Foundation provides funding in one miscellaneous and four specific categories: global health, education, libraries, and the Pacific Northwest. Its outreach, particularly in health, is worldwide, with special emphasis on improving medical facilities, training medical personnel, and enhancing medical education. It emphasizes prevention through education, inoculation, and therapeutic management of such endemic diseases as acquired immunodeficiency syndrome (AIDS), malaria, and poliomyelitis.

ORGANIZATION AND MANAGEMENT

Despite its size and complexity, the Gates Foundation controls overhead expenses scrupulously. Its emphasis is on assisting those who most need help, with minimal bureaucratic interference. With a worldwide toll of over a million deaths yearly from malaria, two million from tuberculosis, and three million from HIV/AIDS, a daunting task faces the Gateses' global health outreach.

Buffett's contribution stipulates that the foundation must continue qualifying as a charitable organization and must distribute an annual amount at least 5 percent more than the previous year's Berkshire contribution. Federal laws governing charitable foundations require them to distribute 5 percent or more of their assets every year.

Even before Buffett's contribution, this government regulation forced the Gates Foundation to distribute approximately a billion dollars every year. When Buffett's total contribution is added to the original endowment, the foundation will be required to distribute over two billion dollars a year to qualify as a charitable foundation.

As the foundation was originally organized, Bill and Melinda Gates were actively involved as cofounders, although the demands on Bill Gates as CEO of Microsoft limited the time that he could spend overseeing the foundation. On June 15, 2006, Gates announced that after July 31, 2008, he would reduce his involvement in the day-to-day operation of Microsoft and would direct most of his energies toward overseeing the foundation.

Gates's father, William H. Gates, Sr., has served as co-chairperson of the foundation since its founding, as has Patty Stonesifer who, besides being co-chairperson, is president and CEO of the Gates Foundation. The foundation in mid-2006 had 241 full-time employees, a modest number for such a complex organization.

SCOPE AND IMPACT

Because Microsoft's corporate center is in Seattle, one of the Gates Foundation's priorities, to sponsor projects affecting America's Northwest, reflects the Gateses' loyalty to that area. The overall scope of the organization, however, is truly global with special emphasis on the Third World, with its daunting health problems, notably HIV-AIDS, malaria, diabetes, and polio.

In October, 2000, the Gates Cambridge Scholarship Program, established with a grant of more than $200

million, enabled promising graduate students from outside the United Kingdom to study at Cambridge University, a program that every year subsidizes one hundred new scholars. The Gates Millennium Scholars' Program, with funding of one billion dollars, is administered by the United Negro College Fund and provides scholarships for minority students in the United States.

The students in these programs frequently pursue careers related to world health. The foundation's awards of $800 million a year for global health almost equals the annual budget of the United Nations' World Health Organization (WHO). The greatest international impact of the Gates Foundation clearly is in global health.

On October 25, 2005, the foundation gave the Global Alliance for Vaccines and Immunization $750 million to underwrite its vaccination programs. A grant of $30 million helped to establish a new Department of Global Health at the University of Washington aimed at preparing health professionals—physicians, paramedics, nurses, social workers, and psychologists—to work with the impoverished on the prevention and treatment of diseases prevalent among them. This grant enabled the University of Washington to hire fourteen new faculty members and to support more than four hundred graduate students and staff.

The Gates Foundation has contributed nearly $300 million to be divided among sixteen teams doing HIV/AIDS research throughout the world. This gift requires that all these teams share their findings with other teams.

The foundation provides funds to help organizations dealing with emergencies such as the 2004 Indian Ocean tsunami and the 2005 earthquake in Kashmir. This funding enables medical professionals to deal with the health problems that accompany such disasters.

Some conservative critics fear that the money the foundation awards will fall into the hands of unscrupulous politicians. The wisdom of throwing money at problems in the Third World, where graft is rampant and distribution is questionable, has been viewed with skepticism in some quarters. Critics suggest that helping Third World nations develop stronger infrastructures and work opportunities for the unemployed might help more than bestowing money upon them.

—R. Baird Shuman, Ph.D.

See also Acquired immunodeficiency syndrome (AIDS); Education, medical; Malaria; Poliomyelitis; Tropical medicine; Tuberculosis; World Health Organization.

FOR FURTHER INFORMATION:

Ashraf, Haroon. "Bill Gates Throws Down the Gauntlet to Medical Researchers." *The Lancet* 361 (February 1, 2003): 404.

Birn, Anne-Emanuelle. "Gates's Grandest Challenge: Transcending Technology as Public Health Ideology." *The Lancet* 366 (August 6, 2005): 514-519.

Chase, Marilyn. "Gates Won't Fund AIDS Researchers Unless They Pool Data." *The Wall Street Journal, Eastern Edition*, July 20, 2006, pp. B1-B2.

Check, Erika. "Global Vaccine Project Gets a Shot in the Arm." *Nature*, January 27, 2005, pp. 345.

Enserink, Martin. "Gates Pledges $168 Million for Malaria Research." *Science* 301 (September 26, 2003): 1828.

Service, Robert F. "Gates Grows UW's Genome Program." *Science* 300 (May 2, 2003): 723.

GAUCHER'S DISEASE

DISEASE/DISORDER

ANATOMY OR SYSTEM AFFECTED: Abdomen, bones, cells, liver, lymphatic system, spleen

SPECIALTIES AND RELATED FIELDS: Biochemistry, cytology, genetics, internal medicine, pediatrics, toxicology

DEFINITION: A congenital disorder caused by a defect in lipid metabolism and characterized by cell hyperplasia in the liver, spleen, and bone marrow.

KEY TERMS:

enzyme: a protein that catalyzes a biological reaction in the body

hyperplasia: enlargement

CAUSES AND SYMPTOMS

Gaucher's disease is an inherited disorder resulting from a mutation in the gene that encodes the enzyme glucocerebrosidase, one of a class of enzymes that functions in the breakdown (hydrolysis) of glucosyl ceramide lipids. The result is an accumulation of a class of lipids known as glucosyl ceramide sphingolipids, primarily in cells of the liver, spleen, or bone marrow. Normally, these lipids are hydrolyzed within digestive organelles called lysosomes, found within these cells. The buildup of lipids within these structures classifies Gaucher's disease as a form of lysosomal storage disease; cells in which these pathologies are presented are known as Gaucher cells.

Gaucher's disease is not common in the general population, affecting approximately 1 in 100,000 persons, although three to four times that number probably carry

INFORMATION ON GAUCHER'S DISEASE

CAUSES: Genetic enzyme deficiency

SYMPTOMS: Varies with type; may include liver and spleen enlargement, bone marrow abnormalities, severe anemia, severe bleeding, central nervous system damage

DURATION: Chronic

TREATMENTS: Enzyme replacement therapy, genetically engineered drugs

one copy of the defective gene. However, in the ethnic population of Ashkenazi (Eastern European) Jews, approximately 1 in 450 persons is afflicted with the disease, making it among the most common genetic disorders in this group. In 2003, the National Gaucher Foundation, an organization that monitors the disorder, estimated that approximately 2,500 Americans had the disease.

Three different types of Gaucher's disease have been described, differing in their severity, in the presence or absence of neurological defects, and in the general demographics of the disorder. The most common form is type I, characterized by hyperplasia of the liver and spleen and accompanied by bone marrow abnormalities; neurological problems are not observed in this form. Its symptoms include severe anemia, attributable to pathological events among the bone marrow precursors; low numbers of platelets, resulting in severe bleeding; and significant hyperplasia in the spleen and liver. The disease, when observed, is generally found in the adult population, though not all persons with this genetic mutation actually experience all, or even any, of the symptoms. Type II (infantile) disorder, a neuropathic or malignant presentation, is a significantly more severe form that affects children under the age of six months; rarely do these children survive beyond two years as a result of significant central nervous system damage, especially among the cranial nerves. The third form, type III (juvenile), is less severe than Type II, and significantly more variable in its prognosis; children can usually grow into their adult years.

TREATMENT AND THERAPY

Until the 1990's, control of Gaucher's disease involved a combination of splenectomy and repeated blood transfusions. The development of enzyme replacement therapy in 1991 provided a means of controlling the disease through the direct presentation of the missing enzyme glucocerebrosidase to the patient's system. The enzyme was obtained and purified from human placentas collected following hospital births. The initial studies using the natural form of glucocerebrosidase were disappointing, but a chemically modified product proved more successful. The modified form of the enzyme was presented intravenously to persons on an outpatient basis approximately twice each month. Though costly, the process proved effective in controlling most forms of type I disease, the most common, but less effective for other forms of the disease. In those patients for whom therapy had proven effective, other aspects of the disorder such as cell hyperplasia were often reversed.

Treatments developed in the late 1990's included genetically engineered forms of drugs that could be taken orally. This form of treatment has proven highly effective with those expressing the type I form and to a lesser extent the type III form. In addition to replacement of the defective enzyme, a new class of drugs was also developed that inhibited the actual synthesis of the potentially toxic lipids by blocking the action of the enzyme glucosylceramide synthase.

No effective treatment exists for the type II form of Gaucher's disease, and central nervous system damage is not reversible, even if the disease does respond to therapy.

PERSPECTIVE AND PROSPECTS

Since the chromosomal site of Gaucher's disease is known—chromosome 1q21, or the long arm of chromosome number 1—prenatal testing is possible to determine whether the developing fetus carries the defective gene. The course, or any decision with regard to treatment, is difficult because of the variable nature of many forms of the disease. Carriers can be observed through the use of molecular techniques, such as restriction fragment length polymorphisms (RFLPs), which detect the presence of abnormal forms of the affected gene. However, even within the population affected, such as Ashkenazi Jews, multiple forms of mutations can be found. The significance of different mutations within the same gene remains confusing, in that different persons with even similar defects may manifest the disease in a variety of forms. Clearly, the role of other factors in the expression of Gaucher's disease remains to be clarified.

The disease is not manifested in every individual carrying the mutation; genetic testing of parents in at-risk groups, or the testing of normal parents who have a child with the disorder, may also provide a means of screening during pregnancy for the possibility of illness in the developing child. Given the variable nature of the disease, the issue of screening remains controversial.

Ideally, gene replacement remains the only method, in theory, which could cure the disease. The systemic aspect of the disorder, however, means that even if possible, replacement would have to be carried out at the level of the fetus. For the near future, treatment and control rest upon an increasingly effective use of oral drugs to compensate for the absent enzyme.

—*Richard Adler, Ph.D.*

See also Enzyme therapy; Enzymes; Genetic counseling; Genetic diseases; Glycogen storage diseases; Lipids; Metabolic disorders; Metabolism; Mucopolysaccharidosis (MPS); Niemann-Pick disease; Screening; Tay-Sachs disease.

FOR FURTHER INFORMATION:

Bellenir, Karen, ed. *Genetic Disorders Sourcebook: Basic Consumer Information About Hereditary Diseases and Disorders*. 3d ed. Detroit: Omnigraphics, 2004.

Futerman, Anthony H., and Ari Zimran, eds. *Gaucher Disease*. Boca Raton, Fla.: CRC/Taylor & Francis, 2007.

Parker, James N., and Philip M. Parker, eds. *The Official Parent's Sourcebook on Gaucher's Disease*. San Diego, Calif.: Icon Health, 2002.

GENE THERAPY

TREATMENT

ALSO KNOWN AS: Gene transfer

ANATOMY OR SYSTEM AFFECTED: Cells

SPECIALTIES AND RELATED FIELDS: Biotechnology, cytology, genetics

DEFINITION: The delivery of genetic material into a cell for the purpose of either correcting a genetic problem or giving the cell a new biochemical function.

KEY TERMS:

gene: the deoxyribonucleic acid (DNA) instructions necessary for the manufacture of a functional protein in a cell

genome: the total genetic information found within a virus, cell, or organism

germ cells: cells involved in the process of sexual reproduction and inheritance; also called gametes *somatic cells:* cells that make up the majority of the human body and that are not passed on from generation to generation

stem cells: cells that are undifferentiated, meaning that they have the potential to develop into a variety of cell and tissue types

vector: in genetics, a system (usually a virus) that is used to carry a gene into the cell for gene therapy

virus: an infectious agent that consists of a protein coat enclosing a small piece of genetic material; viruses are usually less than one-thousandth the size of the living cell

INDICATIONS AND PROCEDURES

The overall goal of gene therapy is to correct an undesirable trait or disease by introducing a modified copy of a gene into a target cell. In most cases, the purpose is not to replace a defective gene in the host cell but rather to provide a new copy so that the correct protein can be expressed and the detrimental effects of the defective gene neutralized. While technically any genetic disorder may be treated by gene therapy, currently there are some limitations. First, the precise genetic mechanism of the disorder must be known, and it must be a single-gene defect. Second, scientists must know the complete genetic sequence of the gene, including regulatory regions, so that a functional copy can be delivered to the cell. Third, there needs to be an effective vector, or delivery system, for administering the correct copy to the target cells.

Generally, scientists classify forms of gene therapy as belonging to one of three types. Theoretically, the most effective form of this procedure is in situ gene therapy, which means that the genetic material is administered directly to the target cells. Unfortunately, it has been difficult to ensure that only target cells receive the genetic material, but there have been some successes. A second method injects the vector containing the genetic material into the fluids of the body. In this method, called in vivo gene therapy, the vector travels throughout the body until it reaches the target cells. A third mechanism, called ex vivo gene therapy, removes cells from the body to be exposed to the vector and then reintroduced back into the body. This method works especially well with undifferentiated stem cells.

Scientists have developed several mechanisms by which the genetic information can be introduced into the target cell. The most common is the viral vector. Viruses are used because typically they are very specific in the types of cells that they infect. Furthermore, their

genomes are usually very small and well understood by scientists. The viruses that are chosen are derived almost exclusively from nonpathogenic strains or have been genetically engineered so that pathogenic portions of the genome have been removed. Common viral vectors are adenoviruses, retroviruses, and herpes simplex viruses. The choice of vector depends on the target and size of gene to be replaced. In each case, after the virus infects the target cell, the DNA is either incorporated directly into the host genome or becomes extrachromosomal.

Medical researchers are also investigating the use of nonviral vectors to deliver DNA into target cells. As is the case with viral vectors, these mechanisms must not disrupt the normal metabolic machinery of the target cell. One system, called plasmid DNA, utilizes small circular pieces of DNA called plasmids to deliver the genetic material. If small enough, the plasmids can pass through the cell membrane. Although they do not integrate into the host genome in the same way as viral vectors do, they are a simple mechanism and lack the potential problems associated with viral vectors. Another mechanism being studied is the packaging of the genetic material within a lipid-based vector called a liposome to ease transport across the membrane. In trials, however, both liposomes and plasmids have displayed a low efficiency in delivering genetic material into target cells.

USES AND COMPLICATIONS

Since the early 1990's, numerous scientific studies have examined the potential effectiveness of gene therapy in treating diseases in mammalian model species, such as mice and monkeys. Using gene therapy, researchers have demonstrated that it may be possible to treat diseases such as Parkinson's disease, sickle cell anemia, and some forms of cancer. Weekly scientific journals such as *Gene Therapy* report the status of these tests. Gene therapy trials in humans are a relatively recent development and represent the next stage in the treatment of human diseases. Severe combined immunodeficiency syndrome (SCID) was the first human disorder for which successful gene therapy was reported, and clinical trials of gene therapy for the treatment of Canavan disease, adenosine deaminase (ADA) deficiency, and cystic fibrosis have begun. Medical researchers have suggested that, in the future, almost any genetic defect may be treatable using gene therapy.

While gene therapy may appear to be the "silver bullet" for diseases such as cancer and Parkinson's dis-

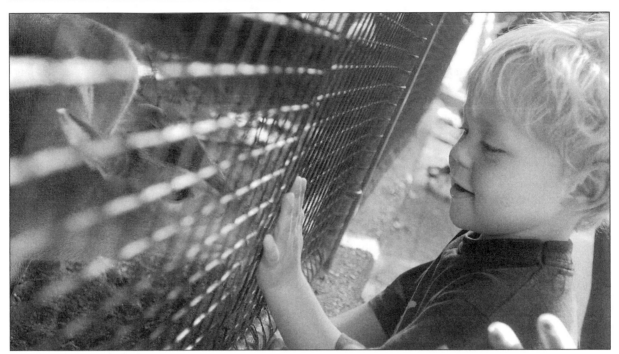

A three-year-old child who received experimental gene therapy to cure severe combined immunodeficiency syndrome (SCID), so-called bubble boy disease, visits a zoo in Amsterdam in 2002. (AP/Wide World Photos)

ease, the procedure is not without its risks. Since gene therapy using viral vectors was first proposed, scientists have recognized the inherent problems with the procedure. Since the technology does not yet exist to target the virus to insert its DNA directly into the specific gene of interest, the chances are that the viral vector will integrate the genetic information into the genome at some site other than the location of the defective gene. This means that the potential exists for the virus to insert itself into a regulatory or structural region of a gene and either render it unusable or impart a new function to the protein. Because of the size of the human genome (more than three billion bases) and the fact that less than 2 percent of the genome is believed to produce functional proteins, the odds of such an event occurring are relatively low. Given the large numbers of vectors used, however, this risk remains a real possibility.

Two cases illustrate the dangers associated with viral vectors. First was the death of a gene therapy trial volunteer at the University of Pennsylvania in 1999. The volunteer, Jesse Gelsinger, suffered from a form of liver disorder called ornithine transcarbamylase deficiency (OTC). OTC is identified as being the result of a single defective gene in a five-step metabolic pathway. Using an adenovirus, researchers sought to re-place the defective gene causing OTC in Gelsinger. Shortly after the gene therapy was begun, Gelsinger developed a systemic immune response to the vector and died.

The second case is actually a story of both success and failure. A French research team at the Necker Hospital for Sick Children in Paris effectively used a retrovirus vector to treat a group of young boys with SCID. Also called "bubble boy disease," SCID is a rare disorder in which the immune system is rendered inoperative. One form of the disease has been traced to a gene on the X chromosome. Using the procedure of ex vivo gene therapy, the researchers removed stem cells from the bone marrow of the boys and, using a retrovirus vector, delivered a functional copy of the defective gene into the cells. The cells were then reinserted back into the bone marrow. The procedure was successful in that all boys were cured of the disease. Thirty months later, however, one of the boys developed leukemia, which was followed four months later by a second case. Analysis of the boys' DNA indicated that the inserted gene had disrupted a gene in which mutations had previously been shown to cause cancer.

While the number of individuals that have developed complications from gene therapy is relatively small, these cases do indicate the potential hazards of using a viral system and have accelerated the research into using nonviral systems such as liposomes and plasmids. Additional research is underway to develop a means of targeting a specific host gene for the insertion of the therapeutic DNA. Scientists are also investigating the possibility of developing a so-called suicide gene, or "off switch," for the procedure that could terminate treatment if an error in insertion were detected.

PERSPECTIVE AND PROSPECTS

The process of gene therapy represents one of the more recent advances in the life sciences. Since James Watson and Francis Crick proposed the structure of DNA in 1953, scientists have been suggesting the possibility of correcting genetic defects in a cell. It has been only since the early 1990's, however, that advances in biotechnology have enabled the actual procedure to be conducted.

The science of gene therapy actually began as enzyme replacement therapy. For patients suffering from diseases in which an enzyme in a metabolic pathway is defective, enzyme replacement therapy provides a temporary cure. In these cases, however, the therapy must be administrated continuously since presence of a defective gene means that the body lacks the ability to manufacture new enzymes.

In the 1980's, enzyme replacement therapy was being used to treat a number of diseases including ADA deficiency, in which an enzyme in a biochemical pathway that converts toxins in the body to uric acid is defective. As a result, the toxins accumulate and eventually render the immune system ineffective. The modern era for gene therapy began in the early 1990's as scientists began to treat ADA deficiency with gene therapy. Through a series of trials, researchers learned that ex vivo treatment of stem cells proved to be the most effective mechanism for treating ADA deficiency with gene therapy. In 1993, researchers obtained stem cells from the umbilical cords of three babies who were born with ADA deficiency. After the correct genes were inserted into these stem cells, the altered cells were inserted back into the donor babies. After years of monitoring, it appears that the process has worked and the potentially fatal effects of ADA deficiency in these children have been reversed.

Cystic fibrosis is a serious respiratory disease that results from a missing protein that forms calcium channels in the membranes of the cells lining the respiratory tract. Affected individuals collect mucus in these respiratory cells and are susceptible to life-threatening respiratory infections. Gene therapy has been used with modest success to replace the defective gene in these cases. The major problem is that these cells have a relatively short life span, so that the relief is only temporary and these expensive treatments must be repeated every few months. The targeting of the replacement gene to only those cells in the respiratory tract where it is needed has also been a considerable technological hurdle to overcome.

Another promising area of gene therapy is the treatment of cancer. Cancer treatment using gene therapy would probably not involve replacing defective genes but rather "knocking out" those genes that are causing uncontrolled cell division within cancer cells. By arresting cell division, scientists can halt the spread of the cancer. This treatment would be especially useful in areas of the body where surgery is risky, such as brain tumors. The primary challenge at this stage is the targeting of the vector. A knockout vector would need to infect only cancer cells and not the other dividing cells of the human body.

A potential area of gene therapy that has yet to be exploited is germ-line gene therapy. Germ cells are those that are responsible for the formation of gametes, or egg and sperm cells. Since a germ cell contains only half the genetic information of an adult cell, it is relatively easy to replace genes using available procedures learned from biotechnology. Furthermore, since following fertilization the genetic material in the germ cells is responsible for the formation of all the remaining more than sixty-three trillion cells in the human body, any genetic change in the germ cells has the ability to be inherited by subsequent generations. Somatic cell therapy, such as that used to treat ADA deficiency and SCID, has the ability to influence only the affected individual, since these cells are not normally part of the reproductive process. Gene therapy in germ cells is currently considered unethical, but many consider it to be the mechanism of eliminating certain diseases from the human species.

While the use of gene therapy to correct human diseases may be stalled temporarily until technical obstacles are overcome, little doubt exists in the biomedical community that gene therapy represents the procedure of the future. At a fundamental level, gene therapy has the potential to be the ultimate cure for many ailments and diseases of humankind. For most of recorded history, medicine has been confined to the treatment of symptoms. Since the start of the twentieth century, advances have enabled enhanced surgical procedures, pharmaceutical drugs that alter or interact with the biochemistry of the cell, improved diagnostic techniques, and a deeper understanding of genetic inheritance. Gene therapy represents the ultimate preventive procedure.

—Michael Windelspecht, Ph.D.;
updated by Jeffrey A. Knight, Ph.D.

See also Bionics and biotechnology; Cancer; Cells; Clinical trials; DNA and RNA; Enzyme therapy; Enzymes; Ethics; Genetic diseases; Genetic engineering; Genetics and inheritance; Genomics; Mutation; Severe combined immunodeficiency syndrome (SCID); Stem cells; Viral infections.

FOR FURTHER INFORMATION:

Gorman, Jessica. "Delivering the Goods: Gene Therapy Without the Virus." *Science News* 163 (January, 2003): 43-44. A short but informative examination of research into nonviral mechanisms of gene therapy, including bioengineered liposomes and naked DNA.

Kresina, Thomas F., ed. *An Introduction to Molecular Medicine and Gene Therapy.* New York: Wiley-Liss, 2001. Covers the entire spectrum of the evolving field of molecular medicine, from nuclear transplantation to gene therapy. Includes specific discussions of cancer and human immunodeficiency virus (HIV), as well as other diseases. Sections also cover ethical considerations and federal regulation.

Lewis, Ricki. *Human Genetics: Concepts and Applications.* 7th ed. New York: McGraw-Hill, 2007. This clearly written text contains an entire chapter dedicated to the history of gene therapy, including specific examples of successes and setbacks.

Panno, Joseph. *Tracking Disease by Repairing Genes.* New York: Facts On File, 2005. A good, well-illustrated basic introduction to the principles and possibilities of gene therapy.

Templeton, Nancy Smyth, ed. *Gene Therapy: Therapeutic Mechanisms and Strategies.* 2d ed. New York: Marcel Dekker, 2004. Provides a review of the various mechanisms of gene therapy, from the established viral vectors to research into less risky systems. Slightly more advanced than some titles, it can be used as a reference for both the general public and scientists.

GENETIC COUNSELING

SPECIALTY

ANATOMY OR SYSTEM AFFECTED: Cells, reproductive system, uterus

SPECIALTIES AND RELATED FIELDS: Cytology, embryology, genetics, obstetrics, preventive medicine, psychology

DEFINITION: The scientific field that uses several biochemical and imaging techniques, as well as family histories, to provide information about genetic conditions or diseases in order to help individuals make medical and reproductive decisions.

KEY TERMS:

chromosomal abnormality: any change to the number, shape, or appearance of the forty-six chromosomes in each human cell; the presence of many such abnormalities will prevent the normal development of an individual and lead to a miscarriage

dominant genetic disease: a disease caused by a mutation in a gene that can be inherited from only one parent

genetic screening: a program designed to determine whether individuals are carriers of or are affected by a particular genetic disease

karyotype: a photograph of the chromosomes taken from the cells of an individual; a karyotype can be used to predict the sex of a fetus or the presence of a large chromosomal abnormality

mutation: an alteration in the DNA sequence of a gene that usually leads to the production of a nonfunctional enzyme or protein and, thus, a lack of a normal metabolic function; this defect may cause a medical condition called a genetic disease

recessive genetic disease: a disease caused by a mutation in a gene that must be inherited from both parents in order for an individual to show the symptoms of the disease; such a disease may show up only occasionally in a family history, especially if the mutation is rare

SCIENCE AND PROFESSION

Genetic counseling is a process of communicating to a couple the medical problems associated with the occurrence of an inherited disorder or birth defect in a family. Included in this process is a discussion of the prognosis and treatment of the problem. Specific reproductive options include abortion of an ongoing pregnancy, birth control or sterilization to prevent additional pregnancies, artificial insemination, the use of surrogate mothers, embryo transplantation, and adoption.

In all cases, the role of the counselor is to provide unbiased information and options to the couple seeking advice. The counselor must not only discuss the medical implications of a condition but also help to alleviate the emotional impact of positive diagnoses and, in particular, to assuage the guilt or denial that a diagnosis may elicit in parents.

The two major categories of medical problems covered by counselors are birth defects and genetic diseases. The first group includes Down syndrome and spina bifida, while the latter includes hemophilia, sickle cell disease, and Tay-Sachs disease. Although the distinction between these two categories can sometimes blur, the key difference involves the clear pattern of inheritance shown by the genetic diseases.

Humans have between thirty thousand and thirty-five thousand genes. Genes are segments of deoxyribonucleic acid (DNA) that are arranged in linear fashion along the forty-six chromosomes. Most genes contain the information necessary for the cells to produce a specific protein, which often is involved in controlling some critical physiological function. For example, the beta globin gene produces a protein called beta globin that makes up half of the hemoglobin that carries oxygen in the red blood cells.

A genetic disease can occur when the DNA changes in structure. Such a change is also known as a mutation. A mutation can lead to the production of a defective protein that cannot carry out its normal function, thus causing a physiological defect. In the case of beta globin, changing only one of the 106 molecules that make up this protein leads to a form of hemoglobin that can produce nonfunctional protein aggregates in red blood cells. These aggregates can cause the red blood cells to collapse and take on a sickle shape. Such cells lose their function, and the tissues are starved for oxygen—a condition known as anemia. This defect, which is called sickle cell disease, is a fatal, heritable disease. As with all genetic disease, such mutations are relatively rare. Certain diseases may, however, be more prevalent within certain ethnic groups; for example, African Americans have a high incidence of sickle cell disease, and Ashkenazic Jews have a high incidence of Tay-Sachs disease.

Humans have two of each kind of chromosome; one set of twenty-three is inherited from the mother, and the other set of twenty-three is inherited from the father. Thus, each person has two copies of each gene, once located on a maternal chromosome, the other on a paternal one. Many types of defects, such as sickle cell disease, require that both genes have mutations in order for the disease to have an effect. Individuals who have one normal gene and one with a mutation are normal but carry the disease; they can pass the mutation on to the next generation in their eggs and sperm. This type of disease is called a recessive genetic disease. The only way a child can have sickle cell disease is if both parents are carriers, since it is unlikely that a person affected by the disease will live long enough to have children.

Since it is equally likely for each parent to pass on the normal gene in eggs or sperm as to pass on the mutation, the laws of probability predict that, on the average, one-fourth of such a couple's offspring should have the disease. One of the major tasks of a genetic counselor is to advise couples of these probabilities if the diagnoses and family histories suggest that they are carriers. Since the laws of genetics involve random occurrences, however, it is possible that in a family with three or four children, all the children will be normal, or that in another family, all the children will have the disease. This degree of uncertainty produces stress and anxiety in couples who seek counseling only to hear that they indeed are at risk. Discussing concepts that involve sophisticated genetic or biochemical themes or issues of probable risk with couples untrained in scientific thinking is difficult, especially considering the highly emotional atmosphere of such discussions.

Other diseases, such as Huntington's chorea, also known as Woody Guthrie's disease for the folksinger who was afflicted by it, are caused by a dominant mutation. A mutation is dominant when an individual needs to inherit only one copy of the mutation in order to have the disease. Unlike recessive diseases that can disappear from a family for generations, a dominant mutation can be inherited only from a person who has the disease. In most cases, such a person has one normal gene and one with the mutation, which means that there is a 50 percent chance that the gene will be passed on. Huntington's chorea is a particularly insidious genetic disease, because the symptoms usually begin to show only in middle age, often after childbearing decisions have been made. Thus, the children of an afflicted parent may have had children before knowing whether they have inherited the mutation from their parents.

There are no cures for the permanent physiological defects that result from genetic disease. In some cases, the disease symptoms can be controlled by supplementing the protein that is lacking. Some forms of insulin-dependent diabetes and most cases of hemophilia can be treated in this way. In other cases, as with the disease phenylketonuria (PKU), special diets can prevent the severe neurological problems that inevitably lead to childhood death if the disease is left untreated.

DNA technology and genetic engineering offer potential cures for some diseases in which the primary defect caused by the mutation is well understood. Gene therapy is a process by which an additional copy of a normal gene is inserted into the cells of an affected individual or the defective gene is replaced by a normal one. Successful experiments with animals have given scientists confidence that these techniques will provide cures for many genetic diseases. These same DNA technologies are making better diagnosis possible and, as in the case of cystic fibrosis, are helping to extend the lives and enhance the quality of life of individuals afflicted with incurable diseases.

One of the more controversial aspects of genetic counseling is the procedure of screening. In this procedure, individuals suspected to be at risk are tested for the presence of a mutation. Screening can let people know whether they have a disease as well as whether they are carriers of the disease and therefore can pass the disease on to their children. Screening can be extended to all individuals, regardless of family or ethnic history. For example, in the United States, most states require that all newborn infants undergo a PKU test. This simple test involves taking a small sample of blood by pricking the heel of the baby. Although the costs of this screening are not insignificant, the benefit is that those infants found to have the disease can be treated immediately by being placed on a special diet so as to avoid the debilitating effects of the disease.

Other screening procedures are targeted at specific groups. The screening program for Tay-Sachs disease focuses on ethnic Jewish populations. This successful, voluntary program has reduced the incidence of Tay-Sachs disease significantly in the United States. The key to the success of the program was the money spent to educate the targeted group. In addition, key members of the population played a leading role in designing the overall program. Because of the much larger size of the potential group at risk, similar efforts to screen African American populations for sickle cell disease have been much less successful. Ethical concerns about the motivations behind government-sponsored or government-encouraged screening of minority populations make these programs difficult to implement. In addition, in mandatory programs, concerns about confidentiality and information release become major obstacles.

DIAGNOSTIC AND TREATMENT TECHNIQUES

Genetic counseling usually begins when a couple or an individual seeks the advice of a family physician or obstetrician regarding the medical risks associated with having a child. Motivating this request may be a previous birth of a child with a defect, a general uneasiness on the part of a couple worried about environmental exposure to potentially harmful agents, a family history of genetic disease, or advanced maternal age (which can be a factor in certain chromosomal abnormalities). Often, the family is referred to a genetic counseling clinic where most of the actual diagnosis and counseling will occur.

Arriving at a proper diagnosis for any obvious condition, as well as giving advice about potential risks, involves obtaining as much family history as possible with respect to the trait, as well as diagnostic information from the couple. If pregnant already, the woman may undergo a prenatal diagnostic procedure that could include ultrasound, blood tests, amniocentesis, and chorionic villus sampling.

Ultrasound is a technique that uses sound waves to visualize the exterior of the developing fetus. This widely used procedure is almost routine in many large urban hospitals. Ultrasound can be used to detect the presence of twins as well as of some profound birth defects such as hydrocephalus (water on the brain) or spina bifida. The latter defect, which involves the failure of the neural tube to close properly during development, leads to weakness, paralysis, and lack of function in lower body areas. The severity of the defect is hard to predict, and, unlike genetic disease, the incidence of recurrence is no higher than normal for subsequent children.

Supplementing ultrasound in the detection of spina bifida is a simple blood test that looks for a protein that the fetus spills into the amniotic fluid in higher quantities if the neural tube fails to close properly. The protein, which is called alpha-fetoprotein, crosses the placenta to circulate in the mother's blood. The amount of this normal protein in the mother's blood correlates with the developmental age of the fetus; therefore, an abnormal level might indicate a problem. Older-than-calculated fetuses and twins can both cause increased levels of alpha-fetoprotein, so care must be taken in this diagnosis. If abnormally high levels of the protein are found, amniocentesis would then be used to measure the protein level in the amniotic fluid, thus increasing the reliability of the diagnosis. In amniocentesis, a few teaspoonfuls of amniotic fluid are removed from the sac that surrounds and protects the developing fetus. Ultrasound is used to visualize the exterior of the fetus to allow the safe removal of this fluid, which contains some fetal cells. Biochemical tests can be performed directly on the fluid and results obtained quickly. Tay-Sachs disease is an example of a genetic disease that can be detected in this fashion, since fetuses with the disease fail to make an enzyme that their normal counterparts do make.

Many techniques, however, require obtaining large numbers of fetal cells and/or DNA. In these cases, the cells must be cultured for one to two weeks in a laboratory in order to get enough material to test. The delay between taking the sample and discussing the results with the clients is a source of stress and anxiety for parents undergoing counseling.

Preparing a karyotype, a photograph showing the numbers and sizes of the chromosomes of the fetus, is a commonly performed procedure following amniocentesis. Normal fetuses contain forty-six chromosomes, and any change in chromosome number, shape, or size can be detected by a skilled clinician. A large percentage of miscarriages involve fetuses with chromosomal abnormalities, so this diagnosis can be critical. A relatively common type of birth defect that can be diagnosed with a karyotype is Down syndrome. Most children born with Down syndrome have forty-seven chromosomes instead of forty-six; thus, this diagnosis is very accurate. In addition, the sex of the fetus can be determined from a karyotype, since male fetuses have an X and a Y chromosome while females have two X chromosomes. This information can be valuable to couples who are at risk for carrying a sex-linked genetic disease such as hemophilia, which could not affect any female offspring. Such information could potentially be used inappropriately for sexual selection of offspring, however, and the counselor must provide this information cautiously.

Amniocentesis is usually performed in the sixteenth week of pregnancy to allow the fetus to grow to a size at which the removal of a small amount of amniotic fluid would not be harmful. Although there is little risk to mother or fetus in this procedure, the delay associated with laboratory culturing means that results are often known in the eighteenth week of pregnancy or even later. At this stage, abortion becomes a more traumatic medical procedure. Chorionic villus sampling, on the other hand, can actually sample small amounts of fetal tissue directly. Since the procedure can safely obtain enough tissue to diagnose most problems and can be performed as early as the ninth or tenth week of pregnancy, abortion becomes a medically less traumatic option.

DNA technology provides the counselor with a battery of new diagnostic procedures that can look directly for the presence of a mutation in the DNA of the fetus. These tests can be performed on parents who are worried about being carriers for a particular disease or can be used on DNA obtained from fetal cells grown in a laboratory. Such tests have very high reliability and can give information about diseases such as sickle cell disease, Huntington's chorea, muscular dystrophy, and cystic fibrosis.

The counselor's task is to take the diagnostic results and interpret them in the context of the medical history and particular family situation. The counselor must point out the options available, both for further diagnosis to confirm or rebut less-sensitive preliminary tests and to discuss potential medical interventions such as the special diets available for children born with PKU. In cases in which no medical intervention is possible, the severity of the problem should be discussed honestly so that the parents can choose either to continue or to abort the pregnancy. Other options, including adoption, artificial insemination, and embryo transplants, can also be evaluated. Finally, the risk of recurrence of the problem in future pregnancies should be discussed.

Counselors need to realize that their clients are often in emotionally fragile states. They must guard against using bias or interjecting their own personal beliefs or values when counseling their clients. Full disclosure of information, both verbally and in a carefully written report, is usually provided.

Compounding the tasks of the counselor is the fact that, in many cases, exact diagnoses are not yet possible. Sometimes, only the relative risks associated with another pregnancy can be determined. Different couples will perceive risks very differently depending on their own religious and moral backgrounds, as well as on the expected severity of the defect. In the case of a genetic disease such as Tay-Sachs, which is 100 percent fatal and requires extensive hospitalization of the child, a modest risk may be considered unacceptable, while in the case of a birth defect such as Down syndrome, whose severity cannot be predicted, and in which case the child may lead a long and rich life, a modest risk may be considered quite differently.

PERSPECTIVE AND PROSPECTS

The need for centers specializing in genetic counseling arose when it became clear that certain diseases and birth defects had a hereditary component. Many families request the services of counselors from these centers, and the centers are also involved in both voluntary and mandatory screening programs. In the United States, about 4 percent of all newborns suffer from a defect that is recognized either at birth or shortly thereafter. This group includes 0.5 percent who have a chromosomal abnormality that results in an obvious medical problem, 0.5 to 1 percent who have classical genetic diseases, and 2 percent who suffer from a birth defect that may have a heritable component. Estimates vary, but more than one-third of all children in pediatric hospitals are there because of some association with a genetic disease.

Physicians have always served as counselors to families, but the rapid advances made in genetics and molecular science during the second half of the twentieth century have clearly surpassed the abilities of most physicians to keep current with treatments and diagnoses. The first formal clinic for genetic counseling was established at the University of Michigan in the 1940's. Most clinics specializing in this field were based at large medical centers; first in major metropolitan areas, and later in smaller population centers.

Genetic counseling clinics usually employ a range of specialists, including clinicians, geneticists, laboratory personnel for performing diagnostic testing, and public health and social workers. In 1969, Sarah Lawrence College instituted a master's-level program in genetic counseling to train candidates formally in the scientific, medical, and counseling skills required for this profession. Since that time, many other programs have been established in the United States. Today, most large counseling programs at medical centers use these specially trained personnel. In rural areas, however, family physicians are still a primary source of counseling; thus, genetic training is an important component of basic medical education.

The sophisticated medical diagnostic tools described above allow a counselor to provide abundant information to couples requesting counseling, but the power of DNA technology has expanded and will continue to expand the scope of current practice. Soon, counselors will not have to give advice in terms of probabilities and likelihoods of risk; molecular detection techniques will make possible the absolute identification of not only individuals with a disease but also related carriers.

As these DNA tools become more widely available, counseling will become a more integral part of preventive medicine. A DNA diagnostic procedure for a heritable form of breast cancer is available that allows women who have the mutation to monitor their health closely in order to receive prompt, lifesaving medical intervention. An important ethical issue here is that some women who have been diagnosed as having the mutation are undergoing preventive mastectomies without having developed any growths in order to ensure that they will not develop cancer. This radical therapy carries with it considerable emotional stress and should be undertaken only after consultation with a physician. As DNA-based diagnostic procedures, perhaps coupled with mandatory screening, become more commonplace, concerns about the release of this information to potential employers or health insurers will become more critical.

—Joseph G. Pelliccia, Ph.D.

See also Abortion; Amniocentesis; Birth defects; Blood testing; Chorionic villus sampling; DNA and RNA; Down syndrome; Ethics; Gene therapy; Genetic diseases; Genetic engineering; Genetics and inheritance; Hemophilia; Laboratory tests; Mutation; Niemann-Pick disease; Phenylketonuria (PKU); Screening; Sickle cell disease; Spina bifida; Tay-Sachs disease; Ultrasonography.

FOR FURTHER INFORMATION:

Davis, Dena S. *Genetic Dilemmas: Reproductive Technology, Parental Choices, and Children's Futures.* New York: Routledge, 2001. Explores real-life medical cases as a means to discuss ethical dilemmas raised by the availability of new reproductive technologies.

Filkins, Karen, and Joseph F. Russo, eds. *Human Prenatal Diagnosis.* Rev. 2d ed. New York: Marcel Dekker, 1990. An advanced sourcebook that describes the procedures of prenatal diagnosis in great detail. Contains information on such issues as risk, reliability, and cost.

Harper, Peter S. *Practical Genetic Counselling.* 6th ed. New York: Oxford University Press, 2004. A good overview of all aspects of genetic counseling, including a discussion of the types of diagnoses, treatments, risks, and emotional strains associated with counseling. Also gives a history of counseling as a discipline.

Jorde, Lynn B., et al. *Medical Genetics.* Rev. 3d ed. St. Louis: Mosby, 2006. An introductory text that covers basic molecular genetics, chromosomal and single gene disorders, immunogenetics, cancer genetics, multifactorial disorders, and fetal therapy.

King, Richard A., Jerome I. Rotter, and Arno G. Motulsky, eds. *Genetic Basis of Common Diseases.* 2d ed. New York: Oxford University Press, 2002. Covers advances in the understanding of molecular processes involved in genetic susceptibility and disease mechanisms. Examines a range of diseases in detail and includes a chapter on genetic counseling.

Lewis, Ricki. *Human Genetics: Concepts and Applications.* 7th ed. New York: McGraw-Hill, 2007. A very accessible undergraduate text that covers the fundamentals, transmission genetics, DNA and chromosomes, and the latest genetic technology, among other topics.

Martin, Richard J., Avroy A. Fanaroff, and Michele C. Walsh, eds. *Fanaroff and Martin's Neonatal-Perinatal Medicine: Diseases of the Fetus and Infant.* 2 vols. 8th ed. Philadelphia: Mosby Elsevier, 2006. Comprehensively covers the fetus, pregnancy disorders, provisions for neonatal care, risk factors, and development and disorders of organ systems, among many other topics.

Moore, Keith L., and T. V. N. Persaud. *The Developing Human.* 7th ed. Philadelphia: W. B. Saunders, 2003. An outstanding textbook on human embryonic development, with specific information about the causes of congenital malformations and common defects occurring in each of the body's systems.

Pierce, Benjamin A. *The Family Genetic Sourcebook.* New York: John Wiley & Sons, 1990. Good background reading on genetics and genetic diseases. The book gives short, clear descriptions of a number of genetic diseases, along with their diagnosis and treatment.

GENETIC DISEASES
DISEASE/DISORDER

ANATOMY OR SYSTEM AFFECTED: All

SPECIALTIES AND RELATED FIELDS: Embryology, genetics, internal medicine, neonatology, obstetrics, pediatrics

DEFINITION: A variety of disorders transmitted from parent to child through chromosomal material; most people experience disease related to genetics in some form, and research into this area is yielding greater understanding of the relationship between disease and hereditary proclivities toward disease, as well as new strategies for early detection and prevention or therapy.

KEY TERMS:

autosomal recessive disease: a disease that is expressed only when two copies of a defective gene are inherited, one from each parent; present on non-sex-determining chromosomes

chromosomes: rod-shaped structures in each cell that contain genes, the chemical elements that determine traits

deoxyribonucleic acid (DNA): the chemical molecule that transmits hereditary information from generation to generation

dominant gene: a gene that can express its effect when an individual has only one copy of it

gene: the hereditary unit, composed of DNA, that resides on chromosomes

inheritance: the passing down of traits from generation to generation

X-linked: a term used to describe genes or traits that are located on the X chromosome; a male needs only one copy of an X-linked gene for it to be expressed

CAUSES AND SYMPTOMS

Hereditary units called genes determine the majority of the physical and biochemical characteristics of an organism. Genes are composed of a chemical compound called deoxyribonucleic acid (DNA) and are organized into rod-shaped structures called chromosomes that reside in each cell of the body. Each human cell carries forty-six chromosomes organized as twenty-three pairs, each composed of several thousand genes. Twenty-two of the chromosome pairs are homologous pairs; that is, similar genes are located at similar sites on each chromosome. The remaining chromosomes are the sex chromosomes. Human females bear two X chromosomes, and human males possess one X and one Y chromosome.

During the formation of the reproductive cells, the chromosome pairs separate and one copy of each pair is randomly included in the egg or sperm. Each egg will contain twenty-two autosomes (non-sex chromosomes) and one X chromosome. Each sperm will contain twenty-two autosomes and either one X or one Y chromosome. The egg and sperm fuse at fertilization, which restores the proper number of chromosomes, and the genes inherited from the baby's parents will determine its sex and much of its physical appearance and future health and well-being.

Genetic diseases are inherited as a result of the presence of abnormal genes in the reproductive cells of one or both parents of an affected individual. There are two broad classifications of genetic disease: those caused by defects in chromosome number or structure, and those resulting from a much smaller flaw within a gene. Within the latter category, there are four predominant mechanisms by which the disorders can be transmitted from generation to generation: autosomal dominant inheritance, in which the defective gene is inherited from one parent; autosomal recessive inheritance, in which defective genes are inherited from both parents, who themselves show no signs of the disorder; X-linked chromosomal inheritance (often called sex-linked), in which the flawed gene has been determined to reside on the X chromosome; and multifactorial inheritance, in which genes interact with each other and/or environmental factors.

Errors in chromosome number include extra and missing chromosomes. The most common chromosomal defect observed in humans is Down syndrome, which is caused by the presence of three copies of chromosome 21, instead of the usual two. Down syndrome occurs at a frequency of about one in eight hundred live births, this frequency increasing with increasing maternal age. The symptoms of this disorder include mental retardation, short stature, and numerous other medical problems. The most common form of Down syndrome results from the failure of the two copies of chromosome 21 to separate during reproductive cell formation, which upon fusion with a normal reproductive cell at fertilization produces an embryo containing three copies of chromosome 21.

Gross defects in chromosome structure include duplicated and deleted portions of chromosomes and broken and rearranged chromosome fragments. Prader-Willi syndrome results from a deletion of a small portion of chromosome 15. Children affected with this disorder are mentally retarded, obese, and diabetic. Cri du chat (literally, cat cry) syndrome is associated with a large deletion in chromosome 5. Affected infants exhibit facial abnormalities, are severely retarded, and produce a high-pitched, kittenlike wail.

Genetic diseases caused by defects in individual genes result when defective genes are propagated through many generations or a new genetic flaw develops in a reproductive cell. New genetic defects arise from a variety of causes, including environmental assaults such as radiation, toxins, or drugs. More than four thousand such gene disorders have been identified.

Manifestation of an autosomal dominant disorder requires the inheritance of only one defective gene from

> ## INFORMATION ON GENETIC DISEASES
>
> **CAUSES:** Abnormal genes in the reproductive cells of one or both parents, environmental factors causing mutations
>
> **SYMPTOMS:** Varies widely; can include mental retardation, respiratory dysfunction, neurological deterioration, progressive muscle deterioration, cleft palate, spina bifida, anencephaly, heart abnormalities
>
> **DURATION:** Typically lifelong
>
> **TREATMENTS:** Typically alleviation of symptoms through surgery, drug therapy, hormone therapy, dietary regulation

one parent who is afflicted with the disease. Inheritance of two dominant defective genes, one from each parent, is possible but generally creates such severe consequences that the child dies while still in the womb or shortly after birth. An individual who bears one copy of the gene has a 50 percent chance of transmitting that gene and the disease to his or her offspring.

Among the most common autosomal dominant diseases are hyperlipidemia and hypercholesterolemia. Elevated levels of lipids and cholesterol in the blood, which contribute to artery and heart disease, are the consequences of these disorders, respectively. Onset of the symptoms is usually in adulthood, frequently after the affected individual has had children and potentially transmitted the faulty gene to them.

Huntington's chorea causes untreatable neurological deterioration and death, and symptoms do not appear until affected individuals are at least in their forties. Children of parents afflicted with Huntington's chorea may have already made reproductive decisions without the knowledge that they might carry the defective gene; they risk a 50 percent chance of transmitting the dread disease to their offspring.

Autosomal recessive genetic diseases require that an affected individual bear two copies of a defective gene, inheriting one from each parent. Usually the parents are simply carriers of the defective gene; their one normal copy masks the effect of the one flawed copy. If two carriers have offspring, 25 percent will receive two copies of the flawed gene and inherit the disease, and 50 percent will be asymptomatic carriers.

Cystic fibrosis is an autosomal recessive disease that occurs at a rate of about one in two thousand live births among Caucasians. The defective gene product causes improper chloride transport in cells and results in thick mucous secretions in lungs and other organs. Sickle cell disease, another autosomal recessive disorder, is the most common genetic disease among African Americans in the United States. Abnormality in the protein hemoglobin, the component of red blood cells that carries oxygen to all the body's tissues, leads to deformed blood cells that are fragile and easily destroyed.

X-linked genetic diseases are transmitted by faulty genes located on the X chromosome. Females need two copies of the defective gene to acquire such a disease, and in general women carry only one flawed copy, making them asymptomatic carriers of the disorder. Males, having only a single X chromosome, need only one copy of the defective gene to express an X-linked disease. Males with X-linked disorders inherit the defective gene from their mothers, since fathers must contribute a Y chromosome to male offspring. Half of the male offspring of a carrier female will inherit the defective gene and develop the disease. In the rare case of a female with two defective X-linked genes, 100 percent of her male offspring will inherit the disease gene, and, assuming that the father does not carry the defective gene, 50 percent of her female offspring will be carriers. There are more than 250 X-linked disorders, some of the more common being Duchenne's muscular dystrophy, which results in progressive muscle deterioration and early death; hemophilia; and red-green color blindness, which affects about 8 percent of Caucasian males.

Multifactorial inheritance, which accounts for a number of genetic diseases, is caused by the complex interaction of one or more genes with each other and with environmental factors. This group of diseases includes many disorders which, anecdotally, "run in families." Representative disorders include cleft palate, spina bifida, anencephaly, and some inherited heart abnormalities. Other diseases appear to have a genetic component predisposing an individual to be susceptible to environmental stimuli that trigger the disease. These include cancer, hypertension, diabetes, schizophrenia, alcoholism, depression, and obesity.

DIAGNOSIS AND DETECTION

Most, but not all, genetic diseases manifest their symptoms immediately or soon after the birth of an affected child. Rapid recognition of such a medical condition and its accurate diagnosis are essential for the proper treatment and management of the disease by parents

and medical personnel. Medical technology has developed swift and accurate diagnostic methods, in many cases allowing testing of the fetus prior to birth. In addition, tests are available that determine the carrier status of an individual for many autosomal recessive and X-linked diseases. These test results are used in conjunction with genetic counseling of individuals and couples who are at risk of transmitting a genetic disease to their offspring. Thus, such individuals can make informed decisions when planning their reproductive futures.

Errors in chromosome number and structure are detected in an individual by analyzing his or her chromosomes. A small piece of skin or a blood sample is taken, the cells in the sample are grown to a sufficient number,

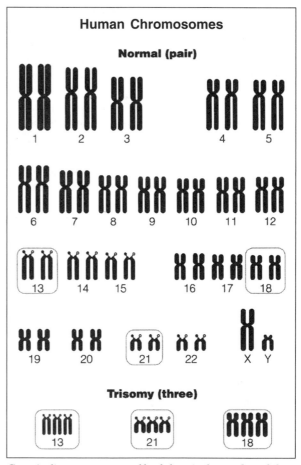

Genetic diseases are caused by defects in the number of chromosomes, in their structure, or in the genes on the chromosome (mutation). Shown here is the human complement of chromosomes (23 pairs) and three errors of chromosome number (trisomies) that lead to the genetic disorders Patau's syndrome (trisomy no. 13), Edward's syndrome (trisomy no. 18), and the more common Down syndrome (trisomy no. 21).

and the chromosomes within each cell are stained with special dyes so that they may be viewed with a microscope. A picture of the chromosomes, called a karyotype, is taken, and the patient's chromosome array is compared with that of a normal individual. Extra or missing chromosomes or alterations in chromosome structure are determined, thus identifying the genetic disease. The analysis of karyotypes is the method used to determine the presence of Down, Prader-Willi, and cri du chat syndromes, among others.

Defects in chromosome number and structure can also be identified in the fetus, prior to birth, using two different sample collecting methods: amniocentesis and chorionic villus sampling. In amniocentesis, a needle is inserted through the pregnant woman's abdomen and uterus, into the fluid-filled sac surrounding the fetus. A sample of this fluid, the amniotic fluid, is withdrawn. The amniotic fluid contains fetal cells sloughed off by the fetus. The cells are grown for several weeks until there are enough to perform chromosome analysis. This procedure is performed only after sixteen weeks' gestation, in order to ensure adequate amniotic fluid for sampling.

Chorionic villus sampling relies on a biopsy of the fetal chorion, a membrane surrounding the fetus that is composed of cells that have the same genetic constitution as the fetus. A catheter is inserted through the pregnant woman's vagina and into the uterus until it is in contact with the chorion. The small sample of this tissue that is removed contains enough cells to perform karyotyping immediately, permitting diagnosis by the next day. Chorionic villus sampling can be performed between the eighth and ninth week of pregnancy. This earlier testing gives the procedure an advantage over amniocentesis, since the earlier determination of whether a fetus is carrying a genetic disease allows safer pregnancy termination if the parents choose this course.

Karyotype analysis is limited to the diagnosis of genetic diseases caused by very large chromosome abnormalities. The majority of hereditary disorders are caused by gene flaws that are too small to see microscopically. For many of these diseases, diagnosis is available through either biochemical testing or DNA analysis.

Many genetic disorders cause a lack of a specific biochemical necessary for normal metabolism. These types of disorders are frequently referred to as "inborn errors of metabolism." Many of these errors can be detected by the chemical analysis of fetal tissue. For ex-

ample, galactosemia is a disease which results from the lack of galactose-1-phosphate uridyl transferase. Infants with this disorder cannot break down galactose, one of the major sugars in milk. If left untreated, galactosemia can lead to mental retardation, cataracts, kidney and liver failure, and death. By analyzing fetal cells obtained from amniocentesis or chorionic villus sampling, the level of this important chemical can be assessed, and, if necessary, the infant can be placed on a galactose-free diet immediately after birth.

DNA analysis can be used to determine whether a genetic disease has been inherited when the chromosomal location of the gene is known, when the chemical sequence of the DNA is known, and/or when particular DNA sequences commonly associated with the gene in question, called markers, are known.

A sequence of four chemical elements of DNA—adenine (A), guanine (G), thymine (T), and cytosine (C)—make up genes. Sometimes the proper DNA sequence of a gene is known, as well as the changes in the sequence that cause disease. Direct analysis of the DNA of the individual suspected of carrying a certain genetic disorder is possible in these cases. For example, in sickle cell disease, it is known that a change in a single DNA chemical element leads to the disorder. To test for this disease, a tissue sample is obtained from prenatal sources (amniocentesis or chorionic villus sampling). The DNA is isolated from the cells and analyzed with highly specific probes that can detect the presence of the defective gene that will lead to sickle cell disease. Informed action may be taken regarding the future of the fetus or the care of an affected child.

Occasionally a disease gene itself has not been precisely isolated and its DNA sequence determined, but sequences very near the gene of interest have been analyzed. If specific variations within these neighboring sequences are always present when the gene of interest is flawed, these nearby sequences can then be used as a marker for the presence of the defective gene. When the variant sequences, called restriction fragment length polymorphisms, are present, so is the disease gene. Prenatal testing for cystic fibrosis has been done using restriction fragment length polymorphisms.

Individuals who come from families in which genetic diseases tend to occur can be tested as carriers. In this way, they will know the risk of passing a certain disease to offspring. For example, individuals whose families have a history of cystic fibrosis, but who themselves are not affected, may be asymptomatic carriers. If they have children with individuals who are also cystic fibrosis carriers, they have a 25 percent chance of passing two copies of the defective gene to their offspring. DNA samples from the potential parents can be analyzed for the presence of one defective gene. If both partners are carriers, their decision about whether to have children will be made with knowledge of the possible risk to their offspring. If only one or neither of them is a carrier, their offspring will not be at risk of inheriting cystic fibrosis, an autosomal recessive disease. Carrier testing is possible for many genetic diseases, as well as for disorders that appear late in life, such as Huntington's chorea.

Many of the gene flaws of multifactorial diseases, those that interact with environmental factors to produce disease, have been identified and are testable. Individuals armed with the knowledge of having a gene that puts them at risk for certain disorders can incorporate preventive measures into their lifestyle, thus minimizing the chances of developing the disease. For example, certain cancers, such as colon and breast cancer, have a genetic component. Individuals who test positive for the genes that predispose them to develop cancer can modify their diets to include cancer-fighting foods and receive frequent medical checkups to detect cancer development at its earliest, most treatable stage. Those with genes that contribute to arteriosclerosis and heart disease can modify their diets and increase exercise, and those with a genetic predisposition for alcoholism could avoid the consumption of alcohol.

PERSPECTIVE AND PROSPECTS
The scientific study of human genetics and genetic disease is relatively new, having begun in the early twentieth century. There are many early historical records, however, which recognize that certain traits are hereditarily transmitted. Ancient Greek literature is peppered with references to heredity, and the Jewish book of religious and civil laws, the Talmud, describes in detail the inheritance pattern of hemophilia and its ramifications for circumcision.

The Augustinian monk Gregor Mendel worked out many of the principles of heredity by manipulating the pollen and eggs of pea plants over many generations. His work was conducted from the 1860's to the 1870's but was unrecognized by the scientific community until 1900.

At about this time, many disorders were being recognized as genetic diseases. Pedigree analysis, a way to trace inheritance patterns through a family tree, has been used since the mid-1800's to track the incidence of hemophilia in European royal families. This analysis indicates that the disease was transmitted through females (indeed, hemophilia is an X-linked disorder). In the early 1900's, Sir Archibald Garrod, a British physician, recognized certain biochemical disorders as genetic diseases and proposed accurate mechanisms for their transmission.

In 1953, Francis Crick and James D. Watson discovered the structure of DNA; thus began studies on the molecular biology of genes. This research resulted in the monumental discovery in 1973 that pieces of DNA from animals and bacteria could be cut and spliced together into a functional molecule. This recombinant DNA technology fostered a revolution in genetic analysis, in which pieces of human DNA could be removed and put into bacteria. The bacteria then replicate millions of copies of the human DNA, permitting detailed analysis. These recombinant molecules also produced the human gene product, thereby facilitating the analysis of normal and aberrant genes.

The recombinant DNA revolution spawned the development of the DNA tests for genetic diseases and carrier status. Knowledge of what a normal gene product is and does is exceptionally helpful in the treatment of genetic diseases. For example, Duchenne's muscular dystrophy is known to be caused by the lack of a protein called dystrophin. This suggests that a possible treatment of the disease is to provide functional dystrophin to the affected individual. Ultimately, medical science seeks to treat genetic diseases by providing a functional copy of the flawed gene to the affected individual. While such gene therapy would not affect the reproductive cells—the introduced gene copy would not be passed down to future generations—the normal gene product would alleviate the genetic disorder.

—Karen E. Kalumuck, Ph.D.

See also Albinos; Amniocentesis; Batten's disease; Birth defects; Breast cancer; Cerebral palsy; Chorionic villus sampling; Colon cancer; Color blindness; Congenital heart disease; Cornelia de Lange syndrome; Cystic fibrosis; Diabetes mellitus; DiGeorge syndrome; DNA and RNA; Down syndrome; Dwarfism; Embryology; Environmental diseases; Fragile X syndrome; Fructosemia; Gaucher's disease; Gene therapy; Genetic counseling; Genetic engineering; Genetics and inheritance; Genomics; Gigantism; Glycogen storage diseases; Hemochromatosis; Hemophilia; Huntington's disease; Immunodeficiency disorders; Klinefelter syndrome; Klippel-Trenaunay syndrome; Laboratory tests; Leukodystrophy; Maple syrup urine disease

(MSUD); Marfan syndrome; Metabolic disorders; Mental retardation; Mucopolysaccharidosis (MPS); Muscular dystrophy; Mutation; Neonatology; Neurofibromatosis; Niemann-Pick disease; Oncology; Pediatrics; Phenylketonuria (PKU); Polycystic kidney disease; Porphyria; Prader-Willi syndrome; Progeria; Proteomics; Rubinstein-Taybi syndrome; Screening; Severe combined immunodeficiency syndrome (SCID); Sickle cell disease; Spina bifida; Tay-Sachs disease; Thalassemia; Thrombocytopenia; Turner syndrome; Von Willebrand's disease; Wilson's disease; Wiskott-Aldrich syndrome.

FOR FURTHER INFORMATION:

Alliance of Genetic Support Groups. http://www .geneticalliance.org. Site provides information on an international coalition of individuals, professionals, and genetic support organizations working together to enhance the lives of everyone affected by genetic conditions.

Bellenir, Karen, ed. *Genetic Disorders Sourcebook*. 3d ed. Detroit: Omnigraphics, 2004. This nontechnical sourcebook offers basic information about lifestyle expectations, disease management techniques, and current research initiatives for the most common types of genetic disorders, including a resource list of three hundred genetic disorders and related topics.

GeneTests. http://www.genetests.org/. Site contains genetics disease database and information relating genetic testing to diagnosis, management, and counseling of individuals and families with inherited disorders.

Gormley, Myra Vanderpool. *Family Diseases: Are You at Risk?* Baltimore: Genealogical, 2002. The author, a certified genealogist and syndicated columnist, explores the relationship between family trees and genetic diseases. Written in popular language, this book gives instruction on how to assess a family's genetic risk, information on the latest scientific breakthroughs, and directions for obtaining further information.

Grant Cooper, Necia, ed. *The Human Genome Project: Deciphering the Blueprint of Heredity*. Rev. ed. Mill Valley, Calif.: University Science Books, 1994. Written to be accessible to the general reader, this book provides a basic introduction to the ideas underlying classical and molecular genetics before going on to describe the purpose of the Human Genome Project.

Hereditary Disease Foundation. http://www .hdfoundation.org/. Site describes the mission of this non-profit, basic science organization dedicated to the cure of genetic disease.

Jorde, Lynn B., John Carrey, and Michael J. Bamshed. *Medical Genetics*. 3d ed. New York: Elsevier, 2003. An introductory text that covers basic molecular genetics, chromosomal and single gene disorders, immunogenetics, cancer genetics, multifactorial disorders, and fetal therapy.

King, Richard A., Jerome I. Rotter, and Arno G. Motulsky, eds. *Genetic Basis of Common Diseases*. 2d ed. New York: Oxford University Press, 2002. Covers advances in the understanding of molecular processes involved in genetic susceptibility and disease mechanisms. Examines a range of diseases in detail and includes a chapter on genetic counseling.

Lewis, Ricki. *Human Genetics: Concepts and Applications*. 7th ed. New York: McGraw-Hill, 2007. A very accessible undergraduate text that covers the fundamentals, transmission genetics, DNA and chromosomes, and the latest genetic technology, among other topics.

McCance, Kathryn L., and Sue M. Huether. *Pathophysiology: The Biologic Basis for Disease in Adults and Children*. 5th ed. St. Louis: Elsevier Mosby, 2006. A text that explores the myriad cellular and genetic causes of disease. Topics include cell injury, immunity, inflammation and wound healing, coping and illness, and ontogenesis.

Marshall, Elizabeth L. *The Human Genome Project: Cracking the Code Within Us*. New York: Franklin Watts, 1997. Describes the Human Genome Project and its process of gene mapping, including concerns of critics of the project. Suitable for grades eight through twelve. Includes an extensive glossary and a bibliography.

Milunsky, Aubrey, ed. *Genetic Disorders of the Fetus: Diagnosis, Prevention, and Treatment*. 5th ed. Baltimore: Johns Hopkins University Press, 2004. This source treats a number of issues, from fetal cells in the maternal circulation to ethical issues surrounding a misdiagnosis, in chapters written by experts in the field. Recommended for clinicians in training and scientists working on the laboratory side of prenatal genetic testing.

Shaw, Michael, ed. *Everything You Need to Know About Diseases*. Springhouse, Pa.: Springhouse Press, 1996. This well-illustrated consumer reference, compiled by more than one hundred doctors and medical experts, describes five hundred illnesses and conditions, their causes, symptoms, diagnosis, treatment,

quired immunodeficiency syndrome (AIDS), the treatment of various cancers, and the synthesis of biopharmaceuticals for a variety of metabolic, growth, and development diseases. In general, biosynthesis is a process in which the gene coding for a particular product is isolated, cloned into another organism (mostly bacteria), and later expressed in that organism (the host). By cultivating the host organism, large quantities of the gene products can be harvested and purified. A few examples can illustrate the useful features of biosynthesis.

Insulin is essential for the treatment of insulin-dependent diabetes mellitus, the most severe form of diabetes. Historically, insulin was obtained from a cow or pig pancreas. Two problems exist for this traditional supply of insulin. First, large quantities of the pancreas are needed to extract enough insulin for continuous treatment of one patient. Second, insulin so obtained is not chemically identical to human insulin, hence some patients may produce antibodies that can seriously interfere with treatment. Human insulin produced through genetic engineering is quite effective yet without any side effects. It has been produced commercially and made available to patients since 1982.

Another successful story in biosynthesis is the production of human growth hormone (HGH), which is used in the treatment of children with growth retardation called pituitary dwarfism. The successful biosynthesis of HGH is important for several reasons. The conventional source of HGH was human pituitary glands removed at autopsy. Each child afflicted with pituitary dwarfism needs twice-a-week injections until the age of twenty. Such a treatment regime requires more than a thousand pituitary glands. The autopsy supply could hardly keep up with the demand. Furthermore, as a result of a small amount of virus contamination in the extracted HGH, many children receiving this treatment developed virus-related diseases.

Other biopharmaceuticals under development or in preclinical or clinical trials through genetic engineering include anticancer drugs, antiaging agents and possible vaccines for AIDS and malaria.

Broadly speaking, three types of gene therapy exist: germ line therapy, enhancement gene therapy, and somatic gene therapy. All gene therapy trials currently underway or in the pipeline are restricted to the somatic cells as targets for gene transfer. Germ line therapy involves the introduction of novel genes into germ cells, such as eggs or in early embryos. Although it has the potential for correcting defective genes completely, germ line therapy is highly controversial. Enhancement gene therapy, through which human potential might be enhanced for some desired traits, raises an even greater ethical dilemma. Both germ line and enhancement gene therapies have been banned based on the unresolved ethical issues surrounding them.

Somatic gene therapy is designed to introduce functional genes into body cells, thus enabling the body to perform normal functions and providing temporary correction for genetic abnormalities. The cloned human gene is first transferred into a viral vector, which is used to infect white blood cells removed from the patient. The transferred normal gene is then inserted into a chromosome and becomes active. After growth to enhance their numbers under sterile conditions, the cells are reimplanted into the patient, where they produce a gene product that is missing in the untreated patient, allowing the individual to function normally. Several disorders are currently being treated with this technique, including severe combined immunodeficiency disease (SCID). Individuals with SCID have no functional immune system and usually die from infections that would be minor in normal people. While several young boys with SCID remarkably showed almost complete recovery following gene therapy, a high percentage of them have subsequently developed leukemias following the introduction of genetically engineered bone marrow stem cells. Gene therapy is also being used or tested as a treatment for cystic fibrosis, skin cancer, breast cancer, brain cancer, and AIDS.

Most of these treatments are only partially successful, and they are prohibitively expensive. Over a ten-year period, from 1990 to 2000, more than four thousand people were treated through gene therapy. Unfortunately, most of these trials were failures that led to some loss of confidence in gene therapy. These failures have been attributed to inefficient vectors and the inability in many cases to specifically target the required host tissues. In the future, as more efficient vectors are engineered, gene therapy is expected to be a common method for treating a large number of genetic disorders.

Genetic Engineering in Agriculture, Forensics, and Environmental Science

As the use of genetic engineering expands rapidly, it is difficult to generate an exhaustive list of all possible applications, but three other areas are worth noting: forensic, environmental, and agricultural applications. Although these areas are not directly related to medicine, they certainly have profound impacts on human well-being. There are numerous ways that genetic engineering may be used to benefit agriculture and food production. First, the production of vaccines and the application of methods for transferring genes is likely to benefit animal husbandry, as scientists can alter commercially important traits such as milk yield, butterfat, and proportion of lean meat. For example, the bovine growth hormone produced through genetic engineering has been used since the late 1980's to boost milk production by cows. A mutant form of the myostatin gene has been identified and found to cause heavy muscling after this gene was introduced first into a mouse and later into the Belgian Blue bull. This technique marks the first step toward breeding cows and meat animals with lower fat and a higher proportion of lean meat. Other examples of using genetic engineering in animal husbandry include hormones for a faster growth rate in poultry and the production of recombinant human proteins in the milk of livestock.

Second, genetic engineering is expected to alter dramatically the conventional approaches of developing new strains of crops through breeding. The technology allows the transferring of genes for nitrogen fixation; the improvement of photosynthesis (and therefore yield); the promotion of resistance to pests, pathogens, and herbicides and tolerance to frost, drought, and increased salinity; and the improvement of nutritional value and consumer acceptability. Genetically engineered tobacco plants have been grown to produce the protein phaseolin, which is naturally synthesized by soybeans and other legume crops.

The first genetically engineered potato was approved for human consumption by the U.S. government in 1995 and by Canada in 1996. This NewLeaf potato, developed by corporate giant Monsanto, carries a gene from the bacterium *Bacillus thuringiensis*. This gene produces a protein toxic to the Colorado potato beetle, an insect that causes substantial loss of the crop if left uncontrolled. The production of this protein by potato plants equips them with resistance to beetles, hence alleviating crop loss, saving on the cost on pesticides, and reducing the risk of environment contamination.

Antiviral genes have been successfully transferred and expressed into cotton, and the release of new cotton strains with resistance to multiple viruses is a matter of time. At least five transgenic corn strains with resistance to herbicides or pathogens had been developed and commercially produced by U.S. farmers by 2002.

Some genes coding tolerance to drought and to subfreezing temperatures have been cloned and transferred into or among crop plants, some of which have already made a great impact on agriculture in developing countries. Initial effort has been made to replace chemical fertilizers with more environment friendly biofertilizers. Secondary metabolites produced naturally by plants have also been purified and used as biopesticides. Soon, there will be more grain, produce, milk, and meat produced by animals or plants that have been genetically engineered in some manner.

Genetic engineering is also useful in forensics. DNA fingerprints from samples collected at crime scenes provide strong evidence in trials, thus helping to solve many violent crimes. DNA can be isolated easily from tissue left at a crime scene, a splattering of blood, a hair sample, or even skin left under a victim's fingernails. A variety of techniques can be used routinely to determine the probability of matching between sample DNA and that of a suspect. DNA fingerprints are also useful in paternity and property disputes and in the study of the genealogy of various species.

The metabolism of microorganisms can be altered through genetic engineering, which enables them to absorb and degrade waste and hazardous material from the environment. The growth rate and metabolic capabilities of microorganisms offer great potential for coping with some environmental problems. Sewage plants can use engineered bacteria to degrade many organic compounds into nontoxic substances. Microbes may be engineered to detoxify specific substances in waste dumps or oil spills. Many bacteria can extract heavy metals (such as lead and copper) from their surroundings and incorporate them into compounds that are recoverable, thus cleaning them from the environment. Many more such applications have yet to be tested or discovered.

PERSPECTIVE AND PROSPECTS

Since the discovery of the double-helical structure of DNA by Francis Crick and James Watson in 1953, human curiosity regarding this amazing molecule has propelled the advancement of biological sciences in an unprecedented fashion. The first successful experiment in genetic engineering was described in 1972 when DNA fragments from two different organisms were joined together to produce a biologically functional hybrid DNA molecule. The next milestone came in 1975, when Dr. Edward Southern introduced Southern blotting, a technique that has many applications and has proved invaluable for the subsequent development of genetic engineering. This technique is used to identify a particular gene or DNA fragment from a mixture of thousands of different genes or DNA fragments. Later, the automated DNA sequencers, which can rapidly churn out letter sequences from DNA fragments, and the discovery of reverse transcriptase and PCR further improved the capabilities of scientists in studying and manipulating DNA molecules and the genes that they carry.

Using these techniques, the first prenatal diagnosis of a genetic disease was made in 1976 for alpha-thalassemia, a genetic disorder caused by the absence of globin genes. This represented a monumental step forward in the use of genetic tools in the medical field. It paved the way for the later development in which mutations in many genes could be detected in early pregnancy. Three years later, insulin was first synthesized through genetic engineering. In 1982, the commercial production of genetically engineered human insulin became a reality.

Gene therapy trials began in 1990, first with SCID. The first complete human genetic map was published in 1993, and various new techniques in DNA fingerprinting and the isolation of specific genes were developed. Also, an increasing number of pharmaceuticals have been produced through genetic engineering. Two versions of the draft copy of the human genome were published in 2001, launching the genomic revolution, and by 2006 complete DNA sequences of the genomes of over two hundred model research organisms, from bacteria to mice, were publically available for researchers. In the twenty-first century, genetic engineering will continue to offer more benefits in medicine and in agriculture in undreamed of ways.

In retrospect, genetic engineering presents a mixed blessing of invaluable benefits and dilemmas that science and technology have always offered humankind. There are those who would like to restrict the uses of genetic engineering and who might prefer that such technology had never been developed. Others believe that the benefits far outweigh the possible risks and that any potential threat can be overcome easily through government regulation or legislation. Others do not take sides on the debate in general but are greatly concerned with some specific applications.

Obviously, the power of genetic engineering demands a new set of decisions, both ethical and economical, by individuals, government, and society. Considerable concern has been expressed by both scientists and the general public regarding possible biohazards from genetic engineering. What if engineered organisms prove resistant to all known antibiotics or carry cancer genes that might spread throughout the community? What if a genetically engineered plant becomes an uncontrollable super weed? Would these kinds of risks outweigh the potential benefits? Others argue that the risk has been exaggerated and therefore do not want to impose limits on research. Genetic engineering has also generated legal issues concerning intellectual properties and patents for different aspects of the technology.

Even more controversial are the many ethical issues. Perhaps the most obvious ethical issue surrounding genetic engineering is the objection to some applications that are considered socially undesirable and morally wrong. One example is bovine growth hormone. Some vigorously opposed its use in boosting milk production for two main reasons. First, the recombinant hormone could change the composition of the milk. However, this view was dismissed by experts from the National Institutes of Health (NIH) and the Food and Drug Administration (FDA) after a thorough study. Second, many dairy farmers feared that greater milk production per cow would drive prices down even further and put some small farmers out of business.

Numerous aspects of the application of genetic engineering to humans also present ethical challenges. In some couples, both people carry a defective gene and have an appreciable chance of having an affected child. Should they refrain entirely from having children of their own? For genetic disorders caused by chromosomal abnormalities, such as Tay-Sachs disease, prenatal diagnosis can detect the defect in a fetus with great precision. Should the fetus be aborted if the screening result is positive? Should screening tests of infants for genetic disorders be required? If so, would such a requirement infringe the rights of the individual by the government? Perhaps the greatest concern of all is the possibility of designing or cloning a human being through genetic engineering. The debate over the ethical, legal, and social implications of genetic engineering should help in the formulation and optimization of public policy and laws regarding this technology, and genetic engineering research and its applications should proceed with caution.

—Ming Y. Zheng, Ph.D.;
updated by Jeffrey A. Knight, Ph.D.

See also Bacteriology; Bionics and biotechnology; Cancer; Cells; Chemotherapy; Cloning; Cytology; Diabetes mellitus; DNA and RNA; Enzyme therapy; Enzymes; Ethics; Fetal tissue transplantation; Gene therapy; Genetic counseling; Genetics and inheritance; Genomics; Hormones; Immunization and vaccination; Mutation; Pharmacology; Screening; Stem cells.

FOR FURTHER INFORMATION:

Brungs, Robert S. J., and R. S. M. Postiglione, eds. *The Genome: Plant, Animal, Human.* St. Louis: ITEST Faith/Science Press, 2000. A collection of excellent scientific, ethical, educational, and theological papers focuses on the genomic revolution and the application of genetic engineering to plants, humans, and other animals.

Daniell, H., S. J. Streatfield, and K. Wycoff. "Medical Molecular Farming: Production of Antibodies, Biopharmaceuticals, and Edible Vaccines in Plants." *Trends in Plant Science* 6 (2001): 219-226. A contemporary review of the production of plant-based medicinal products through genetic engineering and related biotechnology.

Frankel, M. S., and A. Teich, eds. *The Genetic Frontier.* Washington, D.C.: American Association for the Advancement of Science, 1994. A wonderful collection of essays from many experts and organizations dealing with the ethics, laws, and policies of genetic engineering.

Gerdes, Louise I., ed. *Genetic Engineering: Opposing Viewpoints.* Farmington Hills, Mich.: Greenhaven Press, 2004. Presents balanced and well-thought-out opposing views on genetic engineering by proponents and opponents from various angles.

Holland, Suzanne, Karen Lebacqz, and Laurie Zoloth, eds. *The Human Embryonic Stem Cell Debate.* Cambridge, Mass.: MIT Press, 2001. Very thoughtful reflections on debates regarding stem cell research and potential pros and cons by a number of extraordinary people from diverse disciplines.

Kilner, John F., R. D. Pentz, and F. E. Young, eds. *Genetic Ethics: Do the Ends Justify the Genes?* Grand Rapids, Mich.: Wm. B. Eerdmans, 1997. An assembly of experts addresses three dimensions of the genetic challenge: perspective, information, and intervention. A wonderful collection of useful and informative guiding principles on genetic engineering.

Panno, Joseph. *Tracking Disease by Repairing Genes.* New York: Facts On File, 2005. A well-illustrated basic introduction to the principles and possibilities of gene therapy.

Pasternak, Jack J. *An Introduction to Human Molecular Genetics.* 2d ed. Bethesda, Md.: Fitzgerald Science Press, 2005. An excellent primer on many technologies as applied to humans, including genetic engineering, stem cell research, cloning, and gene therapy.

Primrose, S. B., R. M. Twyman, and R. W. Old. *Principles of Genetic Manipulation: An Introduction to Genetic Engineering.* 6th ed. Palo Alto, Calif.: Blackwell Science, 2002. A resource that provides foundational knowledge on the principles and processes of genetic engineering.

Tal, J. "Adeno-Associated Virus-Based Vectors in Gene Therapy." *Journal of Biomedical Science* 7 (2000): 279-291. A good summary of gene therapy and the outlook on recent developments.

GENETIC SEQUENCING. *See* GENOMICS.

GENETICS AND INHERITANCE
BIOLOGY
ANATOMY OR SYSTEM AFFECTED: All

SPECIALTIES AND RELATED FIELDS: Embryology, forensic medicine, genetics, pediatrics

DEFINITION: The passage of traits from parents to offspring in discrete units called genes.

KEY TERMS:

allele: a version of a gene; different alleles of a gene have slightly different nucleotide sequences, resulting in differences in the protein encoded in the gene

chromosome: one of the DNA molecules of a nucleus; in humans, chromosomes occur in twenty-three pairs, with each member of a pair having the same genes but possibly having different alleles of the genes

deoxyribonucleic acid (DNA): the hereditary molecule, in which sequences of nucleic acids encode genetic information

dominant allele: the version of a gene that can produce a recognizable trait in offspring when present in only one of the two chromosomes of a pair

fertilization: the process by which chromosome pairs, separated in production of egg and sperm cells, are rejoined

gene: a sequence of nucleotides in DNA encoding a protein

meiosis: a division mechanism in which homologous chromosomes are separated and delivered singly to egg or sperm cells; as a part of meiosis, recombination generates new combinations of alleles

nucleotide: a chemical subunit of DNA; different sequences of linked nucleotides spell out instructions for the assembly of proteins

recessive allele: a version of a gene that must be present on both chromosomes of a pair in order to produce a recognizable trait in offspring

recombination: the reciprocal exchange of segments between the two chromosomes of a pair, producing new combinations of alleles

THE RULES OF INHERITANCE

The primary genes of interest to heredity consist of a set of coded directions for making proteins. Each gene codes for a protein; distinct versions of a gene, which encode slightly different versions of the protein, may be carried in the same or different individuals. The distinct versions of a gene, called alleles, are responsible for differences in hereditary traits among individuals. Each individual receives a combination of alleles encoding proteins that directly or indirectly determine traits such as eye, skin, and hair color; height; and, to a degree, characteristics such as personality, behavior, and intelligence.

In molecular terms, genes consist of a sequence of chemical units called nucleotides, linked end to end in long, linear deoxyribonucleic acid (DNA) molecules. There are four kinds of nucleotides in DNA; each gene has its own nucleotide sequence. The alleles of a gene differ slightly in nucleotide sequence—some alleles differ in the substitution of only a single nucleotide. There are many thousands of genes arranged in tandem on the DNA molecules of a human cell; each DNA molecule is known as a chromosome. In humans, the chromosomes occur in twenty-three pairs, for a total of forty-six chromosomes. The two members of a chromosome pair contain the same genes in the same order, but different alleles of a gene may be present in the two members of a pair. One member of a chromosome pair is derived from the female parent of the individual; the other member is derived from the male parent. These are called the maternal and paternal chromosomes of the pair.

Inheritance, and the variation in traits among individuals, depends on two processes that separate and rejoin the chromosome pairs in sexual reproduction. One is a division mechanism, meiosis, which occurs in cell lines leading to egg or sperm cells. Meiosis separates the chromosome pairs and places one member of each pair in an egg or sperm cell. The particular combination of maternal and paternal chromosomes delivered to an egg or sperm cell is random. This random segregation,

as it is called, is one source of the variability among offspring in a family. Because there are so many chromosomes, the possibility that two egg or sperm cells produced by the same individual could receive the same combination of maternal and paternal chromosomes is very small—equivalent to one chance in 8.4 million. Another important source of variability comes from a mechanism that occurs before the pairs are separated in meiosis. In this mechanism, called recombination, the two members of a chromosome pair line up side by side and exchange segments perfectly and reciprocally. As a result, alleles are exchanged between the pairs, generating new combinations of alleles. The variability generated by recombination adds to that produced by independent segregation of maternal and paternal chromosomes, so that it is essentially impossible for an individual to produce two egg or sperm cells that are genetically the same.

The second process underlying inheritance is fertilization, in which a sperm and an egg cell fuse, rejoining the twenty-three pairs of chromosomes. Fertilization is another random process, in which any of the millions of sperm cells ejaculated by a male and any of the hundreds of egg cells carried in a female may join. The total variability generated by independent segregation of alleles, recombination, and random union of gametes is such that each human individual, except identical twins, receives a unique combination of alleles. Thus the possibility that any individual has or will ever have a genetic double in the human population, except for an identical twin, is essentially zero. (In the case of identical twins, a single fertilized egg divides to produce two separate, genetically identical cells; instead of remaining together to produce a two-celled embryo, as is normally the case, the cells separate to create two embryos, which develop into genetically identical individuals.)

Because chromosomes occur in pairs, each individual receives two alleles of every gene of the human complement. The two alleles may be the same or different. Some alleles are dominant in their effects, so that one copy of the allele on either chromosome is sufficient to produce the trait encoded in the allele. Other alleles are recessive, so that both chromosomes of the pair must carry the allele for the trait to appear in offspring. In humans, few physical traits are determined by a single gene. Most are the result of complex interactions between several genes, as well as environmental influences. Nonetheless, some traits do tend to follow certain inheritance patterns, but there are exceptions. For example, brown eyes tend to be dominant to blue eyes. If either chromosome carries the brown eye allele, the individual will usually have brown eyes. To have blue eyes, an individual usually carries two genes for blue eyes. Human traits that tend toward dominant inheritance include nearsightedness and farsightedness, astigmatism, dark or curly hair, early balding in males, normal body pigment (as compared to albinism), supernumerary fingers or toes, short fingers or toes, and webbing between fingers and toes. Alleles that tend to be expressed in a recessive fashion include blond hair, straight hair, and congenital deafness.

Although each individual normally carries a maximum of two alleles of any gene, several or many alleles of a gene may exist in the human population as a whole.

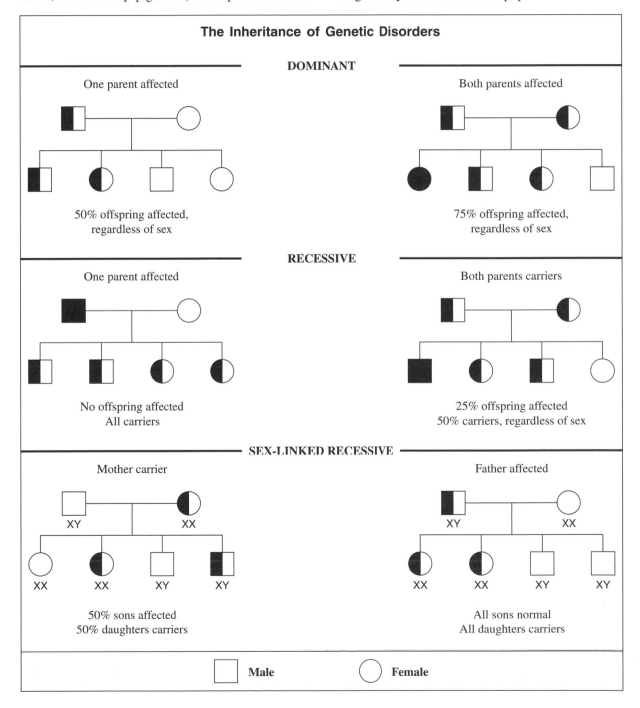

The Inheritance of Genetic Disorders

DOMINANT

One parent affected

50% offspring affected, regardless of sex

Both parents affected

75% offspring affected, regardless of sex

RECESSIVE

One parent affected

No offspring affected
All carriers

Both parents carriers

25% offspring affected
50% carriers, regardless of sex

SEX-LINKED RECESSIVE

Mother carrier

XY   XX

XX   XX   XY   XY

50% sons affected
50% daughters carriers

Father affected

XY   XX

XX   XX   XY   XY

All sons normal
All daughters carriers

☐ **Male**   ◯ **Female**

The major histocompatibility complex (MHC), for example, occurs in hundreds of different alleles throughout the human population—so many that unrelated individuals are unlikely to carry the same combination of MHC alleles. The proteins encoded in these alleles are recognized by the immune system as "self" or "foreign." Unless the same, or a very similar, combination of MHC alleles is present, cells are recognized by the immune system as foreign, and the cells are destroyed. Therefore, MHC combinations recognized as foreign are the primary factor in the rejection of tissue or organ transplants among humans. If the transplant does not come from an individual with the same or a very similar MHC combination, rejection is likely unless the immune system is suppressed by drugs such as cyclosporine. The best donor for a transplant is a close relative, who is most likely to have a similar MHC combination. Because identical twins have the same MHC combination, tissues and organs can be transplanted between them with no danger of rejection.

Sex is determined by a pair of chromosomes that is different in males and females. Females have two members of the pair, the X chromosomes, which have the same genes in the same order but which may have different alleles of the genes. One member of the XX pair was derived from the female's father, and the other from her mother. Males have only one member of this pair, a single X. In addition, males have a small, single chromosome, the Y, which is not present in females. Thus females are XX, and males are XY. During meiosis in females, the XX pair is separated, so that an egg cell may receive either member of the pair. In males, the X and Y are separated, so that a sperm cell receives either an X or a Y. In fertilization, the X chromosome carried by the egg may be joined with an X-carrying sperm, producing a female (XX), or, the egg may be fertilized by a sperm cell carrying a Y, producing a male (XY). Thus, in humans the sex of the offspring is determined by the type of sperm cell, an X or a Y, fertilizing the egg. Most genes carried on an X chromosome have no counterparts on the Y chromosome. Therefore, traits encoded in genes on the X chromosomes (almost none are carried on the Y) are inherited differently from traits carried on other chromosomes of the set, in a pattern known as sex-linked inheritance.

DISORDERS AND DISEASES

Many human diseases, involving every system in the body, depend on the presence of particular dominant or recessive alleles and are directly inherited. Only the

disposition for development of other diseases is inherited—that is, some individuals inherit a combination of alleles that increases the possibility that a genetically based disease will develop during their lifetimes.

The list of diseases contracted through inheritance of a dominant allele is long and impressive. Among the more important of these diseases are achondroplasia, in which individuals are short-statured; familial hypercholesterolemia, in which cholesterol concentration in the blood is abnormally high, leading to vascular disease, particularly of the coronary arteries; Huntington's disease, a disease characterized by dementia, delusion, paranoia, and abnormal movements that begins in persons between twenty and fifty years of age and progresses steadily to death in about fifteen years; Marfan syndrome, a disease of connective tissues involving the skeleton, eyes, and cardiovascular system, characterized by elongated limbs, abnormal position of the eye lens, and structural weakness of blood vessels, particularly of the aorta; neurofibromatosis, characterized by tumors dispersed throughout the body and coffee-colored skin lesions; polycystic kidney disease, in which dilated cysts grow in the kidneys and interfere with kidney function, leading to hypertension and chronic renal failure; spherocytosis, another disease in which blood cells are fragile and easily broken during travel through the circulatory system, producing anemia and jaundice; and thalassemia, a group of diseases most common in persons of Mediterranean descent in which hemoglobin production is faulty, leading to anemias that range from mild to severe.

Diseases caused by recessive genes also appear in the human population. Although many persons are carriers for these diseases, affected persons are rare because both alleles must be present in the recessive form for the disease to develop. Diseases in this category include albinism; sickle cell disease, common in persons of African descent, in which hemoglobin is faulty, leading to fragility of red blood cells, anemia, blockage of blood vessels, and susceptibility to infection; phenylketonuria (PKU), in which the amino acid phenylalanine accumulates in excess in the bloodstream, leading to nervous system damage including mental retardation; Tay-Sachs disease, most common in persons of Jewish descent, characterized by accumulation of lipid molecules in nerve cells leading to motor incoordination, blindness, and mental deterioration; and glycogen storage diseases, with symptoms ranging from cramps to serious muscular and cardiac disease and convulsions. Sickle cell disease is recessively inherited. A person with one copy of the sickle cell gene makes sufficient normal hemoglobin that symptoms of the disease occur only under extreme low oxygen conditions. Cystic fibrosis, one of the most common of genetically determined diseases in Caucasians, is probably also attributable to a recessive allele. In this disease, sweat and mucus-secreting glands are affected; the most serious effects are caused by the secretion of unusually thick and viscid mucus, leading to blockage of ducts in the lungs, liver, pancreas, and salivary glands. Most critical to survival is blockage of passages in the lungs, producing a chronic cough and persistent pulmonary infections. The average life expectancy of persons with cystic fibrosis is twenty years of age.

A number of diseases are caused by recessive genes carried on the X chromosomes and are inherited in sex-linked patterns. Among these are one form of diabetes (diabetes insipidus) in which glucose uptake by cells is faulty, leading to the accumulation of glucose in the blood; hemophilia, in which the blood-clotting mechanism is deficient, making afflicted persons subject to uncontrolled bleeding; and some forms of muscular dystrophy, characterized by progressive muscular weakness. The Duchenne muscular dystrophy appears early in life, progresses rapidly, and leads to death in most cases by the age of twenty.

Because males receive only one copy of the X chromosome, recessive genes are fully expressed in males—there is no chance for a normal allele to compensate for the effects of the recessive gene. For a sex-linked disease to appear in females, both X chromosomes must carry the recessive allele. For these reasons, sex-linked recessive diseases are much more common in males than in females; for some, appearance of the disease is limited almost exclusively to males.

The molecular basis for some genetically based diseases is known. In familial hypercholesterolemia, for example, receptors for cholesterol on cell surfaces are faulty or not produced, preventing the normal uptake of cholesterol from the bloodstream. As a result, cholesterol accumulates and reaches a dangerously high concentration in the blood. In persons carrying dominant alleles for familial hypercholesterolemia on both chromosomes of the pair, coronary arterial disease advances so rapidly that death from heart attack by the age of twenty is frequent. The disease is among the most common of genetically based defects—about 1 in 500 persons has at least one allele for hypercholesterolemia and develops premature coronary artery disease. In PKU, individuals lack an enzyme normally produced in the liver. The enzyme, phenylalanine hydroxylase, converts excess phenylalanine into another amino acid, tyrosine. Without the enzyme, phenylalanine taken in the diet accumulates to dangerously high levels in the body. Some forms of PKU are treatable by restricting dietary intake of phenylalanine from infancy onward.

Some persons have a genetically determined predisposition to develop certain cancers with greater frequency than the average in the population. About 5 percent of cancers are strongly predisposed—that is, individuals inherit a marked tendency to develop the cancer. Among these are familial retinoblastoma, in which retinal tumors develop; familial adenomatous polyps of the colon; and multiple endocrine neoplasia, in which tumors develop in the thyroid, adrenal medulla, and parathyroid glands. Often underlying these strongly predisposed cancers is the inheritance of a faulty gene (called an oncogene) that promotes uncontrolled cell division, or the opposite—inheritance of a faulty gene that in its normal form suppresses cell division (called a tumor suppressor gene). Typically, oncogenes are inherited as dominant genes, and tumor suppressor genes as recessives. In addition, some cancers, including breast, ovarian, and colon cancers other than familial adenomatous polyps, show a degree of predisposition in family lines.

PERSPECTIVE AND PROSPECTS

The primary features of meiosis and fertilization, random segregation of chromosome pairs in meiosis and random rejoining of pairs in fertilization, makes heredity subject to analysis by mathematical techniques. In fact, mathematical analysis of heredity was carried out successfully before there was any understanding concerning meiosis or DNA. The groundwork for this analysis was laid down in the 1860's by an Austrian monk, Gregor Mendel. Mendel's research approach and his conclusions were so advanced that they were misunderstood and unappreciated during his lifetime.

Mendel chose garden peas for his research because they could be grown easily and they possessed several hereditary traits that were known to breed true—that is, to appear dependably in offspring. Mendel crossed pea plants with different traits in various combinations. On analyzing the results of his crosses, Mendel realized that the numbers of offspring exhibiting different traits could be explained mathematically if he assumed that parents contain a pair of factors governing the inheritance of each trait. Furthermore, he concluded that the factors separate, or segregate, independently as gametes are formed and are reunited randomly at fertilization. He also discovered that some traits are inherited as dominant and some as recessive. Mendel's factors were later called genes.

Until Mendel's time, inheritance was commonly believed to occur through a blending of maternal and paternal characteristics. Mendel's work showed instead that traits are passed on as units; depending on whether a trait is dominant or recessive, it may appear in all offspring or only in a definite, predictable percentage. Some time after Mendel's discoveries, in the early 1900's, meiosis was discovered. At this time, Walter Sutton pointed out that Mendel's genes and chromosomes behave similarly in meiosis and fertilization: Both genes and chromosomes occur in pairs that separate randomly in meiosis and are rejoined at fertilization. Genes were therefore concluded to be carried on the chromosomes. Further genetic research confirmed that Mendel's findings with plant genes also apply to animals, including humans, and worked out many additional features of inheritance, including genetic recombination and sex linkage. Later, in the 1950's, almost one hundred years after Mendel's findings, James D. Watson and Francis Crick discovered the structure of DNA and deduced the fact that hereditary information is encoded in the sequence of nucleotides in DNA.

Research in human genetics differs from genetic investigation in other organisms because, for obvious reasons, it is impossible to set up experimental crosses to test whether particular diseases are inherited. Instead, human family lines are analyzed carefully in pedigrees to trace the appearance of disease over several generations. If a disease is genetically determined, it shows up in definite patterns as dominant, recessive, or sex-linked among parents and offspring in the pedigrees. On this basis, prospective parents can be counseled on the chances that their offspring will develop a hereditary disease.

In June of 2000, Francis Collins, director of the National Human Genome Research Initiative, and J. Craig Venter, of Celera Genomics, announced that they had jointly sequenced the entire human genome and that the first working draft was available. Sequencing the human genome will allow scientists to directly compare healthy DNA to DNA harboring disease genes. Discovering the disease genes and studying them will lead to much more rapid understanding of disease processes, as well as the development of diagnostic procedures and potential therapy and cures, than allowed by the techniques available before the completion of this initiative.

—Stephen L. Wolfe, Ph.D.;
updated by Karen E. Kalumuck, Ph.D.

See also Aging; Amniocentesis; Bioinformatics; Biostatistics; Birth defects; Chorionic villus sampling; Cloning; DNA and RNA; Embryology; Environmental diseases; Gene therapy; Genetic counseling; Genetic diseases; Genetic engineering; Genomics; Laboratory tests; Metabolic disorders; Multiple births; Mutation; Neonatology; Obstetrics; Oncology; Pediatrics; Pregnancy and gestation; Preventive medicine; Proteomics; Screening; Sexual differentiation; Sexuality.

For Further Information:

Campbell, Neil A., et al. *Biology: Concepts and Connections.* 5th ed. San Francisco: Pearson/Benjamin Cummings, 2006. This classic introductory textbook provides an excellent discussion of essential biological structures and mechanisms. Of particular interest are the chapters "Mendel and the Gene Idea," "The Chromosomal Basis of Inheritance," and "The Molecular Basis of Inheritance."

Lewin, Benjamin. *Genes IX.* 9th rev. ed. Sudbury, Mass.: Jones & Bartlett, 2007. A college textbook that discusses the entire field of molecular biology and genetics, with many references to the structure and activity of the cell nucleus. Although written at the college level, it is readable and accessible to a general audience. Many highly informative illustrations and diagrams are included.

Lewis, Ricki. *Human Genetics: Concepts and Applications.* 7th ed. New York: McGraw-Hill, 2007. A very accessible undergraduate text that covers the fundamentals, transmission genetics, DNA and chromosomes, and the latest genetic technology, among other topics.

Marieb, Elaine N. *Essentials of Human Anatomy and Physiology.* 8th ed. San Francisco: Pearson/Benjamin Cummings, 2006. This introductory anatomy and physiology textbook, easily accessible to those with little science background, is richly illustrated with diagrams and photographs, which help to illuminate body systems and processes. In-depth discussions of prevalent diseases and disorders and of current areas of research make this an all-around useful reference work.

Moore, Keith L., and T. V. N. Persaud. *The Developing Human.* 7th ed. Philadelphia: W. B. Saunders, 2003. An outstanding textbook on human embryonic development, with specific information about the causes of congenital malformations and common defects occurring in each of the body's systems.

Ridley, Matt. *Nature Via Nurture: Genes, Experience, and What Makes Us Human.* New York: Harper-Collins, 2003. Accessible, engaging discussion of genes, what they contribute to the development of the human brain and neurons, and how that contribution is changed or modified by the environment in which they are expressed.

Wolfe, Stephen L. *Molecular and Cellular Biology.* Belmont, Calif.: Wadsworth, 1993. Chapter 25, "Meiosis and Genetic Recombination," describes these mechanisms. The book, written at the college level, is highly readable and illustrated with many informative diagrams and photographs.

GENITAL DISORDERS, FEMALE
DISEASE/DISORDER

ANATOMY OR SYSTEM AFFECTED: Genitals, reproductive system, uterus

SPECIALTIES AND RELATED FIELDS: Family medicine, gynecology, obstetrics, oncology, urology

DEFINITION: All maladies affecting the reproductive organs of women.

KEY TERMS:

cervix: the narrow portion of the uterus situated at the upper end of the vagina

cyst: a closed sac having a distinct border that develops abnormally within a body space or structure

estrogen: the hormone responsible for female sexual characteristics, produced primarily by the ovaries

Fallopian tubes: tiny tubes that connect the ovaries to the uterus; after ovulation, the egg travels through these tubes, and its fertilization by sperm occurs here

hormone: a chemical compound produced at one site in the body which travels to other parts of the body to exert its effect

hysterectomy: the surgical removal of the uterus; in a total hysterectomy, the uterus, ovaries, and Fallopian tubes are removed

laparoscopy: a surgical procedure in which an instrument is inserted into the body through tiny incisions; usually performed without hospitalization

CAUSES AND SYMPTOMS

Diseases and disorders of the female genitals, both internal organs and outward anatomical structures, encompass a huge number of different types of conditions that can range in severity from merely physically an-

noying to life-threatening. These disorders affect the vulva, vagina, uterus, ovaries, and Fallopian tubes. Many develop from unknown causes, and others have clear-cut origins, such as sexually transmitted diseases. Some have immediately recognizable symptoms, while others are silent until the disease has progressed to a serious stage. Early recognition of symptoms or abnormalities and proper treatment can alleviate pain and save lives.

Endometriosis is a chronic, recurring disease in which the tissue that lines the uterus grows into the abdominal cavity. This tissue normally thickens with blood vessels in preparation for receiving a fertilized egg. In endometriosis, the tissue overgrows the uterus, invades the Fallopian tubes, and reaches the abdominal cavity, where it continues to grow. This abnormally growing tissue will attach to any nearby internal organs, such as the ovaries, bladder, Fallopian tubes, and rectum. The endometrial tissue responds to the same hormonal cues that signal the sloughing off of the uterine lining during menstruation; however, the blood from the endometrial tissue cannot leave the abdominal cavity, leading to inflammation. As the inflammation subsides, it is replaced with scar tissue. This process will repeat with each menstrual cycle, and the scarring can result in infertility, organ malfunction, or adhesions that bind organs together. Some women with endometriosis experience no symptoms, while many experience severe abdominal pain before, during, and after their menstrual periods. Endometrial tissue sometimes can be diagnosed with a pelvic examination, but a definitive diagnosis can be reached only with laparoscopy. The cause of endometriosis is unknown, but some evidence suggests an inherited tendency to develop endometriosis.

Vaginitis is a general term for infections of the vagina. The most common of these is commonly called a yeast infection, caused by the fungus *Candida albicans.* This fungus is usually a harmless organism that lives in nearly everyone's intestinal tract and in the vagina of 20 to 40 percent of American women. Symptoms are caused when the organism grows at an accelerated rate and include severe itching, vaginal discharge, and burning upon urination. Many situations may cause the enhanced growth of the fungus, including use of antibiotics, which disturb the acid balance within the vagina; stress; use of oral contraceptives and corticosteroids; and the low estrogen levels that accompany the menopause.

Uterine fibroids are benign tumors made mainly of

Information on Female Genital Disorders

Causes: Endometriosis, hormonal imbalances, infection, disease, uterine fibroids, sexually transmitted diseases

Symptoms: Varies; can include abdominal pain, pain during menstruation or sexual intercourse, vaginal itching, vaginal discharge, burning upon urination

Duration: Acute or chronic, often with recurrent episodes

Treatments: Depends on cause; may include oral contraceptives, corticosteroids, hormone therapy, anti-inflammatory drugs, surgery, radiation therapy, chemotherapy, immunotherapy

muscle tissue that can grow inside the uterus or along its outer surface. They grow slowly and are dependent on the hormone estrogen for continued growth. They are usually not problematic, but if they become very large they may cause extremely heavy bleeding during menstruation and can interfere with pregnancy and childbirth. Their cause is unknown, but they will shrink or disappear after the menopause.

Uterine prolapse occurs when the pelvic muscles are no longer able to support the pelvic organs, and the uterus "falls" into the vagina. A feeling of one's "insides falling out" is typical of this disorder, which is often precipitated by one or more difficult births.

Ovarian cysts form when an egg developing inside a follicle within the ovary does not ovulate but instead keeps growing. Small cysts will be painless, but larger ones (up to 7.5 centimeters in diameter) may cause abdominal pain. Most cysts will go away on their own, but some can rupture and cause severe pain.

The hallmark of cancer is uncontrolled cell growth. Cancer may prove fatal by causing destruction of a particular organ at the site of origin or by spreading throughout the body and damaging other organs and systems. All the organs of the female reproductive system can be affected by cancer. Cervical cancer begins in superficial layers of the cervix but may spread rapidly through the vagina and throughout the body. Cervical cancer can be detected in its early, most curable stages by a Pap smear. Endometrial cancer affects the glands that line the uterus. It can occur at any age, but the most common age of onset is sixty. Abnormal bleeding accompanies this disorder, which is diagnosed by examination of a biopsy of uterine tissue.

Sarcomas of the uterus are malignant tumors of muscle tissue frequently confused with benign fibroids. This rare cancer is aggressive and difficult to treat. Ovarian cancer constitutes about 25 percent of female reproductive tract cancers, is difficult to detect and cure, and therefore has a high mortality rate. There are no early symptoms, and the cancer seems to occur frequently in those with a family history of the disease. Cancers of the Fallopian tubes and vagina are very rare, but vaginal cancer occurs with greater frequency in women whose mothers were treated with the synthetic estrogen diethylstilbestrol (DES) during the 1940's through the 1960's with the intent of preventing miscarriages. Cancer of the vulva, a form of skin cancer, is relatively easy to treat and has a high cure rate.

Sexually transmitted diseases (STDs) can involve any part of the female genital system. STDs of bacterial origin include gonorrhea and chlamydia, which are major precursors to pelvic inflammatory disease (PID) and syphilis. Untreated, these diseases can lead to serious complications. STDs with a viral cause include genital herpes, genital warts, and acquired immunodeficiency syndrome (AIDS). The causative agent of trichomoniasis is a protozoan. Each STD can be transmitted through direct sexual contact with an infected person, and each has its own set of symptoms and diagnostic criteria.

Treatment and Therapy

A variety of treatments are available for endometriosis, depending on the severity of the disorder. Over-the-counter or prescription anti-inflammatory drugs may give immediate relief of pain, but the condition itself is frequently treated with hormone therapy. Birth control pills that are high in the hormone progestin and low in estrogen can help shrink endometriosis. Danazol, a synthetic male hormone, suppresses the production of estrogen by the ovaries, thereby helping to eliminate the condition, but it has undesirable side effects. In some cases, surgical removal of the tissue is necessary. In laparoscopy, an instrument is inserted through tiny abdominal incisions and used to remove the tissue. In the most severe cases, a complete hysterectomy (removal of the uterus and ovaries) is performed.

Yeast infections that result in vaginitis must be properly diagnosed by a physician. Two medications for yeast infections are available without a prescription: miconazole and clotrimazole, available under brand names in most pharmacies. If a severe infection does not respond to this treatment, cortisone may be prescribed. Yeast infections have a tendency to recur, and taking precautions to prevent additional episodes is advised. Some ways in which to reduce the chance of re-infection include eating a cup of yogurt daily, avoiding sweets, reducing stress, wearing cotton underwear, avoiding tight-fitting clothing, avoiding feminine hygiene sprays, and using vinegar-and-water or povidone-iodine douches.

If no major discomfort is experienced by the woman when uterine fibroids are first detected, usually no treatment beyond regular observation is necessary. For those experiencing pain or difficulty in conception or pregnancy, the fibroids may be surgically removed in an operation called a myomectomy; in severe cases, a hysterectomy is performed. A laparoscope can be used to remove tumors on the outside of the uterus, or a hysteroscope can be inserted through the cervix, which uses a laser to burn away internal fibroids. Synthetic hormones called gonadotropin-releasing hormone agonists block the ovaries' production of estrogen, which leads to shrinking of the fibroids and the possible avoidance of surgery. A new treatment that shows promise is uterine artery embolization (UAE), in which the arteries that supply the fibroids are blocked.

A prolapsed uterus is frequently treated by hysterectomy, but other therapies are possible. Kegel exercises, designed to strengthen the muscles of the pelvic floor, are effective if done regularly for an extended period of time. A pessary, a ring-shaped device that fits around the cervix and props up the uterus, is another alternative, though an inconvenient one. Major surgery to resuspend the uterus is a surgical option to hysterectomy.

Ovarian cysts will usually be resorbed into the ovary within one to three menstrual cycles. Proper monitoring by a physician is needed to determine if the cysts have cleared. If the cyst does not disappear within three months or if it increases in size, ultrasound and/or laparoscopy will be used to determine if a different type of ovarian tumor is present, which would necessitate surgical removal.

Cancer treatment is highly specialized for the particular variety of the disease, its severity, and consideration of the affected individual. Typical treatments include surgical removal of the tumor and/or affected organ, radiation therapy, chemotherapy, and immunotherapy (the reinforcement of the immune system, generally administered after radiation or chemotherapy). When diagnosed in premalignant stages, cervical ab-

normalities may be treated by cryosurgery (freezing and killing the abnormal cells) or laser destruction of the abnormal cells. Advanced cervical cancer is treated by hysterectomy. Endometrial cancer is treated with total hysterectomy, including the uterus, ovaries, and Fallopian tubes, and if the cancer has spread, radiation and/or chemotherapy. The only known cure for uterine sarcoma is total hysterectomy, and removal of both the ovaries and the Fallopian tubes is performed for ovarian cancer. The tumors of vaginal cancer are eliminated surgically or with laser treatment.

Sexually transmitted diseases of bacterial origin are treated successfully with antibiotics. Drug therapy can also eliminate trichomoniasis. There are no cures for the virally transmitted STDs. Certain drugs can reduce the frequency of outbreaks of genital herpes, and genital warts may be removed by freezing, burning, or surgery. No cure exists for AIDS, although drugs are available to prolong life.

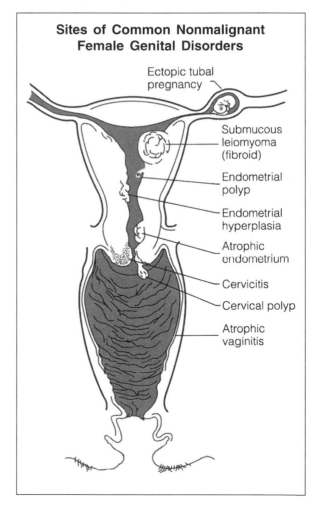

Sites of Common Nonmalignant Female Genital Disorders

Ectopic tubal pregnancy

Submucous leiomyoma (fibroid)

Endometrial polyp

Endometrial hyperplasia

Atrophic endometrium

Cervicitis

Cervical polyp

Atrophic vaginitis

surrounds the sperm-producing tubules, and accessory cells (the Leydig cells). The production of sperm, spermatogenesis, is controlled by hormones from the brain's hypothalamus and pituitary glands. It begins with the secretion of testosterone, the main male hormone, by Leydig cells. Brain hormone and testosterone actions cause the metamorphosis of cells called spermatogonia into sperm during a two-month passage through the seminiferous tubules.

The highly coiled seminiferous tubules, tiny in diameter and more than 200 meters long, coalesce into the efferent tubules, which release sperm into the epididymis. In a twelve-day trip through the highly coiled, 4.5-meter-long epididymis, sperm attain the ability to move (motility) and to fertilize a human egg cell, or ovum. Next, they enter the vas deferens, paired structures that connect the epididymis of each testis to its ejaculatory duct and the urethra. The only known vas function is to transport sperm, as a result of the action of nearby nerves and muscles, into the latter structures. The vas are cut in bilateral vasectomy surgery, which is often used for male sterilization.

The prostate, seminal vesicles, and bulbourethral glands produce the secretions that constitute most sperm-containing semen, which is ejaculated during intercourse. The prostate gland is situated immediately below the urinary bladder and surrounds the portion of the urethra closest to the bladder. It is a fibromuscular gland that empties into the male urethra on ejaculation. Prostate secretions contain important enzymes and make up a quarter of the seminal fluid.

The seminal vesicles are 7.5 centimeters long and empty into the ejaculatory ducts. They produce more than half of the liquid portion of semen, contributing fluid rich in fructose, the main nutrition source of sperm. The tiny, paired bulbourethral (or Cowper's) glands are located below the prostate. They secrete lubricants into the male urethra that ease semen passage.

The male urethra passes from the urinary bladder, through the prostate, and then through the penis. At the end of the penis, it reaches the outside of the body, to pass semen and urine. The penis, a cylindrical erectile organ, surrounds most of the male urethra and contains three cavernous regions. One, the corpus spongiosum, is found around the urethra. The others, the paired corpora cavernosa, are erectile tissues that fill with blood to produce an erection upon male sexual arousal. Erection is a complex reflex that involves both the sympathetic and parasympathetic portions of the human nervous system.

At the time of erection, nerve impulses dilate blood vessels that communicate with the corpora cavernosa and allow them to fill with blood. Sphincters then close off the portion of the urethra closest to the urinary bladder. At the same time, sperm, prostate secretions, bulbourethral gland secretions, and seminal vesicle secretions enter the urethra. Next, muscle contractions propel the ejaculate out of the urethra. The blood then leaves the corpora cavernosa, and the penis resumes its unexcited state.

Complications and Disorders

Proper male sexual function involves several closely coordinated hormonal, nervous, and chemical processes. After a discussion of the male genital system, it thus becomes clear that many factors can cause male genital problems and diseases. Male infertility, for example, can be attributable to inadequate sperm production; undersecretion by the seminal vesicles, Cowper's glands, and/or prostate; malfunction of other endocrine glands or of the nervous system; and dysfunction or lack of the epididymis. Impotence, the inability to have or maintain a satisfactory erection for intercourse, is another frequent male genital problem. It may be psychogenic or caused by anatomic dysfunction, disease, or medications used to treat health problems.

The male sexual response cycle is mediated by the complex interplay of parasympathetic and sympathetic nerves. For example, penis erection is mostly parasympathetic, while ejaculation is largely attributable to sympathetic enervation. Dysfunction disorders include low sexual desire, impotence (erectile dysfunction), and lost orgiastic control (premature ejaculation). Impotence is the most frequent of these problems.

Erectile dysfunction is said to occur when the failure to complete successful intercourse occurs at least 25 to 30 percent of the time. Most often, it is short term (secondary impotence) and related to individual partners or to temporary damage to male self-esteem. Secondary impotence may also be caused by diseases such as diabetes mellitus, medications such as tranquilizers and amphetamines, alcoholism and other psychoactive drug addictions, and minor genital abnormalities. Aging is not necessarily a cause of impotence, even in octogenarians.

Long-lasting (or primary) impotence that occurs despite corrective medical treatment is generally attributable to severe psychopathology and must be treated by psychotherapy and counseling. Psychogenic impotence is implicated when an erection can be achieved by masturbation. The treatment of impotence caused by organic problems may include testosterone administration, the discontinuation of drug therapy or addictive drugs, or corrective surgery, which may include inflatable penis implants.

Male infertility is a problem found in about a third of all cases in which American couples are unable to have children. The problem is thus estimated to occur in 4 to 5 percent of American men. There are a wide number of causes for male infertility, which is always caused by the failure to deliver adequate numbers of mature sperm into the female reproductive tract as a result of organic problems. Impaired spermatogenesis, a frequent cause of male infertility, may have numerous causes. Examples include severe childhood mumps, brain and/or testicular hormone imbalances, drug abuse, obstruction or anatomic malformation of the seminal tract (especially the seminiferous tubules and epididymis), and a defective prostate gland.

Diagnosis includes careful physical examination by a urologist and evaluation of ejaculated semen to identify the number, activity, and potential for fertilization of its sperm. Blood tests will identify hormone imbalances and other possible causative agents. Many treatments are possible for male infertility, ranging from medications, to corrective surgery, to artificial insemination with sperm collected and frozen until enough are on hand to effect fertilization.

Cancer of the male genital organs may occur in the prostate, urethra, penis, or testis. The most important of these is prostate cancer. Urethral cancer is rare. More common is carcinoma of the penis, which occurs most often in uncircumcised men who practice poor genital hygiene. It is very often located beneath the foreskin and does not spread quickly. Total or partial removal of the penis is often required in advanced cases that have been ignored for long periods. Testicular cancers account for most solid genital malignancies in young men. These cancers appear as painful scrotal masses which increase rapidly in size. Any large, firm mass arising from a testis is suspicious and should be examined immediately by X ray, computed tomography (CT) scan, and tests for various tumor markers seen in the blood. Treatment of these tumors includes surgery, radiation, and chemotherapy. Survival rates vary greatly and depend upon the cancer type. Cancer of the prostate and other male genital organs is not clearly understood and may have hormonal and chemical bases. It is believed that periodic self-examination is the most valuable preventive methodology.

Common disorders of the male genital organs include priapism, hydrocele and spermatocele, testicular torsion, and varicocele. Priapism is persistent, painful erection not accompanied by sexual arousal. It is caused by a poorly understood mechanism and is characterized by both pain and much-thickened blood in the corpora cavernosa. Priapism often occurs after prolonged sexual activity and may accompany prostate problems, genital infections such as syphilis, and addictive drug use. Treatment of priapism includes spinal anesthesia, anticoagulants, and surgery. In the absence of prompt, effective treatment, priapism may end male sexual function permanently.

Hydrocele is a common, noncancerous scrotum lesion most common in men over forty. The problem is caused by fluid accumulation resulting from testis inflammation. Hydrocele is not painful and is removed surgically only if excessive in size. Closely related in appearance is a spermatocele, which contains sperm and occurs adjacent to an epididymis. Both hydroceles and spermatoceles are said to transilluminate: They are both so transparent that a flashlight beam will pass through them. Testicular torsion is a twisting of the vas deferens, which causes pain and swelling; surgery is required to return blood flow to the testis. Varicocele describes varicose veins of the testis, which is common and usually harmless.

Sexually transmitted diseases can also affect the male genitals. These diseases include herpes, gonorrhea, syphilis, chlamydia, and genital warts. For the prevention of sexually transmitted diseases, abstention, the careful choice of sexual partners, and the use of male or female condoms are useful.

PERSPECTIVE AND PROSPECTS

Treatment of the various types of male genital disorders and diseases has evolved greatly. Particularly valuable are the strides made in the treatment of impotence. It has been realized that such sexual dysfunction is often a consequence of organic problems that may be remedied by the cessation of causative medication use or by minor surgery. In addition, the utilization of inflatable penis implants in the cases where insoluble psychogenic or organic problems occur has been a milestone in the treatment of this emotionally devastating male genital problem.

Wide examination of the entire spectrum of male genital problems has led to numerous advantageous treatments and to an understanding that withholding unneeded medical treatments can be beneficial. For example, information regarding spermatoceles, hydroceles, and many related nonacute male genital problems has decreased the incidence of unnecessary male genital surgery, and its related risks, for patients.

Another important concept is that of frequent self-examination of the male genitals. This practice has led to a shortening of the time lag between the appearance of a suspicious mass in the scrotum, testes, or other male sex organ and medical attention from professionals (such as urologists) trained both to evaluate their seriousness and to treat them. Early detection has diminished the severity of many genital cancers and facilitated their treatment. Moreover, several clinical tests for such lesions have become more available and more widely used by the public.

It is hoped that these avenues and others, as well as further advances in both diagnostic techniques and treatment possibilities, will eventually eradicate male genital diseases and disorders. Two areas in need of advancements are priapism and prostate cancer, which is an effective killer.

—*Sanford S. Singer, Ph.D.*

See also Aphrodisiacs; Behçet's disease; Candidiasis; Chlamydia; Circumcision, male; Gonorrhea; Herpes; Hydrocelectomy; Hypospadias repair and urethroplasty; Infertility, male; Men's health; Orchitis; Penile implant surgery; Prostate cancer; Prostate enlargement; Prostate gland; Prostate gland removal; Reproductive system; Sexual dysfunction; Sexuality; Sexually transmitted diseases (STDs); Sterilization; Stones; Syphilis; Testicles, undescended; Testicular cancer; Testicular surgery; Testicular torsion; Urology; Urology, pediatric; Vasectomy; Warts.

FOR FURTHER INFORMATION:

American Psychiatric Association. *Diagnostic and Statistical Manual of Mental Disorders: DSM-IV-TR*. Rev. 4th ed. Washington, D.C.: Author, 2000. This compilation includes diagnostic criteria and other useful facts about mental problems associated with male genital diseases. It thus provides insight into the psychogenic aspects of these afflictions.

Beers, Mark H., et al. *The Merck Manual of Diagnosis and Therapy*. 18th ed. Whitehouse Station, N.J.: Merck Research Laboratories, 2006. This book abounds with useful data on the characteristics, etiology, diagnosis, and treatment of male genital disorders and diseases. Written for physicians, it is also quite useful to general readers.

Ellsworth, Pamela, and Bob Stanley. *One Hundred Questions and Answers About Erectile Dysfunction*. Sudbury, Mass.: Jones and Bartlett, 2002. A patient-oriented guide that covers basic questions about the condition, such as causes, symptoms, and diagnosis; available treatments and how to choose among them; and ways of coping with common emotional and physical difficulties associated with the diagnosis and treatment.

Milsten, Richard, and Julian Slowinski. *The Sexual Male: Problems and Solutions*. New York: W. W. Norton, 2001. Accessible discussion of impotence and its causes, effects, and treatments.

Montague, Drogo K. *Disorders of Male Sexual Function*. Chicago: Year Book Medical, 1988. This medical text is useful to all readers wishing detailed information on aspects of men's health, including male reproductive anatomy and physiology, terminology, clinical evaluation, pharmacology, and the treatment of male sexual diseases.

Parker, James N., and Philip M. Parker, eds. *The Official Patient's Sourcebook on Impotence*. San Diego, Calif.: Icon Health, 2002. Draws from public, academic, government, and peer-reviewed research to provide a wide-ranging handbook for patients with impotence.

_____. *The Official Patient's Sourcebook on Testicular Cancer: A Revised and Updated Directory for the Internet Age*. San Diego, Calif.: Icon Health, 2002. Draws from public, academic, government, and peer-reviewed research to provide a wide-ranging handbook for patients with testicular cancer.

Sherwood, Lauralee. *Human Physiology: From Cells to Systems*. 6th ed. Belmont, Calif.: Thomson/Brooks/Cole, 2007. This college text contains useful information on the male genital system, background endocrinology, spermatogenesis, aspects of sexual dysfunction, and sexually transmitted diseases in men. Also a source of many explanatory illustrations.

Taguchi, Yosh, and Merrily Weisbord, eds. *Private Parts: An Owner's Guide to the Male Anatomy.* 3d ed. Toronto: McClelland & Stewart, 2003. A guide to male genital and sexual health, covering topics such as prostate trouble, erectile dysfunction, infertility, cancer, sexually transmitted diseases, vasectomies, and artificial insemination.

Genomics
Specialty

Anatomy or system affected: All

Specialties and related fields: Bacteriology, biochemistry, biotechnology, cytology, embryology, ethics, genetics, microbiology, pharmacology

Definition: The study of whole genomes; a genome is the complete set of genetic information found in a particular organism.

Key terms:

bioinformatics: a computational discipline that provides the tools needed to study whole genomes and proteomes

DNA microarrays: solid supports which contain many or all genes from a given genome, enabling the expression of these genes to be monitored simultaneously

DNA sequencing: determining the order of deoxyribonucleic acid (DNA) bases in a particular unit of genetic information

orthologues: similar genes from different species that are thought to be related by evolution

proteomics: the study of proteomes; a proteome is the complete set of proteins in a particular cell type

synteny: when whole regions of chromosomes from different species are similar in structure

A New Scientific Discipline

Genomics grew out of the field of genetics, the study of heredity. Until the late twentieth century, it had not been possible to study the complete set of hereditary information in a living organism. So, while the field of genetics traces its roots to the 1860's, when the Austrian monk Gregor Mendel performed experiments on the mechanism of heredity in pea plants, the field of genomics is much younger, dating from the 1980's, when American geneticist Thomas Roderick used this term

to name a new scientific journal that dealt with the analysis of genomic information. In Mendel's time, while organisms were seen to exhibit certain traits, it was not known how these traits were determined. By the early 1900's, it was recognized that traits are inherited in units of information called genes, although the chemical nature of the gene was still unknown. It took until the middle of that century to recognize that genes were made up of deoxyribonucleic acid (DNA), the structure of which was first identified by American biologist James Watson and British biophysicist Francis Crick in 1953.

DNA is made up of four different deoxyribonucleotides, commonly referred to as bases: adenine (A), cytosine (C), guanine (G), and thymine (T). Together, they spell out a chemical code that is used by the cell to make proteins. Since it is the set of proteins contained within a cell that gives that cell its unique properties, determining the order of DNA bases in a given genetic unit will reveal what types of proteins are encoded by this information, a procedure known as DNA sequencing. While a gene has been defined as the amount of DNA needed to encode one protein, a genome is the entire set of genes found in an organism, including any noncoding DNA found between genes. The number of genes that have been found to be present in an organism varies from fewer than two hundred in some obligately parasitic bacteria to about twenty-three thousand (in the simple flowering plant *Arabidopsis*); humans were found to have slightly less than this number.

During the 1980's, a public consortium was formed with the goal of sequencing the human genome by 2005, the International Human Genome Sequencing Consortium. The Human Genome Project, as this effort was called, also had the goal of sequencing the genomes of a number of model organisms that have been used by scientists to help understand biological complexity. These model organisms, which included the *Escherichia coli* bacterium, yeast, *Caenorhabditis elegans* (a roundworm), *Drosophila* (the fruit fly), and mouse, also served as steps by which the efficiency of DNA sequencing could be improved over time. *E. coli*, like most bacteria, has a genome that numbers in the millions of bases—usually abbreviated bp (for base pair), since each base in DNA is paired with its complementary base, A to T and G to C—while yeast has a genome of approximately ten million bp and the next three organisms have genomes that number in the hundreds of millions of bp. Mice, like humans, have genomes that are three billion bp in size. Around the turn

using a scanner and recorded directly into a computer. Some have claimed that Sanger and colleagues were actually the first group to sequence a genome, since they published the sequence of a viral genome in the same year that they described their revolutionary technique. Viruses, however, are not free-living organisms, and their genomes are thousands of times smaller than the typical bacterial genome.

The Human Genome Project was first proposed in 1986 and was funded two years later at an expected cost of three billion dollars. The project officially got underway in 1990 as sequencing began in earnest on some of the smaller model genomes. In 1995, as some of these sequencing efforts were nearing completion, American pharmacologist Craig Venter and his colleagues at a private not-for-profit institute, the Institute for Genome Research, published the genome sequence of the bacterium *Haemophilus influenzae*, the first free-living organism to have its genome sequenced.

While the public consortium had been working on sequences using established techniques, Venter and colleagues had developed a faster technique for determining the sequence of whole genomes. While this technique still used the basic Sanger-style chain termination procedure, it simplified an earlier step in the process in which large numbers of clones of genomic fragments were made before sequencing could begin. Venter had circumvented this cloning step; he called his approach whole-genome shotgun sequencing. During the next two years, the public consortium published the sequences of yeast and *E. coli*, respectively, and in 1998 announced that the sequence of *C. elegans* was complete. That same year, Venter announced that he was starting a for-profit company, Celera Genomics, which would complete the human genome within three years using shotgun sequencing. Up until this time, however, Venter had only demonstrated this approach using bacterial genomes. In order to demonstrate the validity of the shotgun approach on large genomes, and to gear up for sequencing the human genome, Celera sequenced the 170 million bp genome of the fruit fly in 2000, at that time the largest genome ever sequenced.

During the final years of the twentieth century, spurred on by the competition from the private sector, the public consortium had redoubled its efforts on the human genome. In February, 2001, the race to sequence the human genome ended in a tie. Both sequencing efforts, public and private, published their draft sequence of the human genome at this time, and in April, 2003, the two efforts together announced the final completed sequence. The mouse genome sequence was also published in 2003. In fact, by mid-2003, about 150 genomic sequences had been determined (the vast majority of which were bacterial genomes) and almost 600 more were underway, including many more multicellular organisms.

Are the time, effort, and money that have been spent on various genome-sequencing projects really worth it? One promise that genomics may hold for the future is the identification of all human disease genes. While this has been one of the main justifications for the Human Genome Project, one should keep in mind that identifying the gene that causes a particular disease is not always equivalent to finding a cure for that disease. Another potential benefit of genomic research is the development of better treatments for bacterial and parasitic infections. A number of disease-causing bacteria have already been the subject of genome sequencing efforts, including the causative agents of bubonic plague, anthrax, and tuberculosis, to name a few. Some indirect benefits of genomics (which may, in time, prove just as valuable) include a better understanding of evolutionary relationships between species as well as a firmer grasp on basic cellular function. In all, the field of genomics promises to be a powerful means of scientific inquiry well into the future.

—James S. Godde, Ph.D.;
updated by Jeffrey A. Knight, Ph.D.

See also Bioinformatics; Biostatistics; Cloning; DNA and RNA; Gene therapy; Genetic counseling; Genetic diseases; Genetic engineering; Genetics and inheritance; Laboratory tests; Mutation; Screening.

For Further Information:

Brown, Terence A. *Genomes 3*. New York: Garland Science, 2007. A comprehensive and sophisticated study of genomics and all applicable techniques and applications.

Campbell, A. Malcolm, and Laurie J. Heyer. *Discovering Genomics, Proteomics, and Bioinformatics*. 2d ed. San Francisco: Benjamin/Cummings, 2007. An introduction to genomics and the techniques used to study genomic data. Contains many Internet-based exercises in bioinformatics.

Clark, M. S. "Comparative Genomics: The Key to Understanding the Human Genome Project." *BioEssays* 21 (1999): 121-130. An in-depth discussion of comparative genomics and its significance to the field as a whole.

Collins, Francis S., et al. "A Vision for the Future of

Genomics Research." *Nature* 422 (April, 2003): 835-847. Upon the completion of the Human Genome Project, the director of the public consortium and his colleagues wrote this article, which presents a plan for the future of genomics.

DeRisi, Joseph L., and Vishwanath R. Iyer. "Genomics and Array Technology." *Current Opinion in Oncology* 11 (1999): 76-79. A review of how DNA microarrays are used in genomic research.

Klug, William S., and Michael R. Cummings. "Genomics, Bioinformatics, and Proteomics." In *Concepts of Genetics.* 8th ed. Upper Saddle River, N.J.: Prentice Hall, 2007. A chapter that details the differences between genomes among the various model organisms that have been sequenced.

Snustad, D. Peter, and Michael J. Simmons. "Genomics." In *Principles of Genetics.* 4th ed. New York: John Wiley & Sons, 2006. A chapter from a textbook which describes the history of genomics as well as its various permutations.

Wei, Liping, et al. "Comparative Genomics Approaches to Study Organism Similarities and Differences." *Journal of Biomedical Informatics* 35 (2002): 142-150. A review of how comparative genomics has been used in both structural and functional studies.

GERIATRICS AND GERONTOLOGY

SPECIALTIES

ANATOMY OR SYSTEM AFFECTED: All

SPECIALTIES AND RELATED FIELDS: All

DEFINITION: Geriatrics refers to the social and health care of the elderly; gerontology is the study of the aging process.

KEY TERMS:

decubitus ulcer: ulceration of the skin and subcutaneous tissues, resulting from protein deficiency and prolonged, unrelieved pressure on bony prominences

dementia: a deterioration or loss of intellectual faculties, reasoning power, memory, and will that is caused by organic brain disease

glaucoma: an eye disease characterized by increased intraocular pressure, which can lead to degeneration of the optic nerve and ultimately blindness if left untreated

Medicare: the popular designation for 1965 amendments to the U.S. Social Security Act, providing hospitalization and certain other benefits to people over the age of sixty-five

polypharmacy: the prescription of many drugs at one time, often resulting in excessive use of medications and adverse drug interactions

prostate: in men, the organ surrounding the neck of the urinary bladder and beginning of the urethra; its secretions make up about 40 percent of semen

THE STUDY OF AGING

The field of geriatrics deals with the care of the elderly. The U.S. government's definition of elderly includes persons sixty-five years of age or older. Geriatricians are physicians with specialized training in geriatric medicine who restrict their practices to caring for persons seventy-five years of age or older. These patients are most likely to suffer from specific geriatric syndromes, including dementia, delirium, urinary incontinence, malnutrition, osteoporosis, falls and immobility, decubitus ulcers, polypharmacy, and sleep disorders. The majority of older persons in the United States live in family settings with their spouses or children. Approximately 30 percent of older persons live alone, the majority of them being women. According to the U.S. Census Bureau, in 2000 the proportion of older persons (those over sixty-five) who lived in nursing homes was about 4.5 percent. Those aged eighty-five and over had a higher proportion, at 18.2 percent, thus indicating that the number of elderly people residing in nursing homes increases strikingly with age. However, the overall percentage of the elderly living in nursing homes is declining. While one may attribute this change to improvements in health care, it may also be attributable to the use of home health aides who provide assisted living to seniors.

The focus of geriatric medicine is on improving functional disability and treating chronic disease conditions that impair a person's ability to perform such activities of daily living as bathing and dressing, maintaining urinary and bowel continence, and eating. A more objective measure of an older person's ability to live independently is the instrumental activities of daily living scale. This scale measures an individual's ability to use the telephone, obtain transportation, go shopping, prepare meals, do housework and laundry, self-administer medicines, and manage money.

The maximum life span of an organism is the theoretical longest duration of that organism's life, excluding premature, unnatural death. The maximum life span of humans is unknown, although most experts believe it to be approximately 120 years. Most people will die of disease or accident, however, before they reach this biological limit. Attempts to understand why this occurs have led to the development of several theories of aging. The aging process is controlled, in large part, by genetic mechanisms. Aging is a biologic process characterized by a progressive development and maturation leading to senescence and death. There are profound changes in cells, tissues, and organs as well as in physiological, cognitive, and psychological processes. Aging is not the acquisition of disease, although aging and disease can be related. In the absence of disease, normal aging is a slow process. It involves the steady decline of organ reserves and homeostatic control mechanisms, which is often not apparent unless there is maximal exertion or stress on an individual system or on the total organism.

Numerous changes in the body occur as people age. For example, one can expect to lose two inches in height from age forty to age eighty. This shrinkage results from a decrease in vertebral bone mass and in the thickness of intervertebral disks, as well as from postural alterations with increased flexion or bending at the hips and knees. Total body fat increases as one ages, accompanied by decreases in muscle mass and total body water. Such changes in body composition have important implications for drug treatments and nutritional plans. For example, fat-soluble medications exhibit a longer duration of action in the elderly. Older persons also experience a thinning of the dermal layer of the skin, with thinner blood vessels, decreased collagen, and less skin elasticity. Sun damage can accelerate these changes. Graying of the hair reflects a progressive loss of functional melanocytes from the hair bulbs. The number of hair follicles of the scalp decreases, as does the growth rate of remaining follicles. The brain also alters with age: The weight of the brain declines, blood flow to the brain decreases, and there is a loss of neurons in specific areas of the brain. These changes in brain structure are highly variable and do not necessarily affect thinking and behavior.

Many changes occur in the vision of the older person. Loss of elasticity in the lens leads to presbyopia, the most common visual problem associated with aging. Presbyopia is a condition in which the distance that is needed to focus on near objects increases. Cataracts increase in prevalence with age, although unprotected exposure of the eyes to ultraviolet rays has been implicated in the pathogenesis as well. Glaucoma also occurs more often in the elderly.

Older persons often experience hearing loss from degenerative processes, including atrophy of the external auditory canal and thickening of the tympanic membrane. The result is presbycusis, a bilateral hearing loss for pure tones. Higher frequencies are more affected than lower ones, and the condition is more severe in men than in women. Pitch discrimination also declines with age, which may account for an increased difficulty in speech discrimination.

The heart alters with age, although the significance of these changes is unclear in the absence of disease. There are declines in intrinsic contractile function and electrical activity. The resting heart rate and cardiac output do not change, but the maximum heart rate decreases in a linear fashion and may be estimated by subtracting a person's age from 220. There are also modest increases in systolic blood pressure.

Minor changes occur in the gastrointestinal system. The liver and pancreas maintain adequate function throughout life, although the metabolism of specific drugs is prolonged in older people. Kidney function declines with age, with a 30 percent loss in renal mass and a decrease in renal blood flow. A linear decline in the ability of the kidneys to filter blood after the age of forty can lead to a decrease in the clearance of some drugs from the body.

In the endocrine system, the blood glucose level before meals changes minimally after the age of forty, although the level of blood glucose after meals increases. These changes may be related to decreases in muscle mass and a decreased insulin secretion rate. Glucose intolerance with aging must be distinguished from the hyperglycemia that can accompany diabetes mellitus; the latter requires treatment. No clinically significant alterations in the levels of the thyroid hormone occur, although the end organ response to thyroid hormones may be decreased. The hypothalamic-pituitary-adrenal axis remains intact. Plasma basal and stimulated norepinephrine levels are higher in healthy elderly individuals than in the young. The secretion of hormones such as androgens and estrogens falls sharply as a result of the loss of endocrine cells.

DISEASES AFFECTING THE ELDERLY

One of the chronic diseases frequently seen in elderly people is osteoporosis. Osteoporosis is defined as a decreased amount of bone per unit of volume; mineralization of the bone remains normal. Many studies have shown that bone mass decreases with age. Vertebral fractures resulting from osteoporosis cause deformity of the spine, loss in height, and pain. The absolute number of vertebral fractures that occur in older persons has been difficult to estimate, as some of these fractures go undiagnosed. The approximately 300,000 hip fractures that the elderly in the United States suffer annually have much more serious consequences. The lifetime risk of hip fracture by the age of eighty is approximately 15 percent for white women and 7 percent for white men. The risk of hip fracture by this age is significantly less in African Americans, with a 6 percent risk for women and a 3 percent risk for men.

One approach to preventing osteoporosis is to maximize the amount of bone that is formed during adolescence. Under normal circumstances, people begin to experience a net bone loss after the age of thirty-five. In women, the onset of menopause accelerates bone loss because of the decline in estrogen levels. Relative calcium deficiency has also been implicated in age-related osteoporosis. By definition, age-related osteoporosis is a diagnosis of exclusion. An older patient who has suffered a fracture first should be evaluated for other causes of osteoporosis, including hyperparathyroidism, hyperthyroidism, diabetes, glucocorticoid excess, or, in men, hypogonadism. Other secondary causes of osteoporosis include malignancy, such as multiple myeloma, leukemia, or lymphoma, and the drug-related effects of alcohol or steroids. Any identifiable causes should be corrected.

People at increased risk for age-related osteoporosis include those with a family history of the disease; light hair, skin, and eyes; and a small body frame. Bone densitometry or quantitative computed tomography (CT) scanning can be performed to provide the most accurate estimates of the risk of an initial fracture. There are a number of prevention and treatment strategies for patients. One should ensure an adequate calcium intake; the current recommendation is a daily intake of 1,200 milligrams of calcium for postmenopausal women. Weight-bearing exercise should be performed throughout the life span. In postmenopausal women, estrogen treatment is often given. While estrogen has not been shown conclusively to increase bone density, it does prevent further bone loss. In patients who cannot take estrogen, an alternative treatment is the hormone calcitonin. Calcitonin works by inhibiting osteoclast function, thereby halting the otherwise normal breakdown of bone.

A disorder that is commonly seen in elderly men is benign prostatic hyperplasia (BPH), or prostate enlargement. The incidence of this disease increases in a progressive fashion, with approximately 90 percent of men aged eighty affected by this condition. The pathogenesis of BPH is hormonal, caused by increased levels of dihydrotestosterone formed from the testosterone within the gland itself. The usual symptoms are those of urinary obstruction, which include hesitancy, straining, and decreased force and dimension of the urinary stream. Screening for benign prostatic hypertrophy includes two parts. The first is a blood test for prostate-specific antigens. The second is a digital rectal exam to inspect the prostate gland. Patients with positive findings will require further evaluation. A significant increase in prostatic tissue may need to be removed surgically. In patients with minimal disease, drug treatment may be used. Finesteride is an inhibitor of the enzyme 5-alpha reductase that is responsible for the conversion of testosterone to dihydrotestosterone. It slows the rate of increase in prostate tissue mass.

Depression is a common problem in both men and women as they get older. The elderly can experience transient mood changes that are the result of an identifiable stress or loss. In older persons, however, depression may be related to some medical condition, particularly dementia, which is associated with multiple strokes or Parkinson's disease. Major depression is more common in hospital and long-term care settings, where the prevalence is about 13 percent. The symptoms of depression include significant weight change, insomnia or hypersomnia, psychomotor agitation or retardation, decreased energy and easy fatigability, feelings of worthlessness or excessive guilt, decreased ability to think or concentrate, and recurrent thoughts of death or suicide. The diagnosis of major depression can be made if at least five of these symptoms are present for at least two weeks. Depressive symptoms must be taken seriously in the elderly. The rate of suicide in older persons is higher than for other groups, with older white males having the highest rates of any age, racial, or ethnic group.

Another depressive disorder experienced by the elderly is dysthymia. Dysthymic disorders are characterized by less severe symptoms than those associated with major depression and by a duration of at least two years. The symptoms generally include at least two of the following: poor appetite or overeating, insomnia or hypersomnia, low energy and fatigue, low self-esteem, poor concentration or difficulty in making decisions, and feelings of hopelessness. Dysthymia may be primary or secondary to a preexisting chronic psychiatric or medical illness, with accompanying loss of function and debilitation.

Adjustment disorders with depressed mood are also seen in older persons. Such disorders occur within three months of a stressful situation and last up to six months. The prototypical situation is the depressive reaction that follows an acute medical illness. In the elderly, the four most common stressors are physical illness, reactions to the death of family and friends, retirement, and moving to an institutional setting. In dealing with depressive symptoms, however, it is important to consider other diagnoses, such as underlying medical illnesses, drug reactions to prescribed or over-the-counter medicines, hypochondriasis, alcohol abuse, and dementias. In older patients, the disorder most often associated with depression is dementia.

Incontinence affects a vast number of elders yet is often unaddressed during a clinic visit because of either lack of the patient's knowledge about potential treatments or embarrassment regarding the issue. Incontinence has a major impact on an elder's quality of life, and, as it is often a treatable condition, it should be discussed by patients with their physicians.

Another topic frequently not discussed involves the issue of remaining sexually active as an elder. Over half of married elders continue to have sex, although sometimes this activity is complicated by fears such as having a heart attack or stroke as a result of the exertion. In addition, medical problems and medication side effects can affect the elder's sexual abilities. Some potential treatments for sexual dysfunction include phosphodiesterase inhibitors and, in the case of low testosterone or low estrogen, hormone replacement therapies, which can aid in increasing the sexual satisfaction of elders.

A thorough diagnostic evaluation can help in the diagnosis of a depressive disorder and can rule out other complicating problems. A careful history is elicited from the patient and from a family member or caretaker. A formal mental status examination is conducted to uncover abnormalities in concentration, speech, psychomotor skills, cognitive ability, and memory. Laboratory blood tests often include a complete blood count, chemical analysis, and thyroid function tests. Abbreviated neuropsychological tests can differentiate between patients with dementia and those with depression alone. The treatment of depression includes psychotherapy and pharmacotherapy. Behavioral interventions, such as special weekly activities and assignments, can be helpful. Most often, some kind of antidepressant medication is effective.

PERSPECTIVE AND PROSPECTS

In the United States, there has been increasing interest in the fields of geriatrics and gerontology because of the country's changing demographics. In 2000, 35 million Americans were sixty-five years of age or older. Because of the very large numbers in the baby-boom age group—that is, people born between 1946 and 1964—it was expected that the number of elderly people would increase dramatically by the year 2030 to 71.5 million, more than doubling the amount of elderly people in 2000. By 2050, it is expected that this number will reach 86.7 million. Those individuals aged sixty-five and over made up approximately 12.5 percent of the U.S. population in 2000. In 2030, this percentage could increase to an incredible 19.5 percent.

Another reason for the increase in the size of the older population in the United States is an increase in life expectancy. Life expectancy is defined as the average number of years a person is expected to live, given population mortality rates. It can be calculated for any age category but is usually given as life expectancy from birth. The life expectancy in the United States is much higher than in undeveloped countries and in most other developed countries as well. This figure rose steadily throughout the twentieth century. A child born in 2000 could expect to live seventy-five years, while someone born in 1900 could expect to live only fifty years. Most of this increase in life expectancy is attributable to a decreased death rate for infants and children resulting from improvements in sanitation, active immunization against childhood diseases, and advances in medical treatments. For persons aged sixty-five, there was an increase in life expectancy over that same time period of only five years, probably the result of improved medical therapies. While the geriatric population is dramatically increasing, the availability of geriatricians is not. As the population continues to grow, the shortage will increase.

Making healthy lifestyle modifications, receiving appropriate medical screening exams, and partaking in numerous prevention strategies may improve the quality of life of the elderly. These actions may also lead to preventing serious accidents and disabling conditions. Lifestyle modifications that should be attempted include alcohol and smoking cessation, as well as diet and exercise programs. With the increasing awareness of obesity as a major problem in society, it is important to keep the geriatric population at a healthy weight that will not lead to adverse health effects.

With the decline in vision and hearing that may be

experienced by the older population, audio/visual screening should be performed and proper corrective measures taken. This may help avoid accidents around the home and while driving. Vaccinations should be up to date to help prevent disease. Unless contraindicated, the elderly should consider obtaining the annual flu vaccine. The pneumococcal vaccine should also be considered. In addition, screening tests are available to assess some of the common conditions affecting the elderly. Those preventive services covered by Medicare as of 2006 include a "Welcome to Medicare Physical Exam" once during the first six months of enrollment, serum cholesterol levels every five years, annual mammograms in women aged forty and over, biannual Pap smears and pelvic exams, fecal occult blood tests starting at age fifty and then annually, a flexible sigmoidoscopy at age fifty and then every four years, a colonoscopy at age fifty and then every ten years, serum prostate specific antigen levels and digital rectal exams starting at age fifty and then annually, glaucoma screening if over fifty and then annually, and bone densitometry testing in women over fifty or at high risk and then biannually. Medicare will also cover the following vaccines: pneumococcal one time, hepatitis B vaccine series one time, and influenza vaccines annually.

Because elders may be taking multiple medications, it is important that they occasionally review these medications with their doctors. By doing so, side effects can be discussed and any drug interactions may be avoided. All dosages and correct use should be reviewed to make sure that the appropriate medications are taken daily and that accidental overdose may be avoided. Pillboxes are an excellent tool to make sure that medications are taken correctly. In addition, it is advisable that elders keep a list of all medications and allergies on their person should an emergency arise.

With the popularity of herbal supplements, it is essential that the elderly discuss their use with a physician. Some of these regimens may have adverse effects of which patients are unaware. In addition, herbal supplements may interact with some of the medications that their physicians have prescribed.

As Americans live longer, the length of time that older persons will rely on society for their care increases as well. This situation places a greater burden on those persons who are working, as they must support greater numbers of people receiving Social Security and Medicare benefits, and requires a rethinking of the age requirements to be eligible for these programs. In

1997, while older persons represented 13 percent of the population, they accounted for 38 percent of the total costs for health care. Other factors adding to the cost of health care include such new technologies as specialized imaging equipment, complex laboratory procedures, and new therapeutic drugs. The goal of much research in geriatric medicine is to prevent or slow down the effects of aging so that the elderly may live in good health. Further research to understand better the mechanisms involved in human aging will help to design preventive and treatment strategies.

—RoseMarie Pasmantier, M.D.;
L. Fleming Fallon, Jr., M.D., Ph.D., M.P.H.;
updated by Kenneth Dill, M.D.,
and Elaine M. Schaefer, D.O.

See also Aging; Aging: Extended care; Alzheimer's disease; Appetite loss; Arthritis; Bed-wetting; Blindness; Bone disorders; Brain disorders; Cardiac arrest; Cataract surgery; Cataracts; Critical care; Deafness; Death and dying; Dementias; Depression; Domestic violence; Emergency medicine; Endocrinology; Euthanasia; Family medicine; Fatigue; Hearing loss; Hip fracture repair; Hormone replacement therapy (HRT); Hospitals; Incontinence; Memory loss; Nursing; Nutrition; Ophthalmology; Orthopedics; Osteoporosis; Pain management; Paramedics; Parkinson's disease; Pharmacology; Physician assistants; Pick's disease; Polypharmacy; Prostate enlargement; Psychiatry; Psychiatry, geriatric; Rheumatology; Sleep; Sleep disorders; Spinal cord disorders; Spine, vertebrae, and disks; Suicide; Vision disorders.

FOR FURTHER INFORMATION:

Beerman, Susan, and Judith Rappaport-Musson. *Eldercare 911: The Caregiver's Complete Handbook for Making Decisions.* Amherst, N.Y.: Prometheus Books, 2002. A practical guide for elder care. Includes topics such as locating services, managing medications, understanding benefits, choosing a nursing home, coping with memory loss, hiring and handling in-home help, helping a parent who refuses help, and recognizing signs of elder abuse.

Beers, Mark H., and Robert Berkow, eds. *The Merck Manual of Geriatrics.* 3d ed. Whitehouse Station, N.J.: Merck Research Laboratories, 2000. Addresses the challenges of geriatric care. Provides diagnosis and treatment information specific to aging patients.

Birren, James E., and K. Warner Schaie, eds. *Handbook of the Psychology of Aging.* 6th ed. Boston: Elsevier Academic Press, 2006. Twenty-four contributions from international researchers explore topics such as the genetics of behavioral aging, environmental influences on aging, gender roles, mental health, declining motor control, wisdom, and technological change and the older worker.

Centers for Disease Control and Prevention. Injury Center. http://www.cdc.gov/ncipc/. This site includes a suggestion of fall precautions that can be implemented by the elderly population to help reduce the risk of fracture.

Coni, Nicholas, et al. *Lecture Notes on Geriatrics*. 6th ed. Malden, Mass.: Blackwell Science, 2003. Easy-to-read study notes on geriatric medicine. Discusses the different changes that occur in the patient during the aging process and characterizes the different diseases seen in the elderly.

Ferri, Fred F., Marsha Fretwell, and Tom J. Wachtel. *Practical Guide to the Care of the Geriatric Patient*. 2d ed. St. Louis: Mosby Year Book, 1997. An excellent resource. The text is clearly written, and the index is especially useful. Nonprofessional readers will have no trouble understanding this book.

Hampton, Roy, and Charles Russell. *The Encyclopedia of Aging and the Elderly*. New York: Facts On File, 1992. Much well-stated information is presented. The scope is broad—lifestyle, myths and misconceptions, medical and legal concerns, death and dying. Statistical information is presented in charts and tables, appendices list organizations, and the bibliography is useful.

He, Wan, et al. *65+ in the United States: 2005*. Washington, D.C.: U.S. Government Printing Office, 2005. A special report that is also available at http://www.census.gov/prod/2006pubs/p23-209.pdf.

Hooyman, Nancy, and H. Asuman Kayak. *Social Gerontology: A Multidisciplinary Perspective*. 7th ed. Boston: Allyn and Bacon, 2005. Contributions from social workers, psychologists, gerontology professionals, and professors examine the ways in which age-related changes in the biological, functional, and psychological domains can influence the older person's interactions with his/her social and physical environment.

Hoyer, William, and Paul A. Roodin. *Adult Development and Aging*. 5th ed. Boston: McGraw-Hill, 2003. An interdisciplinary exploration of the biological, social, and cultural contexts in which change occurs during the adult years.

Isaacs, Bernard. *The Challenge of Geriatric Medicine*. London: Oxford Medical, 1992. This volume presents the issues associated with geriatric medicine and the care of older citizens. It is well written and should be of interest to most readers who want additional information on this subject.

Margolis, Simeon, and Hamilton Moses III, eds. *The Johns Hopkins Medical Handbook: The One Hundred Major Medical Disorders of People over the Age of Fifty*. Rev. ed. Garden City, N.Y.: Random House, 1999. This definitive home medical reference for adults offers an in-depth guide to the most common medical problems occurring in adults over fifty. The directory of hospitals and other health care resources, from support groups to treatment centers, is comprehensive.

Masoro, Edward J., and Steven N. Austad, eds. *Handbook of the Biology of Aging*. 6th ed. Boston: Elsevier Academic Press, 2006. Part of a three-volume series that includes the biological, psychological, and social aspects of aging. Focuses on research approaches to understanding aging, including genetic studies, cellular and molecular biology, neurobiology, and nutrition.

Stenchever, Morton A. *Health Care for the Older Woman*. New York: Chapman and Hall, 1996. A reference that provides medical practitioners and students with comprehensive, current information specific to the care of middle-aged and advanced-aged women. It covers health maintenance issues, including diet, exercise, safety, psychological and psychosocial problems, social problems, and grief and loss.

GERMAN MEASLES. *See* CHILDHOOD INFECTIOUS DISEASES; RUBELLA.

GESTATION. *See* PREGNANCY AND GESTATION.

GESTATIONAL DIABETES
DISEASE/DISORDER

ANATOMY OR SYSTEM AFFECTED: Endocrine system, reproductive system

SPECIALTIES AND RELATED FIELDS: Endocrinology, nutrition, obstetrics

DEFINITION: A medical condition in which diabetes, or unregulated blood glucose, first occurs during pregnancy.

KEY TERMS:

diabetes: a group of disorders characterized by hyperglycemia caused by a lack of insulin secretion or ineffective insulin action

hyperglycemia: high blood glucose

insulin: a hormone secreted by the pancreas whose primary function is to maintain blood glucose levels within a normal range

CAUSES AND SYMPTOMS

Gestational diabetes is the medical term describing a type of diabetes mellitus that is first diagnosed during a woman's pregnancy. Diabetes is a condition where blood glucose is not kept within a normal range. Normally, insulin is a key regulator of blood glucose. In diabetes, insulin may be absent, be present in insufficient amounts, or be ineffective. Gestational diabetes occurs in about 4 percent of all pregnancies in the United States. There is variance in incidence rates as a result of ethnicity, age, and genetic predisposition. Hispanic and African American women have a higher incidence than do Asian and Caucasian women, and older women have a higher incidence than do those who are younger. In general, women with a family history of diabetes are more likely to develop gestational diabetes.

Gestational diabetes normally develops midway through pregnancy. Testing is typically scheduled for between twenty-four and twenty-eight weeks into the pregnancy. A two-step approach is used to screen women who are not at high risk for diabetes. The first step is the 50-gram oral glucose tolerance test. For this test, the woman is given 50 grams of glucose in solution after having fasted overnight. Her blood glucose is tested one hour after drinking the solution. If her blood glucose is above a normal range, the next step is a 100-gram three-hour oral glucose tolerance test. Normally, a person's insulin would react to the ingested glucose to keep the blood glucose within a normal range. If that does not occur, and blood glucose remains high, then a diagnosis of gestational diabetes is made. Additionally, even when a diagnosis of gestational diabetes is not made during the pregnancy, when a baby is born weighing over 10 pounds, a diagnosis of gestational diabetes is made de facto.

As maternal blood glucose rises, so does the risk of fetal complications. The most common complication is fetal macrosomia, or having a birth weight greater than or equal to 4,500 grams. Fetal macrosomia is associated with an increased risk of birth trauma, especially to the head, shoulders, and throat area. Infants born this large often require a cesarean section, which itself has greater health risks than a vaginal birth. Additionally, higher maternal glucose levels lead to poorer placental functioning at an earlier point in pregnancy. While the

> ## INFORMATION ON GESTATIONAL DIABETES
>
> **CAUSES:** Unknown; risk increases with family history of diabetes
> **SYMPTOMS:** Often none for mother; excessive fetal size; hypoglycemia, heart and lung problems, sometimes coma or death in newborn
> **DURATION:** Gestational period and shortly after birth
> **TREATMENTS:** Diet restriction in mother to achieve stable blood glucose levels, insulin use if necessary

placenta is designed to work as a filtering mechanism for between thirty-eight and forty-two weeks, in gestational diabetics it often begins to malfunction by thirty-seven weeks. Therefore, infants of diabetic mothers (IDMs) are delivered early (at thirty-seven weeks) in order to avoid placental malfunction.

When maternal blood glucose levels are elevated above normal, the fetus is stimulated to increase production of insulin. Although this manages the problem of the increased blood glucose for the fetus, it also has negative consequences. If the mother's blood glucose has been elevated just preceding delivery, then the infant's insulin level will be elevated. After delivery, the infant's insulin level may remain elevated, although there is no longer a need for it. This can lead to hypoglycemia, or low blood glucose. Continued hypoglycemia can lead to coma or death for the newborn. In addition, high insulin levels and poor control of the mother's blood glucose is associated with problems with the infant's heart and lung function.

TREATMENT AND THERAPY

Diet is the primary treatment for gestational diabetes. Depending on the meal planning approach, a certain number of calories and/or a certain amount of carbohydrates is prescribed. The total carbohydrates to be eaten is about 40 to 45 percent of total daily calories. Calories should be prescribed to allow for recommended weight gain during pregnancy and to prevent blood glucose from being either too high or too low. If caloric intake is too high, then the blood glucose level will rise, which is detrimental to the fetus. If caloric intake is too low, then the body will break down the mother's body fat or protein reserves to supply the needed energy. When this occurs, breakdown products called ketones are produced. Ketones in the mother's blood are also detrimental to the fetus.

Consistency, in the form of eating the same amount of food at the same time each day, is important. This is most likely to occur if the individal eats small, frequent meals throughout the day. The diet must support three outcomes: blood glucose levels within a target range, adequate nutrient intake to support the pregnancy, and appropriate weight gain for pregnancy. If these three outcomes cannot be achieved by diet alone, then insulin will be used to achieve the desired blood glucose level. Oral hypoglycemic medications have not been tested for use in pregnancy and are not recommended.

Because achieving a normal or near-normal blood glucose level is so critical, the woman will monitor her blood glucose at home using a fingerstick blood sample and a home glucometer. Blood glucose levels are usually tested three to four times a day, although some women will need to test their blood glucose six times each day. Decisions about adjustments in diet and insulin will be based on blood glucose levels.

Usually blood glucose levels normalize postpartum, and continued diet or medication therapy is not needed. However, women who develop gestational diabetes have a higher likelihood of developing Type II diabetes mellitus later in life. For women who have developed gestational diabetes, an oral glucose tolerance test is administered six to eight weeks postpartum and then at three-year intervals. These women should maintain an optimal weight, since obesity is strongly associated with Type II diabetes onset.

PERSPECTIVE AND PROSPECTS

Observations in the 1950's and 1960's that infants born to mothers who had an elevated blood glucose level had a higher rate of morbidity and mortality led to the screening, diagnosis, and treatment guidelines used today. Adherence to these guidelines has greatly improved the health of infants born to mothers with gestational diabetes. However, these infants do have a greater risk of becoming obese and/or developing diabetes in adolescence. Additionally, daughters of mothers who have had gestational diabetes have a greater likelihood of developing gestational diabetes themselves.

—*Karen Chapman-Novakofski, R.D., L.D., Ph.D.;*
updated by Robin Kamienny Montvilo, Ph.D.
See also Cesarean section; Childbirth; Childbirth complications; Diabetes mellitus; Endocrine disorders;

Endocrinology; Endocrinology, pediatric; Hormones; Hypoglycemia; Insulin resistance syndrome; Neonatology; Obesity; Perinatology; Pregnancy and gestation; Women's health.

FOR FURTHER INFORMATION:

American Diabetes Association. *Gestational Diabetes: What to Expect.* 5th ed. Alexandria, Va.: Author, 2005.

Jovanovic-Peterson, Lois. *Managing Your Gestational Diabetes: A Guide for You and Your Baby's Good Health.* New York: John Wiley & Sons, 1998.

Nicholson, W. K., et al. "Maternal Race, Procedures, and Infant Birth Weight in Type 2 and Gestational Diabetes." *Obstetrics and Gynecology* 108, no. 3 (2006): 626-634.

Ross, Tami, Jackie Boucher, and Belinda O'Connell, eds. *American Dietetic Association Guide to Diabetes Medical Nutrition Therapy and Education.* Chicago: American Dietetic Association, 2005.

GIARDIASIS

DISEASE/DISORDER

ANATOMY OR SYSTEM AFFECTED: Gastrointestinal system

SPECIALTIES AND RELATED FIELDS: Family medicine, gastroenterology, pediatrics

DEFINITION: An acute or chronic parasitic infection of the gastrointestinal system.

CAUSES AND SYMPTOMS

The parasite *Giardia lamblia*, which causes giardiasis, is a protozoan acquired through the ingestion of contaminated food or water. This organism can also be spread by person-to-person contact involving fecal contamination. It is the most frequent parasite acquired by children in day care centers and preschools.

After exposure, the incubation period before the onset of symptoms is one to two weeks. After infection, only 25 to 50 percent of affected individuals become symptomatic. The disease is characterized by abdominal pain, cramps, flatulence, weight loss, and diarrhea, which in many cases may be chronic (of a duration longer than fifteen days).

TREATMENT AND THERAPY

Some cases of giardiasis are self-limited. Symptomatic cases, however, in which the diagnosis has been confirmed by laboratory studies, need to be treated. Fura-

INFORMATION ON GIARDIASIS

CAUSES: Parasitic infection
SYMPTOMS: Often asymptomatic; can include abdominal pain, cramps, flatulence, weight loss, diarrhea
DURATION: One to two weeks; occasionally chronic
TREATMENTS: Medication (furazolidone, metronidazole, paromomycin)

zolidone, metronidazole, and paromomycin are effective drugs in the treatment of giardiasis. Furazolidone and metronidazole are equally efficacious; the first may be more practical in children because of its availability in liquid form.

Giardiasis can be prevented by strict hand-washing, especially in those individuals who are in close contact with patients with diarrhea or children in diapers at day care centers. Another important consideration in the prevention of giardiasis resides in the purification of drinking water, which can be achieved through boiling or chemical decontamination. It has been demonstrated that breast-feeding protects infants against symptomatic infection.

PERSPECTIVE AND PROSPECTS

G. lamblia was first observed by microscopist Antoni van Leeuwenhoek in 1675. It was once considered a harmless organism, but its pathogenic role was clearly established in the 1960's. This parasite is one of the most common protozoans able to infect humans in the United States and other developed countries.

—*Benjamin Estrada, M.D.*

See also Diarrhea and dysentery; Food poisoning; Gastroenterology; Gastroenterology, pediatric; Gastrointestinal system; Parasitic diseases; Protozoan diseases.

FOR FURTHER INFORMATION:

Berger, Stephen A., and John S. Marr. *Human Parasitic Diseases Sourcebook*. Sudbury, Mass.: Jones and Bartlett, 2006.

Biddle, Wayne. *A Field Guide to Germs*. 2d ed. New York: Anchor Books, 2002.

Despommier, Dickson D., et al. *Parasitic Diseases*. 5th ed. New York: Apple Tree Productions, 2005.

Kreier, Julius P., ed. *Parasitic Protozoa*. Vol. 10. 2d ed. San Diego, Calif.: Academic Press, 1995.

Roberts, Larry S., and John Janovy, Jr., eds. *Gerald D. Schmidt and Larry S. Roberts' Foundations of Parasitology*. 7th ed. Boston: McGraw-Hill Higher Education, 2005.

GIGANTISM

DISEASE/DISORDER

ALSO KNOWN AS: Acromegaly

ANATOMY OR SYSTEM AFFECTED: Arms, bones, brain, circulatory system, endocrine system, eyes, hands, hair, legs, musculoskeletal system, reproductive system

SPECIALTIES AND RELATED FIELDS: Biochemistry, cardiology, endocrinology, family medicine, general surgery, internal medicine, neurology

DEFINITION: A rare congenital disease that begins in children with pituitary gland tumors that make too much growth hormone, which yields pituitary giants who often die at relatively young ages. After adolescence, the disease is manifested as acromegaly, which is quite serious over the long term.

KEY TERMS:

acromegaly: a disease of adults initially characterized by pathological enlargement of bones of the hands, feet, and face; caused by chronic pituitary gland overproduction of growth hormone by tumors

congenital: referring to a condition (such as a health problem) present or occurring at birth

growth hormone: a hormone produced by the pituitary gland that mediates overall growth

pituitary gland: a peanut-sized gland at the base of the vertebrate brain; its hormone secretions control many other hormone-producing (endocrine) glands and hence control growth, gender maturation, and many other life processes

CAUSES AND SYMPTOMS

Gigantism is a rare disease caused by the presence of tumors of the peanut-sized pituitary gland, located at the base of the brain. Such tumors produce an excess of growth hormone, the biomolecule responsible for overall growth. In children or adolescents having these tumors, excess growth hormone results in overgrowth of all parts of the body. Gigantism occurs because the bones of the arms and legs have not yet calcified and can grow much longer than usual. Hence, an afflicted child becomes very large in size and very tall, often reaching a height of more than 6 feet, 6 inches.

A young child afflicted with pituitary gigantism grows in height as much as 6 inches per year. Thus, an important symptom that identifies the problem is that such children are much taller and larger than others of the same age. In many cases, this great size difference may lead to individuals who are more than twice the height of their playmates. Excessive growth of this sort should lead parents to seek the immediate advice of their family physician, who can aid in the selection of a specialist to identify the problem and develop an appropriate treatment.

As gigantism proceeds, pituitary tumors often invade and replace the rest of the pituitary gland. This is unfortunate, because the pituitary gland produces several other hormones—called trophic hormones—which control mental processes, gender maturation, and healthy overall growth. Consequently, prolonged, untreated gigantism may yield a huge individual who is mentally ill, possessed of various psychoses, sexually immature, and quite unhealthy. In addition, the human musculoskeletal system is not designed to accommodate individuals attaining the great heights of many postadolescent pituitary giants. Hence, it is fairly common that the giants have great difficulty standing and walking; some can do so only with the aid of canes. Moreover, the average life expectancy of a full-sized pituitary giant is shorter than that of individuals of normal stature, and many die by the middle of the third decade of their lives.

In cases where pituitary tumors that oversecrete growth hormone occur after calcification of the long bones is complete—after adolescence—gigantism will not occur. Such individuals develop acromegaly. This often-fatal disease, progressive throughout life, thickens bones and causes the overgrowth of all body organs. Hands and feet grow larger, and the lower jaw, brow ridges, nose, and ears enlarge, coarsening the features. More damaging is the development of head-

aches, high blood pressure that can lead to heart attacks, irritability, and even cancer over the long run. It should be noted that these disabilities are rarely seen in pediatric patients and most often begin in the fourth decade of life. Many medical scientists believe that pituitary gigantism and acromegaly are the basis for the legends about giants and ogres.

TREATMENT AND THERAPY

If a diagnosis of gigantism or acromegaly seems probable, the physician or specialist involved will order a blood test to identify the amount of growth hormone present in the body. Computed tomography (CT) and magnetic resonance imaging (MRI) scans will also be carried out, especially in those suspected of having acromegaly, to identify possible organ changes away from normal size. In cases where growth hormone levels are high and cannot be reduced by chemotherapy—for example, with antigrowth hormone drugs such as somatostatin and bromocriptine—and/or a tumor is identified as being present via CT and MRI, surgery or radiation therapy to destroy the tumor will be attempted.

PERSPECTIVE AND PROSPECTS

It must be recognized that the success of any therapeutic regimens or their combination will prevent additional gigantism or symptoms of acromegaly from occurring. It is not possible, however, to reverse preexisting consequences of the pituitary tumors on young children and adolescent pituitary giants or older giants and acromegalics.

For this reason, it is essential for worried parents or adult patients to visit an appropriate physician as quickly as possible. Such foresight will usually minimize problems associated with either manifestation of pituitary tumors and enable an afflicted individual to have the best possible future life. In addition to extirpating causative tumors, it will then become possible, after additional blood tests plus the thorough examination of CT and MRI data, to identify which body organs need to be treated and to arrest or minimize health complications, such as those associated with the reproductive, cardiovascular, and musculoskeletal systems.

—Sanford S. Singer, Ph.D.

See also Birth defects; Bones and the skeleton; Congenital heart disease; Dwarfism; Endocrine disorders; Endocrine system; Endocrinology; Endocrinology, pediatric; Growth; Hormones; Orthopedics, pediatric.

INFORMATION ON GIGANTISM

CAUSES: Congenital endocrine disorder resulting in pituitary gland tumors

SYMPTOMS: Enlargement of bones of hands, feet, and face; excessive growth and height; sometimes mental illness; sexual immaturity; difficulty walking and standing

DURATION: Lifelong

TREATMENTS: Chemotherapy, antigrowth hormone drugs, surgery, radiation therapy

FOR FURTHER INFORMATION:

Bar, Robert S., ed. *Early Diagnosis and Treatment of Endocrine Disorders*. Totowa, N.J.: Humana Press, 2003. Reviews the early signs and symptoms of endocrine diseases, surveys the clinical testing needed for a diagnosis, and presents recommendations for therapy.

Beers, Mark H., et al. *The Merck Manual of Diagnosis and Therapy*. 18th ed. Whitehouse Station, N.J.: Merck Research Laboratories, 2006. This book abounds with useful data on the characteristics, etiology, diagnosis, and treatment of gigantism. Written for physicians, it is also quite useful to general readers.

Griffin, James E., and Sergio R. Ojeda, eds. *Textbook of Endocrine Physiology*. 5th ed. New York: Oxford University Press, 2004. A detailed account of normal and abnormal functioning of the endocrine system. Written by specialists.

Henry, Helen L., and Anthony W. Norman, eds. *Encyclopedia of Hormones*. 3 vols. San Diego, Calif.: Academic Press, 2003. A comprehensive overview of the role of hormones, the major physiological systems in which they operate, and the biological consequences of an excess or deficiency of a particular hormone.

Imura, Hiroo, ed. *The Pituitary Gland*. 2d ed. New York: Raven Press, 1994. Discusses such topics as the physiology of the pituitary gland, pituitary hormones, the hypothalamo-hypophyseal system, and the diagnosis of pituitary diseases.

Landau, Elaine. *Standing Tall: Unusually Tall People*. New York: Franklin Watts, 1997. This respectful treatment of a sensitive subject opens with actual, personal stories. It explores the role of unusually sized characters in folklore, then explains the causes and challenges of uncommon growth patterns.

Melmed, Schlomo, ed. *The Pituitary*. 2d ed. Boston: Blackwell Science, 2002. Text covering the biochemistry, molecular biology, physiology, pathophysiology, and clinical aspects of the pituitary. Sections include hypothalamic-pituitary function, hypothalamic-pituitary dysfunction, pituitary tumors, pituitary disease in systemic disorders, and diagnostic procedures.

GINGIVITIS

DISEASE/DISORDER

ANATOMY OR SYSTEM AFFECTED: Gums, mouth, teeth

SPECIALTIES AND RELATED FIELDS: Bacteriology, biochemistry, dentistry

DEFINITION: A gum disease that begins when plaque and calculus cause gum inflammation and bleeding. It can lead to periodontitis, which is associated with tooth loss, cardiovascular disease, and diabetes.

KEY TERMS:

collagen: a fibrous protein of bone, cartilage, and connective tissue

epithelium: a tissue made of closely arranged cells that covers most internal surfaces and organs

gingiva: tissue surrounding the teeth

periodontitis: gum disease that causes bone and tooth loss

CAUSES AND SYMPTOMS

Healthy pink gingiva (gums) end at tooth bases in epithelium-covered connective tissue, detached from teeth for 0.15 to 0.30 millimeter. This free gingiva is demarcated from the next gum portion, attached gingiva, by a gingival groove. The space between free gingiva and a tooth is the gingival sulcus. Attached gingiva is bound to the bone that it covers and is 3 to 6 millimeters deep. Free gingiva between teeth, interdental papillae, extend upward in the front of teeth and make the gums look scalloped. All gingival epithelium covers connective tissue holding collagen fibers. Gingival sulcus epithelium holds oral crevicular and junctional epithelium (JE). JE forms a tooth collar, joined to tooth surfaces. Each collar girdles the neck of a tooth and prevents marginal gingivitis and periodontitis.

Gingivitis begins when plaque and calculus irritate free gingiva, causing inflammation and bleeding. Unchecked, it leads to the more serious periodontitis, re-

---

INFORMATION ON GINGIVITIS

CAUSES: Irritation of the gums by dental plaque and tartar; sometimes occurs with colds and influenza or with hormonal changes

SYMPTOMS: Inflammation and bleeding of gums, which become red or reddish-purple

DURATION: Chronic; sometimes acute

TREATMENTS: Removal of plaque and tartar

sulting in tooth loss, cardiovascular disease, and diabetes. Plaque starts as aggregates of bacteria and their capsules on tooth surfaces. It forms in a protein film deposited on the surfaces and thickens as bacteria become established in a growing matrix of protein and capsule polysaccharide, extending into attached gingiva. Plaque and bacterial toxins damage tissue, producing gingivitis by irritating free gingiva, loosening collars around teeth, and causing the detachment of attached gingiva. Plaque is best identified via disclosing solutions of dyes (such as erythrosin). Many view it as the main factor in initial gingival inflammation. Plaque calcification produces calculus, which is most problematic when it causes irritation if gingiva push up against it.

Acute gingivitis of several types is short term and of minor interest. Nonspecific acute gingivitis occurs with colds and influenza. It causes diffuse redness, swelling, and discomfort but resolves quickly upon recovery. Localized acute gingivitis arises from gingival trauma (such as hard food). Removing its causes promotes rapid healing. Ulcerative acute gingivitis, called trench mouth, occurs widely, mostly in the teens or twenties. Patients report soreness, eating difficulty, facile gum bleeds, and headache. It also occurs in heavy smokers as a result of chemical and thermal irritation.

Chronic marginal gingivitis, which accounts for most cases, begins with the reddening and swelling of interdental papilla and/or the gingival margin. Attempts to explore a sulcus cause bleeding. Enlargement, as a result of edema or hyperplasia, may be extensive and followed, after years of disease, by chronic periodontitis where supporting bone is lost. The initial symptoms of chronic marginal gingivitis reported most often are gingival bleeding, either spontaneous or caused by brushing or chewing; gingival margin recession; gums coming away from teeth; gingival enlargement; and color change to red or reddish-purple.

Three types of chronic marginal gingivitis are associated with sex hormones in people who do not practice good oral hygiene: chronic marginal gingivitis of puberty, pregnancy, and menopause. In the puberty type, the hormone changes come with approaching adult-

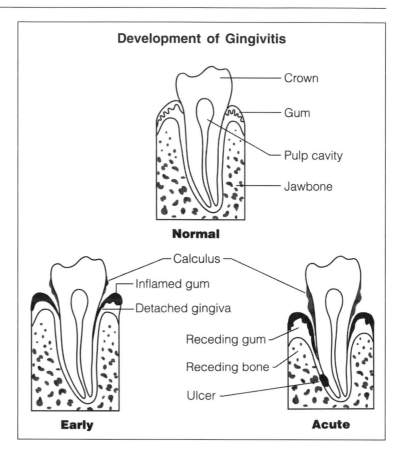

Development of Gingivitis

Crown
Gum
Pulp cavity
Jawbone

Normal

Calculus
Inflamed gum
Detached gingiva
Receding gum
Receding bone
Ulcer

Early   **Acute**

hood are causative. Puberty gingivitis is often accompanied by hyperplasia of interdental papillae. Pregnancy gingivitis occurs in women whose chronic marginal gingivitis worsens after the first trimester. The culprits here, changed blood-vessel permeability and increased inflammation, are the result of hormone changes. The condition produces severe inflammation, marked edema, gingival enlargement, and loose teeth. With good oral hygiene, these problems disappear by the third trimester or birth. Menopausal chronic marginal gingivitis, which can occur at and after the menopause, causes blotchy, reddened attached gingiva, starting as blisters. It may be immunological, the result of patients developing antibodies to their own epithelia.

Treatment and Therapy

Trench mouth is treated with bacteria-killing penicillin or peroxide. The key to treating chronic marginal gingivitis begins by determining gum health from gingival sulcus depth. To obtain this measurement, a metal probe is inserted into the gingiva at several mouth sites until slight resistance is felt. Sulcus depths under 0.30 millimeter indicate healthy gums. Greater depths indicate chronic marginal gingivitis. The deeper the sulcus, the more serious is the gingivitis. The first gingivitis-related dental visit begins with sulcus examination.

When chronic marginal gingivitis is apparent, most plaque and calculus is removed, and the patient is quizzed on oral hygiene habits. The information gained is used to plan several more visits to prove that the patient practices good oral hygiene and to remove any remaining plaque and calculus. The larger and deeper the deposits and the longer exposure to poor hygiene, the more visits are required.

Most chronic marginal gingivitis disappears after dental cleaning and ensuing good oral hygiene. Calculus and plaque removal eliminates the source of irritation and causes healing. Gums become healthy in a few weeks. Mild periodontitis requires more extensive treatment: Bacterial pockets are cleaned out, and antiseptic mouthwash or toothpaste is prescribed. Severe periodontitis may require surgery.

PERSPECTIVE AND PROSPECTS

The best current way to treat gingivitis is preventing it via good oral hygiene, which consists of regular brushing and periodic dental cleaning to prevent plaque and calculus buildup. It is best to brush all teeth and gums with a soft-bristled brush and fluoride toothpaste. Brushing should be done at least twice daily, in the morning and at bedtime. Daily flossing is also recommended. Floss is used to scrape the underside of each tooth, just below the gum line, to remove interdental plaque and to massage the gums. In addition to good daily oral hygiene, annual or semiannual dental visits for cleaning and checkup are valuable.

Curing chronic marginal gingivitis and preventing periodontitis are now thought to diminish the risk of heart disease and stroke, as relationships between oral bacteria and clogged arteries have arisen from recent research. A relationship also exists between diabetes mellitus and chronic marginal gingivitis or periodontitis: Diabetes increases the risk of developing periodontitis, and oral infection makes blood glucose harder to control. People having serious periodontitis and lung problems may inhale mouth bacteria and develop pneumonia. It is believed that susceptibility to gingivitis differs between individuals, so study of the genetics and immunology of gingivitis may have the potential to provide better treatments as well as vaccines.

—*Sanford S. Singer, Ph.D.*

See also Cavities; Dental diseases; Dentistry; Endodontic disease; Gum disease; Periodontal surgery; Periodontitis; Root canal treatment; Teeth; Tooth extraction; Toothache.

FOR FURTHER INFORMATION:

Cook, Allan R., ed. *Oral Health Sourcebook: Basic Information About Diseases and Conditions Affecting Oral Health.* Detroit: Omnigraphics, 1998. Includes much information on oral disease, including gingivitis and periodontitis.

Cross, William G. *Gingivitis.* 2d ed. Bristol, England: J. Wright, 1977. This classic work contains many facts on the disease, as well as excellent illustrations.

Icon Health. *Gingivitis: A Medical Dictionary, Bibliography, and Annotated Research Guide to Internet References.* San Diego, Calif.: Author, 2004. Designed for physicians, medical students, researchers, and patients.

Wilson, Thomas G., and Kenneth S. Kornman, eds. *Fundamentals of Periodontics.* 2d ed. Chicago: Quintessence, 2003. A complete source on periodontics and periodontal diseases of all types.

GLANDS

ANATOMY

ANATOMY OR SYSTEM AFFECTED: Breasts, endocrine system, gastrointestinal system, genitals, nervous system, pancreas, reproductive system, skin

SPECIALTIES AND RELATED FIELDS: Biochemistry, dermatology, endocrinology, gastroenterology, gynecology, vascular medicine

DEFINITION: Organs or areas of the body that produce, store, and secrete fluids, exerting a profound effect on growth, energy production, chemical balance, reproduction, and health.

KEY TERMS:

adrenal glands: the endocrine glands on top of the kidneys that produce a large number of hormones involved in metabolism and in response to stress

endocrine system: the system of glands located throughout the body that produces hormones and secretes them directly into the blood for delivery by the circulatory system

hormone: a product of the endocrine glands transported throughout the bloodstream which controls and regulates other glands or organs by chemical stimulation

pancreas: the gland located under the stomach that produces insulin and glucagon, the hormones responsible for control of the body's blood sugar level *parathyroid glands:* four tiny structures on the back of the thyroid, chiefly concerned with the regulation of calcium and phosphorus

pituitary gland: a tiny gland located under the brain which controls the thyroid, adrenal, and sex glands

sex glands: the ovaries in the female and the testes in the male, which secrete hormones involved in reproduction

thyroid gland: an endocrine gland located in the neck, which regulates the rate of energy production throughout the body

STRUCTURE AND FUNCTIONS

A gland is any tissue or organ that produces and releases a fluid. Some, such as digestive or sweat glands, secrete their juices through a duct or tube. These glands are known as exocrine glands, meaning "externally secreting." Other glands pass their secretions directly into the blood that flows through them. Known as endocrine or "internally secreting" glands, these are the ones that produce hormones. This article will focus only on the endocrine glands and their hormones that control, stimulate, and regulate almost every important function in the body.

Although there are hundreds of known or suspected hormones, there are only several major endocrine glands to produce them. They include the pituitary, pineal gland, and hypothalamus in the brain; the thyroid, parathyroid glands, and thymus in the neck; and the adrenal glands and pancreas in the abdomen. In addition, the female ovaries in the pelvic cavity and the male testes in the scrotum contribute their hormones to the widespread work of the endocrine system.

The largest endocrine organ, the thyroid, is quite small, weighing only about an ounce. It is butterfly-shaped and wrapped around the windpipe in the throat. By means of the two iodine-containing hormones that it produces, called thyroxine (T_4) and triiodothyronine (T_3), this gland controls the rate of the body's metabolism; that is, these hormones control the speed at which energy-producing chemical reactions occur in all the cells of the body. They also play a crucial role in oxygen use, protein synthesis, and the development of the central nervous system. A third thyroid secretion, calcitonin, has a completely different role. By opposing the work of the parathyroids discussed below, it prevents the existence of too much calcium in the blood.

The four tiny parathyroid glands on the back of the thyroid are each only 0.25-inch wide. They supply parathyroid hormone, which maintains the proper balance of calcium in various parts of the body. It is very important to the bones, nerves, muscles, and blood that each contain the exact amount of calcium needed to function correctly. If there is not enough calcium, parathyroid hormone instructs the intestine to absorb more calcium and the kidneys to retain more. If the blood still has an insufficient level of calcium, parathyroid hormone causes it to be released from storage in the bones.

The pancreas, found behind the stomach, is unusual because it is both an exocrine gland, producing digestive enzymes for the intestine, and an important endocrine gland. Its major hormones, insulin and glucagon, are the major regulators of the blood sugar level. Soon after a meal is digested, insulin is released, enabling all cells in general but liver cells in particular to take excess sugar out of the blood at a rapid rate. The liver's stored sugar is then released steadily into the blood between meals because of the steady glucagon production in the pancreas. The careful balancing of these two hormones enables the body to have just the right sugar content in the blood at all times.

The hormones that bring about the most striking changes in both anatomy and behavior are known as the sex hormones. Because sex hormone levels are high in the fetus, they directly influence the development of its sex organs.

Somewhere around the age of eleven, the level of a girl's estrogens rises sharply, causing female puberty. These hormones, produced in the two ovaries (located in the pelvic cavity), cause breast development, the growth of pubic and underarm hair, and the broadening of hips and thighs. Each month of the woman's life until the menopause, the ovarian estrogen and progesterone levels rise and fall, controlling the release of an egg or ovum from her ovary. These same hormones have prepared the uterus to support and nourish a developing embryo if the egg is fertilized.

The two testes, located in the scrotal sac, by their production of testosterone and other androgens bring about male puberty around the age of thirteen. These hormones are responsible for such male secondary sex characteristics as facial hair, deepening of the voice, and heavier muscles and bones. The testes' secretions seem also to cause the greater aggressiveness of men compared to women. Their prime function, however, is aiding the production of healthy sperm.

The two-inch-long adrenal glands, perched on top of the kidneys, are actually two glands in one. The outer 80 percent is called the cortex, while the inner part is named the medulla. The adrenals produce dozens of hormones, most of which are involved in some way with one's ability to cope with stress. One of the major adrenal cortex hormones is cortisol. It helps maintain blood pressure, regulates fluid levels, directs protein and sugar metabolism, increases or decreases body fat reserves, and affects the immune system. A second area of the cortex secretes aldosterone, which directs the kidney to retain sodium and excrete potassium, controlling their levels in the blood. The third cortex area, surprisingly, produces some testosterone and estrogen in both males and females.

The adrenal medulla responds to sudden stress by pouring epinephrine, formerly called adrenaline, into the blood. Dramatic changes in the working of the heart, lungs, liver, muscles, and many other organs then enable the body to cope with sudden emergencies.

The thymus gland, behind the breastbone, is very unusual because it is quite large in a newborn, grows

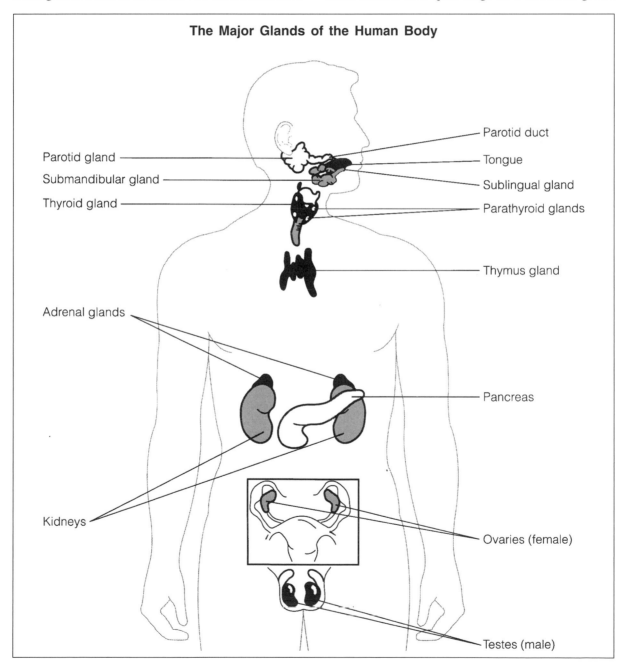

The Major Glands of the Human Body

Parotid gland
Submandibular gland
Thyroid gland

Parotid duct
Tongue
Sublingual gland
Parathyroid glands

Thymus gland

Adrenal glands

Pancreas

Kidneys

Ovaries (female)

Testes (male)

throughout childhood, but shrinks drastically from puberty onward. It is the source of several important secretions, including thymosin, which activates the T cells and B cells. These lymphocytes, a type of white blood cell, provide immunity to disease by destroying invading organisms.

The tiny pineal gland, less than a quarter of an inch long, is embedded close to the very center of the brain. Although the exact function of this pinecone-shaped structure is a mystery, it appears to be the only gland producing melatonin. Proven to be involved in seasonal reproduction in other mammals, melatonin seems to be related to puberty in humans.

The careful and precise control of most of these glands is the work of the pituitary, causing it to be called "the master gland." This small gland, about 0.5 inch in size, has three distinct parts: the front or anterior pituitary, the back or posterior pituitary, and a tiny middle section.

The anterior pituitary sends thyroid-stimulating hormone (TSH) to the thyroid, causing it to release T_3 and T_4. It also secretes adrenocorticotropic hormone (ACTH), which causes the adrenal cortex to give off its many secretions. In the female, the follicle-stimulating hormone (FSH) that the anterior pituitary sends to the ovary causes an egg to mature, while in the male it fosters sperm development. Luteinizing hormone (LH), from the anterior pituitary, triggers the monthly release of an egg and then coaxes the ovary to produce progesterone. The male's LH causes clusters of cells in the testes, called interstitial cells, to produce testosterone. As if these were not enough important jobs for the anterior pituitary to have, it also secretes growth hormone (GH) to stimulate body growth until maturity and secretes prolactin or lactogenic hormone to cause the female breast to produce milk for a nursing baby.

The posterior pituitary secretes only two hormones: oxytocin, which brings about labor and birth, and antidiuretic hormone (ADH), which is also known as vasopressin. ADH causes the kidney to reabsorb the proper amount of water needed by the body, a most important function.

Long after the anterior pituitary was named "the master gland," it was learned that the hypothalamus is the master of the master. This small area of tissue below the brain produces a number of releasing hormones and inhibiting hormones which, in turn, carefully control the anterior pituitary's secretion of FSH, LH, TSH, ACTH, prolactin, and growth hormone. The hypothalamus is also the source of oxytocin and ADH, which is

then stored by the posterior pituitary until it is needed by the body.

Disorders and Diseases

In 1970, only a few dozen hormones from the endocrine glands were known to medical science. By 1990, at least two hundred had been discovered. An understanding of their actions and interactions has generated numerous helpful medical applications.

These complex interactions, involving the concept of feedback, have made possible many treatments for defective glands. Feedback means that healthy glands are self-regulating. For example, more calcium in the blood causes less parathyroid hormone to be released, and then the lowered amount of blood calcium causes more parathyroid hormone production. All glands have these feedback loops, but those involving the hypothalamus, pituitary, and one of its target glands are particularly complicated.

Appropriate medical treatment of thyroid disease, for example, requires careful understanding of its feedback mechanism. An increase in thyroid-stimulating hormone releasing hormones (TRH) from the hypothalamus normally causes the pituitary to give off its thyroid-stimulating hormone. This in turn triggers the production of thyroxine and triiodothyronine.

The type of thyroid disease in which insufficient thyroid hormones are produced is called hypothyroidism. It is quite common, with one in every one thousand men and two in every one hundred women afflicted at some time during life. It is often caused by an inability of the thyroid gland to produce enough hormone, the result of a disease of the pituitary that prevents it from producing TSH or a disease of the hypothalamus that prevents it from producing TRH. Surprisingly, an underactive thyroid is often enlarged but still unable to produce enough T_3 or T_4. This enlargement is called a goiter. In the type called Hashimoto's disease, the hypothyroidism develops because the body mistakenly produces antibodies that destroy the thyroid tissue.

Because of the complexity of the chemical feedback loop involved in thyroid gland control, many cases of hypothyroidism have been caused inadvertently by drugs given for other conditions. Among these medicines are lithium carbonate, used to treat manic depressives; expectorants containing potassium iodide, prescribed for respiratory infections; and a host of other drugs. Physicians prescribing these drugs and patients using them need to watch carefully for the development of symptoms such as intolerance to cold, puffy face and back of hands, weight gain, high blood pressure, yellowed skin, and loss of hair.

Adults afflicted with hypothyroidism, no matter what the cause, also commonly suffer some disturbances to their nervous system, experiencing lethargy, slowness of thought, poor memory, and slowness of reaction to events occurring around them. Even more disastrous are the effects of an underactive thyroid in infants, where it causes mental retardation and stunted physical growth. If diagnosed early enough, the infant can be successfully treated in the same manner as an adult, with lifelong daily doses of TSH, T_3, and T_4 in individually and carefully adjusted amounts.

In addition, like any gland, the thyroid can oversecrete as well as undersecrete. Hypersecretion is also quite common, with three or four out of one thousand people having this disease, the majority being women. The resulting excessive rate of metabolism causes many possible symptoms including intolerance to heat, irritability, excessive perspiration, heart palpitations, rapid weight loss, weakness, shortness of breath, and sore, bulging eyes.

There are two main types of hyperthyroidism. By far the most common is called Graves' disease. It is brought about when the patient's own immune system creates antibodies that cause continuous excess hormone production by the thyroid even though the pituitary is sending the normal amount of TSH. The less common cases of hyperthyroidism involve lumps or nodules that form in the thyroid and oversecrete T_3 and T_4 for no apparent reason. One of three treatments is usually used to cure hyperthyroidism: Radioactive iodine is given to destroy part of the overactive gland, surgery is used to remove part of the gland, or certain drugs are prescribed that prevent the thyroid from producing its hormones.

As common as thyroid disorders are, there is no endocrine disorder as common as diabetes mellitus, which afflicts one out of every one thousand people. When certain cells of the pancreas are destroyed and cannot produce insulin, the person is said to have insulin-dependent diabetes (IDD). This type is most often found in children and young adults. Non-insulin-dependent diabetes (NIDD) occurs more frequently in middle-aged and older people. This condition occurs because the person's tissues become resistant to the insulin; no matter how much the pancreas tries to produce it, sugar is not able to enter the tissues properly. IDD patients are suspected to have been born with genes that make their immune systems destroy their insulin-producing pancreatic cells by mistake, after they have been exposed to certain viruses. NIDD also seems to be inherited, but stress, various illnesses, and obesity rather than viruses trigger the lack of response to insulin as the person ages.

Patients who develop either type of diabetes mellitus usually soon exhibit some if not all of the following symptoms: constant thirst and urination; loss of weight, strength, and energy; frequent hunger pains; and the inability of cuts or bruises to heal. The long-term effects of the very high blood sugar level of diabetics vary from patient to patient. They often include heart disease and high blood pressure, unhealed wounds which become gangrenous, kidney failure, endless infections, nerve damage, and possible coma.

Treatment for diabetes attempts to make the body's cells absorb sugar normally. This can often be achieved through diet, medicines that stimulate insulin production, other drugs that make the tissues more responsive to the work of insulin, and, if necessary, injections of insulin itself. These traditional methods may or may not ever be completely replaced by exciting possibilities explored in the early 1990's: insulin pumps to deliver a steady supply and full or partial pancreas transplants.

Although no one objects to attempts to aid sufferers of thyroid disorders or diabetes mellitus, ethical questions have arisen concerning defects in some endocrine glands. A striking example involves a lack of growth hormone from the pituitary. Doctors, parents, and youngsters often disagree over whether GH therapy should be given to a child who is noticeably shorter than peers at a given age. Because GH, like any hormone, may produce many unwanted side effects, there is much controversy over this particular medical application of endocrine gland research.

PERSPECTIVE AND PROSPECTS

Glands, together with the nervous system, are the body's means of control and coordination. Given this fact, the discovery of each gland's functions had ramifications for medical science as a whole.

Although the ancient Greeks, Romans, and Chinese suspected the importance of some glands, it was only in the seventeenth century that scientists began to acquire useful knowledge of them. At that time, the Englishman Thomas Wharton first recognized the difference between duct and ductless glands. In the 1660's, Théophile Bordeu, a Frenchman regarded by many as the founder of endocrinology, declared that some parts of the body gave off "emanations" that had dramatic effects on other parts of the body. Following Bordeu's lead, the Dutchman Fredrik Ruysch claimed in the 1690's that the thyroid poured important substances into the bloodstream.

Then, in 1775, Percival Platt made an unusual discovery in London while repairing a hernia in a female patient. When he inadvertently removed her ovaries, the woman's menstrual period ceased. This led John Davidge to realize the importance of the ovaries in controlling menstruation. Also in the late 1700's, doctors began to associate a swollen neck, bulging eyes, and a racing pulse with a swollen thyroid gland; they suspected a cause-and-effect relationship.

Thomas Addison, an English physician, found diseased adrenals by autopsy in a group of patients who had exhibited all the same symptoms. He published in 1849 that he definitely suspected another cause-and-effect relationship. That same year, the first experimental proof of the functions of a hormone was found by A. A. Berthold in Germany. Roosters whose testes he had removed lost all usual male characteristics. Testes that had been left free in the abdomens of other birds soon attached themselves, grew blood vessels, and produced the expected rooster characteristics.

Two major breakthroughs occurred in the late 1800's when Paul Langerhans found the actual pancreas cell clusters, called islets, that produce insulin and when Charles-Edouard Brown-Séquard developed a technique to use extracts from glands to determine their function.

The year 1900 brought three major discoveries: William Bayliss and Ernest Starling found that a chemical messenger from the intestine causes the pancreas to excrete digestive juice; Jokichi Takamine discovered that adrenaline increases heart rate and blood pressure; and Alfred Frölich described dwarfed individuals who had suffered previous pituitary damage.

In 1914, in Minnesota, Edward Kendall obtained the chemical he named thyroxine from animal thyroids. Similarly, in 1921, Frederick Banting and Charles Best isolated insulin from the pancreases of animals. By 1948, Kendall and many other workers had isolated two dozen adrenal cortex hormones; Philip Hench made medical news when he first used the one named cortisone to relieve, though not cure, arthritis.

By the mid-1970's, Rosalind Yalow and her colleagues had perfected a technique called radioimmunoassay, which uses radioactive materials to measure minute quantities of hormones. This enables physicians to measure the circulating level of nearly every hormone and diagnose anyone with an excess or deficiency. Many hormones such as insulin, growth hormone, and estrogen can then be given to supplement what the body is underproducing; they have been very expensive and hard to obtain in quantity from animals or deceased humans. By the 1980's, however, recombinant DNA technology and the polymerase chain reaction (PCR) offered unlimited, pure, and readily accessible hormones.

—Grace D. Matzen

See also Abscess drainage; Abscesses; Addison's disease; Adrenalectomy; Brain; Breasts, female; Corticosteroids; Cyst removal; Cysts; Diabetes mellitus; Dwarfism; Endocrine disorders; Endocrinology; Endocrinology, pediatric; Gigantism; Goiter; Hashimoto's thyroiditis; Hormone replacement therapy (HRT); Hormones; Hyperparathyroidism and hypoparathyroidism; Hypoglycemia; Mastectomy and lumpectomy; Mumps; Pancreas; Parathyroidectomy; Prostate enlargement; Prostate gland; Prostate gland removal; Sjögren's syndrome; Systems and organs; Testicular cancer; Testicular surgery; Thyroid disorders; Thyroid gland; Thyroidectomy.

FOR FURTHER INFORMATION:

Brook, Charles G. D., and Nicholas J. Marshall. *Essential Endocrinology.* 4th ed. Malden, Mass.: Blackwell Science, 2001. This text addresses the field of endocrinology, describing the physiology of the endocrine glands and the hormones that they produce. Includes an index.

Goodman, H. Maurice. *Basic Medical Endocrinology.* 3d ed. Boston: Academic Press, 2003. Focuses on research advances in the understanding of hormones involved in regulating most aspects of bodily functions. Includes in-depth coverage of individual glands and regulatory principles.

Henry, Helen L., and Anthony W. Norman, eds. *Encyclopedia of Hormones.* 3 vols. San Diego, Calif.: Academic Press, 2003. A comprehensive overview of the role of hormones, the major physiological systems in which they operate, and the biological consequences of an excess or deficiency of a particular hormone.

Larsen, P. Reed, et al., eds. *Williams Textbook of Endocrinology.* 10th ed. Philadelphia: W. B. Saunders, 2003. Text that covers the spectrum of information related to the endocrine system, including thyroid disorders, diabetes, endocrinology and aging, female reproduction and fertility control, sexual function and dysfunction, kidney stones, and endocrine hypertension.

Little, Marjorie. *The Endocrine System*. Rev. ed. New York: Chelsea House, 2000. This volume is intended not only to provide basic knowledge but also to enable the general reader to pursue the subject through its lengthy bibliography. Also includes a helpful glossary and an extensive list of organizations that will provide further information.

Ruggieri, Paul, and Scott Isaacs. *A Simple Guide to Thyroid Disorders: From Diagnosis to Treatment*. Omaha, Nebr.: Addicus Books, 2003. A user-friendly guide that covers how the thyroid gland works, and explains common disorders, including hypothyroidism and hyperthyroidism. Special attention is given to how thyroid diseases affect specific populations such as women, children, and the elderly.

Scanlon, Valerie, and Tina Sanders. *Essentials of Anatomy and Physiology*. 5th ed. Philadelphia: F. A. Davis, 2007. A text designed around three themes: the relationship between physiology and anatomy, the interrelations among the organ systems, and the relationship of each organ system to homeostasis.

GLAUCOMA
DISEASE/DISORDER

ANATOMY OR SYSTEM AFFECTED: Eyes

SPECIALTIES AND RELATED FIELDS: Ophthalmology, optometry

DEFINITION: A group of eye diseases characterized by an increase in the eye's intraocular pressure; early diagnosis through regular eye examinations can manage the effects of the disease, while late diagnosis may result in impaired vision or blindness.

KEY TERMS:

aqueous humor: the liquid filling the space between the lens and the cornea of the eye, which nourishes and lubricates them

ciliary body: a structure built of muscle and blood vessels which produces the aqueous humor

cornea: the curved, transparent membrane forming the front of the outer coat of the eyeball that serves primarily as protection and focuses light onto the lens

intraocular pressure: the degree of firmness of the eyeball, as controlled by the proper secretion and drainage of the aqueous humor

lens: a transparent, flexible structure, convex on both surfaces and lying directly behind the iris of the eye; it focuses light rays onto the retina

ophthalmic laser: a high-intensity beam of light that permits a surgeon to cut tissue precisely in the treatment of eye diseases

optic disc: the portion of the optic nerve at its point of entrance into the rear of the eye

peripheral vision: side vision, or the visual perception to all sides of the central object being viewed

retina: the thin, delicate, and transparent sheet of nerve tissue that receives visual stimuli and transmits them to the brain through the optic nerve

tonometer: an instrument used to measure the eye's intraocular pressure, thus checking for the presence of glaucoma

CAUSES AND SYMPTOMS

Glaucoma is an eye disease caused by higher-than-normal pressure inside the eye. The intraocular pressure can increase slowly or suddenly for various reasons but always with detrimental results. Of all the causes of blindness, glaucoma is among the most common, but it is also the most preventable. If diagnosed early, it can be controlled and the loss of sight avoided. What complicates the problem is that the most common form of glaucoma shows no symptoms until extensive, irreversible damage has occurred. There is no pain, and the first sign that something is amiss may be that peripheral vision and seeing out of the corner of the eye is diminished, while frontal vision remains clear.

To understand this disease, it is necessary to know what occurs within the eye when the intraocular pressure increases. The inner surface of the cornea is nourished by the aqueous humor, which is also called the aqueous fluid. This secretion from the ciliary body flows into the space behind the iris and then through the pupil into the space in front of the iris. Where the front of the iris joins the back of the cornea is a point called the venous sinus, at the anterior drainage angle. Here

---

INFORMATION ON GLAUCOMA

CAUSES: Congenital or hereditary factors

SYMPTOMS: Often asymptomatic; eye pressure; slow progression toward blindness; at times, terrible pain, nausea, vomiting, severe headaches

DURATION: Ranges from acute to chronic

TREATMENTS: Eyedrops, ointments, pills, surgery

the aqueous humor is reabsorbed and transported to the bloodstream. In a normal eye, this drainage process works correctly and the balance between the amount secreted and the amount reabsorbed maintains a constant intraocular pressure. In glaucoma, the drainage part of the process works inefficiently. For a variety of reasons, some of which are not fully understood, the drainage mechanism is defective. The upset balance in secretion drainage causes the unwanted increase in intraocular pressure in one eye or, more commonly, in both. The iris is pushed forward, further inhibiting drainage of the aqueous fluid.

Even a very small elevation in intraocular pressure will affect the eye adversely, causing damage to its particularly delicate parts. Although the eye as a whole is quite tough, the optic nerve is vulnerable to increased pressure. This vital connection between the eye and the brain is damaged by the stress within the harder eyeball. The delicate nerve fibers and blood vessels of the optic disc, as the beginning of the optic nerve is called, then die. Once they die, they can never be regenerated or replaced, and blindness is the result. The destruction of the optic disc causes a condition called cupping. A normal optic disc is quite level with the retina. Glaucoma causes it to collapse, creating a genuine indentation. Thus, cupping is a definite sign of glaucoma.

The damage that glaucoma inflicts is progressive. The defect in drainage does not necessarily worsen, and the pressure, once elevated, does not necessarily continue to increase. Once begun, however, the killing of the optic nerve cells continues until the resulting loss of vision progresses to total blindness. The first nerve fibers to die are the ones near the outer edge of the optic disc, which originates near the periphery of the retina. The first decrease in vision, therefore, is in one's peripheral vision. Then, as each layer of nerve fibers dies, the visual field narrows and narrows.

This slow, progressive route to blindness is typical of chronic simple glaucoma, or primary open-angle glaucoma (POAG), which accounts for 90 percent of glaucoma cases in the United States. It is called "simple" because the rise in intraocular pressure does not result from any known underlying reason. Although individuals with a family history of glaucoma are more prone to the disease, it is not directly hereditary. Moreover, not everyone with a family history of glaucoma will develop the disease. For reasons that are not well understood, people of African ancestry have glaucoma in much greater numbers than those of European ancestry. In the United States, the incidence of glaucoma among African Americans is three times that of Caucasians. Glaucoma is the second-leading cause of adult blindness in the United States.

In persons of all races, chronic simple glaucoma usually begins after the age of forty; however, the aging process does not seem to be a direct cause of glaucoma. Unlike the formation of senile cataracts, which result from inevitable eye changes as one grows older, glaucoma's development is not explained by the aging process. It can safely be said that glaucoma seems to occur in persons who have a tendency toward inadequate aqueous fluid drainage. As those persons grow older and their bodies lose their resiliency in general, the drainage problem reaches a point where it begins to raise the intraocular pressure beyond the normal range. Those with untreated chronic simple glaucoma are seldom aware of the disease before considerable damage has been done. The progressive death of nerve fibers is ordinarily very slow because the elevation of pressure is slight and causes no pain or blurriness of sight.

Chronic simple glaucoma makes up about 95 percent of all cases of the disease. Several other rare types together make up the other 5 percent. In chronic secondary glaucoma, the drainage defect is caused by some complication of a different eye problem. The causes of chronic secondary glaucoma include inflammation from an eye infection, an allergic reaction, trauma to the eye, a tumor, or even the presence of a cataract. Medications such as corticosteroids can sometimes cause this type of glaucoma to develop. Whatever the cause, chronic secondary glaucoma exhibits the same increased pressure, slow nerve destruction, and ultimate loss of vision as chronic simple glaucoma.

A third variety, acute glaucoma, is both rare and dramatic in its onset. The increase in intraocular pressure is many times higher than that in chronic glaucoma. It also occurs very rapidly, sometimes within hours. The anterior drainage angle where drainage is accomplished is almost totally blocked. The eyeball becomes so hard that the elevated pressure can often be felt simply by touching the front of the eye. The great pressure causes terrible pain and immediate damage to the eye. When nausea, vomiting, and severe headaches accompany eye pressure, acute glaucoma should be suspected. Immediate treatment is required to prevent blindness. Acute glaucoma can be either simple or secondary. It is termed simple when a drainage area that has always been abnormally narrow suddenly becomes totally blocked. It is called secondary when it is precipitated by some other eye condition.

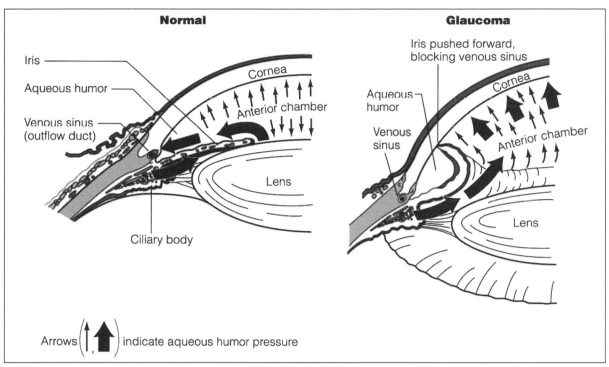

Normal

Iris

Aqueous humor

Venous sinus
(outflow duct)

Cornea

Anterior chamber

Lens

Ciliary body

Glaucoma

Iris pushed forward,
blocking venous sinus

Aqueous
humor

Venous
sinus

Cornea

Anterior chamber

Lens

Arrows indicate aqueous humor pressure

A normal eye versus an eye affected by glaucoma.

The rarest type of glaucoma, congenital glaucoma, is present at birth or develops during early infancy. It results from the incorrect formation of drainage canals while the eye is developing. Because a baby's eyeball is much smaller and softer than an adult's, this glaucoma is often recognized by the bulging of the eyes.

It is quite easy for an eye doctor to detect even the apparently symptomless chronic glaucoma, and the rate of successful treatment is high. It is unfortunate, then, that glaucoma is responsible for innumerable cases of permanent loss of vision. In the vast majority of these patients, the destruction of the eye could have been prevented. If everyone over the age of forty had an annual eye examination, blindness caused by glaucoma could essentially be eliminated.

TREATMENT AND THERAPY

The treatments available for glaucoma include eyedrops, ointments, pills, and surgery, using both scalpels and lasers. In both acute and congenital glaucoma, there is no time for the use of medications. Patients need to be admitted to the hospital and operated on immediately if their eyesight is to be saved. For open-angle glaucoma, medications may be topical—eye drops or ointments, or inserts, thin medicated strips put in to the corner of the eye—or oral (pills and tablets).

Some of the more recent medications are unoprostone isopropyl/ophthalmic solution, brinzolamide ophthalmic suspension, dorzdamide hydrochloride-timolo meleate ophthalmic solution, and brimonidine tartrate ophthalmic solution. Studies in the 1970's that suggested that marijuana might be an effective treatment agent have since been shown to be no more effective than are a number of drugs already on the market.

If diagnosed early, cases of both chronic simple and chronic secondary glaucoma can often be effectively treated by medications. The first drug given in the form of eyedrops was discovered in the nineteenth century. Called pilocarpine, it is obtained from the leaves or roots of a South American bush. The drug is classified as a miotic because it constricts the pupil of the eye. Constriction of the pupil draws it away from the drainage angle, automatically increasing the drainage of aqueous fluid and therefore decreasing the pressure. To be effective, it is generally used four times a day. Other glaucoma drugs act to decrease the secretion of the fluid, which also decreases the intraocular pressure. Timolol maleate, the most frequently prescribed drug for glaucoma, works in this fashion. It usually needs to be used twice a day. Some ophthalmologists prefer to use some of both types of drops for the same patient, decreasing pressure by both mechanisms. Others prescribe one medication that produces both effects. Dipivefrin is one such medication.

In either case, to avoid possible unpleasant side effects the most dilute concentration, to be used the fewest times each day, is prescribed first. If this does not control the pressure, more concentrated drops, to be used more times daily, must then be prescribed. The medications in these eyedrops can often be used more easily by elderly patients in the form of a gel, an ointment, or a tiny disc which is placed on the cornea. Although considerably more costly than frequent drops, these methods are less of a nuisance. The gels and ointments need only be used once a day, while the discs are time-released over an entire week.

If drops or gels do not produce the desired reduction in pressure, pills can be used, not to replace the drops but to supplement them. These tablets are essentially diuretics that decrease the production of aqueous humor. Taken once a day, or less frequently in a time-release capsule, acetazolamide is the drug most often prescribed.

There are also several fast-acting drugs that can be injected into a vein to lower pressure by rapidly pulling some aqueous fluid into blood vessels in the eye, bypassing the drainage angle. These are not used in the treatment of chronic glaucoma except as preparation for a planned surgery. They are, however, often used when patients are admitted to the hospital for acute glaucoma to prevent damage until emergency surgery can be performed.

In the great number of patients, chronic glaucoma can be controlled by one of these medications. In those rare cases when it cannot, surgery must be performed. Although initially successful, such surgeries must often be repeated in the future. As with the above medications, glaucoma surgery aims to decrease the intraocular pressure by decreasing secretion or increasing effective drainage.

Although surgery can never reverse the optic nerve damage that has already occurred, it is often effective in preventing further destruction. The first of these surgical procedures was developed in the mid-nineteenth century. Called an iridectomy or iridotomy, it attempts to provide a better access to the patient's drainage angle by removing part of the iris. A second type of surgical procedure, known as a trabeculectomy or filtering operation, attempts to control intraocular pressure by creating a new, wider drainage outlet for the aqueous humor. Until the use of lasers, both of these operations were performed manually by a surgeon with steady hands using sharp blades on a tiny part of the eye.

To perform an iridectomy, the surgeon must cut a tiny hole into the edge of the iris with surgical scissors, allowing aqueous fluid to flow into the space between the iris and the cornea. Covered by the upper eyelid, this small hole is visible only by close examination and should not let in unwanted extra light or cause any discomfort to the patient.

The filtering operation, or trabeculectomy, can be performed in several different ways, but each involves the eye surgeon's use of a scalpel to create an artificial canal through the outer wall of the patient's eye. The passageway created, known as a fistula or filtering bleb, permits the aqueous humor to drain properly from the inner eye. By removing a part of the abnormal tissue from the drainage angle, the surgeon unclogs the drainage mechanism.

A different approach to glaucoma control does not involve cutting. It attempts to help the patient by destroying part of the source of the excess fluid, the oversecreting ciliary body. When a cold probe is applied to the ciliary body, the procedure is termed cryotherapy; when a hot probe is used, the method is called cyclodiathermy. No incision is required in either case because the probes are applied externally. A very common side effect of these two procedures, however, is fairly severe inflammation. Even when inflammation does not occur, the desired result may be only partially achieved. Both cryotherapy and cyclodiathermy are less commonly used than either iridectomy or trabeculectomy, and the procedures are usually performed only on older patients.

Many of these manual procedures are being replaced by several types of laser therapy. A laser is a precisely directed beam of high-intensity light that can function as a surgical knife. Laser surgery is generally safer than the older methods because it is less invasive to the body, as no incision is made in the eye. It can be done on an outpatient basis with only a local anesthetic. Recovery time, the likelihood of complications, and postoperative discomfort are all lessened. Patients with acute glaucoma, chronic simple glaucoma, and certain types of secondary glaucoma (depending on the cause) can be successfully treated with lasers.

Both iridotomy and trabeculectomy can be performed using an instrument called the argon laser. This particular laser is relatively low-powered, but it is efficient and very popular with ophthalmologists. After a drop of anesthetic is placed in the eye, the surgeon aims the highly focused argon beam at a precise location within the affected eye. The beam need only be directed into the eye for one-tenth of a second to achieve its effect. In an iridotomy, the laser simply drills a tiny hole in the iris for the fluid to circulate freely, while in a trabeculectomy several laser cuts are made on the clogged drainage angle to open it. A more sophisticated ophthalmic laser is the YAG laser. After a drop of anesthetic is placed on the eye, a weak "aiming beam" of helium-neon laser light is shone directly into the afflicted eye to pinpoint the area to be treated. This is followed by two to five bursts of the YAG laser, which drills a hole for better drainage.

All the above treatments for glaucoma, whether pharmaceutical or surgical, have the potential for serious side effects and complications. Consequently, research continues to seek therapies with better rates of success and fewer complications. Some of the possible complications include infection, bleeding, undesirable changes in the intraocular pressure, and loss of vision. Side effects include stinging or redness of the eyes, blurred vision, headache, changes in heart rate, mood changes, tingling of the fingers and toes, drowsiness, and loss of appetite.

Perspective and Prospects

The development of ways to diagnose glaucoma has paralleled the general development of the ophthalmologist's tools. These devices in turn reflect the links between the science of those branches of physics that study pressure, lenses, mirrors, and light and the science that studies the normal and abnormal functioning of the eye.

In 1851, the German doctor Hermann von Helmholtz invented the ophthalmoscope, which enables one to study the interior of the eye. His instrument focuses a beam of light into the patient's eye and then magnifies its reflection. If this test reveals early signs of cupping of the optic disc, glaucoma can be diagnosed long before other symptoms have appeared.

Intraocular pressure can be measured with an instrument called a tonometer. The two basic varieties are called Schiötz tonometry and applanation tonometry. Both only became possible after biochemists developed anesthetic drops to put in the eye so that the patient would not feel the device touching the very sensitive cornea. The earlier of the two devices, developed in 1905 by the Norwegian physician Hjalmar Schiötz, is a very simple device that is still the most widely used tonometer in the world. With the patient lying down

and looking upward, the physician places the hand-sized instrument directly on the cornea. A simple lever is moved by the pressure within the eye to indicate whether that pressure is within the normal range or dangerously high. The Goldman applanation tonometer is considered even more accurate and is often used to confirm the results of the simpler Schiötz device. An orange dye called fluorescein is added to the anesthetic. The patient, in a sitting position, rests the head against a bar to steady it. The doctor uses a tonometer to touch the cornea while simultaneously peering into it with a well-illuminated microscope.

More specialized glaucoma examination may require gonioscopy, visual field tests, or tonography. The gonioscope has mirrors and facets to provide an illuminated view of the drainage angle, a normally dark corner at a 90 degree angle from the examiner. Excessive narrowing of the angle is an indication of glaucoma. There are many kinds of visual field tests, but all give a map of the central area where vision is sharp and more acute, versus the peripheral area where it is weaker. Since damage to the optic nerve always causes a narrowing of the visual field, this mapping is very important. The ability to measure the field has grown from oculokinetic perimetry—using an inexpensive test chart, pencil, record sheet, and human examiner—to the expensive and sophisticated automated perimetry, which generates a computer analysis. Tonography does not measure the visual field but again attacks the problem by measuring the intraocular pressure. Unlike the ordinary use of tonometry, which involves momentary contact with the cornea, tonography uses the tonometer for four minutes to massage the eye. In a normal eye, pressure will drop; in a glaucoma patient, it will not.

All these tests, developed through years of ophthalmic research, have given medical science invaluable tools to diagnose glaucoma and prevent blindness.

—Grace D. Matzen;
updated by Victoria Price, Ph.D.

See also Blindness; Cataract surgery; Cataracts; Eye infections and disorders; Eye surgery; Eyes; Laser use in surgery; Ophthalmology; Optometry; Sense organs; Vision disorders.

For Further Information:

Buettner, Helmut, ed. *Mayo Clinic on Vision and Eye Health: Practical Answers on Glaucoma, Cataracts, Macular Degeneration, and Other Conditions.* Rochester, Minn.: Mayo Foundation for Medical Education and Research, 2002. A helpful handbook on all the medical, social, and emotional facets of vision impairment.

Eden, John. *The Physician's Guide to Cataracts, Glaucoma, and Other Eye Problems.* Yonkers, N.Y.: Consumer Reports Books, 1992. This excellent book provides the reader with nontechnical yet truly accurate explanations of the functioning of the normal eye and of the disease conditions glaucoma and cataracts.

Epstein, David L., et al., eds. *Chandler and Grant's Glaucoma.* 4th ed. Baltimore: Williams & Wilkins, 1997. A standard text on glaucoma. Includes bibliographic references and an index.

Galloway, N. R., et al. *Common Eye Diseases and Their Management.* 3d ed. London: Springer, 2006. While this text may be difficult for the general reader, it is useful for obtaining more precise medical information. Intended for medical students but accessible to nonscientists because of the author's writing style.

Glaucoma Research Foundation. http://www.glaucoma.org/. A group that strives to maintain the sight and independence of individuals with glaucoma through research and education with the ultimate goal of finding a cure.

Marks, Edith. *Coping with Glaucoma.* Garden City Park, N.Y.: Avery, 1997. Following an explanation of glaucoma, offers a discussion of diagnosis, medication, and complementary therapies and diets. References support services and makes suggestions about choosing a doctor and aiming for mutual participation in management of the disease.

Morrison, John C., and Irvin P. Pollack. *Glaucoma: A Clinical Guide.* New York: Thieme, 2003. A clinical text that is nonetheless helpful for the lay reader covering such topics as genetics, gonioscopy, perimetry, childhood glaucoma, retinal disorders, neuroprotection, and ocular hypotony.

Samz, Jane. *Vision.* New York: Chelsea House, 1990. Contains a rather brief treatment of the topic of glaucoma. This volume is useful for understanding the normal eye, eye tests in general, and a diversity of other eye diseases. Includes lists of helpful organizations and further readings, as well as a brief glossary.

Sutton, Amy, ed. *Eye Care Sourcebook: Basic Consumer Health Information About Eye Care and Eye Disorders.* 2d ed. Detroit: Omnigraphics, 2003. A complete guide to eye care that includes such topics as eye anatomy, preventive vision care, refractive disorders and eye diseases, current research and clinical trials, and a list of organizations.

GLOMERULONEPHRITIS. *See* NEPHRITIS.

GLYCOGEN STORAGE DISEASES
DISEASE/DISORDER

ANATOMY OR SYSTEM AFFECTED: Heart, liver, muscles

SPECIALTIES AND RELATED FIELDS: Biochemistry, biotechnology, nutrition, pediatrics, perinatology

DEFINITION: Inherited metabolic disorders that lead to the accumulation of an abnormal amount or type of glycogen in the liver, muscles, and heart.

KEY TERMS:

autosomal recessive trait: a genetic trait coded on an autosomal chromosome (not an X or Y chromosome) that is expressed only when two copies are inherited, one from each parent

cirrhosis: the abnormal formation of connective tissue in an organ, resulting in loss of function; usually refers to the liver

enzyme: a protein that catalyzes a biological reaction in the body

glycogen: the storage form of carbohydrate in the body; a polymer of glucose units that has a highly branched, treelike structure

lysosome: an organelle inside cells that contains a variety of enzymes for breaking down cellular constituents

nasogastric tube: a tube fed through the nose to the stomach

X-linked trait: a genetic trait coded on the X chromosome; predominantly affects males, who have only one X chromosome

CAUSES AND SYMPTOMS

Glycogen storage diseases are caused by inherited defects in the enzymes involved in the synthesis or breakdown of glycogen and are characterized by the accumulation of an abnormal type or amount of glycogen. At least twelve such diseases have been identified; they can be diagnosed by enzymatic analysis of a biopsy tissue sample. Prenatal diagnosis of most of these conditions is possible but, because their overall frequency is estimated at 1 in 20,000 to 25,000 live births, is generally not performed unless warranted. Most of these diseases are inherited as autosomal recessive traits, although phosphorylase kinase deficiency is X-linked. In many cases, the causative deoxyribonucleic acid (DNA) mutations have been identified. These diseases primarily affect the liver and muscles, which normally contain most of the glycogen in the body.

Maintaining normal blood glucose levels is essential for the function of various tissues and particularly the brain, which depends on blood glucose as a source of energy. In the fed state, when dietary carbohydrate is digested, blood glucose levels rise and are used to replenish liver glycogen. In the fasted state, when blood glucose levels otherwise fall, liver glycogen is broken down and used to maintain normal blood glucose levels. This cycling in the storage and breakdown of liver glycogen is essential to permit the body to survive periods without meals, especially overnight.

In liver glycogen storage diseases, this cycling is disrupted. Most cases are attributed to defects in four enzymes: glucose-6-phosphatase, glycogen branching enzyme, glycogen debrancher enzyme, and glycogen phosphorylase (or phosphorylase kinase). Because glucose-6-phosphatase is responsible for converting the breakdown product of glycogen (glucose-6-phosphate) to free glucose for release into the blood, its deficiency does not allow stored liver glycogen to restore depleted blood glucose, as during an overnight fast. If untreated, this condition, also known as von Gierke's disease, results in seizures, coma, and death. Inadequately treated patients may survive but experience growth retardation and develop kidney problems and liver cancer.

Muscle glycogen is also synthesized in the fed state, but it is broken down to provide energy for muscle contraction. Glycogen storage diseases of muscle usually cause intolerance to exercise and susceptibility to fatigue. Most of these cases are attributed to defects in three enzymes: lysosomal glucosidase, glycogen phosphorylase, and phosphofructokinase. The glucosidase found in lysosomes is responsible for breaking down any glycogen that accumulates in these intracellular organelles. When this enzyme is missing, the lyso-

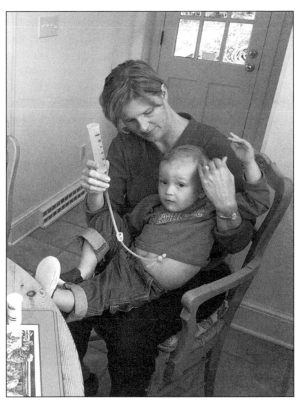

A mother pours liquid cornstarch solution into her young child's feeding tube. He has a rare glycogen storage disease and must have cornstarch every four hours in order to avoid seizures. (AP/Wide World Photos)

somes become engorged with glycogen, disrupting their normal function and other cellular metabolism. In the most severe cases, glycogen accumulation in the heart is pronounced, resulting in an enlarged heart and death from heart failure before age two. Glycogen phosphorylase in muscle breaks down glycogen for its use in contraction. When this enzyme is deficient, muscle tissues lack the fuel to provide for extensive exercise, resulting in cramping; the avoidance of heavy exercise prevents symptoms. Phosphofructokinase is a crucial enzyme in the metabolism of glucose; in the muscle, its deficiency has a consequence much like that of glycogen phosphorylase, namely the inability to engage in strenuous exercise.

When glycogen is synthesized, the branching enzyme inserts branchpoints to give it a treelike structure. A defect in this enzyme leads to an abnormal, long, unbranched glycogen. Because it folds back on itself in a way that makes it difficult for glycogen breakdown enzymes to act on it, it is not broken down. While this condition generally does not lead to low fasting blood

---

Information on Glycogen Storage Diseases

Causes: Genetic enzyme defects

Symptoms: In liver diseases, may include seizures, coma, growth retardation, kidney problems, and liver cancer; in muscle diseases, may include exercise intolerance, susceptibility to fatigue, heart enlargement, and heart failure

Duration: Lifelong

Treatments: Varies by type; includes continuous glucose intake

glucose, as alternative pathways are available, the accumulated abnormal glycogen, apparently considered a foreign object, leads to liver cirrhosis and death by age five; no treatment is available other than liver transplantation. A defect in the debranching enzyme that removes the branchpoints during the breakdown of glycogen severely restricts the yield of glucose to those units beyond a branchpoint. Glycogen phosphorylase is the main enzyme that breaks down glycogen to monomeric units, and its deficiency or that of an enzyme controlling its activity (phosphorylase kinase) result in variable manifestation, depending on the severity of the condition. Most patients with the latter diseases usually require no specific treatment.

TREATMENT AND THERAPY

A defect in glucose-6-phosphatase can be treated by providing continuous sources of glucose during the day (snacks between meals) and especially overnight (nightly nasogastric infusions of glucose or eating slowly digested carbohydrate, such as uncooked cornstarch, before sleep). If this condition is detected early and treated properly, then normal growth and development are observed. No effective treatment is available for muscle glycogen storage disease involving a defect in lysosomal glucosidases.

PERSPECTIVE AND PROSPECTS

The first observation of a defect in glycogen metabolism was made in 1928. In 1929, Edgar von Gierke first noted glucose-6-phosphatase deficiency and, in 1932, J. C. Pompe first reported the lysosomal glucosidase deficiency; their names remain associated with these conditions. As normal glycogen metabolism came to be understood, the enzymatic basis for at least twelve glycogen storage disorders were identified. Each is a candidate for enzyme replacement therapy or gene replacement therapy, although these treatments remained experimental at the beginning of the twenty-first century.

—*James L. Robinson, Ph.D.*

See also Enzyme therapy; Enzymes; Fatty acid oxidation disorders; Food biochemistry; Metabolic disorders; Metabolism; Niemann-Pick disease.

FOR FURTHER INFORMATION:

Chen, Y.-T. "Glycogen Storage Diseases." In *The Metabolic and Molecular Bases of Inherited Disease*, edited by Charles R. Scriver et al. 8th ed. New York: McGraw-Hill, 2001.

Hirschhorn, R., and A. J. J. Reuser. "Glycogen Storage Disease Type II: Acid-Glucosidase (Acid Maltase) Deficiency." In *The Metabolic and Molecular Bases of Inherited Disease*, edited by Charles R. Scriver et al. 8th ed. New York: McGraw-Hill, 2001.

Professional Guide to Diseases. 8th ed. Ambler, Pa.: Lippincott Williams & Wilkins, 2005.

GLYCOLYSIS

BIOLOGY

ANATOMY OR SYSTEM AFFECTED: Blood, cells, muscles, musculoskeletal system

SPECIALTIES AND RELATED FIELDS: Biochemistry, cytology, exercise physiology, pharmacology, sports medicine

DEFINITION: The chemical process of splitting a molecule of glucose in order to obtain energy for other cellular processes; at times of intense activity, glycolysis produces most of the energy used by muscles.

KEY TERMS:

adenosine triphosphate (ATP): an important biological molecule that represents the energy currency of the cell; the energy in a special high-energy bond in ATP is used to drive almost all cellular processes that require energy

aerobic: occurring in the presence of oxygen

anaerobic: occurring in the absence of oxygen

cellular respiration: a complex series of chemical reactions by which chemical energy stored in the bonds of food molecules is released and used to form ATP

chemical energy: the energy locked up in the chemical bonds that hold the atoms of a molecule together; food molecules, such as glucose, contain much energy in their bonds

creatine phosphate: an energy-containing molecule present in significant quantities in muscle tissue; energy is stored in a high-energy bond similar to that of ATP

enzyme: a biological catalyst that speeds up a chemical reaction without itself being used up; enzymes are made of protein, and a single enzyme can usually only catalyze a single chemical reaction

nicotinamide adenine dinucleotide (NAD): a molecule used to hold pairs of electrons when they have been removed from a molecule by some biological process; the empty molecule is denoted by NAD+, while it is denoted as NADH when it is carrying electrons

STRUCTURE AND FUNCTIONS

Glycolysis is the first step in the process that cells use to extract energy from food molecules. Although energy can be extracted from most types of food molecule, glycolysis is usually considered to begin with glucose. In fact, the term "glycolysis" actually means the splitting (*lysis*) of glucose (*glyco*). This is a good description for the process, since the glucose molecule is split into two halves. The glucose molecule consists of a backbone of six carbon atoms to which are attached, in various ways, twelve hydrogen atoms and six oxygen atoms. The glucose molecule is inherently stable and unlikely to split spontaneously at any appreciable rate.

When the energy is extracted from a glucose molecule, it is stored, for the short term, in a much less stable molecule called adenosine triphosphate (ATP). The ATP molecule consists of a complex organic molecule (adenosine) to which are attached three simple phosphate groups (see figure).

found anywhere else in the molecule. While the first phosphate is attached by what one could call a "normal" chemical bond, the second and third phosphates are attached by high-energy bonds. These are chemical bonds that require a considerable amount of energy to create. Thus ATP is an ideal energy storage molecule that provides readily available energy for the biosynthetic reactions of the cell and other energy-requiring processes.

When one of the high-energy bonds of ATP is broken, a large amount of energy is released. Usually, only the bond holding the last phosphate is broken, producing a molecule of adenosine diphosphate (ADP) and a free phosphate group. The phosphate group is only split from ATP at the precise moment when energy is required by some other process in the cell. This breaking of ATP provides the energy to drive cellular processes. The processes include activities such as the synthesis of molecules, the movement of molecules, and the contraction of muscle. The third phosphate can be reattached to ADP using energy released from glycolysis, or by other components of cellular respiration. The production of ATP can be diagrammed as follows: "energy from glycolysis + ADP + phosphate → ATP." Similarly, the breakdown of ATP can be diagrammed as "ATP → ADP + phosphate + usable energy." With this understanding of how ATP works, one can look at how it is generated in the cell by glycolysis.

The first step in the production of energy from sugar is really an energy-consuming process. Since glucose is inherently a stable molecule, it must be activated before it will split. It is activated by attaching a phosphate group to each end of the six-carbon backbone. These phosphate groups are supplied by ATP. Therefore, glycolysis begins by using the energy from two ATP molecules. The atoms of the glucose molecule are also rearranged during the activation process so that it is changed into a very similar sugar, fructose. A fructose molecule with a phosphate group on either end is called fructose 1,6-diphosphate. Thus one can summarize the activation process as "glucose + 2 ATP → fructose 1,6-diphosphate + 2 ADP."

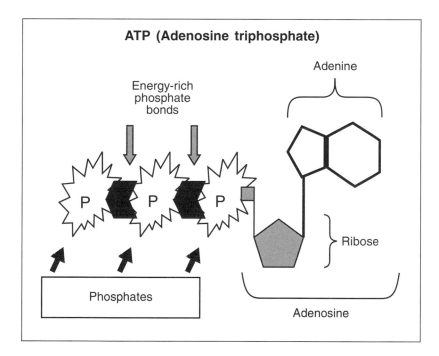

ATP (Adenosine triphosphate)

Energy-rich phosphate bonds

Adenine

P   P   P

Phosphates

Ribose

Adenosine

ATP consists of a five-carbon sugar called ribose, linked on one side to the nitrogenous base adenine and on the other side to a linear chain of phosphate groups. The molecule formed by the attachment of adenine to ribose is called adenosine, and the linkage of three phosphates generates adenosine triphosphate. The first phosphate is attached to the ribose sugar by means of a chemical bond whose energy is no greater than those bonds

Fructose 1,6-diphosphate is a much more reactive molecule and can be readily split by an enzyme called aldolase into two three-carbon compounds called dihydroxyacetone phosphate (DHAP) and glyceraldehyde 3-phosphate (G3P). DHAP is converted into G3P by an enzyme called triose phosphate isomerase, which makes G3P the starting point for all the following steps of glycolysis. Each G3P undergoes several reactions, but only the more consequential reactions will be mentioned. G3P undergoes an oxidation reaction, catalyzed by an enzyme called glyceraldehyde 3-phosphate dehydrogenase. Oxidation reactions involve the loss of high-energy electrons. Electrons are highly energetic and have a negative electrical charge. They are picked up and carried by molecules specially designed for this purpose.

These energy-carrying molecules are called nicotinamide adenine dinucleotide (NAD). Biologists have agreed on a conventional notation for this molecule to allow the reader to know whether the molecule is carrying electrons or is empty. Since the empty molecule has a net positive charge, it is denoted as NAD^+. When full, it holds a pair of electrons. One electron would neutralize the positive charge, while two result in a negative charge. The negative charge attracts one of the many hydrogen ions (H^+) in the cell. Thus when carrying electrons the molecule is denoted NADH. G3P surrenders two high-energy electrons to NAD^+. The G3P molecule also picks up a free phosphate group at the end opposite from where one is already attached to form 1,3-bisphosphoglycerate. One can summarize the reaction as "2 Glyceraldehyde 3-phosphate + 2 NAD^+ + 2 inorganic phosphates → ? 2 1,3-bisphosphoglycerate + NADH + H^+." The following reactions merely transfer the energy in these chemical bonds to high-energy bonds by transferring these phosphate groups to ADP molecules to produce ATP. Since each G3P eventually produces two ATPs, and two G3Ps are produced from each original glucose molecule, glycolysis produces four ATP molecules all together. However since two ATPs were used to activate the glucose, the cell has a net gain of two ATP molecules for each glucose molecule used.

The rearrangement of the atoms leaves them in a form called pyruvate. Pyruvate still contains much energy locked up in its chemical bonds. In most of the cells of the body and most of the time, pyruvate will be further broken down and all of its energy released. This further breakdown of pyruvate requires oxygen and is beyond the scope of this topic. It should be pointed out,

however, that the complete breakdown of two molecules of pyruvate can produce more than thirty additional ATP molecules. With the addition of oxygen, the end products are the simple molecules of carbon dioxide and water.

The oxidative pathways that completely break down pyruvate are limited by the lack of oxygen in very active muscles. The ability to deal with electrons from NADH is also drastically reduced. Glycolysis can continue even in the absence of oxygen, but the electrons produced by glycolysis must be dealt with.

There is a very limited amount of NAD+ in each cell. NAD+ is designed to hold electrons briefly, while they are transferred to some other system. In the absence of oxygen, the electrons are transferred to pyruvate. Since pyruvate cannot be broken down without oxygen, there is an ample supply. Transferring electrons from NADH to pyruvate allows the empty NAD+ to pick up more electrons produced by glycolysis. Therefore, glycolysis can continue producing two ATP molecules from each glucose molecule used. While two ATPs per glucose molecule is a small amount compared to the more than thirty ATPs produced by oxidative metabolism, it is better than none at all.

The process of generating energy (ATPs) in the absence of oxygen is referred to as fermentation. Most people are familiar with the fermentation of grapes to produce wine. Yeast has the enzymes to transfer electrons from NADH to a derivative of pyruvate and to convert the resulting molecule into alcohol and carbon dioxide. No further energy is obtained from this process. Alcohol still contains much of the energy that was in glucose. Humans and other mammals have different enzymes than yeast cells. These enzymes transfer the electrons from NADH to pyruvate, producing lactate.

GLYCOLYSIS AND MUSCLE ACTIVITY

When yeast is fermented anaerobically (without oxygen), it will continue producing alcohol until it poisons itself. Most yeast cannot tolerate more than about 12 percent alcohol, the concentration found in most wine. The lactate produced by fermentation in humans is also poisonous. People, however, do not respire completely anaerobically. The two ATPs produced per glucose molecule used are simply not enough to supply the energy needs of most human cells. Muscle cells have to be somewhat of an exception. There are times when one asks the muscle cells to use energy much faster than one can supply them with oxygen. One may consider a muscle working under various levels of physical activity and examine its oxygen requirements and waste products.

At rest, a muscle requires very little ATP energy. For an individual sitting on the couch watching television, energy demands are minimal. The lungs inhale and exhale slowly and take in enough oxygen to keep its concentration in the blood high. A relatively slow heart rate can pump enough of this oxygen-rich blood to the muscles to supply their very minimal needs. As soon as one uses a muscle, however, its ATP consumption increases dramatically. Even if an individual simply walks as far as the refrigerator, large quantities of ATP are required to cause the leg muscles to contract. Muscle cells maintain a constant level of ATP so that, as soon as one asks a muscle to contract, it can do so. The ATP that is broken down is almost instantly regenerated from an additional energy store peculiar to muscle cells. Creatine phosphate is a molecule similar to ATP, in that the phosphate group is attached by a high-energy bond. There is more creatine phosphate in muscle cells than ATP. As soon as ATP is broken down, phosphates, and their high-energy bonds, are transferred from creatine phosphate. Within the first few seconds of activity, the ATP concentration in a muscle cell remains almost constant, but the creatine phosphate level begins to drop.

As soon as the creatine phosphate concentration drops, the aerobic (oxygen-requiring) respiratory processes speed up. These processes break down glucose all the way to carbon dioxide and water and release plenty of ATP. This ATP can then be used for muscle contraction. If the muscle has now stopped contracting, the new ATP produced will be used to rebuild the store of creatine phosphate.

Within the first minute or so of muscle contraction, the use of oxygen can be quite high. The circulatory system has not yet responded to this increased oxygen demand. Muscle tissue, however, has a reserve of oxygen. The red color of most mammalian muscles is attributable to the presence of myoglobin, which is similar to hemoglobin in that it has a strong affinity for oxygen. The myoglobin stores oxygen directly in the muscle, so that the muscle can operate aerobically while the circulatory and respiratory systems adjust to the increased oxygen demand.

At low or moderate muscle activity, the carbon dioxide produced by aerobic respiration in muscles will trigger an increase in the activity of both the circulatory and the respiratory systems. The increased demand for oxygen by the muscles is supplied by an increased blood flow. Jogging around a track or participating in aerobic exercises would be considered low to moderate muscular activity. Respiration rate and pulse rate both increase with jogging. This increase in oxygen supply to the muscles provides all that they need. The level of creatine phosphate will be lower than that in resting muscles, but it will soon be replenished when the activity is stopped. The muscle cells have a good supply of food molecules in the form of glycogen. Glycogen is simply a long string of glucose molecules connected together for convenient storage. At a rate of activity such as that created by jogging, the glycogen supply can last for hours. Even after it is used up, glycogen stored in the liver can be broken down to glucose and carried to the muscles by the blood. An individual will probably want to stop jogging before his or her muscles will want to quit.

High levels of muscular activity pose a different set of problems. After more than about a minute of vigorous exercise, the muscles begin to use ATP faster than oxygen can be supplied to regenerate it. The additional ATP is supplied by lactic acid fermentation. Glucose is only broken down as far as pyruvate, then converted to lactate by the addition of electrons from NADH. Lactate begins to accumulate in the muscle tissue. Since the body is still using large amounts of ATP but not taking in enough oxygen, it is said to enter a state of oxygen debt. When the muscular activity ends, the oxygen debt is repaid.

One can use an example of someone running to catch a bus, sprinting for 50 yards at full speed. That is not enough time for the circulation and lungs to respond to the increased demand for oxygen. The muscles have made up the difference between supply and demand with lactic acid fermentation. The individual now sits down in the bus and pants—to repay his or her oxygen debt.

Some of the oxygen will go to replenish the store in muscle myoglobin. Some of it will be used in oxidative metabolism in the muscle to replenish the reserves of creatine phosphate. The rest will be used to deal with the accumulated lactate. The lactate is not all dealt with in the muscle where it was produced. Being a small molecule, it easily enters the bloodstream. In muscles throughout the body, it can be converted back to pyruvate. Pyruvate can then reenter the oxidative pathway and be used to generate ATP, with the use of oxygen. The lactate, then, is being used as a food molecule to supply the needs of resting muscle. Much of the lactate is metabolized in the liver. Some of it will be metabolized with oxygen to produce the energy to convert the rest of it back to glucose. The glucose can then be circulated in the blood or stored in the liver or muscles as glycogen. A minimal amount of lactate is excreted in the urine or in sweat.

If the subject of the preceding example kept running at full speed, having missed the bus and run all the way to the office, lactate would build up in the muscles and in the blood. If the office was far enough away, the subject would eventually reach the point of exhaustion and stop running. At that point, the level of lactate in the leg muscles would be high enough to inhibit the enzymes of glycolysis. Glycolysis would slow down so that lactate would not become any more concentrated. The muscles' supply of creatine phosphate would be almost exhausted, but the ATP supply would be only slightly lower than in a resting muscle. The body is protected from damaging itself: Too much lactate would lower the pH to dangerous levels, and the absolute lack of ATP causes muscles to lock, as in rigor mortis. The body's self-protection mechanisms force one to stop before either of these conditions exists. Once the subject stops running, and pants long enough, he or she can continue. The additional oxygen taken in by increased respiration will have metabolized a sufficient amount of lactate to allow the muscles to start working again.

In cases where an individual has an inherited deficiency of particular enzymes of glycolysis, the consequences for muscle tissue are rather dire. Muscles, which depend heavily on glycolysis when operating under conditions of oxygen debt, fail to perform well if any of the glycolytic enzymes are defective. Symptoms include frequent muscle cramps, easy fatigability, and evidence of heavy muscle damage after strenuous exertion.

GLYCOLYSIS AND RED BLOOD CELL FUNCTION

Red blood cells are the oxygen-ferrying units of the bloodstream and are filled with an iron-containing protein called hemoglobin. Hemoglobin binds oxygen tightly when oxygen concentrations are high and releases oxygen when oxygen concentrations are low. In order to perform their task successfully, red blood cells must maintain the health and functionality of their hemoglobin stores, and glycolysis helps them do that. In red blood cells, approximately 90 to 95 percent of the glucose that enters the cell is metabolized to lactate by means of glycolysis and lactate dehydrogenase. The ATP generated by glycolysis is used to bring charged atoms into the cell such as calcium, potassium, and others. The NADH generated by glycolysis is also used to

maintain the iron found in hemoglobin in a state that allows it to bind oxygen. Glycolysis is also used to form the metabolite 2,3-DPG (2,3-Diphosphoglycerate). 2,3-DPG binds to hemoglobin and forces it to release oxygen more readily when oxygen concentrations are low. Thus 2,3-DPG aids hemoglobin delivery of oxygen to the tissues.

Abnormalities in the enzymes that catalyze the reactions of glycolysis are inherited. Individuals who inherit two copies of a gene that encodes a mutant form of a glycolytic enzyme experience uncontrolled destruction of red blood cells (hemolysis). The red blood cell destruction that results from defects in glycolytic enzymes is chronic and not ameliorated by drugs. An enlarged spleen is a typical symptom of glycolytic enzyme abnormalities as the spleen tends to fill with dying red blood cells. The red blood cell destruction can be so severe that blood transfusions might be necessary. Removal of the spleen reduces red blood cell destruction.

INSULIN, DIABETES, AND GLYCOLYSIS

Glycolysis is heavily regulated by the hormones insulin and glucagon. Insulin, a hormone made and released by the beta cells of the pancreatic islets, stimulates the insertion of the GLUT4 glucose transporter into the membranes of cells. People with Type I diabetes mellitus, who are incapable of making sufficient quantities of insulin, tend to have very high blood sugar readings, since their cells cannot receive the signal to insert the glucose transporter into their membranes and take up glucose from the blood. This prevents the removal of glucose from the blood, and in Type I diabetics the blood glucose level climbs to abnormally high levels. GLUT4 allows the uptake of glucose without the input of energy. Therefore, glycolysis occurs as fast as the cells can take up glucose.

Insulin also stimulates the synthesis of a metabolite called fructose 2,6-bisphosphate. Fructose 2,6-bisphosphate is a potent activator of phosphofructokinase, and activation of this enzyme ensures the activation of glycolysis. Insulin also activates the expression of genes that encode the protein involved in glycolysis. During uncontrolled diabetes, reduced glucose transport in muscle inhibits muscle cell glycolysis. In liver cells, reduced glycolytic gene expression and attenuation of the levels of fructose 2,6-bisphosphate reduce glycolysis. This contributes to the voluntary muscle weakness, liver dysfunction, and heart problems that are sometimes observed in diabetics.

GLYCOLYSIS AND CANCER

The uptake of glucose and its degradation by glycolysis occurs ten times faster in tumor cells than in nontumor cells. This phenomenon, called the Warburg effect, seems to benefit tumor cells, since they lack an extensive capillary network to feed them oxygen and must rely on anaerobic glycolysis to generate ATP.

Oxygen-poor conditions also induce the synthesis of a protein called hypoxia-inducible factor (HIF). HIF is a transcription factor that helps turn on the expression of specific genes that help cells survive oxygen-poor conditions. The synthesis of at least eight glycolytic enzymes are activated by HIF. These fundamental observations of cancer cells have shown that glycolytic enzymes are excellent potential drug targets for anticancer agents.

PERSPECTIVE AND PROSPECTS

Cellular respiration is the process by which organisms harvest usable energy in the form of ATP molecules from food molecules. Lactic acid fermentation is the form of respiration used by human muscles when oxygen is in limited supply. Glycolysis is the energy-producing component of lactic acid fermentation, which is much less efficient than aerobic cellular respiration. Fermentation harvests only two molecules of ATP for every glucose molecule used, while aerobic respiration produces a yield of more than thirty molecules of ATP. Most forms of life will only resort to fermentation when oxygen is absent or in short supply. While higher forms of life such as humans can obtain energy by fermentation for short periods, they incur an oxygen debt that must eventually be repaid. The yield of two molecules of ATP for each glucose molecule used is simply not enough to sustain their high demand for energy.

Nevertheless, lactic acid fermentation is an important source of ATP for humans during strenuous physical exercise. Even though it is an inefficient use of glucose, it can provide enough ATP for a short burst of activity. After the activity is over, the lactate produced must be dealt with, which usually requires the use of oxygen.

Most popular exercise programs focus on aerobic activity. Aerobic exercises do not place stress on muscles to the point where the blood cannot supply enough oxygen. These exercises are designed to improve the efficiency of the oxygen delivery system so that there is less need for anaerobic metabolism. Training programs in general attempt to tune the body so that the need for

lactic acid fermentation is reduced. They concentrate on improving the delivery of oxygen to the muscles, storing oxygen in the muscles, or increasing the efficiency of muscular contraction.

Insulin signaling activates glycolysis whereas another pancreatic peptide hormone, glucagon, inhibits glycolysis. Diabetics can suffer from inadequate glycolytic activity in particular organs, which can result in organ dysfunction. Expression of mutant forms of various glycolytic enzymes or supporting enzymes in transgenic mice has elucidated the link between abnormalities in glycolysis and the pathology of diabetes mellitus.

Over eighty years ago, the German biochemist Otto Warburg demonstrated that cancer cells voraciously take up glucose and metabolize to lactate. Glycolysis is very active in cancer cells and helps them flourish under low-oxygen conditions. The development of new glycolytic inhibitors may constitute a new class of anticancer drugs that have wide-ranging therapeutic applications.

—James Waddell, Ph.D.;
updated by Michael A. Buratovich, Ph.D.
See also Cells; Enzymes; Exercise physiology; Food biochemistry; Metabolism; Muscles; Sports medicine.

FOR FURTHER INFORMATION:

Alberts, Bruce, et al. *Essential Cell Biology*. 2d ed. New York: Garland, 2004. Lively, well-written introduction to cell structure and function, packed with exceptionally high quality diagrams.

Campbell, Neil A., et al. *Biology: Concepts and Connections*. 5th ed. San Francisco: Pearson/Benjamin Cummings, 2006. This classic introductory textbook provides an excellent discussion of essential biological structures and mechanisms. Its extensive and detailed illustrations help to make even difficult concepts accessible to the nonspecialist.

Fox, Stuart I. *Human Physiology*. 9th ed. New York, McGraw-Hill, 2006. A college-level human physiology textbook that is richly illustrated and so well written that even high school students could benefit from it. Chapter 5 has a very good discussion of glycolysis and its physiological uses and consequences.

Nelson, David L. and Michael A. Cox. *Lehninger Principles of Biochemistry*. 4th ed. New York, W. H. Freeman, 2005. Chapters 14 and 15 explain glycolysis, its regulation, mechanisms and physiological consequences in extreme detail but with perspicuous clarity.

Sackheim, George I., and Dennis D. Lehman. *Chemistry for the Health Sciences*. 8th ed. Upper Saddle River, N.J.: Prentice-Hall, 1998. An accessible guide to the chemical processes involved in human health. Stresses the relationship between inorganic chemistry and the life processes.

Shephard, Roy J. *Biochemistry of Physical Activity*. Springfield, Ill.: Charles C Thomas, 1984. Chapter 3, "Carbohydrates and Phosphagen," provides a detailed description of energy production and use in muscles.

Wu, Chaodong, et al. "Regulation of Glycolysis: The Role of Insulin." *Experimental Gerontology* 40 (2005): 894-899. The positive regulation of glycolysis by insulin and how perturbation of the insulin pathway decreases glycolysis in various tissues.

GOITER

DISEASE/DISORDER

ANATOMY OR SYSTEM AFFECTED: Endocrine system, glands, neck

SPECIALTIES AND RELATED FIELDS: Endocrinology

DEFINITION: An enlargement of the thyroid gland that is noncancerous and not caused by a temporary condition such as inflammation.

KEY TERMS:

goitrogenic: referring to a factor (typically food or chemicals) that produces goiter

hypersection: the excess production and secretion of a hormone or other chemical

CAUSES AND SYMPTOMS

Goiter is often a painless medical condition. Its only visible symptoms may be a slight but visible enlargement of the thyroid that creates a swelling at the base of the neck. In severe cases, the swelling becomes massive and the patient experiences difficulty breathing or swallowing as the enlarged thyroid compresses against the windpipe or esophagus. Other symptoms that may indicate goiter include weight loss, increased heart rate, elevated blood pressure, hair loss, and tremors. Goiter can be confirmed by ultrasound scan of the thyroid, blood tests for abnormal levels of thyroxine or thyroid-stimulating hormone, or low rates of iodine excretion in the urine.

The several types of medical goiter fall into two broad categories, simple goiter and toxic goiter. Simple goiter is caused by a dietary deficiency of iodine. In response, one or both lobes of the thyroid gland enlarge in an attempt to produce more of the iodine-containing

---

INFORMATION ON GOITER

CAUSES: Of simple goiter, iodine deficiency or hormonal changes (adolescence, pregnancy); of toxic goiter, excessive production of thyroxine from oversecretion of thyroid-stimulating hormone by pituitary

SYMPTOMS: Thyroid enlargement ranging from slight to massive, with difficulty breathing or swallowing

DURATION: Acute or chronic

TREATMENTS: Iodine tablets, sometimes surgical removal of all or part of thyroid

---

hormone thyroxine. Two types of simple goiter are recognized, endemic goiter and sporadic goiter.

Endemic goiter typically occurs in land-locked geographic regions or in areas where farm soils are iodine-depleted. Simple goiter was once common in areas of central Asia, central Africa, and the so-called Goiter Belt of the United States, which extended from the Great Lakes to the Intermountain West (between the Rockies and the Sierras).

Simple goiter most often appears in adolescence, but it may sometimes occur during pregnancy. This condition should be corrected in pregnant women to ensure the healthy development of the fetus and the birth of a healthy infant. Simple goiter readily responds to treatment via iodine tablets, but in some patients surgical removal of all or part of the enlarged thyroid may be necessary. Public health measures undertaken to eliminate or prevent simple goiter include the addition of iodine to table salt and also to water reservoirs in certain areas.

Sporadic goiter occurs in some individuals because of an excessive consumption of goitrogenic (goiter-causing) foods, such as cabbage, soybeans, spinach, and radishes. Sporadic goiter has also been linked with exposure to certain medications, such as aminoglutethimide or lithium. Although this type of goiter is considered nontoxic, it does produce impaired thyroid activity. Sporadic goiter can be treated by limiting the consumption of goitrogenic foods.

Toxic goiter is caused by an excessive production of thyroxine hormone by the thyroid gland. This type of goiter is also called hyperthyroid goiter, exopthalmic goiter, or Graves' disease. Toxic goiter results from an oversecretion (hypersecretion) of thyroid-stimulating hormone by the pituitary. In turn, the thyroid gland responds by enlarging and secreting excess amounts of

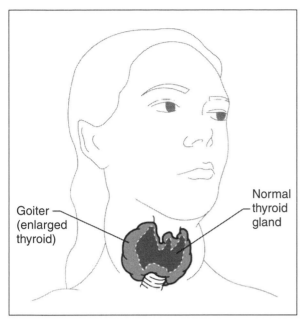

Goiter (enlarged thyroid); dashed lines show relative size of normal thyroid.

thyroxine, resulting in goiter. Symptoms of Graves' disease include elevated metabolic rate, higher body temperature, rapid weight loss, nervousness, and irritability. In some patients, this type of goiter results in protrusive eyeballs and the appearance of staring.

Euthyroid goiter occurs when dietary levels of iodine are only slightly below normal. The pituitary gland responds to lowered thyroxine levels in the blood by producing additional thyroid-stimulating hormone. The thyroid gland responds to the elevated thyroid-stimulating hormone by enlarging in an effort to increase thyroxine production.

TREATMENT AND THERAPY

Most goiters can be treated effectively through dietary supplements of iodine. The administration of iodine supplements must be very carefully regulated, however, to prevent a so-called thyroxin storm resulting from excess thyroxine production by the enlarged thyroid gland. Some patients may choose alternative natural herbal therapies taken in tablet form, but these substances should be used only in consultation with a physician.

—Dwight G. Smith, Ph.D.

See also Endocrine disorders; Endocrinology; Endocrinology, pediatric; Hyperparathyroidism and Hypoparathyroidism; Malnutrition; Thyroid disorders; Thyroid gland; Thyroidectomy.

FOR FURTHER INFORMATION:

DeMaeyer, E. M. *The Control of Endemic Goiter.* Washington, D.C.: World Health Organization, 1988. Informational booklet published by the World Health Organization.

Gaitan, Eduardo, ed. *Environmental Goitrogenesis.* Boca Raton, Fla.: CRC Press, 1989. Comprehensive and balanced treatment of all forms of factors that affect thyroid condition and function.

Hall, R., and J. Köbberling, eds. *Thyroid Disorders Associated with Iodine Deficiency and Excess.* New York: Raven Press, 1985. Provides an extensive treatment of the types of goiter associated with dietary deficiency of iodine.

Hamburger, J. I. *Nontoxic Goiter: Concept and Controversy.* Springfield, Ill.: Charles C Thomas, 1973. A classic review of the medicinal science of goiter.

Icon Health. *Goiter: A Medical Dictionary, Bibliography, and Annotated Research Guide to Internet References.* San Diego, Calif.: Author, 2004. Designed for physicians, medical students, researchers, and patients.

GONORRHEA

DISEASE/DISORDER

ANATOMY OR SYSTEM AFFECTED: Eyes, genitals, reproductive system, throat, urinary system

SPECIALTIES AND RELATED FIELDS: Gynecology, microbiology

DEFINITION: A common treatable sexually transmitted disease which primarily infects the reproductive tract and which is caused by the bacterium *Neisseria gonorrhea.*

KEY TERMS:

contact tracing: also known as partner referral; a process that consists of identifying the sexual partners of infected patients, informing these partners of their exposure to disease, and offering resources for counseling and treatment

screening procedures: tests that are carried out in populations which are usually asymptomatic and at high risk for a disease in order to identify those in need of treatment

sexually transmitted disease: an infection caused by organisms transferred through sexual contact (genital-genital, oral-genital, oral-anal, or anal-genital); the transmission of infection occurs through exposure to lesions or secretions that contain the organisms

CAUSES AND SYMPTOMS

Gonorrhea is the second most common sexually transmitted disease (STD) in the United States, the most common being chlamydia. In the United States, the incidence of gonorrhea has fallen. In 1995, the incidence was about 150 cases out of every 100,000 population, down from the mid-1970's of more than 400 cases. The highest incidence of gonorrhea is in sexually active men and women under twenty-five years of age.

Gonorrhea is caused by the bacterium *Neisseria gonorrhea*, a gram-negative diplococcus. The bacterium infects the mucous membranes with which it comes in contact, most commonly the urethra and the cervix but also the throat, rectum, and eyes. Some men will be asymptomatic, but most will experience urinary discomfort and a purulent urethral discharge. Long-term complications of this infection in men include epididymitis, prostatitis, and urethral strictures (scarring). In women, the disease is more likely to be asymptomatic. Women with symptoms may have purulent vaginal discharge, urinary discomfort, urethral discharge, lower abdominal discomfort, or pain with intercourse. Pelvic inflammatory disease (PID) and its consequences may occur if gonorrheal infection ascends past the cervix into the upper genital tract (uterus, Fallopian tubes, ovaries, and pelvic cavity) in women. Complications of PID include infertility and an increased risk of ectopic pregnancy.

In rare cases, gonorrhea can enter the bloodstream and disseminate throughout the body, causing fever, joint pain, and skin lesions. Gonorrhea can infect the heart valves, pericardium, and meninges as well. When it infects the joints, a condition known as septic arthritis occurs, characterized by pain and swelling of the joints and potential destruction of the joints.

Gonorrhea can be transmitted to infants through the birth canal, leading to an eye infection that can damage the eye and impair vision. Fortunately, erythromycin eye drops are routinely given to newborns to prevent eye infection. These eyedrops are effective against *Neisseria gonorrhea* as well as *Chlamydia trachomatis*.

TREATMENT AND THERAPY

Treatment for gonorrhea consists of antibiotics. With the development of penicillin-resistant strains of gonorrhea, effective therapy relies on antibiotics to which gonorrhea remains susceptible, such as cef-triaxone. In uncomplicated cases of gonorrheal infection, such as cervicitis, a single dose is given.

A patient who has risk factors for STDs and a clinical picture suggestive of gonorrhea may receive treatment presumptively, before confirmatory laboratory test results for gonorrhea are available. Because a large number of patients with gonorrhea also have chlamydia, patients are treated concomitantly with an antibiotic directed against chlamydia, such as doxycycline. Once laboratory test results confirm the diagnosis of gonorrhea, the patient is tested for other STDs, such as human immunodeficiency virus (HIV), hepatitis B and C, and syphilis.

As with all STDs, a key component of therapy includes counseling regarding safe sex. This includes the use of barrier contraceptives, such as condoms, and the avoidance of high-risk sexual behaviors. Contact tracing is another important element to STD treatment. It notifies the patient's sexual partners of their exposure to gonorrhea or other STDs. Contact tracing also involves offering resources to these partners for medical attention. Contact tracing can prevent both reinfection of the patient through subsequent sexual encounters and the spread of STDs to other sexual partners that the patient's partner may have.

PERSPECTIVE AND PROSPECTS

The symptoms of gonorrhea have been described in numerous cultures in the past, including those dating back to the ancient Chinese, Egyptians, and Romans. The actual gonorrhea bacterium was first identified by Albert Neisser in the 1870's, and it was one of the first bacteria ever discovered. *Neisseria gonorrhea* has continued to be well-studied on both the molecular and the epidemiological level.

INFORMATION ON GONORRHEA

CAUSES: Bacterial infection through intercourse

SYMPTOMS: In men, sometimes urinary discomfort and discharge, with long-term complications of epididymitis, prostatitis, and urethral scarring; in women, sometimes vaginal discharge, urinary discomfort, urethral discharge, lower abdominal discomfort, and pain with intercourse, with possible pelvic inflammatory disease, infertility, and increased risk of ectopic pregnancy

DURATION: Acute

TREATMENTS: Antibiotics, counseling regarding safe sex

Antibiotic therapy, in the form of sulfanilamide, was first used to combat *N. gonorrhea* in the 1930's. By the 1940's, however, gonococcal strains resistant to this antibiotic appeared, and the therapy of choice became penicillin. Over the next several decades, *N. gonorrhea* evolved the ability to resist penicillin, forcing clinicians to use other drugs to combat the bacterium, such as ceftriaxone and ciprofloxacin. In the 1980's, the Centers for Disease Control instituted surveillance programs to monitor antibiotic resistance patterns in different United States cities. Continued success in combating *N. gonorrhea* will depend on the ability to minimize the development of antibiotic resistance.

Finally, since many patients with gonorrhea infection have no symptoms, screening programs of asymptomatic patients who are in high-risk groups (those younger than twenty-five and/or with multiple sexual partners) play a vital role in decreasing the incidence of *N. gonorrhea* infections.

—*Anne Lynn S. Chang, M.D.*

See also Blindness; Conjunctivitis; Eyes; Genital disorders, female; Genital disorders, male; Gynecology; Reproductive system; Sexually transmitted diseases (STDs); Urology.

FOR FURTHER INFORMATION:

Centers for Disease Control and Prevention. *Sexually Transmitted Diseases Treatment Guidelines 2006.* Atlanta: Author, 2006.

Holmes, King K., et al., eds. *Sexually Transmitted Diseases.* 3d ed. New York: McGraw-Hill, 1999.

Kasper, Dennis L., et al., eds. *Harrison's Principles of Internal Medicine.* 16th ed. New York: McGraw-Hill, 2005.

Ryan, Kenneth J., and C. George Ray, eds. *Sherris Medical Microbiology: An Introduction to Infectious Diseases.* 4th ed. New York: McGraw-Hill, 2004.

Sutton, Amy L., ed. *Sexually Transmitted Diseases Sourcebook.* 3d ed. Detroit: Omnigraphics, 2006.

GOUT

DISEASE/DISORDER

ALSO KNOWN AS: Gouty arthritis

ANATOMY OR SYSTEM AFFECTED: Feet, joints

SPECIALTIES AND RELATED FIELDS: Internal medicine, podiatry, rheumatology

DEFINITION: A form of arthritis of the peripheral joints, often characterized by painful, recurrent acute attacks and resulting from deposits of uric acid in joint spaces.

KEY TERMS:

acute gout: a very painful gout attack, most common in the left big toe; usually the first indicator of occurrence of the disease

arthritis: any of more than a hundred related diseases, including gout, that are characterized by joint inflammation

cartilage: a tough, white, fibrous connective tissue attached to the bone surfaces that is involved in movement

corticosteroid: a fatlike steroid hormone made by the adrenal glands, or similar synthetic chemicals manufactured by pharmaceutical companies

gene: a piece of the hereditary material deoxyribonucleic acid (DNA) that carries the information needed to produce an inheritable characteristic

genetic engineering: also called recombinant DNA research; a group of scientific techniques that allow scientists to alter genes

hyperuricemia: the presence of abnormally high uric acid levels, which usually leads to gout symptoms

rheumatologist: a physician who studies rheumatoid arthritis and related diseases

secondary gout: gout symptoms caused by other diseases and by therapeutic drugs

synovial fluid: the thick, clear, lubricating fluid that bathes joints and helps them to move smoothly

tophaceous gout: chronic gout that may be characterized by tophi, severe joint degeneration, and/or serious kidney problems

tophi: lumps in the cartilage and joints of chronic gout sufferers, caused by crystals of uric acid

CAUSES AND SYMPTOMS

Gout, once called the affliction of kings, is a hereditary disease that causes inflammation of the peripheral joints. It is also called gouty arthritis because arthritis means joint inflammation and describes more than a hundred related diseases. Gout has afflicted humans since antiquity, and it was first described by Hippocrates in the fifth century B.C.E. It usually first presents itself as an extremely painful swelling of the big toe of the left foot in men over the age of forty. Gout attacks, termed acute gout, are quite rare in premenopausal women. In fact, more than 90 percent of all gout sufferers are men. The prevalence of gout is extremely high in Pacific Islanders, with 10 percent of adult males afflicted. One characteristic portrayal of gout sufferers, which may come from the "affliction of kings" concept, is of obese and obviously affluent individuals.

INFORMATION ON GOUT

CAUSES: Heredity, female hormones, disease, medications (chemotherapy, diuretics, some antibiotics)

SYMPTOMS: Joint inflammation (particularly the big toe), scarring, and deformity

DURATION: Chronic with acute episodes

TREATMENTS: Drugs, surgery, dietary changes

This is partly a misconception because gout is a very democratic disease, found in the poor as often as in the wealthy. Nevertheless, acute gout attacks are often brought on by very rich meals or by drinking sprees, so obesity is accurately portrayed as a contributing factor.

An acute gout attack may occur in almost any joint, with the most common sites after the big toe being the ankles, fingers, feet, wrists, elbows, and knees. Such attacks are not often seen in the shoulders, hips, or spine and, if they do occur, appear only after a gout sufferer has had many previous attacks in other joints. Acute gout of the big toe occurs so often that it has been given its own name, podagra. Common explanations for the very frequent occurrence of podagra are that considerable pressure is placed on the big toe in the process of walking and that most people are right-handed and are therefore "left-footed," putting more pressure on the left foot than on the right one in walking or in sports.

An acute gout attack is preceded by feelings of weakness, nausea, chills, and excessive urination. Then, the area that is affected becomes red to purple, swollen, and so tender that the slightest touch is very painful. This pain is so severe that many sufferers describe it as being crushing, or even excruciating. Acute gout attacks come on suddenly, and many victims report suddenly being jolted awake by pain in the night. Fortunately, such attacks are few and far between and usually last only from a few days to a week. In addition, more than half of those who have one attack of podagra will never have another gout attack.

The problems associated with acute gout are attributable to a chemical called uric acid. Uric acid does not dissolve well in the blood and other biological fluids, such as the synovial fluid in joints. When overproduced by the body or excreted too slowly in urine, undissolved uric acid forms sharp crystals. These crystals and their interactions with other joint components cause the pain felt by gout sufferers. It is interesting to note that gout is caused by the overproduction of uric acid in some individuals and by uric acid underexcretion in others. Many of the foods that seem to cause gout are rich in chemicals called purines, which are converted to uric acid in the course of preparation for excretion by the kidneys.

Much more dangerous to gout victims than the acute attacks is leaving the disease untreated. When this happens, crystals of uric acid produce lumps or masses in the joints throughout the body and in the kidneys. In the joints, the masses, called tophi, lead to inflammation, scarring, and deformity that can produce an irreversible degenerative process. Tophi are most common in the fingers and the cartilage of various parts of the body, and external tophi are found in the cartilage of the ears of gout sufferers. The visible tophi, however, are only representative, and undetected uric acid masses may be widely spread throughout the body. Such untreated gout is called chronic or tophaceous gout.

Tophaceous gout is another disease with a long history. It was first described by the Greek physician Galen in the second century C.E. Another extremely dangerous aspect of tophaceous gout is unseen kidney stones, which will cause great pain on urination, produce high blood pressure, and even cause fatalities in 3 to 5 percent of afflicted persons.

The prime indicator of gout is high blood levels of uric acid, called hyperuricemia; however, this condition, without other symptoms, does not always signal existent, symptomatic gout. Therefore, the best indicator of the presence of the disease is a combination of hyperuricemia, acute attacks, and observed uric acid in the synovial fluid of all troublesome, gouty joints.

Some investigators propose that gout sufferers are highly intelligent because such famous individuals as Michelangelo, Leonardo da Vinci, Martin Luther, Charles Darwin, and Benjamin Franklin were afflicted with the disease. This trend, however, may indicate that famous people are usually able to afford a lifestyle that causes the predilection to high uric acid levels (for example, the eating of purine-rich foods and high alcohol consumption). Rheumatologists who have studied gout would argue that alcoholism is a better predictor for the disease because gout is very common in heavy drinkers. In fact, studies in which gout patients were given purine-rich diets or purine-rich diets plus alcoholic beverages showed that alcohol increased the number and severity of gout attacks.

Gout is also associated with a number of other diseases, including Down syndrome, lead poisoning, some types of diabetes, psoriasis, and kidney disease.

Furthermore, a number of therapeutic drugs used in chemotherapy for cancer, diuretics, and some antibiotics can cause acute gout symptoms. These types of gout are differentiated from the hereditary disease already described—so-called primary gout—by the term "secondary gout." Drug-induced secondary gout goes away quickly when administration of the offending drug is stopped.

Another group of diseases that have symptoms somewhat similar to gout are called pseudogout. They have an entirely different cause (mineral crystals in the joints), occur in men and women with equal frequency, usually begin in extreme old age, and are treated quite differently.

It is also interesting that while premenopausal women are nearly gout-free, the disease becomes fairly common after the menopause. This fact supports a role for female hormones in preventing the disease. Primary gout in women is usually much more severe and destructive than gout in men. In those families in which maternal gout is observed, it is likely that occurrence of the disease in male offspring will occur earlier than is usual, such as near the age of thirty.

TREATMENT AND THERAPY

Once primary gout has been diagnosed, three methods are available for treating it: therapeutic drugs, surgery, and special diets. Most often, gout treatment uses therapeutic drugs, with the drug of choice being colchicine. Colchicine treatment can be traced back for thousands of years, to Egypt in 1500 B.C.E. Originally, it was given as an extract of the meadow saffron plant, *Colchicum autumnale*. In modern times, the pure chemical has been isolated for medicinal use.

Colchicine is reportedly a specific remedy for gout and has no effect on any other type of arthritis. In fact, the reversal of severe joint pain with colchicine is often used as a diagnostic tool that tells physicians that the joint disease being treated is indeed gout. Colchicine can be utilized to treat acute gout attacks or can be taken routinely for long periods of time. Its actions in the handling of acute attacks are quick and profound. In some cases, however, colchicine will have side effects, including severe stomach cramps, nausea, and diarrhea. When these effects occur, colchicine use is discontinued until they disappear and then its use is reinstituted.

Most of the basis for colchicine action is its decrease of the inflammation that causes the pain of gout attacks. This action is believed to be attributable to colchicine's interaction with white blood cells that destroy uric acid crystals and subsequent prevention of the cells from releasing inflammatory factors. Other drugs that work in this way are nonsteroidal anti-inflammatory drugs (NSAIDs) such as aspirin, ibuprofen, indomethacin, naproxen, and phenylbutazone. Colchicine and NSAIDs are usually given by mouth. In some cases, anti-inflammatory steroid hormones called corticosteroids, such as prednisone and prednisolone, are used to treat acute gout. The corticosteroids are given by injection into the gouty joint. Despite the rapid, almost miraculous effects of these steroids, they are best avoided unless absolutely necessary because they can lead to serious medical problems.

Another group of antigout medications consists of the uricosuric drugs. Two favored examples of such drugs are probenecid (Benemid) and sulfinpyrazone (Anturane). The uricosuric drugs prevent the occurrence of hyperuricemia and eventual tophaceous gout by increasing uric acid excretion in the urine, therefore lowering the uric acid levels in the blood. This lowering has two effects: the prevention of the attainment of uric acid levels in the blood and joints that lead to crystal or tophus formation and the eventual dissolution of crystals and tophi as blood levels of uric acid drop.

Uricosuric drugs have no effect, however, on an acute gout attack and can sometimes make such attacks even more painful. For this reason, uricosuric drug

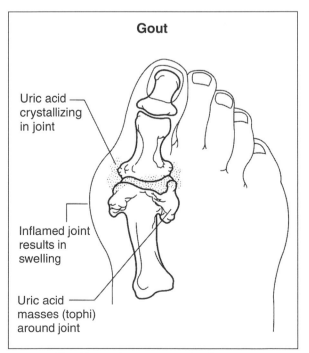

The big toe is a common site for gout.

therapy is always started after all acute gout attack symptoms have subsided. Aspirin blocks the effects of the uricosuric drugs and should be replaced with acetaminophen (for example, Tylenol) whenever they are utilized for chemotherapeutic purposes. Side effects of excessive doses of uricosuric drugs can include headache, nausea and vomiting, itching, and dizziness. Their use should be discontinued immediately when such symptoms occur. Later reuse of the uricosuric drugs is usually possible.

The third category of antigout drugs is a single chemical, allopurinol (usually, Lopurin or Zyloprim). This drug lowers the body's ability to produce uric acid. It is highly recommended for all gout-afflicted people who have kidney disease that is severe enough for kidney stones to form. It has undesired side effects, however, that include skin rashes, drowsiness, a diminished blood count, and severe allergic reactions. As a result, the use of allopurinol is disqualified for many patients. One advantage of allopurinol chemotherapy over the use of uricosuric agents is the fact that it can be taken along with aspirin.

The end result of a chemotherapeutic regimen with uricosuric drugs and/or allopurinol is the lowering of the blood and urinary uric acid levels so that crystals and tophi do not form or, where formed, redissolve. Often, their combination with colchicine is useful for preventing the occurrence of gout attacks during the initial chemotherapy period.

While surgery is not a common treatment for gout, people who have large tophi that have opened up, become infected, or interfere with joint mobility may elect to have them removed in this fashion. In some cases, severe disability or joint pain caused by the degenerative effects of long-term tophaceous gout is also corrected surgically. Care should be taken, however, to evaluate the consequences of such surgery carefully because the postoperative healing process is often quite slow and many other problems can be encountered.

Media sources often praise special diets in treating gout, without firm proof of their effectiveness. The finding that gout is usually a hereditary disease resulting from metabolic defects that either prevent uric acid excretion or cause its accumulation has pointed out that most dietary factors have a relatively small effect on the disease. Consequently, chemotherapy is much more effective than dietary intervention for diminishing gout symptoms. Nevertheless, there are several incontestable dietary aspects essential to the well-being of persons afflicted with gout.

First, dieting is quite useful, and overweight gout sufferers should lose weight. Such action is best taken slowly and under medical supervision. In fact, excessively fast weight loss can temporarily worsen gout symptoms by elevating blood uric acid levels. In addition, excesses of a number of foods should be avoided by gout sufferers because they are overly rich in the purines that give rise to uric acid when the body processes them. Some examples are the organ meats (liver, kidneys, and sweetbreads), mushrooms, anchovies, sardines, caviar, gravy and meat extracts, shellfish, wine, and beer. Modest intake of these foods is allowable. For example, the daily intake of one can of beer, a glass of wine, or an ounce or two of hard liquor is permissible. The gout sufferer should remember that excessive alcohol intake often brings on acute gout attacks and, even worse, will contribute to worsening tophus and kidney stone formation.

Another adjunct to the prevention or diminution of gout symptoms is the daily intake of at least a half gallon of water or other nonalcoholic beverages. This will help to flush uric acid out of the body, in the urine, and may help to dissipate both tophi and kidney stones. Plain water is best, as it contains no calories that will increase body weight, potentially aggravating gout and leading to other health problems.

Perspective and Prospects

Many sources agree that primary gout is under control in most afflicted people, who can look forward to a normal life without permanent adverse effects from the disease. Those individuals who seek medical treatment at the first appearance of gout symptoms may combine chemotherapy, an appropriate diet regimen, and alcohol avoidance to prevent all but a few acute attacks of the disease. In addition, they will not develop tophi or kidney problems.

Even those afflicted persons who put off treatment until kidney stones or tophi appear can be helped easily. Again, an appropriate diet and the wise choice of chemotherapy agents will prevail. Only the patients who neglect all gout treatment until excessive joint damage and severe kidney disease occur are at serious risk, yet even with these individuals, remission of most severe symptoms is usually possible. The long-term neglect of gout symptoms is unwise, however, because severe tophaceous gout can be both deforming and fatal.

Currently, the eradication of most primary gout, not gout treatment, is seen as the desired goal of research. It is believed that a prime methodology for the eradication of gout will be the use of genetic engineering for gene replacement therapy. Primary gout sufferers are victims of gene lesion diseases: Their bodies lack the ability, because of defective genes, to control either the production or the excretion of uric acid. It is hoped that gene replacement technology will enable medical science to add the missing genes back into their bodies. Other research aspects viewed worthy of exploration in the attempts to vanquish primary gout are the understanding of how to cause white blood cells to destroy uric acid crystals in the joints more effectively and safely and to decode the basis for the gout-preventing effects of female hormones related to their presence in premenopausal women.

—*Sanford S. Singer, Ph.D.*

See also Alcoholism; Arthritis; Down syndrome; Feet; Foot disorders; Lead poisoning; Obesity; Podiatry; Rheumatology; Urinary disorders.

FOR FURTHER INFORMATION:

Beers, Mark H., et al. *The Merck Manual of Diagnosis and Therapy*. 18th ed. Whitehouse Station, N.J.: Merck Research Laboratories, 2006. Contains a useful exposition of the characteristics, etiology, diagnosis, and treatment of gout and its relationship to other forms of arthritis. Designed for physicians, the material is also useful for less specialized readers. Information on related topics is also included.

Devlin, Thomas M., ed. *Textbook of Biochemistry: With Clinical Correlations*. 6th ed. Hoboken, N.J.: Wiley-Liss, 2006. This college textbook presents considerable information on gout, hormones, genetic engineering, and related topics. Includes chemical structures, diagrams, and references useful to the reader. All descriptions are simple but scholarly.

Fries, James F. *Arthritis: A Take-Care-of-Yourself Health Guide for Understanding Your Arthritis*. 5th ed. Reading, Mass.: Addison-Wesley, 1999. Covers gout and pseudogout in a chapter on crystal arthritis, discussing the features, prognosis, and treatments of both problems. Crystal arthritis types are very well differentiated and integrated into the consideration of arthritis.

Parker, James N., and Philip M. Parker, eds. *The 2002 Official Patient's Sourcebook on Gout*. San Diego, Calif.: Icon Health, 2002. Draws from public, academic, government, and peer-reviewed research to provide a wide-ranging handbook for patients with gout.

PDR Guide to Drug Interactons, Side Effects, and Inductions 2007. Montvale, N.J.: Thomson Healthcare, 2007. This atlas of prescription drugs includes those used against gout—their manufacturers, useful dose ranges, metabolism and toxicology, and contraindications. This text, found in most public libraries, is useful for both physicians and patients.

Scriver, Charles R., et al., eds. *The Metabolic Basis of Inherited Disease*. 8th ed. 2 vols. New York: McGraw-Hill, 2001. This classic medical text contains excellent information on gout—it descibes the symptoms, diagnosis, biochemistry, and genetics of the disease in great detail. Aimed at health science professionals, the book contains much important information for the diligent general reader as well. Pictures, diagrams, and large number of handy references are included.

GRAFTS AND GRAFTING
PROCEDURE

ANATOMY OR SYSTEM AFFECTED: All

SPECIALTIES AND RELATED FIELDS: Critical care, dermatology, emergency medicine, general surgery, genetics, immunology, neurology, physical therapy, plastic surgery

DEFINITION: The transplantation of tissue from one part of the body to another or from one individual to another in order to treat disease or injury; such surgery requires careful genetic matching in order to avoid a harmful immune response.

KEY TERMS:

allograft: a graft of tissue from one individual to another individual (usually between close relatives)

autograft: a graft of tissue from one part of an individual's body to another part

graft-versus-host disease (GVHD): a genetic incompatibility between tissues in which immune system cells from the grafted tissue attack host tissue

histocompatibility: tissue compatibility, as determined by histocompatibility protein antigens present on the cell membranes of all tissue cells

histology: the study of tissues and their development, roles, and locations within the body

host-versus-graft disease (HVGD): a tissue rejection in which the immune system cells of the graft recipient attack the grafted tissue from a donor individual

immune response: the reaction of an intricate system of cells that identify, attack, immobilize, and remove foreign tissue from the body through chemical signals

leukocytes: white blood cells, immune system cells which either produce antibodies or phagocytically consume cells and tissues that are genetically foreign in nature

tissue: a specialized region of cells that forms organs within the body; the four principal types are epithelial, connective, nervous, and muscular

totipotence: the capacity for cells of a given tissue type to regenerate and replace killed or damaged cells within a given body region

INDICATIONS AND PROCEDURES

In medicine, a graft is a tissue region which is transferred from one part of the body to another body part (autograft) or from one individual to another individual (allograft). Grafts between individuals of differing species (xenografts) also are possible. The actual transfer of tissue is called a transplant. The identification and matching of appropriate tissue types and the surgical connection of the tissue constitute grafting.

Examples of autografts include the use of leg veins to reconstruct the coronary arteries during heart bypass surgery, skin transplants during reconstructive facial surgery, and thumb/big toe interposable transplants following the loss of a hand or foot digit. Examples of allografts include major organ transplantations (including that of the heart, liver, and kidney), bone marrow transplantation, and blood transfusions between two genetically matched individuals. Xenograft examples include the grafting of animal tissue such as skin or stomach epithelia to the equivalent body parts in humans.

Genetic matching of donor and recipient tissues in grafting and transplantation is critical to the success of the tissue graft. Thus, tissue compatibility, termed histocompatibility, is of primary importance for successful grafting. Autografts are the most successful grafts because they occur on the same individual, and consequently there is no genetic difference between donor and recipient cells. As the genetic difference between donors and graft recipients increases, however, the probability decreases that a graft will be successful.

For example, grafts between identical twins are highly successful because the donor and recipient are genetically identical; hence, the situation is the same as an autograft. Grafts between siblings are likely to succeed. Allografts between people having distinct genetic differences, however, are less likely to succeed. Xenografts are extremely difficult except for basic mammalian tissues, such as epithelial tissue.

Histology is the study of tissues and their development within the human body. The four principal tissue types within the human body and within other mammalian species are epithelial tissue, which lines the inside and outside surfaces of organs throughout the body; connective tissue (such as cartilage, bone, fat, and blood), which provides structure or transport throughout the body; nervous tissue, which conducts electrical impulses as information networks throughout the body; and muscular tissue, which provides contractility and movement for various body parts. All organs consist of a specific pattern of these four tissues: Epithelial tissue provides cover and protection, connective tissue provides support, nervous tissue provides information from the central control regions of the brain, and muscular tissue allows responses to localized change in the organ. In addition, the cells of tissues subspecialize for unique roles within the tissue of which they are a part. For example, nervous system cells may specialize to form receiving sensory neurons or transmitting motor neurons.

Regardless of tissue type, each of the thousand trillion cells in an individual possesses the same basic genes as the others, and therefore many of the same proteins are expressed throughout the body. All cells within an individual have proteins located within the lipid bilayers of their cell membranes. Several of these proteins are located on every single cell of the individual and thus serve as genetic identification markers for the individual's immune system. These cell surface identification proteins are called histocompatibility proteins.

The histocompatibility proteins, of which there are many, are encoded by a battery of human genes called the major histocompatibility complex (MHC). These proteins ensure tissue compatibility for all cells in an individual with respect to that individual's immune system. The cells of the immune system recognize the specific histocompatibility proteins of one's own cells as "self" markers. Foreign cells, which are missing a few or many of the individual's specific set of histocompatibility proteins, are recognized by the immune system as "nonself" and are attacked. This self-versus-nonself reaction is how the immune system distinguishes its own cells from any invading foreign cells and tissues. Therefore, the histocompatibility proteins play a critical role in the successful identification of one's own cells and the destruction of infections, such as those caused by bacterial or fungal cells.

An immune response occurs when immune system cells called leukocytes (white blood cells) cannot locate the specific "self" histocompatibility proteins on a sampled cell. A type of leukocyte called a T lymphocyte will release a protein called immunoglobulin to immobilize the foreign "nonself" cell lacking the correct histocompatibility antigens (the proteins on the cell membranes). Immunoglobulins, also called antibodies, are proteins secreted by T lymphocytes to immobilize foreign antigens.

After the T lymphocyte antibodies have immobilized the antigens on the foreign cells, another type of leukocyte called a B lymphocyte produces antibodies that attack the foreign antigens. Furthermore, the B lymphocytes will multiply themselves, creating millions of copies to produce a clone army of B lymphocytes, all of which make the same antibodies targeted at the same foreign antigens. These specialized clones constitute a memory cell line, which will attack these antigens again if the organism is exposed to them in the future. This reaction is the basis of immunization.

Furthermore, after the T and B lymphocyte antibodies immobilize the foreign antigens, phagocytic leukocytes such as neutrophils and macrophages migrate to the region to ingest and completely destroy the foreign cells. This process will continue until either the foreign cells are vanquished or the immune system is exhausted.

The immune response just described may appear simple, but it is very complicated. In addition to the complex chemical identification of histocompatibility proteins on all of an individual's cells, the production of specific antibodies by T and B lymphocytes involves an extraordinary rearrangement of genes within these immune cells that is still poorly understood.

The immune response directly affects grafts and grafting. For transplants performed between two individuals, most tissues require a close genetic match between the donor and the recipient. They should be as closely related to each other as possible so that they share a common genetic heritage and, therefore, a high probability that their respective cells have most, if not all, of the same histocompatibility proteins. A close genetic relationship between the graft donor and recipient maximizes the chance that a graft will succeed and that an immune response against nonself tissues will not occur.

USES AND COMPLICATIONS

Grafts, grafting, and transplants between individuals are extremely important in the treatment of maiming or disfiguring accidents and life-threatening diseases. A huge demand exists for grafted tissue, not merely organ transplants, for use in a variety of medical conditions and procedures.

The most common and successful types of grafts are autografts from one part of an individual's body to another part, or from one identical twin to her or his sibling. In autograft cases, there is a perfect match for the histocompatibility proteins on all the cells and tissues. Thus, an immune response will not occur unless the immune system is abnormal in some way, as with such autoimmune diseases as lupus erythematosus and rheumatoid arthritis.

An example of an autograft is the transfer of a vein from the leg to the heart in a patient suffering from coronary artery disease; the grafted vein serves as a replacement coronary artery, supplying blood, nutrients,

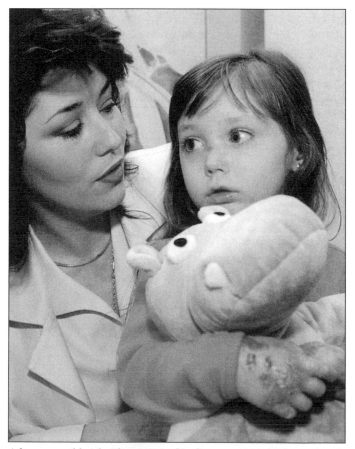

A four-year-old girl with a genetic skin disease waits to undergo a grafting procedure using laboratory-grown skin. (AP/Wide World Photos)

and oxygen to the heart muscle. Another type of autograft is the transfer of skin from the abdomen or pelvic region to the face as part of reconstructive plastic surgery. A severed thumb can be replaced by the big toe, its equivalent digit on the foot.

Allografts, those between different individuals, can be successful if there is careful genetic matching between the donor and recipient tissues. Because of the specificity of matching for certain tissue and cell types, donor-recipient matching may mean an average of any two people out of a thousand or, with more critical tissue lines such as stem cells, two people out of ten million. Often, siblings will serve as tissue donors. Otherwise, the lengthy process of finding possible tissue donors and determining their specific histocompatibility profiles must be conducted before the graft can take place between a recipient and a matched tissue donor.

Grafts are simple between generalized surface tissue such as epithelial and connective tissues. Pig epithelial tissue has been used for skin and stomach tissue grafts on human recipients. Bone marrow transplants for aplastic anemia and leukemia patients, however, require more difficult histocompatibility matching. The use of fetal nervous tissue grafts into the brain tissue of Alzheimer's disease patients has yielded promising results in regenerating brain tissue and slowing the acceleration of this debilitating disease, which generally strikes the elderly.

Grafts are useful for tissue lines lacking totipotence, the ability to regenerate damaged or dead cells. The example cited above of fetal tissue being used to treat Alzheimer's disease is a clear illustration of such tissue-grafting applications. Mature brain tissue in adult humans cannot regenerate. Fetal tissue grafts, however, have facilitated the regenerative capacity of some brain tissue in these patients.

Likewise, stem cell lines such as the red bone marrow of flat bones, where white blood cells (leukocytes) and red blood cells (erythrocytes) are manufactured, are important targets for tissue grafting. In leukemia, a patient's bone marrow is rapidly producing malignant leukocytes. It is clear that the stem cell line producing these cells is aberrant in such patients. Consequently, a small graft of bone marrow tissue from a histocompatible donor's bone marrow may lead to the establishment of a healthy stem cell line in the patient to stop the overproduction of aberrant cells.

In any grafting process, the donor tissue is surgically inserted and secured into the recipient's tissue site. There, the tissue, if the graft is successful, can grow and expand into the localized organ region to perform its correct function in the individual's body. In the event that there is not a histocompatible match between the donor tissue within the recipient's body, two possible rejection mechanisms can ensue. In host-versus-graft disease (HVGD), which is the most common type, the recipient's immune system releases antibodies and eventually destroys the donor tissue. In graft-versus-host disease (GVHD), immune system cells transplanted with the donor tissue into the recipient migrate into the recipient's tissues and attack the cells; the recipient will become ill and may die. The grafted tissue has rejected the entire body into which it has been transferred.

PERSPECTIVE AND PROSPECTS

In 1990, the Nobel Prize in Physiology or Medicine was awarded to American medical researchers Joseph E. Murray of the Harvard Medical School and E. Donnall Thomas of Seattle's Fred Hutchinson Cancer Research Center. These two scientists were pioneers in the use of grafts, grafting, and tissue transplants to save people's lives. Murray performed the first successful kidney transplant, between two identical twins, in 1954. Murray teamed with Thomas at Harvard to study methods for preventing host-versus-graft rejections. During the 1960's at the University of Washington, Thomas developed the technique of destroying a potential bone marrow recipient's immune system using radiation, followed by the grafting of donor bone marrow tissue into the patient, thereby increasing the chances that the transplant will succeed before the patient's immune system can become active again. Both scientists also made important discoveries concerning the major histocompatibility proteins.

Grafts and grafting play a vital role in medicine. Grafts can save the lives of people with such diseases as leukemia, anemia, and cancer. Grafts also can be useful in reconstructing damaged organs and skin, especially for burn victims. Still, much research is needed to understand histocompatibility better and to reduce the chance of tissue rejection.

—*David Wason Hollar, Jr., Ph.D.*

See also Alzheimer's disease; Amputation; Bone grafting; Bone marrow transplantation; Breast surgery; Burns and scalds; Cleft lip and palate repair; Corneal transplantation; Critical care; Critical care, pediatric; Dermatology; Dermatopathology; Emergency medicine; Facial transplantation; Fetal tissue transplantation; Hair transplantation; Heart transplantation; Heart valve replacement; Immune system; Kidney transplantation; Laceration repair; Leukemia; Liver transplantation; Pigmentation; Plastic surgery; Skin; Skin lesion removal; Transplantation; Xenotransplantation.

FOR FURTHER INFORMATION:

Adelman, Daniel C., et al., eds. *Manual of Allergy and Immunology.* 4th ed. Philadelphia: Lippincott Williams & Wilkins, 2002. Examines research developments and the clinical diagnosis and treatment of allergies and immune disorders. Covers transplantation immunology.

Alberts, Bruce, et al. *Molecular Biology of the Cell.* 4th ed. New York: Garland, 2002. Describes the evolution of cells and introduces cell structure and function. The text is clearly written at the college level and is illustrated by numerous diagrams and photographs. Section on the immune system contains an excellent discussion of the immune system, grafts, rejection, and histocompatibility.

Beck, William S., Karel F. Liem, and George Gaylord Simpson. *Life: An Introduction to Biology.* 3d ed. New York: HarperCollins, 1991. An outstanding introductory textbook for biology majors that is clearly written and beautifully illustrated. Chapter 23, "Immunity," is a good discussion of basic concepts, including descriptions of immune reactions and various types of transplants such as blood type ABO and Rh factor matchups.

Cohen, Barbara J. *Memmler's The Human Body in Health and Disease.* 10th ed. Philadelphia: Lippincott Williams & Wilkins, 2005. This book is a thorough but brief introduction to human anatomy, physiology, and disease that is written specifically for the layperson. Chapter 17, "Body Defenses, Immunity, and Vaccines," describes the immune system, transplants, and graft rejection.

Eisen, Herman N. *General Immunology: An Introduction to Molecular and Cellular Principles of the Immune Response.* 3d ed. Philadelphia: J. B. Lippincott, 1990. This incredibly thorough and concise work describes in great detail the various workings of animal immune systems, including types of antibodies, immune system cells, grafts, graft rejection, histocompatibility proteins, and the genetic basis of the immune response.

Kindt, Thomas J., Richard A. Goldsby, and Barbara A. Osborne. *Kuby Immunology.* 6th ed. New York: W. H. Freeman, 2007. The section on hypersensitiv-

ity in this immunology textbook is well written and includes a mixture of detail and overview of the subject. Particularly useful are discussions of the various types of hypersensitivity reactions.

Palca, Joseph. "Overcoming Rejection to Win a Nobel Prize." *Science* 250 (October 19, 1990): 378. Palca's article is an announcement of the 1990 Nobel Prize in Physiology or Medicine awarded to Americans Joseph E. Murray and E. Donnall Thomas, pioneers in grafting and transplant medical research. Palca discusses the careers of these two scientists and the major experiments leading to their momentous discoveries.

GRAM STAINING

PROCEDURE

ANATOMY OR SYSTEM AFFECTED: Cells, immune system

SPECIALTIES AND RELATED FIELDS: Bacteriology, biochemistry, cytology, microbiology

DEFINITION: A staining process used as a means of differentiating microorganisms, which are classified as either gram-positive or gram-negative.

KEY TERMS:

cell wall: a structure outside the cell membrane of most bacteria, composed of varying amounts of carbohydrates, lipids, and amino acids

gram-negative: referring to microorganisms that appear pink following the Gram-staining procedure

gram-positive: referring to microorganisms that appear violet following the Gram-staining procedure

Gram's stain: a method of staining bacteria as a primary means of differentiation and identification

lipopolysaccharide (LPS): a major component of the cell wall of gram-negative bacteria; the toxicity of LPS is associated with illnesses caused by gram-negative organisms

mordant: a chemical that acts to fix a stain within a physical structure; the role played by iodine in Gram's stain

peptidoglycans: repeating units of sugar derivatives that make up a rigid layer of bacterial cell walls; found in both gram-positive and gram-negative cells

INDICATIONS AND PROCEDURES

The observation and identification of bacteria are of obvious primary importance in the study of microorganisms. Even with the use of powerful microscopes, direct observation of unstained bacteria is difficult. The use of stains to increase their contrast with the background allows bacteria to be observed more easily.

As a result of resident acidic groups—polysaccharides or nucleic acids—the surfaces of bacteria tend to be negatively charged. Conversely, the dye portion of common stains such as methylene blue or crystal violet consists of positively charged ions. For staining purposes, a sample of bacteria is placed on a glass slide and allowed to dry. The solution of stain is flooded over the bacterial "smear" for about a minute, and the slide is then rinsed. The main purpose of such simple stains is to allow the cells to be observed.

In contrast with simple stains, differential staining methods do not stain all cells in the same manner. Bacteria grown under different environmental conditions, or bacteria that may differ from one another in their physical structure, will exhibit different staining properties when treated with differential stains. Gram staining (also called Gram's stain) is an example of a differential stain.

Gram staining is a relatively simple procedure and is among the first practices learned by students in microbiology laboratories. The process begins with the preparation of a bacterial smear on the slide. A stain, crystal violet, is allowed to flood the dried smear. The slide is rinsed, and a solution of iodine is dropped over the smear. The iodine functions as a mordant, fixing the crystal violet into a complex insoluble in water. Following another rinse, the smear is covered with either an alcohol or an acetone "destaining" solution for several seconds, rinsed again, and counterstained with the red dye safranin. After a last wash, the bacteria are observed with a microscope. If they were not destained by the alcohol step, retaining the blue or violet color, they are considered gram-positive; if they have stained pink because of the counterstain safranin, they are considered gram-negative.

The precise means by which Gram staining works is not entirely clear. The cell wall structure of gram-positive bacteria either prevents the alcohol/acetone solution from removing the crystal violet-iodine complex from the cell or prevents the solution from having access to the complex. Though the question remains whether the cell wall structure is the sole determining factor in the differential procedure, there is no doubt that the cell wall features are primary factors in the determination of Gram-staining results. Therefore, the structure of the cell wall in most bacteria reflects the Gram-staining characteristics.

The cell wall structure found in gram-positive bacteria differs significantly from that in gram-negative cells. While both contain a rigid layer called the peptidoglycan, the peptidoglycan layer is much thicker and makes up a significantly larger portion of the cell wall in gram-positive bacteria. In contrast, a significant portion of the cell wall found in gram-negative bacteria is composed of lipid derivatives.

The peptidoglycan portion of the cell is composed of repeating units of two sugar derivatives: N-acetylglucosamine and N-acetylmuramic acid. The peptidoglycan within the wall is in the form of sheets, layered on top of one another. In gram-positive bacteria, approximately 90 percent of the cell wall material consists of peptidoglycan; among gram-negative bacteria, about 10 percent of the wall is represented by this rigid layer.

These cell wall structures are stabilized by short chains of amino acids that cross-link the layers of peptidoglycan. Formation of the cross bridges is an enzymatic process called transpeptidation. The antibiotic penicillin inhibits the enzyme that carries out the formation of such cross-links. The result is a weakening in the cell wall, and possibly cell death. Since the peptidoglycan layer of gram-negative bacteria represents a much smaller proportion of the cell wall, such microorganisms are often more resistant to the action of penicillin than are gram-positive bacteria.

During the Gram-staining procedure, decolorization of the cell is carried out during the wash with alcohol or acetone. The thick peptidoglycan layer found in gram-positive bacteria, however, prevents movement of the crystal violet-iodine complex from the cell. Thus, the cells do not decolorize; they retain their violet appearance.

The peptidoglycan layer is a small proportion of the gram-negative cell wall. Much of the outer wall in these bacteria is a layer of lipopolysaccharide (LPS), which acts as a physical barrier but also contains pharmacological properties. The LPS layer is a complex structure containing a lipid portion (lipid A), a core polysaccharide consisting of a variety of sugars, and an outer layer of branched sugars called the O-region (O-polysaccharide). The LPS layer is anchored to the thin peptidoglycan portion of the cell wall through a lipoprotein complex. The LPS portion of gram-negative cell walls is often termed the endotoxin because of its pharmacological activity. Release of LPS as a result of cell death during certain types of infection can result in high fever or shock.

Since the cell wall of gram-negative bacteria contains proportionately little peptidoglycan, the crystal violet-iodine complex is easily removed during the

Gram-staining procedure. Following the alcohol step, the cells again appear colorless. Therefore, when they are counterstained with the safranin, the bacteria will appear pink.

An evaluation of Gram-staining characteristics is generally the first step in the identification of newly isolated bacteria. Most bacteria can be classified as either gram-positive or gram-negative, and this step, along with characterization of the shape of the organism, is of immense importance in narrowing down the possible identities of an isolate.

Further means of identification generally involve the use of selective or differential types of media. These processes utilize the biochemical properties of bacteria for their identification. A selective medium is one in which chemical compounds have been added that inhibit the growth of certain forms of bacteria but allow the growth of others. For example, the chemical dye eosin-methylene blue (EMB) inhibits the growth of gram-positive bacteria while allowing gram-negative bacteria to grow. If a mixed culture of bacteria is inoculated onto EMB medium, only the gram-negative microorganisms will grow. A differential medium will allow a variety of bacteria to grow, but different types of bacteria may produce different reactions on the medium. Since EMB agar contains lactose as a carbon source, it is also a differential medium. Bacteria that ferment lactose produce a green metallic color of colony on EMB; bacteria that do not ferment lactose produce a pink colony.

Biochemical tests are more useful for the identification of organisms that are gram-negative than for those that are gram-positive. Biochemical variations among both genera and species of gram-positive bacteria tend to be too variable for effective identification of these organisms. By contrast, such biochemical results among gram-negative bacteria generally do not vary significantly within the species and hence are useful means of further identification.

The biochemical tests used for identification of gram-negative bacteria can be summarized in the form of a flowchart. Such charts represent the series of tests that divide bacteria into smaller and smaller groups. For example, following a determination of morphological and Gram-staining characteristics, differential tests may be carried out to observe the ability of the bacteria to ferment various types of carbohydrates. A series of broths containing such sugars as glucose, lactose, or sucrose are inoculated. Generally, a pH indicator such as the chemical phenol red is included, as is an inverted glass tube (Durham tube) for observation of gas production. If the organism can ferment lactose and produces acid and gas, the broth tube of lactose will appear yellow and there will be a gas bubble in the Durham tube. If the organism does not ferment lactose, no growth or change from the red color of the broth will be observed in that tube.

Further differentiation of either lactose-positive or lactose-negative organisms, to continue with this particular example, can be carried out with other biochemical tests. Certain species of bacteria are capable of removing a molecule of carbon dioxide from amino acids; others are not. In some cases, multiple tests can be run at the same time. For example, a common differential test for gram-negative bacteria utilizes a medium called triple sugar iron (TSI) agar. TSI agar contains a small amount of glucose and larger amounts of lactose and sucrose, hence the designation of triple sugar. Iron is also contained in the medium. The agar is prepared in a test tube and allowed to harden on a slant. Organisms are inoculated onto the surface of the slant and stabbed into the butt of the slant. If glucose alone is fermented, only enough acid is produced to turn the butt yellow. If either lactose or sucrose is fermented, both the slant and butt of the agar will turn yellow. Production of hydrogen sulfide gas is indicated by a black precipitate from iron sulfide; other gas production is indicated by bubble formation in the region of the stab. In this manner, inoculation of a single type of medium can provide multiple tests for identification.

At one time, each of these differential tests had to be carried out individually. Beginning in the 1970's, however, a variety of media kits became available that allow fifteen to twenty tests to be run simultaneously. These kits consist of strips of miniaturized versions of biochemical tests that permit the rapid identification of gram-negative bacteria.

Even though some biochemical tests are less helpful in the identification of gram-positive bacteria, some characteristics of these organisms can be used. These organisms may be round (cocci) or rod-shaped (bacilli). If bacilli, they may be aerobic (they utilize oxygen) or anaerobic (they do not utilize oxygen). By testing for coagulase, an enzyme which will cause the coagulation of plasma, cocci can be further differentiated.

Finally, serological methods can be used in the identification of either gram-positive or gram-negative organisms. In these tests, a fluorescent dye is attached to molecules of antibodies, proteins directed against the surface molecules of specific bacteria. The ability of the antibodies to attach to bacteria is indicative of the species.

USES AND COMPLICATIONS

The use of Gram-staining methodology is arguably the single most important step in the identification of microorganisms; its applications are far-ranging. Most diseases of humans and other animals, as well as of plants, are caused by microorganisms. Isolation and identification of disease-causing bacteria are key aspects in understanding the etiology of such diseases. Many aspects of technology, from the discovery or development of new antibiotics to the development of new strains of microbes, utilize such methodologies as Gram's stain in the identification of fresh isolates.

Clinical methods for the identification of infectious agents follow a series of defined steps. The particular material involved depends on the type and site of infection and can include such fluids as blood, urine, pus, or saliva. The specific symptoms of the illness may also provide clues as to the particular agents involved.

For example, among the most common infections are those of the urinary tract. These are particularly common nosocomial, or hospital-acquired, infections. Samples are taken with a sterile swab, which is used to inoculate special types of selective or differential media. Generally speaking, such infections are usually associated with gram-negative bacteria. The majority of these infections, about 90 percent, are caused by *Escherichia coli* (*E. coli*), a common intestinal organism. To a lesser extent, such infections may be associated with other genera such as *Klebsiella*, *Pseudomonas*, *Proteus*, or *Streptococcus*. All but *Streptococcus* are gram-negative bacilli.

Confirmation of the Gram morphology follows growth on selective media. The media of choice in this example are those selective for gram-negative bacteria: either eosin-methylene blue or MacConkey agars. Both inhibit the replication of bacteria such as *Staphylococcus*, commonly found on the surface of the skin and a possible contaminant during the swabbing of the site of infection.

The presence of the sugar lactose in either MacConkey or EMB agar allows these media to be differential in addition to being selective. Lactose fermenters such as *Escherichia*, *Klebsiella*, or *Enterobacter* will produce pink colonies on MacConkey agar, while gram-negative organisms such as *Proteus*, *Pseudomonas*, or *Salmonella*, which do not ferment lactose, will produce colorless colonies on this medium. Analogous results can be seen with other differential enteric agars. More detailed types of analysis using other forms of media or utilizing immunological methods may be necessary to fine-tune the diagnosis, or antibiotic susceptibility tests may simply be conducted to determine the treatment of choice.

In some instances, Gram morphology may be sufficient for the identification of a microorganism. For example, the presence of gram-negative cocci in a cervical smear from a patient suspected of having contracted a sexually transmitted disease is indicative of a *Neisseria gonorrhea* infection. The identification can be confirmed using immunological methods or through growth on selective media such as Thayer-Martin agar, which contains antibiotics inhibitory to most other gram-negative bacteria.

If the clinical sample consists of blood or cerebrospinal fluid, both of which are normally sterile, either gram-negative or gram-positive organisms may be involved. The initial step toward identification is a Gram's stain of the material. Gram-negative bacteria can be identified using methods already described. Generally speaking, the bacterial content of blood during bacteremia will be too low for ready observation. For this reason, blood samples are inoculated into bottles of nonselective growth media, one of which is grown under aerobic conditions and one under anaerobic conditions. If and when growth becomes apparent, smears are prepared for Gram staining.

Gram-positive cocci will almost always be members of either of two genera: *Staphylococcus* or *Streptococcus*. The two can be differentiated on the basis of catalase production, an enzyme which degrades hydrogen peroxide; staphylococci produce the enzyme, while streptococci do not. A variety of commercial kits are available for rapid identification of species. These contain a battery of tests based on biochemical properties of the organisms, including tolerance of high salt, fermentation of unusual sugars, and growth characteristics on blood agar plates (nutrient agar containing sheep red blood cells).

The identification of gram-positive bacilli is more difficult, given their biochemical variation even within the genus. The major subdivisions of this group are based on their tolerance of oxygen. Obligate gram-positive anaerobes, organisms that cannot tolerate oxygen, include the genus *Clostridium*, members of which cause tetanus, gangrene, and food poisoning. Aerobes and facultative anaerobes, which are oxygen-tolerant, include the genera *Bacillus*, *Corynebacterium*, and *Listeria*. Further identification often requires immunological means.

The gram-negative bacillus *E. coli* is frequently used as a marker for sewage contamination of water supplies. Since it is a common intestinal organism and rarely found in soil, its presence in water samples is indicative of possible fecal contamination of that water. Testing for the presence and level of *E. coli* utilizes the biochemical properties of the microbe. Various quantities of the water sample are placed in tubes of lactose broth; growth is indicative of a lactose fermenter and is presumptive for the presence of *E. coli*. A sample of the lactose culture is then streaked on EMB agar. The development of metallic green-colored colonies of gram-negative bacilli confirms the presence of *E. coli*. The smaller the volume of the water sample that produced growth in lactose, the higher the level of *E. coli* in that sample. In a sense, *E. coli* serves as a surrogate marker in these tests. It may not itself be a pathogen (though some strains of *E. coli* may indeed cause severe intestinal infections), but other gram-negative intestinal pathogens such as *Salmonella*, *Shigella*, or *Vibrio*, even if present in water supplies, may be in a concentration too low for ready detection. Therefore, the presence of *E. coli* suggests possible fecal contamination, allowing for proper sewage treatment. Conversely, the absence of *E. coli* in the water sample indicates that fecal contamination, and therefore the presence of other intestinal pathogens, is unlikely.

PERSPECTIVE AND PROSPECTS

During the latter portion of the nineteenth century, the role of bacteria as etiological agents of disease became apparent. Eventually the experimental observations linking the presence of bacteria with various illnesses coalesced in the so-called germ theory of disease. During the early 1880's, the German physician Robert Koch, along with his colleagues and students, developed an experimental method that could be applied to associate a particular organism with a specific disease. These procedures eventually became known as Koch's postulates. Inherent in Koch's postulates was the necessity to observe the microbial agent, either in tissue or following growth in the laboratory. Staining methods, however, were often crude or imprecise. The best one might hope for was to be able to at least observe the organism.

Hans Christian Gram, a Danish physician working with C. Friedlander in Berlin during the early 1880's,

was able to introduce a highly effective method of staining bacteria. Gram's method was a modification of that developed earlier by Paul Ehrlich. The procedure began by first staining the sample with Gentian Violet in aniline water, followed by treatment with iodine in a potassium iodide solution. Gram found that when tissue sections or smears treated in such a manner were washed with dilute alcohol, certain types of bacteria (or schizomycetes, as they were then known) became decolorized (gram-negative), while other forms of bacteria retained their violet appearance (gram-positive). The procedure, published in 1884, was shown to be applicable for most types of bacteria. As a result, a process for differentiation between various types of bacteria became available. In addition, the ability to detect smaller quantities of bacteria in tissue increased significantly.

—Richard Adler, Ph.D.

See also Bacterial infections; Bacteriology; Cells; Cytology; *E. coli* infection; Laboratory tests; Microbiology; Salmonella infection; Shigellosis; Staphylococcal infections; Streptococcal infections.

FOR FURTHER INFORMATION:

Alcamo, I. Edward. *Microbes and Society: An Introduction to Microbiology.* Sudbury, Mass.: Jones and Bartlett, 2002. A nonscientific text for the liberal arts student that explores the importance of microbes to human life and their role in food production and agriculture, in biotechnology and industry, in ecology and the environment, and in disease and bioterrorism.

Alcamo, I. Edward, and Lawrence M. Elson. *Microbiology Coloring Book.* New York: HarperCollins, 1996. This volume is one in a series of "coloring books" that are excellent sources of information. Detailed instructions help the reader navigate the intricacies of the world of microbes through observation and reading. This book is jammed with useful facts about the biology of microorganisms and the methods used to study them.

Goodsell, David. *The Machinery of Life.* New York: Springer-Verlag, 1993. A short book on the biology of the cell for the general reader. The section on *Escherichia coli* as the prototype for bacteria is well written and easy to understand. Especially striking are the large number of computer graphics illustrating molecular structures.

Madigan, Michael T., and John M. Martinko. *Brock Biology of Microorganisms.* 11th ed. Upper Saddle

River, N.J.: Pearson Prentice Hall, 2006. An outstanding microbiology text. The authors provide a thorough description of bacteria and the means by which they are studied. Relevant to this topic are chapters on methods of isolation and characterization.

Singleton, Paul. *Bacteria in Biology, Biotechnology, and Medicine.* 6th ed. New York: John Wiley & Sons, 2004. The author has written a concise description of bacteria and their roles in nature. Included are chapters on bacterial structure, staining, and methods of classification and identification. Portions of the book cover molecular aspects of cells.

Snyder, Larry, and Wendy Champness. *Molecular Genetics of Bacteria.* 2d ed. Washington, D.C.: ASM Press, 2002. A text that introduces the field of bacterial molecular genetics and describes the mechanisms of mutations and gene exchange in bacteria and phages. Concentrates specifically on the bacterium *E. Coli* while using examples from other bacteria as appropriate.

Wilson, Michael, Brian Henderson, and Rod McNab. *Bacterial Virulence Mechanisms.* New York: Cambridge University Press, 2002. Basing their discussion on research advances in microbiology, molecular biology, and cell biology, the authors describe the interactions that exist between bacteria and human cells both in health and during infection.

Winn, Washington C., Jr., et al. *Koneman's Color Atlas and Textbook of Diagnostic Microbiology.* 6th ed. Philadelphia: Lippincott Williams & Wilkins, 2006. Presents methods of identification for most organisms likely to appear in a clinical laboratory. Of particular interest are the large number of color photographs illustrating results for major staining methods and biochemical tests.

GRAY HAIR
DISEASE/DISORDER

ANATOMY OR SYSTEM AFFECTED: Hair
SPECIALTIES AND RELATED FIELDS: Dermatology
DEFINITION: The reduction in hair pigmentation that is a natural by-product of aging.

CAUSES AND SYMPTOMS

Hair color is produced by tiny pigment cells in hair follicles called melanocytes. Each melanocyte has long, armlike extensions that carry the pigment granules known as melanin to the hair cells. In the course of a

---

INFORMATION ON GRAY HAIR

CAUSES: Aging; also hyperthyroidism, anemia, autoimmune disease, severe stress, vitamin B$_{12}$ deficiency, skin pigmentation disorders (vitiligo)
SYMPTOMS: Change in hair color; drier, coarser, more wiry hair
DURATION: Chronic
TREATMENTS: Masking via chemical and vegetable rinses and dyes

---

lifetime, the production of pigment-forming enzymes drops, and the activity of the melanocytes in each follicle begins to wane, resulting in gray hair. Each individual's melanocyte clock is different, but in Caucasians the reduction of melanocyte activity usually occurs earlier than in other ethnic groups. On the average, graying starts at age thirty-four in Caucasians, in the late thirties in Asians, and at age forty-four in African Americans.

Pigment loss starts at the root, with some strands of hair gradually fading in color, while others may grow in gray or white. Initial graying can be accelerated by hyperthyroidism, anemia, autoimmune disease, severe stress, or vitamin B$_{12}$ deficiency. Disorders of skin pigmentation, such as vitiligo, can also result in the loss of hair pigmentation.

Once gray hair begins to appear, the rate at which it progresses over the rest of the head depends entirely upon each individual. It does not appear to be a function of the original hair color or texture, ethnic background, or the condition of the scalp. By age fifty, 50 percent of Caucasians are significantly gray. As hair loses its pigment, it often gets drier, resulting in coarser, wirier hair.

TREATMENT AND THERAPY

For some individuals, gray hair is a symbol of maturity, while for others it is an embarrassing sign associated with the aging process. In most cases, graying can be readily masked if so desired. Effective chemical and vegetable rinses and dyes are available.

—*Alvin K. Benson, Ph.D.*

See also Aging; Hair; Hair loss and baldness; Hair transplantation; Pigmentation; Skin; Skin disorders.

FOR FURTHER INFORMATION:

Feinberg, Herbert S. *All About Hair.* Alpine, N.J.: Wallingford Press, 1978.

Greenwood-Robinson, Maggie. *Hair Savers for Women: A Complete Guide to Preventing and Treating Hair Loss*. New York: Crown, 2000.

Jewell, Diana Lewis. *Going Gray, Looking Great! The Modern Woman's Guide to Unfading Glory*. New York: Fireside, 2004.

Levine, Norman, ed. *Pigmentation and Pigmentary Disorders*. Boca Raton, Fla.: CRC Press, 1993.

Schneider, Edward L., and John W. Rowe. *Handbook of the Biology of Aging*. 5th ed. San Diego, Calif.: Academic Press, 2001.

Scott, Susan Craig, and Karen W. Bressler. *The Hair Bible*. New York: Simon & Schuster, 2003.

GRIEF AND GUILT

DISEASE/DISORDER

ANATOMY OR SYSTEM AFFECTED: Psychic-emotional system

SPECIALTIES AND RELATED FIELDS: Family medicine, psychiatry, psychology

DEFINITION: Grief and accompanying guilt are common reactions to the fact or eventuality of serious losses of various kinds, especially death; every person eventually experiences grief, and while grief is normal, its effects can be incapacitating.

KEY TERMS:

abnormal grief: an unhealthy response to a loss, which may include anger, an inability to feel loss, withdrawal, and deterioration in health

grief: a multifaceted physical, emotional, psychological, spiritual, and social reaction to loss

guilt: a cognitive and emotional response often associated with the grief experience in which a person feels a sense of remorse, responsibility, and/or shame regarding the loss

loss: the sudden lack of a previously held possession, physical state, or social position or the death of a loved one

CAUSES AND SYMPTOMS

During life, people unavoidably experience a variety of losses. These may include the loss of loved ones, important possessions or status, or health and vitality, and ultimately the loss of self through death. "Grief" is the word commonly used to refer to an individual's or group's shared experience following a loss. The experience of grief is not a momentary or singular phenomenon. Instead, it is a variable, and somewhat predictable, process of life. Also, as with many phenomena within the range of human experience, it is a multidimensional process including biological, psychological, spiritual, and social components.

The biological level of the grief experience includes the neurological and physiological processes that take place in the various organ systems of the body in response to the recognition of loss. These processes, in turn, form the basis for emotional and psychological reactions. Various organs and organ systems interact with one another in response to the cognitive stimulation resulting from this recognition. Human beings are self-reflective creatures with the capacity for experiencing, reflecting upon, and giving meaning to sensations, both physical and emotional. Consequently, the physiological reactions of grief that take place in the body are given meaning by those experiencing them.

The cognitive and emotional meanings attributed to the experience of grief are shaped by and influence interactions within the social dimensions of life. In other words, how someone feels or thinks about grief influences and is influenced by interactions with family, friends, and helping professionals. In addition, the individual's religious or spiritual frame of reference may have a significant influence on the subjective experience and cognitive-emotional meaning attributed to grief.

The grief reactions associated with a loss such as death vary widely. While it is very difficult and perhaps unfair to generalize about such an intensely personal experience, several predictors of the intensity of grief have become evident. The amount of grief experienced seems to depend on the significance of the loss, or the degree to which the individual subjectively experiences a sense of loss. This subjective experience is partially dependent on the meaning attributed to the loss by the survivors and others in the surrounding social

---

INFORMATION ON GRIEF AND GUILT

CAUSES: Loss of loved ones, important possessions or status, health and vitality, and ultimately the loss of self through death

SYMPTOMS: Anxiety and/or depression; difficulty sleeping; feeling sad and/or that life has lost its meaning; feelings of loss, shock, shame, rage, numbness, relief, anger, and/or guilt; social isolation, withdrawal, or alienation

DURATION: Varies widely

TREATMENTS: Counseling, antidepressants

context. This meaning is in turn shaped by underlying belief systems, such as religious faith. Clear cognitive, emotional, and/or spiritual frameworks are helpful in guiding people constructively through the grief process.

People in every culture around the world and throughout history have developed expectations about life, and these beliefs influence the grief process. Some questions are common to many cultures. Why do people die? Is death a part of life, or a sign of weakness or failure? Is death always a tragedy, or is it sometimes a welcome relief from suffering? Is there life after death, and if so, what is necessary to attain this afterlife? The answers to these and other questions help shape people's experience of the grief process. As Elisabeth Kübler-Ross states in *Death: The Final Stage of Growth* (1975), the way in which a society or subculture explains death will have a significant impact on the way in which its members view and experience life.

Another factor that influences the experience of grief is whether a loss was anticipated. Sudden and/or unanticipated losses are more traumatic and more difficult to explain because they tend to violate the meaning systems mentioned above. The cognitive and emotional shock of this violation exacerbates the grief process. For example, it is usually assumed that youngsters will not die before the older members of the family. Therefore, the shock of a child dying in an automobile crash may be more traumatic than the impact of the death of an older person following a long illness.

Death and grief are often distasteful to human beings, at least in Western Judeo-Christian cultures. These negative, fearful reactions are, in part, the result of an individual's difficulty accepting the inevitability of his or her own death. Nevertheless, in cultures which have less difficulty accepting death and loss as normal, people generally experience more complicated grief experiences. The Micronesian society of Truk is a death-affirming society. The members of the Truk society believe that a person is not really grown up until the age of forty. At that point, the individual begins to prepare for death. Similarly, some native Alaskan groups teach their members to approach death intentionally. The person about to die plans for death and makes provisions for the grief process of those left behind.

In every culture, however, the grief-stricken strive to make sense out of their experience of loss. Some attribute death to a malicious intervention from the outside by someone or something else; death becomes frightening. For others, death is in response to divine intervention or is simply the completion of "the circle of life" for that person. Yet for most people in Western societies, even those who come to believe that death is a part of life, grief may be an emotional mixture of loss, shock, shame, sadness, rage, numbness, relief, anger, and/or guilt.

Kübler-Ross points out in her timeless discourse "On the Fear of Dying" (*On Death and Dying*, 1969) that guilt is perhaps the most painful companion of death and grief. The grief process is often complicated by the individual's perception that he or she should have prevented the loss. This feeling of being responsible for the death or other loss is common among those connected to the deceased. For example, parents or health care providers may believe that they should have done something differently in order to detect the eventual cause of death sooner or to prevent it once the disease process was detected.

Guilt associated with grief is often partly or completely irrational. For example, there may be no way that a physician could have detected an aneurysm in her patient's brain prior to a sudden and fatal stroke. Similarly, a parent cannot monitor the minute-by-minute activities of his adolescent children to prevent lethal accidents. Kübler-Ross explains a related phenomenon among children who have lost a parent by pointing out the difficulty in separating wishes from deeds. A child whose wishes are not gratified by a parent may become angry. If the parent subsequently dies, the child may feel guilty, even if the death is some distance in time away from the event in question.

The guilt may also involve remorse over surviving someone else's loss. People who survive an ordeal in which others die often experience "survivor's guilt." Survivors may wonder why they survived and how the deceased person's family members feel about their survival, whether they blame the survivors or wish that they had died instead. As a result, survivors have difficulty integrating the experience with the rest of their lives in order to move on. The feelings of grief and guilt may be exacerbated further if survivors believe that they somehow benefited from someone else's death. A widow who is suddenly the beneficiary of a large sum of money attached to her husband's life insurance policy may feel guilty about doing some of the things that they had always planned but were unable to do precisely because of a lack of money.

Last, guilt may result when people believe that they did not pay enough attention to, care well enough for, or deserve the love of the person who died. These feelings and thoughts are prompted by loss—loss of an ongoing relationship with the one who died, as well as part of the empathetic response to what it might be like to die oneself.

Feelings of guilt are not always present, even if the reaction is extreme. If individuals experience guilt, however, they may "bargain" with themselves or a higher power, review their actions to find what they did wrong, take a moral inventory to see where they could have been more loving or understanding, or even begin to act self-destructively. Attempting to resolve guilt while grieving loss is doubly complicated and may contribute to the development of what is considered an abnormal grief reaction.

The distinctions between normal and abnormal grief processes are not clear-cut and are largely context-dependent; that is, what is normal depends on standards that vary among different social groups and historical periods. In addition, at any particular time the variety of manifestations of grief depend on the individual's personality and temperament; family, social, and cultural contexts; resources for coping with and resolving problems; and experiences with the successful resolution of grief.

Despite this diversity, the symptoms that are manifested by individuals experiencing grief are generally grouped into two different but related diagnostic categories: depression and anxiety. It is normal for the grieving individual to manifest symptoms related to anxiety and/or depression to some degree. For example, a surviving relative or close friend may temporarily have difficulty sleeping, or feel sad or that life has lost its meaning. Relative extremes of these symptoms, however, in either duration or intensity, signal the possibility of an abnormal grief reaction.

In *Families and Health* (1988), family therapist William Doherty and family physician Thomas Campbell identify the signs of abnormal grief reactions as including periods of compulsive overactivity without a sense of loss; identification with the deceased; acquisition of symptoms belonging to the last illness of the deceased; deterioration of health in the survivors; social isolation, withdrawal, or alienation; and severe depression. These signs may also include severe anxiety, abuse of substances, work or school problems, extreme or persistent anger, or an inability to feel loss.

TREATMENT AND THERAPY

There is no set time schedule for the grief process. While various ethnic, cultural, religious, and political groups define the limits of the period of mourning, they cannot prescribe the experience of grief. Yet established norms do influence the grief experience inasmuch as the grieving individuals have internalized these expectations and standards. For example, the typical benefit package of a professional working in the United States offers up to one week of paid "funeral" leave in the event of the death of a significant family member. On the surface, this policy begins to prescribe or define the limits of the grief process.

Such a policy suggests, for example, that a mother or father stricken with grief at the untimely death of a child ought to be able to return to work and function reasonably well once a week has passed. Most individuals will attempt to do so, even if they are harboring unresolved feelings about the child's death. Coworkers, uncomfortable with responding to such a situation and conditioned to believe that people need to "get on with life," may support the lack of expression of grief.

Helpful responses to grief are as multifaceted as is grief itself. Ultimately, several factors ease the grief process. These include validating responses from significant others, socially sanctioned expression of the experience, self-care, social or religious rituals, and possibly professional assistance. Each person responds to grief differently and requires or is able to use different forms of assistance.

Most reactions to loss run a natural, although varied, course. Since grief involves coming to grips with the reality of death, acceptance must eventually be both intellectual and emotional. Therefore, it is important to allow for the complete expression of both thoughts and feelings. Those attempting to assist grief-stricken individuals are more effective if they have come to terms with their own feelings, beliefs, and conflicts about death, and any losses they personally have experienced.

Much of what is helpful in working through grief involves accepting grief as a normal phenomenon. Grief-related feelings should not be judged or overly scrutinized. Supportive conversations include time for ventilation, empathic responses, and sharing of sympathetic experiences. Helpful responses may take the form of "To feel pain and sadness at this time is a normal, healthy response" or "I don't know what it is like to have a child die, but it looks like it really hurts" or "It is understandable if you find yourself thinking that life has lost its purpose." In short, people must be given permission to grieve. When it becomes clear that the person is struggling with an inordinate amount of feelings based on irrational beliefs, these underlying beliefs—not the feelings—may need to be challenged.

People tend to have difficulty concentrating and focusing in the aftermath of a significant loss. The symptoms of anxiety and depression associated with grief may be experienced, and many of the basic functions of life may be interrupted. Consequently, paying attention to healthy eating and sleeping schedules, establishing small goals, and being realistic about how long it may take before "life returns to normal" are important.

While the prescription of medication for the grief-stricken is fairly common, its use is recommended only in extreme situations. Antianxiety agents or antidepressants can interfere with the normal experiences of grief that involve feeling and coming to terms with loss. Sedatives can help bereaved family members and other loved ones feel better over the short term, with less overt distress and crying. Many experts believe, however, that they inhibit the normal grieving process and lead to unresolved grief reactions. In addition, studies suggest that those who start on psychotropic medication during periods of grief stay on them for at least two years.

The grief process is also eased by ritual practices that serve as milestones to mark progress along the way. Some cultures have very clearly defined and well-established rituals associated with grief. In the United States, the rituals practiced continue to be somewhat influenced by family, ethnic, and regional cultures. Very often, however, the rituals are confined to the procedures surrounding the preparation and burial of the body (for example, viewing the body at the mortuary, a memorial service, and interment). As limited as these experiences might be, they are designed to ease people's grief. Yet the grief process is often just beginning with the death and burial of the loved one. Consequently, survivors are often left without useful guidelines to help them on their way.

Another common, although unhelpful, phenomenon associated with the process is for the grief-stricken person initially to receive a considerable amount of empathy and support from family, friends, and possibly professionals (such as a minister or physician) only to have this attention drop off sharply after about a month. The resources available through family and other social support systems diminish with the increasing expectation that the bereaved should stop grieving and "get on with living." If this is the case, or if an individual never did experience a significantly supportive response from members of his or her social system, the

role of psychotherapy and/or support groups should be explored. Many public and private agencies offer individual and family therapy. In addition, in many communities there are a variety of self-help support groups devoted to growth and healing in the aftermath of loss.

PERSPECTIVE AND PROSPECTS

The grief process, however it is shaped by particular religious, ethnic, or cultural contexts, is reflective of the human need to form attachments. Grief thus reflects the importance of relationships in one's life, and therefore it is likely that people will always experience grief (including occasional feelings of guilt). Processes such as the grief experience, with its cognitive, emotional, social, and spiritual dimensions, may affect an individual's psychological and physical well-being. Consequently, medical and other health care and human service professionals will probably always be called upon to investigate, interpret, diagnose, counsel, and otherwise respond to grief-stricken individuals and families.

In the effort to be helpful, however, medical science has frequently intervened too often and too invasively into death, dying, and the grief process—to the point of attempting to disallow them. For example, hospitals and other institutions such as nursing homes have become the primary places that people die. It is important to remember that it has not always been this way. Even now in some cultures around the world, people die more often in their own homes than in a "foreign" institution.

In the early phases of the development of the field of medicine, hospitals as institutions were primarily devoted to the care of the dying and the indigent. Managing the dying process was a primary focus. More recently, however, technological advances and specialty development have shifted the mission of the hospital to being an institution devoted to healing and curing. The focus on the recovery process has left dying in the shadows. Death has become equated with failure and associated with professional guilt.

It is more difficult for health care professionals to involve themselves or at least constructively support the grief process of individuals and families if it is happening as a result of the health care team's "failure." In a parallel fashion, society has become unduly fixated on avoiding death, or at least prolonging its inevitability to the greatest possible extent. The focus of the larger culture is on being young, staying young, and recoiling from the effects of age. As a result, healthy grief over the loss of youthful looks, stamina, health, and eventually life is not supported.

Medical science can make an important contribution in this area by continuing to define the appropriate limits of technology and intervention. The struggle to balance quantity of life with quality of life (and death) must continue. In addition, medical science professionals need to redouble their efforts toward embracing the patient, not simply the disease; the person, not simply the patient; and the complexities of grief in death and dying, not simply the joy in healing and living.

—Layne A. Prest, Ph.D.

See also Antidepressants; Death and dying; Depression; Emotions: Biomedical causes and effects; Midlife crisis; Neurosis; Phobias; Postpartum depression; Psychiatric disorders; Psychiatry; Psychiatry, child and adolescent; Psychiatry, geriatric; Psychoanalysis; Stress; Suicide.

FOR FURTHER INFORMATION:

Canfield, Jack L., and Mark Victor Hansen. *Chicken Soup for the Grieving Soul: Stories About Life, Death and Overcoming the Loss of a Loved One.* Deerfield Beach, Fla.: Health Communications, 2003. Part of a popular series. Offers personal stories of loss and grief and explores coping strategies and healing from the loss of a loved one.

Corr, Charles A., Clyde M. Nabe, and Donna M. Corr. *Death and Dying, Life and Living.* 5th ed. Belmont, Calif.: Wadsworth, 2005. This book provides perspective on common issues associated with death and dying for family members and others affected by life-threatening circumstances.

Doka, Kenneth J., ed. *Living with Grief After Sudden Loss: Suicide, Homicide, Accident, Heart Attack, Stroke.* Washington, D.C.: Taylor & Francis, Hospice Foundation of America, 1997. Provides information that will be useful for individuals dealing with the different kinds of adjustment related to the death of a loved one or the loss of functioning or abilities.

Greenspan, Miriam. *Healing Through the Dark Emotions: The Wisdom of Grief, Fear, and Despair.* Boston: Shambhala, 2003. Examines grief from a cultural perspective and argues that grief, fear, and despair are not pathologies to be medicated away but emotions that foster psychological and spiritual growth.

GriefNet. http://griefnet.org/. An Internet community of persons dealing with grief, death, and major loss. Offers more than forty e-mail support groups for adults and children.

James, John K., and Russell Friedman. *When Children Grieve: For Adults to Help Children Deal with Death, Divorce, Pet Loss, Moving, and Other Losses.* New York: HarperCollins, 2002. Provides excellent guidelines for helping children develop a lifelong, healthy response to loss.

Klass, Dennis, Phyllis R. Silverman, and Steven L. Nickman, eds. *Continuing Bonds: New Understandings of Grief.* Washington, D.C.: Taylor & Francis, 1996. Examines cross-cultural manifestations of bereavement, particularly the psychological aspects. Includes a bibliography and an index.

Kübler-Ross, Elisabeth, and David Kessler. *On Grief and Grieving: Finding the Meaning of Grief Through the Five Stages of Loss.* New York: Scribner, 2005. A book from the author of the classic *On Death and Dying* (1970).

Staudacher, Carol. *Beyond Grief: A Guide for Recovering from the Death of a Loved One.* New York: Barnes & Noble Books, 2000. A clear and readable guide to the grief process. The author provides specific examples relevant for some of the most painful grief experiences: those following the death of a spouse, child, or parent at an early age.

GROWTH

BIOLOGY

ANATOMY OR SYSTEM AFFECTED: All

SPECIALTIES AND RELATED FIELDS: Embryology, endocrinology, obstetrics, orthopedics, pediatrics

DEFINITION: The development of the human body from conception to adulthood; growth occurs at different rates for different systems over this period, and varies by sex and individual as well.

KEY TERMS:

accretion: a type of growth in which new, nongrowing material is simply added to the surface

allometric growth: unequal rates of growth of different body parts, or in different directions

developmental biology: broadly, the study of ontogeny; narrowly, the study of how gene action is controlled

embryonic stage: that part of ontogeny during which organs are formed

fetal stage: that part of ontogeny after the organs are formed but before birth takes place

interstitial growth: growth throughout a structure, usually in all directions *isometric growth:* equal rates of growth of all parts, or in all directions

ontogeny: the entire developmental sequence, from conception through the various embryonic stages, birth, childhood, maturity, senescence, and death; also, the study of this sequence

ossification: the formation of bone tissue

PROCESS AND EFFECTS

The human body grows from conception until adult size is reached. Adult size is reached in females around the age of eighteen and in males around twenty or twenty-one, but there is considerable variation in either direction. (Nearly all numerical measurements of growth and development are subject to much variation.) On the average, males end up with a somewhat larger body size than females because of these two or three extra years of growth.

Growth begins after conception. The first phase of growth, including approximately the first month after conception, is called embryonic growth, and the growing organism is called an embryo. During embryonic growth, the most important developmental process is differentiation, the formation of the various organs and tissues. After the organs and tissues are formed, the rest of prenatal growth is called fetal growth and the developing organism is called a fetus. Respiratory movements begin around the eighteenth week of gestation,

during the fetal stage; limb movements (such as kicking) begin to be felt by the mother around the twenty-fourth week, with a considerable range of variation. At birth, the average infant weighs about 3.4 kilograms (7.5 pounds) and measures about 50 centimeters (20 inches) in length.

Growth continues after birth and throughout childhood and adolescence. From the perspective of developmental biology, childhood is defined as the period from birth to puberty, which generally begins at twelve years of age, and adolescence continues from that point to the cessation of skeletal growth at around the age of eighteen in females and twenty or twenty-one in males. The long period of adulthood that follows is marked by a stable body size, with little or no growth except for the repair and maintenance of the body, including the healing of wounds. After about age sixty, there may be a slight decline in body height and in a few other dimensions.

By one year of age, the average baby is 75 centimeters (30 inches) long and weighs 10 kilograms (22 pounds). (There is actually a slight decline in weight in the first week of postnatal life, but this is usually regained by age three weeks.) For ages one to six, the average weight (in kilograms) can be approximated by the equation "weight = age × 2 + 8." For ages seven to twelve, growth takes place more rapidly: Average weight (in kilograms) can be approximated by "weight =

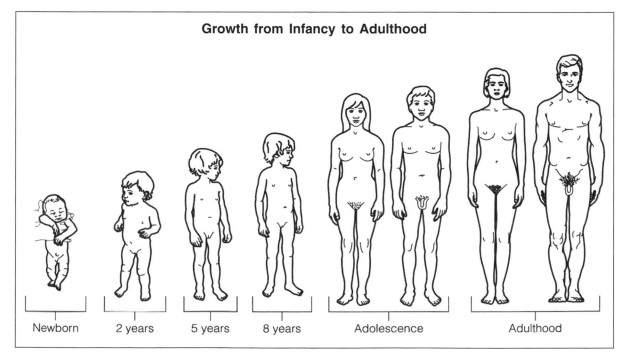

Growth from Infancy to Adulthood

Newborn   2 years   5 years   8 years   Adolescence   Adulthood

age × 3.5 – 2.5," while average height (in centimeters) can be approximated for ages two to twelve by the equation "height = age × 6 + 77." Head circumference has a median value of about 34.5 centimeters at birth, 46.3 centimeters at an age of one year, 48.6 centimeters at age two, and 49.9 centimeters at age three. All these figures are about 1 centimeter larger in boys than in girls, with considerable individual variation. Median heights and weights, when differentiated by sex, reveal that boys and girls are generally similar until age fourteen, after which boys continue to gain in both dimensions.

Growth of the teeth takes place episodically. In most children, the first teeth erupt between five and nine months of age, beginning with the central incisors, the lower pair generally preceding the upper pair. The lateral incisors (with the upper pair first), the first premolars, the canines, and the second premolars follow, in that order. All these teeth are deciduous teeth ("baby teeth") that will eventually be shed, to be replaced during late childhood by the permanent teeth. At one year of age, most children have between six and eight teeth.

Growth takes place in several directions. Growth at the same rate in all directions is called isometric growth, which maintains similar proportions throughout the growth process. Isometric growth occurs in nautilus shells and a variety of other invertebrates. Most of human growth, however, is allometric growth, which takes place at different rates in different directions. Allometric growth results in changes in shape as growth proceeds. Moreover, different parts of the body grow at different rates and in different directions. During fetal development, for example, the head develops in advance of the fore and hind limbs, and the fetus at about six months of age has a head which is about half its length. The head of a newborn baby is about one-third of its body length, compared to about one-seventh for an adult. In contrast, the legs make up only a small part of the body length in either the six-month-old fetus or the newborn baby, and their absolute length and proportionate length both increase throughout childhood and adolescence.

Growth of the skeleton sets the pace for growth of the majority of the body, except for the nervous system and

MEDIAN HEIGHTS AND WEIGHTS FROM CHILDHOOD TO ADULTHOOD

Age	Boys Height (cm)	Boys Weight (kg)	Girls Height (cm)	Girls Weight (kg)
2	87	12	87	12
3	95	15	94	14
4	103	17	102	16
5	110	19	108	18
6	117	21	115	20
7	122	23	121	22
8	127	25	127	25
9	132	28	132	28
10	138	31	138	33
11	143	35	145	37
12	150	40	152	42
13	157	45	157	46
14	163	51	160	50
15	169	57	162	54
16	174	62	162	56
17	176	66	163	57
18	177	69	164	57

reproductive organs. Most parts of the skeleton begin as fast-growing cartilage. The process in which cartilage tissue turns into bone tissue is called ossification, which begins at various centers in the bone. The first center of ossification within each bone is called the diaphysis; in long bones, this ossification usually takes place in the center of the bone, forming the shaft. Secondary centers of ossification form at the ends of long bones and at certain other specified places; each secondary center of ossification is called an epiphysis. In a typical long bone, two epiphyses form, one at either end. Capping the end of the bone, beyond the epiphysis, lies an articular cartilage. Between the epiphysis and the diaphysis, the cartilage that persists is called the epiphyseal cartilage; this becomes the most rapidly growing region of the bone. During most of the growth of a long bone, the increase in width occurs by accretion, a gradual process in which material is added at a slow rate only along a surface. In the case of a bone shaft, increase in width takes place only at the surface, beneath the surrounding membrane known as the periosteum. By contrast, the epiphyseal cartilage grows much more rapidly, and it also grows by interstitial growth, meaning that growth takes place throughout the growing tissue in all directions at once. As the epiphyseal cartilage grows, parts of it slowly become bony, and those bony portions grow more slowly.

During the first seven or eight years of postnatal life, the growth of the epiphyseal cartilage takes place faster than its replacement by bone tissue, causing the size of the epiphyseal cartilage to increase. Starting around age seven, the interstitial growth of the epiphyseal cartilage slows down, while the replacement of cartilage by bone speeds up, so that the epiphyseal cartilage is not growing as fast as it turns into bone tissue; the size of the epiphyseal cartilage therefore starts to decrease. At the time of puberty, the hormonal influences create an adolescent growth spurt during which the individual's bone growth increases for about a one-year period. In girls, the adolescent growth spurt takes place about two years earlier than it does in boys—the average age is around twelve in girls, versus about fifteen in boys—but there are tremendous individual variations both in the extent of the growth spurt and in its timing. At age fourteen, most girls have already experienced most of their adolescent growth spurt, while most boys are barely beginning theirs. Consequently, the average fourteen-year-old girl is a bit taller than the average fourteen-year-old boy.

At around eighteen years of age in females and twenty or twenty-one years of age in males, the replacement of the epiphyseal cartilage by bone is finally complete, and bone growth ceases. The age at which this occurs and the resulting adult size both vary considerably from one individual to another. For the rest of adult life, the skeleton remains more or less constant in size, diminishing only slightly in old age.

Most of the other organs of the body grow in harmonious proportion with the growth of the skeleton, reaching a maximum growth rate during the growth spurt of early adolescence and reaching a stable adult size at around age eighteen in women and age twenty or twenty-one in men. The nervous system and reproductive system, however, constitute major exceptions to this rule. The nervous system and brain grow faster at an earlier age, reaching about 90 to 95 percent of their adult size by one year of age. The shape of the head, including the shape of the skull, keeps pace with the development of the brain and nervous system. For this reason, babies and young children have heads that constitute a larger proportion of their body size than do the heads of adults.

The growth of the reproductive system also follows its own pattern. Most reproductive development is delayed until puberty. The reproductive organs of the em-

bryo form slowly and remain small. The reproductive organs of children, though present, do not reach their mature size until adolescence. These organs, both the internal ones and the external ones, remain small throughout childhood. Their period of most rapid growth marks the time of puberty, which spans ages eleven through thirteen, with a wide range of variation. At this time, the pituitary gland begins secreting increased amounts of the follicle-stimulating hormone (FSH), which stimulates the growth and maturation of the gonads (the ovaries of females and the testes of males). The ovaries or testes then respond by producing increased amounts of the sex hormones testosterone (in males) or estrogen (in females), which stimulate the further development of both primary and secondary sexual characteristics. Primary sexual characteristics are those which are functionally necessary for reproduction, such as the presence of a uterus and ovaries in females or the presence of testes and sperm ducts in males. Secondary sexual characteristics are those which distinguish one sex from another, but which are not functionally necessary for reproduction. Examples of secondary sexual characteristics include the growth of breasts or the widening of the hips in females, the growth of the beard and deepening of the voice in males, and the growth of hair in the armpits and pubic regions of both sexes.

Growth takes place psychologically and socially as well as physically. Newborn babies, though able to respond to changes in their environment, seem to pay attention to such stimuli only on occasion. At a few weeks of age, the baby will respond to social stimuli (such as the sound of the mother's voice) by smiling. Babies usually can grasp objects by five months of age, depending on the size and shape of the object. By six months, most babies will show definite signs of pleasure in response to social stimulation; this may include an open-mouth giggle or laugh. At seven months of age, most babies will respond to adult facial expressions and will show different responses to familiar adults as opposed to strangers. The age at which babies learn to crawl varies greatly, but most infants learn the technique by nine or ten months of age. Social imitation begins late in the first year of life. Also, by this time, children learn object permanence, meaning that they will search for a missing object if they have watched it being hidden. Walking generally develops around eighteen months of age, but the time of development varies greatly.

Jean Piaget (1896-1980) was a pioneer in the study

of the social and cognitive development of children. Piaget identified four stages of cognitive and social growth, which he called sensorimotor, preoperational, concrete operational, and formal operational. In the sensorimotor stage, from birth to about two years of age, infants begin with reflexes such as sucking or finger curling (in response to touching their palms). Starting with these reflexes, they gradually learn to understand their senses and apply the resulting information in order to acquire important adaptive motor skills that can be used to manipulate the world (as in picking up things) or to navigate about and explore the world (as in walking). Socially, infants develop ways to make desirable stimuli last by such acts as smiling. In the preoperational stage, which lasts from about two to six years of age, children acquire a functional use of their native language. Their imagination flourishes, and pretending becomes an important and frequent activity. Most of the thinking at the preoperational stage is egocentric, however, which means that the child perceives the world only from his or her own point of view and has difficulty seeing other points of view.

The concrete operational stage spans the years from about seven to eleven years of age. This is the stage at which children learn to apply logic to concrete objects. For example, they realize that liquid does not change volume when poured into a taller glass, and they develop the ability to arrange objects in order (for example, by size) or to classify them into groups (for example, by color or shape). The final stage is called the formal operational stage, beginning around age twelve. This is the stage of adolescence and adulthood, when the person learns to manipulate abstract concepts in such areas as ethical, legal, or mathematical reasoning. This is also the stage at which people develop the ability to construct hypothetical situations and to use them in arguments.

COMPLICATIONS AND DISORDERS

Disorders of growth include dwarfism, gigantism, and several other disorders such as achondroplasia (chondrodystrophy). Dwarfism often results from an insufficiency of the pituitary growth hormone, also called somatostatin or somatotrophic hormone. Some short-statured individuals are normally proportioned, while others have proportions differing from those of most other people. An overabundance of growth hormone causes gigantism, a condition marked by unusually rapid growth, especially during adolescence. In some individuals, the amount of growth hormone remains normal during childhood but increases to excessive amounts during the teenage years; these individuals are marked by acromegaly, a greater than normal growth which affects primarily the hands, feet, and face.

Achondroplasia, also called chondrodystrophy, is a genetically controlled condition caused by a dominant gene. In people having this condition, the epiphyseal cartilages of the body's long bones turn bony too soon, so that growth ceases before it should. Those exhibiting chondrodystrophy therefore have short stature and childlike proportions but rugged faces that look older than they really are.

Inadequate growth can often result from childhood malnutrition, particularly from insufficient amounts of protein. If a child is considerably shorter or skinnier than those of the same age, that child's diet should be examined for the presence of malnutrition. Intentional malnutrition is one of the characteristic features of anorexia nervosa. The opposite problem, overeating, can lead to obesity, although obesity can also result from many other causes, including diabetes and other metabolic problems.

By the late twentieth century, human growth hormone, a drug used since the 1950's to help very short children grow, was being used for "off-label" purposes that included anti-aging and body-building. In 2002, researchers suggested an apparent link between the use of the hormone and cancer, specifically Hodgkin's disease and colorectal cancer.

PERSPECTIVE AND PROSPECTS

As a phenomenon, growth of both wild and domestic animals was well known to ancient peoples. Hippocrates (c. 460-c. 370 B.C.E.), considered the father of medicine, wrote a treatise on embryological growth, and Aristotle (384-322 B.C.E.) wrote a longer and more complete work on the subject. During the Renaissance, Galileo Galilei (1564-1642) studied growth mathematically and distinguished between isometric and allometric forms of growth, arguing that the bones of giants would be too weak to support their weight.

The most important era in the study of human embryonic development was ushered in by the Estonian naturalist Karl Ernst von Baer (1792-1876), who discovered the human ovum. From this point on, detailed studies of human embryonic and postnatal development proceeded at a rapid pace, especially in Germany. Much of the modern understanding of growth in more general or mathematical terms derives from the classic studies of the British anatomist D'Arcy Wentworth

Thomson (1860-1948). In the twentieth century, Piaget became a leader in the study of childhood social and cognitive growth phases.

—Eli C. Minkoff, Ph.D.

See also Aging; Childbirth; Conception; Dwarfism; Embryology; Endocrine disorders; Endocrinology; Endocrinology, pediatric; Failure to thrive; Gigantism; Glands; Hormones; Hypertrophy; Malnutrition; Menopause; Menstruation; Nutrition; Prader-Willi syndrome; Pregnancy and gestation; Puberty and adolescence; Sexuality; Vitamins and minerals; Weight loss and gain.

FOR FURTHER INFORMATION:

Bar, Robert S., ed. *Early Diagnosis and Treatment of Endocrine Disorders*. Totowa, N.J.: Humana Press, 2003. Reviews the early signs and symptoms of endocrine diseases, surveys the clinical testing needed for a diagnosis, and presents recommendations for therapy.

Behrman, Richard E., Robert M. Kliegman, and Hal B. Jenson, eds. *Nelson Textbook of Pediatrics*. 17th ed. Philadelphia: Saunders, 2004. Text covering all medical and surgical disorders in children with authoritative information on genetics, endocrinology, aetiology, epidemiology, pathology, pathophysiology, clinical manifestations, diagnosis, prevention, treatment, and prognosis.

Goodman, H. Maurice. *Basic Medical Endocrinology*. 3d ed. Boston: Academic Press, 2003. Focuses on research advances in the understanding of hormones involved in regulating most aspects of bodily functions. Includes in-depth coverage of individual glands and regulatory principles.

McMillan, Julia A., et al., eds. *Oski's Pediatrics: Principles and Practice*. 4th ed. Philadelphia: Lippincott Williams & Wilkins, 2006. Contains many good descriptions and illustrations of different stages of development, various disorders common in children, and several treatments for these disorders.

Marieb, Elaine N. *Essentials of Human Anatomy and Physiology*. 8th ed. San Francisco: Pearson/Benjamin Cummings, 2006. This introductory anatomy and physiology textbook, easily accessible to those with little science background, is richly illustrated with diagrams and photographs, which help to illuminate body systems and processes.

Moore, Keith L., and T. V. N. Persaud. *The Developing Human*. 7th ed. Philadelphia: W. B. Saunders, 2003. An outstanding textbook on human embryonic development, with specific information about the causes of congenital malformations and common defects occurring in each of the body's systems.

Rosse, Cornelius, and Penelope Gaddum-Rosse. *Hollinshead's Textbook of Anatomy*. 5th ed. Philadelphia: Lippincott-Raven, 1997. A very thorough, up-to-date, detailed reference work. Provides helpful descriptions and illustrations, including descriptions of the immature stages of growth.

Standring, Susan, et al., eds. *Gray's Anatomy*. 39th ed. New York: Elsevier Churchill Livingstone, 2005. The classic work on anatomy, containing the most thorough descriptions. The excellent color illustrations provide much realistic detail in most cases and well-selected highlights in a few. Developmental stages are covered in detail.

Tsiaras, Alexander, and Barry Werth. *From Conception to Birth: A Life Unfolds*. New York: Doubleday, 2002. Using state-of-the-art medical imaging technology, traces the development of a human life from conception through birth in spectacular, highly detailed photographs.

GUILLAIN-BARRÉ SYNDROME

DISEASE/DISORDER

ALSO KNOWN AS: Acute inflammatory demyelinating polyneuropathy

ANATOMY OR SYSTEM AFFECTED: Immune system, muscles, musculoskeletal system, nerves, nervous system

SPECIALTIES AND RELATED FIELDS: Internal medicine, neurology

DEFINITION: An acute degeneration of peripheral motor and sensory nerves, known to physicians as acute inflammatory demyelinating polyneuropathy, a common cause of acute generalized paralysis.

KEY TERMS:

antibody: a substance produced by plasma cells which usually binds to a foreign particle; in Guillain-Barré syndrome, antibodies bind to myelin protein

antigen: any substance that stimulates white blood cells to mount an immune response

areflexia: loss of reflex

autoimmune disorder: a condition in which the immune system attacks the body's own tissue instead of foreign tissue

B cell: a type of white blood cell that produces antibodies

CSF protein: a protein in the cerebrospinal fluid which is usually very low

demyelination: a loss of the myelin coating of nerves

electromyogram: the external recording of electrical impulses from muscles

macrophage: a white blood cell that engulfs foreign protein; in Guillain-Barré syndrome, it also attacks myelin

motor weakness: muscle weakness resulting from the failure of motor nerves

nerve conduction velocity: the speed at which a nerve impulse travels along a nerve

neurogenic atrophy: shrinkage of muscle caused by a loss of nervous stimulation

neuropathy: a condition in which nerves are diseased, are inflamed, or show abnormal degeneration

phagocytosis: the process of engulfing particles

polyneuropathy: neuropathy found in many areas

CAUSES AND SYMPTOMS

Guillain-Barré syndrome (GBS) is an acute disease of the peripheral nerves, especially those that connect to muscles. It causes weakness, areflexia (loss of reflex), ataxia (difficulty in maintaining balance), and sometimes ophthalmoplegia (eye muscle paralysis). GBS demonstrates a variable, multifocal pattern of inflammation and demyelination of the spinal roots and the cranial nerves, although the brain itself is not obviously affected. By the 1990's, it was the most common cause of generalized paralysis in the United States, averaging two cases per 100,000 people per year. The disease was first described in the early 1900's by Georges Guillain and Jean-Alexander Barré, two French neurologists. Little was known of the cause of GBS or the mechanism for its symptoms, however, until the 1970's. Since then, symposia sponsored by the National Institute of Neurological and Communicative Disorders and Stroke have shed more light on this condition.

Most individuals with GBS have a rapidly progressing muscular weakness in more than one limb and also experience paresthesia (tingling) and numbness in the hands and feet. These sensations have the effect of reducing fine muscle control, balance, and one's awareness of limb location. The prevailing scientific opinion regarding GBS is that it is an autoimmune disorder involving white blood cells, which for some unknown reason attack nerves and/or produce antibodies against myelin, the insulating covering of nerves. The weakness is usually ascending in nature, beginning with numbness in the toes and fingers and progressing to total limb weakness. The demyelination is more prominent in the nerves of the trunk and occurs to a lesser extent in the more distal nerves. The brain and spinal cord

are protected from GBS by the blood-brain barrier, although antibodies to myelin have been found in the cerebrospinal fluid of some patients.

With GBS, there is often a precipitating event such as surgery, pregnancy, upper respiratory infection, viral infection (such as cytomegalovirus), or vaccination. Preexisting debilitating illnesses such as systemic lupus erythematosus (SLE) or Hodgkin's disease also seem to predispose a person to GBS. GBS has been diagnosed in patients having heart transplants in spite of the fact that they are receiving immunosuppressive drugs. The increased risk with such surgery may be attributable to the stress associated with the procedure. Most patients who come down with GBS have had some prior condition that placed stress on the immune system prior to the appearance of GBS.

The patient with GBS is frequently incapable of communicating as a result of paralysis of the vocal cords. Typically, motor paralysis will worsen rapidly and then plateau after four weeks, with the patient bedridden and often in need of respiratory support. Autonomic nerves can also be affected, causing gastrointestinal disturbances, adynamic ileus (loss of function in the ileum of the small intestine), and indigestion. Other, less common symptoms include pupillary disturbances, pooling of blood in limbs, heart rhythm disturbances, and a decrease in the heart muscle's strength. These patients are usually hypermetabolic because considerable caloric energy goes into an immune response that is self-destructive and into mechanisms that are attempting to repair the damage.

In addition to the loss of myelin, cell body damage

**INFORMATION ON
GUILLAIN-BARRÉ SYNDROME**

CAUSES: Autoimmune disorder; often with precipitating event such as surgery, pregnancy, upper respiratory infection, viral infection (such as cytomegalovirus), vaccination

SYMPTOMS: Weakness; loss of reflex; difficulty maintaining balance; eye muscle paralysis; tingling and numbness in hands and feet; reduced fine motor control, balance, and awareness of limb location; paralysis of vocal cords

DURATION: Chronic with acute episodes

TREATMENTS: Plasmapheresis, administration of cyclosporine or corticosteroids

to nerves may result and may be associated with permanent deficits. If the nerve cell itself is not severely damaged, regrowth and remyelination can occur. Antibodies to myelin proteins and to acidic glycolipids are seen in a majority of patients. Blood serum taken from patients with GBS has been shown to block calcium channels in muscle, and experiments in Germany have found that cerebrospinal fluid from GBS patients blocks sodium channels.

Like most autoimmune conditions, GBS is cyclic in nature; the patient will have "good" days and "bad" days because the immune system is sensitive to the levels of steroid hormones in the body, which are known to fluctuate. In addition to paralysis, there is significant pain with GBS. Many of the nerve fibers that register the pain response (nociceptors) are nonmyelinated and therefore are not interrupted in GBS. Pain management can be difficult, requiring the use of such drugs as fentanyl, codeine, morphine, and other narcotics. The course of the disease is variable and is a function of the level of reactivity of the patient's immune system. The autoimmune attack is augmented in those patients experiencing activation of serum complement protein induced by antibodies. Recovery usually takes months, and frequently the patient requires home health care. Complications can lead to death, but most patients recover fully, though some have residual weakness.

The physician must be careful to distinguish GBS from lead poisoning, chemical or toxin exposure, polio, botulism, and hysterical paralysis. Diagnosis can be confirmed using cerebrospinal fluid (CSF) analysis. GBS patients have protein levels greater than 0.55 gram per deciliter of CSF. Macrophages are frequently found in the CSF, as well as some B cells. Nerve conduction velocity will be decreased in these patients to a value that is 50 percent of normal in those nerves that are still functioning. These changes can take several weeks to develop.

With GBS, macrophages and T cells have been shown to be in contact with nerves, as evidenced in electron micrographs. T-cell and macrophage activation in these individuals point to an immune response gone awry, possibly precipitated by a virus or exposure to an antigen that is foreign but similar in appearance to one of the proteins in myelin. T cells, upon encountering an unrecognizable antigen, will produce interleukin 2, initiate attack, and recruit macrophages to participate. The use of an anti-T-cell drug theoretically should improve nerve function, but researchers at the University of Western Ontario failed to find any benefit from the infusion of an anti-T-cell monoclonal antibody. Unexpectedly, GBS has been found in patients testing positive for the human immunodeficiency virus (HIV) who are asymptomatic, in spite of the fact that their T cells are under attack from the HIV virus and are diminished in number. Although myelin proteins are thought to be the immunogens, other candidates include gangliosides in the myelin. Antiganglioside antibodies have been seen in a majority of the GBS patients. This trait may distinguish GBS from amyotrophic lateral sclerosis (Lou Gehrig's disease) and multiple sclerosis, which seem to involve different myelin proteins as antigens.

In GBS, the white blood cells attack peripheral motor nerves more often than other types of nerves, implying a biochemical difference between motor and sensory nerves that has yet to be discovered. One possible cause of this disease is a similarity between a protein or glycolipid that is present normally in myelin and coincidentally on an infectious agent, such as a virus. The immune system responds to the agent, resulting in a sensitization of the macrophages and T cells to that component of myelin. B cells are then stimulated to produce antibodies against this antigen, and they unfortunately cross-react with components of the myelin protein. The severity of the disease will depend on the number of macrophages and lymphocytes activated and whether serum complement-binding antibodies are being produced. Serum complement proteins are activated by a particular class of antibodies, resulting in the activation of enzymes in the blood that potentiate tissue destruction and neurogenic atrophy. Serum complement levels can be determined by a serum complement fixation test.

In severe cases of GBS, intercostal muscles are more severely compromised and respiratory function needs to be monitored closely. The immune response will subside when T-suppressor cells have reached their peak levels. Halting the autoimmune response will not reverse the symptoms immediately, since it takes time for antibody levels to decrease and for the nerves to regrow and remyelinate, which occurs at the rate of 1 to 2 millimeters per day. Some nerves will undergo retrograde degeneration and be lost from the neuronal pool. Other nerves will have more closely spaced nodes and conduct impulses at a lower velocity. Nerve sprouting will also occur, which will result in one nerve's being responsible for more muscle fibers or serving a larger sensory area and in decreased fine motor control.

TREATMENT AND THERAPY

In Guillain-Barré syndrome, the amount of muscle and nerve involvement can be assessed by performing an electromyogram, which can reveal the amount of motor nerve interruption and the conduction velocity of the nerves that continue to function. Based upon the assumption that an autoimmune response is in progress, corticosteroids such as prednisolone and methylprednisolone are sometimes administered in high doses. The benefits of such drugs have been shown to be marginal, while the side effects are considerable.

More recently, a procedure known as plasmapheresis has been tried with better results, especially when performed in the first two weeks. This procedure involves removing 250 milliliters (a little more than a pint) of plasma from the blood every other day and replacing this volume with a solution containing albumin, glucose, and appropriate salts. Six treatments are typical and usually result in a faster recovery of muscle control than for those not receiving plasmapheresis. Because relapses may occur if the patient produces new antibodies to myelin, immunosuppressants are given to the patient after plasmapheresis. Another procedure, intravenous immunoglobulin therapy, is in the clinical trial stage and is based on the strategy of blocking the binding of antibodies to nerves.

Cyclosporine, a T-cell inhibitor, is also being tried, with some promising results. Some researchers note, however, that transplant patients, who routinely take cyclosporine, have a higher-than-normal risk of developing GBS. Others emphasize that no one knows what their risk for GBS would be without the administration of cyclosporine. Because of the variability of the body's immune response, the benefits of this drug will depend on whether, in a given individual, it is an antibody response or T-cell response. Cyclosporine will benefit those who have a strong T-cell response. T-cell reactivity can be tested with the mixed lymphocyte assay, and T-cell counts can be done.

Cerebrospinal fluid filtration is also being tried in order to remove reactive white blood cells and antibodies. Serum so filtered loses its nerve-inhibiting effect, as evidenced by its application to in vitro nerve and muscle cells. GBS has been mimicked in animal models, which show antibody and T-cell reactivity to myelin protein. Guillain-Barré syndrome has many of the characteristics of an autoimmune disease and could serve as a model for an acquired autoimmune condition.

PERSPECTIVE AND PROSPECTS

Guillain-Barré syndrome is an example of a delicate physiological balance gone awry. The immune system has the difficult task of distinguishing between self and enemy, and if it detects the latter it must either inactivate or eliminate the intruder. Mistakes in recognition or communication between immune cells can cause either an unintended attack or the failure to attack when appropriate. GBS probably represents an unnecessary attack on self tissue, in this case myelin, and may be considered a form of hyperimmunity. Many diseases fall into this category. They include rheumatoid arthritis, juvenile diabetes, Crohn's disease, ulcerative colitis, Graves' disease, multiple sclerosis, amyotrophic lateral sclerosis, ankylosing spondylitis (inflammation of the joints between the vertebrae), and systemic lupus erythematosus. The other type of response, hypoimmune, is seen in cancer and immunodeficiency diseases such as acquired immunodeficiency syndrome (AIDS).

Questions that arise with GBS are the same ones that arise in many other diseases. It must be determined why the immune system chose this time to initiate an attack against a self-antigen. The answer could be a mistake in recognition, an error in translating the deoxyribonucleic acid (DNA) code in the bone marrow cells, an alteration of the antigen by some environmental factor, or an alteration of an antigen-detector protein on a white blood cell. Researchers also try to discover if there is a genetic predisposition for GBS. Seeking answers about GBS may shed light on other conditions as well, and treatments beneficial to GBS patients have a high probability of benefiting patients with other immune disorders. GBS is a reminder that physiological stress can translate to immunological stress, and under stress the immune system can make mistakes. Failure to react can result in diseases such as cancer, and unnecessary action can lead to diseases such as GBS.

—William D. Niemi, Ph.D.

See also Ataxia; Autoimmune disorders; Immune system; Immunology; Motor neuron diseases; Nervous system; Neuralgia, neuritis, and neuropathy; Neurology; Neurology, pediatric; Numbness and tingling; Paralysis; Stress.

FOR FURTHER INFORMATION:

Abbas, Abul K., and Andrew K. Lichtman. *Basic Immunology: Functions and Disorders of the Immune System.* 2d ed. Philadelphia: Elsevier Saunders, 2006. Provides introductory text on the basics of immunology and describes the primary disorders that impair immunological function. Illustrations, case studies, review questions, key point summaries, and a glossary are included.

Adelman, Daniel C., et al., eds. *Manual of Allergy and Immunology*. 4th ed. Philadelphia: Lippincott Williams & Wilkins, 2002. Examines research developments and the clinical diagnosis and treatment of allergies and immune disorders.

Baron-Faust, Rita, and Jill P. Buyon. *The Autoimmune Connection*. Chicago: Contemporary Books, 2003. Examines myriad health issues in women and investigates their possible environmental triggers. Each chapter includes signs, diagnosis and tests, current and future treatments, and looks at the role of female hormones, menstruation, pregnancy, and menopause in affecting the course of each disease.

Guillain-Barré Syndrome Foundation International. http://www.gbsfi.com/. A Web site focused on providing informative support and increasing the opportunities for patients, family, and friends to network and communicate.

Kierman, John A. *Barr's The Human Nervous System: An Anatomical Viewpoint*. 8th ed. Philadelphia: Lippincott Williams & Wilkins, 2005. A softbound text designed for a medical school introductory course in the basic sciences. Provides a good foundation for understanding the nervous system, with some discussion of demyelination.

Lechtenberg, Richard. *Synopsis of Neurology*. Philadelphia: Lea & Febiger, 1991. A pocket-sized book with summary descriptions of the most common neurological syndromes. Covers diagnostic techniques and symptoms associated with neurological problems, including Guillain-Barré syndrome.

Nicholls, John G., A. Robert Martin, and Bruce G. Wallace. *From Neuron to Brain*. 4th ed. Sunderland, Mass.: Sinauer Associates, 2000. An excellent and detailed neurobiology text that can help the reader understand the basis and consequences of demyelinating conditions such as Guillain-Barré syndrome.

Noback, Charles R., et al. *The Human Nervous System: Structure and Function*. 6th ed. Totowa, N.J.: Humana Press, 2005. A concise, easy-to-read paperback that offers a good balance of physiology and anatomy. Well illustrated.

Parker, James N., and Philip M. Parker, eds. *The Official Patient's Sourcebook on Guillain-Barré Syndrome*. San Diego, Calif.: Icon Health, 2002. Draws from public, academic, government, and peer-reviewed research to provide a wide-ranging handbook for patients with Guillain-Barré syndrome.

Pearlman, Alan L., and Robert C. Collins. *Neurobiology of Disease*. New York: Oxford University Press, 1990. An advanced text that provides detailed descriptions of most neurological abnormalities. Contains a good description of Guillain-Barré syndrome and a chapter devoted to demyelinating disease.

Sticherling, Michael, and Enno Christophers. *Treatment of Autoimmune Disorders*. New York: Springer, 2003. Explores the basic mechanisms of autoimmune disorders; neurological, gastrointestinal, ophthalmological, and skin diseases; and current and future therapeutic options.

GULF WAR SYNDROME
DISEASE/DISORDER

ANATOMY OR SYSTEM AFFECTED: Blood, brain, cells, chest, eyes, gastrointestinal system, gums, hair, immune system, joints, muscles, psychic-emotional system, skin

SPECIALTIES AND RELATED FIELDS: Biochemistry, environmental health, epidemiology, ethics, occupational health, psychology, public health

DEFINITION: A popular term used to describe collectively a variety of symptoms, not a specific disease, suffered by veterans of the Persian Gulf War.

KEY TERMS:

cytokines: proteins which are used by white blood cells to communicate with similar cells

organophosphates: chemical pesticides

pyridostigmine bromide: a chemical that prevents damage from possible nerve gas exposure

sarin: a nerve gas that can cause convulsions and death

CAUSES AND SYMPTOMS

This condition is characterized by flulike symptoms, which sufferers complain of experiencing simultaneously but which do not indicate any specific known disease. Such physical symptoms include chronic fatigue, fever, muscle and joint pain and weakness, and intense headaches. Some patients report episodes of memory loss, insomnia, nightmares, and limited attention spans as well as neuropsychological disorders, such as depression, anxiety attacks, and mood swings. Respiratory problems, diarrhea and gastrointestinal distress, blurred vision, arthritis, bleeding gums, hair loss, and skin rashes sometimes accompany other symptoms.

Physicians disagree about the causal factors of Gulf War syndrome. While some medical professionals diagnose veterans' symptoms as resulting from exposure to wartime toxins, bacteria, or viruses, other doctors state that the symptoms are psychosomatic and due to post-traumatic stress disorder. Gulf War syndrome has not been attributed to any infectious disease that veterans might have contracted in the Persian Gulf. Significantly, it has been difficult for researchers to prove any laboratory abnormality or unique characteristic for this disorder or to isolate any organ system as the primary system affected by this condition. Most medical professionals say that Gulf War syndrome is a condition representing factors of several diseases but is not a separate disease.

Many Persian Gulf War veterans believe their ailments are service related. Approximately 800,000 coalition forces were deployed to the Persian Gulf after Iraq invaded Kuwait in August, 1990. About 10 percent of these veterans have claimed to have Gulf War syndrome (statistics vary according to sources). Soldiers hypothesize that exposure to sarin caused the syndrome. Other possible causes include germ and chemical warfare (although no evidence of either has been verified), antianthrax and botulism vaccines, pyridostigmine bromide (PB) tablets, and exposure to radiation from depleted uranium, fumes from burning oil wells, and organophosphates.

TREATMENT AND THERAPY

Because they do not think their concerns are being seriously addressed, many veterans rely on self-diagnosis based on other veterans' accounts exchanged orally, in the press, or on the Internet. Self-medication with over-the-counter pain relievers is a common treatment on which veterans depend for the soothing of symptoms. Physicians prescribe more potent pharmaceuticals and physical therapy to alleviate symptoms and reinforce patients' immune systems. The American, Canadian, and British governments have established medical programs through publicly funded veterans' administrations and privately endowed medical institutions to research the syndrome's causes, ascertain its etiology, identify derivative presentations of the syndrome, develop effective treatment methods, and offer medical care for veterans exhibiting Gulf War syndrome symptoms.

Physicians recommend that some veterans suffering Gulf War syndrome undergo counseling to address neuropsychological symptoms and assist readjustment

---

INFORMATION ON GULF WAR SYNDROME

CAUSES: Unclear; possibly exposure to wartime toxins, bacteria, or viruses; psychosomatic factors; post-traumatic stress disorder

SYMPTOMS: Varies widely; can include chronic fatigue, fever, muscle and joint pain and weakness, intense headaches, episodes of memory loss, insomnia, nightmares, anxiety attacks, mood swings, respiratory problems, blurred vision, rashes

DURATION: Chronic

TREATMENTS: Self-medication with over-the-counter pain relievers, prescribed drug and physical therapy, counseling

---

to peacetime or civilian life and frustration with enduring chronic sickness. Exercise, a nutritional diet, and support groups are also helpful to many veterans suffering Gulf War syndrome. Genetic testing of veterans and their spouses is also sometimes pursued to determine causation of birth defects in some veterans' children, which are often incorrectly attributed to Gulf War service. Complications associated with treatment of Gulf War syndrome include possible common side effects of pain relievers, such as drowsiness. Patients also risk becoming addicted to pain relievers that they use to numb the ever-present aches associated with chronic illnesses.

PERSPECTIVE AND PROSPECTS

Originally identified when some American, British, and Canadian Gulf War veterans complained of various ailments after returning home in 1991, Gulf War syndrome was sensationalized in the press as a mystery illness. Physicians familiar with military medical history recognized similarities with symptoms documented in soldier populations as early as the American Civil War. This awareness suggested that the syndrome was indicative of a common wartime factor rather than a unique occurrence in the Gulf War.

Gulf War syndrome became politicized as government officials and veterans disagreed regarding description of and funding for treatment of the syndrome. After clinical investigations of twenty thousand Gulf War veterans, the Institute of Medicine declared that no Gulf War syndrome existed, although some soldiers did suffer nonchronic illnesses, such as malaria. Five independent panels confirmed the conclusion that no unique case of an illness had been proven.

Physicians and scientists representing the Departments of Defense, Veterans Affairs, and Health and Human Services stated that the rates of incidence of Gulf War veterans' symptoms, hospitalization, and mortality are not greater than those reported for the general population and that many veterans may have already been genetically predisposed to certain physiological conditions. They also questioned why veterans from other countries, especially Arab nations, did not report syndrome symptoms, nor were any similar reports issued after World War II soldiers returned from the Persian Gulf.

In 2002, in what veterans called a "stunning reversal," the U.S. Department of Defense admitted that there is increasing evidence that neural damage affects some veterans of the Gulf War and doubled research funding. The change in stance was partly in response to research emanating from the University of Texas Southwestern Medical Center in Dallas and the U.S. Department of Veterans Affairs. Using a statistical technique called factor analysis, researchers at these facilities identified unusual clusters of symptoms that could be divided into syndromes. Syndrome 1 involved sleep and memory disturbances, syndrome 3 involved joint and muscle pain, while syndrome 2, the most serious, involved confusion and dizziness. Using magnetic resonance spectroscopy (MRS), the research team found that veterans with syndrome 2 had lost nerve cells in the brain structures that are involved with the symptoms of the syndrome. Moreover, syndrome 2 veterans were also approximately eight times more likely as healthy veterans to have had a bad reaction to the PB tablets. Researchers surmise that chemical weapons and the PB tablets that were designed to protect against them affect the same physiological pathway. The increasing scientific evidence of real physiological damage among veterans has helped spur the U.S. government to begin more strenuous investigation into its causes. In 2002, the Department of Veterans Affairs appointed a Research Advisory Committee on Gulf War veterans.

Determined to understand Gulf War syndrome, some researchers hypothesize how variables possibly affected veterans' immune symptoms to cause physiochemical responses, such as increased cytokine production and brain cell damage. Others claim that chemical exposure contaminated soldiers' bloodstreams and is to blame for renal failure and cancers. Unless addi-

tional research determines a singular illness, Gulf War syndrome will remain a puzzling, vague, controversial condition with no specific cure or prevention for future military forces. A Veterans Administration Persian Gulf Health Registry and Department of Defense Persian Gulf Health Surveillance System were also created to monitor veterans' health status and to detect patterns that might possibly provide further insights about the complexities of Gulf War syndrome.

—*Elizabeth D. Schafer, Ph.D.*

See also Biological and chemical weapons; Environmental diseases; Environmental health; Epidemiology; Poisoning; Toxicology.

FOR FURTHER INFORMATION:

Blanck, Ronald R., and members of the Persian Gulf Veterans Coordinating Board. "Unexplained Illnesses Among Desert Storm Veterans: A Search for Causes, Treatment, and Cooperation." *Archives of Internal Medicine* 155 (February 13, 1995): 262-268.

Bloom, Saul, et al. *Hidden Casualties: Environmental, Health, and Political Consequences of the Persian Gulf War.* Berkeley, Calif.: Arms Control Research Center, North Atlantic Books, 1994.

Eddington, Patrick G. *Gassed in the Gulf: The Inside Story of the Pentagon-CIA Cover-up of Gulf War Syndrome.* Washington, D.C: Insignia, 1997.

Gulf War Veteran Resource Pages. http://www.gulfweb.org/.

Hersh, Seymour M. *Against All Enemies: Gulf War Syndrome, the War Between America's Ailing Veterans and Their Government.* New York: Ballantine Books, 1998.

Office of the Secretary of Defense. National Defense Research Institution. *A Review of the Scientific Literature as It Pertains to Gulf War Illnesses.* 8 vols. Santa Monica, Calif.: Rand, 1998-2001.

Wheelwright, Jeff. *The Irritable Heart: The Medical Mystery of the Gulf War.* New York: W. W. Norton, 2000.

GUM DISEASE
DISEASE/DISORDER
ANATOMY OR SYSTEM AFFECTED: Gums, mouth, teeth
SPECIALTIES AND RELATED FIELDS: Dentistry
DEFINITION: Inflammation of the soft tissue that surrounds the teeth; in advanced disease, there is also loss of bone that holds the teeth in place.

Causes and Symptoms

Bacterial infection is the most common cause of gum disease. In early stages of the disease, only the soft tissues—the gums, or gingiva—are affected, but in later stages bacteria also attack the hard tissues underlying the gums.

The bacteria responsible for gum disease accumulate in plaque, which is a sticky biofilm of bacteria that forms on the teeth, both above and below the gum line. Plaque that remains on the teeth for more than about seventy-two hours may harden into tartar, which cannot be removed completely except by a professional. Plaque accumulation is usually the result of inadequate tooth brushing and flossing.

Plaque contains many different kinds of bacteria. Bacteria that live below the gum line, where oxygen is low or lacking, are the main culprits in gingivitis, an inflammation of the soft gum tissues. Toxins produced by the bacteria destroy the collagen fibers that make up the connective tissue between the gum and the tooth, causing the gum to loosen and detach from the tooth. The widening and deepening of the space between tooth and gum produces a pocket. Whereas in healthy gums there is a crevice about 1 to 3 millimeters deep between the gum and tooth, in gingivitis there is a pocket up to 4 millimeters deep. The gum becomes movable instead of clinging to the tooth. The gum also swells, is red rather than a healthy pink, and bleeds when brushed or probed. At this early stage, there is little or no pain.

From a gum pocket, bacteria can advance to the bone and to the other hard tissues that support the tooth: the cementum, which covers the roots of the tooth, and the periodontal ligament, which anchors the tooth to the jawbone. Gum disease that has progressed to the bone is referred to as periodontitis. It usually results from a long-term accumulation of plaque and tartar.

In early periodontitis, the crests or peaks of the bone between the teeth have begun to erode. The patient may as yet be unaware of the problem because there is no pain. As the inflammation destroys the fibers of the periodontal ligament and further dissolves the bone, the pocket often deepens to between 4 and 8 millimeters. In advanced stages, most of the bone surrounding the tooth is destroyed and the tooth loosens. Abscesses and pain are common at this point. Advanced periodontitis can cause teeth to fall out or require extraction and is one of the main causes of tooth loss in adults.

In both gingivitis and periodontitis, the damage may be localized. Furthermore, the disease does not pro-

---

INFORMATION ON GUM DISEASE

Causes: Bacterial infection
Symptoms: Red, swollen gums that bleed easily; may progress to bone loss. loose teeth, abscesses, and pain
Duration: Chronic and sometimes progressive
Treatments: Removal of plaque and tartar, antibiotics (oral and inserted into gum pockets), surgery

---

gress at a uniform rate but instead advances episodically, with periods of remission. Most adults have had gingivitis at one time or another, but some individuals are especially susceptible, including those who smoke, have certain medical conditions, or take particular medications.

Treatment and Therapy

Gum disease is treatable. To diagnose the disease, the dentist may use X rays to determine the extent of bone loss, and a dental probe to measure the depth of pockets. The dentist removes plaque and tartar by scaling the surfaces of the teeth and planing the surfaces of the roots. An ultrasonic scaler, which cleans the teeth with high-frequency vibrations, may also be used. Once the bacterial biofilm has been removed, the gums are able to heal and reattach to the teeth, thereby shrinking the pockets.

Oral antibiotics are also useful in fighting periodontitis, though they are not effective for gingivitis. In addition, antibiotic-impregnated materials inserted into deep gum pockets can deliver high concentrations of antibiotic directly to the infected area.

Surgery is performed on some patients, either by a general dentist or by a periodontist. Under local anesthesia, flaps of gum tissue are cut away from the underlying bone, thus allowing better access for scraping and cleaning the tooth roots and for correcting bone defects caused by the infection. Some of the infected gum tissue is also removed, and the remaining gum is sutured back in place.

An important tool in the fight against gum disease is good oral hygiene. The patient should brush and use dental floss daily to remove plaque. In addition to toothpastes, effective cleaning agents include baking soda, peroxide, and some mouth rinses. A regular schedule of teeth cleaning by a dental professional is also essential. Depending on how fast a patient accu-

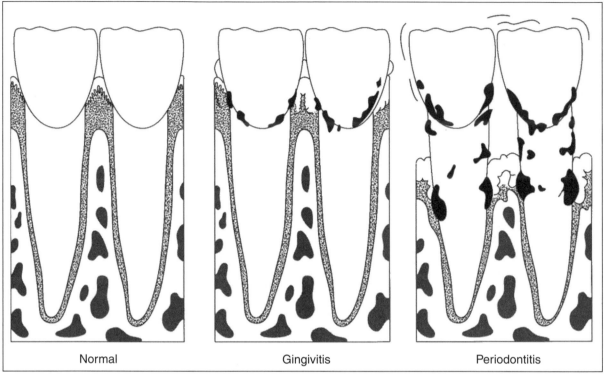

Normal | Gingivitis | Periodontitis

Gum disease begins with poor oral hygiene; if unchecked, it leads to gingivitis (inflammation and infection of the gums) and periodontitis (erosion of supporting bone and tooth loss).

mulates tartar, professional cleaning may be required every three to six months.

PERSPECTIVE AND PROSPECTS

Humans have attempted to clean their teeth since prehistoric times. Early humans fashioned implements out of twigs and bone splinters to remove bits of food trapped between their teeth. Later, the toothpick became the main tooth-cleaning tool. The Chinese are credited with inventing the toothbrush around 1000 A.D. It was not until the late 1930's, however, that an inexpensive toothbrush became available.

Research on the causes, prevention, and treatment of gum disease is being conducted at dental schools and at the National Institute of Dental and Cranio-Facial Research. Research areas include attempts to regenerate periodontal tissues. Bone grafting can help restore lost bone, and guided tissue regeneration may help recreate periodontal ligament.

—*Jane F. Hill, Ph.D.*

See also Cavities; Dental diseases; Dentistry; Endodontic disease; Gingivitis; Periodontal surgery; Periodontitis; Root canal treatment; Teeth; Tooth extraction; Toothache.

FOR FURTHER INFORMATION:

Beers, Mark H., et al., eds. *The Merck Manual of Medical Information, Second Home Edition.* Whitehouse Station, N.J.: Merck Research Laboratories, 2003.

Christensen, Gordon J. *A Consumer's Guide to Dentistry.* 2d ed. St. Louis: Mosby, 2001.

Marsh, P. D. "Dental Plaque." In *Microbia Biofilms,* edited by Hilary Lappin-Scott and J. William Costerton. New York: Cambridge University Press, 1995.

Serio, Francis G. *Understanding Dental Health.* Jackson: University of Mississippi Press, 1998.

Smith, Rebecca W. *The Columbia University School of Dental and Oral Surgery's Guide to Family Dental Care.* New York: W. W. Norton, 1997.

GYNECOLOGY

SPECIALTY

ANATOMY OR SYSTEM AFFECTED: Breasts, genitals, reproductive system, uterus

SPECIALTIES AND RELATED FIELDS: Endocrinology, family medicine, obstetrics, oncology, psychiatry, psychology

DEFINITION: The branch of medicine concerned with the diseases and disorders that are specific to women, particularly those of the genital tract, as well as women's health, endocrinology, reproductive physiology, family planning, and contraceptive use.

KEY TERMS:

menarche: the onset of menstrual cycles in a woman

menopause: the permanent cessation of menstrual cycles, signifying the conclusion of a woman's reproductive life

menstruation: the cyclic bleeding that normally occurs, usually in the absence of pregnancy, during the reproductive period of the human female; typically occurs at twenty-eight-day intervals

Papanicolau (Pap) smear: a screening test for precancer and cancer of the cervix; it is performed by placing a sample of cervical cells on a microscope slide along with a preservative solution or by placing the cells into a small container filled with preservative solution

puberty: the physiological sequence of events by which a child acquires the reproductive capacities of an adult; the growth of secondary sexual characteristics occurs, reproductive functions begin, and the differences between males and females are accentuated

SCIENCE AND PROFESSION

Gynecology is the branch of medical science that treats the functions and diseases unique to women, particularly in the nonpregnant state. A gynecologist is a licensed medical doctor who has obtained specialty training. Unlike many fields in medicine which are clearly defined by surgical or nonsurgical practice, gynecology involves both. In the early 1800's, gynecology was closely tied to general surgery. In fact, one of the first reported cases of abdominal surgery in which the patient survived and was cured of a condition occurred in 1809, with the successful removal of a massive ovarian tumor by Ephraim McDowell (without the benefit of anesthesia or antibiotics).

Today, gynecology is much more than just a surgical field. With the tremendous progress made in the basic sciences and medical sciences by the twenty-first century, gynecology now involves a broad spectrum of medical fields, including developmental and congenital disorders relating to puberty and adolescence, sexually transmitted diseases (STDs) and other infectious diseases, contraception, menstrual disturbances, endocrinology, early pregnancy issues, infertility, preventive health, menopausal problems, incontinence, and oncology, specifically dealing with cancers of the reproductive system such as the ovaries, uterus, and breasts.

Many of the medical problems dealt with in gynecology have far-reaching social, ethical, and legal consequences. Among the most controversial issues in medicine today involve abortion and STDs (such as human immunodeficiency virus, or HIV), both of which are conditions commonly managed by gynecologists. Another example of a common problem managed by gynecologists with important social implications is contraception. Female steroid hormones were among the first biological substances to be purified in the laboratory in the twentieth century. These hormones were then intentionally fed to animals for their contraceptive effect and eventually given to human beings as well in the form of the birth control pill. The birth control pill is an invention that has been widely credited with providing women with a relatively easy means to control their own fertility. Many social scholars would argue that women's ability to harness their own fertility was key in enabling women to delay childbearing, pursue education and careers, and take roles in society that were formerly occupied almost exclusively by men.

To understand gynecology, it is first necessary to have a working knowledge of relevant female anatomy and physiology. Broadly, the female reproductive organs are divided into two groups, external and internal. Within each group are many specific components, most of which are analogous to structures in the male because they are derived from the same sources during embryological development. The external organs are the vulva (the fleshy "lips" covered with skin), vagina, and clitoris; the internal organs are the uterus (including the cervix), Fallopian tubes, and ovaries. These organs mature during puberty and communicate with regions of the brain, specifically the hypothalamus and pituitary, to coordinate function.

The vagina is a tube of tissue that connects the vulva with the uterus. In adult females, it is 9 to 10 centimeters in length. When a woman is standing upright, the vagina extends upward and backward from the opening to the uterus. There is a slight cuplike expansion near the uterus. It is here that the actual connection between the vagina and uterus is made through a muscular structure called the cervix. The muscles of the vagina are normally constricted, thus closing the tube. The vagina can stretch to accommodate a penis during intercourse and a fetus during birth.

The cervix is a ring of muscle; the central opening is called the cervical os. Throughout most of the month, the cervical os forms a tight barrier. When the lining of the uterus is sloughed during a menstrual period, the cervix relaxes slightly. During childbirth, the cervix dilates to 10 centimeters (about 4 inches).

The uterus is a hollow, thick-walled, muscular organ. It normally forms a right angle with the vagina, angling upward and anteriorly. The bladder is immediately anterior to the uterus. In a nonpregnant woman, the uterus is pear-shaped. In a woman who has never been pregnant, it is 8 centimeters in length, 6 centimeters wide, and 4 centimeters thick. It increases in size during pregnancy; after birth, it shrinks but does not quite return to its size prior to pregnancy. The lining of the uterus is shed approximately every twenty-eight days during a normal menstrual period.

The Fallopian tubes are two canals that transport eggs from the ovaries to the uterus. The Fallopian tube is the site where sperm meet the egg and fertilization occurs. The tubes are wide near the ovaries and become narrow toward the uterus. The ovaries are two almond-shaped bodies found in the pelvic cavity, and they brush up against the Fallopian tubes. The ovaries are about 3.5 by 2 by 1.5 centimeters in size, although there can be much variation. The ovaries contain eggs, which are released at monthly intervals between puberty and the menopause.

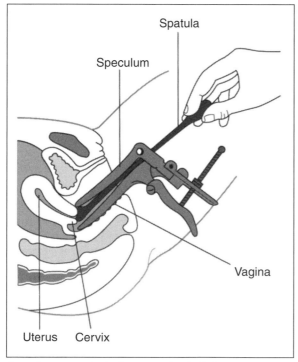

A routine gynecological examination includes a Pap smear, in which a spatula is used to perform a biopsy of the cervix for laboratory analysis.

DIAGNOSTIC AND TREATMENT TECHNIQUES

As with all medical problems, a good history from the patient regarding the nature of the problem is crucial for diagnosis. The history is almost always followed by a physical examination. Probably the best known diagnostic technique in gynecology is the bimanual pelvic examination. Any woman who is sexually active or age eighteen should receive one from a physician. The purpose of the examination is to confirm normal anatomy, rule out pathological conditions, and prevent the development of cancers through screening tests such as the Pap smear.

The pelvic examination is typically performed with the woman on her back, knees apart, with feet and legs supported by stirrups. Visual inspection of the external genitalia is performed; this involves inspecting the pubic region to ensure normal secondary sexual development as well as to look for abnormalities such as unusual lesions on the labia, which may indicate infections (by fungi, bacteria, viruses, or parasites), skin conditions (such as eczema), or cancer. The next portion is a bimanual examination. The examiner places one hand on the patient's abdomen and gently inserts two fingers of the other hand into the patient's vagina; gloves are worn at all times. The examiner proceeds to feel the uterus and ovaries by gently pushing them toward the anterior abdomen. The external hand on the abdomen serves as a counterforce to enable the examiner to feel the contours of the uterus and ovaries and hence to assess their size.

The last portion of the examination is a visual inspection of the interior of the vagina and the surface of the cervix. Because the vagina is normally closed, a device called a speculum is carefully placed in the vaginal canal. The speculum has two "blades"; each blade is analogous to a tongue depressor, which pushes the tongue out of the way to enable inspection of the throat. The blades are then slowly opened to part the vaginal tissues and enable visualization of the vaginal canal and cervix. The vaginal walls and cervix are inspected for abnormalities, and the consistency of vaginal fluid is noted. If any abnormalities are noted, cultures or biopsies may taken to facilitate diagnosis. When indicated, a Pap smear is performed by swabbing the exterior of the cervix as well as the cervical canal. The cells that are obtained from the swab can then be sent to the pathology laboratory for analysis to screen for precancer or cancer of the cervix.

Although the bimanual examination is the mainstay of office practice, this examination is but a small fraction of diagnostic modalities commonly employed by gynecologists. A complete physical examination, including breast examination, is often performed for a comprehensive survey to aid in diagnosis. When abnormalities are suspected, a vast array of imaging techniques and laboratory tests can be invaluable in diagnosis. For instance, when a pelvic mass is felt on bimanual examination, the gynecologist may order an ultrasound to better characterize the mass. Laboratory tests such as CA-125 levels may be indicated to help differentiate the pelvic mass from a benign growth versus a malignancy, such as of the ovary.

Other diagnostic tests commonly employed by gynecologists in office practice are blood and urine tests for pregnancy, blood or culture tests (for STDs such as HIV, syphilis, gonorrhea, chlamydia, and herpes), and biopsies of the external genitalia, which may assist in diagnosing skin conditions such as lichen sclerosus or precancers. If an endocrinologic abnormality is suspected, then blood tests to check the levels of various hormones (such as thyroid hormone, follicle-stimulating hormone, or prolactin) can help pinpoint the problem. In a patient with urinary incontinence, urodynamic testing, which records the pressures of the bladder and abdomen under different conditions, may help diagnose and characterize the type of incontinence.

A number of diagnostic tests commonly employed by gynecologists require going to an operating room, most often because of the need for patient sedation or anesthesia. One example is hysteroscopy, whereby a small camera mounted on a cannula is introduced through the cervix to visualize the cervical canal and uterine lining. Hysteroscopy can be useful in the diagnosis of polyps or fibroids (benign tumors of the uterus) which may be causing abnormal vaginal bleeding. Another example is diagnostic laparoscopy, whereby a small camera mounted on a cannula is introduced into the abdominal and pelvic cavity to inspect for abnormalities such as pelvic scarring, masses, or endometriosis, a condition in which cells resembling the uterine lining are found in the pelvic or abdominal cavities.

Gynecologists have a vast array of treatment options available to them. In the office setting, common treatment modalities include the use of antibiotics for uncomplicated pelvic infections, such as chlamydia, gonorrhea, or trichomoniasis. Another problem commonly treated in the office setting is undesired fertility. A number of contraceptive modalities exist, including the prescription of birth control pills, the placement of an intrauterine device (IUD), or the injection of sustained-release hormones. In women experiencing menopausal symptoms such as hot flashes, hormonal pills or other medications may be prescribed. Women with chronic pelvic pain may be treated with medications such as antidepressants. Urinary incontinence may respond to bladder training, pessaries, or medications.

In the operating room, procedures may be carried out in a controlled setting to treat disease. A woman with abnormal vaginal bleeding caused by fibroids who no longer desires childbearing may receive a hysterectomy, with or without removal of the ovaries. If a woman is interested in retaining her uterus, the fibroids can be isolated and removed surgically through a common surgical procedure called a myomectomy. In women who desire permanent sterilization, a common surgical procedure performed by gynecologists is tubal ligation. Another common surgical procedure is the removal of pelvic masses such as ovarian cysts. Endometriosis or pelvic scars can be removed or destroyed through laparotomy (also known as abdominal surgery) or laparoscopy (minimally invasive abdominal surgery). When a Pap smear or biopsy indicates noninvasive cancer of the cervix, treatment is possible through excision of the part of the cervix surrounding the cancer. In women with urinary incontinence not helped by medical management, surgery may be indicated to treat the problem. Women who are infertile as a result of blocked Fallopian tubes can be treated with in vitro fertilization. In this procedure, eggs are harvested from the woman in the operating room, and fertilization is performed in the laboratory. When the embryos are sufficiently developed, they are placed in the uterine cavity through an office procedure.

Perspective and Prospects

The formation of a medical field specific to women's diseases largely began in the nineteenth century. At the time, the treatment of women's diseases was inextricably linked with the role of women in society. In the nineteenth century, women were often viewed as frail and limited by their cyclical physiology and childbearing role. Consequently, they were excluded from the male-dominated spheres of politics, professional careers, and education. For instance, influential psychiatrist Henry Maudsley (1835-1918) wrote about the harm that higher education would cause to the physiologic development of postpubescent girls. Edward Clarke (1820-1877), a Harvard Medical School professor, wrote in 1873 that higher education might develop the intellect, but at the expense of the reproductive organs, leading to painful menstrual periods and abnormal uterine function.

The field has evolved dramatically since then, with much of the evolution tied to changes in the role of women in society as well as to technological and scientific advances. Today, one of the major forces changing gynecological practice (as well as many other fields of medicine) is the concept of evidence-based medicine. This movement is based on the idea that medical practice must be guided by scientific evidence as well as good intentions. Without objective evidence that a treatment is effective, even the best of intentions can result in patient harm. Although a physician may practice evidence-based medicine, this does not mean that clinical judgment and the tailoring of treatments to fit individual patients should be ignored. In fact, applying scientific evidence in an automatic way to all patients is not endorsed. Gynecologists today most often practice evidence-based medicine either by examining the available literature themselves, by using evidence-based medical summaries developed by others, or by using evidence-based protocols developed by others.

One example of evidence-based medicine guiding clinical practice involves Pap smear screening. Although the classical teaching had been that Pap smears were recommended on a yearly basis, this frequency was not based on any direct evidence that this protocol would lead to better outcomes than screening less frequently. Consequently, both the U.S. Preventative Services Task Force and the American Cancer Society have suggested lengthening the period between successive Pap smears in women thirty years of age or older who have had negative results on three or more consecutive Pap smears. In fact, the U.S. Preventative Services Task Force recommends Pap smears be performed "at least every three years" rather than every year.

Among the studies cited for this recommendation is one that followed more than 100,000 women at community-based clinics throughout the United States who had previously received three years of normal Pap smears. There was no statistically significant difference in the number of precancers or cancers of the cervix found on the new Pap smear based on the time interval since the last Pap smear (that is, one year versus three years). In an era where the optimum use of limited resources is of concern to patients, physicians, health maintenance organizations (HMOs), and insurance companies alike, the careful application of evidence-based medicine to appropriate situations in medical practice can result in the best overall benefit for all parties involved.

—*Anne Lynn S. Chang, M.D.*

See also Abortion; Amenorrhea; Assisted reproductive technologies; Biopsy; Breast biopsy; Breast cancer; Breast disorders; Breasts, female; Cervical, ovarian, and uterine cancers; Cervical procedures; Chlamydia; Circumcision, female, and genital mutilation; Conception; Contraception; Culdocentesis; Cyst removal; Cystectomy; Cystitis; Cysts; Dysmenorrhea; Electrocauterization; Endocrinology; Endometrial biopsy; Endometriosis; Endoscopy; Episiotomy; Gamete intrafallopian transfer (GIFT); Genital disorders, female; Glands; Gonorrhea; Herpes; Hormone replacement therapy (HRT); Hot flashes; Human papillomavirus (HPV); Hysterectomy; In vitro fertilization; Incontinence; Infertility, female; Laparoscopy; Mammography; Mastectomy and lumpectomy; Mastitis; Menopause; Menorrhagia; Menstruation; Myomectomy; Nutrition; Obstetrics; Ovarian cysts; Pap smear; Pelvic inflammatory disease (PID); Placenta; Postpartum depression; Preeclampsia and eclampsia; Pregnancy and gestation; Premenstrual syndrome (PMS); Reproductive system; Sex change surgery; Sexual dysfunction; Sexuality; Sexually transmitted diseases (STDs); Sterilization; Syphilis; Toxic shock syndrome; Tubal ligation; Ultrasonography; Urethritis; Urinary disorders; Urology; Warts; Women's health.

FOR FURTHER INFORMATION:

Berek, Jonathan S., ed. *Berek and Novak's Gynecology.* 14th ed. Philadelphia: Lippincott Williams & Wilkins, 2007. A standard text covering all aspects of gynecology, with an emphasis on diagnosis and treatment. Topics include biology and physiology, family planning, sexuality, evaluation of pelvic infections, early pregnancy loss, benign breast disease, benign gynecologic conditions, malignant diseases of the reproductive tract, and breast cancer.

Boston Women's Health Collective. *Our Bodies, Ourselves: A New Edition for a New Era.* 35th anniversary ed. New York: Simon & Schuster, 2005. Contains in-depth discussions of topics related to gynecology. This book was written by women for women and is one of the best reference works available on this subject for the general reader.

Doherty, Gerard M., and Lawrence W. Way, eds. *Current Surgical Diagnosis and Treatment.* 12th ed. New York: Lange Medical Books/McGraw-Hill,

2006. Provides information on the surgical aspects of women's health and gynecology.

Kasper, Dennis L., et al., eds. *Harrison's Principles of Internal Medicine*. 16th ed. New York: McGraw-Hill, 2005. Contains many good chapters on women's major health problems.

Rushing, Lynda, and Nancy Joste. *Abnormal Pap Smears: What Every Woman Needs to Know*. Amherst, N.Y.: Prometheus Books, 2001. Explains the causes of cervical neoplasia and the treatment procedures used. Numerous diagrams show the stages of cervical disease.

Scott, James R., et al., eds. *Danforth's Obstetrics and Gynecology*. 9th ed. Philadelphia: Lippincott Williams & Wilkins, 2003. A basic textbook that describes many common gynecological problems, along with their diagnosis, management, and treatment.

Speroff, Leon, and Marc A. Fritz. *Clinical Gynecologic Endocrinology and Infertility*. 7th ed. Philadelphia: Lippincott Williams & Wilkins, 2005. The authoritative textbook on the normal role of hormones in women, hormonal disturbances and the medical diseases to which they can lead, and the evaluation and treatment of infertility.

Stenchever, Morton A., et al. *Comprehensive Gynecology*. 4th ed. St. Louis: Mosby, 2006. The definitive textbook on gynecological problems.

Stewart, Elizabeth Gunther, and Paula Spencer. *The V Book: A Doctor's Guide to Complete Vulvovaginal Health*. New York: Bantam Books, 2002. Covers a wealth of information related to vulvovaginal health, including picking a good gynecologist and asking the right questions, vulvovaginal hygiene, the safe use of tampons, common ailments and their symptoms, and which medical tests to insist upon from one's doctor.

Tierney, Lawrence M., Stephen J. McPhee, and Maxine A. Papadakis, eds. *Current Medical Diagnosis and Treatment 2007*. New York: McGraw-Hill Medical, 2006. An easy-to-read medical textbook with good chapters related to women's health.

Weschler, Toni. *Taking Charge of Your Fertility*. Rev. ed. New York: HarperCollins, 2001. An excellent book that encourages women to become responsible for their own reproductive health. Includes discussions of infertility, natural birth control, and achieving pregnancy.

GYNECOMASTIA

DISEASE/DISORDER

ANATOMY OR SYSTEM AFFECTED: Breasts, chest, endocrine system, glands

SPECIALTIES AND RELATED FIELDS: Endocrinology

DEFINITION: An enlargement of the glandular part of the male breast that may affect one or both breasts and be painless or painful.

CAUSES AND SYMPTOMS

True gynecomastia must be distinguished from malignant or benign breast tumors and from enlargement of the fatty part of the breast because of obesity. Causes of gynecomastia include normal physiological changes, endocrine diseases, other diseases such as chronic liver or kidney disease, tumors, and many drugs.

Some newborn boys may have swollen breasts as a result of the maternal estrogen to which they are exposed during pregnancy. This enlargement may be accompanied by the secretion of milk, known as galactorrhea. Up to 70 percent of boys experience gynecomastia as they go through puberty, usually between the ages of twelve and fifteen. It is usually one-sided, but it may involve both breasts either at the same time or sequentially. This normally subsides within a year; the only treatment is reassurance that it will resolve on its own.

In athletes who take androgens and anabolic steroids, about half will develop gynecomastia. Other drugs that can cause this problem include alcohol, cimetidine, diazepam, diethylstilbestrol, digitalis, estrogens, some tranquilizers, many of the drugs used to treat schizophrenia, marijuana, methadone, synthetic narcotics, growth hormone, and tricyclic antidepressants.

Elderly men, particularly if they gain weight, may also develop gynecomastia because of the changes in the balance between male and female hormones that come with aging.

Types of cancer leading to gynecomastia include lung and testicular cancers. Likewise, tumors of the adrenal gland may cause this problem. Sometimes the enlargement of the breast tissue is the first sign of some serious underlying disease, but often it occurs for no apparent reason.

Men who develop gynecomastia where the cause is not obvious should have a radiographic study of the chest performed, along with blood studies to measure hormones such as prolactin, testosterone, luteinizing hormone, estradiol, and thyroid hormones. Some men may require genetic testing to determine the cause of

---

INFORMATION ON GYNECOMASTIA

CAUSES: Normal physiological changes, endocrine diseases, diseases such as chronic liver or kidney disease, tumors, maternal estrogen during pregnancy, certain drugs (androgens, anabolic steroids, alcohol, cimetidine, diazepam, DES, digitalis, estrogens, some tranquilizers, schizophrenia drugs, marijuana, methadone, synthetic narcotics, growth hormone, tricyclic antidepressants)

SYMPTOMS: Enlargement of breasts in males, sometimes with milk secretion

DURATION: Within one year

TREATMENTS: None (self-resolving), cessation of drug use

---

their gynecomastia. Finally, a needle biopsy may be necessary.

TREATMENT AND THERAPY

The treatment of gynecomastia depends upon the cause. In the case of infant or pubertal boys, nothing is required but time for the problem to resolve on its own. When the condition is the result of a drug, it will usually resolve once the drug is stopped. Weight loss is indicated where the appearance of gynecomastia is attributable to obesity. Treating endocrine disorders, other illnesses, and tumors usually resolves the gynecomastia.

When the problem is painful, it may be treated with an antiestrogen drug. Severe or persistent gynecomastia may be treated by surgical means, although the results are not entirely satisfactory. In some cases, liposuction via the armpit and mastectomy performed under the skin may improve the situation.

—*Rebecca Lovell Scott, Ph.D., PA-C*

See also Breast cancer; Breast disorders; Breasts, female; Endocrine system; Endocrinology; Endocrinology, pediatric; Hormones; Men's health; Neonatology; Pediatrics; Puberty and adolescence.

FOR FURTHER INFORMATION:

Beers, Mark H., et al., eds. *The Merck Manual of Medical Information, Second Home Edition*. Whitehouse Station, N.J.: Merck Research Laboratories, 2003.

Komaroff, Anthony, ed. *Harvard Medical School Family Health Guide*. New York: Free Press, 2005.

Masters, William H., Virginia E. Johnson, and Robert C. Kolodny. *Human Sexuality*. 5th ed. New York: HarperCollins College, 1995.

Hair

Anatomy

Anatomy or system affected: Hair, skin

Specialties and related fields: Dermatology

Definition: Threadlike outgrowths of nonliving, mostly proteinaceous material that cover much of the body of humans and other mammals.

Key terms:

alopecia: hair loss, especially if noticeable or significant

alopecia areata: loss of hair in patches

follicle: the structure in skin that manufactures hair

hirsutism: excessive hair growth

Structure and Functions

Humans grow three kinds of hair. The downy hair that covers the fetus is lanugo. Soon after birth, it is replaced by vellus (or villus) hair. Vellus hair covers the entire skin surface except for the palms of the hands and the soles of the feet. It is fine, short, nearly colorless, and slow-growing.

The thick, pigmented hair on the head, eyebrows, and eyelids is terminal hair. Somewhere between 65 and 95 percent (by weight) of terminal hair is protein. Other components include water, fats (lipids), trace elements (minerals), and pigment. Because proteins twist into complex three-dimensional shapes held together by chemical bonds, hair is both rigid and flexible. Terminal hair replaces villus hair on the genitals at puberty. Called pubic hair, it is coarse and curly. Also at puberty, terminal hair begins to grow in the armpits and on the faces of males.

The shaft of a single hair has three layers. The outer casing is the cuticle, made of overlapping layers of proteinaceous material. Inside the cuticle lies the cortex, a column of cells containing keratin, the same protein that hardens tooth enamel and fingernails. The central core of the hair is the medulla. Also called the pith, it is made of small, hardened cells snared in a web of fine filaments.

Hair grows from a tiny pouch below the skin's surface called a follicle. At the bottom of the follicle lies the papilla, an upward-growing finger of connective tissue. The papilla forms the root of the hair shaft. The actively growing part of the hair shaft is the hair bulb. The cells that generate the hair lie just above the hair bulb. As soon as hair cells are manufactured, they harden and die, forming the hair shaft.

Tiny blood vessels around each follicle supply nutrients. Sebaceous glands that open into the follicle produce the oily sebum that lubricates hair and skin. In the papilla of the follicle, melanocytes produce melanin, the same pigment that gives skin its color. There are two kinds of melanin: Eumelanin makes hair black or brown, while pheomelanin makes it red or blond. Melanin is deposited in the cortex of the hair shaft of terminal hair, giving it its color.

Hair helps insulate the body. Arrector pili muscles at the base of the follicle elevate hair in response to environmental stimuli, including cold. The high sulfur content of keratin gives it heat-retaining properties. Hair also retards water loss from the body. Body hair augments the sense of touch. Hair's movement facilitates the detection of light touches and slight temperature changes.

Terminal hair cushions the head against blows and protects the scalp from sunburn. Eyelashes keep dirt, insects, and foreign objects out of the eyes. Eyebrows keep sweat from running down into the eyes. The hair inside the ears is coated with the waxy substance cerumen that traps dirt and prevents infections. Hair in the nose filters dust and bacteria from the air.

Hair growth and replacement occur in three stages. Anagen is the active growth stage. It lasts from two to six years. During catagen, lasting about two weeks, the lower segment of the hair follicle breaks down. A "club hair" separates from the papilla and falls out. Then, during telogen, the follicle "rests." Telogen lasts several weeks or months. At any one time, about 80 to 90 percent of the hairs on the head are in anagen, 3 to 4 percent are in catagen, and the remainder are in telogen.

Disorders and Diseases

While a loss of fifty to one hundred scalp hairs per day is normal, alopecia, or noticeable hair loss, occurs in nearly one-third of women and two-thirds of men. Women typically notice a general thinning of the hair, while men usually experience male pattern baldness: loss at the hairline and crown first, followed by loss at top of the head. The cause is neither a loss of follicles nor a cessation of hair growth. Instead, follicles gradually shrink and become less active, producing shorter, finer vellus hairs. Three interacting factors—heredity, hormones, and aging—cause the change in follicles. Genetic programming controls the age when hair loss begins and how fast it progresses. Male hormones (even in women) must be present for balding to occur.

No drug can reverse baldness in its later stages. However, minoxidil (trade name Rogaine) slows the rate of hair loss or promotes regrowth in about 25 percent of men and 20 percent of women. It received the approval of the U.S. Food and Drug Administration (FDA) in 1988 and became available without a prescription in 1996. Another drug, finasteride (trade name Propecia), was approved in 1997 for use in men only.

Surgical alternatives are available for those bothered by baldness. To transplant or graft hair, surgeons remove segments of scalp from the sides and back of the head (where follicles are less sensitive to hormones) and transfer them to the top. To perform a scalp reduction, surgeons cut away a portion of hairless scalp, then stitch the remaining scalp together, reducing the total area of baldness. Another alternative is flap surgery. A flap of hair-bearing scalp is turned to cover the spot where bald scalp has been removed.

Alopecia areata is the loss of hair in round patches, usually on the scalp, beard, eyebrows, or pubic area. It is thought to be an autoimmune disease. The immune system "mistakes" the hair follicles for invading disease agents and attacks them, reducing their size and decreasing hair production. The disorder may result from fever, stress, surgery, allergies, crash diets, burns, scalds, and tumors. Other possible causes include radiation exposure, an overactive or underactive thyroid gland, liver or kidney disease, and illnesses ranging from influenza to scarlet fever. A deficiency of iron, zinc, or certain vitamins is the cause in some cases, as is chemotherapy for cancer. Hair loss is also a side effect of many drugs. Alopecia areata is seldom serious or permanent, but it can be disturbing. A doctor may prescribe drugs to combat it, but it generally resolves itself within a year.

Hirsutism, excessive hair growth on the face or body, can cause concern, especially for women. Although it can be triggered by tumors, diseases of the ovaries or adrenal glands, contraceptive pills, hormonal drugs, or anabolic steroids, the most common cause is the menopause. As production of the female hormone estrogen declines, the relative concentration of male hormones (produced naturally by the adrenal glands) rises, causing dark hairs to appear on the upper lip, chin, and cheeks. Shaving, tweezing, waxing, sugaring, or using depilatory creams and lotions removes hair temporarily. Electrolysis, in which a needle inserted into the follicle delivers a current that destroys the follicle, removes hair permanently. In severe cases, doctors may prescribe drugs that block the action of male hormones to treat hirsutism in women.

PERSPECTIVE AND PROSPECTS

Since ancient times, people have sought to prevent or reverse the balding process. The Egyptians of the sixteenth century B.C.E. prescribed a blend of iron, red lead, onions, and alabaster, along with prayers to the sun god. In 420 B.C.E., the Greek Hippocrates, often called the founder of modern medicine, recommended a mixture of opium, horseradish, pigeon droppings, beetroot, and spices.

The concept of surgical hair transplantation arose in the early 1800's, and in the twentieth century reliable techniques were developed. Japanese physicians pioneered hair transplantation and grafting in the late 1930's and early 1940's, but it was not until the 1980's that procedures yielding cosmetically acceptable results were achieved in the United States. Drug treatments for baldness were discovered by chance as side effects. Minoxidil originally treated hypertension; finasteride ameliorated prostate enlargement.

Attempts to remove unwanted hair have roots in prehistory. Sharpened rocks and shells used for hair removal have been found in archaeological sites dating back twenty thousand years. The ancient Sumerians invented tweezers, and the Egyptians buried razors and arsenic-based depilatories with their dead. Native American men tweezed facial hair with clamshells, and North American colonists in the seventeenth century used caustic lye to burn hair away. In 1903, the American inventor King Gillette marketed the first razor with a disposable blade. Jacob Schick introduced the electric shaver in 1931.

In the 1960's, lasers were first used to heat and disable hair follicles over large areas, and hair removal entered the arena of medical practice. Early lasers emitted a continuous wave that risked overheating and skin damage. The invention of a switching device allowed light energy to enter the follicle in controlled pulses. In 1995, the FDA approved the first laser device for hair removal. Most developed since that time use water or gel to cool the skin and laser light to target the melanin in the hair. Other strategies are being investigated, and studies of such variables as beam width, pulse duration, and delivery rate may result in laser hair removal treatments that are safe, effective, and permanent.

Basic research on the nature and action of the immune system may lead to treatments for autoimmune disorders including alopecia areata. The cloning of individual hair follicles may facilitate hair transplantation. Gene therapy could, in theory, be used to alter the genetic control of follicles, preventing inherited baldness entirely.

—Faith Hickman Brynie, Ph.D.
See also Dermatology; Gray hair; Hair loss and baldness; Hair transplantation; Laser use in surgery; Plastic surgery; Skin; Skin disorders.

For Further Information:

Anderson, Richard R. "Lasers in Dermatology: A Critical Update." *Journal of Dermatology* 27, no. 11 (November, 2000): 700-705.

Brynie, Faith Hickman. *101 Questions About Your Skin That Got Under Your Skin . . . Until Now.* Brookfield, Conn.: Twenty-first Century Books, 1999.

Burns, Tony, et al., eds. *Rook's Textbook of Dermatology.* 7th ed. Malden, Mass.: Blackwell Science, 2004.

Freedburg, Irwin M., et al., eds. *Fitzpatrick's Dermatology in General Medicine.* 6th ed. 2 vols. New York: McGraw-Hill, 2003.

Kuntzman, Gersh. *Hair! Mankind's Historic Quest to End Baldness.* New York: AtRandom, 2001.

Hair loss and baldness
Disease/disorder

Anatomy or system affected: Hair, head, skin

Specialties and related fields: Dermatology, endocrinology, plastic surgery

Definition: Symptoms of genetic factors, endocrine disorders, and aging which occur in both men and women, although more frequently in men, affecting more than one-half of the male population.

Key terms:

alopecia: a condition in which all hair falls out, not only that on the scalp but also eyebrows, eyelashes, and even body hair

follicle: a small, saclike cavity for secretion or excretion

hair shaft: the hair itself, consisting of the central part (medulla), the middle part (cortex), and the outer part (cuticle)

psoriasis: a chronic skin disease characterized by scaly, reddish patches

seborrhea: a dermatologic condition characterized by an excessively dry skin (seborrhea oleosa) or oily skin (seborrhea sicca)

Causes and Symptoms

The major reason that hair on the scalp thrives more lavishly than on other parts of the body is that scalp hairs are produced by the largest follicles found in human skin. Throughout the early years of infancy, these follicles increase in size, shedding their hairs about every two to six years to clear a path for a new hair that grows thicker and longer than the one that it replaced. In the mid-teens, nearly every follicle in an individual's scalp is generating an actively growing hair, and by the late teens scalp hair reaches its adult size, populating the scalp in numbers that will never again be equaled.

For most adults entering their twenties, this situation reverses, and hair loss begins to occur—either permanently or temporarily. At this stage in their development, nearly every man and more than 80 percent of women find their hairlines receding. As the years progress, the shedding continues, and the density of scalp hair continues to diminish. Nearly all the permanent hair loss that affects the human scalp is produced by the natural aging process and/or common baldness.

Common, or male pattern, baldness (baldness is classified into various groups depending on its pattern on the scalp) affects at least 20 million Americans. The term "baldness" is often used when a definite hairline recession, a bald spot on the crown, thinning over the top of the scalp, or a combination of the three is detected. The sides and rear scalp fringe areas are usually spared, except for the inevitable thinning that accompanies age. These regions appear to be capable of generating enough two-to-six-year hair cycles to keep them well covered for most, if not all, of a male's average life span.

The less frequent causes of permanent hair loss can be categorized into three groups. The first involves injury to follicles created by constant tension or pulling of scalp hair. Tight ponytails or chignons, worn over a number of years, often result in permanent bald patches on the sides of the head. In addition, tight rollers and the process of hair weaving kill follicles. The second infrequent cause of permanent hair loss is physical injury, such as a laceration or burn. If hair is ironed as a method of straightening over a period of years, hair follicles will become damaged. The third cause involves various inflammatory skin disorders and growths that occasionally affect the scalp. For example, a scalp wen, or cyst, tends to occur in families and requires no treatment unless it appears to be growing. Removal involves a simple office procedure and eliminates the bald spot that results from pressure of the enlarging cyst upon adjacent scalp follicles.

Nearly all humans lose some scalp hair every day. The number of falling hairs, however, often varies

considerably from day to day. This daily variation in
hair loss is not an indication of abnormality. An average of thirty to sixty hairs may be shed from the scalp
each day. While days, weeks, and months may pass
with little to no hair loss, large numbers of hairs may be
lost over similar time periods. The yearly average,
however, remains fairly constant.

This daily variation in hair loss merely reflects the
fact that hair follicles act independently of one another.
Their three-year growth and three-month rest cycles
occur randomly. Aside from the tendency to lose more
hair in the autumn, chance dictates the periods when the
scalp will contain more resting hairs (hairs having
small whitish roots).

Dandruff and its two related conditions of seborrhea
and psoriasis, both scaly scalp conditions, may create a
significant diffuse hair loss. Because these conditions
are so common, they account for most of the shedding
that requires medical treatment. In most cases, these
problems can be controlled without medical assistance.

Temporary hair loss can result from alopecia areata,
pregnancy, severe illness, surgery, certain medications, hormonal disorders, or dieting. Alopecia areata is
a condition that usually produces temporary shedding
of scalp—and occasionally body—hair. In most cases,
the hair regrows spontaneously or after medical therapy has ended. Occasionally, if this problem begins
during childhood, all the scalp and body hair may be
lost permanently. Extensive shedding may follow
pregnancy or the discontinuation of birth control pills.
After several months, however, the hair usually begins
to regrow. Hair loss may also result from a severe illness associated with high fever (usually influenza) or
an extensive surgical procedure. In the case of surgery,
the cause is related to changes in body chemistry. Various medications can also create hair loss. The main
offenders are the amphetamines, blood thinners, antithyroid drugs, anticancer drugs (as well as radiation

treatments), and birth control pills. Hormonal disorders, particularly thyroid dysfunction, can create a thinning problem, but this condition is rarely an isolated
symptom. In rare instances, improper nutrition can result in hair loss, such as in the case of dieters who eliminate protein from their daily food intake.

The conditions responsible for temporary shedding
usually create a thinning problem quite rapidly. Aside
from hair breakage or forcible extraction (hair pulling),
the problem is usually one of increased numbers of
resting hairs, resulting in massive hair loss. (The two
conditions primarily responsible for creating permanent hair loss—aging and common baldness—usually
develop slowly, over many years. Thinning occurs simply because the scalp follicles are no longer capable of
producing new hairs.)

If something occurs to double the number of resting
hairs from their normal 15 to 30 percent, then hundreds
of hairs may fall each day. If this lasts for several
months, about one-third of the scalp's hair may be lost.
A loss of about 30 to 40 percent is required before thinning becomes obvious. After the shedding abates, it
may take years for the scalp hair to return to its original
density, since the new hairs can grow only about an
inch every two months.

TREATMENT AND THERAPY

Scientific research in the area of hair loss has produced
a drug that has been relatively effective in some individuals. The drug minoxidil was originally used as an
antihypertensive medication; however, 70 percent of
patients taking it reported unexpected hair growth, occasionally in such undesirable places as the forehead. A
0.2 percent minoxidil solution for external use was devised by a major drug company in the United States and
marketed under the name Rogaine. The Food and Drug
Administration approved Rogaine as the only prescription drug that effectively combats baldness.

Although it is uncertain how the drug works, it is
believed that minoxidil enables shrunken follicles to
grow back to a size capable of producing sturdy, visible
hairs. Minoxidil has been shown to have promising,
though limited, results. It is best at filling in those
patchy gaps that herald the beginnings of baldness. Between one-third and one-half of men in some studies
exhibited "significant" or "cosmetically acceptable"
hair growth. Minoxidil is not a cure, however, and it
requires a lifetime commitment. When the drug is
stopped, hair thins out within months.

Much of the problem with all these chemical inducements aimed at hair regrowth or retarding hair loss is the lack of long-term studies to substantiate short-term treatments. For example, many patients who have tried minoxidil and other chemical stimulants and reported successful regrowth of hair have not continued applications over long enough periods of time to justify some of the claims made for these hair regrowth drugs.

Finasteride is a Food and Drug Administration (FDA) approved drug that is marketed under the brand name Propecia and taken orally. Propecia works by inhibiting DHT production, which shuts down growth of hair follicles. Without certain levels of DHT in the bloodstream, hair follicles continue to grow. Propecia has a reported 29 to 68 percent success rate but is effective only as long as it is taken; all hair gain is lost within six to twelve months if treatment is stopped. Propecia is most effective in promoting hair growth in the crown area of the scalp, which explains its popularity. Finasteride is ineffective for treating hair loss in women and may be harmful to pregnant women. Conversely, the drug works well for women who suffer from follicular sensitivity to androgens and may be prescribed by a physician who ensures that the patient is taking proper birth control measures while the drug is in use.

Another ointment that has gained popularity of use is Revivogen, although this drug has not yet been approved by the FDA. Ingredients in Revivogen consist mostly of a mixture of fatty acids that are derived from the de-estering of natural oils such as linseed oil and oil from seeds of borage plants. As with minoxidil, the mode of action is not completely known, but scientists suspect that Revivogen inhibits DHT levels in the scalp to combat hair loss.

Antiandrogen is applied as a topical medication to block the binding of DHT with hair follicles. Follicles that remain unblocked continue to grow hair. Antiandrogen occurs in Nizoral shampoo and Neutrogena T-Gel, which are readily available. Use of shampoos containing antiandrogen has so far produced mixed results. Some individuals report decreased hair loss rate but no hair regrowth in bald areas. In other individuals, the use of antiandrogens has produced no discernable reduction in loss of hair or hair regrowth in bald areas.

Ketoconazole is a synthetic antifungal drug used to prevent and treat fungal infections of the skin and mouth. Since it is both an antifungal and a 5-alpha reductase inhibitor, it can help to slow the balding process. There is some suggestion that ketoconazole could inhibit testosterone synthesis during embryonic development, which may inhibit genital development of the male fetus.

An herbal extract from the partially dried fruit of the dwarf palm called palmetto has been shown to be an DHT inhibitor producing few or no notable side effects. It is more commonly used to treat symptoms of prostate disorders. Topical applications of saw palmetto herbal extract have produced noted hair growth in six of ten subjects, but the other four test subjects reported no improvement. If further tests are successful, then the use of saw palmetto as a hair restorer may increase dramatically, as it is less expensive and has minor side effects compared to other hair restoration drugs.

Hair follicles contain stem cells that may be employed in hair restoration within a few years, pending the outcome of current studies and funding for programs to support those studies. This treatment method is variously labeled hair multiplication or hair cloning. Several companies are involved in the production of hair multiplication treatments based on follicle stem cells. A United Kingdom study announced success by removing hair follicles from the back of the neck,

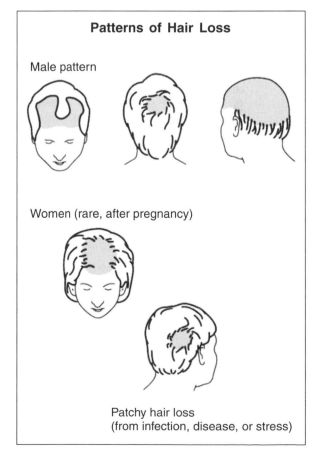

Patterns of Hair Loss

Male pattern

Women (rare, after pregnancy)

Patchy hair loss
(from infection, disease, or stress)

growing them in cultures, and inserting them in the scalp. Test subjects reported a 70 percent success rate using this method, which has stimulated further interest in development and medical approval of this promising hair restoration method.

Another nonsurgical method for achieving permanent hair is hair weaving, a process that originated in the African American culture in the nineteenth century. Weaving hair involves braiding it tightly so that a toupee or smaller weft (section of hair) can be attached permanently. All that is required is a sufficient amount of hair remaining on the scalp to serve as an anchor for a hairpiece.

The braids are usually formed from the thicker hair found on the sides and back of the scalp. A semicircular ridge is created that holds a hairpiece firmly in place. If enough hair is still growing on top of the scalp, it can be twisted into smaller braids to anchor individual wefts. This type of weave permits better aeration and easier cleansing of the scalp.

A hair "fusion," "bonding," or "linking" is exactly like a weave except that the hairpiece or wefts are glued, instead of tied, onto the braided hair. This so-called chemical bond is insoluble in water and quite caustic. Frequent hair breakage has limited the usefulness of this method.

While weaved or fused hair does not grow, it still requires regular care and maintenance to keep it looking acceptable. The scalp hair used to anchor the weave naturally continues to grow. As it grows, the attached hair starts to ride above the scalp. Thus the weave or fusion must be reanchored frequently (as often as every three weeks). In addition, the tension placed on the anchoring scalp hair creates accelerated shedding, and this hair loss is often irreversible.

Hair implants, also known as medical or suture implants, have become the principal method for fixing a hairpiece securely to the scalp. Implants are usually not permanent, are only quasi medical, and are to be distinguished from transplants, with which they share a resemblance in name only. Implants are stitches made from either stainless steel or nylon-type materials that are sewn into the scalp and tied into rings. Like the weave hair braids, the knotted stitches act as anchors, holding a hairpiece or several wefts against the barren scalp. If the implants secure a hairpiece, only two or perhaps six stitches are needed. If the implants anchor many smaller wefts of hair, however, more than a dozen stitches must be sewn into the scalp. A physician must perform this procedure, since only someone with a medical license can inject a local anesthetic and sew stitches into the scalp. The problems generated by sewing and leaving stitches in the scalp, however, are pain, infection, and scarring.

In the 1970's, a surgical procedure known as tunnel grafting was developed. This procedure is not available in implant clinics. A small rectangle of skin is removed from behind each ear. The two pieces are immediately grafted to the front and back of the scalp to form two loops that serve as anchors for a hairpiece. While the operation is relatively simple to perform, extreme care must be taken to ensure proper graft acceptance and healing. Although this method avoids the pitfalls of implanted stitches, it still retains two of the problems common to any kind of artificial anchoring device. Since only two loops are available to fix a hairpiece, the hairpiece can still lift off the scalp. In addition, the skin loops are as vulnerable to injury as suture loops. Scalp lacerations resulting from forcible removal of the hairpiece have occurred.

From the discovery of hair transplants in the 1960's to the late 1970's, it has been estimated that approximately one million people—both men and women— underwent such transplants. As with the implant procedure, a medical license is mandatory in order to inject a local anesthetic into the scalp and make the surgical incisions required for a hair transplant. Doctors who specialize in hair transplants are usually dermatologists; some are plastic surgeons.

Even the baldest scalp contains thousands of transplantable hair follicles. To move them where they are most needed, three surgical methods have been developed, employing scalp grafts known variously as "flaps," "strips," and "plugs." While all three methods are used, most hair transplants are performed with plug grafts because they are the simplest and safest to work with and yield the most satisfying results. The transplant candidate need only be bald enough to justify undergoing the procedure and be endowed with enough side and rear fringe scalp hair to make the procedure worthwhile.

To create a flap or "full thickness" graft, a surgeon cuts out three sides of a rectangular patch of scalp from above the ears and swings it over to the bald area to create a new hairline. This is a major hospital procedure requiring considerable surgical expertise. Although a fairly large portion of bald scalp can be provided with instant hair density, this method is fraught with problems. To ensure a proper take, or graft survival, the blood vessels feeding the transplant must remain intact while they are moved along with it. Because the vessels are quite fragile, they are frequently damaged, resulting in poor graft survival and catastrophic hair loss.

To alleviate this problem, a variation of this type of transplant, known as a free flap procedure, was developed by a team of Japanese surgeons. The free flap is cut out on all four sides, completely severing the blood supply. After setting the graft into its new location, the surgeons meticulously reestablish its blood supply to the recipient blood vessels using a delicate microsurgical technique.

Even if this technical obstacle is surmounted, however, other aesthetic problems remain. The first problem involves the surgical scar that delineates the border between the forehead and the transplanted hairline. Little can be done to minimize this scar. The other problem concerns the unnatural direction in which the newly transplanted hair grows. A flap graft cannot provide hair that will grow in the direction of the hair that has been lost. Hairs growing from the sides of the scalp exit much closer to the surface than in other areas. When transplanted to the frontal area, these hairs lie much too flat against the scalp. Thus, while a flap may provide a faster way to achieve a high-density transplant, the problems of graft survival and poor aesthetic results have limited its usefulness.

A surgical strip graft is a narrow rectangular patch of scalp, cut out on all four sides, that is usually transplanted to create a hairline. Unlike the larger flap, its blood supply need not be moved along with it or be laboriously reestablished. After the strip is placed into its new location, the adjacent bald scalp sends new blood vessels directly into it. Like a flap graft, however, it must be sewn into place. If it is used to create a hairline, an unsightly scar will mark its border with the forehead as well. While this procedure can be performed in an office rather than at a hospital, extreme care must be taken to avoid damaging this delicate graft. Despite the most painstaking precautions, poor takes result quite often. Areas of nongrowth are common, and not infrequently the entire graft becomes almost completely devoid of hair.

A "hair transplant" usually refers to a procedure in which a small cylinder of hair-bearing scalp, or plug, is taken from the rear or side fringe areas and transferred to either the bald crown or the scalp's frontal region. While this transplant method requires several sessions to approach the density of hair acquired with a flap graft, the ease with which it can be performed, coupled with its superior aesthetic results, make it the logical choice for surgically replacing hair.

The surgeon uses a trephine, or "punch," to remove the cylindrical section of scalp, properly called a donor graft rather than a plug. The graft is quite small, measuring about 0.8 centimeter deep by 0.5 centimeter in diameter. The hair follicle is intimately related to all three skin layers. The bulb—or hair-producing portion of the follicle—lies within and is cushioned by the fat, or adipose, layer. The entire follicle is supported by and receives its nourishment from the fibrous portion of skin, or dermis, which is about 0.6 centimeter thick in the scalp. The skin mantle, or epidermis, provides the opening, or "pore," through which the hair exits to the surface of the scalp.

When a donor graft is removed, all three skin layers must be included. The hair is actually superfluous to the procedure: The hair follicle is all that is essential. After removing the hair-bearing donor grafts, the physician next punches out identical sections of bald scalp. The term "plug" actually refers to the hairless cylinder of scalp that is taken from the bald area. The donor graft is placed into the void left by the removal of the bald plug. Light pressure is applied for several seconds to allow the blood to clot and hold the graft in place. Because these grafts are so small and clotting occurs so rapidly, stitches are not required to fix them in place.

Within hours, new blood vessels move into the graft from the surrounding skin to feed the new section. Within several days, as healing continues, the graft and its adjacent host skin become one. Keeping the grafts small facilitates easy penetration by these vital blood vessels. When larger grafts, or strips, are used, the blood supply may not reach all the hair follicles, and they die.

Because of the small size, the grafts' rounded edges blend into the host skin quite evenly, creating an acceptable hairline. While they might appear obvious on close inspection, they are always less noticeable than the borders left by flaps and strips. Because the grafts are small and are taken from the rear half of the scalp, where the hairs grow out in the same manner as the front and crown hairs, they can be directed to duplicate exactly the original pattern of growth in the bald host areas. This method is a minor office procedure that, in the hands of an experienced physician, is considered safe, with little discomfort experienced by the patient.

PERSPECTIVE AND PROSPECTS

The observation that eunuchs are not subject to gout or baldness was made by Hippocrates in the year 400 B.C.E. and is contained in the *Hippocratic Corpus* as a short medical truth or aphorism. Aristotle, himself balding, was interested in the fact that eunuchs did not become bald and were unable to grow hair on their chests. These observations were either forgotten or overlooked for the next twenty-five centuries, and medical science remained baffled by male pattern baldness until James B. Hamilton, an anatomist, in 1949 again made the observation that eunuchs did not become bald. His suggestion that androgens are a prerequisite and incitant in male pattern baldness and his later classification of the patterns and grades of baldness are landmarks in the study of male pattern baldness. Subsequent investigations of hair loss confirmed the significance of androgens in male pattern baldness, and Hamilton's classification remains in use.

Hamilton demonstrated conclusively that the extent and development of male pattern baldness were dependent on the interaction of three factors: androgens, genetic predisposition, and age. In summary, he found that genetic, endocrine, and aging factors are interdependent. No matter how strong the inherited predisposition, male pattern alopecia will not result if androgens are missing. Neither are the androgens able to induce baldness in individuals not genetically predisposed to baldness. The action of aging is demonstrated by the immediate loss of hair upon exposure to androgens in the sixth decade of life, whereas hair in young men exposed to androgens tends to remain much longer.

Over the centuries, men have tried every imaginable approach to retain hair. They have shampooed their scalps with tar, petroleum, goose dung, and cow urine. They have stuck their heads into rubber caps connected to vacuum pumps to suck recalcitrant hairs to the surface. In the 1960's, hair transplants became the most efficient and aesthetically pleasing method of retaining scalp hair. Research in the area of drug treatment continues.

—Genevieve Slomski, Ph.D.;
updated by Dwight G. Smith, Ph.D.

See also Aging; Dermatology; Gray hair; Hair; Hair transplantation; Men's health; Plastic surgery; Pregnancy and gestation; Psoriasis; Skin; Skin disorders.

FOR FURTHER INFORMATION:

"Bothered by Baldness? Here Are Your Options." *Health News* 18, no. 3 (June/July, 2000): 3. The vast majority of men with thinning hair have "male pattern baldness." Some of the treatments available to men to prevent baldness are discussed, including medication and hair transplants.

Greenwood-Robinson, Maggie. *Hair Savers for Women: A Complete Guide to Preventing and Treating Hair Loss.* New York: Crown, 2000. Provides guidelines for dealing with hair loss that stems from stress, hormonal imbalance, illness, chemotherapy, or medical side effects. Medical and natural approaches are covered as baldness remedies.

Harris, James, and Emanuel Marritt. *The Hair Replacement Revolution: A Consumer's Guide to Effective Hair Replacement Techniques.* Garden City Park, N.Y.: Square One, 2003. An easy-to-understand guide that explores the three basic approaches to hair replacement—drug therapies, artificial hair systems, and surgical procedures—and the strengths, weaknesses, and breakthroughs of each.

Regrowth.com. http://www.hairloss.org/. Site dedicated to researching treatments for hair loss and verifying product claims for hair growth.

Scott, Susan Craig, and Karen W. Pressler. *The Hair Bible.* New York: Simon & Schuster, 2003. Covers a wide range of hair-related topics, including basics of hair care, remedies for scalp troubles, female pattern baldness, the emotional effects of hair loss, and hair grafts or scalp reductions that can mitigate hair loss.

Setterberg, Fred. "The Naked Truth About Baldness." *In Health* 3 (September/October, 1989): 112-118. This article summarizes for the general reader the main causes of permanent hair loss and discusses treatment options such as transplants and the drug minoxidil.

Stough, Dow B., and Robert S. Haber, eds. *Hair Replacement: Surgical and Medical.* St. Louis: Mosby, 1996. This book discusses hair loss and its various treatments, such as stimulants and transplantation.

Thompson, Wendy, and Jerry Shapiro. *Alopecia Areata: Understanding and Coping with Hair Loss.* Rev. ed. Baltimore: Johns Hopkins University Press, 2000. Details current research, diagnosis, treatment options, and practical strategies for living with the condition.

HAIR TRANSPLANTATION
PROCEDURE

ANATOMY OR SYSTEM AFFECTED: Hair, head, skin

SPECIALTIES AND RELATED FIELDS: Dermatology, general surgery, plastic surgery

DEFINITION: The surgical relocation of healthy hair follicles to a part of the scalp where shrunken follicles are producing short, thin hair or no hair.

KEY TERMS:

alopecia: a hair restoration technique that involves surgical removal of a bald portion of scalp followed by stretching of hair-covered scalp to restore hair

donor graft: a segment of hair surgically transplanted as a plug or micrograft from one part of the scalp to another

micrograft: a small filament of donor hair typically containing three or four active hair follicles

INDICATIONS AND PROCEDURES

Several types of balding may cause a patient to seek out hair transplantation. Androgenetic alopecia (common baldness) is a condition that can affect both men and women who are genetically predisposed to it. Usually beginning in late adolescence or early adulthood, androgenetic hormones cause hair follicles gradually to grow smaller and eventually to yield hair that can be detected only by a microscope, or no hair at all.

Different patterns of balding have been observed. Frontal recession is a gradual process during which the frontal hairline retreats from the forehead. In vertex thinning, the hair on the crown of the head gradually disappears, exposing the scalp; the denuded area grows slowly in a concentric pattern. With complete balding, progressive frontal recession combines with vertex balding to create a condition in which hair is present only in a rim at the sides and back of the scalp.

Hair transplantation can involve several approaches for the restoration of a full head of hair. In some ways, the simplest surgical procedure for hair restoration is transplanting of the scalp rather than the hair itself. Called alopecia reduction, flap surgery, or scalp reduction, this procedure involves surgically restructuring the forehead to remove the bald areas of scalp, stretching the hair-covered scalp areas to cover the areas that are removed. Good candidates for scalp reduction are individuals with sufficiently thick or dense donor hair immediately adjacent to bald areas. Scalp reduction procedures may be performed in combination with hair transplantation to enhance the resulting hairline following surgery. Scalp reduction is considered to be a good method of hair restoration for some individuals because it is less intrusive and stressful than hair transplantation. However, scalp reduction may have limited use as a hair transplantation methodology for individuals that are experiencing onset of male pattern baldness as the areas of scalp stretched to cover the bald areas may eventually experience hair loss as well.

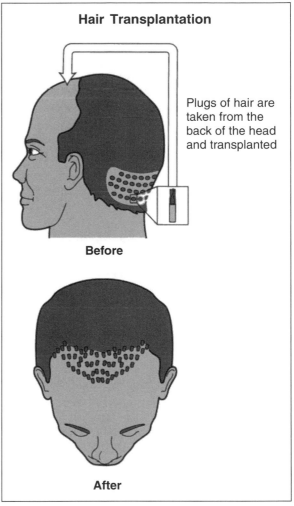

Hair Transplantation

Plugs of hair are taken from the back of the head and transplanted

Before

After

In the punch graft method of hair transplantation, tiny plugs of hair are taken from areas of the scalp where hair growth is still abundant and are inserted into areas where growth has stopped, usually the forehead or the crown.

Hair replacement via hair transplantation involves surgery, which should be performed by a board-certified physician skilled in this procedure. Hair transplantation has the distinct advantage over all other procedures currently in place for hair restoration because the candidate's own hair is used. Candidates for surgical hair transplantation must have healthy hair growth on the back and sides of the head to serve as donor hair, donor grafts, or donor flaps. Choice of location for donor hair will also be influenced by factors such as hair color, hair texture, and growth direction.

The type of hair transplantation method is generally determined by the extent of hair loss and the quality of donor hair available. If minimal hair restoration is necessary, then punch grafts, slit grafts, and strip grafts are typically the hair transplantation method. More extensive hair restoration may require scalp reduction procedures and extensive hair grafts.

All hair transplantation procedures involve the application of anesthesia. It may be administered as local anesthesia applied topically to the donor and recipient areas of the scalp or as general anesthesia if more extensive transplants are undertaken or if the hair transplantation process is more complex.

Following the introduction of anesthesia, the surgeon removes small micrografts of hair typically containing several follicles. They are inserted in narrow slits in the bald areas of scalp or are simply inserted as very small microplugs. Earlier procedures that have largely been discontinued excised plugs containing several dozen hair follicles, which were then inserted into areas of bald scalp, but this left visible and unsightly bumps or plugs from which hair grew in clumps. Some individuals who underwent this earlier plug procedure have since had all or part of their hair restored with modern micrograft or microfollicle procedures.

For many patients, hair transplantation processes can be accomplished as an outpatient procedure requiring no more than a single day. More extensive and more complicated hair transplantation cases will require additional sessions that may extend over several months.

The procedure begins with the hair trimmed short. A special instrument called a punch tube removes round donor grafts, while donor strips are surgically excised by scalpel. These donor grafts may be separated into individual hair follicles and then inserted into strips or holes in the scalp, washed with a saline solution, and closed with one or more stitches. Following the transplant session, the scalp is cleaned, washed, and covered with gauze.

USES AND COMPLICATIONS

All hair restoration procedures require surgery, which may not be suitable for everyone, and patients seeking hair transplantation are cautioned to consult a physician, and perhaps a psychiatrist as well, to determine whether their mental and physical health are optimal for the surgical procedure.

Patients desiring hair transplantation must be cautioned that despite the claims of proponents, there is no certainty that the procedure will be successful. Problems with unsuccessful hair transplantation have led doctors to require patients to sign a form which specifically indicates that the procedure is not guaranteed.

PERSPECTIVE AND PROSPECTS

More than fifty thousand hair transplantation procedures are performed each year in the United States, and that number is expected to increase as more practitioners are trained and the cost, which often amounts to several thousand dollars, is reduced.

—Russell Williams, M.S.W.;
updated by Dwight G. Smith, Ph.D.

See also Dermatology; Grafts and grafting; Hair; Hair loss and baldness; Men's health; Plastic surgery; Skin; Transplantation.

FOR FURTHER INFORMATION:

Hannapel, Coriene E. "Hair Transplant Advances Add Up to Better Results." *Dermatology Times* 21, no. 6 (June, 2000): 35. Dr. Walter P. Unger, codirector of dermatologic surgery at the University of Toronto, discusses the shift to using only follicular units for transplanting, as opposed to using both follicular units and minigrafts.

Regrowth.com. http://www.hairloss.org/. Site dedicated to researching treatments for hair loss and verifying product claims for hair growth.

Sams, W. Mitchell, Jr., and Peter J. Lynch, eds. *Principles and Practice of Dermatology*. 2d ed. New York: Churchill Livingstone, 1996. A dermatology reference guide and text emphasizing accurate diagnosis by succinct discussions in eighty-five presentations featuring color photographs. The contributing dermatologists detail all major topics in the field of dermatology.

Scott, Susan Craig, and Karen W. Pressler. *The Hair Bible*. New York: Simon & Schuster, 2003. Covers a wide range of hair-related topics, including basics of hair care, remedies for scalp troubles, female pattern baldness, the emotional effects of hair loss, and hair transplantations or scalp reductions that can mitigate hair loss.

Segell, Michael. "The Bald Truth About Hair." *Esquire* 121, no. 5 (May 1, 1994): 111-117. A guide to avoiding baldness is offered. Baldness can occur in three ways: vertex baldness (the top of the head), frontal recession, or a combination of both.

Thompson, Wendy, and Jerry Shapiro. *Alopecia Areata: Understanding and Coping with Hair Loss*. Rev. ed. Baltimore: Johns Hopkins University Press, 2000. Details current research, diagnosis, treatment options, and practical strategies for living with the condition.

HALITOSIS

DISEASE/DISORDER

ANATOMY OR SYSTEM AFFECTED: Gums, lungs, mouth, nose, stomach, teeth, throat

SPECIALTIES AND RELATED FIELDS: Dentistry, gastroenterology, microbiology, otorhinolaryngology

DEFINITION: Bad breath that is often caused by bacterial activity in the mouth.

CAUSES AND SYMPTOMS

The primary cause of halitosis stems from anaerobic bacteria that reside in the back of the mouth, particularly on the back of the tongue. These bacteria break down proteins and generate smelly gases, especially hydrogen sulfide and methyl mercaptan. More than twenty-two different bacteria have been identified as producing bad odors in the mouth. Periodontal disease, decayed teeth, and infected tonsils are also sources of bad breath. Dry mouth caused by a decreased flow of saliva can produce halitosis. Foods such as onions, garlic, and hot peppers produce chemical odors that are expelled in the breath. In general, particles of food that remain in the mouth on the tongue or between teeth collect bacteria and can cause bad breath. Tobacco products cause halitosis, stain teeth, and irritate gum tissues.

Outside the mouth, chronic infections of the sinuses or lungs can also cause halitosis. Kidney failure has been associated with ammonia-smelling breath, while inadequate diabetic control results in sweet-smelling breath. Halitosis originating from the stomach is very rare, since the esophagus is a closed tube that connects the stomach with the mouth.

Symptoms associated with halitosis include foul-smelling breath, a bad taste in the mouth, a white-to-yellow coating on the tongue, and bleeding gums. For many people, the problem of bad breath is manifest only when they begin to talk. To detect bad breath, one should ask a family member, close friend, or dentist how one's breath smells.

TREATMENT AND THERAPY

The basic treatment for halitosis includes brushing the teeth, tongue, and gums properly after each meal; flossing the teeth at least once a day; visiting the dentist regularly; drinking adequate fluids; and eating fresh, fibrous fruits and vegetables. Although it may take time and patience to overcome the gagging reflex, it is important periodically to clean the back of the tongue thoroughly and gently with a toothbrush or a scraper.

Some mouthwashes have been clinically proven to reduce bad breath effectively, as have some toothpastes. Chewing sugarfree gum, mint, cloves, or fennel seeds for a short time can likewise reduce the odor. Dentures should be cleaned properly every day and should not be kept in the mouth overnight. Nose and throat infections resulting in halitosis may need medical treatment.

PERSPECTIVE AND PROSPECTS

More than fifty million people in the United States suffer some degree of halitosis. It originates in the mouth in more than 90 percent of the cases. Although Islamic and Jewish teachings implicate the stomach as a source of bad breath, it almost never originates there. In almost all cases, halitosis is treatable. Rarely is it an indication of a significant general health problem.

—Alvin K. Benson, Ph.D.

See also Alcoholism; Bacterial infections; Cavities; Dental diseases; Dentistry; Dentures; Endodontic disease; Food biochemistry; Gastroenterology; Gastroenterology, pediatric; Gastrointestinal disorders; Gastrointestinal system; Gum disease; Nasopharyngeal disorders; Otorhinolaryngology; Pharyngitis; Sense organs; Sinusitis; Smell; Smoking; Sore throat; Taste; Tonsillitis.

INFORMATION ON HALITOSIS

CAUSES: Anaerobic bacteria; also periodontal disease, decayed teeth, infected tonsils, certain foods (onions, garlic, hot peppers), tobacco products

SYMPTOMS: Foul-smelling breath, bad taste in mouth, white-to-yellow coating on tongue, bleeding gums

DURATION: Chronic

TREATMENTS: Brushing of the teeth, tongue, and gums after each meal; flossing; mouthwash; regular dentist visits; adequate fluids; fresh fruits and vegetables

---

FOR FURTHER INFORMATION:

Icon Health. *Halitosis: A Medical Dictionary, Bibliography, and Annotated Research Guide to Internet References.* San Diego, Calif.: Author, 2004.

Miller, Richard A. *Beating Bad Breath: Your Complete Guide to Eliminating and Preventing Halitosis.* Baltimore: Noble House, 1995.

Rosenberg, Mel, and Daniel van Steenberghe, eds. *Bad Breath: A Multidisciplinary Approach*. Leuven, Belgium: Leuven University Press, 1996.

HALLUCINATIONS
DISEASE/DISORDER

ANATOMY OR SYSTEM AFFECTED: Brain, nervous system, psychic-emotional system

SPECIALTIES AND RELATED FIELDS: Neurology, psychiatry, psychology

DEFINITION: The perception of sensations without relevant external stimuli.

Society often associates hallucinations with psychotic behavior, because schizophrenia and other forms of mental illness frequently involve hallucinations. Another widely publicized example of these symptoms is the use of hallucinogenic drugs, for example, LSD (lysergic acid diethylamide) or marijuana. One must also consider the role of hallucinations in religious experiences and megalomania; such perceptions occur when ordinary people are subjected to extraordinary stimuli.

Medical science has resisted the study of hallucinations and treated them as symptoms of mental illness. Increasing evidence shows, however, that they arise from specific brain and nervous system structures involving specific biological experiences and common reactions to stimuli. Consequently, people suffering from drug abuse, alcoholism, and disorders similar to Alzheimer's disease, in which severe loss of memory can provoke illusions, are subject to hallucinations.

Since a hallucination can be the result of physical causes as well as the traditional mental unbalance of schizophrenia or manic depression, it is difficult to categorize its symptoms. An individual experiencing hallucinations at times other than waking or falling asleep should see his or her doctor. If the incidents are attributable to a serious illness, early detection is possible. If they are an effect of a particular medication, the prescription should be changed immediately.

—*K. Thomas Finley, Ph.D.*

See also Addiction; Alcoholism; Alzheimer's disease; Bipolar disorders; Brain; Brain disorders; Delusions; Dementias; Intoxication; Narcolepsy; Neurology; Neurology, pediatric; Paranoia; Pick's disease; Poisonous plants; Psychiatric disorders; Psychiatry; Psychiatry, child and adolescent; Psychiatry, geriatric; Psychosis; Schizophrenia; Sleep disorders; Stress.

INFORMATION ON HALLUCINATIONS

CAUSES: Psychological disorders, various diseases, use of hallucinogenic drugs
SYMPTOMS: Varies; can include depression, insomnia, maniclike mood swings
DURATION: Short-term to chronic
TREATMENTS: Counseling, drug therapy

FOR FURTHER INFORMATION:

Asaad, Ghazi. *Hallucinations in Clinical Psychiatry: A Guide for Mental Health Professionals*. New York: Brunner/Mazel, 1990. Discusses the diagnosis and treatment of hallucinations. Includes bibliographical references and an index.

Bloom, Floyd E., M. Flint Beal, and David J. Kupfer, eds. *The Dana Guide to Brain Health*. New York: Simon & Schuster, 2003. An easy-to-understand health guide to the brain from neuroscience, neurology, and psychiatry perspectives. More than seventy psychiatric and neurological disorders, their diagnoses, and their treatments are covered.

Lennox, Belinda R., et al. "Spatial and Temporal Mapping of Neural Activity Associated with Auditory Hallucinations." *The Lancet* 353, no. 9153 (February 20, 1999): 644. Results show the strong association of the right middle temporal gyrus with the experience of auditory hallucination in the patient studied, supporting the hypothesis that auditory hallucinations reflect abnormal activation of the auditory cortex.

Nolte, John. *Human Brain: An Introduction to Its Functional Anatomy*. 5th ed. New York: Mosby, 2002. Text covering major concepts and structure-function relationships in the human neurological system.

Sadock, Benjamin James, and Virginia A. Sadock. *Kaplan and Sadock's Synopsis of Psychiatry: Behavioral Sciences/Clinical Psychiatry*. 9th ed. Philadelphia: Lippincott Williams & Wilkins, 2003. Integrates biological, psychological, and sociological perspectives to provide a comprehensive overview of the field of psychiatry.

Siegel, Ronald K. *Fire in the Brain: Clinical Tales of Hallucination*. New York: Plume, 1992. This textbook describes clinical case studies of patients suffering from hallucinations. Includes bibliographical references.

Slade, Peter D., and Richard P. Bentall. *Sensory Deception: A Scientific Analysis of Hallucinations*. Baltimore: Johns Hopkins University Press, 1988. Discusses the mechanisms of hallucination. Includes bibliographical references and an index.

Stephens, G. Lynn, and George Graham. *When Self-Consciousness Breaks: Alien Voices and Inserted Thoughts.* Cambridge, Mass.: MIT Press, 2003. Utilizes a number of case studies to explain alienated self-consciousness. Includes bibliographical references and an index.

HAMMERTOE CORRECTION
PROCEDURE

ANATOMY OR SYSTEM AFFECTED: Blood vessels, bones, feet, musculoskeletal system, nervous system, tendons

SPECIALTIES AND RELATED FIELDS: General surgery, orthopedics, podiatry

DEFINITION: The surgical removal of ligaments and joining of the middle joints in the toes to correct hammertoe, a deformity in which the toes bend downward abnormally.

INDICATIONS AND PROCEDURES

A hammertoe is a painful deformity that usually affects the second toe. The clawlike appearance of the toe results from malignancy of the joint surface or shortening and weakening of the foot and toe muscle. People with diabetes mellitus are prone to hammertoe development because of the nerve and muscle damage frequently associated with the disease. In other cases, hammertoe results from the wearing of shoes that are too short and do not fit properly. High-heeled shoes, which place pressure on the front of the foot and compress the smaller toes tightly together, can contribute to hammertoe formation. Painful calluses form on the tops of toes when the deformed toe rubs against the top of the shoe. Special orthotics and pads are often used to redistribute pressure and relieve pain. In severe cases, surgery may be required.

Before the operation, blood and urine studies are conducted and X rays are taken of both feet. Hammertoe correction surgery begins with the injection of a local anesthetic. To prevent bleeding in the surgical area, a tourniquet is applied above the ankle. An incision is made through the skin above the affected joint. The tendons that attach to the toes are located and cut free of the connective tissue to the foot bone. The tendons are then divided, enabling the toe to straighten. To keep the toe from bending, the middle joints are permanently connected together with fine pins and wires. Fine sutures are used to close the skin, and the tourniquet is removed. After the surgery, additional blood studies are taken. Sutures are usually removed seven to ten days after the procedure.

USES AND COMPLICATIONS

The correction of hammertoe usually arises out of a need to correct severe deformity or relieve persistent pain. During recovery, flat, comfortable shoes should be worn. After recovery, shoes should be worn that fit well and do not cramp the toes or put undue stress on the front of the foot. Though full recovery from surgery is expected in four weeks, vigorous exercise should be avoided for six weeks after surgery. Once the time for healing has passed, the affected toe will appear in a normal position, and pain will be relieved. Because of the connecting of joints in the toe, however, movement of the toes will be limited.

Possible complications associated with hammertoe correction include excessive bleeding and surgical wound infection.

—Jason Georges

See also Bone disorders; Bones and the skeleton; Feet; Foot disorders; Hammertoes; Lower extremities; Orthopedic surgery; Orthopedics; Podiatry.

FOR FURTHER INFORMATION:

Copeland, D. P. M. Glenn, and Stan Solomon. *The Foot Doctor: Lifetime Relief for Your Aching Feet.* Emmaus, Pa.: Rodale Press, 1986.

Currey, John D. *Bones: Structures and Mechanics.* Princeton, N.J.: Princeton University Press, 2002.

Lippert, Frederick G., and Sigvard T. Hansen. *Foot and Ankle Disorders: Tricks of the Trade.* New York: Thieme, 2003.

Lorimer, Donald L., et al., eds. *Neale's Disorders of the Foot.* 7th ed. New York: Elsevier Churchill Livingstone, 2006.

Van De Graaff, Kent M., and Stuart I. Fox. *Concepts of Human Anatomy and Physiology.* 5th ed. Dubuque, Iowa: Wm. C. Brown, 2000.

HAMMERTOES
DISEASE/DISORDER

ANATOMY OR SYSTEM AFFECTED: Feet

SPECIALTIES AND RELATED FIELDS: Orthopedics, podiatry

DEFINITION: Toes that are bent permanently at the joint nearest to the foot; the closely related term "clawtoe" denotes a toe that is bent at both joints.

CAUSES AND SYMPTOMS

Hammertoes and clawtoes can occur in one or more of the four smaller toes on each foot, with the second toe being the most common site for these deformities. Hammertoes and clawtoes are thought to be caused by muscle imbalance, contraction of the tendons, and enlargement of the toe joints. Although anyone can develop these conditions, they are felt to be caused primarily by wearing high heels or shoes that are too tight. It is common for people to develop painful corns and calluses in association with these conditions, particularly on the top or on the tip of the toe where it is most likely to rub against the shoe. Furthermore, people with hammertoes or clawtoes may experience considerable pain if the toe gets inflamed and may also develop skin ulcers from the rubbing of their shoes against the bent toe. These ulcers can become infected and develop abnormal channels to the skin surface called sinus tracts. These conditions may also cause significant problems with walking for the affected individual.

TREATMENT AND THERAPY

Treatment of hammertoes or clawtoes depends on the severity of the condition and whether there are secondary complications such as corns or ulcers. The simplest treatment is to change to shoes with broad toes and soft soles that cushion the foot and to avoid wearing high heels and shoes that pinch the toes. Accompanied by excellent foot care such as callus and corn removal, this may be all that is required to prevent pain and irritation of the toes. In cases that are more advanced, various inserts can be added to the shoes. These include metatarsal bars, orthotics, and other devices. A metatarsal bar supports the ball of the foot, spreading the pressure normally put on this area over a greater part of the foot. Orthotics are specially molded plastic devices that serve much the same purpose. In some cases, podiatrists (foot doctors) or orthopedists recommend toe caps, padded sleeves that help prevent friction between the toe and the shoe. In a few cases, it may be necessary to cut the tendons in the toe or to perform arthroplasty (repair of the joint itself) to provide relief.

—*Rebecca Lovell Scott, Ph.D., PA-C*

See also Bone disorders; Bones and the skeleton; Corns and calluses; Foot disorders; Hammertoe correction; Lower extremities; Skin; Skin disorders.

FOR FURTHER INFORMATION:

Copeland, D. P. M. Glenn, and Stan Solomon. *The Foot Doctor: Lifetime Relief for Your Aching Feet.* Emmaus, Pa.: Rodale Press, 1986.

Currey, John D. *Bones: Structures and Mechanics.* Princeton, N.J.: Princeton University Press, 2002.

Levy, Leonard A., and Vincent J. Hetherington, eds. *Principles and Practice of Podiatric Medicine.* New York: Churchill Livingstone, 1990.

Lippert, Frederick G., and Sigvard T. Hansen. *Foot and Ankle Disorders: Tricks of the Trade.* New York: Thieme, 2003.

Lorimer, Donald L., et al., eds. *Neale's Disorders of the Foot.* 7th ed. New York: Elsevier Churchill Livingstone, 2006.

HAND-FOOT-AND-MOUTH DISEASE
DISEASE/DISORDER

ANATOMY OR SYSTEM AFFECTED: Gastrointestinal system, mouth, skin

SPECIALTIES AND RELATED FIELDS: Dermatology, pediatrics, virology

DEFINITION: An enteroviral disease which usually affects children, causing vesicular eruptions on the hands, feet, oral mucosa, and tongue.

CAUSES AND SYMPTOMS

Hand-foot-and-mouth disease is usually caused by Coxsackievirus A16, but it may also be associated with a number of other coxsackieviruses and enterovirus 71. Young children, ages one to five, are most commonly infected in the summer or early fall. They often become infected through contact with the nasal and oral secretions of infected children, and nursery school outbreaks may occur. Skin lesions and fecal material may also contribute to the spread of the virus. The incubation period is three to six days.

The illness commences with a low-grade fever (100 to 101 degrees Fahrenheit) and a sore mouth. Oral lesions begin as small, red macules and evolve rapidly

---

INFORMATION ON HAMMERTOES

CAUSES: Muscle imbalance, tendon contraction, enlargement of toe joints, improper footwear

SYMPTOMS: Pain, inflammation, corns and calluses, skin ulcers

DURATION: Typically short-term

TREATMENTS: Change of footwear, use of corrective inserts or devices, sometimes arthroplasty or cutting of affected tendon

INFORMATION ON HAND-FOOT-AND-MOUTH DISEASE

CAUSES: Viral infection
SYMPTOMS: Low-grade fever, sore mouth, oral lesions that rupture into painful ulcers, skin lesions on hands and feet
DURATION: Seven to ten days
TREATMENTS: None (self-resolving); topical anesthetic agents for mouth lesions

into fragile vesicles that rupture, leaving painful ulcers. Any part of the mouth may be involved, but the hard palate buccal mucosa and tongue are mainly affected with an average of five to ten lesions. Similar lesions develop on the skin over the next one to two days; they usually number twenty to thirty, but there may be as many as one hundred. Discrete macular lesions, about 4 millimeters in diameter, appear on the hands and feet and sometimes the buttocks. These lesions often occur along skin lines and progress to become papules and white or gray flaccid vesicles containing infective virus. The lesions may be painful or tender. The fever occurs during the first one to two days of the illness, which resolves in seven to ten days. Rarely, the viral infection is complicated by meningoencephalitis, carditis, or pneumonia.

TREATMENT AND THERAPY

There is no specific treatment for hand-foot-and-mouth disease. The infection usually resolves without complications in about one week. Topical anesthetic agents, such as viscous lidocaine, may be used to soothe the discomfort of the mouth lesions. Popsicles and cool sherbets may be given to young children to help soothe a sore mouth. Acetaminophen given at an appropriate dosage for the body weight of the child may also help to relieve the pain of this condition. Some pediatricians recommend a blend of Benadryl and liquid antacid to relieve the stinging sensation of the mouth lesions.

PERSPECTIVE AND PROSPECTS

The first described outbreak of this disease occurred in Toronto, Canada, in 1957. British authors first coined the term "hand-foot-and-mouth disease" when they reported an outbreak in Birmingham, England, in 1959. While there currently are no medications available for treating enteroviral infections, a number of antiviral agents are being studied and might be useful for com-

plicated forms of this disease, such as meningoencephalitis.

—*H. Bradford Hawley, M.D.;*
updated by Lenela Glass-Godwin, M.WS.
See also Childhood infectious diseases; Dermatology, pediatric; Encephalitis; Fever; Meningitis; Rashes; Skin; Skin disorders; Viral infections.

FOR FURTHER INFORMATION:

Barnhill, Raymond, and A. Neil Crowson, eds. *Textbook of Dermatopathology*. 2d ed. New York: McGraw-Hill, 2004.

Belshe, Robert B., ed. *Textbook of Human Virology*. 2d ed. St. Louis: Mosby Year Book, 1991.

Freedberg, Irwin M., et al., eds. *Fitzpatrick's Dermatology in General Medicine*. 6th ed. 2 vols. New York: McGraw-Hill, 2003.

Mandell, Gerald L., John E. Bennett, and Raphael Dolin, eds. *Mandell, Douglas, and Bennett's Principles and Practice of Infectious Diseases*. 6th ed. New York: Elsevier/Churchill Livingstone, 2005.

HANTAVIRUS

DISEASE/DISORDER

ANATOMY OR SYSTEM AFFECTED: Kidneys, lungs, respiratory system

SPECIALTIES AND RELATED FIELDS: Critical care, environmental health, epidemiology, internal medicine, public health, pulmonary medicine, virology

DEFINITION: An often-fatal viral infection carried by rodents that causes influenza-like symptoms and respiratory failure.

CAUSES AND SYMPTOMS

Hantavirus, which is distantly related to Ebola virus, is transmitted through contact with the urine and droppings of wild rodents, such as the deer mouse and cotton rat. Contact usually involves the inhalation of contaminated particles in dust. Hantavirus is not transmissible between humans.

Infection takes two major forms. In South America, one strain causes hemorrhagic fever with renal syndrome, involving kidney failure, hemorrhaging, and shock. In the United States, another strain results in hantavirus pulmonary syndrome. Early symptoms mimic influenza; they include fever, chills, muscle aches, nausea and vomiting, malaise, and a dry cough. After initial improvement, increasing shortness of breath follows and may progress to pulmonary edema, internal bleeding, respiratory failure, and death.

TREATMENT AND THERAPY

Diagnosis of hantavirus pulmonary syndrome involves physical examination for hypoxia, hypotension, and adult respiratory distress syndrome. Laboratory tests show an elevated white blood cell count and a decreasing platelet count, and chest X rays may reveal edema. The presence of hantavirus is confirmed through serological testing.

There is no cure for hantavirus pulmonary syndrome; treatment is focused on alleviating the symptoms. This condition must be treated in the intensive care unit (ICU) of a hospital, as careful monitoring of respiratory function and blood gases is essential. In severe cases, the use of an endotracheal tube and a ventilator becomes necessary. Experiments have been performed with intravenous ribavirin therapy; the efficacy of this treatment is being evaluated. Unfortunately, even with aggressive measures, the death rate ranges from 50 to 80 percent.

PERSPECTIVE AND PROSPECTS

The incidence of hantavirus pulmonary syndrome seemed to rise sharply in the 1990's. Epidemiologists were uncertain whether the number of cases increased or more cases were reported following identification of the virus in the United States in 1993.

Because much remains to be learned about the transmission, development, and treatment of hantavirus infection, public health efforts have been in education and prevention. Hikers and campers are thought to be at a greater risk; they are urged to avoid exposure to rodent droppings and questionable water sources. People entering cabins, sheds, or other buildings that have not been used recently should air out the building first and use disinfectant on all surfaces.

—*Tracy Irons-Georges*

See also Edema; Environmental diseases; Environmental health; Epidemiology; Lungs; Pulmonary diseases; Pulmonary medicine; Respiration; Viral infections; Zoonoses.

FOR FURTHER INFORMATION:

Cockrum, E. Lendell. *Rabies, Lyme Disease, Hanta Virus, and Other Animal-Borne Human Diseases in the United States and Canada*. Tucson, Ariz.: Fisher Books, 1997.

Kumar, Vinay, et al., eds. *Robbins Basic Pathology*. 8th ed. Philadelphia: Saunders/Elsevier, 2007.

Meyer, Andrea S., and David R. Harper. *Of Mice, Men, and Microbes: Hantavirus*. San Diego, Calif.: Academic Press, 1999.

Murray, Patrick R., Ken S. Rosenthal, and Michael A. Pfaller. *Medical Microbiology*. 5th ed. Philadelphia: Elsevier/Mosby, 2005.

Pan American Health Organization. *Hantavirus in the Americas: Guidelines for Diagnosis, Treatment, Prevention, and Control*. Washington, D.C.: Author, 1999.

Sompayrac, Lauren. *How Pathogenic Viruses Work*. 5th ed. Boston: Jones and Bartlett, 2002.

Strauss, James, and Ellen Strauss. *Viruses and Human Disease*. San Diego, Calif.: Academic Press, 2001.

HARELIP. *See* CLEFT LIP AND PALATE.

HASHIMOTO'S THYROIDITIS
DISEASE/DISORDER

ALSO KNOWN AS: Struma lymphomatosa, lymphadenoid goiter, chronic lymphocytic thyroiditis, autoimmune thyroiditis

ANATOMY OR SYSTEM AFFECTED: Endocrine system, glands, immune system, neck

SPECIALTIES AND RELATED FIELDS: Endocrinology

DEFINITION: An autoimmune disease that results in inflammation of the thyroid gland caused when abnormal blood antibodies and white blood cells infiltrate and attack thyroidal cells.

CAUSES AND SYMPTOMS

Hashimoto's thyroiditis is a common type of hypothyroidism. The cause and etiology of this disorder is not fully understood; however, it is thought to have an autoimmune origin, in which abnormal blood antibodies and white blood cells, called lymphocytes, infiltrate and attack thyroid cells. The combative interplay between the lymphocytes and the thyroid may lead to a complete absence of thyroid cells. A family history of thyroid disease is commonly traced.

INFORMATION ON HANTAVIRUS

CAUSES: Viral infection spread through contact with urine and droppings of wild rodents

SYMPTOMS: Fever, chills, muscle aches, nausea and vomiting, malaise, dry cough, kidney failure, hemorrhaging, shock

DURATION: Acute

TREATMENTS: None; alleviation of symptoms

The highest incidence of the disease is observed in young or middle-aged women, but it may occur at any age. The onset is very slow, and the disease may progress for many months or years before it is fully detected. The symptoms may vary, but the condition is usually characterized by a mild pressure on the thyroid gland. In some cases, a firm, slightly irregular, and sometime tender goiter (enlarged thyroid gland) may develop in the neck region. In more severe cases, the disease may cause symptoms related to low thyroid function (hypothyroidism), such as fatigue, weight gain, intolerance to cold, constipation, and hair loss.

The symptomology of Hashimoto's thyroiditis may resemble other medical conditions. Therefore, in addition to a full medical examination, the diagnostic procedure must also include blood tests to determine the levels of thyroid hormone and thyroid antibodies. If a patient has developed the classic symptoms that accompany Hashimoto's thyroiditis but has a normal blood test, then a biopsy in which a needle is inserted into the thyroid and some cells are removed may be performed to confirm the diagnosis.

TREATMENT AND THERAPY

Though a specific treatment is not yet available, the hypothyroidism resulting from Hashimoto's thyroiditis can be treated with hormones. Medical practitioners opt to commence hormone therapy, in the form of thyroxine, as soon as a diagnosis is made, even if thyroid function is normal at the time. The hormone therapy is expected to shrink any goiter that has developed. If there is no response, then surgery may be required.

The prognosis for a full recovery is usually very good because the disease remains dormant or stable for many years.

—*Nicholas Lanzieri; updated by Sharon W. Stark, R.N., A.P.R.N., D.N.Sc.*

See also Endocrine disorders; Endocrinology; Glands; Goiter; Hormones; Hyperparathyroidism and hypoparathyroidism; Metabolism; Parathyroidectomy; Thyroid disorders; Thyroid gland; Thyroidectomy.

FOR FURTHER INFORMATION:

Bayliss, R. I. S., and W. M. Tunbridge. *Thyroid Disease: The Facts*. 3d ed. New York: Oxford University Press, 1999.

Burrow, Gerard N., Jack H. Oppenheimer, and Robert Volpé. *Thyroid Function and Disease*. Philadelphia: W. B. Saunders, 1990.

Larsen, P. Reed, et al., eds. *Williams Textbook of Endocrinology*. 10th ed. Philadelphia: W. B. Saunders, 2003.

Shannon, Joyce Brennfleck, ed. *Thyroid Disorders Sourcebook: Basic Consumer Health Information About Disorders of the Thyroid and Parathyroid Glands*. Detroit: Omnigraphics, 2005.

MedlinePlus. *Chronic Thyroiditis (Hashimoto's Disease)*. Edited by Robert Hurd. http://www.nlm.nih.gov/medlineplus/ency/article/000371.htm.

Wood, Lawrence C., David S. Cooper, and E. Chester Ridgway. *Your Thyroid: A Home Reference*. 4th rev. ed. New York: Ballantine Books, 2005.

HAY FEVER

DISEASE/DISORDER

ALSO KNOWN AS: Seasonal allergic rhinitis

ANATOMY OR SYSTEM AFFECTED: Eyes, immune system, lungs, lymphatic system, nose, respiratory system, throat

SPECIALTIES AND RELATED FIELDS: Immunology, otorhinolaryngology

DEFINITION: A damaging immune response to otherwise harmless foreign substances such as pollen grains and mold spores.

CAUSES AND SYMPTOMS

Allergic rhinitis, popularly known as hay fever, represents the most common allergic disorder, affecting approximately 10 percent of the population; the most common source of the allergy is wind-dispersed pollen. These tiny grains are produced in phenomenal numbers to ensure transfer of the pollen (which contains the plant's sperm) to other flowers of the same plant species. Trees, grasses, and certain forbs (especially the ragweeds) are the most common culprits. The first time that a susceptible person is exposed, the pollen acts to sensitize the immune system. On second and subsequent exposures, the pollen triggers an allergic response.

This response is triggered by the formation of a specific class of antibody known as IgE against the proteins on the pollen grains (generally called antigens and in this case called allergens). Immunoglobulin E (IgE) attaches to tissue cells called mast cells by one end and to the pollen grains at the other end. This attachment causes the mast cells to release defensive substances, the best known of which is histamine. These substances cause increased permeability of capillaries and the production and release of mucous and watery substances from the nasal passages and eyes. Itching and sneezing accompany the release. The tendency to produce IgE against pollen allergens is an inherited trait; persons with one or both parents who have allergies toward certain substances are more likely to exhibit the same allergies than persons whose parents do not exhibit such responses.

TREATMENT AND THERAPY

It is generally agreed that avoidance of the allergen is the most effective therapy for hay fever. Staying inside a building with air conditioning or well-filtered air during the worst allergy season helps. However, avoiding an allergen completely, such as ragweed pollen during ragweed's flowering season, is essentially impossible.

The most common treatments employed are desensitization and drugs. Desensitization involves a series of injections of slowly increasing concentrations of the allergen, in the hope of turning the patient's immune system from the production of IgE to the production of immunoglobulin G (IgG), which does not trigger the mast cells. Drugs such as antihistamines, which block the action or the release of histamine and the other substances released by mast cells, are commonly recommended, either in prescription strength or over the counter. Steroid and decongestant sprays have also been successful in relieving the symptoms of hay fever in some individuals.

PERSPECTIVE AND PROSPECTS

For many persons, long-term avoidance of allergens such as pollen may be difficult. Current drugs such as antihistamines are directed primarily at relieving symptoms without removing the cause: the binding of IgE to the allergen. Future drugs may address the variety of steps involved in the allergic response while causing fewer side effects such as sleepiness. Other treatments may involve augmentation of IgG production in response to immunization with the allergen, since IgG competes with IgE in binding to the allergen.

—*Carl W. Hoagstrom, Ph.D.;*
updated by Richard Adler, Ph.D.

See also Allergies; Antihistamines; Autoimmune disorders; Decongestants; Immune system; Nasopharyngeal disorders; Otorhinolaryngology; Over-the-counter medications; Sense organs; Sinusitis; Smell; Sneezing.

FOR FURTHER INFORMATION:

Abbas, Abul K., and Andrew K. Lichtman. *Basic Immunology: Functions and Disorders of the Immune System.* 2d ed. Philadelphia: Elsevier Saunders, 2006.

Delves, Peter J., et al. *Roitt's Essential Immunology.* 11th ed. Malden, Mass.: Blackwell, 2006.

Janeway, Charles A., Jr., et al. *Immunobiology: The Immune System in Health and Disease.* 6th ed. New York: Garland Science, 2005.

Kindt, Thomas J., Richard A. Goldsby, and Barbara A. Osborne. *Kuby Immunology.* 6th ed. New York: W. H. Freeman, 2007.

Rabson, Arthur, et al. *Really Essential Medical Immunology.* 2d ed. Malden, Mass.: Blackwell Science, 2005.

HEAD AND NECK DISORDERS
DISEASE/DISORDER

ANATOMY OR SYSTEM AFFECTED: Bones, brain, head, muscles, musculoskeletal system, neck, nervous system, respiratory system, spine, throat

SPECIALTIES AND RELATED FIELDS: Dentistry, emergency medicine, neurology, otolaryngology, sports medicine

DEFINITION: Physical trauma or neurological problems affecting the head and neck, including the spinal cord.

The head and neck region of the human body houses a sophisticated collection of structures including the special sense organs (structures for breathing, speaking, and eating) and the brain, brain stem, and cervical (neck) portion of the spinal cord. A multitude of disorders or injuries can occur in this complex region.

Trauma to the head and neck. Head or neck trauma can result from a harsh blow on the head, as can occur in a fall or with a strike from an object. These injuries are commonly seen in young, basically healthy persons who come to emergency rooms during evenings or weekends as a result of sports accidents, automobile accidents, or domestic or street violence. In the older age group, strokes and aneurysms are more common problems. Some of these accidents or events can cause permanent nerve and brain damage to the injured person.

Concussions and contusions of the head are common results of head trauma, which induces an internal neurological response. A concussion is a loss of consciousness or awareness of one's surroundings that may last a few minutes or days. Sometimes a concussion appears only as a moderately decreased level of awareness and not a total loss of consciousness. There is no evidence of a change in the brain's structure but, oddly, there is a change in the way in which the brain operates so that alertness is altered. Concussion is presumably a temporary change in brain chemistry, and the damage is reversible unless repeated head blows, such as a professional boxer may experience, are endured. Concussions may occur from other trauma, such as loss of blood flow to the brain, but such trauma is more closely associated with the more urgent threat of permanent brain damage. A contusion is popularly referred to as a bruise. The color associated with a fresh bruise is attributable to an aggregation of blood in an area that was damaged, causing many small blood vessels to rupture and release blood into the surrounding tissue. A bruise around the eye, temple, or forehead causes a black eye.

Automobile accidents rank as one of the common causes of head and neck injury. One of the more famil-

iar complaints after a car accident is the condition called whiplash. Whiplash is the layperson's term for hyperextension of the neck, whereby the head is thrust backward (posteriorly) abruptly and beyond the normal range of neck motion. Hyperflexion occurs when the head is abruptly thrust in the forward (anterior) direction—sometimes as a recoil from hyperextension. The pain of whiplash originates from the damage to the anterior longitudinal ligament along the neck region of the spinal cord. This ligament can be overly stretched or even torn as a result of a sudden snap or jerk of the neck. Furthermore, the bony vertebrae may also grind against one another after the trauma, causing additional irritation, swelling, and pain in the neck area.

One of the common troubles of a gun or knife wound to the head and neck region is superficial and deep lacerations (cuts). If left unsutured, a deep scalp wound can cause death by hemorrhage. Superficial lacerations to the face may also cause considerable bleeding; such wounds generally are not life-threatening, but they often require stitches in order to heal.

Trauma to the head and neck area can arise from spontaneous internal events such as a stroke, an embolus, or an aneurysm. Each of these conditions is serious and potentially life-threatening because of the risk of losing blood flow to the brain and other vital tissues of the head and neck region.

Neurological problems of the head and neck. Although the bony cranium offers some protection to the head, the neck is, in some regards, more vulnerable to intrusion. Breathing can be interrupted by severing the left or right phrenic nerve, each of which innervates its corresponding half of the most important muscle of breathing, the diaphragm.

The left or right vagus nerve may also be severed. The vagus nerves supply the sympathetic system of the thorax and abdomen, and they also innervate the vocal cords. Severance of one of the vagus nerves causes a hoarseness of the voice as a result of the loss of function of one-half of the vocal cords. If both vagus nerves are damaged—a rare event—then the ability to speak is forever lost.

The sympathetic trunk is another nerve at risk in the neck. Severance of this nerve leads to Horner's syndrome, which consists of a group of signs including ptosis (drooping eyelids), constricted pupils, a flushed face as a result of vasodilation, and dry skin on the face and neck because of the inability to sweat.

Transection (the complete severance) of the lower cervical spinal cord causes upper and lower limb paral-

---

INFORMATION ON HEAD AND NECK DISORDERS

CAUSES: Injury, neurological problems
SYMPTOMS: Pain, bruising, whiplash, alignment problems, inflammation
DURATION: Short-term to chronic
TREATMENTS: Surgery, drug therapy, corrective devices

ysis and trouble with urination, and damage to the upper cervical cord can cause death because of loss of innervation to the muscles of respiration. Hemisection (partial severance) of the cervical spinal cord can also cause Horner's syndrome. Damage to the spinal cord can occur from a knife or gun wound or from crushing or snapping the cord by sudden impact, as with an injury from an earthquake or an automobile accident.

—*Mary C. Fields, M.D.*

See also Amnesia; Aneurysmectomy; Aneurysms; Ataxia; Botox; Brain; Brain damage; Brain disorders; Cluster headaches; Coma; Computed tomography (CT) scanning; Concussion; Craniosynostosis; Craniotomy; Dementias; Dizziness and fainting; Electroencephalography (EEG); Embolism; Encephalitis; Epilepsy; Hallucinations; Headaches; Hemiplegia; Hydrocephalus; Laryngitis; Memory loss; Meningitis; Migraine headaches; Nasal polyp removal; Nasopharyngeal disorders; Neuralgia, neuritis, and neuropathy; Neuroimaging; Neurology; Neurology, pediatric; Neurosurgery; Numbness and tingling; Palsy; Paralysis; Paraplegia; Pharyngitis; Quadriplegia; Seizures; Shunts; Sinusitis; Spinal cord disorders; Sports medicine; Strokes; Thrombosis and thrombus; Torticollis; Transient ischemic attacks (TIAs); Unconsciousness; Voice and vocal cord disorders; Whiplash.

FOR FURTHER INFORMATION:

American Medical Association. *American Medical Association Family Medical Guide*. 4th rev. ed. Hoboken, N.J.: John Wiley & Sons, 2004. The perfect beginner's guide, not only to head and neck medicine but also to any common medical topic.

Litin, Scott C., ed. *Mayo Clinic Family Health Book*. 3d ed. New York: HarperResource, 2003. A good general medical text for the layperson that covers the entire medical field. While the information is derived from a wide variety of highly technical sources, the articles are written to be easily understood by a general audience.

Marieb, Elaine N. *Essentials of Human Anatomy and Physiology*. 8th ed. San Francisco: Pearson/Benjamin Cummings, 2006. This introductory anatomy and physiology textbook, easily accessible to those with little science background, is richly illustrated with diagrams and photographs, which help to illuminate body systems and processes.

Moore, Keith L., and Arthur F. Dalley II. *Clinically Oriented Anatomy*. 5th ed. Philadelphia: Lippincott Williams & Wilkins, 2006. Moore addresses the normal human anatomy and offers clinical commentary for the sake of relevance. Enhanced by multicolored, detailed sketches. Expertly written.

Nicholls, John G., A. Robert Martin, and Bruce G. Wallace. *From Neuron to Brain*. 4th ed. Sunderland, Mass.: Sinauer Associates, 2000. An excellent and detailed neurobiology text that can help the reader understand the basis and consequences of conditions arising from head injuries.

Noback, Charles R., et al. *The Human Nervous System: Structure and Function*. 6th ed. Totowa, N.J.: Humana Press, 2005. A concise, easy-to-read paperback that offers a good balance of physiology and anatomy. Well illustrated.

Scanlon, Valerie, and Tina Sanders. *Essentials of Anatomy and Physiology*. 5th ed. Philadelphia: F. A. Davis, 2007. A text designed around three themes: the relationship between physiology and anatomy, the interrelations among the organ systems, and the relationship of each organ system to homeostasis.

HEADACHES
DISEASE/DISORDER

ANATOMY OR SYSTEM AFFECTED: Brain, head, nervous system, psychic-emotional system

SPECIALTIES AND RELATED FIELDS: Family medicine, internal medicine, neurology

DEFINITION: A general term referring to pain localized in the head and/or neck, which may signal mere tension or serious disorders.

KEY TERMS:

cluster headache: a severe type of headache, characterized by excruciating pain; attacks occur in groups, or clusters

migraine headache: a type of headache characterized by pain on one side of the head, often accompanied by disordered vision and gastrointestinal disturbances

prophylactic treatment: a treatment focusing on preventing disease, illness, or their symptoms from occurring

symptomatic treatment: a treatment focusing on aborting disease, illness, or their symptoms once they have occurred

tension-type headache: a type of headache characterized by bandlike or caplike pain over the head

CAUSES AND SYMPTOMS

In 1988, an ad hoc committee of the International Headache Society developed the current classification system for headaches. This system includes fourteen exhaustive categories of headache with the purpose of developing comparability in the management and study of headaches. Headaches most commonly seen by health care providers can be classified into four main types: migraine, tension-type, cluster, and "other" acute headaches.

Migraine headaches have been estimated to affect approximately 12 percent of the population. The headaches are more common in women, and they tend to run in families; they are usually first noticed in the teen years or young adulthood. For the diagnosis of migraine without aura ("aura" refers to visual disturbances or hallucinations, numbness and tingling on one side of the face, dizziness, or impairment of speech or hearing—symptoms that occur twenty to thirty minutes prior to the onset of the headache), the person must experience at least ten headache attacks, each lasting between four and seventy-two hours with at least two of the following characteristics: The headache is unilateral (occurs on one side), has a pulsating quality, is moderate to severe in intensity, or is aggravated by routine physical activity. Additionally, one of the following symptoms must accompany the headache: nausea and/or vomiting, or sensitivity to light or sounds. The person's medical history, a physical examination, and (where appropriate) diagnostic tests must exclude other organic causes of the headache, such as brain tumor or infection. Migraine with aura is far less common.

Migraines may be triggered or aggravated by physical activity, by menstruation, by relaxation after emotional stress, by ingestion of alcohol (red wine in particular) or certain foods or food additives (chocolate, hard cheeses, nuts, fatty foods, monosodium glutamate, or nitrates used in processed meats), by prescription medications (including birth control pills and hypertension medications), and by changes in the weather. Yet the precise pathophysiology of migraines is unknown. It had been posited that spasms in the blood vessels of the brain, followed by the dilation of these same blood vessels, cause the aura and head pain; however, studies using sophisticated brain and cerebral blood-flow scanning techniques indicate that this is likely not the case and that some type of inflammatory process may be involved related to the permeability of cerebral blood vessels and the resultant release of certain neurochemicals.

The tension-type headache is the most common type of headache; its prevalence is approximately 79 percent. Tension-type headaches are not hereditary, are found more frequently in females, and are first noticed in the teen years of young adulthood, although they can appear at any time of life. For the diagnosis of tension-type headaches, the person must experience at least ten headache attacks lasting from thirty minutes to seven days each, with at least two of the following characteristics: The headache has a pressing or tightening (nonpulsating) quality, is mild or moderate in intensity (may inhibit but does not prohibit activities), is bilateral or variable in location, and is not aggravated by physical activity. Additionally, nausea, vomiting, and light or sound sensitivity are absent or mild. Furthermore, the patient's medical history and physical or neurological examination exclude other organic causes for the headache apart from the following: oral or jaw dysfunction, muscular stress, or drug overuse. Tension-type headache sufferers describe these headaches as a bandlike or caplike tightness around the head, and/or muscle tension in the back of the head, neck, or shoulders. The pain is described as slow in onset with a dull or steady aching.

Tension-type headaches are believed to be precipitated primarily by emotional factors but can also be stimulated by muscular and spinal disorders, jaw dysfunction, paranasal sinus disease, and traumatic head injuries. The pathophysiology of tension-type headaches is controversial. Historically, tension-type headaches were attributed to sustained muscle contractions of the pericranial muscles. Studies indicate, however, that most patients do not manifest increased pericranial muscle activity and that pericranial muscle blood flow and/or central pain mechanisms might be involved in the pathophysiology of tension-type headaches. It is also believed that muscle contraction and scalp muscle ischemia play some role in tension-type headache pain.

Cluster headaches are the least frequent of the headache types and are thought to be the most severe and painful. Cluster headaches are more common in males, with estimates of 0.4 to 1.0 percent of males being affected. Traditionally, these headaches first appear at about thirty years of age, although they can start later in life. There is no genetic predisposition to these headaches. For the diagnosis of cluster headaches, the person must experience at least ten severely painful headache attacks, typically on one side of the face and lasting from fifteen minutes to three hours. One of the following symptoms must accompany the headache on the painful side of the face: a bloodshot eye, tearing, nasal congestion, nasal discharge, forehead and facial sweating, contraction of the pupils, or drooping eyelids. Physical and neurological examination and imaging must exclude organic causes for the headaches, such as tumor or infection. Cluster headaches often occur once or twice daily, or every other day, but can be as frequent as ten attacks in one day, recurring on the same side of the head during the cluster period. The temporal "clusters" of these headaches give them their descriptive name.

A cluster headache is described as a severe, excruciating, piercing, sharp, and burning pain through the eye. The pain is occasionally throbbing but always unilateral. Radiation of the pain to the teeth has been reported. Duration of a headache can range from ten minutes to three hours, with the next headache in the cluster occurring sometime the same day. Cluster headache sufferers are often unable to sit or lie still and are in such pain that they have been known, in desperation, to hit their heads with their fists or to smash their heads against walls or floors.

Cluster headaches can be triggered in susceptible patients by alcohol consumption, subcutaneous injections of histamine, and sublingual use of nitroglycerine. Because these agents all cause the dilation of blood vessels, these attacks are believed to be associated with dilation of the temporal and ophthalmic arteries and other extracranial vessels. There is no evidence that intracranial blood flow is involved. Cluster headaches have been shown to occur more frequently during the weeks before and after the longest and shortest days of the year, lending support for the hypothesis of a link to seasonal changes. Additionally, cluster headaches often occur at about the same time of day in a given sufferer, suggesting a relationship to the circadian rhythms of the body. Vascular changes, hormonal changes, neurochemical excesses or deficits, histamine levels, and autonomic nervous system changes are all being studied for their possible role in the pathophysiology of cluster headaches.

Acute headaches, using the International Headache Society's classification scheme, constitute many of the headaches not mentioned above. Distinct from the other headache types, which are often considered to be chronic in nature, acute headaches often signify underlying disease or a life-threatening medical condition. These headaches can display pain distribution and quality similar to those seen in chronic headaches. The temporal nature of acute headaches, however, often points to their seriousness. Acute headaches of concern are usually the first or worst headache the patient has had or are headaches with recent onset that are persistent or recurrent. Other signs that cause a high index of suspicion include an unremitting headache that steadily increases without relief, accompanying weakness or numbness in the hands or feet, an atypical change in the quality or intensity of the headache, headache upon exertion, recent head trauma, or a family history of cardiovascular problems. Such headaches can point to hemorrhage, meningitis, stroke, tumor, brain abscess, hematoma, and infection, which are all potentially life-threatening conditions. A thorough evaluation is necessary for all patients exhibiting the danger signs of acute headache.

Treatment and Therapy

Because there are several hundred causes of headaches, the evaluation of headache complaints is crucial. Medical science offers myriad evaluation techniques for headaches. The initial evaluation includes a complete history and physical examination to determine the factors involved in the headache complaint, such as the general physical condition of the patient, neurological functioning, cardiovascular condition, metabolic status, and psychiatric condition. Based on this initial evaluation, the health care professional may elect to perform a number of diagnostic tests to confirm or reject a diagnosis. These tests might include blood studies, X rays, computed tomography (CT) scans, psychological evaluation, electroencephalograms (EEGs), magnetic resonance imaging (MRI), or studies of spinal fluid.

Once a headache diagnosis is made, a treatment plan is developed. In the case of acute headaches, treatment may take varying forms, from surgery to the use of prescription medications. For migraine, tension-type, and cluster headaches, there are several common treatment options. Headache treatment can be categorized into two types: abortive (symptomatic) treatment or prophylactic (preventive) treatment. Treatment is tailored to the type of headache and the type of patient.

A headache is often a highly distressing occurrence for patients, sometimes causing a high level of anxiety, relief-seeking behavior, and a dependency on the health care system. The health care provider must consider not only biological elements of the illness but also possible resultant psychological and sociological elements as well. An open, communicative relationship with the patient is paramount, and treatment routinely begins with soliciting patient collaboration and providing patient education. Patient education takes the form of normalizing (or "decatastrophizing") the headache experience for patients, thereby reducing their fears concerning the etiology of the headache or about being unable to cope with the pain. Supportiveness, understanding, and collaboration are all necessary components of any headache treatment.

There are a number of abortive pharmacological treatments for migraine headaches. Ergotamine tartrate (an alkaloid or salt) is effective in terminating migraine symptoms by either reducing the dilation of extracranial arteries or in some way stimulating certain parts of the brain. Isomethaptine, another effective treatment for migraine, is a combination of chemicals that stimulates the sympathetic nervous system, provides analgesia, and is mildly tranquilizing. Another class of medications for migraines are nonsteroidal anti-inflammatory drugs (NSAIDs); these drugs, as the name implies, work on the principle that inflammation is involved in migraine. Both narcotic and nonnarcotic pain medications are often used for migraines, primarily for their analgesic properties; the concern in prescribing potent narcotic pain medications is the potential for their overuse. Antiemetic medications prevent or arrest vomiting and have been used in the treatment of migraines. Sumatriptan, a vasoactive agent that increases the amount of the neurochemical serotonin in the brain, shows promise in treating migraines that do not respond to other treatments.

Prophylactic treatments for migraines include beta-blockers, methysergide, and calcium channel blockers, which are believed to interfere with the dilation or contraction of extracranial arteries by acting on the sympathetic nervous system or on the central nervous system

itself. Antidepressants, medications used typically for the treatment of depression, have also been found to prevent migraine attacks; there appears to be an analgesic effect from certain antidepressants that is effective for chronic migraines. Antiseizure medications have been found to be useful for some migraine patients, although the mechanism of action is unknown. NSAIDs have also been used as a preventive measure for migraines.

There are several nonpharmacological treatment options for migraine headaches. These include stress management, relaxation training, biofeedback (a variant of relaxation training), psychotherapy (both individual and family), and the modification of headache-precipitating factors (such as avoiding certain dietary precipitants). Each of these treatments has been found to be effective for certain patients, particularly those with chronic migraine complaints. For some patients, they can be as effective as pharmacological treatments. The exact mechanism of action for their effect on migraines has not been established. Other self-management techniques include lying quietly in a dark room, applying pressure to the side of the head or face on which the pain is experienced, and applying cold compresses to the head.

The abortive treatment options for tension-type headaches include narcotic and nonnarcotic analgesics, because of their pain-reducing properties. More often with tension-type headaches, the milder over-the-counter pain medications (such as aspirin or acetaminophen) are used. NSAIDs, simple muscle relaxants, or antianxiety drugs can also be used. Muscle relaxants and antianxiety drugs are believed to relax smooth muscles, reducing scalp muscle ischemia and therefore head pain.

Prophylactic treatments for tension-type headaches include antidepressants, narcotic and nonnarcotic analgesics, muscle relaxants, and antianxiety drugs. Occasionally, "trigger-point injections" are used to relieve tension-type headaches. Trigger points are areas within muscles, primarily in the upper back and neck, that are hypersensitive; when stimulated, they can cause headaches. These trigger points can be injected with a local anesthetic or steroid to decrease their sensitivity or to eliminate possible inflammation in the area.

Nonpharmacological treatment of tension-type headaches is similar to that for migraines and includes stress management, relaxation training, biofeedback, and psychotherapy. Psychotherapy has been found to be a very important adjunct to any treatment of tension-type headaches because the illness, particularly when chronic, can lead to a pain syndrome characterized by family dysfunction, medication overuse, and vocational disruptions. Other self-management techniques include taking a hot shower or bath, placing a hot water bottle or ice pack on the head or back of the neck, exercising, and sleeping.

For cluster headaches, one of the most excruciating types of headache, the most common abortive treatment is administering pure oxygen to the patient for ten minutes. The exact mechanism of action is unknown, but it might be related to the constriction of dilated cerebral arteries. Ergotamine tartrate or similar alkaloids given orally, intramuscularly, or intravenously can also abort the attack in some patients. Nasal drops of a local anesthetic (lidocaine hydrochloride) or cocaine have been used to interrupt the activity of the trigeminal nerve that is believed to be involved in cluster attacks. The efficacy of these treatments is inconclusive.

Prophylactic treatment of this headache type is crucial. Ergotamine, methysergide, calcium channel blockers, antiseizure medications, and steroidal anti-inflammatory medications have been used with some success in the prevention of cluster attacks. The mechanism of action for these medications is unknown. Lithium carbonate, a drug commonly prescribed for bipolar disorders, has been found to be effective for some cluster patients. This medication is believed to affect certain regions of the brain, possibly the hypothalamus.

While no nonpharmacological treatment strategies are routinely offered to cluster headache patients, surgery is an option in severe cases, particularly if the headaches are resistant to all other available treatments. Percutaneous radio frequency thermocoagulation of the trigeminal ganglion is a surgical procedure that destroys the trigeminal nerve pathway, the chief nerve pathway to the face. Modest successes have been found with this extreme treatment option.

PERSPECTIVE AND PROSPECTS

Headaches are among the most common complaints to physicians and quite likely have been a problem since the beginning of humankind. Accounts of headaches can be found in the clinical notes of Arateus of Cappadocia, a first century physician. Descriptions of specific headache subtypes can be traced to the second century in the writings of the Greek physician Galen. Headaches are prevalent health problems that affect all ages and sexes and those from various cultural, social, and educational backgrounds.

The lifetime prevalence estimates of headaches is 93 percent for males and 99 percent for females. Studies in the United States estimate that 65 to 85 percent of the population will experience a headache within a year. Data from cross-cultural studies echo the significance of this public health problem: Frequent, severe headaches are reported by 10.4 percent of men and 35.3 percent of women in Thailand; 17.6 percent of men and 20.2 percent of women in urban Africa report a history of recurrent headaches; 57 percent of men and 73 percent of women in Finland report at least one headache in the previous year; and 39 percent of men and 60 percent of women in New Zealand also report an annual headache frequency.

As these data indicate, the prevalence of headaches is greater in women, although the reason is unknown. Age seems to be a mediating factor as well, with significantly fewer people sixty-five years of age or older reporting headache problems. There are no socioeconomic differences in prevalence rates, with persons in high-income and low-income brackets having similar rates. There are data to suggest that people with college educations or higher report headaches more often than those with only some high school education. The only vocational area that has been tied to increased rates of headaches are people who work at computer terminals.

The total economic costs of headaches are staggering. Headaches constitute approximately 1.7 percent of all visits to physician offices. Of visits to hospital emergency rooms, 2.5 percent are for headaches. The expenses associated with advances in assessment techniques and routine health care have risen rapidly. The cost in lost workdays adds to this economic picture. Thirty-six percent of headache sufferers in one study reported missing one or more days of work in the previous year because of headaches. The scientific study of headaches is necessary to understand this prevalent illness. Efforts, such as those by the International Headache Society, to develop accepted definitions of headaches will greatly assist efforts to identify and treat headaches.

—Oliver Oyama, Ph.D.

See also Anxiety; Brain; Brain disorders; Caffeine; Cluster headaches; Head and neck disorders; Migraine headaches; Multiple chemical sensitivity syndrome; Neuralgia, neuritis, and neuropathy; Neuroimaging; Neurology; Neurology, pediatric; Sinusitis; Stress; Stress reduction; Tumor removal; Tumors.

FOR FURTHER INFORMATION:

Blanchard, Edward B., and Frank Andrasik. *Management of Chronic Headaches: A Psychological Approach*. New York: Pergamon Press, 1985. The authors review the evaluation and treatment of headaches from a psychological perspective. Alternative, nonpharmacological treatments for headaches are described in detail.

Diamond, Seymour. "Migraine Headaches." *The Medical Clinics of North America* 75, no. 3 (May 1, 1991): 545-566. Diamond is one of the world's authorities on headaches. His article is well organized and comprehensively addresses the subject of migraines in a readable and interesting format. A practical guide to treating the headache patient.

Ivker, Robert S. *Headache Survival: The Holistic Medical Treatment Program for Migraine, Tension, and Cluster Headaches*. New York: Putnam, 2002. A guide that surveys nutritional and holistic remedies that aim to treat the cause, as well as the symptoms, of headaches.

Lang, Susan, and Lawrence Robbins. *Headache Help: A Complete Guide to Understanding Headaches and the Medications That Relieve Them*. Boston: Houghton Mifflin, 2000. Discusses a wide range of topics related to headaches including treatment options for migraines, cluster headaches, and tension headaches; the actions and side effects of over-the-counter and prescription medications; how hormones affect migraines; and alternative treatments, including herbs and acupuncture.

National Headache Foundation. http://www.headaches.org/. Operates local support groups and provides information for headache sufferers, their families, and physicians.

Paulino, Joel, and Ceabert J. Griffith. *The Headache Sourcebook*. Chicago: Contemporary Books, 2001. Reviews types of headaches, provides information on diagnosis and treatment, and offers advice on effectively communicating one's symptoms to doctors to expedite correct care.

Rapoport, Alan M., and Fred D. Sheftell. *Headache Relief*. New York: Simon & Schuster, 1991. The book takes the often-complicated theory, evaluation, and treatment of headaches and explains each area in very understandable terms for the layperson. The authors describe a "how-to" approach to treating headaches.

Saper, Joel R., et al. *Handbook of Headache Management: A Practical Guide to Diagnosis and Treatment of Head, Neck, and Facial Pain*. 2d ed. Philadelphia: Lippincott Williams & Wilkins, 1999. A manual for doctors with patients complaining of headache pain.

HEALING

BIOLOGY

ANATOMY OR SYSTEM AFFECTED: All

SPECIALTIES AND RELATED FIELDS: Alternative medicine, cytology, dermatology, family medicine, hematology, histology, immunology, plastic surgery, vascular medicine

DEFINITION: The process of mending damaged tissue by which an organism restores itself to health.

KEY TERMS:

collagen: a white fibrous protein produced by the body to fill in areas destroyed by injury; the healing component more commonly thought of as scar tissue

delayed primary closure: a procedure in which the wound is left open four to six days and then sewn closed; used for infected or contaminated wounds

healing by primary intention: the most desirable healing in the least amount of time, with minimal scar tissue formation; the edges of the wound close together

healing by secondary intention: less desirable healing of a wound, with replacement of damaged area by granulation tissue; delayed healing and excessive scar formation occur

regeneration: the renewal, regrowth, or restoration of destroyed or missing tissue; the production of new tissue

tensile strength: the greatest stress that can be placed on a tissue without tearing it apart; relative to the strength of a tissue

wounds: injuries classified as open or closed depending on whether the skin is broken; types of open wounds include abrasions, lacerations, avulsions, punctures, and incisions

THE HEALING PROCESS

The human body is not able to reproduce injured parts during the healing process. Most injured tissue in the body is replaced with collagen, a white protein known as scar tissue. Body areas capable of reproducing, or regenerating, include the outer layer of skin and the inner layers of the intestines.

The human body is involved in a continuous process of self-healing every day. The outer layer of the skin is constantly rubbed off, yet the body is able to replace (regenerate) new skin to take its place. Another body area capable of regeneration is the innermost layer of the intestine. All other types of tissue, however, such as muscle, fat, blood vessels, or even bones, must rely on other ways to heal when injured. How quickly the body heals depends on many factors, but the process is a predictable one. The healing process includes three phases: the acute inflammatory phase, the repair or regeneration phase, and the remodeling phase.

The first phase of healing, the immediate inflammatory phase, includes the first three or four days after the injury. This process, carried out by vascular, chemical, and cellular events, leads to the repair of tissue, to regeneration, or to scar tissue formation. If the hand is sliced open by a piece of broken glass, the first healing response would be a temporary decrease in blood flow, known as vasoconstriction, that lasts from a few seconds up to several minutes. This narrowing of the blood vessels occurs because of a decrease in the diameter of

the blood vessels at the injury site and prevents the person from bleeding to death. With extensive vessel damage, however, the body is unable to close off enough vessels, and life-threatening hemorrhaging may occur.

When only a small amount of tissue is cut, the blood begins to seal the broken vessels by coagulation, also known as blood clot formation. The next step is activation of the chemicals needed in the healing process, which is possible only after the blood vessel diameter increases in a process called vasodilation. During vasodilation, the blood flow is slowed and the blood becomes thicker, resulting in swelling. At this point, a buildup or accumulation of fluid results from the seeping of plasma, the fluid portion of the blood, through the vessel walls. This seeping or leakage results from the difference in pressure within the vessel and outside its walls. The amount of swelling at the injury site de-

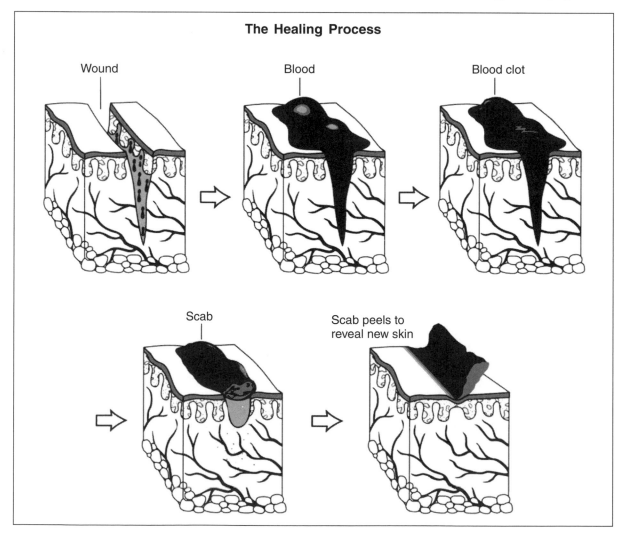

The Healing Process

Wound

Blood

Blood clot

Scab

Scab peels to reveal new skin

pends on the amount of seeping, which in turn depends on how much tissue damage has occurred.

Because the blood flow is slower, the concentration of red blood cells and white blood cells is increased. The white blood cells line up and adhere to the inside walls of small blood vessels, known as venules. These white blood cells then pass through the venule walls and are chemically attracted to the injury site over the next several hours. A specialized connective tissue cell, known as a mast cell, is also sent to the injury site. Mast cells contain heparin and histamine. Heparin prolongs the clotting time of blood by temporarily preventing coagulation, while histamine causes dilation of the capillaries. During this earliest phase, both heparin and histamine are important factors, since their actions allow other specialized cells to move into the injured area. The amount of bleeding and fluid buildup at the injury site depends on the extent of damage and how easily materials can cross the walls of intact vessels. Both of these conditions influence the healing process.

The second phase of healing can be called the repair or regeneration phase. For tissue capable of regeneration, this phase involves the restoration of destroyed or missing tissue. For other types of tissue, this second phase would entail the repair process. The healing of a deep cut in the hand would not be considered regeneration, since the body is not able to remake all the different layers of skin and muscle injured. This healing phase would extend forward from the previously described inflammatory phase. During this phase, the cut is naturally cleaned through the body's ability to remove cellular waste, the help of the red blood cells, and the formation of a blood clot.

Two types of healing can occur. Primary healing, or healing by primary intention, could take place in the hand laceration example, since the edges are even and close together. If this injury resulted in a large piece of tissue being removed, then the body would fill the gap with scar tissue. The replacement of tissue with scar tissue is an example of secondary healing, or healing by secondary intention. A torn muscle would be an example of secondary healing if it is allowed to heal on its own by the formation of scar tissue within the muscle.

No matter which type of healing occurs, several factors regulate how quickly and how completely this process takes place. Because blood vessels and cells are deprived of oxygen and die from the injury, this new cellular waste or debris must be cleaned from the area before repair or regeneration can take place. This tissue death promotes the formation of new capillary buds on the walls of the intact vessels. As these mature, the injury site is newly supplied with oxygenated blood and the healing process continues into the third phase.

The third phase of healing, known as the remodeling phase, includes the laying down of young scar tissue that increases in strength over the next year. Although the healing process has no distinct time frame, it is believed that three to six weeks are needed for the production of scar tissue. There must be a balance between the toughness and the elasticity of the scar. The amount of stress placed on a newly formed scar will determine the tensile strength of the collagen content. If stress or strain is placed on this forming scar tissue too early, the healing process will take longer. A desirable outcome would be a scar of adequate collagen content through the development of sufficient mature collagen fibers of proper tensile strength. Adequate tensile strength is also affected by how long inflammation is present.

If an injury site has inflammation that lasts up to one month, it is considered a subacute inflammation. When it lasts for months or years, it is then called chronic inflammation. Chronic inflammation is a condition where small traumas happen repeatedly; it is often seen in overuse injuries. Because this type of injury lasts longer, different types of chemicals try to initiate complete healing. The role of some of these special chemicals is not completely understood.

The healing of a broken bone, similar in many ways to the healing of the skin, is somewhat easier to understand. The first phase shows the same acute inflammation that lasts about four days, involving clotting blood, dead bone cells, and soft tissue damage around the injury site. The second phase, the repair and regeneration phase, differs slightly when a bone is broken, since the blood clot (hematoma) becomes granulated and builds between the two bone ends. The bone produces a specialized cell that turns into a soft or hard fibrous callus, matures into cartilage, and finally becomes bone with a firmly woven network of cells.

The beginning soft callus is a network of unorganized bone that forms at the two broken edges and is later absorbed and replaced by a hard callus. With appropriate care, a broken bone will develop a new network in the center and eventually become primary bone. The amount of oxygen available in the area determines this development. It is important to keep in mind that when the injury is severe enough to break a bone, then the blood supply is interrupted, lowering the amount of oxygen that is available. Low oxygen could result in the formation of only fibrous tissue or carti-

IN THE NEWS:
ROLE OF GROWTH HORMONE IN HEALING

Growth hormone (GH) has been shown to be a stimulating, but not an essential, factor in healing of the colon in dwarf rats. In the September, 2006, issue of the *Scandanavian Journal of Surgery*, researchers investigated the physiological role of growth hormone deficiency on the healing of colonic anastomoses and whether any reduced healing capacity in growth-hormone-deficient rats could be reversed by treatment with growth hormone.

Dwarf rats were treated with recombinant human growth hormone (rhGH) for seven days prior to surgery and for four days postoperatively. The surgery involved cutting out a one-centimeter-wide portion of rat intestine and reconnecting the cut ends in a procedure called end-to-end anastomosis. Researchers measured the strength of the anastomoses of the dwarf rats compared to control groups as an indication of the degree of healing. It was found that treatment with rhGH stimulated healing of the colonic anastomoses in dwarf rats, compared to dwarf rats not treated with rhGH and untreated normal rats that have normal pituitary function. Although healing also occurred in the dwarf rats not treated with rhGH and untreated normal rats, it was not as extensive as the healing that occurred in dwarf rats treated with rhGH.

An interesting finding is that there was no difference in healing between the untreated dwarf rats and the untreated normal rats. This indicates that, although growth hormone plays a role in healing in dwarf rats, growth hormone is not essential to the healing process and other factors may be involved in regulation of healing. Further studies will be needed to examine the possibility of using growth hormone in a clinical setting to stimulate postsurgery healing and to determine the appropriate patient population to treat.

Jason J. Schwartz, Ph.D., J.D.

is extremely important that oxygen levels are adequate for proper healing. If the blood supply is not sufficient, then the tissue may die, especially in broken bone fragments. Fortunately, most tissues of the body have a good blood supply, as demonstrated by the amount of bleeding that takes place when the skin and underlying tissues are injured.

The second condition that interferes with healing is excessive movement because the body part was not immobilized. In order for the scar tissue or even new bone to become well organized, the two edges of the injured tissue must be kept close together.

The third reason for poor healing is infection. Although the body has many defenses against infection, foreign material can slow healing. If this infectious material invades the space between the two bone ends of a fracture, the necessary building materials may not reach the site. Infection invading the hand tissue cut by the glass could prevent the edges from healing together because of pus, scab formation, or the interference of germs.

lage. Strong, healthy bone results when oxygen and the correct amount of compression are available. The third phase, the remodeling phase, describes the time when the callus has been reabsorbed and special intersecting bone fibers cover the broken area. It may take many years for this entire process to be completed, until the bone has regained its normal shape and ability to withstand stresses.

DISORDERS AND TREATMENT

Any of the three stages of healing can be delayed or prevented. The three main causes for failed healing are poor blood supply, poor immobilization, or infection.

The healing process within the body can be seriously hampered if the blood supply is poor, since the delivery of nutrients, chemicals, hormones, and specialized building materials to the injury site is hampered. It

There are many different types of injuries, and several steps must be taken in caring for each type. Soft tissues, the first line of defense against injuries, can be used to describe all tissues other than bone. Soft tissue injuries are classified as either closed or open. In a closed wound, the damage lies below the surface of the skin and the skin remains intact. A sprained ankle or a bruised knee are classified as closed wounds. In an open wound, the skin or mucous membranes, such as the lining of the mouth, are broken or torn.

There are four types of open soft tissue injuries; each has specific characteristics and heals differently. The first type is an abrasion, in which part of the outer layer of the skin and some underlying tissue is rubbed or scraped off. A common injury of this type is a scraped knee resulting from a fall on the sidewalk. The second type, the laceration, results from a sharp object cutting the skin, such as the previous example of a piece of glass cutting the skin either superficially or very deeply. The third type, an avulsion, results when a piece of skin or even an entire fingertip is torn off or left loosely hanging by a small flap of skin. It is important that this flap not be removed since a physician can sometimes reattach the part. The last type of soft tissue injury is the puncture wound, which results when a sharp object penetrates the skin and into a body part. Such an injury could be a stab from a knife or an ice pick, a splinter stuck in the foot, or even a bullet shot into the leg. The initial management is the same for all four types of injury.

Management of open wounds must include control of bleeding, infection prevention, and immobilization. Two of the above injuries, an avulsion and a puncture wound, require additional special care. In the case of an avulsed body part, the amputated part should be saved; wrapped in a dry, sterile piece of gauze; and placed in a plastic bag. If this bag is kept in something cool, such as a bucket of ice, the possibility of reattachment is increased. An impaled object remaining in a puncture wound should never be removed but held in place and all movement restricted until medical care can be given.

Several medical treatments can aid in promoting the healing process, as can commonsense first aid measures taken immediately after an injury occurs. For example, with a glass cut to the hand one should immediately stop the bleeding by placing a sterile piece of gauze, or a very clean cloth, directly over the laceration. By adding direct pressure over the gauze, the circulation is reduced. If the cut is deep, if the bleeding cannot be controlled, or if a piece of glass remains in the wound, then it is advisable to seek medical attention. A physician would then thoroughly clean the injury site and stitch the two edges together. Immobilizing the two flaps of skin together by sewing them will allow the first two phases of healing to progress. By having the wound inspected and cleaned by medical personnel, the risk of infection is reduced. A small injury can be cared for at home, but infection must be prevented through proper cleansing. Even soap and water, along with a bandage or dressing, will help to ward off infections.

PERSPECTIVE AND PROSPECTS

Many strategies to improve the healing of human tissue have evolved over time—from ancient times, when healers packed mud on the top of sores to draw out the infection, to modern alternative medicines. Every person, at one time or another, receives a cut, scrape, bump, or bruise. Therefore, there is much interest in speeding up the healing process.

Renewed interests in nontraditional approaches to medicine explore the healing powers locked within the human body. The use of homeopathy, acupuncture, and acupressure are examples of alternatives to antibiotics and standard first aid measures to help an injury heal. Holistic health care, hypnosis, and osteopathic medicine offer other areas of exploration. The practice of Chinese medicine includes the use of herbs, crystals, massage, and meditation to allow healing to proceed quickly but through natural means. Even the use of aromatherapy—treatment through the inhalation of specific smells—has gained a foothold in the medical world. The manipulations done by chiropractic doctors offer other possibilities. Some seek cures in nature, from sources below the sea or deep in the forest. Yet, many untapped resources remain. The continuing research in genetics offers vast possibilities, and the link between mental attitude and the immune system presents a rich area for further exploration. Even innovations as simple as a special glue, used to replace sutures or staples for closing wounds, would have an important influence on the future of the healing process.

—*Maxine M. Urton, Ph.D.*

See also Antibiotics; Aromatherapy; Bleeding; Blood and blood disorders; Chiropractic; Circulation; Dermatology; Grafts and grafting; Histology; Host-defense mechanisms; Hyperbaric oxygen therapy; Immune system; Immunology; Infection; Inflammation; Laceration repair; Meditation; Skin; Surgery, general; Vascular system; Wounds.

FOR FURTHER INFORMATION:

American Academy of Orthopaedic Surgeons. *Emergency Care and Transportation of the Sick and Injured.* Edited by Benjamin Gulli, Les Chatelain, and Chris Stratford. 9th ed. Sudbury, Mass.: Jones and Bartlett, 2005. Covers soft tissue injuries. Offers graphic photographs of actual injuries and discusses care and management. This text is often used in the training of emergency medical technicians, yet chapters are easily understood by the nonmedical layperson.

American Medical Association. *Handbook of First Aid and Emergency Care.* Rev. ed. New York: Random House, 2000. Provides a listing of injuries, illnesses, and medical emergencies accompanied by easy-to-follow instructions and illustrations.

DiPietro, Luisa A., and Aime L. Burns, eds. *Wound Healing: Methods and Protocols*. Totowa, N.J.: Humana Press, 2003. A clinical text that describes classic and contemporary laboratory methods for studying tissue repair and examines systemic and genetic conditions that influence the healing process.

Eisenberg, David. *Encounters with Qi*. New York: W. W. Norton, 1995. Extensive explanations of the Chinese principles in medicine are covered, from ancient practices through current uses. Examines the uses of herbs, acupuncture, and psychic healing to restore the body's inner balance.

Gach, Michael R. *Acupressure's Potent Points: A Guide to Self-Care for Common Ailments*. New York: Bantam Books, 1990. An extensively illustrated book showing the self-use of acupressure to relieve physical problems by activating the body's natural self-healing processes.

Goldberg, Linn, and Diane L. Elliot. *The Healing Power of Exercise: Your Guide to Preventing and Treating Diabetes, Depression, Heart Disease, High Blood Pressure, Arthritis, and More*. New York: Wiley, 2002. This book explains how exercise can reduce your risk of certain diseases as well as alleviate symptoms.

Handal, Kathleen A. *The American Red Cross First Aid and Safety Handbook*. Boston: Little, Brown, 1992. A comprehensive, fully illustrated guide outlining basic first aid and emergency care steps to be taken until medical assistance can be obtained. Updated materials can also be obtained directly from local Red Cross Association chapters listed in telephone books.

Kemper, Kathi J. *The Holistic Pediatrician: A Pediatrician's Comprehensive Guide to Safe and Effective Therapies for the Twenty-five Most Common Ailments of Infants, Children, and Adolescents*. New York: HarperCollins, 2002. Integrates mainstream and alternative medicine to aid parents in dealing with the most common childhood health problems and injuries.

Woodham, Anne, and David Peters. *The Encyclopedia of Healing Therapies*. New York: DK, 1997. This book explains holistic and complementary medicine and offers a guide to well-being. Also contains information on finding practitioners, a directory of associations, a glossary, and a bibliography.

HEALTH MAINTENANCE ORGANIZATIONS (HMOs)

ORGANIZATIONS

ALSO KNOWN AS: Competitive medical plans

DEFINITION: A business competitor within a free market economy that provides health care insurance and services to group and individual clients for an established, prepaid monthly premium and that generally attempts to provide care at a lower cost than traditional fee-for-service insurance programs by transferring financial risk to physicians through capitation and other incentives.

KEY TERMS:

disability insurance: a health coverage policy that protects against loss of income resulting from sickness or accident, whereby benefits are structured to pay approximately 40 to 60 percent of earnings up to a maximum total amount

group model HMO: an HMO organized by physicians whereby a private professional corporation is established which then individually contracts with an HMO to provide services exclusively for its subscribers

independent practice association model HMO: a flexible arrangement whereby several office physicians in a community form a networked professional corporation that seeks group contracts among local employers and provides all medical care for a capitated rate per client per month to subscribers, who often choose a personal primary care physician

managed care: the techniques by which an HMO, a health insurance carrier, or a self-insuring employer makes certain that the health care services it is endorsing are cost-effective and of a high quality

point-of-service model HMO: also called an open-ended HMO; a model that includes an option which allows subscribers to seek medical care outside the established network and receive partial reimbursement, with all remaining expenses paid out-of-pocket

preferred providers: physicians and other health care providers and hospitals who choose to provide health care at a reduced cost for subscribers to an HMO

staff model HMO: an HMO that is directly controlled at its headquarters, with all physicians and other health care workers being full-time, salaried employees

ROLE IN THE HEALTH CARE INDUSTRY

A health maintenance organization (HMO) in a free market economy functions in a dual role as both a health insurance company and a provider of health services, roles that were previously separated within the U.S. health care system. HMOs—also known as competitive medical plans, managed care plans, or alternative delivery systems—are generally organized by an employer, physician group, union, consumer group, insurance company, or for-profit health care agency. They were originally formed from one, or a mixture, of the following models: point of service, staff, group, and independent practice association.

The role of an HMO as an insurer is to seek group contracts with employers and individual clients and to negotiate premiums to be prepaid in exchange for covering preagreed benefits. Its role in service delivery is to affiliate with or hire directly physicians to provide the expected volume of care that is required for all subscribers under contract. An HMO owns or contracts with one or more health centers for ambulatory care and with hospitals for inpatient care. Within its private health center or in contracts with freestanding providers, an HMO will furnish services from other health care providers such as physical and occupational therapy, pharmacy, and mental health care, which are rapidly increasing in their level of responsibility.

HMOs are attractive to employers because the annual medical bill for the average subscriber-patient consistently has proved to be approximately 30 percent less than that of conventional insurers. One advantage of HMO membership is that all medical expenses, from routine and emergency care to hospitalization, are covered within a single, fixed monthly premium. In addition, presenting an HMO membership card at time of services with a small copayment means no forms to fill out, no deductibles to pay, and no bills to submit. Disadvantages include that new subscribers often cannot keep a trusted physician they have had for years, providers become extremely busy when they are assigned hundreds of patients in exchange for a fixed fee, and subscribers often must accept fewer choices in treatment options.

PRACTICES AND PROCEDURES

The term "managed care" describes the techniques by which an HMO, a health insurance carrier, or a self-insuring employer makes certain that the health care services that it endorses are high in quality and cost-effective. This system was once used in many countries. Workers joined a mutual aid association and paid premiums, and the association was responsible for hiring enough quality full-time or part-time physicians to

provide the required services. These restrictive arrangements could not survive within a country that has a national health insurance law because every covered citizen would then have the right to choose any provider and subsequently bill the system. Managed care is able to survive in the United States only because a compulsory national health insurance law has not been enacted, as has been done in other industrialized countries.

The headquarters of an HMO competitively markets its services to employer groups and individuals and administers the revenue and payments. An HMO generally contracts or directly hires a limited number of physicians in addition to building, staffing, and equipping the necessary number of health centers and hospitals. Its marketing claim is to provide good quality care within the employer's group premium, without seeking further supplements from the employer. Because an HMO and its providers are at personal financial risk, the organization directly imposes financial discipline upon its physicians, hospitals, and other health care providers. The HMO retains a percentage of the premiums paid from employers for its administrative and facility costs and pays a monthly "capitated rate" per client to the providers. HMOs have historically had persistent difficulty in recruiting and retaining physicians, and patients have consistently informed the HMOs that they prefer private offices to health centers.

Managed care procedures generally involve the HMO establishing a network of physicians with superior reputations in each region, with these physicians agreeing to bill the carriers according to limited reimbursement rules. Each client is assigned to a "primary care gatekeeper" who is expected to provide most care in his or her private office for limited fees. When a referral to a specialist, laboratory, or hospital is necessary, authorization is required from the headquarters of the managed care organization. Hospitals contract with these organizations to limit their charges and follow established rules about economical care and prompt discharge. The managed care organization reviews utilization by physicians and hospitals, attempts to correct wasteful practices, and subsequently drops health care providers with expensive and/or poor practice styles.

In contrast to more traditional HMOs, point-of-service plans have more recently emerged. These plans enable clients to have freedom of choice with respect to providers and some treatment options but requires them personally to pay the balance for their chosen higher-priced services. If the patient goes to physicians, hospitals, and other providers within the network and follows rules about utilization and authorization, the out-of-pocket financial costs are minimal. The patient retains the option to go to an out-of-plan provider, pay the bill in full, and then be reimbursed for the limited amount established in the individual plan. The employer's group contract with the managed care organization provides for limited and predictable premiums. The considerable costs of out-of-plan services thus are shifted from the group contract to the individual patient.

Managed care plans will continue to monitor closely the treatment patterns of physicians and encourage them to prescribe cheaper medications, to develop standards that physicians are expected to follow in treatment of various diseases, and to hold utilization review panels that review patient records and decide which treatments a patient's health plan will cover and which it will not. Because of the numerous consumer complaints that arose from actions resulting from the decisions of case managers, who often do not have any medical training, nineteen states had passed comprehensive managed care laws by 1997. In the year 1997 alone, states passed a record 182 laws related to managed care, up from 100 in 1996. Legislation during the late 1990's and into the twenty-first century focused on issues such as adopting measures to ban physician gag clauses, establishing consumer grievance procedures, requiring disclosure of financial incentives for physicians to withhold care, holding external reviews of internal decisions to deny care, and ensuring the ability to sue an HMO for malpractice. In 2001, many of these issues were addressed via a legislative "Bill of Rights" for patients. The bill led to a contentious debate over whether and how to regulate managed care plans. The bill was passed, but critics claim its provisions do not apply to all of the more than 160 million people enrolled in health insurance plans and fail to give unhappy patients the right to sue their health plans for punitive damages. Several states have also attempted—with some, like Washington State, succeeding—to implement their own managed care reforms.

PERSPECTIVE AND PROSPECTS

The first HMOs in the United States were established in the 1930's with the pioneering efforts of the Ross-Loos Medical Group in California, but most experienced only minimal growth until the 1970's. Beginning in the early 1970's, HMOs proliferated rapidly, primarily as a result of escalating costs for health care services and in-

creasing competition among a growing number of physicians. The Health Maintenance Organizations Act of 1973 provided federal grants and loans for the establishment of HMOs and required many employers to offer HMO membership to employees as a health insurance alternative. The federal government began to promote the HMO concept as a means by which to control costs by discouraging physicians from performing unnecessary and costly procedures, to meet the increased demand for health insurance particularly in underserved areas, and to foster preventive medicine. Monetary incentives, which are strongly supported by numerous politicians, are in theory the major forces behind personal freedom of choice, containment of costs, and assurance of quality. Innovated by the Kaiser Foundation Health Plan in California, the Health Insurance Plan of Greater New York, and the Group Health Cooperative of Puget Sound, greater numbers of preferred provider organizations began to appear in the 1980's and 1990's as a more flexible alternative to standard HMOs. Many major health insurers such as Blue Cross and Blue Shield then began exerting control over the daily operations of both HMOs and preferred provider organizations. Managed care was spread rapidly across the United States by the large health insurance companies, largely stimulated by the ongoing difficulties experienced by national policy in containing medical costs. In 1970, there were approximately thirty different managed care plans; by 1997, this number had grown to more than fifteen hundred. In 1997, more than 80 percent of HMOs were for-profit organizations. The significance of this figure is that an increasing amount of money that could be spent on medical care is now being spent on marketing costs and stockholder dividends.

The largest looming question regarding the future of HMOs is whether physicians and other health care workers, as well as client subscribers, will continue to enroll in and thus support the system. Managed care necessarily adds substantial administrative overhead, with the ongoing question of whether the final result is greater efficiency for the entire system or simply for subscribing employers. Another controversial topic of discussion involves the responsibility of an HMO to provide disability insurance, which becomes necessary when a client incurs loss of income resulting from sickness or an accident that is not covered by workers' compensation. An organization that will exert considerable influence in future HMO developments is the American Association of Retired Persons (AARP), a large, nonprofit advocacy group for Americans over the age of fifty with more than 30 million members. It has begun giving endorsements to HMOs that meet its standards of quality and price.

In other industrialized nations, both the services covered and the extent of coverage equal or exceed the coverage of a standard HMO within the United States. Several countries have universal health care insurance coverage, although in many industrialized nations certain categories of residents may be exempt. Notable examples include Germany, which requires the purchase of private health insurance by law; Canada and Sweden, which have public insurance coverage for essentially any citizen; and Great Britain, which has a majority of medical services located within the public sector.

—*Daniel G. Graetzer, Ph.D.*

See also Allied health; Ethics; Law and medicine; Malpractice.

FOR FURTHER INFORMATION:

Birenbaum, Aaron. *Wounded Profession: American Medicine Enters the Age of Managed Care.* Westport, Conn.: Greenwood Press, 2002. Traces the evolution of health care in the United States during the 1990's and examines the rising costs, consumer backlash, and new legislation.

Brink, Susan, and Nancy Shute. "Are HMOs the Right Prescription?" *U.S. News and World Report* 123, no. 4 (October 13, 1997): 60-65. Covered in this well-researched article is the growing dissatisfaction of subscribers with the quality of health care received, with a rating of the best HMOs in the United States.

Dranove, David. *The Economic Evolution of American Health Care: From Marcus Welby to Managed Care.* Princeton, N.J.: Princeton University Press, 2002. Traces the economic, technological, and historical forces that have transformed the health care field.

Freeborn, Donald K., and Clyde R. Pope. *Promise and Performance in Managed Care: The Prepaid Group Practice Model.* Rev. ed. Baltimore: Johns Hopkins University Press, 2000. This excellent text highlights the evolution of several common promises of HMOs that employ the prepaid practice model and evaluates their performance based on relevant criteria.

Johnsson, Julie. "HMOs Dominate, Shape the Market." *American Medical News* 39, no. 4 (1996): 1-3. A well-written article that outlines the competition among HMOs and how they attempt to obtain lower prices from providers as premiums continue to drop.

Kongstvedt, Peter R. *Managed Care: What It Is and How It Works.* 2d ed. Gaithersburg, Md.: Aspen, 2002. Provides a historical overview of managed care and covers organizational structures, concepts, and practices of the managed care industry.

Lairson, D. R., et al. "Managed Care and Community-Oriented Care: Conflict or Complement?" *Journal of Health Care for the Poor and Underserved* 8, no. 1 (1997): 36-55. This informative article evaluates models for community health planning and health care reform designed for the medically indigent, including programs that receive support from the U.S. government and programs that do not.

Ludmerer, Kenneth M. *Time to Heal: American Medical Education from the Turn of the Century to the Managed Care Era.* New York: Oxford University Press, 2001. Ludmerer looks at the future of medicine in America and reveals some very disturbing trends in managed care, education, and research funding. Contains a wealth of factual details and insightful questions.

Zelman, W. A. *The Changing Health Care Marketplace.* San Francisco: Jossey-Bass, 1996. An excellent evaluation of past trends in HMOs and predictions of what the future might hold.

HEARING AIDS

TREATMENT

ANATOMY OR SYSTEM AFFECTED: Ears

SPECIALTIES AND RELATED FIELDS: Audiology, otorhinolaryngology

DEFINITION: Electromechanical devices meant to improve ease of communication and minimize listening fatigue. Patients with profound sensorineural hearing loss receive little or no benefit from conventional hearing aids but may use a cochlear implant, an electronic prosthetic device surgically placed in the inner ear to deliver electrical signals to the brain, where they are interpreted as sounds.

KEY TERMS:

assistive listening devices: earphones or a headset with amplification to supplement or substitute for traditional hearing aids

audiogram: a graph used to display one's hearing ability for average speech sounds, in which decibels have been converted from sound pressure levels to hearing levels

audiologist: a diagnostician who administers hearing tests and dispenses hearing aids *cochlea:* an inner ear cavity shaped like a snail surrounded by fluid; when set in motion, this fluid displaces rows of thousands of microscopic hair cells, each of which functions to receive electrical activity and transfer it to the central auditory system

presbycusis: a hearing loss of unknown cause, often attributed to aging

INDICATIONS AND PROCEDURES

Hearing loss is one of the most common conditions affecting older adults, but it is not limited to that age group. In the early twenty-first century, it was estimated that about one in ten individuals in the United States had a significant hearing loss and that 120 million people worldwide had hearing loss significant enough to interfere with communication. In the United States, approximately one million people each year purchase hearing aids. These devices were developed to help those people affected by hearing loss ranging from mild to severe and resulting from a number of causes. The most common type of hearing loss, sensorineural, is linked to a variety of physical and psychosocial dysfunctions (isolation, depression, hypertension, and stress), as well as illnesses such as ischemic heart disease and arrhythmias.

Over the years, hearing aids have evolved in several ways. Two major trends have been in signal processing and size. In the 1960's, the best available hearing aids were limited to help in quiet only; in loud situations, they made things worse. Therefore, it was common practice to remove them around noise. They produced sound like cheap transistor radios. Starting in the 1980's and 1990's, advanced circuitry has offered consumers improved quality of hearing in quiet as well as some increased ability to hear in noise; sound distortion is now minimal. Certain hearing aids can be electronically adjusted for individual users; for example, they can be reprogrammed to accommodate increased hearing loss. Certain hearing aids have volume controls; others adjust automatically. Research has shown that consumers report greater satisfaction with sound quality than they did in the past, and people with hearing loss in both ears tend to be more satisfied with two hearing aids, enabling them to determine the direction of sounds.

Prior to the 1940's, hearing aids were large and re-

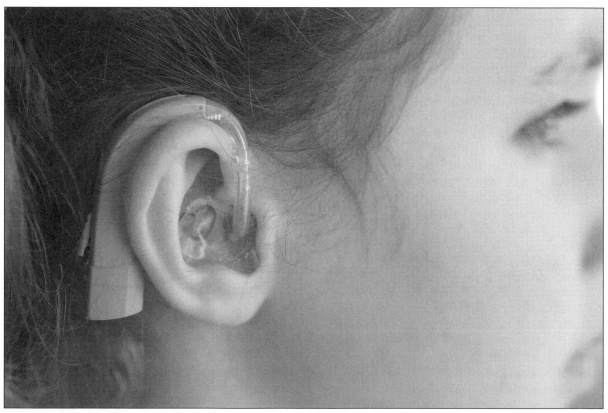

A girl with a hearing aid that extends behind the ear. (©Oktay Ortakcioglu/iStockphoto.com)

quired carrying a battery pack strapped to one's body. In the 1940's, vacuum tubes reduced the size of hearing aids to that of a transistor radio. Hearing aids in the ear or on the head were not available until the 1960's. Because of the size reduction of hearing aids, they have become more comfortable and less noticeable.

For patients with bilateral profound sensorineural hearing loss, which does not respond to traditional hearing aids, a cochlear implant is now possible. A cochlear implant is an electronic prosthesis surgically implanted in the inner ear. It has external parts that are worn outside the ear, including a microphone, speech processor, headpiece antenna, and cable. It is not a hearing aid. A cochlear implant delivers electrical signals to the brain, where they are interpreted as sounds. Potential candidates for these implants include both children and adults in a wide age range. Generally, children should be at least eighteen months old, and many successful implant recipients are in their eighties. Adults who become deaf later in life, and who have fully developed speech and language before their hearing loss, have better results with the implant than do those who were born deaf or who lost their hearing early in life. It has been shown, however, that the child who is born deaf who is given a cochlear implant early in life can receive great benefit from it. In adults, the memory of sound appears to be one of the most important factors for success. For children, early implantation and placement in an educational program that emphasizes the development of auditory skills appear to be important factors for success.

USES AND COMPLICATIONS

One of the biggest impediments to hearing aid use is patient reactions to hearing loss. Many people try to cover up the fact that they have hearing difficulties, and when hearing loss is confirmed, they experience a wide range of emotions, from horror, denial, disbelief, and withdrawal to embarrassment, sadness, resentment, and gradual acceptance and coping. People's coping skills and behavior patterns vary, in part because hearing loss generally occurs gradually and may take a long time to be recognized.

For those who embrace hearing aids, a variety of technological and cosmetic choices are available. A number of options exist regarding hearing aid style: behind-the-ear, custom in-the-ear, in-the-canal, and the smallest, the completely in-canal hearing aid. In addition to aesthetic considerations and sound fidelity, one's anatomy and manual dexterity may dictate the

style that is most effective and efficient. The degree of hearing loss and other medical conditions are also important factors when evaluating the best hearing aid.

PERSPECTIVE AND PROSPECTS

Hearing aid technology has improved such that patients with mild to moderate hearing loss will be candidates for hearing aids and those with severe loss will be candidates for hearing aids or cochlear implants, depending upon how well they function with a particular device. Patients with profound hearing loss will benefit best from cochlear implants.

Initially, only those patients who were completely deaf in both ears were considered candidates for cochlear implants. With significant improvements in implant technology, however, the benefits gained by implanted patients, both children and adults, have markedly improved. This, in turn, has led to a broadening of criteria for implant patients. Select patients with severe hearing loss who receive some benefit from hearing aids are considered possible implant candidates.

—Marcia J. Weiss, M.A., J.D.

See also Aging; Audiology; Deafness; Ear infections and disorders; Ear surgery; Ears; Hearing loss; Hearing tests; Otorhinolaryngology; Sense organs.

FOR FURTHER INFORMATION:

Biderman, Beverly. *Wired for Sound: A Journey into Hearing.* Toronto: Trifolium Books, 1998.

Carmen, Richard, ed. *The Consumer Handbook on Hearing Loss and Hearing Aids: A Bridge to Healing.* 2d rev. ed. Sedona, Ariz.: Auricle Ink, 2004.

Dillon, Harvey. *Hearing Aids.* New York: Thieme, 2001.

Romoff, Arlene. *Hear Again: Back to Life with a Cochlear Implant.* New York: League for the Hard of Hearing, 1999.

HEARING LOSS
DISEASE/DISORDER

ANATOMY OR SYSTEM AFFECTED: Brain, ears

SPECIALTIES AND RELATED FIELDS: Audiology, speech pathology

DEFINITION: Loss of sensitivity to sound as a result of disease, infection, injury, noise, or aging.

KEY TERMS:

conductive hearing loss: hearing loss resulting from interference with sound vibration; occurs in the external and middle ear *sensorineural hearing loss:* hearing loss resulting from disease or aging; occurs in the inner ear

hearing aid: a hearing device that amplifies sounds

CAUSES AND SYMPTOMS

The causes of hearing loss vary, although three major factors enhance the progression of loss as one ages: exposure to noise, previous middle-ear disease, and vascular disease. There are basically two types of hearing loss, conductive hearing loss and sensorineural hearing loss. Conductive hearing loss results from interference with sound vibration through the external and middle ear. In other words, the sound cannot get to the inner ear. In some types of conductive hearing loss, if the sound amplitude is increased enough, then the person may be able to hear. Possible reasons for conductive hearing loss include impacted or large amounts of cerumen (wax) in the ear, foreign bodies (such as soap, food, or insects) in the ear canal, otitis media (middle-ear infection), rheumatoid arthritis, and otosclerosis, in which the stapes becomes fixed to the oval window of the cochlea.

Earwax buildup is a common and treatable cause of conductive hearing loss. There have been reports that as much as 25 percent of nursing home residents have impacted cerumen. Older adults can be taught how to remove the wax on their own. Cerumenex (by prescription only) and Debrox (sold without a prescription) can be used as directed, followed by lavage to remove the wax and residual medication. Some health care providers recommend the instillation of mineral oil into the ear canal twenty-four hours before removal to help soften the wax, followed by lavage with one part hydrogen peroxide to three parts water at room temperature.

Sensorineural hearing loss means the presence of disease anywhere from the organ of Corti to the brain. The result is loss of hearing high-tones, for it is the hair cells in the basal curvature of the organ of Corti that are sensitive to high tones. Presbycusis is sensorineural hearing loss caused by aging of the inner ear. The onset of presbycusis may begin anytime from the third to the sixth decade of life, depending on type. Presbycusis affects 60 percent of individuals over age sixty-five in the United States. Older adults suffering from these disturbances show distinct and differing audiograms, which are used clinically to diagnose types of impairment. The standard type of presbycusis with hearing loss at high Hertz is often associated with sensory and neural presbycusis. There are four types of presbycusis: sensory, neural, metabolic, and cochlear conductive.

INFORMATION ON HEARING LOSS

CAUSES: Buildup of earwax, perforated eardrum, disease, congenital malformation, swelling of external ear canal, otitis media, traumatic injury, long-term exposure to loud and continuous noise, tumors

SYMPTOMS: Difficulty understanding speech, difficulty hearing in presence of background noise, social isolation

DURATION: Ranges from short-term to chronic

TREATMENTS: Rehabilitation programs, use of hearing aids, surgery

---

The elderly first start to lose hearing in the high frequency range. High frequency consonants and sibilants become more difficult to recognize—for example, *f*, *g*, *l*, *t*, *s*, *ch*, *sh*, and *th*. In presbycusis, high frequency sounds become unintelligible. Understanding spoken words depends largely on the clear perception of high frequency consonants rather than low frequency vowel sounds. This is why words starting with the above letters or combinations become unintelligible. Many times, older adults have both conductive and sensorineural frequency losses. The precise cause of the defect requires help from a specialist and the use of sophisticated audiometric testing.

The sound waves that travel through the ear have two main characteristics, frequency and amplitude. Frequency is related to the pitch of a sound and is measured by the number of vibrations or cycles per second. The higher the vibration frequency, the higher the perceived pitch of the sound. Hertz (Hz) is the unit of measurement to denote cycles per second. Amplitude is related to the loudness of a sound. The greater the intensity with which a sound strikes the eardrum, the louder the tone. The unit of measurement of intensity of sound is decibels (dB).

Among the offenders to hearing are radio headphones, lawn mowers, diesel trucks, and loud music. A single very loud noise can damage the middle ear. An eardrum can be broken by sounds reaching 160 decibels to 1,000 Hertz. Also, continuous noise of more than 80 to 85 decibels can cause harm to hearing. Normal conversation is measured at 60 decibels. A noisy restaurant, a vacuum cleaner, an electric shaver, and a screaming child can reach decibels between 80 and 85 decibels. Louder everyday noises include a blow-dryer (100 decibels), a subway train (100 decibels), and a car horn (110 decibels). Anyone exposed to noise in the 80 decibel range should wear hearing protection.

Another common hearing problem is tinnitus (ringing in the ears). Medications such as aspirin, aminoglycoside antibiotics, and diuretics can cause toxic effects to the hair cells of the organ of Corgi, thereby resulting in sensorineural hearing loss. Tinnitus, an internal noise generated within the hearing system, occurs in many types of hearing disorders at all ages, but it is reported more frequently in the elderly. Tinnitus affects seven million people, of which 10 to 37 percent are elderly, and that number is growing. The ringing sound is generally increased pitched with sensorineural loss and low pitched with conductive hearing loss. However, tinnitus may be present with or without hearing loss. Some types of tinnitus do not usually awaken people out of sleep, nor does it interfere with leisure activities. Older adults can attempt to alleviate the condition through biofeedback or by disguising the sound. Soft radio music and other distracting sounds may offer some comfort.

TREATMENT AND THERAPY

There are many treatments for hearing loss, and depending on the type of loss, some treatments work better than others. For example, with conductive hearing loss, if the cause is excessive earwax buildup, then the results can be remarkable when the wax is removed. For both types of hearing loss, conductive and sensorineural, simple measures can be used to facilitate better communication.

One technique that can help in communicating with someone with hearing loss is facing the person when speaking, so that he or she can see one's face and lips. Using simple, short sentences or phrases and speaking slowly in a low voice can be helpful. Loudness is not helpful and can be irritating, whereas a low voice enables people to hear lower frequencies, which usually can be heard more easily.

Although hearing aids may help certain types of hearing loss, many people do not like to use them. Vanity plays a role in keeping people away from hearing devices. People may not use hearing aids because they may think of themselves as getting old, and hearing loss may be seen as a normal and inevitable event as one grows older. The cost of purchasing a hearing aid is a concern for many. On average, one in-the-ear hearing aid can cost $2,500 to $3,000, and most people need two hearing aids. Medicare does not provide reimbursement. The hearing aid itself can create problem for the user. A person wearing such a device for the first

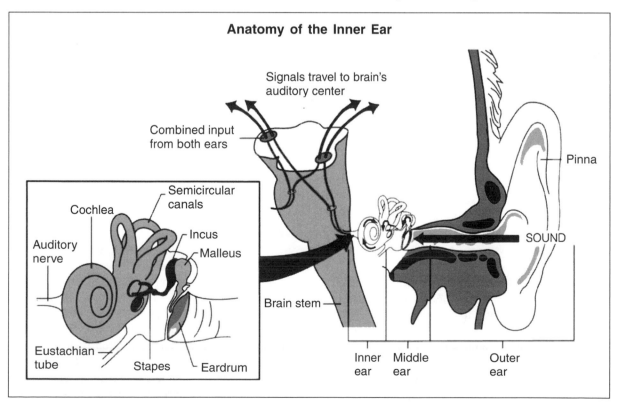

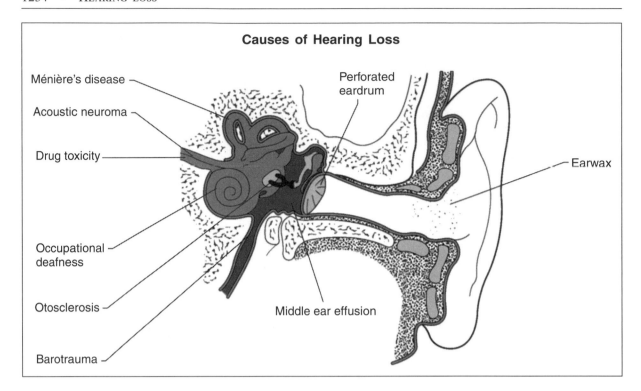

Causes of Hearing Loss

Ménière's disease

Acoustic neuroma

Drug toxicity

Occupational deafness

Otosclerosis

Barotrauma

Perforated eardrum

Earwax

Middle ear effusion

time needs to go through an adjustment period, and some older adults do not give themselves enough time to get used to the hearing aid. Some hearing aids have been known to cause irritation to the external ear. Also, the increased humidity within the external auditory canal may cause infectious otitis externa.

There are basically three kinds of hearing aids: the body type, the behind-the-ear-type, and in-the-ear type. The body type resembles a handheld amplifier with a wire that attaches to an earpiece. The behind-the-ear type is worn behind and in the ear. A person with poor eyesight and rheumatoid arthritis would probably benefit from the body type or behind the-ear type. These types are easier to see and handle because of their larger size. The in-the-ear devices are small and cosmetically more acceptable, but they are more difficult to manipulate. The selection often depends on the wearer's personal preference, vision capabilities, and manual dexterity.

It takes time to adjust to using a hearing aid. Sounds and voices are made louder, not clearer. The wearer must become accustomed to the background noise. Often, the user must be encouraged to continue using the hearing aid during this adjustment period. The greatest satisfaction is achieved with hearing aids if hearing loss is between 55 and 80 decibels. There is only partial benefit if the loss is greater than 80 decibels.

Perspective and Prospects

Hearing is regarded by some to be the most important of the five senses. It is imperative for people to protect their hearing for as long as they can. In today's world, where excessive noises are bombarding eardrums everyday, people need to protect themselves.

Hearing loss occurs when hair cells in the ear are damaged or destroyed by excessively loud noise or moderately loud noise for prolonged periods of time. Hearing loss usually occurs gradually and without pain. Over time, sounds become muffled and higher frequency sounds become hard to distinguish. Normal conversation occurs around 60 decibels. Anything higher than 60 decibels for extended periods of time may lead to hearing loss. According to the Ear Institute in Los Angeles, about 30 percent of hearing loss is due to exposure to loud sounds.

There are ways to reduce excessive noise levels in the environment. First, the time exposed to loud noises should be limited. This can be accomplished by removing the sound or decreasing the volume. The popular audio products now on the market can pose a risk to hearing. Most people are not aware of the potential dangers of listening to music at high volumes. A person listening to music by wearing earphones should not be heard by the person standing next to them. Similarly, a loud device such as a vacuum cleaner should be operated for no more than ten minutes at a time, with a five-minute break between uses.

It is interesting to note that hearing loss results from both loudness and time exposure. For example, a one-time gunshot noise near the ear can be just as damaging as extended exposure to loud music at 120 decibels for fifteen minutes or more. Anyone working in an environment that reaches noise levels of more than 85 decibels for extended periods of time should wear protective devices. Earplugs and hearing protection devices are needed for construction workers, traffic personal, musicians, disc jockeys, air traffic personnel, nightclub employees and patrons, or anyone exposed to loud noises.

Scientists are conducting research to discover whether damaged hair cells of the ear are capable of rebuilding their structure over a forty-eight-hour period (the time that it takes for hearing to return after a temporary loss). Researchers speculate that permanent hearing loss may occur when self-repair mechanisms are compromised.

Scientists are studying blood flow in the cochlear section of the ear to evaluate how drugs may affect hair cells. Researchers are also examining blood flow to the cochlea when people are exposed to conversational sound and loud sounds. It seems that when a person is exposed to loud sounds, the blood flow in the cochlea drops. Drugs that are used to treat blood flow problems, such as in peripheral vascular disease, may show a benefit to maintaining blood flow to the cochlea. These and other drug therapies may show promising results in helping people with hearing loss. Finally, with a reduction in harmful noise, hearing loss will decrease.

—*Janet Mahoney, R.N., Ph.D., A.P.R.N.*

See also Aging; Audiology; Deafness; Ear infections and disorders; Ear surgery; Ears; Hearing aids; Hearing tests; Ménière's disease; Nasopharyngeal disorders; Neuralgia, neuritis, and neuropathy; Otorhinolaryngology; Sense organs; Speech disorders.

FOR FURTHER INFORMATION:

Carmen, Richard, ed. *The Consumer Handbook on Hearing Loss and Hearing Aids: A Bridge to Healing*. 2d rev. ed. Sedona, Ariz.: Auricle Ink, 2004. This book has received rave reviews within the hearing profession. A consumer author for more than twenty years, clinical audiologist Carmen brings together the most renowned audiologists, scientists, physicians, thinkers, and experts in the field. Discusses the emotions involved in hearing loss, where and how to find help, self-assessment for those who do not yet admit a loss, and effective transition from hearing loss to hearing aids.

Craine, Michael. *Hear Well Again: A Step by Step Program to Better Hearing*. Chapel Hill, N.C.: Professional Press, 1999. An easy-to-read, comprehensive review of hearing aid technology, hearing health care, and solutions to alleviate hearing problems.

Gallo, Joseph J., et al., eds. *Handbook of Geriatric Assessment*. 4th ed. Sudbury, Mass.: Jones & Bartlett, 2006. Emphasizes material that has practical application in primary care settings in order to encourage a multidimensional approach for the care of the aged.

Mahoney, Janet. "Hearing Loss and Assessment: A Concern for All." *Nursing Spectrum* 13, no. 1 (January 10, 2000). Updates nurses' knowledge about assessment techniques and treatment options for patients with various types of hearing loss.

Paterson, J. "What You Need to Know About Hearing Loss." *USA Weekend*, November, 21, 1997. An article that gives valuable insight into the topic of hearing loss. Included is a self-quiz about hearing loss.

Shelp, Scott G. "Your Patient Is Deaf, Now What?" *RN* 60, no. 2 (February, 1997): 37-41. This article illustrates the use of American Sign Language (ASL). Includes a comprehensive Signed English Dictionary that represents both ASL, the national language of the deaf in the United States, and manually signed English, another type of sign language that resembles ASL but has a structure similar to written or spoken English.

Tabloski, Patricia A. *Gerontological Nursing*. Upper Saddle River, N.J.: Pearson Prentice Hall, 2006. Tabloski is a gerontological nurse practitioner who has provided primary care to older patients in a variety of settings. She has taught graduate and undergraduate students about gerontology.

HEARING TESTS

PROCEDURE

ANATOMY OR SYSTEM AFFECTED: Ears, nervous system

SPECIALTIES AND RELATED FIELDS: Audiology, neurology, occupational health, otorhinolaryngology, pediatrics, speech pathology

DEFINITION: Evaluation techniques for determining the type and severity of hearing loss in children and adults.

KEY TERMS:

auditory brainstem response: measurement of the nervous discharge produced by the central auditory system as a response to sound stimulation; also known as brainstem auditory evoked response (BAER) or auditory brainstem potentials (ABR)

auditory nerve: the nerve that conducts sound stimuli to the brain for interpretation

behavioral audiometry: a technique that the audiologist employs to evaluate hearing in infants, toddlers, or uncooperative patients (both children and adults) with developmental deficits

cochlea: the organ localized in the inner portion of the auditory system that detects sound

mastoid: referring to the bone behind the ear

middle ear: the part of the auditory system, consisting of the ossicular chain and the auditory tube, that serves as a conductor of and transducer of sound

otoacoustic emissions: sound produced in the middle ear as a response to the vibration produced by the cochlea when it is stimulated by external sounds

INDICATIONS AND PROCEDURES

Hearing tests are done to establish the presence, type, and severity of hearing impairment in children and adults. Such tests are conducted by an audiologist, although screening tests can also be done by a technician under the supervision of an audiologist. The severity of hearing loss is classified as mild, moderate, moderately severe, severe, and profound. It is also classified according to the anatomic region affected: conductive, sensorineural, or mixed hearing loss.

The selection of tests to evaluate hearing will depend on the patient's age and ability to follow directions and the ability of the audiologist to elicit responses from the patient. When a patient cannot follow instructions such as lifting a hand or pressing a button, a test that does not require the patient's cooperation is used. Two tests that do not require the patient's cooperation are the auditory brainstem potential (ABR) test and the evoked otoacoustic emissions (EOAE) test. Both tests require only that the patient be quiet. For this purpose, the patient may need sedation if normal sleep cannot be induced.

The ABR test requires the placement of four electrodes in the child's head: in both mastoid regions and in the mid forehead and upper center of the head. A stimulus is sent through a small microphone placed in the patient's external ear canal or via headphones. The instrument records the average of the electrical discharges generated by the auditory nerve in response to sound stimuli and produces a tracing of waves that correspond to the different electrical potentials generated in response to the stimuli. Analysis of the waves can determine the presence of hearing loss and measure its severity. The ABR test may be used for screening, to determine whether the subject can hear, or for the clinical evaluation of hearing loss. It can be done at any age. An automated method of ABR testing is available for screening newborn infants for hearing loss; it automatically determines if the patient has passed or failed. The clinical ABR test requires specially trained personnel and takes from forty-five to fifty minutes to perform. The automated method can be applied by a technician.

The EOAE test involves recording the sound produced by hair cells within the cochlea by way of a microphone placed in the outer ear canal. Normally, when sound enters the cochlea, the hair cells produce a sound that bounces backward and can be recorded. This sound correlates with the sound sent to the auditory nerve. If there is damage to the hair cells in the cochlea, then no sound is elicited. The EOAE test can be performed without sedation if the patient cooperates by staying quiet. It can be done by a technician and takes approximately ten minutes or less. The EOAE test is used for universal screening of newborn infants. It can be done at all ages to help determine the integrity of the cochlea and thus whether an observed hearing defect is within the cochlea.

Behavioral techniques are the most practical, cost-effective, and time-efficient methods for the accurate assessment of hearing. They give more complete information on the child's hearing as well as functional information about how the child uses his or her hearing. The simplest test is behavioral observation audiometry, in which the audiologist records the behavioral response to an applied sound stimuli of a known frequency. This test can be done with infants up to six months of age, toddlers, and uncooperative patients, such as children or adults with developmental delays. Visual reinforcement audiometry (VRA) is done with infants and toddlers from six months to twenty-four months of age. It is also used with uncooperative patients. In this test, the patient is submitted to sounds of different intensity and trained to respond to the sound stimuli by means of an attractive stimulus. Every time that the sound appears, the stimulus illuminates. When the patient hears the sound, he or she will look for the reinforcement. Play audiometry is a test that can be used in children over two years of age. The child is taught to move a block or place a puzzle piece every time he or she hears a sound.

In 2002, Ruth Litovsky, an University of Wisconsin-Madison communicative disorders professor, introduced a binaural hearing test to evaluate how people respond to sounds in a noisy environment resembling public areas and schools. Using computers showing images related to words being broadcasted on loudspeaker, her test assesses which sounds people ignore and which sounds secure their attention.

In 2003, the *Ear, Nose, and Throat Journal* provided information describing the Otogram from Tympany, a Sonic Innovation subsidiary. This device enables patients to test their hearing at sites using automated technology. During the twenty-minute testing period, patients undergo an audiogram that thoroughly evaluates their acoustic capabilities with tympanometry and other standard diagnostic tests, responding to the tests via touchscreens with results recorded by computer.

In 2005, Bio-Logic Systems Corporation and House Ear Institute researchers introduced the hearing in noise test (HINT), which assesses how hearing functions in police and emergency personnel whose hearing is vital to their work. The test involves subjects repeating sentences while exposed to a variation of noise and quiet. The source azimuth identification in noise test (SAINT) evaluates subjects' ability to detect where sounds are located.

Perspective and Prospects

Early detection of hearing loss has become a priority among intervention services because it has devastating effects on language development and consequently on social adaptation. It has been found that the mean age at which deafness is diagnosed is around three, which is after speech development should have occurred. Thus, children with hearing loss are placed at a disadvantage with their peers.

In 1993, the National Institutes of Health (NIH) developed a consensus statement by which all newborn infants in the United States were to be screened for hearing loss. The aim was that by the year 2000, all newborns would have been screened before being discharged from the hospital. By 1999, many U.S. states had passed legislation requiring hearing screening of newborns, but a study described in the July, 1999, issue of *The American Journal of Otology* recommended screening only babies with a risk for impaired hearing, stating that pediatricians and child care providers would detect deafness in infants and toddlers.

The October, 2001, the *Journal of the American Medical Association* evaluated nineteen studies, emphasizing that screening newborns was not superior to tests by pediatricians when infants were several months old and stressing that determining the value of newborn screening required additional study. In October, 2005, the *Archives of Pediatrics & Adolescent Medicine* estimated that more than half of children whose hearing test results revealed that they needed additional tests never underwent such testing.

The role of otitis media (middle-ear infections) in producing hearing impairment is an area of great concern and controversy. Special attention to the hearing evaluation of children with recurrent and chronic otitis media is indicated.

*—Gloria Reyes Báez, M.D.,
and Hilda Velez Rodriguez, M.S.;
updated by Elizabeth D. Schafer, Ph.D.*

See also Deafness; Ear infections and disorders; Ears; Hearing loss; Neonatology; Physical examination; Screening; Sense organs.

For Further Information:

Bess, Fred H., and Judith S. Gravel, eds. *Foundations of Pediatric Audiology*. San Diego, Calif.: Plural, 2006. Focuses on testing infants and children and how medical personnel can provide effective treatment for young deaf patients. Includes a bibliography.

Dobie, Robert A. and Susan B. Van Hemel, eds. *Hearing Loss: Determining Eligibility for Social Security Benefits*. Washington, D.C.: National Academies Press, 2005. Includes a chapter describing various tests and offers suggestions to improve testing. Discusses how impaired hearing affects employees and their work capacity. Includes illustrations, tables, and a glossary.

Elder, Nina. "Now Hear This—Check Your Baby's Hearing." *Better Homes and Gardens* 78, no. 5 (May, 2000): 264. One out of every three hundred U.S. babies is born with a hearing problem, yet only 25 percent of newborns get hearing tests. If a hearing problem is detected within the first six months of life, a child has a good chance of catching up with his or her peers.

Glaser, Gabrielle. "Pediatricians Urge Hearing Tests at Birth." *The New York Times*, April 6, 1999, p. 7. Hearing impairment in infants can cause delays in speech, language, and cognitive development, according to Dr. Philip Ziring. Often, hearing loss is not diagnosed in children until they are two or three years old and are not speaking properly.

Hall, James W., III. *New Handbook of Auditory Evoked Responses*. Boston: Pearson Education, 2006. An exhaustive study of auditory evoked response aimed at the medical professional. Includes bibliographical references and an index.

Hearing Exchange. http://www.hearingexchange.com/ An online community designed to foster the exchange of information and the provision of support for the hearing impaired.

Koike, Kazunari J. *Everyday Audiology: A Practical Guide for Health Care Professionals*. San Diego, Calif.: Plural, 2006. Explains tests such as the tympanogram, VRA, ABR, and Stenger for medical personnel.

McCormick, Barry, ed. *The Medical Practitioner's Guide to Paediatric Audiology*. New York: Cambridge University Press, 1995. A handbook of hearing disorders in infancy and childhood. Includes discussion of the various hearing tests and aids available.

Martin, Frederick N., and John Greer Clark. *Introduction to Audiology*. 9th ed. Boston: Pearson/Allyn and Bacon, 2006. In addition to providing thorough coverage of the physics of sound, anatomy, and physiology of the auditory system, covers the causes and treatment of hearing disorders and the relevant diagnostic and therapeutic techniques. This edition includes a CD-ROM.

Northern, Jerry L., and Marion P. Downs. *Hearing in Children*. 5th ed. Philadelphia: Lippincott Williams & Wilkins, 2002. Topics covered include hearing and hearing loss, auditory mechanics, medical aspects of hearing loss, deviation of auditory behavior, and amplification.

Roush, Jackson, ed. *Screening for Hearing Loss and Otitis Media in Children*. San Diego, Calif.: Singular, 2001. Although clinical in nature, describes myriad hearing tests in great detail.

Sataloff, Robert T., and Joseph Sataloff. *Hearing Loss*. 4th ed. New York: Taylor & Francis, 2005. Several chapters focus on diagnostic testing methods and how to administer and evaluate tests, discussing incorrect procedures. Illustrations include figures of audiograms, word lists for speech tests, and sample patient hearing records. Appendices describe ear anatomy and diseases.

HEART

ANATOMY

ANATOMY OR SYSTEM AFFECTED: Blood, blood vessels, chest, circulatory system

SPECIALTIES AND RELATED FIELDS: Cardiology, exercise physiology

DEFINITION: The muscle that pumps blood through the body by means of rhythmic contractions.

KEY TERMS:

arteries: vessels that take blood away from the heart and toward the tissues

atria: the upper receiving chambers of the heart that lie above the ventricles

atrioventricular (A-V) node: a small region of specialized heart muscle cells that receives the electrical impulse from the atria and begins its transmission to the ventricles

coronary arteries: the arteries that supply blood to the heart muscle

diastole: the period of relaxation of the heart between beats

sinoatrial (S-A) node: a small region of specialized heart muscle cells that spontaneously generates and sends an electrical signal that gives the heart an automatic rhythm for contraction

systole: the period of contraction of the heart when blood moves out of the heart chambers and into the arteries

veins: vessels that take blood to the heart and from the tissues

ventricles: the lower pumping chambers of the heart located below the atria; they force blood into the arteries

STRUCTURE AND FUNCTIONS

All the cells in the human body are dependent on the blood in the cardiovascular system (the heart and blood vessels) for the transport of gases, nutrients, hormones, and other factors. Likewise, the tissues must have a way to dispose of waste products so that they do not build to harmful levels. All these substances are dissolved in the blood, but something must provide the force to transport the blood to all parts of the body at all times—the heart. This organ must beat continuously from early in development to death. It beats without conscious control and can vary how quickly it moves blood throughout the body depending on the needs and activities of the tissues.

In humans, an individual's heart is about the size of his or her fist and is enclosed in the center of the chest cavity between the lungs. The heart contains specialized muscle cells known as cardiac muscle. These cardiac cells make up most of the thickness of the walls of the heart; they are responsible for moving blood out of the heart and are also involved in maintaining the rhythm of the heartbeat. This heavily muscled layer is referred to as the myocardium. The inner lining of the heart is called the endocardium; it is continuous with the lining of all the blood vessels in the body. The outermost layer of the heart is the epicardium, which covers the myocardium. The heart moves as it beats and is contained within a fluid-filled bag called the pericardial sac. The rhythmically beating heart has the potential to rub against adjacent structures (such as the lungs), harming itself and those structures. Therefore,

it is important that the heart be encased in the pericardial sac, with its lubricating fluid.

The human heart has four separate chambers. These internal cavities can be identified by their location and function. The upper pair of smaller chambers are known as atria, and the lower larger chambers are called ventricles. Because the atria and ventricles have a muscular wall which separates them into right and left halves, one can refer to the individual chambers as the right atrium and left atrium, and the right ventricle and left ventricle. The wall that separates the right and left halves of the heart is called the septum. The septum prevents any mixing of blood from the right and left sides of the heart. The atria and ventricles on the same side, however, must allow blood to pass between them

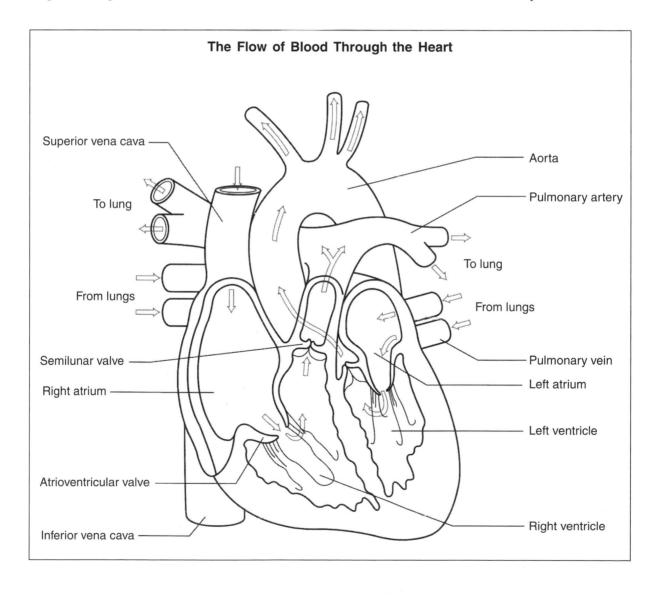

The Flow of Blood Through the Heart

Superior vena cava

To lung

From lungs

Semilunar valve

Right atrium

Atrioventricular valve

Inferior vena cava

Aorta

Pulmonary artery

To lung

From lungs

Pulmonary vein

Left atrium

Left ventricle

Right ventricle

in a single direction. This action is accomplished by one-way valves between the atria and ventricles. The valve that allows blood to pass from the right atrium to the right ventricle is called the tricuspid valve because it is made of three flaps. On the left side of the heart is the bicuspid valve (with two flaps), which is also known as the mitral valve. The bicuspid valve allows blood from the left atrium to flow only into the left ventricle. This rather complex anatomy is necessary because the heart must pump blood in one direction and into two separate systems.

The anatomy of the heart often makes more sense if one understands its function or physiology. As an example, one may consider an active cell in the body, perhaps a muscle cell that moves the foot. This cell utilizes oxygen to help metabolize food for energy. During this process, carbon dioxide is produced as a waste product, and high levels of carbon dioxide can be harmful to cells. Therefore, one of the jobs of the cardiovascular system is to deliver oxygen and take away carbon dioxide. Once the carbon dioxide is picked up by the blood, it travels back to the heart via veins and enters the right atrium. From the right atrium, the blood passes the tricuspid valve and enters the right ventricle. The right ventricle then sends the blood past a one-way valve called the semilunar valve into blood vessels that transport it to the lungs. At the lungs, the blood loses carbon dioxide and picks up oxygen. This oxygenated blood must now be delivered to the tissues. First, the blood returns to the heart and enters the left atrium. From the left atrium, blood is pushed past the bicuspid valve into the left ventricle. The blood is then pumped from the powerful left ventricle through another set of semilunar valves into the blood vessels that will carry the blood to all the tissues of the body, including the heart itself. The blood vessels that feed the heart directly are known as coronary vessels.

The orderly pattern by which blood flows through the heart, lungs, and body requires the chambers of the heart to work in a coordinated fashion. The atria contract together to help send blood into the ventricles. The ventricles then contract together so that blood flows through the lungs from the right ventricle and through the tissues of the body from the left ventricle. The tricuspid and bicuspid valves prevent a backflow of blood into the atria when the ventricles contract, and the semilunar valves prevent blood from returning to the ventricles after they have contracted.

Something must coordinate the contraction of the heart so that the atria contract together before the ventricles do so. Highly specialized cells of the myocardium have the ability to conduct electrical impulses rapidly and to discharge spontaneously at a certain rate. These properties allow the heart to be stimulated in a synchronous way and for it to generate its own rate and rhythm. One region of the right atrium is known as the sinoatrial (S-A) node; it functions as the heart's pacemaker. The S-A node has the ability to generate spontaneously an electrical signal with a relatively rapid rhythm. Therefore, it serves to "pace" the heart rate. When the S-A node sends its electrical impulse throughout the atria, the atria contract. There is a slight delay before the impulse reaches the ventricles, which allows the atria to contract fully before the ventricles. The atrioventricular (A-V) node will then pick up the electrical signal and send it through both ventricles via specialized conductive heart muscle fibers known as Purkinje's fibers. Purkinje's fibers transmit the electrical signal ensuring that all the ventricular muscle cells contract at nearly the same time. The ventricles contract in such a way that the bottom tip of the heart (apex) contracts slightly before the region of the ventricles next to the atria (base). Additionally, the ventricles contract in a somewhat twisting motion that causes the heart to "wring out" the blood.

This rather complex system allows the heart to contract at its own rate and in a highly synchronous fashion. Nevertheless, one's heart rate varies depending on one's physical activity or emotional state. For example, during exercise or when an individual is under stress, the heart rate goes up. When one is relaxed, the heart does not beat as rapidly. Therefore, the body must have a way to regulate the rate at which the S-A node signals the heart to contract.

The autonomic nervous system, which functions without one's conscious control, regulates the heart rate. It is divided into two systems: parasympathetic and sympathetic. The parasympathetic nervous system is active during periods of rest and has the ability to slow the heart. During periods of physical or emotional stress, the sympathetic nervous system stimulates the heart to contract more forcefully and at a more rapid rate. The parasympathetic and sympathetic systems communicate with the heart via chemical messengers known as neurotransmitters. The parasympathetic nervous system uses the neurotransmitter acetylcholine to slow the heart, while norepinephrine and epinephrine are the chemicals used by the sympathetic nervous system to increase the heart rate.

DISORDERS AND DISEASES

Even though the heart seems to be adaptable to a variety of situations throughout one's life, it can malfunction. In fact, diseases of the heart and blood vessels are the number-one killer in the United States. One common disease that affects the heart directly is coronary artery disease, which can lead to life-threatening heart attacks. Although medical researchers are still investigating the causes of coronary artery disease, most of the evidence points to hypertension (high blood pressure) and atherosclerosis (a buildup of fatty plaque in the walls of arteries).

Hypertension is usually defined as a blood pressure greater than 140/90 millimeters of mercury (mmHg) at rest. A typical blood pressure for a young, healthy adult is 120/80 mmHg. The top number measures the force of blood against an artery wall during the contraction of the heart; this is referred to as the systolic pressure. The bottom number, the diastolic pressure, is a measurement of force when the heart is relaxed. If either systolic or diastolic pressure exceeds 140/90 mmHg, the patient is considered hypertensive. The cause of hypertension has not been determined, but it is known that with hypertension the heart must work harder to push the blood through the arteries, including the coronary arteries. Physicians treat hypertension by prescribing drugs that block the effect of the sympathetic nervous system on the heart, such as metoprolol (Lopressor). They may also prescribe drugs such as prazosin (Minipress) that prevent the arteries from becoming too narrow.

Hypertension is also seen in patients who have atherosclerosis. This buildup of fatty materials such as cholesterol under the lining of the artery causes the plaque to protrude, narrowing the diameter of the vessel. This can lead to blood clot formation on artery walls which are irregular. This clot, also known as a thrombus, may dislodge and travel in the bloodstream. Eventually, it may block a small artery, thereby preventing the flow of blood to the tissue. If this happens in a coronary artery, a myocardial infarction (heart attack) will result.

A heart attack occurs when a portion of the heart dies because of a lack of oxygen or a buildup of waste products. Heart muscle has no way of repairing itself, and the resulting damage is permanent. If the patient is transported to the hospital immediately, the emergency room physician may give drugs to prevent further blood clot formation (aspirin and heparin) and to help dissolve the already formed clot (streptokinase and tis-

sue plasminogen activator, or TPA). If the coronary artery is only partially blocked, the patient may suffer from angina pectoris, a chest pain that radiates down the left arm. These patients usually take drugs such as nitroglycerin, which help dilate (widen) blood vessels, reestablishing adequate flow to the heart.

Another devastating disease of the heart is congestive heart failure, a condition in which the heart fails to pump enough blood to meet the demands of the body's tissues. The heart becomes enlarged because of the resulting excessive increase in blood volume. There are several causes of heart failure, most of which stem from the fact that the heart loses its ability to pump efficiently. For example, a patient who has had a heart attack may have lost significant function as a result of heart damage. Even without a heart attack, some individuals may have malfunctioning heart valves or other problems that cause an inefficient ejection of blood and thus heart failure.

The cardiovascular system attempts to compensate for heart failure in several ways. The sympathetic nervous system increases the heart rate, and the kidneys retain more fluid to increase blood volume. These compensatory mechanisms help to reestablish adequate blood flow for a while. Because of the increase in blood volume, however, more blood enters the chambers of the heart and causes them to stretch. At some point, the ventricles can no longer force out the increased amount of blood entering them, and they enlarge. This increase in the size of the heart chamber further enlarges the heart and strains the heart muscle. The heart will continue to weaken, unable to keep up with the body's demands. Compensatory mechanisms attempt to meet the body's need for continuous blood flow but in doing so further overload the heart. This vicious circle may lead to complete heart failure and death.

Congestive heart failure may involve only one side of the heart, perhaps because of a heart attack which affected that side. If the heart failure occurs on the left side, the right ventricle is pumping blood to the lungs in an efficient manner but the left ventricle cannot pump all the blood returning from the lungs. Therefore, blood backs up and pools in the lung tissues. Similarly, if the right ventricle begins to fail and the left ventricle is normal, blood begins to pool throughout the body since the right side of the heart cannot keep up in its pumping.

Physicians are able to slow the progression of congestive heart failure by prescribing drugs such as digoxin that increase the force of heart muscle contraction and thereby the amount of blood ejected with each beat. Therapeutic agents such as captopril (Capoten) help to reduce the fluid retention in the kidneys.

Coronary artery disease and heart failure are related to the inability of the heart to contract. In addition, the specialized heart muscle cells that provide the heart's rhythm and conduct the electrical signals necessary for a coordinated heartbeat may be affected by disease. In the resting adult, the heart normally beats about seventy to eighty times per minute. Several conditions exist whereby the heart loses control of its normal rate and rhythm, a serious condition.

For example, if the heart begins to beat too rapidly, the ventricles do not have enough time to fill and the movement of blood to the heart muscle and the rest of the body is impaired. The atria or ventricles may contract at a high rate and lose their coordinated sequence of contraction; this is referred to as atrial or ventricular fibrillation. If immediate action is not taken to reestablish the normal rate and conduction sequence, the patient will die. Emergency measures such as electrical defibrillation may shock the heart into reestablishing its normal rhythm and conduction pathways. It is easy to understand how these abnormal patterns of heart activity occur if one imagines more than one pacemaker attempting to control heart function. The cause of these and other, less severe heart rhythms may be heart damage affecting the conductive pathway, drugs, or even psychological distress.

Heart disease is a major cause of death, but most experts agree that many heart problems are preventable. High blood pressure and high blood levels of fat and cholesterol are associated with an increased incidence of coronary artery disease. Cigarette smoking and excessive weight are also correlated with heart disease. Additionally, exercise seems to be critical in maintaining a healthy heart, as sedentary individuals have a twofold increase in their risk of heart disease when compared to active people.

It is likely that individuals who are at risk can lessen the probability of having heart problems by adopting a more healthful lifestyle, including stopping smoking, reducing excessive weight and mental stress, and engaging in enjoyable physical activities (with their physicians' permission).

PERSPECTIVE AND PROSPECTS

The role of the heart in the functioning of the human body was questioned by the ancient Egyptians, who attributed breathing to the heart. It was the Chinese who first documented that the heart is responsible for the pulse and movement of blood. They also believed that the heart was the seat of happiness. The ancient Greeks had a different idea about the function of the heart, believing that it was the region where thinking originated.

It was not until William Harvey (1578-1657), an English physiologist, published his experiments on the heart and circulation that scientists believed blood was pumped continuously by the heart. He observed that both ventricles of the heart contracted and expanded at the same time. Harvey also noted that when the heart was removed from an animal, it continued to contract and relax; that is, it had an automatic rhythm.

More than one hundred years after Harvey published his work, Stephen Hales made the first blood pressure measurements. He did so by inserting a tube into the neck artery of a horse and watching the blood rise 3 meters above the animal. Then early in the twentieth century Willem Einthoven invented an instrument to measure electrical currents. This instrument was used by Thomas Lewis to measure the electrical activity in the heart, the first electrocardiograph (ECG).

By the mid-nineteenth century, heart surgeries were being performed to correct heart defects. These early surgeries had to be done with the heart still beating. In 1953, the heart-lung machine was used to take over the pumping function of the heart during surgery so that the surgeon could stop the heart. In 1967, Christiaan Barnard performed the first heart transplantation in a human. Heart transplants were performed during the next ten years with no long-term survivors, usually because of tissue rejection. In 1982, a completely artificial heart was implanted into a patient. This patient died in the spring of 1983.

Heart transplants have become much more successful, however, mainly because of the use of immunosuppressive drugs that help to prevent rejection of the transplanted heart. Similarly, newer drugs and procedures such as coronary bypass surgery, angioplasty, and atherectomy are becoming more effective in treating heart disease. Nevertheless, perhaps the best approach to maintaining a healthy heart is to practice preventive medicine. Scientists are making comparable strides in finding ways to prevent heart disease as they are in treating already existing conditions.

—*Matthew Berria, Ph.D.*

See also Anatomy; Aneurysmectomy; Aneurysms; Angina; Angiography; Angioplasty; Anxiety; Arrhythmias; Arteriosclerosis; Biofeedback; Blue baby syndrome; Bypass surgery; Cardiac arrest; Cardiac rehabilitation; Cardiology; Cardiology, pediatric;

Cardiopulmonary resuscitation (CPR); Catheterization; Circulation; Congenital heart disease; Echocardiography; Electrical shock; Electrocardiography (ECG or EKG); Embolism; Endocarditis; Exercise physiology; Heart attack; Heart disease; Heart failure; Heart transplantation; Heart valve replacement; Hypertension; Internal medicine; Mitral valve prolapse; Pacemaker implantation; Palpitations; Resuscitation; Reye's syndrome; Rheumatic fever; Shock; Sports medicine; Strokes; Systems and organs; Thoracic surgery; Thrombolytic therapy and TPA; Thrombosis and thrombus; Transplantation; Vascular medicine; Vascular system.

FOR FURTHER INFORMATION:

Hales, Dianne. *An Invitation to Health*. 12th ed. New York: Brooks Cole, 2006. This text should be read by anyone who wishes an overview of health topics. Several chapters deal with the function of the heart and how lifestyle influences its health.

The Incredible Machine. Washington, D.C.: National Geographic Society, 1994. A colorful book that describes in layperson's terms how the body works and how one alters one's own health. The chapter on the cardiovascular system is well written and contains exciting photographs and drawings of the heart.

McGoon, M. *The Mayo Clinic Heart Book*. 2d ed. New York: William Morrow, 2000. One of the most respected texts for laypeople on heart disease. Covers all aspects of anatomy, physiology, diagnosis, treatment, and prevention.

Mackenna, B. R., and R. Callander. *Illustrated Physiology*. 6th ed. New York: Churchill Livingstone, 1996. Provides the reader with a visual explanation of physiology on a basic level. Chapter 5 contains many excellent diagrams, illustrations, and explanations of cardiovascular anatomy and physiology.

Marieb, Elaine N., and Katja Hoehn. *Human Anatomy and Physiology*. 7th ed. San Francisco: Pearson Benjamin Cummings, 2007. Nonscientists at the advanced high school level or above will be able to understand this fine textbook. It includes a complete glossary, index, pronunciation guide, and other helpful features.

Park, Myung K. *The Pediatric Cardiology Handbook*. 3d ed. St. Louis: Mosby, 2003. A text for the medical specialist with discussion of all congenital heart defects, including atrial septal defects, ventricular septal defects, cushion defects, coarctation, and interrupted aortic arch.

Tortora, Gerard J., and Bryan Derrickson. *Principles of Anatomy and Physiology*. 11th ed. Hoboken, N.J.: John Wiley & Sons, 2006. An outstanding textbook of human anatomy and physiology, covering the heart and circulatory system in depth.

HEART ATTACK
DISEASE/DISORDER

ALSO KNOWN AS: Myocardial infarction

ANATOMY OR SYSTEM AFFECTED: Circulatory system, heart

SPECIALTIES AND RELATED FIELDS: Cardiology, critical care, emergency medicine, internal medicine

DEFINITION: Myocardial infarction; the sudden death of heart muscle characterized by intense chest pain, sweating, shortness of breath, or sometimes none of these symptoms.

KEY TERMS:

atherosclerosis: narrowing of the internal passageways of essential arteries caused by the buildup of fatty deposits

atria: the chambers in the right and left top portions of the heart that receive blood from the veins and pump it to the ventricles

fibrillation: wild beating of the heart, which may occur when the regular rate of the heartbeat is interrupted

myocardium: the muscle tissue that forms the walls of the heart, varying in thickness in the upper and lower regions

sinoatrial node: the section of the right atrium that determines the appropriate rate of the heartbeat

ventricles: the chambers in the right and left bottom portions of the heart that receive blood from the atria and pump it to the arteries

CAUSES AND SYMPTOMS

Although varied in origin and effect on the body, heart attacks (or myocardial infarctions) occur when there are interruptions in the delicately synchronized system either supplying blood to the heart or pumping blood from the heart to other vital organs. The heart is a highly specialized muscle whose function is to pump life-sustaining blood to all parts of the body. The heart's action involves the development of pressure to propel blood through arriving and departing channels—veins and arteries—that must maintain that pressure within their walls at critical levels throughout the system.

The highest level of pressure in the total cardiovascular system is to be found closest to the two "pumping" chambers on the right and left lower sections of the heart, called ventricles. Dark, bluish-colored blood, emptied of its oxygen content and laden with carbon dioxide waste instead of the oxygen in fresh blood, flows into the upper portion of the heart via the superior and inferior venae cavae. It then passes from the right atrium chamber into the right ventricle. Once in the ventricle, this blood cannot flow back because of one-way valves separating the "receiving" from the "pumping" sections of the total heart organ.

After this valve closes following a vitally synchronized timing system, constriction of the right ventricle by the myocardium muscle in the surrounding walls of the heart forces the blood from the heart, propelling it toward the oxygen-filled tissue of the lungs. Following reoxygenation, bright red blood that is still under pressure from the thrust of the right ventricle flows into the left atrium. Once channeled into the left ventricle, the pumping process that began in the right ventricle is then repeated on the left by muscular constriction, and oxygenated blood flows out of the aortic valve under pressure throughout the cardiovascular system to nourish the body's cells. Because the force needed to supply blood under pressure from the left ventricle for the entire body is greater than the first-phase pumping force needed to move blood into the lungs, the myocardium surrounding the left ventricle constitutes the thickest muscular layer in the heart's wall.

The efficiency of this process, as well as the origins of problems of fatigue in the heart that can lead to heart attacks and eventual heart failure, is tied to the maintenance of a reasonably constant level of blood pressure. If pulmonary problems (blockage caused by the effects of smoking or environmental pollution, for example) make it harder for the right ventricle to push blood through the lungs, the heart must expend more energy in the first stage of the cardiovascular process. Simi-

larly, and often in addition to the added work for the heart because of pulmonary complications, the efficiency of the left ventricle in handling blood flow may be reduced by the presence of excessive fat in the body, causing this ventricle to expend more energy to propel oxygenated blood into vital tissues.

Although factors such as these may be responsible for overworking the heart and thus contributing to eventual heart failure, other causes of heart attacks are to be found much closer to the working apparatus of the heart, particularly in the coronary arteries. The coronary arteries begin at the top of the heart and fan out along its sides. They are responsible for providing large quantities of blood to the myocardium muscle, which needs continual nourishment to carry out the pumping that forces blood forward from the ventricles. The passageways inside these and other key arteries are vulnerable to the process known as atherosclerosis, which can affect the blood supply to other organs as well as to the heart. In the heart, atherosclerosis involves the accumulation, inside the coronary arteries, of fatty deposits called atheromas. If these deposits continue to collect, less blood can flow through the arteries. A narrowed artery also increases the possibility of a variant form of heart attack, in which a sudden and total blockage of blood flow follows the lodging of a blood clot in one of these vital passageways.

A symptomatic condition called angina pectoris, characterized by intermittent chest pains, may develop if atherosclerosis reduces blood (and therefore oxygen) supply to the heart. These danger signs can continue over a number of years. If diagnosis reveals a problem that might be resolved by preventive medication, exercise, or recommendations for heart surgery, then this condition, known as myocardial ischemia, may not necessarily end in a full heart attack.

A full heart attack occurs when, for one of several possible reasons including a vascular spasm suddenly constricting an already clogged artery or a blockage caused by a clot, the heart suddenly ceases to receive the necessary supply of blood. This brings almost immediate deterioration in some of the heart's tissue and causes the organ's consequent inability to perform its vital functions effectively.

Another form of attack and disruption of the heart's ability to deliver blood can come either independently of or in conjunction with an arterially induced heart attack. This form of attack involves a sustained interruption in the rate of heartbeats. The necessary pace or rate of myocardial contractions, which can vary depending

---

INFORMATION ON HEART ATTACK

CAUSES: Pulmonary problems, atherosclerosis, smoking, high blood pressure, diabetes mellitus

SYMPTOMS: Varies but often includes intense chest pain, sweating, shortness of breath

DURATION: Acute

TREATMENTS: Drug therapy, surgery, preventive medication, exercise, dietary change, medical devices

on the organism's rate of physical exertion or age, is regulated in the sinoatrial node in the right atrium, which generates its own electrical impulses. The ultimate sources for the commands to the sinoatrial node are to be found in the network of nerves coming directly from the brain. There are, however, other so-called local pacemakers located in the atria and ventricles. If these sources of electrical charges begin giving commands to the myocardium that are not in rhythm with those coming from the sinoatrial node, then dysrhythmic or premature beats may confuse the heart muscle, causing it to beat wildly. In fact, the concentrated pattern of muscle contractions will not be coordinated and instead will be dispersed in different areas of the heart. The result is fibrillation, a series of uncoordinated contractions that cannot combine to propel blood out of the ventricles. This condition may occur either as the aftershock of an arterially induced heart attack or suddenly and on its own, caused by the deterioration of the electrical impulse system commanding the heart rate. In patients whose potential vulnerability to this form of heart attack has been diagnosed in advance, a heart physician may decide to surgically implant a mechanical pacemaker to ensure coordination of the necessary electrical commands to the myocardium.

TREATMENT AND THERAPY

Extraordinary medical advances have helped reduce the high death rates formerly associated with heart attacks. Many of these advances have been in the field of preventive medicine. The most widely recognized medical findings are related to diet, smoking, and exercise. Although controversy remains, there is general agreement that cholesterol absorbed by the body from the ingestion of animal fats plays a key role in the dangerous buildup of platelets inside arterial passageways. It has been accepted that regular, although not necessarily strenuous, exercise is an essential long-term preventive strategy that can reduce the risk of heart attacks. Exercise also plays a role in therapy after a heart attack. In both preventive and postattack contexts, it has been medically proven that the entire cardiovascular system profits from the natural muscle-strengthening process (in the heart's case) and general cleansing effects (in the case of oxygen intake and stimulated blood flow) that result from controlled regular exercise.

The actual application of medical scientific knowledge to assist in the campaign against the deadly effects of heart disease involves multiple fields of specializa-

Pain Associated with Heart Attack

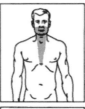
Pain radiating up into jaw and through to back

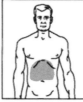
Pain felt in upper abdomen

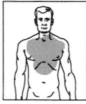
Pressure in the central chest area, from mild to severe

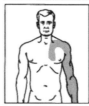
Pain radiating down left arm; may cause sensation of weakness in the arm

tion. These may range from the sophisticated use of electrocardiograms (ECGs) to monitor the regularity of heartbeats, to specialized drug therapies aimed at preventing heart attacks in people who have been diagnosed as high-risk cases, to coronary bypass surgery or even heart transplants. In the 1980's, highly specialized surgeons at several university and private hospitals began performing operations to implant artificial hearts in human patients.

In the case of ECGs, it has become possible, thanks to the use of portable units that record the heartbeat patterns of persons over an extended period of time, to gain a much more accurate impression of the actual functioning of the heart. Previous dependence on electrocardiographic data gathered during an appointed and limited examination provided only minimal information to doctors.

In 2003, the Food and Drug Administration (FDA) approved a simple blood test that, when used with ECGs, could greatly improve the ability of doctors to

IN THE NEWS:
LOW-GRADE INFLAMMATION AS A TRIGGER

Researchers have suspected for some time that the body's inflammatory response may play a critical role in heart attacks and strokes. It is well known that risk factors for heart attack and stroke include obesity, high cholesterol levels, high blood pressure, and smoking. Blood tests in a 1988 study in Finland, however, showed the presence of a bacterium called *Chlamydia pneumoniae* inside the cells of people with coronary artery disease. It seemed apparent, however, that *C. pneumoniae* alone was not a risk factor or cause of heart disease.

Researchers in the Helsinki Heart Study also looked for the presence of human heat-shock protein 60 (hHsp60), indicating an immune response which could possibly lead to atherosclerosis, and of C-reactive protein (CRP), which sends white blood cells to the site of injury or infection but can cause harm if prolonged or excessive. An eight-year follow-up of this study showed that the risk for heart disease increased when levels of *C. pneumoniae* or hHsp60 antibodies were high. However, the risk was greatest when all three factors were elevated, indicating a possible synergistic effect. It was concluded that chronic infection, autoimmunity, and inflammation in combination contributed to coronary events in the study population.

The research of Dr. Paul Ridker of Boston's Brigham and Women's Hospital further showed that levels of CRP over 3 milligrams per liter of blood more than doubled the risk of heart attack and stroke. A test for CRP levels is available, but there are questions of who should be tested and when.

High CRP levels have also been associated with being overweight, a known risk factor for heart disease. Adjusting for age, smoking, and other chronic diseases, the association was especially strong for obese women, who were six times as likely to have elevated CRP levels, while obese men were twice as likely. One theory to explain this outcome would be that many overweight or obese persons have persistent low-grade inflammation. This may be the result of another protein, interleukin 6, produced by fat tissue, which in turn stimulates the production of CRP by the liver.

Scientific research continues to establish definitive links between heart disease and chronic infections, inflammation, and autoimmune conditions. These links could lead to attacking the basic processes of atherosclerosis, to treatment with anti-inflammatory drugs, and to the prevention of heart attacks and stroke.

—*Martha Oehmke Loustaunau, Ph.D.*

an attack, helped rule out a heart attack 70 percent of the time when used with standard heart attack tests during initial studies.

The domains of preventive surgery and specialized drug treatment to prevent dangerous blood clotting are vast. Statistically, the most important and widely practiced operations that were developed in the later decades of the twentieth century were replacement of the aortic valve, the coronary bypass operation, and, with greater or lesser degrees of success, the actual transplantation of voluntary donors' hearts in the place of those belonging to heart disease patients. Coronary bypass operations involve the attachment to the myocardium of healthy arteries to carry the blood that can no longer pass through the patient's clogged arterial passageways; these healthy arteries are taken by the heart surgeon from other areas of the patient's own body.

Another sphere of medical technology, that of balloon angioplasty, held out a major nonsurgical promise of preventing deterioration of the arteries leading to the heart. This sophisticated form of treatment involves the careful, temporary introduction of inflatable devices inside clogged arteries, which are then stretched to increase the space within the arterial passageway for blood to flow. By the 1990's, however, doctors recognized one disadvantage of balloon angioplasty. By stretching the essential blood vessels being treated, this procedure either stretches the plaque with the artery or breaks loose debris that remains behind, creating a danger of renewed clogging. Thus another technique, called atherectomy, was developed to clear certain coronary arteries, as well as arteries elsewhere in the body.

confirm or rule out a heart attack in patients visiting emergency rooms (ERs). Nearly five million Americans visit ERs each year with possible heart attack symptoms but only about one in five actually is experiencing a heart attack. The test, which uses the metal cobalt to hunt changes in a blood protein that occur during

Atherectomy involves a motorized catheter device resembling a miniature drill that is inserted into clogged arteries. As the drill turns, material that is literally shaved off the interior walls of arteries is retrieved through a tiny collection receptacle. Early experimentation, especially to treat the large anterior descending coronary artery on the left side of the heart, showed that atherectomy was 87 percent effective, whereas, on the average, angioplasty removed only 63 percent of the blockage. In addition, similar efforts to provide internal, nonsurgical treatment of clogged arteries using laser beams were being made by the early 1990's.

PERSPECTIVE AND PROSPECTS

The modern conception of cardiology dates from William Harvey's seventeenth century discovery of the relationship between the heart's function as a pump and the circulatory "restoration" of blood. Harvey's much more scientific views replaced centuries-old conceptions of the heart as a blood-warming device only.

Although substantial anatomical advances were made over the next two centuries that helped explain most of the vital functions of the heart, it was not until the early decades of the twentieth century that science developed therapeutic methods to deal with problems that frequently cause heart attacks. Drugs that affect the liver's production of substances necessary for normal coagulation of blood, for example, were discovered in the 1930's. A large variety of such anticoagulants have since been developed to help thin the blood of patients vulnerable to blood clotting. Other drugs, including certain antibiotics, are used to treat persons whose susceptiblitity to infection is known to be high. In these cases, the simple action of dislodging bacteria from the teeth when brushing can cause an invasion of the vital parts of the heart by an infection. This bacterial endocarditis, the result of the actual destruction of heart tissue or the sudden release of clots of infectious residue, could lead to a heart attack in such individuals although they have no other symptoms of identifiable heart disease.

The most spectacular advance in the scientific treatment of potential heart attack victims, however, has been in the field of cardiac surgery. Many advances in open heart surgery date from the late 1950's, when the development of heart and lung replacement machines made it safe enough to substitute electronic monitors for some of the organism's normal body functions. Before the 1950's, operations had been limited to surgical treatment of the major blood vessels surrounding the heart.

Various technical methods have also been developed that help identify problems early enough for drug therapy to be attempted before the decision to perform surgery is made. The use of catheters, which are threaded into the coronary organ using the same vessels that transport blood, became the most effective way of locating problematic areas. The process known as angiography, which uses X rays to trace the course of radio-opaque dyes injected through a catheter into local heart areas under study, can actually tell doctors if drug therapy is having the desired effects. In cases where such tests show that preventive drug therapy is not effective, an early decision to perform surgery can be made, preventing the source of coronary trouble from multiplying the patient's chances of suffering a heart attack.

—Byron D. Cannon, Ph.D.

See also Angina; Arrhythmias; Arteriosclerosis; Bypass surgery; Cardiac arrest; Cardiac rehabilitation; Cardiology; Cardiopulmonary resuscitation (CPR); Cholesterol; Circulation; Critical care; Echocardiography; Electrocardiography (ECG or EKG); Embolism; Emergency medicine; Heart; Heart disease; Heart failure; Heart transplantation; Heart valve replacement; Hypercholesterolemia; Hyperlipidemia; Hypertension; Ischemia; Mitral valve prolapse; Pacemaker implantation; Palpitations; Phlebitis; Resuscitation; Thrombolytic therapy and TPA; Thrombosis and thrombus.

FOR FURTHER INFORMATION:

American Heart Association. http://www.american heart.org/. Site provides comprehensive information on heart disease and conditions, healthy lifestyles, and resources, and provides interactive health tools.

Baum, Seth J. *The Total Guide to a Healthy Heart: Integrative Strategies for Preventing and Reversing Heart Disease.* New York: Kensington, 2000. This book brings together the practices of both conventional and alternative approaches to reversing heart disease and maintaining heart health. Offers great insight into why the integrative approach to maintaining a healthy heart will be the medicine of the new millennium.

Berra, Kathleen, et al. *Heart Attack! Advice for Patients by Patients.* New Haven, Conn.: Yale University Press, 2002. After an introductory chapter detailing diagnosis, treatment, and rehabilitation, offers eleven other chapters authored by heart attack survivors—including several medical professionals—and their lessons learned. Diet and nutrition, advances in treatment, and cardiac rehabilitation programs are covered.

Crawford, Michael, ed. *Current Diagnosis and Treatment in Cardiology.* 2d ed. New York: Lange Medical Books/McGraw-Hill, 2003. Discusses advances in cardiac diagnostics, treatments, and prognostic indicators and includes extensive information on prevention techniques.

Eagle, Kim A., and Ragavendra R. Baliga. *Practical Cardiology: Evaluation and Treatment of Common Cardiovascular Disorders.* Philadelphia: Lippincott Williams & Wilkins, 2003. Details advances in cardiac medicine.

Gersh, Bernard J., ed. *The Mayo Clinic Heart Book.* 2d ed. New York: William Morrow, 2000. One of the most respected texts for laypeople on heart disease. Covers all aspects of anatomy, physiology, diagnosis, treatment, and prevention.

Gillis, Jack. *The Heart Attack Prevention and Recovery Handbook.* Point Roberts, Wash.: Hartley & Marks, 1997. Using simple, brief explanations, Gillis's text covers essential information that heart attack victims and families need immediately for reassurance and recovery. Presents excellent discussions of emotional effects on patients, medications, and treatments.

Kligfield, Paul. *The Cardiac Recovery Handbook: The Complete Guide to Life After Heart Attack or Heart Surgery.* 2d ed. Long New York: Hatherleigh Press, 2006. A clearly written book that details all aspects of cardiac recovery, including the initial diagnosis of heart disease, medications and surgical options, hospitalization, rehabilitation, diet and exercise, and financial planning.

Yannios, Thomas A. *The Heart Disease Breakthrough: The Ten-Step Program That Can Save Your Life.* Rev. ed. New York: Wiley, 1999. Yannios, associate director of critical care and nutritional support at Ellis Hospital in Schenectady, New York, describes the smallest components of cholesterol, which can do more damage to the heart than the overall LDL levels that concern so many people.

Zaret, Barry L., Marvin Moser, and Lawrence S. Cohen, eds. *Yale University School of Medicine Heart Book.* New York: William Morrow, 1992. Discusses the prevention and control of heart disease. Illustrated, with a bibliography and an index.

HEART DISEASE
DISEASE/DISORDER

ANATOMY OR SYSTEM AFFECTED: Blood vessels, circulatory system, heart

SPECIALTIES AND RELATED FIELDS: Cardiology, family medicine, internal medicine

DEFINITION: One of the leading causes of death in many industrialized nations; heart diseases include atherosclerotic disease, coronary artery disease, cardiac arrhythmias, and stenosis, among others.

KEY TERMS:

cardiac arrhythmia: a disturbance in the heartbeat

coronary arteries: blood vessels surrounding the heart that provide nourishment and oxygen to heart tissue

nodes: areas of electrochemical transmission within the heart that regulate the heartbeat

plaque: an accumulation of matter within artery walls that can impede blood flow

CAUSES AND SYMPTOMS

The heart is a fist-sized organ located in the upper left quarter of the chest. It consists of four chambers: the right and left atria on top and the right and left ventricles at the bottom. The chambers are enclosed in three layers of tissue: the outer layer (epicardium), the middle layer (myocardium), and the inner layer (endocardium). Surrounding the entire organ is the pericardium, a thin layer of tissue that forms a protective covering for the heart. The heart also contains various nodes that transmit electrochemical signals, causing heart muscle tissue to contract and relax in the pumping action that carries blood to organs and cells throughout the body.

Signals from the brain cause the heart to contract rhythmically in a sequence of motions that move the blood from the right atrium down through the tricuspid valve into the right ventricle. From here, blood is pushed through the pulmonary valve into the lungs, where it fulfills one of its major functions: to pick up oxygen in exchange for carbon dioxide. From the lungs, the blood is pumped back into the heart, entering the left atrium from which it is pumped down through the mitral valve into the left ventricle. Blood is then pushed through the aortic valve into the main artery of the body, the aorta, from which it starts its journey to the organs and cells. As it passes through the arteries of the gastrointestinal system, the blood picks up nutrients which, along with the oxygen that it has taken from the lungs, are brought to the cells and exchanged for waste products and carbon dioxide. The blood then enters the veins, through which it is eventually returned to the heart. The heart nourishes and supplies itself with oxygen through the coronary arteries, so called because they sit on top of the heart like a crown and extend down the sides.

The heart diseases collectively include all the disorders that can befall every part of the heart muscle: the pericardium, epicardium, myocardium, endocardium, atria, ventricles, valves, coronary arteries, and nodes. The most significant sites of heart diseases are the coronary arteries and the nodes; their malfunction can cause coronary artery disease and cardiac arrhythmias, respectively. These two disorders are responsible for the majority of heart disease cases.

Coronary artery disease occurs when matter such as cholesterol and fibrous material collects and stiffens on the inner walls of the coronary arteries. This plaque that forms may narrow the passage through which blood flows, reducing the amount of blood delivered to the heart, or may build up and clog the artery entirely, shutting off the flow of blood to the heart. In the former case, when the coronary artery is narrowed, the condition is called ischemic heart disease. Because the most common cause of ischemia is narrowing of the coronary arteries to the myocardium, another designation of the condition is myocardial ischemia, referring to the fact that blood flow to the myocardium is impeded. Accumulation of plaque within the coronary arteries is referred to as coronary atherosclerosis.

As the coronary arteries become clogged and then narrow, they can fail to deliver the required oxygen to the heart muscle, particularly during stress or physical effort. The heart's need for oxygen exceeds the arteries' ability to supply it. The patient usually feels a sharp, choking pain, called angina pectoris. Not all people who have coronary ischemia, however, experience anginal pain; these people are said to have silent ischemia.

The danger in coronary artery disease is that the accumulation of plaque will progress to the point where the coronary artery is clogged completely and no blood is delivered to the part of the heart serviced by that artery. The result is a myocardial infarction (commonly called a heart attack), in which some myocardial cells die when they fail to receive blood. The rough, uneven texture of the plaque instead may cause the formation of a blood clot, or thrombus, which closes the artery in a condition called coronary thrombosis.

Although coronary ischemia is usually thought of as a disease of middle and old age, in fact it starts much earlier. Autopsies of accident victims in their teens and twenties, as well as young soldiers killed in battle, show that coronary atherosclerosis is often well advanced in young persons. Some reasons for these findings and for why the rates of coronary artery disease and death began to rise in the twentieth century have been proposed. While antibiotics and vaccines reduced the mortality of some bacterial and some viral infections, Western societies underwent significant changes in lifestyle and eating habits that contributed to the rise of coronary heart disease: high-fat diets, obesity, and the stressful pace of life in a modern industrial society. Further, cigarette smoking, once almost a universal habit, has been shown to be highly pathogenic (disease-causing), contributing significantly to the development of heart disease, as well as lung cancer, emphysema, bronchitis, and other disorders. In the early and middle decades of the twentieth century, coronary heart disease was considered primarily an ailment of middle-aged and older men. As women began smoking, however, the incidence shifted so that coronary artery disease became almost equally prevalent, and equally lethal, among men and women.

Other conditions such as hypertension or diabetes mellitus are considered precursors of coronary artery disease. Hypertension, or high blood pressure, is an extremely common condition that, if unchecked, can contribute to both the development and the progression of coronary artery disease. Over the years, high blood pressure subjects arterial walls to constant stress. In response, the walls thicken and stiffen. This "hardening" of the arteries encourages the accumulation of fatty and fibrous plaque on inner artery walls. In patients with diabetes mellitus, blood sugar (glucose) levels rise either because the patient is deficient in insulin or because the

---

INFORMATION ON HEART DISEASE

CAUSES: Pulmonary problems, atherosclerosis, smoking, diabetes, hypertension, infection, high-fat diet and obesity, stress

SYMPTOMS: Varies; can include pain, sweating, shortness of breath, inability to exercise, irregular heartbeat, dizziness, loss of consciousness

DURATION: Acute or chronic

TREATMENTS: Drug therapy, surgery, preventive medication, exercise, dietary change, medical devices

insulin that the patient produces is inefficient at removing glucose from the blood. High glucose levels favor high fat levels in the blood, which can cause atherosclerosis.

Cardiac arrhythmias are the next major cause of morbidity and mortality among the heart diseases. Inside the heart, an electrochemical network regulates the contractions and relaxations that form the heartbeat. In the excitation or contraction phase, a chain of electrochemical impulses starts in the upper part of the right atrium in the heart's pacemaker, the sinoatrial or sinus node. The impulses travel through internodal tracts (pathways from one node to another) to an area between the atrium and the right ventricle called the atrioventricular node. The impulses then enter the bundle of His, which carries them to the left atrium and left ventricle. After the series of contractions is complete, the heart relaxes for a brief moment before another cycle is begun. On the average, the process is repeated sixty to eighty times a minute.

This is normal rhythm, the regular, healthy heartbeat. Dysfunction at any point along the electrochemical pathway, however, can cause an arrhythmia. Arrhythmias range greatly in their effects and their potential for bodily damage. They can be completely unnoticeable, merely annoying, debilitating, or frightening. They can cause blood clots to form in the heart, and they can cause sudden death.

The arrhythmic heart can beat too quickly (tachycardia) or too slowly (bradycardia). The contractions of the various chambers can become unsynchronized, or out of step with one another. For example, in atrial flutter or atrial fibrillation, the upper chambers of the heart beat faster, out of synchronization with the ventricles. In ventricular tachycardia, ventricular contractions increase, out of synchronization with the atria. In ventricular fibrillation, ventricular contractions lose all rhythmicity and become uncoordinated to the point at which the heart is no longer able to pump blood. Cardiac death can then occur unless the patient receives immediate treatment.

An arrhythmic disorder called heart block occurs when the impulse from the pacemaker is "blocked." Its progress through the atrioventricular node and the bundle of His may be slow or irregular, or the impulse may fail to reach its target tissues. The disorder is rated in three degrees. First-degree heart block is detectable only on an electrocardiogram (ECG), in which the movement of the impulse from the atria to the ventricles is seen to be slowed. In second-degree heart block,

only some of the impulses generated reach from the atria to the ventricles; the pulse becomes irregular. Third-degree heart block is the most serious manifestation of this disorder: No impulses from the atria reach the ventricles. The heart rate may slow dramatically, and the blood flow to the brain can be reduced, causing dizziness or loss of consciousness.

Disorders that affect the heart valves usually involve stenosis (narrowing), which reduces the size of the valve opening; physical malfunction of the valve; or both. These disorders can be attributable to infection (such as rheumatic fever) or to tissue damage, or they can be congenital. If a valve has narrowed, the passage of blood from one heart chamber to another is impeded. In the case of mitral stenosis, the mitral valve between the left atrium and the left ventricle is narrowed. Blood flow to the left ventricle is reduced, and blood is retained in the left atrium, causing the atrium to enlarge as pressure builds in the chamber. This pressure forces blood back into the lungs, creating a condition called pulmonary edema, in which fluid collects in the air sacs of the lungs. Similarly, malfunctions of the heart valves that cause them to open and close inefficiently can interfere with the flow of blood into the heart, through it, and out of it. This impairment may cause structural changes in the heart that can be life-threatening.

Heart failure may be a consequence of many disease conditions. It occurs primarily in the elderly. In this condition, the heart becomes inefficient at pumping blood. If the failure is on the right side of the heart, blood is forced back into the body, causing edema in the lower legs. If the failure is on the left side of the heart, blood is forced back into the lungs, causing pulmonary edema. There are many manifestations of heart failure, including shortness of breath, fatigue, and weakness.

Numerous diseases afflict the tissues of the heart wall—the epicardium, myocardium, and endocardium, as well as the pericardium. They are often caused by bacterial or viral infection, but they may also result from tissue trauma or a variety of toxic agents.

TREATMENT AND THERAPY

The main tools for diagnosing heart disease are the stethoscope, the electrocardiograph (ECG), and the X ray. With the stethoscope the doctor listens to heart sounds, which provide information about many heart functions such as rhythm and the status of the valves. The doctor can determine whether the heart is functioning normally in pumping blood from one chamber into the other, into the lungs, and into the aorta. The ECG gives the doctor a graph representation of heart function. Twelve to fifteen electrodes are placed on various parts of the body, including the head, chest, legs, and arms. The activities of the heart are printed on a strip of paper as waves or tracings. The doctor analyzes the printout for evidence of heart abnormalities, changes in heart function, signs of a heart attack, or other problems. Generally, the electrocardiographic examination is conducted with the patient at rest. In some situations, however, the doctor wishes to view heart action during physical stress. In this case, the electrodes are attached to the patient and the patient is required to exercise on a treadmill or stationary bicycle. The physician can see what changes in heart function occur when the cardiac workload is increased. The X ray gives the doctor a visual picture of the heart. Any enlargements or abnormalities can be seen, as well as the status of the aorta, pulmonary arteries, and other structures.

Another standard diagnostic tool is the echocardiograph. High-frequency sound waves are pointed at the heart from outside the body. The sound waves bounce against heart tissue and are shown on a monitor. The general configuration of the heart can be seen, as well as the shape and thickness of the chamber walls, the valves, and the large blood vessels leading to and from the heart. Velocity and direction of blood flow through the valves can be determined.

Various procedures can help the doctor assess the degree of ischemia within the heart. In one test, a radioactive isotope is injected into a vein and its dispersion in the heart is read by a scanner. This procedure can show which parts of the heart are being deprived of oxygen. In another test using a radioactive isotope, the reading is made while the patient exercises, in order to detect any changes in expansion and contraction of the heart wall that would indicate impaired circulation. The coronary angiogram gives a picture of the blockage within the coronary arteries. A thin tube called a catheter is threaded into a coronary artery, and a dye that is opaque to X rays is released. The X-ray picture will reveal narrowings in the artery resulting from plaque buildup.

The main goals of therapy in treating heart diseases are to cure the condition, if possible, and otherwise help the patient live a normal life and prevent the condition from becoming worse. In coronary artery disease, the physician seeks to maintain blood flow to the heart and to prevent heart attack. Hundreds of medications are available for this purpose, including vasodilators (agents that relax blood vessel walls and increase their capacity to carry blood). Chief among the coronary vasodilators are nitroglycerin and other drugs in the nitrate family. Also, calcium channel blockers are often used to dilate blood vessels. Beta-blocking agents are used because they reduce the heart's need for oxygen and alleviate the symptoms of angina. In addition, various support measures are recommended by physicians to stop plaque buildup and halt the progress of the disease. These include losing weight, reducing fats in the diet, and stopping smoking. The physician also treats concomitant illnesses that can contribute to the progress of coronary artery disease, such as hypertension and diabetes.

Sometimes medications and diet are not fully successful, and the ischemia continues. The cardiologist can unblock a clogged artery by a procedure called angioplasty. The physician threads a catheter containing a tiny balloon to the point of the blockage. The balloon is inflated to widen the inner diameter of the artery, and blood flow is increased. This procedure is often successful, although it may have to be repeated. In atherectomy, a miniature drill shaves off the plaque, which is then removed. If neither procedure is successful, coronary bypass surgery may be indicated. In this procedure, clogged coronary arteries are replaced with healthy blood vessels from other parts of the body.

When coronary artery disease progresses to a heart attack, the patient should be treated in the hospital or similar facility. The possibility of sudden death is high during the attack and remains high until the patient is stabilized. Emergency measures are undertaken to minimize the extent of heart damage, reduce heart work, keep oxygen flowing to all parts of the body, and regulate blood pressure and heartbeat.

Cardiac arrhythmias can be managed by a variety of medications and procedures. Digitalis, guanidine, procainamide, tocanamide, and atropine are widely used to restore normal heart rhythm. In acute situations, the patient's heart rhythm can be restored by electrical cardioversion, in which an electrical stimulus is applied from outside the body to regulate the heartbeat. When a slowed heartbeat cannot be controlled by medication, a pacemaker may be implanted to regulate heart rhythm.

Treatment of heart valve disorders and disorders of the heart wall is directed at alleviating the individual condition. Antibiotics and/or valve replacement surgery may be required. In many cases, valve disorders can be completely corrected. Cardiac transplantation remains a possible treatment for some heart patients.

This is an option for comparatively few patients because there are ten times as many candidates for heart transplants as there are available donor hearts.

PERSPECTIVE AND PROSPECTS

Heart disease became a major killer in the United States in the twentieth century. In the early decades, the best that the medical community could do was to treat symptoms. Since then, the emphasis has shifted to prevention. Hundreds of investigative studies have been undertaken to determine the causes of the most prevalent heart dysfunction, coronary artery disease. Many of these studies have involved tens of thousands of subjects, and they point to a general consensus that coronary artery disease is a multifactorial disorder, the primary elements of which are cholesterol and other fatty substances circulating in the bloodstream, smoking, diabetes, high blood pressure, stress, and obesity.

The reasons that mortality from heart disease is declining include improved medications and treatment modalities, and much credit has to be given to the success of preventive measures. Millions of Americans have stopped smoking and have begun watching their diets. Entire industries are devoted to helping Americans eat more intelligently. While fast-food outlets continued to offer high-fat standards, such as hot dogs and hamburgers, they have also added salads and leaner selections.

Perhaps most important, medical and sociological authorities have turned their attention to children. Because advanced atherosclerosis has been detected in young men and women, cholesterol-watching has become a major preoccupation with parents and school dieticians. In addition, national programs have been instituted to discourage smoking among the young. Whether the rates of coronary heart disease will be lower in these individuals than in their parents remains to be seen, but the success of these measures in the older populations indicates that the prognosis is good.

The prognosis is also good for other heart diseases. New drugs continue to be licensed for the treatment of arrhythmias, and more versatile and reliable pacemakers increase the prospects of a normal life for many patients. Improvements in heart surgery have been particularly impressive, especially those for managing congenital heart defects in neonates and infants. Heart transplants have been successfully performed on these patients, and numerous other procedures promise significant improvement in the prospects of young people with heart disease.

Rheumatic fever, however, one of the major causes of heart disease in children, remains a threat. No vaccine is available for immunization against the streptococcus strains that cause rheumatic fever, but fortunately there are effective antibiotics to control infection in these patients. Rheumatic fever usually develops subsequent to a throat infection. Careful monitoring of the child with a sore throat can avoid progression of the infection to rheumatic fever.

—C. Richard Falcon

See also Aneurysms; Angina; Arrhythmias; Arteriosclerosis; Blue baby syndrome; Bypass surgery; Cardiac arrest; Cardiac rehabilitation; Cardiology; Cardiology, pediatric; Cholesterol; Circulation; Claudication; Congenital heart disease; Diabetes mellitus; Echocardiography; Electrocardiography (ECG or EKG); Embolism; Endocarditis; Heart; Heart attack; Heart failure; Heart transplantation; Heart valve replacement; Hypercholesterolemia; Hyperlipidemia; Hypertension; Ischemia; Mitral valve prolapse; Obesity; Pacemaker implantation; Palpitations; Phlebitis; Pulmonary hypertension; Thrombolytic therapy and TPA; Thrombosis and thrombus; Varicose veins; Venous insufficiency.

FOR FURTHER INFORMATION:

American Heart Association. http://www.american heart.org/. Site provides comprehensive information on heart disease and conditions, healthy lifestyles, and resources, and provides interactive health tools.

Baum, Seth J. *The Total Guide to a Healthy Heart: Integrative Strategies for Preventing and Reversing Heart Disease.* New York: Kensington, 2000. This book brings together the practices of both conventional and alternative approaches to reversing heart disease and maintaining heart health. Offers great insight into why the integrative approach to maintaining a healthy heart will be the medicine of the new millennium.

Gersh, Bernard J., ed. *The Mayo Clinic Heart Book.* 2d ed. New York: William Morrow, 2000. One of the most respected texts for laypeople on heart disease. Covers all aspects of anatomy, physiology, diagnosis, treatment, and prevention.

Goldberg, Nieca. *Women Are Not Small Men: Life-Saving Strategies for Preventing and Healing Heart Disease in Women.* New York: Random House, 2002. Written by the founder and chief of the Women's Heart Program at New York's Lenox Hill Hospital, details the way in which women experience heart disease and recovery in fundamentally different ways than men do. Physiology, symptoms, and treatment and medications are scrutinized.

Kramer, Gerri Freid, and Shari Mauer. *Parent's Guide to Children's Congenital Heart Defects: What They Are, How to Treat Them, How to Cope with Them.* New York: Three Rivers Press, 2001. Experts in pediatric cardiology provide easy-to-understand answers to help parents coping with a child's heart disease. Includes the latest information on diagnosis, treatment options, surgery, aftercare, and growing up with heart defects, as well as stories from parents who have lived through the ordeal.

Litin, Scott C., ed. *Mayo Clinic Family Health Book.* 3d ed. New York: HarperResource, 2003. Perhaps the best general medical text for the layperson, this book covers the entire medical field. The sections on the heart diseases are exemplary for clarity and thoroughness.

Piscatella, Joseph, and Barry Franklin. *Take a Load Off Your Heart: 109 Things You Can Do to Prevent or Reverse Heart Disease.* New York: Workman, 2002. Easy-to-follow guide that details such preventive measures as managing stress, improving diet, and exercising and offers more than one hundred practical tips for preventing, stabilizing, and reversing heart disease.

Taylor, George J., ed. *Primary Care Management of Heart Disease.* St. Louis: Mosby, 2000. A resource on the therapy and diagnosis of heart disease. Includes bibliographical references and an index.

Yannios, Thomas A. *The Heart Disease Breakthrough: The Ten-Step Program That Can Save Your Life.* Rev. ed. New York: Wiley, 1999. Yannios, associate director of critical care and nutritional support at Ellis Hospital in Schenectady, New York, describes the smallest components of cholesterol, which can do more damage to the heart than the overall LDL levels that concern so many people.

Zaret, Barry L., Marvin Moser, and Lawrence S. Cohen, eds. *Yale University School of Medicine Heart Book.* New York: William Morrow, 1992. This text will give the reader a clear understanding of the various heart diseases, as well as of methods of treating and preventing them.

Zipes, Douglas P., et al., eds. *Braunwald's Heart Disease: A Textbook of Cardiovascular Medicine.* 7th ed. Philadelphia: Elsevier Saunders, 2005. A comprehensive reference work for students, residents, and clinicians.

HEART FAILURE
DISEASE/DISORDER

ANATOMY OR SYSTEM AFFECTED: Circulatory system, heart

SPECIALTIES AND RELATED FIELDS: Cardiology, internal medicine, vascular medicine

DEFINITION: A condition in which the heart cannot pump enough blood to meet the needs of the body because its ability to contract is impaired.

KEY TERMS:

congestive heart failure: the stage of heart failure that occurs when a backup of pressure results in accumulation of fluid in the veins and tissues

coronary arteries: the arteries that supply blood to the heart muscle

diuretic: a drug that stimulates the kidneys to eliminate more salt and water from the body

edema: the accumulation of fluid around the cells in tissue

ejection fraction: the ratio of the stroke volume to the residual volume, expressed as a percentage

hormone: a chemical messenger released by a gland which is carried by the blood to its target

inotropic agent: a drug that improves the ability of the heart muscle to contract

optimal length: the length of a heart muscle cell at which stimulation can elicit the maximum possible force development

residual volume: the blood volume left in the heart chamber at the end of a heartbeat

stroke volume: the blood volume leaving either the right or the left side of the heart with each beat; each side usually ejects the same volume per beat

vasodilator: a drug that relaxes blood vessels

CAUSES AND SYMPTOMS

The circulation of the blood has many functions. It is essential for the delivery of oxygen, nutrients, and elements of the immune system to tissues. It also contributes to regulation and communication between different parts of the body by moving chemical messengers from where they are produced to where they have a biological effect. The delivery of warm blood to the surface of the skin is one essential element in temperature control. The blood pressure determines how much water can move across the exchange surfaces in the kidneys, thus affecting water balance in the body. The movement of blood through the kidneys, the lungs, and all tissues is important for waste removal.

All these functions depend on the ability of the heart

INFORMATION ON HEART FAILURE

CAUSES: Varies; can include inherited or acquired diseases, allergic reactions, connective tissue or metabolic abnormalities, high blood pressure, anatomical defects, toxic quantities of drugs, sudden blockage of coronary arteries

SYMPTOMS: Labored breathing; light-headedness; generalized weakness; cold, pale, or even bluish skin tone; accumulation of fluid in extremities and/or lungs; distended neck veins; abnormal heart rate and rhythm; chest pain

DURATION: Acute or chronic

TREATMENTS: Drug therapy, surgery, preventive medication, exercise, dietary change, medical devices

to contract and eject blood. Blood is pumped, in two serial circuits, from the right heart through the lungs into the left heart and from the left heart around the body back to the right heart. In each circuit, the blood travels through large arteries, then to smaller arterioles, to capillaries (where exchange takes place), and back via small venules and veins to the heart. Heart failure describes the situation in which heart function is reduced. While still able to beat, the heart is unable to meet the circulatory needs of the body. That is, the heart muscle is unable to contract enough to pump the blood adequately.

The severity of the heart failure can be gauged by the ejection fraction, a measure of the pumping capacity of the heart. It is the percentage calculated from the stroke volume (the volume of blood leaving a heart chamber with each beat) divided by the residual volume (the volume left in the heart chamber at the end of a heartbeat). Thus the ejection fraction measures how much blood in the heart chamber can actually leave when the heartbeat occurs. In normal, healthy hearts, this value is 100 percent: The amount that stays in the heart is approximately equal to the amount that leaves it. In mild or moderate heart failure, it ranges approximately between 15 and 40 percent: Less blood leaves the heart with each beat, and more blood remains behind.

The pressure inside the heart at the end of a heartbeat is another index of heart performance. If the heart is failing and more blood is left behind in the heart at the end of a beat, the pressure inside the heart at the end of the beat will be increased. In cases of severe failure, the pressure in the arteries outside the heart will fall.

In failure, the heart cannot supply enough blood for all the functions of the circulation. This fact accounts for the variety of symptoms that accompany heart failure: labored breathing; light-headedness; generalized weakness; cold, pale, or even bluish skin tone; and accumulation of fluid in the extremities and/or lungs. Other possible symptoms include distended neck veins, accumulation of fluid in the abdomen, abnormal heart rate and rhythm, and chest pain.

The specific symptoms of the condition depend on the type of failure, its severity, its underlying causes, and the ways in which the body attempts to compensate. There are several ways to categorize types of heart failure: acute or chronic, forward or backward, and right-sided or left-sided.

Acute heart failure refers to a sudden decrease in heart function. It can be caused by toxic quantities of drugs, anesthetics, or metals or by certain disease states, such as infections. Most often, however, it is caused by a sudden blockage of the coronary arteries supplying the heart muscle. A sudden blockage caused by a blood clot can induce a heart attack and subsequent heart failure, causing chest pain and often abnormal heart rate or rhythm. These effects are sometimes so rapid that there is little time for the body to attempt compensation.

Chronic heart failure is a progressive reduction in heart function that develops over time. It can be caused by inherited or acquired diseases, allergic reactions, connective tissue or metabolic abnormalities, high blood pressure, and anatomical defects. The most common cause, however, is coronary artery disease. This disease narrows blood vessels and leads to a reduction in the amount of blood reaching the heart muscle. It causes reduced oxygen availability and, eventually, a reduction in the ability of the heart muscle to contract.

In the early stages of chronic failure, the hormone and nervous systems promote compensation in the heart, blood vessels, and kidneys to help the heart continue to pump enough blood. These systems stimulate the heart muscle directly to make it beat harder. They also take advantage of the fact that modest stretching of the heart muscle increases its ability to contract. By stimulating the blood vessels to contract, more blood moves back toward the heart, causing a cold, pale, or even bluish skin tone. Stimulation of the kidney to retain water and sodium results in an increase in blood volume, which also moves more blood back to the heart. In each case, the heart muscle is stretched by these increases and, therefore, can contract harder.

Yet these reactions do not constitute a long-term solution. The heart muscle can become fatigued from overwork and can become overstretched. A resulting accumulation of fluid in the heart reduces its ability to contract. Compensation fails, and the additional fluid in the blood starts to back up in the circulation. This condition is called backward heart failure. At the same time, the heart is unable to pump hard enough to move the blood forward against the higher resistance caused by the contraction of the blood vessels. This condition is termed forward heart failure. Congestive heart failure is the stage that occurs when the backup of pressure is worsened by fluid retention and blood vessel contraction. The congestion, or accumulation of fluid, occurs in the veins and tissues.

Left-sided or right-sided heart failure can occur

alone or together. The right side of the heart pumps blood to the lungs to be oxygenated, and the left side of the heart pumps oxygenated blood to the organs of the body. Normally, these two sides are well matched so that the same volume moves through each side. When the right heart cannot contract properly, however, blood accumulates upstream in the veins and somewhat less blood reaches the lungs to pick up oxygen, resulting in distended veins and shortness of breath. It is primarily a backward heart failure. Fluid can back up in the veins and increase pressure in the capillaries so that it starts to leak out of the circulation into the surrounding tissues. This leads to an accumulation of fluid (called edema), especially in the liver and lower extremities. In isolated right-sided heart failure, this pressure rarely backs up to such an extent that it causes problems through the rest of the circulation to the left side of the heart.

In contrast, when the left side of the heart cannot

IN THE NEWS:
HOMOCYSTEINE LEVELS AND CONGESTIVE HEART FAILURE

In the January, 2003, issue of the *Journal of the American Medical Association* (JAMA), a team of researchers from the National Heart, Lung, and Blood Institute's Framingham Heart Study, the U.S. Department of Agriculture Human Nutrition Research Center on Aging, and Boston University reported that elevated levels of total homocysteine in the blood are associated with an increased risk for congestive heart failure, a condition in which the heart is unable to maintain adequate blood circulation to the tissues.

The correlation between elevated homocysteine levels and increased risk of cardiovascular disease in general—and specifically myocardial infarction (heart attack), arteriosclerosis, coronary heart disease, and stroke—has been well established, but this was the first study to pinpoint congestive heart failure.

Homocysteine is an amino acid, but unlike most amino acids, it is not a component of proteins. Its primary role seems to be to act as an intermediate in the formation and breakdown of other molecules. Excess levels of homocysteine probably result from its accumulation when its conversion to the next intermediate occurs too slowly, a process often thought to be caused by folic acid deficiency. This conversion

can be accelerated by the administration of folic acid.

The subjects of this eight-year study were 2,491 participants of the Framingham Heart Study, who at the start of the study had no histories of myocardial infarction or congestive heart failure. Their average age was seventy-two years. Patients were examined at various times after the initial measurement of plasma homocysteine, and the examinations included plasma homocysteine measurement, blood pressure measurement, electrocardiogram evaluation, systematic assessment of cardiovascular risk factors, and a review of cardiovascular events in each patient's medical record. There were 156 patients who developed congestive heart failure, and the association between plasma homocysteine levels and the incidence of congestive heart failure was examined. Patients with higher-than-average homocysteine levels were more likely to develop congestive heart failure. Women with higher-than-average homocysteine levels had twice the risk for congestive heart failure when compared to the total female population of the study. Researchers noted, however, that additional studies to evaluate the effect of folic acid supplementation on the risk of congestive heart failure are needed.

—*Lorraine Lica, Ph.D.*

contract properly, it can back up pressure so badly that it creates a pressure overload against which the right side of the heart must pump. This increase in the workload on the right side of the heart frequently leads to two-sided heart failure. This outcome is especially common since the disease conditions that exist in the left side are likely to exist on the right as well. In left-sided heart failure, blood accumulates upstream in the lungs, increasing pressure enough to cause a leakage of fluid into the lungs (pulmonary edema). This leakage interferes with oxygen uptake and therefore causes shortness of breath. It also results in inadequate blood flow to the body's tissues, including the muscles and brain, resulting in generalized weakness and light-headedness. Left-sided heart failure is thus both a backward and a forward failure.

TREATMENT AND THERAPY

Treatments for cardiac failure, like its symptoms, depend on a variety of factors. The first goal of treatment is to avoid any obvious precipitating causes of the failure, such as alcohol, drugs, the cessation of essential medications, acute stress, a salt-loaded diet, overexercise, infection, illness, or surgery. The next approach is to take the simplest measures to reduce distension of the heart by controlling salt and water retention and to decrease the workload of the heart by altering the circulatory needs of the tissues. The former can be achieved by dietary salt restriction, restriction of fluid consumption, or mechanical removal of fluid accumulating around the lungs or abdomen. The latter can be accomplished with bed rest and weight loss.

Typically, drug therapy is also required in order to treat heart failure. No single agent meets all the requirements for optimal treatment, which includes rapid relief of labored breathing and edema, enhanced heart performance, reduced mortality, reduced progression of the underlying disease, safety, and minimal side effects. Therefore, drugs are used in combination to achieve control over sodium and water retention, improve heart contraction, reduce heart work, and protect against blood clots.

The purpose of therapy with diuretic drugs (drugs that increase salt and water loss through the kidneys) is threefold: to reduce the pooling of fluid that can take place in the lungs, abdomen, and lower extremities; to minimize the buildup of back pressure from the accumulation of blood in the veins; and to reduce the circulating blood volume. All these things will lessen the overstretch of the heart muscle and bring it to a level of stretch that is closer to its optimum. Care must be taken, however, not to reduce severely the water content of the blood, which could reduce the stretch on the heart muscle to below the optimum and consequently impair heart contraction. One way to monitor how much water is lost or retained is for patients to empty their bladders and then weigh themselves each day before breakfast. If weight changes steadily or suddenly, then sodium and water loss may be too great or too little. In either case, an adjustment is in order. Some generic diuretic drugs used to treat heart failure include furosemide, ethacrynic acid, the thiazides, and spironolactone.

The purpose of therapy with inotropic drugs (drugs that increase the contractile ability of heart muscle) is to improve the pumping action of the heart. This effect causes an increase in stroke volume (more blood moves out of the heart per beat) and helps compensate for forward failure. The increased output also reduces the backup of blood returning to the heart and thus also compensates for backward failure.

Digitalis, a derivative of the foxglove plant which originated as a Welsh folk remedy, is still the most frequently used inotropic drug for the treatment of chronic heart failure. Because it improves heart muscle contraction, it reverses to some extent all the symptoms of heart failure. Digitalis exerts its effects by increasing the accumulation of calcium inside the heart muscle cells. Calcium interacts with the structure of the shortening apparatus inside the cell to make more contractile interactions within the cell possible. Its disadvantages are that it becomes toxic in high doses and that it can severely damage performance of an already healthy heart.

Other inotropic agents also act to improve contraction by increasing calcium levels within the heart muscle cells. Some of them mimic the naturally produced hormones and neurotransmitters that are released and depleted in early stages of heart failure. These are called the sympathomimetic drugs. They include drugs such as dopamine, terbutaline, and levodopa. While these drugs improve heart performance, they can have serious side effects: increased heart rate, palpitations, and nervousness. One group of inotropic agents improves cardiac contraction while relaxing blood vessels. These drugs, called phosphodiesterase inhibitors, stop the breakdown of an essential cellular messenger molecule which helps to manage calcium levels and other events inside both heart cells and blood vessel cells. Examples of these drugs include amrinone and milrinone. Their use is not common because they can cause stomach upset and fatigue and because they are not clearly superior to other treatments.

The purpose of therapy with vasodilator drugs (drugs that relax the blood vessels) is to decrease the work of the heart. The resulting expansion of the blood vessels makes it easier for blood to be pumped through them. It also leaves room for pooling some of the blood in the veins, decreasing the amount of blood returning to the heart and so reducing overstretching as well. Some of the vasodilators, such as hydralazine, pinacidil, dipyridamole, and the nitrates, act directly on the blood vessels. Other vasodilators, such as angiotensin-converting enzyme (ACE) inhibitors and adrenergic inhibitors, inhibit the release of naturally produced substances that would make the blood vessels contract. Sometimes it is hard to predict the effects of vasodilators because they may act differently in different blood vessels and the body may attempt to offset the effects of the drug by releasing substances that contract blood vessels. Vasodilator drug therapy is usually added to other treatments when the symptoms of heart failure persist after digitalis and diuretic therapy are used.

The purpose of therapy with antithrombotics (blood clot inhibitors) is to prevent any further obstruction of the circulation with blood clots. Because heart failure changes the mechanics of blood flow and is the result of damaged heart muscle, it can increase the formation of blood clots. When blood clots form an obstruction in the large blood vessels of the lungs, it is often fatal. Clots can also lodge in the heart, causing further damage to heart muscle, or in the brain, where they could cause a stroke. Both the short-acting clot inhibitor heparin and oral agents such as aspirin are used to prevent these effects.

The combination of all these drug therapies, while unable to reverse the permanent damage of heart failure, makes it possible to treat the condition. Individuals treated for heart failure can lead comfortable, productive lives.

If the heart failure progresses to acutely life-threatening proportions and the patient is in all other ways healthy, the next alternative is surgical replacement of the heart. Artificial hearts are sometimes used as a transition to heart transplant while a donor is sought. Yet transplantation is not a perfect solution. Transplanted hearts do not have the nervous system input of a normal heart and so their control from moment to moment is different. They are also subject to rejection. Nevertheless, they provide an enormous improvement in quality of life for severe heart failure patients.

PERSPECTIVE AND PROSPECTS

The vital significance of the pulse and heartbeat have been part of human knowledge since long before recorded history. Pulse taking and herbal treatments for poor heartbeat have been recorded in ancient Chinese, Egyptian, and Greek histories. Digitalis has been used in treatment for at least two hundred years. It was first formally introduced to the medical community in 1785 by the English botanist and physician William Withering. He learned of it from a female folk healer named Hutton, who used it with other extracts to treat more than one kind of swelling. Withering identified the foxglove plant as the source of its active ingredient and characterized it as having effects on the pulse as well as on fluid retention. The plant is indigenous to both the United Kingdom and Europe and may well have been employed as a folk remedy for far longer. It is still the most widely used agent for the treatment of heart failure.

The developments in physiology and medicine during the nineteenth century set the stage for greater understanding and further treatments of heart failure. It was then that the stethoscope and blood pressure cuff were created for diagnostic purposes. In basic science, cell theory, hormone theory, and kidney physiology led to a better understanding of how heart muscle contraction and fluid balance might be coordinated in the body. The concepts and techniques required to keep organs and tissues alive outside the body with an artificial circulation system were conceived and introduced. Anesthesia and sterile techniques essential for cardiac surgery were developed.

These ideas and accomplishments contributed to important discoveries in the early twentieth century that greatly enhanced the understanding of the early compensatory responses to heart failure. For example, it was found that when heart muscle is stretched, it will contract with greater force on the next beat and that heart muscle usually operates at a muscle length that is less than optimal. Thus, when the amount of blood returning to the heart increases and stretches the muscle in the walls of the heart, the heart will contract with greater force, ejecting a greater volume of blood. This phenomenon, called the Frank-Starling mechanism, was first demonstrated in isolated heart muscle by the German physiologist Otto Frank and in functional hearts by the British physiologist Ernest Henry Starling in 1914.

Subsequent developments in the second half of the twentieth century, such as more specific vasodilator and diuretic drugs as well as the heart-lung machine, have led to the options of more complete drug therapy, artificial hearts (first introduced to replace a human heart by William DeVries in 1982), and heart transplant (first performed by Christiaan Barnard in 1967) as options for the treatment of heart failure.

—*Laura Gray Malloy, Ph.D.*

See also Arrhythmias; Arteriosclerosis; Cardiac arrest; Cardiology; Cardiology, pediatric; Cholesterol; Circulation; Congenital heart disease; Echocardiography; Edema; Endocarditis; Heart; Heart attack; Heart disease; Heart transplantation; Hypercholesterolemia; Hyperlipidemia; Hypertension; Ischemia; Mitral valve prolapse; Obesity; Palpitations; Vascular medicine; Vascular system.

For Further Information:

Campbell, Neil A., et al. *Biology: Concepts and Connections.* 5th ed. San Francisco: Pearson/Benjamin Cummings, 2006. This classic introductory textbook provides an excellent discussion of essential biological structures and mechanisms, including a chapter on cardiovascular function and disease.

Crawford, Michael, ed. *Current Diagnosis and Treatment in Cardiology.* 2d ed. New York: Lange Medical Books/McGraw-Hill, 2003. Discusses advances in cardiac diagnostics, treatments, and prognostic indicators and includes extensive information on prevention techniques.

Dox, Ida G., et al. *The HarperCollins Illustrated Medical Dictionary.* 4th ed. New York: HarperCollins, 2001. A home medical dictionary with more than 26,000 medical terms and 2,500 illustrations, including all those of most concern to cardiovascular patients. Defines relevant anatomical structures, functional terminology, and some widely used chemical compounds and drugs under generic names. An excellent resource for high school or college students.

Gersh, Bernard J., ed. *The Mayo Clinic Heart Book.* 2d ed. New York: William Morrow, 2000. One of the most respected texts for laypeople on heart disease. Covers all aspects of anatomy, physiology, diagnosis, treatment, and prevention.

Sherwood, Lauralee. *Human Physiology: From Cells to Systems.* 6th ed. Belmont, Calif.: Thomson/Brooks/Cole, 2007. A basic physiology textbook oriented toward an understanding of human function and disease. Superbly well written and offers excellent illustrations. Includes chapters that address car-diovascular function, with specific reference to heart failure and the cardiovascular abnormalities that precipitate it.

Heart transplantation
Procedure

Anatomy or system affected: Chest, circulatory system, heart, lungs, nervous system, respiratory system

Specialties and related fields: Cardiology, critical care, emergency medicine, general surgery

Definition: The removal of a diseased heart and its replacement with a healthy donor heart.

Key terms:

cardiomyopathy: a serious acute or chronic disease in which the heart becomes inflamed; it may result from multiple causes, including viral infection

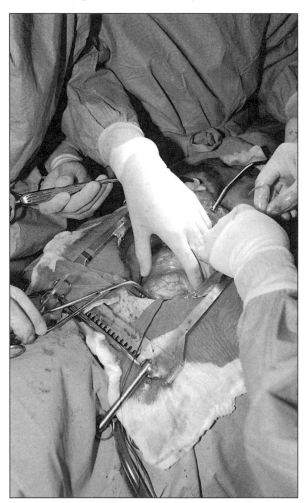

A heart is about to be removed during a transplantation procedure. (PhotoDisc)

congenital: present at birth

congestive heart failure: abnormal heart function characterized by circulatory congestion caused by cardiac disorders, especially myocardial infarction of the ventricles

coronary atherosclerosis: the accumulation of cholesterol, lipids, and other cellular debris in the coronary arteries, thereby limiting circulation in the heart

immunity: a defense function of the body that produces antibodies to destroy invading antigens and other disease-causing organisms

leukocytes: white blood cells that are important in the development of immunity

primary cardiomyopathy: cardiomyopathy that cannot be attributed to a specific cause

secondary cardiomyopathy: cardiomyopathy that is attributable to a specific cause (such as hypertension) and that is often associated with diseases involving other organs

INDICATIONS AND PROCEDURES

Heart transplantation is performed when congestive heart failure or heart injury cannot be treated by other conventional medical or surgical means. It is reserved for patients with a high risk of dying within two years. The procedure involves removal of a diseased heart and its replacement with a healthy human heart or possibly an animal heart. In special cases, the surgeon may place the donor heart next to the diseased heart without removing it; this is called a piggyback transplant.

Patients who are candidates for heart transplantation include those with valvular disease, congenital heart disease, or rare conditions such as tumors. The selection of recipients is based on which patients are likely to exhibit the most pronounced improvement, functional capacity, and life expectancy after surgery. In the United States, the limited availability of donor hearts has necessitated the creation of a national organ procurement and distribution network called the United Network for Organ Sharing (UNOS), which distributes organs based on severity of illness, waiting time, donor and recipient blood types, and body size match.

USES AND COMPLICATIONS

The first human heart transplantation was performed on December 3, 1967, by Christiaan Barnard in Capetown, South Africa. The heart transplantation procedures that were tried soon afterward usually had a low success rate because the patient's body often rejected the new heart when leukocytes and other cells of the

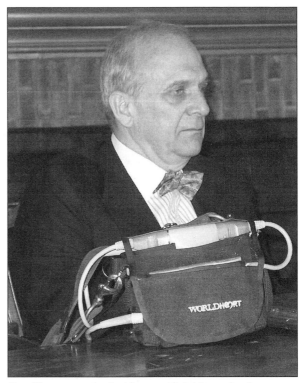

Pete Kenyon survived with an artificial heart for three years until he could receive a donor organ. The pump mechanism is carried in a pouch. (AP/Wide World Photos)

immune system recognized the new heart as foreign material and attacked it. With an improved understanding of immune system functioning and drug intervention, however, survival rates have gradually improved. Currently in the United States, approximately two thousand patients undergo heart transplantation annually in more than 230 heart transplantation centers. The one-year survival rate is 80 percent, the five-year survival rate is 70 percent, the ten-year survival rate is nearly 50 percent, and some patients have lived longer than twenty years, according to statistics from the American Heart Association. About fifteen thousand Americans aged fifty-five or younger (and forty thousand aged sixty-five or younger) would benefit from heart transplantation. Transplantation has been conducted with newborn babies, and adult patients have run marathons and even played professional sports. The average age at which the procedure is performed is forty-seven years for men and thirty-nine years for women.

The complications immediately following this type of surgery include irreversible damage to the heart, because of coronary atherosclerosis or multiple heart attacks, and primary or secondary cardiomyopathy, because the cardiac muscle cells cannot contract normally. Heart transplant recipients must take immunosuppressive (antirejection) medications for the remainder of their lives to prevent rejection; thus they must also cope with the numerous side effects of these drugs.

In the News: The AbioCor Artificial Heart

Scientific efforts at developing an artificial heart have been important because only about two thousand human donor hearts are available in the United States per year, despite many thousands of patients requiring a heart transplant. The initial experimental model, the Jarvik-7 in 1982, required a large pump outside the body and tethered the recipient to its 375-pound machine. Technological advances in miniaturization and energy transfer permitted the creation of the AbioCor, the first implantable artificial heart affording full mobility to the patient.

The AbioCor is made of titanium and a unique plastic designed to withstand being flexed forty million times a year. Before receiving Food and Drug Administration (FDA) approval for a clinical trial with fifteen patients, the makers of the AbioCor heart had to demonstrate that it could beat two hundred million times, enough beats to last five years. The device uses a wireless power transfer system. An external battery worn on the waist connects with an external coil on the chest, which transfers energy via radio waves to a coil inside the chest. No wires break the skin or provide a route for infection. A computer chip inside the chest controls the pumping action, and the external battery can operate four or five hours without recharging. An internal battery, kept continually charged by the external battery, provides thirty minutes of emergency power, permitting the user to disconnect the external power when showering.

Only patients likely to die within thirty days and unable to receive a live heart transplant were eligible to take part in the clinical trial. Success was defined as survival for 60 days with clear improvement in quality of life. On July 2, 2001, the first person to receive an implant lived for 151 days. Five more pumps were implanted in 2001, followed by an additional pump in 2002. Two patients died on the operating table, but the others lived more than 60 days. The longest surviving recipient lived 512 days and spent several months at home with his family before dying on February 7, 2003. The company temporarily suspended implants in 2002 and modified the AbioCor after two patients died of strokes. Clinical trials resumed in 2003, with three patients receiving artificial hearts in January and March of that year.

The dimensions of the AbioCor heart limit its usability. The human heart is about the size of a fist and weighs about 10 ounces. The AbioCor, the size of a grapefruit, weighs 2 pounds, too large for 50 percent of men and 80 percent of women. The developers hope to overcome this problem in future models.

—Milton Berman, Ph.D.

For at least one year after transplantation, the heart is denervated (cut away from the body's nervous system), causing a resting pulse rate of up to 130 beats per minute, as compared to 60 to 80 beats per minute in a normal heart. The chances for long-term success depend in part on the amount of damage or disease in other organs as a result of stroke, chronic obstructive lung disease, and liver or kidney disease. Transplant recipients must also deal with the psychological and emotional strain of the operation and its aftermath. Patients with a history of alcohol and drug abuse or mental illness, and those who lack a social support network of family and friends, are not considered good candidates for heart transplantation.

Perspective and Prospects

The rapid increase in the number of heart transplantations performed worldwide is attributable to specialized medical care and to numerous advances in knowledge regarding surgery, tissue preservation, immunology, and infectious disease. The extraordinary degree of success since the 1970's has enabled many patients who have undergone heart transplantation to live longer and more independent lives. Tremendous strides have been made in diagnosing rejection and developing immunosuppressive medications, and the development of several new antirejection drugs is anticipated soon. New techniques for diagnosing rejection candidates without the performance of a heart biopsy will be a major focus of future research, as will increasing access to donor organs. A better understanding of the immune system may give doctors greater success in transplanting organs from other species (a procedure called a xenograft) instead of human organs. Ongoing research will continue to focus on identifying risk factors for heart disease—such as high blood cholesterol and abnormal lipid subfractions, high blood pressure, diabetes mellitus, family history, and cigarette smoking—as early as possible in order to delay reaching the point at which heart transplantation is necessary.

—*Daniel G. Graetzer, Ph.D.*

See also Cardiac rehabilitation; Cardiology; Cardiology, pediatric; Circulation; Echocardiography; Electrocardiography (ECG or EKG); Grafts and grafting; Heart; Heart disease; Heart failure; Heart valve replacement; Immune system; Immunology; Transplantation; Xenotransplantation.

FOR FURTHER INFORMATION:

American College of Sports Medicine. *ACSM's Guidelines for Exercise Testing and Prescription.* 7th ed. Philadelphia: Lippincott Williams & Wilkins, 2006. Covers the standards of exercise testing and therapy, including instruction for patients suffering from heart disease.

American Heart Association. *Heart and Stroke Facts.* Dallas: Author, 1994. Contains information for the layperson on cardiovascular and cerebrovascular disease. Includes an index.

Baumgartner, William A., et al., eds. *Heart and Lung Transplantation.* 2d ed. Philadelphia: W. B. Saunders, 2002. Discusses organ procurement, evaluation criteria, and long-term patient management, including immunosuppression, complications, and psychological adjustments.

Crawford, Michael, ed. *Current Diagnosis and Treatment in Cardiology.* 2d ed. New York: Lange Medical Books/McGraw-Hill, 2003. Discusses advances in cardiac diagnostics, treatments, and prognostic indicators and includes extensive information on prevention techniques.

Deng, Mario C., et al. "Effect of Receiving a Heart Transplant: Analysis of a National Cohort Entered on to a Waiting List, Stratified by Heart Failure Severity." *British Medical Journal* 321, no. 7260 (September 2, 2000): 540-545. A study of cardiac transplantation in Germany reveals that patients with a predicted low or medium risk of mortality have no reduction in mortality risk as a result of transplantation.

Eagle, Kim A., and Ragavendra R. Baliga. *Practical Cardiology: Evaluation and Treatment of Common Cardiovascular Disorders.* Philadelphia: Lippincott

Williams & Wilkins, 2003. Details advances in cardiac medicine.

Ewert, Ralf, et al. "Relationship Between Impaired Pulmonary Diffusion and Cardiopulmonary Exercise Capacity After Heart Transplantation." *Chest* 117, no. 4 (April, 2000): 968. Diffusion impairment and reduced performance in cardiopulmonary exercise testing have been found in patients after heart transplantation.

HEART VALVE REPLACEMENT
PROCEDURE

ANATOMY OR SYSTEM AFFECTED: Chest, circulatory system, heart

SPECIALTIES AND RELATED FIELDS: Cardiology, general surgery

DEFINITION: A surgical procedure that involves removing a defective heart valve and replacing it with another tissue valve or with a mechanical valve.

KEY TERMS:

anticoagulants: a class of drugs that slow the clotting time of blood

bacterial endocarditis: bacterial infection of the heart, which may scar or destroy a valve

murmur: the sound made by blood flowing backward through a heart valve

regurgitation: the leakage of blood backward through a valve

stenosis: a condition in which valve tissue has hardened and thickened, interfering with blood flow through the valve

INDICATIONS AND PROCEDURES

Valve replacement surgery is a procedure used when a heart valve no longer functions properly. There are several reasons that a heart valve may fail. Sometimes, a major defect present at birth must be repaired immediately. Minor defects present at birth may go undetected for years. When and if these minor defects become worse as a result of aging, valve replacement surgery may be necessary. Another cause of heart valve damage is infection. Rheumatic fever can cause the scarring of a valve. These scars can become more of a problem with age, and surgery may eventually be necessary. Bacterial endocarditis is another type of infection that can damage the heart very quickly. Valve replacement surgery is often needed as a result of this type of infection.

When a heart valve is damaged, the result is usually stenosis or regurgitation. Stenosis occurs when the valve becomes thick and hard. As a result, normal blood flow through the valve is obstructed. A valve that becomes stretched or weak may not close properly, resulting in blood flowing backward through the valve; this is called regurgitation. When the blood flows backward through the valve, a sound is made. This sound, called a murmur, generally can be heard with a stethoscope.

When a heart valve fails to function properly, the ability of the heart to do work is impaired. In an attempt to maintain normal work levels, the heart begins to enlarge, or experience hypertrophy. When further hypertrophy is no longer possible, the heart fails. This condition will result in permanent damage to the heart muscle and eventually death. Some of the symptoms of valve problems include chest pain or tightness, shortness of breath, temporary blindness, slurred speech, weakness, numbness, lack of coordination, unusually rapid weight gain, fatigue, and loss of consciousness.

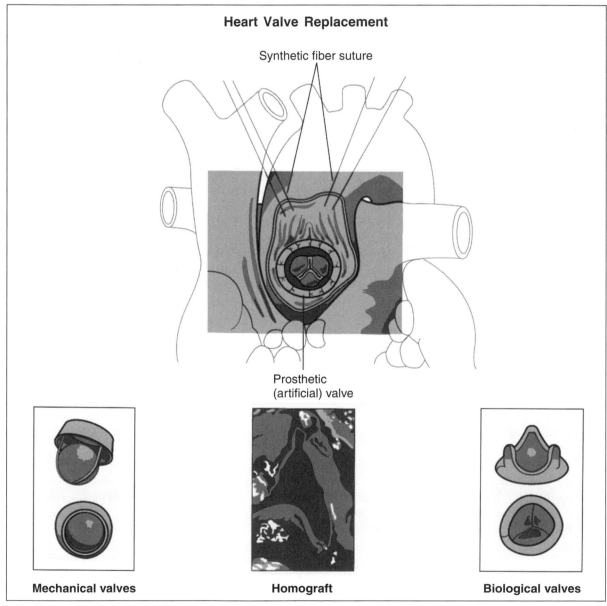

Heart Valve Replacement

Synthetic fiber suture

Prosthetic (artificial) valve

Mechanical valves   **Homograft**   **Biological valves**

When heart valves fail, they can be replaced by mechanical valves, which are made from artificial materials such as plastic, metal, and carbon fibers; by homografts, which are taken from cadavers; or by biological valves, which are either taken from pigs or constructed from the tissues of the patient or of a cow.

These symptoms are typically the result of inadequate blood flow, particularly to the brain.

In some cases, surgery can be used to repair the valve. Many times, however, the damage is too extensive for this type of surgery, and the valve must be replaced. The replacement valve may come from a deceased person's heart or from an animal's heart (usually that of a pig), or it may be a mechanical (prosthetic) valve. Prosthetic valves are made from metal, plastic, or carbon ceramic.

During valve replacement surgery, the chest is opened to expose the heart. Blood flow through the heart is diverted through an oxygenator and a pump that maintains the flow of oxygenated blood throughout the body. The surgeon removes the damaged valve and sutures a replacement valve to the heart. Upon completion of the surgery, if the replaced valve functions effectively, normal blood flow is restored through the heart.

Uses and Complications

Heart valve replacement is a very reliable procedure. Although problems with the new valve are possible, the majority of these surgeries are 100 percent effective. Nevertheless, there are two long-term concerns for the patient. Blood thinners or anticoagulants—drugs that slow the clotting process and may prevent blood clots—are usually required with prosthetic valves. These drugs help prevent blood from coagulating in and around the new valve. Some patients must also take antibiotics to prevent additional infections in the heart. Antibiotics are needed especially when patients visit the dentist, when bleeding is likely. If bleeding occurs, bacteria may enter the blood and become lodged in the replacement valve. The ensuing infection can cause further damage to the heart.

When one compares the use of tissue versus mechanical (prosthetic) valves for replacement, some differences emerge. In general, tissue valves work better. In addition, they are less likely to require drugs to increase blood-clotting time. On the other hand, they are harder to obtain. With more people acting as donors and with better preservation techniques becoming available, tissue replacements are preferred.

Perspective and Prospects

Mechanical valves were first used as replacements for damaged valves in the early 1960's. In 1962, the initial clinical use of tissue valves was described. Tissue valve replacements were conducted simultaneously by Donald Ross in England and Sir Brian Barratt-Boyes in New Zealand. The acceptance of tissue valve use was slow because the number of donors was small and the methods for preserving valves for later use were poor. The result was shorter survival times for the replacement valves used in the 1960's and early 1970's.

By the 1980's, better preservation techniques were developed, which allowed surgeons to use living human tissue. These replacements have been found to be superior to nonliving tissues and mechanical valves. In the future, both mechanical and tissue replacements will continue to be used, based on availability and the specific needs of the patient.

—*Bradley R. A. Wilson, Ph.D.*

See also Angiography; Angioplasty; Bleeding; Blood and blood disorders; Bypass surgery; Cardiac arrest; Cardiac rehabilitation; Cardiology; Cardiology, pediatric; Circulation; Echocardiography; Electrocardiography (ECG or EKG); Endocarditis; Heart; Heart attack; Heart disease; Heart failure; Heart transplantation; Pacemaker implantation; Rheumatic fever; Thrombolytic therapy and TPA.

For Further Information:

Alpert, Joseph S., James E. Dalen, and Shahbudin H. Rahimtoola, eds. *Valvular Heart Disease*. 3d ed. Philadelphia: Lippincott Williams & Wilkins, 2000. Discusses diseases of the heart valve and their treatments. Includes bibliographical references and an index.

Bonhoeffer, Philipp, et al. "Percutaneous Replacement of Pulmonary Valve in a Right-Ventricle to Pulmonary-Artery Prosthetic Conduit with Valve Dysfunction." *The Lancet* 356, no. 9239 (October 21, 2000): 1403-1405. The authors show that percutaneous valve replacement in the pulmonary position is possible. With further technical improvements, this new technique might be used for valve replacement in other cardiac and noncardiac positions.

Crawford, Michael, ed. *Current Diagnosis and Treatment in Cardiology*. 2d ed. New York: Lange Medical Books/McGraw-Hill, 2003. Discusses advances in cardiac diagnostics, treatments, and prognostic indicators and includes extensive information on prevention techniques.

Eagle, Kim A., and Ragavendra R. Baliga. *Practical Cardiology: Evaluation and Treatment of Common Cardiovascular Disorders*. Philadelphia: Lippincott Williams & Wilkins, 2003. Details advances in cardiac medicine.

Kramer, Gerri Freid, and Shari Mauer. *Parent's Guide to Children's Congenital Heart Defects: What They Are, How to Treat Them, How to Cope with Them.* New York: Three Rivers Press, 2001. Experts in pediatric cardiology provide easy-to-understand answers to help parents coping with a child's heart disease. Includes the latest information on diagnosis, treatment options, surgery, aftercare, and growing up with heart defects, as well as stories from parents who have lived through the ordeal.

Mitka, Mike. "Final Report on Mechanical vs. Bioprosthetic Heart Valves." *The Journal of the American Medical Association* 283, no. 15 (April 19, 2000): 1947-1948. A long-term follow-up study presented at the annual meeting of the American College of Cardiology has given surgeons a clear answer to the question of whether to perform heart valve replacement with a mechanical or a bioprosthetic device.

Nauer, Kathleen A., Barbara Schouchoff, and Kathleen Demitras. "Minimally Invasive Aortic Valve Surgery." *Critical Care Nursing Quarterly* 23, no. 1 (May, 2000): 66-71. Heart surgery has seen the emergence of minimally invasive techniques in the quest for less traumatic and less painful surgery. This procedure can be provided without the increased cost of endoscopic instrumentation by use of standard instrumentation, cannulation, and prostheses.

Otto, Catherine M. "Timing of Aortic Valve Surgery." *Heart* 84, no. 2 (August, 2000): 211. The timing of aortic valve surgery is described for patients complaining of two conditions: aortic stenosis and chronic aortic regurgitation.

HEARTBURN

DISEASE/DISORDER

ALSO KNOWN AS: Acid indigestion

ANATOMY OR SYSTEM AFFECTED: Chest, gastrointestinal system, throat

SPECIALTIES AND RELATED FIELDS: Family medicine, gastroenterology, internal medicine

DEFINITION: A feeling of warmth or discomfort in the chest.

CAUSES AND SYMPTOMS

Heartburn occurs when acid travels backward from the stomach to the esophagus. Acid is normally present at very high concentrations in the stomach, where it aids digestion. Contrary to popular belief, most people who

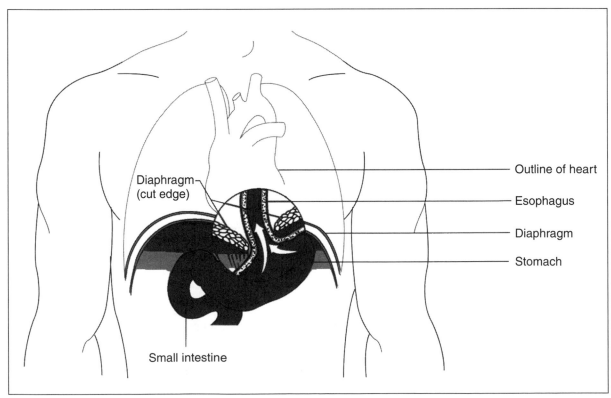

Heartburn is caused by a reflux of stomach acid into the esophagus shortly after eating.

suffer from heartburn do not produce too much acid. Rather, they have a malfunction of the lower esophageal sphincter (LES), a ring of muscle between the stomach and the esophagus. Except when food is being swallowed, the LES stays closed. This keeps acid confined to the stomach. If the LES remains open, or if it is weakened, then stomach acid can travel freely to the esophagus and irritate its inner lining, resulting in heartburn.

Heartburn is described as a hot, burning feeling in the chest. It usually occurs thirty minutes to one hour after eating and lasts for several minutes. It is often worsened by lying down or bending over and is improved by standing up. Other associated symptoms may include a sour taste in the mouth, sore throat, or hoarseness. Some patients develop a dry cough as a result of acid irritating the throat. Heartburn must be distinguished from more ominous causes of chest pain, including a heart attack or other heart-related chest pain. Usually, chest pain attributable to such causes becomes worse with exertion, while heartburn should not.

TREATMENT AND THERAPY

The initial therapy for heartburn includes elimination of dietary and lifestyle factors that weaken the LES: tobacco, excessive alcohol, fatty foods, chocolate, and caffeine. Medications such as calcium-channel blockers and nitrates can also worsen heartburn, but they should not be discontinued without consulting a physician. It has been suggested that avoiding late-night meals and elevating the head of the bed with blocks underneath the headboard can improve heartburn, especially if symptoms occur mostly during nighttime. Occasional heartburn can be treated with over-the-counter antacids or medications such as ranitidine, which reduces acid production. If symptoms do not improve, then prescription medications are also available.

Surgery to reinforce the LES, called a Nissen fundoplication, is another option. Although results are excellent, patients often must take acid-suppressive medications after the procedure. Heartburn that is persistent or accompanied by trouble swallowing, weight loss, or bleeding requires more thorough investigation, as with endoscopy, to exclude the possibility of cancer or other serious medical conditions.

—*Ahmad Kamal, M.D.*

IN THE NEWS: LINK TO ESOPHAGEAL CANCER

Severe heartburn, more properly called gastroesophageal reflux disease (GERD), results when stomach acid refluxes, or backs up, into the lower region of the esophagus. It is more common in older individuals, and the primary cause is the inability of the sphincter (muscle fibers) of the esophagus to close properly, blocking the passage of the acid. Heartburn is among the more common complaints of older persons, with more than sixty million Americans reporting severe heartburn at least once a month. Nearly half of those individuals suffer GERD on a daily basis. The problem is probably universal, as approximately 20 percent of European adults report similar symptoms.

A variety of risk factors or behaviors are associated with GERD, primarily smoking, obesity, or ingestion of fatty foods prior to bedtime. Recent concerns about GERD have centered on its possible association with esophageal cancer. Esophageal cancer is now the eighth most common cancer in the United States, accounting for some twelve thousand deaths each year. The incidence of adenocarcinoma of the esophagus, a type of cancer associated with mucus-secreting cells, has increased nearly eight-fold since the 1970's.

In 1999, Jesper Lagergren and his colleagues reported a long-term study carried out in Sweden in which individuals who reported severe GERD for more than twenty years had a greater than fourfold risk of developing esophageal cancer. In addition to reporting that nearly 90 percent of the patients with esophageal cancer suffered from heartburn prior to diagnosis, a possible indication of a cause and effect relationship, the authors reported a dose-response relationship between severe heartburn and the development of cancer: the more severe the heartburn, the greater the risk of cancer. The authors suggested that GERD might be associated with nearly half of all adenocarcinomas and some 90 percent of adenocarcinomas of persons with severe heartburn.

The strongest evidence to support a link between GERD and esophageal cancer would involve a prospective follow-up among individuals receiving medication to reduce GERD. If indeed an association exists, reduction of GERD should result in a long-term reduction in the incidence of esophageal cancer.

—*Richard Adler, Ph.D.*

See also Acid reflux disease; Caffeine; Chest; Digestion; Gastroenterology; Gastroenterology, pediatric; Gastrointestinal disorders; Gastrointestinal system; Indigestion; Nausea and vomiting; Over-the-counter medications; Pain; Stress; Stress reduction; Ulcer surgery; Ulcers; Vagotomy.

FOR FURTHER INFORMATION:

Cheskin, Lawrence J., and Brian E. Lacy. *Healing Heartburn.* Baltimore: Johns Hopkins University Press, 2002.

Kasper, Dennis L., et al., eds. *Harrison's Principles of Internal Medicine.* 16th ed. New York: McGraw-Hill, 2005.

Minocha, Anil, and Christine Adamec. *How to Stop Heartburn: Simple Ways to Heal Heartburn and Acid Reflux.* New York: John Wiley & Sons, 2001.

Shimberg, Elaine Fantle. *Coping with Chronic Heartburn: What You Need to Know About Acid Reflux and GERD.* New York: St. Martin's Griffin, 2001.

HEAT EXHAUSTION AND HEAT STROKE
DISEASE/DISORDER

ANATOMY OR SYSTEM AFFECTED: Blood vessels, circulatory system, skin

SPECIALTIES AND RELATED FIELDS: Critical care, emergency medicine, family medicine, internal medicine, sports medicine

DEFINITION: Heat-related illnesses in which the body temperature rises to dangerous levels and cannot be controlled through normal mechanisms, such as sweating.

CAUSES AND SYMPTOMS

The human body is well equipped to maintain a nearly constant internal body temperature. In fact, the body temperature of human beings is usually controlled so closely that it rarely leaves a very narrow range of 36.1 to 37.8 degrees Celsius (97 to 100 degrees Fahrenheit) regardless of how much heat the body is producing or what the environmental temperature may be. Humans maintain a constant temperature so that the millions of biochemical reactions in the body remain at an optimal rate. An increase in body temperature of only 1 degree Celsius will cause these reactions to move about 10 percent faster. As internal temperatures rise, however, brain function becomes slower because important proteins and enzymes lose their ability to operate effectively. Most adults will go into convulsions when their temperature reaches 41 degrees Celsius (106 degrees Fahrenheit), and 43 degrees Celsius (110 degrees Fahrenheit) is usually fatal.

A special region of the brain known as the hypothalamus regulates body temperature. The hypothalamus detects the temperature of the blood much like a thermostat detects room temperature. When the body (and hence the blood) becomes too warm, the hypothalamus activates heat-loss mechanisms. Most excess heat is lost through the skin by the radiation of heat and the evaporation of sweat. To promote this heat loss, blood vessels in the skin dilate (open up) to carry more blood to the skin. Heat from the warm blood is then lost to the cooler air. If the increase in blood flow to the skin is not enough, then sweat glands are stimulated to produce and secrete large amounts of sweat. The process, called perspiration, is an efficient means of ridding the body of excess heat as long as the humidity is not too high. In fact, at 60 percent humidity, evaporation of sweat from the skin stops. When the body cannot dissipate enough heat, heat exhaustion and heat stroke may occur.

Heat exhaustion is the most prevalent heat-related illness. It commonly occurs in individuals who have exercised or worked in high temperatures for long periods of time. These people have usually not ingested adequate amounts of fluid. Over time, the patient loses fluid through sweating and respiration, which decreases the amount of fluid in the blood. Because the body is trying to reduce its temperature, blood has been shunted to the skin and away from vital internal organs. This reaction, in combination with a reduced blood volume, causes the patient to go into mild shock. Common signs and symptoms of heat exhaustion include cool, moist skin that may appear either red or pale; headache; nausea; dizziness; and exhaustion. If heat exhaustion is not recognized and treated, it can lead to life-threatening heat stroke.

Heat stroke occurs when the body is unable to eradicate the excess heat as rapidly as it develops. Thus, body temperature begins to rise. Sweating stops because the water content of the blood decreases. The loss of evaporative cooling causes the body temperature to continue rising rapidly, soon reaching a level that can cause organ damage. In particular, the brain, heart, and kidneys may begin to fail until the patient experiences convulsions, coma, and even death. Therefore, heat stroke is a serious medical emergency which must be recognized and treated immediately. The signs and symptoms of heat stroke include high body temperature (41 degrees Celsius or 106 degrees Fahrenheit); loss of consciousness; hot, dry skin; rapid pulse; and quick, shallow breathing.

TREATMENT AND THERAPY

As with most illnesses, prevention is the best medicine for heat exhaustion and heat stroke. When exercising in hot weather, people should wear loose-fitting, lightweight clothing and drink plenty of fluids. When individuals are not prepared to avoid heat-related illness, however, rapid treatment may save their lives. When emergency medical personnel detect signs and symptoms of sudden heat-induced illness, they attempt to do three major things: cool the body, replace body fluids, and minimize shock.

For heat exhaustion, the initial treatment should be to place the patient in a cool place, such as a bathtub filled with cool (not cold) water. The conscious patient is given water or fruit drinks, sometimes containing salt, to replace body fluids. Occasionally, intravenous fluids must be given to return blood volume to normal in a more direct way. Hospitalization of the patient may

be necessary to be sure that the body is able to regulate body heat appropriately. Almost all patients treated quickly and effectively will not advance to heat stroke. The activity that placed the patient in danger should be discontinued until one is sure all symptoms have disappeared and steps have been taken to prevent a future episode of heat exhaustion.

Heat stroke requires urgent medical attention, or the high body temperature will cause irreparable damage and often death. Body temperature must be reduced rapidly. With the patient in a cool environment, the clothing is removed and the skin sprinkled with water and cooled by fanning. Contrary to popular belief, rubbing alcohol should not be used, as it can cause closure of the skin's pores. Ice packs are often placed behind the neck and under the armpits and groin. At these sites, large blood vessels come close to the skin and are capable of carrying cooled blood to the internal organs. Body fluid must be replaced quickly by intravenous administration because the patient is usually unable to drink as a result of convulsions or confusion and may even be unconscious. Once the body temperature has been brought back to normal, the patient is usually hospitalized and watched for complications. With early diagnosis and treatment, 80 to 90 percent of previously healthy people will survive.

—*Matthew Berria, Ph.D.*

See also Critical care; Critical care, pediatric; Dehydration; Emergency medicine; Fever; Hyperthermia and hypothermia; Resuscitation; Shock; Sweating; Unconsciousness.

FOR FURTHER INFORMATION:

American Academy of Orthopaedic Surgeons. *Emergency Care and Transportation of the Sick and Injured.* Edited by Benjamin Gulli, Les Chatelain, and Chris Stratford. 9th ed. Sudbury, Mass.: Jones and Bartlett, 2005. Covers soft tissue injuries. Offers graphic photographs of actual injuries and discusses care and management. This text is often used in the training of emergency medical technicians, yet chapters are easily understood by the nonmedical layperson.

American Medical Association. *Handbook of First Aid and Emergency Care.* Rev. ed. New York: Random House, 2000. Provides a listing of injuries, illnesses, and medical emergencies accompanied by easy-to-follow instructions and illustrations.

Hales, Dianne. *An Invitation to Health.* 12th ed. New York: Brooks Cole, 2006. This text should be read

---

INFORMATION ON HEAT EXHAUSTION AND HEAT STROKE

CAUSES: Dehydration

SYMPTOMS: For heat exhaustion, cool and moist skin that appears either red or pale, headache, nausea, dizziness, exhaustion; for heat stroke, cessation of perspiration, hot and dry skin, rapid pulse, quick and shallow breathing

DURATION: Acute

TREATMENTS: Cooling of body, replacement of body fluids, treatment of shock, emergency resuscitation

by anyone who wishes an overview of health topics.

Leikin, Jerrold B., and Martin S. Lipsky, eds. *American Medical Association Complete Medical Encyclopedia*. New York: Random House Reference, 2003. A concise presentation of numerous medical terms and illnesses. A good general reference.

McArdle, William, Frank I. Katch, and Victor L. Katch. *Exercise Physiology: Energy, Nutrition, and Human Performance*. 6th ed. Philadelphia: Lippincott Williams & Wilkins, 2007. A wide-ranging text on exercise and the human body, covering topics such as nutrition, energy transfer, exercise training, systems of energy delivery and utilization, enhancement of energy capacity, the effect of environmental stress, and the effect of exercise on successful aging and disease prevention.

Marieb, Elaine N., and Katja Hoehn. *Human Anatomy and Physiology*. 7th ed. San Francisco: Pearson Benjamin Cummings, 2007. Nonscientists at the advanced high school level or above will be able to understand this fine textbook. It includes a complete glossary, index, pronunciation guide, and other helpful features.

Heel spur removal

Procedure

Anatomy or system affected: Bones, feet, musculoskeletal system

Specialties and related fields: General surgery, orthopedics, podiatry

Definition: The surgical removal of a heel spur, a hard, bony growth on the heel.

Indications and Procedures

Heel spurs, also known as calcaneal spurs, are hard, bony growths on the heel bone. Pain and tenderness in the sole of the foot under the heel bone are common first indicators of this condition. Painful heel spurs can cause difficulty in walking and standing. Running, jogging, and prolonged standing often contribute to their development, especially when unpadded shoes are worn. When efforts to alleviate pain, such as activity modification and the use of shoes with cushioned heels, have been exhausted, it may be necessary for the spur to be surgically removed.

Most heel spur removal operations are performed at outpatient surgical facilities. Before the operation, blood and urine studies are conducted, and X rays are taken of both feet. Local or spinal anesthetics are administered. The surgeon, orthopedist, or podiatrist conducting the operation will choose a convenient site to make an incision, usually over the spur. Using special instruments, the heel spur is carved free and removed. The opening in the skin is closed with sutures. Barring complications, the sutures can be removed ten to fourteen days later. After the surgery, additional blood studies are taken, and laboratory examination of the removed tissue is performed.

Uses and Complications

Heel spurs form as a result of hard pounding or prolonged stress on the heel of the foot. Shock-absorbing soles in shoes and orthopedic inserts that cushion hard blows to the heel during vigorous exercise can help prevent and aid in recovery from heel spur operations. Following a removal operation, vigorous exercise can be resumed in approximately three months.

Clean cloths or tissues can be pressed against the wound for ten minutes if bleeding occurs within the first twenty-four hours after the surgery. The scar from the incision will recede gradually. Although it is important to keep the foot clean, the wound must be kept dry between baths. For the first two or three days after surgery, the wound should be covered with a dry bandage. Complications associated with heel spur removal surgery can include excessive bleeding and surgical wound infection, which should be examined by a doctor.

—*Jason Georges*

See also Bone disorders; Bones and the skeleton; Feet; Foot disorders; Lower extremities; Orthopedic surgery; Orthopedics; Podiatry.

For Further Information:

Copeland, D. P. M. Glenn, and Stan Solomon. *The Foot Doctor: Lifetime Relief for Your Aching Feet*. Emmaus, Pa.: Rodale Press, 1986.

Currey, John D. *Bones: Structures and Mechanics*. Princeton, N.J.: Princeton University Press, 2002.

Levy, Leonard A., and Vincent J. Hetherington, eds. *Principles and Practice of Podiatric Medicine*. New York: Churchill Livingstone, 1990.

Lippert, Frederick G., and Sigvard T. Hansen. *Foot and Ankle Disorders: Tricks of the Trade*. New York: Thieme, 2003.

Lorimer, Donald L., et al., eds. *Neale's Disorders of the Foot*. 7th ed. New York: Elsevier Churchill Livingstone, 2006.

Van De Graaff, Kent M., and Stuart I. Fox. *Concepts of Human Anatomy and Physiology*. 5th ed. Dubuque, Iowa: Wm. C. Brown, 2000.

MAGILL'S

MEDICAL GUIDE

ENTRIES BY ANATOMY OR SYSTEM AFFECTED

ALL
Accidents
African American health
Aging
Aging: Extended care
Alternative medicine
American Indian health
Anatomy
Antibiotics
Anti-inflammatory drugs
Antioxidants
Asian American health
Autoimmune disorders
Autopsy
Biological and chemical weapons
Bionics and biotechnology
Biophysics
Birth defects
Burkitt's lymphoma
Cancer
Carcinogens
Carcinoma
Chemotherapy
Chronobiology
Clinical trials
Cloning
Critical care
Critical care, pediatric
Cryotherapy and cryosurgery
Cushing's syndrome
Death and dying
Disease
Domestic violence
Drug resistance
Embryology
Emergency medicine
Emergency medicine, pediatric
Environmental diseases
Environmental health
Enzyme therapy
Epidemiology
Family medicine
Fatigue
Fever
Forensic pathology
Gangrene
Gene therapy
Genetic diseases
Genetics and inheritance
Genomics

Geriatrics and gerontology
Grafts and grafting
Growth
Healing
Herbal medicine
Histology
Holistic medicine
Homeopathy
Hydrotherapy
Hyperadiposis
Hyperthermia and hypothermia
Hypertrophy
Hypochondriasis
Iatrogenic disorders
Imaging and radiology
Immunopathology
Infection
Inflammation
Insulin resistance syndrome
Internet medicine
Intoxication
Invasive tests
Ischemia
Leptin
Magnetic resonance imaging
    (MRI)
Malignancy and metastasis
Malnutrition
Massage
Meditation
Men's health
Metabolic disorders
Metabolic syndrome
Mold and mildew
Mucopolysaccharidosis (MPS)
Multiple births
Münchausen syndrome by proxy
Neonatology
Noninvasive tests
Nursing
Occupational health
Oncology
Over-the-counter medications
Pain
Pain management
Paramedics
Parasitic diseases
Pathology
Pediatrics
Perinatology

Physical examination
Physician assistants
Physiology
Phytochemicals
Plastic surgery
Polypharmacy
Positron emission tomography
    (PET) scanning
Preventive medicine
Progeria
Prostheses
Proteomics
Psychiatry
Psychiatry, child and adolescent
Psychiatry, geriatric
Psychosomatic disorders
Puberty and adolescence
Radiation therapy
Radiopharmaceuticals
Reflexes, primitive
Safety issues for children
Safety issues for the elderly
Screening
Self-medication
Sexually transmitted diseases
    (STDs)
Staphylococcal infections
Stem cells
Streptococcal infections
Stress reduction
Sudden infant death syndrome
    (SIDS)
Suicide
Supplements
Surgery, general
Surgery, pediatric
Surgical procedures
Surgical technologists
Systems and organs
Teratogens
Terminally ill: Extended care
Toxic shock syndrome
Tropical medicine
Tumor removal
Tumors
Veterinary medicine
Viral infections
Vitamins and minerals
Well-baby examinations
Women's health

Sciatica
Scoliosis
Slipped disk
Spinal cord disorders
Spine, vertebrae, and disks
Spondylitis
Sympathectomy
Tendon disorders

BLADDER
Abdomen
Bed-wetting
Bladder cancer
Bladder removal
Candidiasis
Catheterization
Cystitis
Cystoscopy
Endoscopy
Fetal surgery
Fistula repair
Incontinence
Internal medicine
Lithotripsy
Pyelonephritis
Schistosomiasis
Sphincterectomy
Stone removal
Stones
Toilet training
Ultrasonography
Urethritis
Urinalysis
Urinary disorders
Urinary system
Urology
Urology, pediatric

BLOOD
Anemia
Angiography
Bleeding
Blood and blood disorders
Blood testing
Bone marrow transplantation
Candidiasis
Circulation
Corticosteroids
Cyanosis
Cytomegalovirus (CMV)
Dialysis
Disseminated intravascular
  coagulation (DIC)
E. coli infection

Ebola virus
Epstein-Barr virus
Ergogenic aids
Facial transplantation
Fetal surgery
Fluids and electrolytes
Gulf War syndrome
Heart
Hematology
Hematology, pediatric
Hemolytic disease of the newborn
Hemolytic uremic syndrome
Hemophilia
Histiocytosis
Host-defense mechanisms
Hyperbaric oxygen therapy
Hyperlipidemia
Hypoglycemia
Immunization and vaccination
Immunology
Insect-borne diseases
Ischemia
Jaundice
Jaundice, neonatal
Laboratory tests
Leukemia
Liver
Malaria
Marburg virus
Nephrology
Nephrology, pediatric
Nosebleeds
Pharmacology
Pharmacy
Phlebotomy
Rh factor
Scurvy
Septicemia
Serology
Sickle cell disease
Sturge-Weber syndrome
Thalassemia
Thrombocytopenia
Thrombolytic therapy and TPA
Thrombosis and thrombus
Toxemia
Toxicology
Transfusion
Transplantation
Ultrasonography
Von Willebrand's disease
Wiskott-Aldrich syndrome
Yellow fever

BLOOD VESSELS
Aneurysmectomy
Aneurysms
Angiography
Angioplasty
Arteriosclerosis
Bleeding
Blood and blood disorders
Blood testing
Bruises
Bypass surgery
Caffeine
Catheterization
Cholesterol
Circulation
Claudication
Diabetes mellitus
Disseminated intravascular
  coagulation (DIC)
Dizziness and fainting
Edema
Electrocauterization
Embolism
Endarterectomy
Hammertoe correction
Heart
Heart disease
Heat exhaustion and heat stroke
Hemorrhoid banding and removal
Hemorrhoids
Hypercholesterolemia
Hypertension
Hypotension
Ischemia
Klippel-Trenaunay syndrome
Necrotizing fasciitis
Neuroimaging
Nosebleeds
Obesity
Obesity, childhood
Phlebitis
Phlebotomy
Polycystic kidney disease
Preeclampsia and eclampsia
Scleroderma
Shock
Stents
Strokes
Sturge-Weber syndrome
Thalidomide
Thrombosis and thrombus
Transient ischemic attacks (TIAs)
Umbilical cord
Varicose vein removal

Varicose veins
Vascular medicine
Vascular system
Venous insufficiency
Von Willebrand's disease

BONES
Amputation
Arthritis
Bone cancer
Bone disorders
Bone grafting
Bone marrow transplantation
Bones and the skeleton
Bowlegs
Bunions
Cells
Cerebral palsy
Chiropractic
Cleft lip and palate
Cleft lip and palate repair
Craniosynostosis
Craniotomy
Disk removal
Dwarfism
Ear surgery
Ears
Ewing's sarcoma
Failure to thrive
Feet
Foot disorders
Fracture and dislocation
Fracture repair
Gaucher's disease
Gigantism
Hammertoe correction
Hammertoes
Head and neck disorders
Heel spur removal
Hematology
Hematology, pediatric
Hip fracture repair
Hip replacement
Histiocytosis
Hormone replacement therapy
  (HRT)
Jaw wiring
Kneecap removal
Knock-knees
Kyphosis
Laminectomy and spinal fusion
Lower extremities
Marfan syndrome
Motor skill development

Neurofibromatosis
Niemann-Pick disease
Nuclear medicine
Nuclear radiology
Orthopedic surgery
Orthopedics
Orthopedics, pediatric
Osgood-Schlatter disease
Osteochondritis juvenilis
Osteogenesis imperfecta
Osteomyelitis
Osteonecrosis
Osteopathic medicine
Osteoporosis
Paget's disease
Periodontitis
Physical rehabilitation
Pigeon toes
Podiatry
Prader-Willi syndrome
Rheumatology
Rickets
Rubinstein-Taybi syndrome
Sarcoma
Scoliosis
Slipped disk
Spinal cord disorders
Spine, vertebrae, and disks
Sports medicine
Teeth
Temporomandibular joint (TMJ)
  syndrome
Tendon disorders
Tendon repair
Upper extremities

BRAIN
Abscess drainage
Abscesses
Addiction
Alcoholism
Altitude sickness
Alzheimer's disease
Amnesia
Anesthesia
Anesthesiology
Aneurysmectomy
Aneurysms
Angiography
Antidepressants
Aphasia and dysphasia
Aromatherapy
Attention-deficit disorder (ADD)
Auras

Batten's disease
Biofeedback
Brain
Brain damage
Brain disorders
Brain tumors
Caffeine
Chronic wasting disease (CWD)
Cluster headaches
Cognitive development
Coma
Computed tomography (CT)
  scanning
Concussion
Cornelia de Lange syndrome
Corticosteroids
Craniotomy
Creutzfeldt-Jakob disease (CJD)
Cytomegalovirus (CMV)
Dehydration
Dementias
Developmental stages
Dizziness and fainting
Down syndrome
Drowning
Dyslexia
Electroencephalography (EEG)
Embolism
Emotions: Biomedical causes and
  effects
Encephalitis
Endocrinology
Endocrinology, pediatric
Epilepsy
Failure to thrive
Fetal alcohol syndrome
Fetal surgery
Fetal tissue transplantation
Fibromyalgia
Fragile X syndrome
Galactosemia
Gigantism
Gulf War syndrome
Hallucinations
Head and neck disorders
Headaches
Huntington's disease
Hydrocephalus
Hypertension
Hypnosis
Hypotension
Intraventricular hemorrhage
Jaundice
Kinesiology

Pacemaker implantation
Pityriasis rosea
Pleurisy
Pneumonia
Pulmonary diseases
Pulmonary medicine
Pulmonary medicine, pediatric
Respiration
Respiratory distress syndrome
Resuscitation
Sneezing
Thoracic surgery
Tuberculosis
Wheezing
Whooping cough

CIRCULATORY SYSTEM
Aneurysmectomy
Aneurysms
Angina
Angiography
Angioplasty
Antihistamines
Apgar score
Arrhythmias
Arteriosclerosis
Biofeedback
Bleeding
Blood and blood disorders
Blood testing
Blue baby syndrome
Bypass surgery
Cardiac arrest
Cardiac rehabilitation
Cardiology
Cardiology, pediatric
Cardiopulmonary resuscitation
   (CPR)
Catheterization
Chest
Cholesterol
Circulation
Claudication
Congenital heart disease
Decongestants
Dehydration
Diabetes mellitus
Dialysis
Disseminated intravascular
   coagulation (DIC)
Dizziness and fainting
Ebola virus
Echocardiography
Edema

Electrocardiography (ECG or EKG)
Electrocauterization
Embolism
Endarterectomy
Endocarditis
Ergogenic aids
Exercise physiology
Facial transplantation
Heart
Heart attack
Heart disease
Heart failure
Heart transplantation
Heart valve replacement
Heat exhaustion and heat stroke
Hematology
Hematology, pediatric
Hemorrhoid banding and removal
Hemorrhoids
Hormones
Hyperbaric oxygen therapy
Hypercholesterolemia
Hypertension
Hypotension
Ischemia
Juvenile rheumatoid arthritis
Kidneys
Kinesiology
Klippel-Trenaunay syndrome
Liver
Lymphatic system
Marburg virus
Marijuana
Mitral valve prolapse
Motor skill development
Nosebleeds
Obesity
Obesity, childhood
Osteochondritis juvenilis
Pacemaker implantation
Palpitations
Phlebitis
Phlebotomy
Placenta
Preeclampsia and eclampsia
Resuscitation
Reye's syndrome
Rheumatic fever
Scleroderma
Septicemia
Shock
Shunts
Smoking
Sports medicine

Stents
Steroid abuse
Strokes
Sturge-Weber syndrome
Systems and organs
Testicular torsion
Thrombocytopenia
Thrombolytic therapy and TPA
Thrombosis and thrombus
Transfusion
Transient ischemic attacks (TIAs)
Transplantation
Typhus
Varicose vein removal
Varicose veins
Vascular medicine
Vascular system
Venous insufficiency

EARS
Altitude sickness
Antihistamines
Audiology
Auras
Biophysics
Cornelia de Lange syndrome
Cytomegalovirus (CMV)
Deafness
Decongestants
Dyslexia
Ear infections and disorders
Ear surgery
Ears
Fragile X syndrome
Hearing aids
Hearing loss
Hearing tests
Histiocytosis
Leukodystrophy
Ménière's disease
Motion sickness
Myringotomy
Nervous system
Neurology
Neurology, pediatric
Osteogenesis imperfecta
Otoplasty
Otorhinolaryngology
Plastic surgery
Quinsy
Rubinstein-Taybi syndrome
Sense organs
Speech disorders
Wiskott-Aldrich syndrome

ENDOCRINE SYSTEM

Addison's disease
Adrenalectomy
Assisted reproductive technologies
Bariatric surgery
Biofeedback
Breasts, female
Contraception
Corticosteroids
Cretinism
Diabetes mellitus
Dwarfism
Eating disorders
Emotions: Biomedical causes and effects
Endocrine disorders
Endocrinology
Endocrinology, pediatric
Ergogenic aids
Failure to thrive
Gestational diabetes
Gigantism
Glands
Goiter
Hashimoto's thyroiditis
Hormone replacement therapy (HRT)
Hormones
Hot flashes
Hyperhidrosis
Hyperparathyroidism and hypoparathyroidism
Hypoglycemia
Klinefelter syndrome
Liver
Melatonin
Nonalcoholic steatohepatitis (NASH)
Obesity
Obesity, childhood
Overtraining syndrome
Pancreas
Pancreatitis
Parathyroidectomy
Placenta
Postpartum depression
Prader-Willi syndrome
Prostate enlargement
Prostate gland
Prostate gland removal
Sex change surgery
Sexual differentiation
Steroid abuse
Steroids
Sweating
Systems and organs
Testicular cancer
Testicular surgery
Thyroid disorders
Thyroid gland
Thyroidectomy
Turner syndrome
Weight loss medications

EYES

Albinos
Antihistamines
Astigmatism
Auras
Batten's disease
Behçet's disease
Blindness
Blurred vision
Botox
Cataract surgery
Cataracts
Chlamydia
Color blindness
Conjunctivitis
Corneal transplantation
Cornelia de Lange syndrome
Cytomegalovirus (CMV)
Diabetes mellitus
Dyslexia
Eye infections and disorders
Eye surgery
Eyes
Face lift and blepharoplasty
Galactosemia
Glaucoma
Gonorrhea
Gulf War syndrome
Jaundice
Juvenile rheumatoid arthritis
Keratitis
Laser use in surgery
Leukodystrophy
Macular degeneration
Marfan syndrome
Marijuana
Microscopy, slitlamp
Motor skill development
Multiple chemical sensitivity syndrome
Myopia
Ophthalmology
Optometry
Optometry, pediatric
Pigmentation
Ptosis
Refractive eye surgery
Reiter's syndrome
Rubinstein-Taybi syndrome
Sense organs
Sjögren's syndrome
Strabismus
Sturge-Weber syndrome
Styes
Toxoplasmosis
Trachoma
Transplantation
Vision disorders

FEET

Athlete's foot
Bones and the skeleton
Bunions
Cornelia de Lange syndrome
Corns and calluses
Cysts
Feet
Flat feet
Foot disorders
Fragile X syndrome
Frostbite
Ganglion removal
Gout
Hammertoe correction
Hammertoes
Heel spur removal
Lower extremities
Nail removal
Nails
Orthopedic surgery
Orthopedics
Orthopedics, pediatric
Osteoarthritis
Pigeon toes
Podiatry
Rubinstein-Taybi syndrome
Sports medicine
Tendinitis
Tendon repair
Thalidomide
Warts

GALLBLADDER

Abscess drainage
Abscesses
Bariatric surgery
Cholecystectomy
Cholecystitis

HANDS

Amputation
Arthritis
Bones and the skeleton
Bursitis
Carpal tunnel syndrome
Cerebral palsy
Cornelia de Lange syndrome
Corns and calluses
Cysts
Fracture and dislocation
Fracture repair
Fragile X syndrome
Frostbite
Ganglion removal
Nail removal
Nails
Neurology
Neurology, pediatric
Orthopedic surgery
Orthopedics
Orthopedics, pediatric
Osteoarthritis
Rheumatoid arthritis
Rheumatology
Rubinstein-Taybi syndrome
Scleroderma
Skin lesion removal
Sports medicine
Tendinitis
Tendon disorders
Tendon repair
Thalidomide
Upper extremities
Warts

HEAD

Altitude sickness
Aneurysmectomy
Aneurysms
Angiography
Antihistamines
Botox
Brain
Brain disorders
Brain tumors
Cluster headaches
Coma
Computed tomography (CT)
    scanning
Concussion
Cornelia de Lange syndrome
Craniosynostosis
Craniotomy

Dizziness and fainting
Electroencephalography (EEG)
Embolism
Epilepsy
Facial transplantation
Fetal tissue transplantation
Fibromyalgia
Hair loss and baldness
Hair transplantation
Head and neck disorders
Headaches
Hydrocephalus
Lice, mites, and ticks
Meningitis
Migraine headaches
Nasal polyp removal
Nasopharyngeal disorders
Neuroimaging
Neurology
Neurology, pediatric
Neurosurgery
Rhinoplasty and submucous
    resection
Rubinstein-Taybi syndrome
Seizures
Shunts
Sports medicine
Strokes
Sturge-Weber syndrome
Temporomandibular joint (TMJ)
    syndrome
Thrombosis and thrombus
Unconsciousness
Whiplash

HEART

Aneurysmectomy
Aneurysms
Angina
Angiography
Angioplasty
Anxiety
Apgar score
Arrhythmias
Arteriosclerosis
Biofeedback
Bites and stings
Blue baby syndrome
Bypass surgery
Caffeine
Cardiac arrest
Cardiac rehabilitation
Cardiology
Cardiology, pediatric

Cardiopulmonary resuscitation (CPR)
Catheterization
Circulation
Congenital heart disease
Cornelia de Lange syndrome
DiGeorge syndrome
Echocardiography
Electrical shock
Electrocardiography (ECG or EKG)
Embolism
Endocarditis
Exercise physiology
Fatty acid oxidation disorders
Glycogen storage diseases
Heart
Heart attack
Heart disease
Heart failure
Heart transplantation
Heart valve replacement
Hemochromatosis
Hypertension
Hypotension
Internal medicine
Juvenile rheumatoid arthritis
Kinesiology
Lyme disease
Marfan syndrome
Marijuana
Mitral valve prolapse
Nicotine
Obesity
Obesity, childhood
Pacemaker implantation
Palpitations
Prader-Willi syndrome
Respiratory distress syndrome
Resuscitation
Reye's syndrome
Rheumatic fever
Rubinstein-Taybi syndrome
Scleroderma
Shock
Sports medicine
Stents
Steroid abuse
Strokes
Thoracic surgery
Thrombolytic therapy and TPA
Thrombosis and thrombus
Toxoplasmosis
Transplantation
Ultrasonography
Yellow fever

HIPS

Aging
Arthritis
Arthroplasty
Arthroscopy
Bone disorders
Bones and the skeleton
Chiropractic
Dwarfism
Fracture and dislocation
Fracture repair
Hip fracture repair
Hip replacement
Liposuction
Lower extremities
Orthopedic surgery
Orthopedics
Orthopedics, pediatric
Osteoarthritis
Osteochondritis juvenilis
Osteonecrosis
Osteoporosis
Physical rehabilitation
Pityriasis rosea
Rheumatoid arthritis
Rheumatology
Sciatica

IMMUNE SYSTEM

Acquired immunodeficiency
    syndrome (AIDS)
Allergies
Antibiotics
Antihistamines
Arthritis
Asthma
Autoimmune disorders
Bacterial infections
Bacteriology
Bites and stings
Blood and blood disorders
Bone grafting
Bone marrow transplantation
Candidiasis
Cells
Chagas' disease
Childhood infectious diseases
Chronic fatigue syndrome
Cornelia de Lange syndrome
Corticosteroids
Cytology
Cytomegalovirus (CMV)
Cytopathology
Dermatology

Dermatopathology
DiGeorge syndrome
Disseminated intravascular
    coagulation (DIC)
E. coli infection
Ebola virus
Emotions: Biomedical causes and
    effects
Endocrinology
Endocrinology, pediatric
Enzyme therapy
Enzymes
Epstein-Barr virus
Facial transplantation
Fungal infections
Grafts and grafting
Gram staining
Guillain-Barré syndrome
Gulf War syndrome
Hashimoto's thyroiditis
Healing
Hematology
Hematology, pediatric
Histiocytosis
Hives
Homeopathy
Host-defense mechanisms
Human immunodeficiency virus
    (HIV)
Immune system
Immunization and vaccination
Immunodeficiency disorders
Immunology
Immunopathology
Juvenile rheumatoid arthritis
Kawasaki disease
Leprosy
Lymphatic system
Magnetic field therapy
Marburg virus
Measles
Microbiology
Monkeypox
Multiple chemical sensitivity
    syndrome
Mumps
Mutation
Myasthenia gravis
Nicotine
Noroviruses
Oncology
Pancreas
Pharmacology
Poisoning

Poisonous plants
Pulmonary diseases
Pulmonary medicine
Pulmonary medicine, pediatric
Rh factor
Rheumatology
Rubella
Sarcoma
Scarlet fever
Scleroderma
Serology
Severe acute respiratory syndrome
    (SARS)
Severe combined immunodeficiency
    syndrome (SCID)
Sjögren's syndrome
Smallpox
Sneezing
Stress
Stress reduction
Systemic lupus erythematosus (SLE)
Systems and organs
Thalidomide
Toxicology
Transfusion
Transplantation
Wiskott-Aldrich syndrome

INTESTINES

Abdomen
Abdominal disorders
Appendectomy
Appendicitis
Appetite loss
Bacterial infections
Bariatric surgery
Bypass surgery
Celiac sprue
Colic
Colitis
Colon and rectal polyp removal
Colon and rectal surgery
Colon cancer
Colon therapy
Colonoscopy and sigmoidoscopy
Constipation
Crohn's disease
Diarrhea and dysentery
Digestion
Diverticulitis and diverticulosis
E. coli infection
Eating disorders
Endoscopy
Enemas

Enterocolitis
Fistula repair
Food poisoning
Gastroenterology
Gastroenterology, pediatric
Gastrointestinal disorders
Gastrointestinal system
Hemorrhoid banding and removal
Hemorrhoids
Hernia
Hernia repair
Hirschsprung's disease
Ileostomy and colostomy
Indigestion
Internal medicine
Intestinal disorders
Intestines
Irritable bowel syndrome (IBS)
Kaposi's sarcoma
Kwashiorkor
Lactose intolerance
Laparoscopy
Malabsorption
Malnutrition
Metabolism
Nutrition
Obesity
Obesity, childhood
Obstruction
Peristalsis
Pinworm
Proctology
Rotavirus
Roundworm
Salmonella infection
Soiling
Sphincterectomy
Stomach, intestinal, and pancreatic
   cancers
Tapeworm
Toilet training
Trichinosis
Tumor removal
Tumors
Typhoid fever
Ulcer surgery
Ulcers
Worms

JOINTS
Amputation
Arthritis
Arthroplasty
Arthroscopy

Braces, orthopedic
Bursitis
Carpal tunnel syndrome
Chlamydia
Corticosteroids
Cyst removal
Cysts
Endoscopy
Exercise physiology
Fracture and dislocation
Fragile X syndrome
Gout
Gulf War syndrome
Hammertoe correction
Hammertoes
Hip fracture repair
Juvenile rheumatoid arthritis
Klippel-Trenaunay syndrome
Kneecap removal
Lyme disease
Motor skill development
Orthopedic surgery
Orthopedics
Orthopedics, pediatric
Osteoarthritis
Osteochondritis juvenilis
Osteomyelitis
Osteonecrosis
Physical rehabilitation
Reiter's syndrome
Rheumatoid arthritis
Rheumatology
Rotator cuff surgery
Scleroderma
Spondylitis
Sports medicine
Systemic lupus erythematosus (SLE)
Temporomandibular joint (TMJ)
   syndrome
Tendinitis
Tendon disorders
Tendon repair
Von Willebrand's disease

KIDNEYS
Abdomen
Abscess drainage
Abscesses
Adrenalectomy
Corticosteroids
Cysts
Dialysis
Galactosemia
Hantavirus

Hemolytic uremic syndrome
Hypertension
Hypotension
Internal medicine
Kidney cancer
Kidney disorders
Kidney transplantation
Kidneys
Laparoscopy
Lithotripsy
Metabolism
Nephrectomy
Nephritis
Nephrology
Nephrology, pediatric
Nuclear medicine
Nuclear radiology
Polycystic kidney disease
Preeclampsia and eclampsia
Pyelonephritis
Renal failure
Reye's syndrome
Scleroderma
Stone removal
Stones
Toilet training
Transplantation
Ultrasonography
Urinalysis
Urinary disorders
Urinary system
Urology
Urology, pediatric

KNEES
Amputation
Arthritis
Arthroplasty
Arthroscopy
Bone disorders
Bones and the skeleton
Bowlegs
Braces, orthopedic
Bursitis
Endoscopy
Exercise physiology
Fracture and dislocation
Kneecap removal
Knock-knees
Liposuction
Lower extremities
Orthopedic surgery
Orthopedics
Orthopedics, pediatric

Endoscopy
Exercise physiology
Fetal surgery
Hantavirus
Heart transplantation
Heimlich maneuver
Hiccups
Histiocytosis
Hyperbaric oxygen therapy
Hyperventilation
Influenza
Internal medicine
Interstitial pulmonary fibrosis
  (IPF)
Kaposi's sarcoma
Kinesiology
Legionnaires' disease
Lung cancer
Lung surgery
Lungs
Marijuana
Measles
Multiple chemical sensitivity
  syndrome
Nicotine
Niemann-Pick disease
Oxygen therapy
Plague
Pleurisy
Pneumonia
Pulmonary diseases
Pulmonary hypertension
Pulmonary medicine
Pulmonary medicine, pediatric
Respiration
Respiratory distress syndrome
Resuscitation
Scleroderma
Severe acute respiratory syndrome
  (SARS)
Smoking
Sneezing
Thoracic surgery
Thrombolytic therapy and TPA
Thrombosis and thrombus
Toxoplasmosis
Transplantation
Tuberculosis
Tularemia
Tumor removal
Tumors
Wheezing
Whooping cough
Wiskott-Aldrich syndrome

LYMPHATIC SYSTEM
Angiography
Bacterial infections
Blood and blood disorders
Breast cancer
Breast disorders
Bruises
Burkitt's lymphoma
Cancer
Cervical, ovarian, and uterine
  cancers
Chemotherapy
Circulation
Colon cancer
Corticosteroids
DiGeorge syndrome
Edema
Elephantiasis
Gaucher's disease
Histology
Hodgkin's disease
Immune system
Immunology
Immunopathology
Kawasaki disease
Klippel-Trenaunay syndrome
Liver cancer
Lower extremities
Lung cancer
Lymphadenopathy and lymphoma
Lymphatic system
Malignancy and metastasis
Mononucleosis
Oncology
Overtraining syndrome
Prostate cancer
Skin cancer
Sleeping sickness
Splenectomy
Stomach, intestinal, and pancreatic
  cancers
Systems and organs
Tonsillectomy and adenoid removal
Tonsillitis
Tularemia
Tumor removal
Tumors
Upper extremities
Vascular medicine
Vascular system

MOUTH
Acid reflux disease
Behçet's disease

Candidiasis
Canker sores
Cavities
Cleft lip and palate
Cleft lip and palate repair
Cold sores
Cornelia de Lange syndrome
Crowns and bridges
Dental diseases
Dentistry
Dentistry, pediatric
Dentures
DiGeorge syndrome
Endodontic disease
Facial transplantation
Fluoride treatments
Gingivitis
Gum disease
Halitosis
Hand-foot-and-mouth disease
Heimlich maneuver
Herpes
Jaw wiring
Kawasaki disease
Lisping
Mouth and throat cancer
Nicotine
Nutrition
Orthodontics
Periodontal surgery
Periodontitis
Reiter's syndrome
Root canal treatment
Rubinstein-Taybi syndrome
Sense organs
Sjögren's syndrome
Taste
Teeth
Teething
Temporomandibular joint (TMJ)
  syndrome
Thumb sucking
Tooth extraction
Toothache
Ulcers
Wisdom teeth

MUSCLES
Acupressure
Amputation
Amyotrophic lateral sclerosis
Anesthesia
Anesthesiology
Apgar score

Ataxia
Back pain
Bed-wetting
Bell's palsy
Beriberi
Biofeedback
Botox
Botulism
Breasts, female
Cerebral palsy
Chest
Childhood infectious diseases
Chronic fatigue syndrome
Claudication
Creutzfeldt-Jakob disease (CJD)
Cysts
Ebola virus
Emotions: Biomedical causes and effects
Ergogenic aids
Exercise physiology
Facial transplantation
Fatty acid oxidation disorders
Feet
Fibromyalgia
Flat feet
Foot disorders
Glycogen storage diseases
Glycolysis
Guillain-Barré syndrome
Gulf War syndrome
Head and neck disorders
Hemiplegia
Hiccups
Kinesiology
Leukodystrophy
Lower extremities
Marburg virus
Mastectomy and lumpectomy
Motor neuron diseases
Motor skill development
Multiple chemical sensitivity syndrome
Multiple sclerosis
Muscle sprains, spasms, and disorders
Muscles
Muscular dystrophy
Necrotizing fasciitis
Neurology
Neurology, pediatric
Numbness and tingling
Orthopedic surgery
Orthopedics

Orthopedics, pediatric
Osgood-Schlatter disease
Osteopathic medicine
Overtraining syndrome
Palsy
Paralysis
Paraplegia
Parkinson's disease
Physical rehabilitation
Poisoning
Poliomyelitis
Ptosis
Quadriplegia
Rabies
Respiration
Rheumatoid arthritis
Rotator cuff surgery
Seizures
Speech disorders
Sphincterectomy
Sports medicine
Steroid abuse
Strabismus
Tattoos and body piercing
Temporomandibular joint (TMJ) syndrome
Tendon disorders
Tendon repair
Tetanus
Tics
Torticollis
Tourette's syndrome
Trembling and shaking
Trichinosis
Upper extremities
Weight loss and gain
Yellow fever

MUSCULOSKELETAL SYSTEM
Acupressure
Amputation
Amyotrophic lateral sclerosis
Anatomy
Anesthesia
Anesthesiology
Arthritis
Ataxia
Back pain
Bed-wetting
Bell's palsy
Beriberi
Biofeedback
Bone cancer
Bone disorders

Bone grafting
Bone marrow transplantation
Bones and the skeleton
Botulism
Bowlegs
Braces, orthopedic
Breasts, female
Cells
Cerebral palsy
Chest
Childhood infectious diseases
Chiropractic
Chronic fatigue syndrome
Claudication
Cleft lip and palate
Cleft lip and palate repair
Craniosynostosis
Cretinism
Cysts
Depression
Dwarfism
Ear surgery
Ears
Emotions: Biomedical causes and effects
Ergogenic aids
Ewing's sarcoma
Exercise physiology
Feet
Fetal alcohol syndrome
Fibromyalgia
Flat feet
Foot disorders
Fracture and dislocation
Fracture repair
Gigantism
Glycolysis
Guillain-Barré syndrome
Hammertoe correction
Hammertoes
Head and neck disorders
Heel spur removal
Hematology
Hematology, pediatric
Hemiplegia
Hip fracture repair
Hip replacement
Hyperparathyroidism and hypoparathyroidism
Jaw wiring
Juvenile rheumatoid arthritis
Kinesiology
Kneecap removal
Knock-knees

Kyphosis
Lower extremities
Marfan syndrome
Marijuana
Mastectomy and lumpectomy
Motor neuron diseases
Motor skill development
Multiple sclerosis
Muscle sprains, spasms, and
    disorders
Muscles
Muscular dystrophy
Myasthenia gravis
Neurology
Neurology, pediatric
Nuclear medicine
Nuclear radiology
Numbness and tingling
Orthopedic surgery
Orthopedics
Orthopedics, pediatric
Osteochondritis juvenilis
Osteogenesis imperfecta
Osteomyelitis
Osteonecrosis
Osteopathic medicine
Osteoporosis
Paget's disease
Palsy
Paralysis
Paraplegia
Parkinson's disease
Periodontitis
Physical rehabilitation
Pigeon toes
Poisoning
Poliomyelitis
Prader-Willi syndrome
Precocious puberty
Quadriplegia
Rabies
Respiration
Rheumatoid arthritis
Rheumatology
Rickets
Sarcoma
Scoliosis
Seizures
Sleepwalking
Slipped disk
Speech disorders
Sphincterectomy
Spinal cord disorders
Spine, vertebrae, and disks

Sports medicine
Systemic lupus erythematosus (SLE)
Systems and organs
Teeth
Tendinitis
Tendon disorders
Tendon repair
Tetanus
Tics
Tourette's syndrome
Trembling and shaking
Trichinosis
Upper extremities
Weight loss and gain
Yellow fever

NAILS
Anemia
Dermatology
Fungal infections
Malnutrition
Nail removal
Nails
Nutrition
Podiatry

NECK
Asphyxiation
Back pain
Botox
Braces, orthopedic
Choking
Cretinism
Endarterectomy
Goiter
Hashimoto's thyroiditis
Head and neck disorders
Heimlich maneuver
Hyperparathyroidism and
    hypoparathyroidism
Laryngectomy
Laryngitis
Mouth and throat cancer
Otorhinolaryngology
Paralysis
Parathyroidectomy
Quadriplegia
Spine, vertebrae, and disks
Sympathectomy
Thyroid disorders
Thyroid gland
Thyroidectomy
Tonsillectomy and adenoid
    removal

Tonsillitis
Torticollis
Tracheostomy
Whiplash

NERVES
Anesthesia
Anesthesiology
Back pain
Bell's palsy
Biofeedback
Brain
Carpal tunnel syndrome
Cells
Creutzfeldt-Jakob disease (CJD)
Cysts
Emotions: Biomedical causes and
    effects
Epilepsy
Facial transplantation
Fibromyalgia
Guillain-Barré syndrome
Hemiplegia
Huntington's disease
Leprosy
Leukodystrophy
Lower extremities
Marijuana
Motor neuron diseases
Motor skill development
Multiple chemical sensitivity
    syndrome
Multiple sclerosis
Nervous system
Neuralgia, neuritis, and neuropathy
Neuroimaging
Neurology
Neurology, pediatric
Neurosurgery
Numbness and tingling
Palsy
Paralysis
Paraplegia
Parkinson's disease
Physical rehabilitation
Poliomyelitis
Ptosis
Quadriplegia
Sciatica
Seizures
Sense organs
Shock therapy
Skin
Spina bifida

Porphyria
Precocious puberty
Preeclampsia and eclampsia
Premenstrual syndrome (PMS)
Prion diseases
Quadriplegia
Rabies
Reye's syndrome
Sciatica
Seasonal affective disorder
Seizures
Sense organs
Shingles
Shock therapy
Shunts
Skin
Sleep
Sleep disorders
Sleeping sickness
Sleepwalking
Smell
Snakebites
Spina bifida
Spinal cord disorders
Spine, vertebrae, and disks
Sports medicine
Stammering
Strokes
Sturge-Weber syndrome
Stuttering
Sympathectomy
Syphilis
Systems and organs
Taste
Tay-Sachs disease
Teeth
Tetanus
Thrombolytic therapy and TPA
Tics
Touch
Tourette's syndrome
Toxicology
Toxoplasmosis
Trembling and shaking
Unconsciousness
Upper extremities
Vagotomy
Wilson's disease
Yellow fever

NOSE
Allergies
Antihistamines
Aromatherapy

Auras
Childhood infectious diseases
Common cold
Cornelia de Lange syndrome
Decongestants
Facial transplantation
Fifth disease
Halitosis
Nasal polyp removal
Nasopharyngeal disorders
Nicotine
Nosebleeds
Otorhinolaryngology
Plastic surgery
Pulmonary medicine
Pulmonary medicine, pediatric
Respiration
Rhinitis
Rhinoplasty and submucous
   resection
Rosacea
Rubinstein-Taybi syndrome
Sense organs
Sinusitis
Skin lesion removal
Smell
Sneezing
Sore throat
Taste
Viral infections

PANCREAS
Abscess drainage
Abscesses
Diabetes mellitus
Digestion
Endocrinology
Endocrinology, pediatric
Fetal tissue transplantation
Food biochemistry
Gastroenterology
Gastroenterology, pediatric
Gastrointestinal disorders
Gastrointestinal system
Glands
Hemochromatosis
Hormones
Internal medicine
Malabsorption
Metabolism
Pancreas
Pancreatitis
Polycystic kidney disease

Stomach, intestinal, and pancreatic
   cancers
Transplantation

**PSYCHIC-EMOTIONAL
   SYSTEM**
Addiction
Aging
Alcoholism
Alzheimer's disease
Amnesia
Anesthesia
Anesthesiology
Anorexia nervosa
Antidepressants
Antihistamines
Anxiety
Aphasia and dysphasia
Aphrodisiacs
Appetite loss
Aromatherapy
Asperger's syndrome
Attention-deficit disorder (ADD)
Auras
Autism
Bariatric surgery
Biofeedback
Bipolar disorders
Bonding
Brain
Brain disorders
Bulimia
Chronic fatigue syndrome
Club drugs
Cluster headaches
Cognitive development
Colic
Coma
Concussion
Corticosteroids
Death and dying
Delusions
Dementias
Depression
Developmental stages
Dizziness and fainting
Domestic violence
Down syndrome
Dyslexia
Eating disorders
Electroencephalography (EEG)
Emotions: Biomedical causes and
   effects
Endocrinology

Nicotine
Obstetrics
Orchitis
Ovarian cysts
Pap smear
Pelvic inflammatory disease (PID)
Penile implant surgery
Placenta
Precocious puberty
Preeclampsia and eclampsia
Pregnancy and gestation
Premature birth
Premenstrual syndrome (PMS)
Prostate cancer
Prostate enlargement
Prostate gland
Puberty and adolescence
Reproductive system
Sex change surgery
Sexual differentiation
Sexual dysfunction
Sexuality
Sexually transmitted diseases
  (STDs)
Sperm banks
Sterilization
Steroid abuse
Stillbirth
Syphilis
Systems and organs
Testicles, undescended
Testicular cancer
Testicular surgery
Testicular torsion
Trichomoniasis
Tubal ligation
Turner syndrome
Ultrasonography
Urology
Urology, pediatric
Vasectomy
Von Willebrand's disease
Warts

RESPIRATORY SYSTEM
Abscess drainage
Abscesses
Altitude sickness
Amyotrophic lateral sclerosis
Antihistamines
Apgar score
Apnea
Asbestos exposure
Aspergillosis

Asphyxiation
Asthma
Bacterial infections
Bronchiolitis
Bronchitis
Cardiopulmonary resuscitation
  (CPR)
Chest
Chickenpox
Childhood infectious diseases
Choking
Chronic obstructive pulmonary
  disease (COPD)
Common cold
Corticosteroids
Coughing
Croup
Cystic fibrosis
Decongestants
Diphtheria
Drowning
Edema
Embolism
Emphysema
Epiglottitis
Exercise physiology
Fetal surgery
Fluids and electrolytes
Fungal infections
Halitosis
Hantavirus
Head and neck disorders
Heart transplantation
Heimlich maneuver
Hiccups
Hyperbaric oxygen therapy
Hyperventilation
Influenza
Internal medicine
Interstitial pulmonary fibrosis (IPF)
Kinesiology
Laryngectomy
Laryngitis
Legionnaires' disease
Lung cancer
Lung surgery
Lungs
Marijuana
Measles
Monkeypox
Mononucleosis
Multiple chemical sensitivity
  syndrome
Nasopharyngeal disorders

Nicotine
Niemann-Pick disease
Obesity
Obesity, childhood
Otorhinolaryngology
Oxygen therapy
Pharyngitis
Plague
Pleurisy
Pneumonia
Poisoning
Pulmonary diseases
Pulmonary hypertension
Pulmonary medicine
Pulmonary medicine, pediatric
Respiration
Resuscitation
Rheumatic fever
Rhinitis
Roundworm
Severe acute respiratory syndrome
  (SARS)
Sinusitis
Sleep apnea
Smallpox
Sneezing
Sore throat
Strep throat
Systems and organs
Thoracic surgery
Thrombolytic therapy and TPA
Thrombosis and thrombus
Tonsillectomy and adenoid removal
Tonsillitis
Toxoplasmosis
Tracheostomy
Transplantation
Tuberculosis
Tularemia
Tumor removal
Tumors
Voice and vocal cord disorders
Wheezing
Whooping cough
Worms

SKIN
Abscess drainage
Abscesses
Acne
Acupressure
Acupuncture
Age spots
Albinos

Orthopedics
Orthopedics, pediatric
Osteoarthritis
Osteogenesis imperfecta
Osteoporosis
Paget's disease
Paralysis
Paraplegia
Physical rehabilitation
Poliomyelitis
Quadriplegia
Sciatica
Scoliosis
Slipped disk
Spina bifida
Spinal cord disorders
Spine, vertebrae, and disks
Spondylitis
Sports medicine
Sympathectomy
Whiplash

SPLEEN
Abdomen
Abdominal disorders
Abscess drainage
Abscesses
Anemia
Bleeding
Gaucher's disease
Hematology
Hematology, pediatric
Immune system
Internal medicine
Jaundice, neonatal
Lymphatic system
Metabolism
Niemann-Pick disease
Splenectomy
Thrombocytopenia
Transplantation

STOMACH
Abdomen
Abdominal disorders
Abscess drainage
Abscesses
Acid reflux disease
Allergies
Bariatric surgery
Botulism
Bulimia
Burping
Bypass surgery

Colitis
Crohn's disease
Digestion
Eating disorders
Endoscopy
Food biochemistry
Food poisoning
Gastrectomy
Gastroenterology
Gastroenterology, pediatric
Gastrointestinal disorders
Gastrointestinal system
Gastrostomy
Halitosis
Heartburn
Hernia
Hernia repair
Indigestion
Influenza
Internal medicine
Kwashiorkor
Lactose intolerance
Malabsorption
Malnutrition
Metabolism
Motion sickness
Nausea and vomiting
Nutrition
Obesity
Obesity, childhood
Peristalsis
Poisoning
Poisonous plants
Pyloric stenosis
Radiation sickness
Rotavirus
Roundworm
Salmonella infection
Stomach, intestinal, and pancreatic
    cancers
Ulcer surgery
Ulcers
Vagotomy
Vitamins and minerals
Weaning
Weight loss and gain

TEETH
Cavities
Cornelia de Lange syndrome
Crowns and bridges
Dental diseases
Dentistry
Dentistry, pediatric

Dentures
Endodontic disease
Fluoride treatments
Forensic pathology
Fracture repair
Gastrointestinal system
Gingivitis
Gum disease
Jaw wiring
Lisping
Nicotine
Nutrition
Orthodontics
Osteogenesis imperfecta
Periodontal surgery
Periodontitis
Prader-Willi syndrome
Root canal treatment
Rubinstein-Taybi syndrome
Teeth
Teething
Temporomandibular joint (TMJ)
    syndrome
Thumb sucking
Tooth extraction
Toothache
Veterinary medicine
Wisdom teeth

TENDONS
Carpal tunnel syndrome
Cysts
Exercise physiology
Ganglion removal
Hammertoe correction
Kneecap removal
Orthopedic surgery
Orthopedics
Orthopedics, pediatric
Osgood-Schlatter disease
Physical rehabilitation
Sports medicine
Tendinitis
Tendon disorders
Tendon repair

THROAT
Acid reflux disease
Antihistamines
Asbestos exposure
Auras
Bulimia
Catheterization
Choking

Croup
Decongestants
Drowning
Epiglottitis
Epstein-Barr virus
Fifth disease
Gastroenterology
Gastroenterology, pediatric
Gastrointestinal disorders
Gastrointestinal system
Goiter
Head and neck disorders
Heimlich maneuver
Hiccups
Histiocytosis
Laryngectomy
Laryngitis
Mouth and throat cancer
Nasopharyngeal disorders
Nicotine
Nosebleeds
Otorhinolaryngology
Pharyngitis
Pulmonary medicine
Pulmonary medicine, pediatric
Quinsy
Respiration
Smoking
Sore throat
Strep throat
Tonsillectomy and adenoid removal
Tonsillitis
Tracheostomy
Voice and vocal cord disorders

URINARY SYSTEM
Abdomen
Abdominal disorders
Abscess drainage
Abscesses
Adrenalectomy
Bed-wetting
Bladder cancer
Bladder removal
Candidiasis
Catheterization
Circumcision, male
Cystitis
Cystoscopy
Cysts
Dialysis

E. coli infection
Endoscopy
Fetal surgery
Fistula repair
Fluids and electrolytes
Geriatrics and gerontology
Hemolytic uremic syndrome
Hermaphroditism and
    pseudohermaphroditism
Host-defense mechanisms
Hypertension
Incontinence
Internal medicine
Kidney cancer
Kidney disorders
Kidney transplantation
Kidneys
Laparoscopy
Lithotripsy
Nephrectomy
Nephritis
Nephrology
Nephrology, pediatric
Pediatrics
Penile implant surgery
Pyelonephritis
Reiter's syndrome
Renal failure
Reye's syndrome
Schistosomiasis
Stone removal
Stones
Systems and organs
Testicular cancer
Toilet training
Transplantation
Trichomoniasis
Ultrasonography
Urethritis
Urinalysis
Urinary disorders
Urinary system
Urology
Urology, pediatric

UTERUS
Abdomen
Abdominal disorders
Abortion
Amenorrhea
Amniocentesis

Assisted reproductive technologies
Cervical, ovarian, and uterine
    cancers
Cervical procedures
Cesarean section
Childbirth
Childbirth complications
Chorionic villus sampling
Conception
Contraception
Culdocentesis
Dysmenorrhea
Ectopic pregnancy
Electrocauterization
Endocrinology
Endometrial biopsy
Endometriosis
Fistula repair
Genetic counseling
Genital disorders, female
Gynecology
Hermaphroditism and
    pseudohermaphroditism
Hysterectomy
In vitro fertilization
Infertility, female
Internal medicine
Laparoscopy
Menopause
Menorrhagia
Menstruation
Miscarriage
Multiple births
Myomectomy
Obstetrics
Pap smear
Pelvic inflammatory disease PID)
Placenta
Pregnancy and gestation
Premature birth
Premenstrual syndrome (PMS)
Prostate enlargement
Reproductive system
Sex change surgery
Sexual differentiation
Sperm banks
Sterilization
Stillbirth
Tubal ligation
Ultrasonography

ENTRIES BY SPECIALTIES AND RELATED FIELDS

ALL
Accidents
African American health
American Indian health
Anatomy
Asian American health
Biostatistics
Clinical trials
Disease
Geriatrics and gerontology
Health maintenance organizations
  (HMOs)
Iatrogenic disorders
Imaging and radiology
Internet medicine
Invasive tests
Laboratory tests
Men's health
Neuroimaging
Noninvasive tests
Pediatrics
Physical examination
Physiology
Polypharmacy
Preventive medicine
Proteomics
Screening
Self-medication
Systems and organs
Telemedicine
Terminally ill: Extended care
Veterinary medicine
Women's health

ALTERNATIVE MEDICINE
Acupressure
Acupuncture
Allied health
Alternative medicine
Antioxidants
Aphrodisiacs
Aromatherapy
Biofeedback
Chronobiology
Club drugs
Colon therapy
Enzyme therapy
Healing
Herbal medicine
Holistic medicine

Hydrotherapy
Hypnosis
Magnetic field therapy
Marijuana
Massage
Meditation
Melatonin
Nutrition
Oxygen therapy
Pain management
Stress reduction
Supplements
Yoga

ANESTHESIOLOGY
Acupuncture
Anesthesia
Anesthesiology
Catheterization
Cesarean section
Critical care
Critical care, pediatric
Dentistry
Hyperbaric oxygen therapy
Hyperthermia and hypothermia
Hypnosis
Pain management
Pharmacology
Pharmacy
Surgery, general
Surgery, pediatric
Surgical procedures
Surgical technologists
Toxicology

AUDIOLOGY
Aging
Aging: Extended care
Audiology
Biophysics
Deafness
Dyslexia
Ear infections and disorders
Ear surgery
Ears
Hearing aids
Hearing loss
Hearing tests
Ménière's disease
Motion sickness

Neurology
Neurology, pediatric
Otoplasty
Otorhinolaryngology
Sense organs
Speech disorders

BACTERIOLOGY
Anthrax
Antibiotics
Bacterial infections
Bacteriology
Biological and chemical weapons
Blisters
Boils
Botulism
Cells
Childhood infectious diseases
Cholecystitis
Cholera
Cystitis
Cytology
Cytopathology
Diphtheria
Drug resistance
E. coli infection
Endocarditis
Fluoride treatments
Gangrene
Genomics
Gonorrhea
Gram staining
Impetigo
Infection
Laboratory tests
Legionnaires' disease
Leprosy
Lyme disease
Mastitis
Microbiology
Microscopy
Necrotizing fasciitis
Nephritis
Osteomyelitis
Pelvic inflammatory disease (PID)
Plague
Pneumonia
Salmonella infection
Scarlet fever
Serology

Shigellosis
Staphylococcal infections
Strep throat
Streptococcal infections
Syphilis
Tetanus
Tonsillitis
Tropical medicine
Tuberculosis
Tularemia
Typhoid fever
Typhus
Whooping cough

BIOCHEMISTRY
Acid-base chemistry
Antidepressants
Autopsy
Bacteriology
Caffeine
Cholesterol
Corticosteroids
Digestion
Endocrinology
Endocrinology, pediatric
Enzyme therapy
Enzymes
Ergogenic aids
Fatty acid oxidation disorders
Fluids and electrolytes
Fluoride treatments
Food biochemistry
Fructosemia
Gaucher's disease
Genetic engineering
Genomics
Glands
Glycogen storage diseases
Glycolysis
Gram staining
Histology
Hormones
Leptin
Leukodystrophy
Lipids
Malabsorption
Metabolism
Nephrology
Nephrology, pediatric
Niemann-Pick disease
Nutrition
Pathology
Pharmacology
Pharmacy

Respiration
Stem cells
Steroids
Toxicology
Urinalysis
Wilson's disease

BIOTECHNOLOGY
Assisted reproductive technologies
Bionics and biotechnology
Biophysics
Cloning
Computed tomography (CT)
    scanning
Dialysis
Echocardiography
Electrocardiography (ECG or EKG)
Electroencephalography (EEG)
Fatty acid oxidation disorders
Gene therapy
Genetic engineering
Genomics
Glycogen storage diseases
Huntington's disease
Hyperbaric oxygen therapy
In vitro fertilization
Magnetic resonance imaging
    (MRI)
Pacemaker implantation
Positron emission tomography
    (PET) scanning
Prostheses
Severe combined immunodeficiency
    syndrome (SCID)
Sperm banks
Stem cells
Xenotransplantation

CARDIOLOGY
Aging
Aging: Extended care
Aneurysmectomy
Aneurysms
Angina
Angiography
Angioplasty
Anxiety
Arrhythmias
Arteriosclerosis
Biofeedback
Blue baby syndrome
Bypass surgery
Cardiac arrest
Cardiac rehabilitation

Cardiology
Cardiology, pediatric
Cardiopulmonary resuscitation
    (CPR)
Catheterization
Chest
Cholesterol
Circulation
Congenital heart disease
Critical care
Critical care, pediatric
DiGeorge syndrome
Dizziness and fainting
Echocardiography
Electrocardiography (ECG or EKG)
Emergency medicine
Endocarditis
Exercise physiology
Fetal surgery
Geriatrics and gerontology
Heart
Heart attack
Heart disease
Heart failure
Heart transplantation
Heart valve replacement
Hematology
Hemochromatosis
Hypercholesterolemia
Hypertension
Hypotension
Internal medicine
Ischemia
Kinesiology
Leptin
Marfan syndrome
Metabolic syndrome
Mitral valve prolapse
Mucopolysaccharidosis (MPS)
Muscles
Neonatology
Nicotine
Noninvasive tests
Nuclear medicine
Pacemaker implantation
Palpitations
Paramedics
Physical examination
Polycystic kidney disease
Prader-Willi syndrome
Progeria
Prostheses
Pulmonary hypertension
Rheumatic fever

Rubinstein-Taybi syndrome
Sports medicine
Stents
Thoracic surgery
Thrombolytic therapy and TPA
Thrombosis and thrombus
Transplantation
Ultrasonography
Vascular medicine
Vascular system
Venous insufficiency

CRITICAL CARE
Accidents
Aging: Extended care
Amputation
Anesthesia
Anesthesiology
Apgar score
Brain damage
Burns and scalds
Catheterization
Club drugs
Coma
Critical care
Critical care, pediatric
Drowning
Echocardiography
Electrical shock
Electrocardiography (ECG or EKG)
Electroencephalography (EEG)
Emergency medicine
Emergency medicine, pediatric
Geriatrics and gerontology
Grafts and grafting
Hantavirus
Heart attack
Heart transplantation
Heat exhaustion and heat stroke
Hospitals
Hyperbaric oxygen therapy
Hyperthermia and hypothermia
Hypotension
Necrotizing fasciitis
Neonatology
Nursing
Oncology
Osteopathic medicine
Pain management
Paramedics
Psychiatry
Psychiatry, child and adolescent
Psychiatry, geriatric
Pulmonary medicine

Pulmonary medicine, pediatric
Radiation sickness
Resuscitation
Safety issues for children
Safety issues for the elderly
Severe acute respiratory syndrome
 (SARS)
Shock
Thrombolytic therapy and TPA
Toxic shock syndrome
Tracheostomy
Transfusion
Tropical medicine
Wounds

CYTOLOGY
Acid-base chemistry
Bionics and biotechnology
Biopsy
Blood testing
Cancer
Carcinoma
Cells
Cholesterol
Cytology
Cytopathology
Dermatology
Dermatopathology
E. coli infection
Enzymes
Fluids and electrolytes
Food biochemistry
Gaucher's disease
Genetic counseling
Genetic engineering
Genomics
Glycolysis
Gram staining
Healing
Hematology
Hematology, pediatric
Histology
Immune system
Immunology
Karyotyping
Laboratory tests
Lipids
Melanoma
Metabolism
Microscopy
Mutation
Oncology
Pathology
Pharmacology

Pharmacy
Sarcoma
Serology
Stem cells
Toxicology

DENTISTRY
Abscess drainage
Abscesses
Aging: Extended care
Anesthesia
Anesthesiology
Canker sores
Cavities
Crowns and bridges
Dental diseases
Dentistry
Dentistry, pediatric
Dentures
Endodontic disease
Fluoride treatments
Forensic pathology
Fracture and dislocation
Fracture repair
Gastrointestinal system
Gingivitis
Gum disease
Halitosis
Head and neck disorders
Jaw wiring
Lisping
Mouth and throat cancer
Nicotine
Orthodontics
Osteogenesis imperfecta
Periodontal surgery
Periodontitis
Plastic surgery
Prader-Willi syndrome
Prostheses
Root canal treatment
Rubinstein-Taybi syndrome
Sense organs
Sjögren's syndrome
Teeth
Teething
Temporomandibular joint (TMJ)
 syndrome
Thumb sucking
Tooth extraction
Toothache
Von Willebrand's disease
Wisdom teeth

DERMATOLOGY

Abscess drainage
Abscesses
Acne
Age spots
Albinos
Anthrax
Anti-inflammatory drugs
Athlete's foot
Biopsy
Birthmarks
Blisters
Boils
Burns and scalds
Carcinoma
Chickenpox
Corns and calluses
Corticosteroids
Cryotherapy and cryosurgery
Cyst removal
Cysts
Dermatitis
Dermatology
Dermatology, pediatric
Dermatopathology
Eczema
Electrocauterization
Facial transplantation
Fungal infections
Ganglion removal
Glands
Grafts and grafting
Gray hair
Hair
Hair loss and baldness
Hair transplantation
Hand-foot-and-mouth disease
Healing
Histology
Hives
Hyperhidrosis
Impetigo
Itching
Laser use in surgery
Lice, mites, and ticks
Light therapy
Melanoma
Moles
Monkeypox
Multiple chemical sensitivity
    syndrome
Nail removal
Nails
Necrotizing fasciitis

Neurofibromatosis
Pigmentation
Pinworm
Pityriasis alba
Pityriasis rosea
Plastic surgery
Podiatry
Poisonous plants
Prostheses
Psoriasis
Puberty and adolescence
Rashes
Reiter's syndrome
Ringworm
Rosacea
Scabies
Scleroderma
Sense organs
Skin
Skin cancer
Skin disorders
Skin lesion removal
Stretch marks
Sturge-Weber syndrome
Sunburn
Sweating
Systemic lupus erythematosus (SLE)
Tattoo removal
Tattoos and body piercing
Touch
Von Willebrand's disease
Warts
Wiskott-Aldrich syndrome
Wrinkles

EMBRYOLOGY

Abortion
Amniocentesis
Assisted reproductive technologies
Birth defects
Blue baby syndrome
Brain damage
Brain disorders
Cerebral palsy
Chorionic villus sampling
Cloning
Conception
Down syndrome
Embryology
Fetal alcohol syndrome
Gamete intrafallopian transfer
    (GIFT)
Genetic counseling
Genetic diseases

Genetics and inheritance
Genomics
Growth
Hermaphroditism and
    pseudohermaphroditism
In vitro fertilization
Karyotyping
Klinefelter syndrome
Miscarriage
Mucopolysaccharidosis (MPS)
Multiple births
Nicotine
Obstetrics
Placenta
Pregnancy and gestation
Reproductive system
Rh factor
Rubella
Sexual differentiation
Spina bifida
Stem cells
Teratogens
Toxoplasmosis
Ultrasonography

EMERGENCY MEDICINE

Abdominal disorders
Abscess drainage
Accidents
Aging
Altitude sickness
Amputation
Anesthesia
Anesthesiology
Aneurysms
Angiography
Appendectomy
Appendicitis
Asphyxiation
Biological and chemical weapons
Bites and stings
Bleeding
Blurred vision
Botulism
Brain damage
Bruises
Burns and scalds
Cardiac arrest
Cardiology
Cardiology, pediatric
Cardiopulmonary resuscitation
    (CPR)
Catheterization
Cesarean section

Choking
Club drugs
Coma
Computed tomography (CT)
    scanning
Concussion
Critical care
Critical care, pediatric
Croup
Diphtheria
Dizziness and fainting
Domestic violence
Drowning
Echocardiography
Electrical shock
Electrocardiography (ECG or EKG)
Electroencephalography (EEG)
Emergency medicine
Emergency medicine, pediatric
Epiglottitis
Food poisoning
Fracture and dislocation
Frostbite
Grafts and grafting
Head and neck disorders
Heart attack
Heart transplantation
Heat exhaustion and heat stroke
Heimlich maneuver
Hospitals
Hyperbaric oxygen therapy
Hyperthermia and hypothermia
Hyperventilation
Hypotension
Intoxication
Jaw wiring
Laceration repair
Lumbar puncture
Lung surgery
Meningitis
Monkeypox
Necrotizing fasciitis
Noninvasive tests
Nosebleeds
Nursing
Osteopathic medicine
Oxygen therapy
Pain management
Paramedics
Peritonitis
Physician assistants
Plague
Plastic surgery
Pneumonia

Poisoning
Pulmonary diseases
Pulmonary medicine
Pulmonary medicine, pediatric
Pyelonephritis
Radiation sickness
Resuscitation
Reye's syndrome
Safety issues for children
Safety issues for the elderly
Salmonella infection
Severe acute respiratory syndrome
    (SARS)
Shock
Snakebites
Spinal cord disorders
Splenectomy
Sports medicine
Staphylococcal infections
Streptococcal infections
Strokes
Sunburn
Surgical technologists
Thrombolytic therapy and TPA
Toxic shock syndrome
Tracheostomy
Transfusion
Transplantation
Unconsciousness
Wheezing
Wounds

ENDOCRINOLOGY
Addison's disease
Adrenalectomy
Anti-inflammatory drugs
Assisted reproductive technologies
Bariatric surgery
Breasts, female
Chronobiology
Corticosteroids
Cretinism
Cushing's syndrome
Diabetes mellitus
Dwarfism
Endocrine disorders
Endocrinology
Endocrinology, pediatric
Enzymes
Ergogenic aids
Failure to thrive
Galactosemia
Gamete intrafallopian transfer
    (GIFT)

Geriatrics and gerontology
Gestational diabetes
Gigantism
Glands
Goiter
Growth
Gynecology
Gynecomastia
Hair loss and baldness
Hashimoto's thyroiditis
Hemochromatosis
Hermaphroditism and
    pseudohermaphroditism
Hormone replacement therapy
    (HRT)
Hormones
Hot flashes
Hyperadiposis
Hyperparathyroidism and
    hypoparathyroidism
Hypertrophy
Hypoglycemia
Hysterectomy
Infertility, female
Infertility, male
Insulin resistance syndrome
Internal medicine
Klinefelter syndrome
Laboratory tests
Laparoscopy
Leptin
Liver
Melatonin
Menopause
Menstruation
Metabolic disorders
Metabolic syndrome
Nephrology
Nephrology, pediatric
Neurology
Neurology, pediatric
Niemann-Pick disease
Nonalcoholic steatohepatitis (NASH)
Nuclear medicine
Obesity
Obesity, childhood
Pancreas
Pancreatitis
Parathyroidectomy
Pharmacology
Pharmacy
Precocious puberty
Prostate enlargement
Prostate gland

Puberty and adolescence
Radiopharmaceuticals
Sex change surgery
Sexual differentiation
Sexual dysfunction
Sleep
Stem cells
Steroids
Testicles, undescended
Testicular cancer
Thyroid disorders
Thyroid gland
Thyroidectomy
Toxicology
Tumors
Turner syndrome
Vitamins and minerals
Weight loss and gain
Weight loss medications

ENVIRONMENTAL HEALTH
Allergies
Asbestos exposure
Asthma
Bacteriology
Biological and chemical weapons
Blurred vision
Cholera
Cognitive development
Elephantiasis
Environmental diseases
Environmental health
Epidemiology
Food poisoning
Frostbite
Gulf War syndrome
Hantavirus
Heat exhaustion and heat stroke
Holistic medicine
Hyperthermia and hypothermia
Insect-borne diseases
Interstitial pulmonary fibrosis (IPF)
Lead poisoning
Legionnaires' disease
Lice, mites, and ticks
Lung cancer
Lungs
Lyme disease
Malaria
Mercury poisoning
Microbiology
Mold and mildew
Multiple chemical sensitivity
    syndrome

Nasopharyngeal disorders
Occupational health
Parasitic diseases
Pigmentation
Plague
Poisoning
Poisonous plants
Pulmonary diseases
Pulmonary medicine
Pulmonary medicine, pediatric
Salmonella infection
Skin cancer
Snakebites
Stress
Stress reduction
Toxicology
Trachoma
Tropical medicine
Tularemia
Typhoid fever
Typhus

EPIDEMIOLOGY
Acquired immunodeficiency
    syndrome (AIDS)
Anthrax
Bacterial infections
Bacteriology
Biological and chemical weapons
Biostatistics
Carcinogens
Childhood infectious diseases
Cholera
Creutzfeldt-Jakob disease (CJD)
Disease
E. coli infection
Ebola virus
Elephantiasis
Environmental diseases
Environmental health
Epidemiology
Food poisoning
Forensic pathology
Gulf War syndrome
Hantavirus
Hepatitis
Influenza
Insect-borne diseases
Laboratory tests
Legionnaires' disease
Leprosy
Lice, mites, and ticks
Malaria
Marburg virus

Measles
Mercury poisoning
Microbiology
Multiple chemical sensitivity
    syndrome
Necrotizing fasciitis
Occupational health
Parasitic diseases
Pathology
Plague
Pneumonia
Poisoning
Poliomyelitis
Prion diseases
Pulmonary diseases
Rabies
Rotavirus
Salmonella infection
Severe acute respiratory syndrome
    (SARS)
Sexually transmitted diseases
    (STDs)
Stress
Trichomoniasis
Tropical medicine
Typhoid fever
Typhus
Viral infections
World Health Organization
Yellow fever
Zoonoses

ETHICS
Abortion
Animal rights vs. research
Assisted reproductive technologies
Circumcision, female, and genital
    mutilation
Circumcision, male
Cloning
Ergogenic aids
Ethics
Euthanasia
Fetal surgery
Fetal tissue transplantation
Gene therapy
Genetic engineering
Genomics
Gulf War syndrome
Hippocratic oath
Law and medicine
Malpractice
Marijuana
Münchausen syndrome by proxy

Sperm banks
Stem cells
Xenotransplantation

EXERCISE PHYSIOLOGY
Back pain
Biofeedback
Bone disorders
Bones and the skeleton
Cardiac rehabilitation
Cardiology
Circulation
Dehydration
Echocardiography
Electrocardiography (ECG or EKG)
Ergogenic aids
Exercise physiology
Glycolysis
Heart
Heat exhaustion and heat stroke
Kinesiology
Lungs
Massage
Metabolism
Motor skill development
Muscle sprains, spasms, and
    disorders
Muscles
Nutrition
Orthopedic surgery
Orthopedics
Orthopedics, pediatric
Oxygen therapy
Overtraining syndrome
Physical rehabilitation
Physiology
Pulmonary diseases
Pulmonary medicine
Pulmonary medicine, pediatric
Respiration
Sports medicine
Steroid abuse
Sweating
Tendinitis
Vascular system

FAMILY MEDICINE
Abdominal disorders
Abscess drainage
Abscesses
Acne
Acquired immunodeficiency
    syndrome (AIDS)
Alcoholism

Allergies
Alzheimer's disease
Amyotrophic lateral sclerosis
Anemia
Angina
Antidepressants
Antihistamines
Anti-inflammatory drugs
Antioxidants
Arthritis
Athlete's foot
Attention-deficit disorder (ADD)
Bacterial infections
Bed-wetting
Bell's palsy
Beriberi
Biofeedback
Birthmarks
Bleeding
Blisters
Blurred vision
Boils
Bronchiolitis
Bronchitis
Bunions
Burkitt's lymphoma
Burping
Caffeine
Candidiasis
Canker sores
Chagas' disease
Chickenpox
Childhood infectious diseases
Chlamydia
Cholecystitis
Cholesterol
Chronic fatigue syndrome
Cirrhosis
Cluster headaches
Cold sores
Common cold
Constipation
Contraception
Corticosteroids
Coughing
Cryotherapy and cryosurgery
Cytomegalovirus (CMV)
Death and dying
Decongestants
Dehydration
Depression
Diabetes mellitus
Diaper rash
Diarrhea and dysentery

Digestion
Dizziness and fainting
Domestic violence
Enterocolitis
Epiglottitis
Exercise physiology
Factitious disorders
Failure to thrive
Family medicine
Fatigue
Fever
Fifth disease
Fungal infections
Ganglion removal
Genital disorders, female
Genital disorders, male
Geriatrics and gerontology
Giardiasis
Grief and guilt
Gynecology
Gynecomastia
Halitosis
Hand-foot-and-mouth disease
Headaches
Healing
Heart disease
Heartburn
Heat exhaustion and heat stroke
Hemorrhoid banding and removal
Hemorrhoids
Herpes
Hiccups
Hirschsprung's disease
Hives
Hyperadiposis
Hypercholesterolemia
Hyperlipidemia
Hypertension
Hypertrophy
Hypoglycemia
Incontinence
Indigestion
Infection
Inflammation
Influenza
Intestinal disorders
Juvenile rheumatoid arthritis
Kawasaki disease
Laryngitis
Leukodystrophy
Malabsorption
Maple syrup urine disease (MSUD)
Measles
Mitral valve prolapse

Glands
Heartburn
Hemochromatosis
Hemolytic uremic syndrome
Hemorrhoid banding and removal
Hemorrhoids
Hernia
Hernia repair
Hirschsprung's disease
Ileostomy and colostomy
Indigestion
Internal medicine
Intestinal disorders
Intestines
Irritable bowel syndrome (IBS)
Lactose intolerance
Laparoscopy
Liver
Liver cancer
Liver disorders
Liver transplantation
Malabsorption
Malnutrition
Metabolism
Nausea and vomiting
Nonalcoholic steatohepatitis (NASH)
Noroviruses
Nutrition
Obstruction
Pancreas
Pancreatitis
Peristalsis
Poisonous plants
Polycystic kidney disease
Proctology
Pyloric stenosis
Rotavirus
Roundworm
Salmonella infection
Scleroderma
Shigellosis
Soiling
Stomach, intestinal, and pancreatic cancers
Stone removal
Stones
Tapeworm
Taste
Toilet training
Trichinosis
Ulcer surgery
Ulcers
Vagotomy
Von Willebrand's disease

Weight loss and gain
Wilson's disease
Worms

GENERAL SURGERY
Abscess drainage
Adrenalectomy
Amputation
Anesthesia
Anesthesiology
Aneurysmectomy
Appendectomy
Bariatric surgery
Biopsy
Bladder removal
Bone marrow transplantation
Breast biopsy
Breast surgery
Bunions
Bypass surgery
Cataract surgery
Catheterization
Cervical procedures
Cesarean section
Cholecystectomy
Circumcision, female, and genital mutilation
Circumcision, male
Cleft lip and palate repair
Colon and rectal polyp removal
Colon and rectal surgery
Corneal transplantation
Craniotomy
Cryotherapy and cryosurgery
Cyst removal
Disk removal
Ear surgery
Electrocauterization
Endarterectomy
Endometrial biopsy
Eye surgery
Face lift and blepharoplasty
Fistula repair
Ganglion removal
Gastrectomy
Grafts and grafting
Hair transplantation
Hammertoe correction
Heart transplantation
Heart valve replacement
Heel spur removal
Hemorrhoid banding and removal
Hernia repair
Hip replacement

Hydrocelectomy
Hypospadias repair and urethroplasty
Hysterectomy
Kidney transplantation
Kneecap removal
Laceration repair
Laminectomy and spinal fusion
Laparoscopy
Laryngectomy
Laser use in surgery
Liposuction
Liver transplantation
Lung surgery
Mastectomy and lumpectomy
Myomectomy
Nail removal
Nasal polyp removal
Nephrectomy
Neurosurgery
Oncology
Ophthalmology
Orthopedic surgery
Otoplasty
Parathyroidectomy
Penile implant surgery
Periodontal surgery
Phlebitis
Plastic surgery
Prostate gland removal
Prostheses
Rhinoplasty and submucous resection
Rotator cuff surgery
Sex change surgery
Shunts
Skin lesion removal
Sphincterectomy
Splenectomy
Sterilization
Stone removal
Surgery, general
Surgery, pediatric
Surgical procedures
Surgical technologists
Sympathectomy
Tattoo removal
Tendon repair
Testicular surgery
Thoracic surgery
Thyroidectomy
Tonsillectomy and adenoid removal
Toxic shock syndrome
Tracheostomy

Transfusion
Transplantation
Tumor removal
Ulcer surgery
Vagotomy
Varicose vein removal
Vasectomy
Xenotransplantation

GENETICS
Aging
Albinos
Alzheimer's disease
Amniocentesis
Assisted reproductive technologies
Attention-deficit disorder (ADD)
Autoimmune disorders
Batten's disease
Bioinformatics
Bionics and biotechnology
Birth defects
Bone marrow transplantation
Breast cancer
Breast disorders
Chorionic villus sampling
Cloning
Cognitive development
Colon cancer
Color blindness
Cornelia de Lange syndrome
Cystic fibrosis
Diabetes mellitus
DiGeorge syndrome
DNA and RNA
Down syndrome
Dwarfism
Embryology
Endocrinology
Endocrinology, pediatric
Enzyme therapy
Enzymes
Failure to thrive
Fetal surgery
Fragile X syndrome
Fructosemia
Galactosemia
Gaucher's disease
Gene therapy
Genetic counseling
Genetic diseases
Genetic engineering
Genetics and inheritance
Genomics
Grafts and grafting

Hematology
Hematology, pediatric
Hemophilia
Hermaphroditism and
    pseudohermaphroditism
Huntington's disease
Hyperadiposis
Immunodeficiency disorders
In vitro fertilization
Insulin resistance syndrome
Karyotyping
Klinefelter syndrome
Klippel-Trenaunay syndrome
Laboratory tests
Leptin
Leukodystrophy
Malabsorption
Maple syrup urine disease (MSUD)
Marfan syndrome
Mental retardation
Metabolic disorders
Motor skill development
Mucopolysaccharidosis (MPS)
Muscular dystrophy
Mutation
Neonatology
Nephrology
Nephrology, pediatric
Neurofibromatosis
Neurology
Neurology, pediatric
Niemann-Pick disease
Obstetrics
Oncology
Osteogenesis imperfecta
Pediatrics
Phenylketonuria (PKU)
Polycystic kidney disease
Porphyria
Prader-Willi syndrome
Precocious puberty
Reproductive system
Rh factor
Rubinstein-Taybi syndrome
Screening
Severe combined immunodeficiency
    syndrome (SCID)
Sexual differentiation
Sexuality
Sperm banks
Stem cells
Tay-Sachs disease
Tourette's syndrome
Transplantation

Turner syndrome
Wiskott-Aldrich syndrome

GERIATRICS AND GERONTOLOGY
Age spots
Aging
Aging: Extended care
Alzheimer's disease
Arthritis
Bed-wetting
Blindness
Blurred vision
Bone disorders
Bones and the skeleton
Brain
Brain disorders
Cataract surgery
Cataracts
Chronic obstructive pulmonary
    disease (COPD)
Corns and calluses
Critical care
Crowns and bridges
Deafness
Death and dying
Dementias
Dentures
Depression
Domestic violence
Emergency medicine
Endocrinology
Euthanasia
Family medicine
Fatigue
Fracture and dislocation
Fracture repair
Gray hair
Hearing aids
Hearing loss
Hip fracture repair
Hip replacement
Hormone replacement therapy
    (HRT)
Hormones
Hospitals
Incontinence
Memory loss
Nursing
Nutrition
Ophthalmology
Orthopedics
Osteoporosis
Pain management

Paramedics
Parkinson's disease
Pharmacology
Pick's disease
Psychiatry
Psychiatry, geriatric
Rheumatology
Safety issues for the elderly
Sleep disorders
Spinal cord disorders
Spine, vertebrae, and disks
Suicide
Vision disorders
Wrinkles

GYNECOLOGY
Abortion
Amenorrhea
Amniocentesis
Assisted reproductive technologies
Biopsy
Bladder removal
Breast biopsy
Breast cancer
Breast disorders
Breast-feeding
Breasts, female
Cervical, ovarian, and uterine
  cancers
Cervical procedures
Cesarean section
Childbirth
Childbirth complications
Chlamydia
Circumcision, female, and genital
  mutilation
Conception
Contraception
Culdocentesis
Cyst removal
Cystitis
Cysts
Dysmenorrhea
Electrocauterization
Endocrinology
Endometrial biopsy
Endometriosis
Endoscopy
Episiotomy
Genital disorders, female
Glands
Gonorrhea
Gynecology

Hermaphroditism and
  pseudohermaphroditism
Herpes
Hormone replacement therapy
  (HRT)
Hormones
Hot flashes
Human papillomavirus (HPV)
Hysterectomy
In vitro fertilization
Incontinence
Infertility, female
Internal medicine
Laparoscopy
Leptin
Mammography
Mastectomy and lumpectomy
Mastitis
Menopause
Menorrhagia
Menstruation
Myomectomy
Nutrition
Obstetrics
Ovarian cysts
Pap smear
Pelvic inflammatory disease (PID)
Peritonitis
Postpartum depression
Preeclampsia and eclampsia
Pregnancy and gestation
Premenstrual syndrome (PMS)
Reiter's syndrome
Reproductive system
Sex change surgery
Sexual differentiation
Sexual dysfunction
Sexuality
Sexually transmitted diseases
  (STDs)
Sterilization
Syphilis
Toxemia
Toxic shock syndrome
Trichomoniasis
Tubal ligation
Turner syndrome
Ultrasonography
Urethritis
Urinary disorders
Urology
Von Willebrand's disease
Warts

HEMATOLOGY
Acid-base chemistry
Acquired immunodeficiency
  syndrome (AIDS)
Anemia
Bleeding
Blood and blood disorders
Blood testing
Bone grafting
Bone marrow transplantation
Bruises
Burkitt's lymphoma
Cholesterol
Circulation
Cyanosis
Cytology
Cytomegalovirus (CMV)
Cytopathology
Dialysis
Disseminated intravascular
  coagulation (DIC)
Ergogenic aids
Fluids and electrolytes
Forensic pathology
Healing
Hematology
Hematology, pediatric
Hemolytic disease of the newborn
Hemolytic uremic syndrome
Hemophilia
Histiocytosis
Histology
Hodgkin's disease
Host-defense mechanisms
Hypercholesterolemia
Hyperlipidemia
Hypoglycemia
Immune system
Immunology
Infection
Ischemia
Jaundice
Jaundice, neonatal
Kidneys
Laboratory tests
Leukemia
Liver
Lymphadenopathy and lymphoma
Lymphatic system
Malaria
Nephrology
Nephrology, pediatric
Niemann-Pick disease
Nosebleeds

Phlebotomy
Rh factor
Septicemia
Serology
Sickle cell disease
Stem cells
Thalassemia
Thrombocytopenia
Thrombolytic therapy and TPA
Thrombosis and thrombus
Transfusion
Vascular medicine
Vascular system
Von Willebrand's disease

HISTOLOGY
Autopsy
Biopsy
Cancer
Carcinoma
Cells
Cytology
Cytopathology
Dermatology
Dermatopathology
Fluids and electrolytes
Forensic pathology
Healing
Histology
Laboratory tests
Microscopy
Nails
Necrotizing fasciitis
Pathology
Tumor removal
Tumors

IMMUNOLOGY
Acquired immunodeficiency
    syndrome (AIDS)
Allergies
Antibiotics
Antihistamines
Arthritis
Aspergillosis
Asthma
Autoimmune disorders
Bacterial infections
Biological and chemical weapons
Bionics and biotechnology
Bites and stings
Blood and blood disorders
Boils
Bone cancer

Bone grafting
Bone marrow transplantation
Breast cancer
Cancer
Candidiasis
Carcinoma
Cervical, ovarian, and uterine
    cancers
Childhood infectious diseases
Chronic fatigue syndrome
Colon cancer
Corticosteroids
Cytology
Cytomegalovirus (CMV)
Dermatology
Dermatopathology
DiGeorge syndrome
Endocrinology
Endocrinology, pediatric
Epstein-Barr virus
Facial transplantation
Fungal infections
Grafts and grafting
Healing
Hematology
Hematology, pediatric
Histiocytosis
Hives
Homeopathy
Host-defense mechanisms
Human immunodeficiency virus
    (HIV)
Hypnosis
Immune system
Immunization and vaccination
Immunodeficiency disorders
Immunology
Immunopathology
Impetigo
Juvenile rheumatoid arthritis
Kawasaki disease
Laboratory tests
Leprosy
Liver cancer
Lung cancer
Lymphatic system
Microbiology
Multiple chemical sensitivity
    syndrome
Myasthenia gravis
Nicotine
Noroviruses
Oncology
Oxygen therapy

Pancreas
Prostate cancer
Pulmonary diseases
Pulmonary medicine
Pulmonary medicine, pediatric
Rheumatology
Sarcoma
Scleroderma
Serology
Severe combined immunodeficiency
    syndrome (SCID)
Skin cancer
Stem cells
Stomach, intestinal, and pancreatic
    cancers
Stress
Stress reduction
Systemic lupus erythematosus (SLE)
Thalidomide
Transfusion
Transplantation
Tropical medicine
Wiskott-Aldrich syndrome
Xenotransplantation

INTERNAL MEDICINE
Abdomen
Abdominal disorders
Anatomy
Anemia
Angina
Anti-inflammatory drugs
Antioxidants
Anxiety
Appetite loss
Arrhythmias
Arteriosclerosis
Aspergillosis
Autoimmune disorders
Bacterial infections
Bariatric surgery
Behçet's disease
Beriberi
Biofeedback
Bleeding
Bronchiolitis
Bronchitis
Burkitt's lymphoma
Burping
Bursitis
Candidiasis
Chickenpox
Childhood infectious diseases
Cholecystitis

Tetanus
Thrombosis and thrombus
Toxic shock syndrome
Tumor removal
Tumors
Ulcer surgery
Ulcers
Ultrasonography
Viral infections
Vitamins and minerals
Weight loss medications
Whooping cough
Wilson's disease
Worms
Wounds

MICROBIOLOGY

Abscesses
Anthrax
Antibiotics
Aspergillosis
Autopsy
Bacterial infections
Bacteriology
Bionics and biotechnology
Drug resistance
E. coli infection
Epidemiology
Fluoride treatments
Fungal infections
Gangrene
Gastroenterology
Gastroenterology, pediatric
Gastrointestinal disorders
Gastrointestinal system
Genetic engineering
Genomics
Gram staining
Immune system
Immunization and vaccination
Immunology
Impetigo
Laboratory tests
Microbiology
Microscopy
Pathology
Pharmacology
Pharmacy
Protozoan diseases
Serology
Severe acute respiratory syndrome
  (SARS)
Smallpox
Toxic shock syndrome

Toxicology
Tropical medicine
Tuberculosis
Urinalysis
Urology
Urology, pediatric
Viral infections

NEONATOLOGY

Apgar score
Birth defects
Blue baby syndrome
Bonding
Cardiology, pediatric
Cesarean section
Childbirth
Childbirth complications
Chlamydia
Cleft lip and palate
Cleft lip and palate repair
Congenital heart disease
Critical care, pediatric
Cystic fibrosis
Disseminated intravascular
  coagulation (DIC)
Down syndrome
E. coli infection
Endocrinology, pediatric
Failure to thrive
Fetal alcohol syndrome
Fetal surgery
Gastroenterology, pediatric
Genetic diseases
Genetics and inheritance
Hematology, pediatric
Hemolytic disease of the newborn
Hydrocephalus
Intraventricular hemorrhage
Jaundice
Jaundice, neonatal
Karyotyping
Malabsorption
Maple syrup urine disease
  (MSUD)
Motor skill development
Multiple births
Neonatology
Nephrology, pediatric
Neurology, pediatric
Nicotine
Nursing
Obstetrics
Orthopedics, pediatric
Pediatrics

Perinatology
Phenylketonuria (PKU)
Physician assistants
Premature birth
Pulmonary medicine, pediatric
Respiratory distress syndrome
Rh factor
Shunts
Sudden infant death syndrome
  (SIDS)
Surgery, pediatric
Tay-Sachs disease
Toxoplasmosis
Transfusion
Trichomoniasis
Tropical medicine
Umbilical cord
Urology, pediatric
Well-baby examinations

NEPHROLOGY

Abdomen
Cysts
Diabetes mellitus
Dialysis
E. coli infection
Edema
Hemolytic uremic syndrome
Internal medicine
Kidney cancer
Kidney disorders
Kidney transplantation
Kidneys
Lithotripsy
Nephrectomy
Nephritis
Nephrology
Nephrology, pediatric
Polycystic kidney disease
Preeclampsia and eclampsia
Pyelonephritis
Renal failure
Stone removal
Stones
Transplantation
Urinalysis
Urinary disorders
Urinary system
Urology
Urology, pediatric

NEUROLOGY

Altitude sickness
Alzheimer's disease

NURSING

Aging: Extended care
Allied health
Anesthesiology
Cardiac rehabilitation
Critical care
Critical care, pediatric
Emergency medicine
Emergency medicine, pediatric
Geriatrics and gerontology
Holistic medicine
Hospitals
Immunization and vaccination
Neonatology
Noninvasive tests
Nursing
Nutrition
Pediatrics
Physical examination
Physician assistants
Surgery, general
Surgery, pediatric
Surgical procedures
Surgical technologists
Well-baby examinations

NUTRITION

Aging: Extended care
Anorexia nervosa
Antioxidants
Appetite loss
Bariatric surgery
Beriberi
Breast-feeding
Bulimia
Cardiac rehabilitation
Cholesterol
Digestion
Eating disorders
Exercise physiology
Fatty acid oxidation disorders
Food biochemistry
Fructosemia
Galactosemia
Gastroenterology
Gastroenterology, pediatric
Gastrointestinal disorders
Gastrointestinal system
Geriatrics and gerontology
Gestational diabetes
Glycogen storage diseases
Hyperadiposis
Hypercholesterolemia
Irritable bowel syndrome (IBS)

Jaw wiring
Kwashiorkor
Lactose intolerance
Leptin
Leukodystrophy
Lipids
Malabsorption
Malnutrition
Metabolic disorders
Metabolic syndrome
Metabolism
Nursing
Nutrition
Obesity
Obesity, childhood
Osteoporosis
Phytochemicals
Scurvy
Sports medicine
Supplements
Taste
Tropical medicine
Ulcers
Vagotomy
Vitamins and minerals
Weaning
Weight loss and gain
Weight loss medications

OBSTETRICS

Amniocentesis
Apgar score
Assisted reproductive technologies
Birth defects
Breast-feeding
Breasts, female
Cervical, ovarian, and uterine
    cancers
Cesarean section
Childbirth
Childbirth complications
Chorionic villus sampling
Conception
Cytomegalovirus (CMV)
Disseminated intravascular
    coagulation (DIC)
Down syndrome
Ectopic pregnancy
Embryology
Emergency medicine
Episiotomy
Family medicine
Fetal alcohol syndrome
Fetal surgery

Gamete intrafallopian transfer
    (GIFT)
Genetic counseling
Genetic diseases
Genetics and inheritance
Genital disorders, female
Gestational diabetes
Gonorrhea
Growth
Gynecology
Hemolytic disease of the newborn
In vitro fertilization
Incontinence
Invasive tests
Karyotyping
Miscarriage
Multiple births
Neonatology
Nicotine
Noninvasive tests
Obstetrics
Perinatology
Placenta
Postpartum depression
Preeclampsia and eclampsia
Pregnancy and gestation
Premature birth
Pyelonephritis
Reproductive system
Rh factor
Rubella
Sexuality
Sperm banks
Spina bifida
Stillbirth
Teratogens
Toxemia
Toxoplasmosis
Trichomoniasis
Ultrasonography
Urology

OCCUPATIONAL HEALTH

Altitude sickness
Asbestos exposure
Asphyxiation
Back pain
Biofeedback
Blurred vision
Carcinogens
Cardiac rehabilitation
Carpal tunnel syndrome
Environmental diseases
Environmental health

Gigantism
Glycogen storage diseases
Growth
Gynecomastia
Hand-foot-and-mouth disease
Hematology, pediatric
Hemolytic uremic syndrome
Hirschsprung's disease
Hives
Hormones
Hydrocephalus
Hypospadias repair and
    urethroplasty
Juvenile rheumatoid arthritis
Kawasaki disease
Klippel-Trenaunay syndrome
Kwashiorkor
Learning disabilities
Leukodystrophy
Malabsorption
Malnutrition
Maple syrup urine disease (MSUD)
Massage
Measles
Menstruation
Metabolic disorders
Motor skill development
Mucopolysaccharidosis (MPS)
Multiple births
Multiple sclerosis
Mumps
Münchausen syndrome by proxy
Muscular dystrophy
Neonatology
Nephrology, pediatric
Neurology, pediatric
Niemann-Pick disease
Nightmares
Nosebleeds
Nursing
Nutrition
Obesity, childhood
Optometry, pediatric
Orthopedics, pediatric
Osgood-Schlatter disease
Osteogenesis imperfecta
Otoplasty
Otorhinolaryngology
Pediatrics
Perinatology
Phenylketonuria (PKU)
Pigeon toes
Pinworm
Poliomyelitis

Porphyria
Prader-Willi syndrome
Precocious puberty
Premature birth
Progeria
Psychiatry, child and adolescent
Puberty and adolescence
Pulmonary medicine, pediatric
Pyloric stenosis
Rashes
Reflexes, primitive
Respiratory distress syndrome
Reye's syndrome
Rheumatic fever
Rickets
Roseola
Rotavirus
Roundworm
Rubella
Rubinstein-Taybi syndrome
Safety issues for children
Scarlet fever
Seizures
Severe combined immunodeficiency
    syndrome (SCID)
Sexuality
Sibling rivalry
Soiling
Sore throat
Steroids
Strep throat
Streptococcal infections
Sturge-Weber syndrome
Styes
Sudden infant death syndrome
    (SIDS)
Surgery, pediatric
Tapeworm
Tay-Sachs disease
Teething
Testicles, undescended
Testicular torsion
Thumb sucking
Toilet training
Tonsillectomy and adenoid removal
Tonsillitis
Trachoma
Tropical medicine
Urology, pediatric
Weaning
Well-baby examinations
Whooping cough
Wiskott-Aldrich syndrome
Worms

PERINATOLOGY
Amniocentesis
Assisted reproductive technologies
Birth defects
Breast-feeding
Cesarean section
Childbirth
Childbirth complications
Chorionic villus sampling
Cretinism
Critical care, pediatric
Embryology
Fatty acid oxidation disorders
Fetal alcohol syndrome
Glycogen storage diseases
Hematology, pediatric
Hydrocephalus
Karyotyping
Metabolic disorders
Motor skill development
Neonatology
Neurology, pediatric
Nursing
Obstetrics
Pediatrics
Perinatology
Pregnancy and gestation
Premature birth
Reflexes, primitive
Shunts
Stillbirth
Sudden infant death syndrome
    (SIDS)
Trichomoniasis
Umbilical cord
Well-baby examinations

PHARMACOLOGY
Acid-base chemistry
Aging: Extended care
Anesthesia
Anesthesiology
Antibiotics
Antidepressants
Antihistamines
Anti-inflammatory drugs
Bacteriology
Blurred vision
Chemotherapy
Club drugs
Corticosteroids
Critical care
Critical care, pediatric
Decongestants

Bunions
Corns and calluses
Feet
Flat feet
Foot disorders
Fungal infections
Hammertoe correction
Hammertoes
Heel spur removal
Lower extremities
Nail removal
Orthopedic surgery
Orthopedics
Physical examination
Pigeon toes
Podiatry
Tendon disorders
Tendon repair
Warts

PREVENTIVE MEDICINE
Acupressure
Acupuncture
Aging: Extended care
Alternative medicine
Aromatherapy
Biofeedback
Braces, orthopedic
Caffeine
Cardiology
Chiropractic
Cholesterol
Chronobiology
Disease
Echocardiography
Electrocardiography (ECG or EKG)
Environmental health
Exercise physiology
Family medicine
Genetic counseling
Geriatrics and gerontology
Holistic medicine
Host-defense mechanisms
Hypercholesterolemia
Immune system
Immunization and vaccination
Immunology
Mammography
Massage
Meditation
Melatonin
Noninvasive tests
Nursing
Nutrition

Occupational health
Osteopathic medicine
Over-the-counter medications
Pharmacology
Pharmacy
Physical examination
Phytochemicals
Preventive medicine
Psychiatry
Psychiatry, child and adolescent
Psychiatry, geriatric
Screening
Serology
Spine, vertebrae, and disks
Sports medicine
Stress
Stress reduction
Tendinitis
Tropical medicine
Yoga

PROCTOLOGY
Bladder removal
Colon and rectal polyp removal
Colon and rectal surgery
Colon cancer
Colonoscopy and sigmoidoscopy
Crohn's disease
Diverticulitis and diverticulosis
Endoscopy
Fistula repair
Gastroenterology
Gastrointestinal disorders
Gastrointestinal system
Genital disorders, male
Geriatrics and gerontology
Hemorrhoid banding and removal
Hemorrhoids
Hirschsprung's disease
Internal medicine
Intestinal disorders
Intestines
Irritable bowel syndrome (IBS)
Physical examination
Proctology
Prostate cancer
Prostate gland
Prostate gland removal
Reproductive system
Urology

PSYCHIATRY
Addiction
Aging

Aging: Extended care
Alcoholism
Alzheimer's disease
Amnesia
Amyotrophic lateral sclerosis
Anorexia nervosa
Antidepressants
Anxiety
Appetite loss
Asperger's syndrome
Attention-deficit disorder (ADD)
Auras
Autism
Bariatric surgery
Bipolar disorders
Bonding
Brain
Brain damage
Brain disorders
Breast surgery
Bulimia
Chronic fatigue syndrome
Circumcision, female, and genital
  mutilation
Club drugs
Corticosteroids
Delusions
Dementias
Depression
Developmental stages
Domestic violence
Eating disorders
Electroencephalography (EEG)
Emergency medicine
Emotions: Biomedical causes and
  effects
Factitious disorders
Failure to thrive
Family medicine
Fatigue
Grief and guilt
Gynecology
Hallucinations
Huntington's disease
Hypnosis
Hypochondriasis
Incontinence
Intoxication
Light therapy
Marijuana
Masturbation
Memory loss
Mental retardation
Midlife crisis

Münchausen syndrome by proxy
Neurosis
Neurosurgery
Nicotine
Nightmares
Obesity
Obesity, childhood
Obsessive-compulsive disorder
Pain
Pain management
Panic attacks
Paranoia
Penile implant surgery
Phobias
Pick's disease
Postpartum depression
Post-traumatic stress disorder
Prader-Willi syndrome
Psychiatric disorders
Psychiatry
Psychiatry, child and adolescent
Psychiatry, geriatric
Psychoanalysis
Psychosis
Psychosomatic disorders
Schizophrenia
Seasonal affective disorder
Separation anxiety
Sex change surgery
Sexual dysfunction
Sexuality
Shock therapy
Sleep
Sleep disorders
Speech disorders
Steroid abuse
Stress
Stress reduction
Sudden infant death syndrome
  (SIDS)
Suicide
Toilet training
Tourette's syndrome

PSYCHOLOGY
Addiction
Aging
Aging: Extended care
Alcoholism
Amnesia
Amyotrophic lateral sclerosis
Anorexia nervosa
Anxiety
Appetite loss

Aromatherapy
Asperger's syndrome
Attention-deficit disorder (ADD)
Auras
Bariatric surgery
Bed-wetting
Biofeedback
Bipolar disorders
Bonding
Brain
Brain damage
Brain disorders
Bulimia
Cardiac rehabilitation
Cirrhosis
Club drugs
Cognitive development
Death and dying
Delusions
Depression
Developmental stages
Domestic violence
Dyslexia
Eating disorders
Electroencephalography (EEG)
Emotions: Biomedical causes and
  effects
Environmental health
Factitious disorders
Failure to thrive
Family medicine
Forensic pathology
Genetic counseling
Grief and guilt
Gulf War syndrome
Gynecology
Hallucinations
Holistic medicine
Hormone replacement therapy
  (HRT)
Huntington's disease
Hypnosis
Hypochondriasis
Juvenile rheumatoid arthritis
Kinesiology
Klinefelter syndrome
Learning disabilities
Light therapy
Marijuana
Meditation
Memory loss
Mental retardation
Midlife crisis
Motor skill development

Münchausen syndrome by proxy
Neurosis
Nightmares
Nutrition
Obesity
Obesity, childhood
Obsessive-compulsive disorder
Occupational health
Overtraining syndrome
Pain management
Panic attacks
Paranoia
Phobias
Pick's disease
Plastic surgery
Postpartum depression
Post-traumatic stress disorder
Psychosomatic disorders
Puberty and adolescence
Separation anxiety
Sex change surgery
Sexual dysfunction
Sexuality
Sibling rivalry
Sleep
Sleep disorders
Sleepwalking
Speech disorders
Sports medicine
Steroid abuse
Stillbirth
Stress
Stress reduction
Sturge-Weber syndrome
Stuttering
Sudden infant death syndrome
  (SIDS)
Suicide
Temporomandibular joint (TMJ)
  syndrome
Tics
Toilet training
Tourette's syndrome
Weight loss and gain
Yoga

PUBLIC HEALTH
Acquired immunodeficiency
  syndrome (AIDS)
Aging: Extended care
Allied health
Alternative medicine
Anthrax
Asbestos exposure

Prader-Willi syndrome
Pulmonary diseases
Pulmonary hypertension
Pulmonary medicine
Pulmonary medicine, pediatric
Respiration
Respiratory distress syndrome
Severe acute respiratory syndrome
  (SARS)
Sleep apnea
Smoking
Thoracic surgery
Thrombolytic therapy and TPA
Tuberculosis
Tumor removal
Tumors
Wheezing

RADIOLOGY
Angiography
Biophysics
Biopsy
Bladder cancer
Bone cancer
Bone disorders
Bones and the skeleton
Brain tumors
Cancer
Catheterization
Computed tomography (CT)
  scanning
Critical care
Critical care, pediatric
Emergency medicine
Ewing's sarcoma
Gallbladder cancer
Imaging and radiology
Kidney cancer
Liver cancer
Lung cancer
Magnetic resonance imaging (MRI)
Mammography
Mouth and throat cancer
Noninvasive tests
Nuclear medicine
Nuclear radiology
Oncology
Positron emission tomography
  (PET) scanning
Prostate cancer
Radiation sickness
Radiation therapy
Radiopharmaceuticals
Sarcoma

Stents
Surgery, general
Testicular cancer
Ultrasonography

RHEUMATOLOGY
Aging
Aging: Extended care
Anti-inflammatory drugs
Arthritis
Arthroplasty
Arthroscopy
Autoimmune disorders
Behçet's disease
Bone disorders
Bones and the skeleton
Bursitis
Corticosteroids
Fibromyalgia
Geriatrics and gerontology
Gout
Hip replacement
Hydrotherapy
Inflammation
Lyme disease
Orthopedic surgery
Orthopedics
Orthopedics, pediatric
Osteoarthritis
Osteonecrosis
Physical examination
Rheumatic fever
Rheumatoid arthritis
Rheumatology
Rotator cuff surgery
Scleroderma
Sjögren's syndrome
Spondylitis
Sports medicine

SEROLOGY
Anemia
Blood and blood disorders
Blood testing
Cholesterol
Cytology
Cytopathology
Dialysis
Fluids and electrolytes
Forensic pathology
Hematology
Hematology, pediatric
Hemophilia
Hodgkin's disease

Host-defense mechanisms
Hyperbaric oxygen therapy
Hypercholesterolemia
Hyperlipidemia
Hypoglycemia
Immune system
Immunology
Immunopathology
Jaundice
Laboratory tests
Leukemia
Malaria
Pathology
Rh factor
Septicemia
Serology
Sickle cell disease
Thalassemia
Transfusion

SPEECH PATHOLOGY
Alzheimer's disease
Amyotrophic lateral sclerosis
Aphasia and dysphasia
Audiology
Autism
Cerebral palsy
Cleft lip and palate
Cleft lip and palate repair
Deafness
Dyslexia
Ear infections and disorders
Ear surgery
Ears
Electroencephalography (EEG)
Hearing loss
Hearing tests
Jaw wiring
Laryngitis
Learning disabilities
Lisping
Paralysis
Rubinstein-Taybi syndrome
Speech disorders
Strokes
Stuttering
Thumb sucking
Voice and vocal cord disorders

SPORTS MEDICINE
Acupressure
Anorexia nervosa
Arthroplasty
Arthroscopy

Athlete's foot
Biofeedback
Blurred vision
Bones and the skeleton
Braces, orthopedic
Cardiology
Critical care
Dehydration
Eating disorders
Emergency medicine
Ergogenic aids
Exercise physiology
Fracture and dislocation
Fracture repair
Glycolysis
Head and neck disorders
Heat exhaustion and heat stroke
Hydrotherapy
Kinesiology
Massage
Motor skill development
Muscle sprains, spasms, and
    disorders
Muscles
Nutrition
Orthopedic surgery
Orthopedics
Overtraining syndrome
Oxygen therapy
Physical examination
Physical rehabilitation
Physiology
Psychiatry
Rotator cuff surgery
Safety issues for children
Spine, vertebrae, and disks
Sports medicine
Steroid abuse
Steroids
Tendinitis
Tendon disorders
Tendon repair

TOXICOLOGY
Biological and chemical weapons
Bites and stings
Blood testing
Botulism
Club drugs
Critical care
Critical care, pediatric
Cyanosis
Dermatitis
Eczema

Emergency medicine
Environmental diseases
Environmental health
Food poisoning
Forensic pathology
Gaucher's disease
Hepatitis
Herbal medicine
Homeopathy
Intoxication
Itching
Laboratory tests
Lead poisoning
Liver
Mold and mildew
Multiple chemical sensitivity
    syndrome
Nicotine
Occupational health
Pathology
Pharmacology
Pharmacy
Poisoning
Poisonous plants
Rashes
Snakebites
Toxicology
Toxoplasmosis
Urinalysis

UROLOGY
Abdomen
Abdominal disorders
Bed-wetting
Bladder cancer
Bladder removal
Catheterization
Chlamydia
Circumcision, male
Cystitis
Cystoscopy
Dialysis
E. coli infection
Endoscopy
Fetal surgery
Fluids and electrolytes
Genital disorders, female
Genital disorders, male
Geriatrics and gerontology
Gonorrhea
Hemolytic uremic syndrome
Hermaphroditism and
    pseudohermaphroditism
Hydrocelectomy

Hypospadias repair and
    urethroplasty
Incontinence
Infertility, male
Kidney cancer
Kidney disorders
Kidney transplantation
Kidneys
Lithotripsy
Nephrectomy
Nephritis
Nephrology
Nephrology, pediatric
Pediatrics
Pelvic inflammatory disease (PID)
Penile implant surgery
Polycystic kidney disease
Prostate cancer
Prostate enlargement
Prostate gland
Prostate gland removal
Pyelonephritis
Reiter's syndrome
Reproductive system
Schistosomiasis
Sex change surgery
Sexual differentiation
Sexual dysfunction
Sexually transmitted diseases
    (STDs)
Sterilization
Stone removal
Stones
Syphilis
Testicles, undescended
Testicular cancer
Testicular surgery
Testicular torsion
Toilet training
Transplantation
Trichomoniasis
Ultrasonography
Urethritis
Urinalysis
Urinary disorders
Urinary system
Urology
Urology, pediatric
Vasectomy

VASCULAR MEDICINE
Amputation
Aneurysmectomy
Aneurysms